T0260127

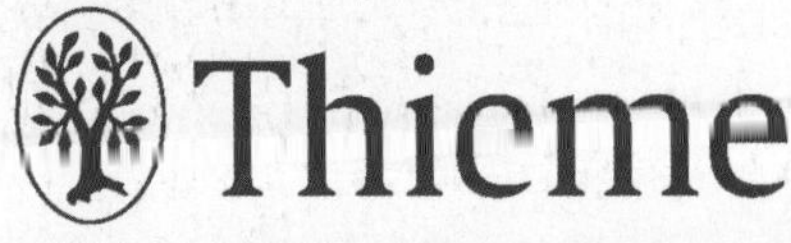
Thieme

Textbook of Pharmacology

Prasan R. Bhandari, MBBS, MD
Professor and Head
Department of Pharmacology
Symbiosis Medical College for Women
Pune, Maharashtra, India

Thieme
Delhi • Stuttgart • New York • Rio de Janeiro

Publishing Director: Ritu Sharma
Senior Development Editor: Dr Nidhi Srivastava
Director-Editorial Services: Rachna Sinha
Project Manager: Gaurav Prabhuzantye
Vice President Sales and Marketing: Arun Kumar Majji
Managing Director & CEO: Ajit Kohli

Thieme Medical and Scientific Publishers Private Limited.
A - 12, Second Floor, Sector - 2, Noida - 201 301,
Uttar Pradesh, India, +911204556600
Email: customerservice@thieme.in
www.thieme.in

Cover design: © Thieme
Cover image source: Composed by Thieme Group using following images: Pill © everythingpossible/stock.adobe.com
Page make-up by RECTO Graphics, India

Printed in India by EIH Limited – Unit Printing Press

5 4 3 2 1

ISBN: 978-93-90553-15-0
eISBN: 978-93-90553-16-7

Dedicated to the Almighty Creator for who, what, and why I am; and to

My parents, Mr Ramchandra G. Bhandari and Mrs Asha R. Bhandari;

My in-laws, Mr Dayanand A. Kamath and Mrs Sharada D. Kamath;

My sister, Mrs Veebha (Lochan) V. Prabhu, and my brother-in-law, Mr Vishnu R. Prabhu;

My sister-in-law, Mrs Savita V. Shanbhag, and my co-brother, Mr Vinayak P. Shanbhag;

My nephews Ramnath V. Prabhu and Siddhant V. Shanbhag;

My guru, guide, and philosopher, Mr Dileep Keskar and Mr Narasimha Bhat (Shri Mahaalasa Narayani temple, Ponda, Goa);

Lastly, but most importantly, my wife, Mrs Sangeeta P. Bhandari, and my two lovely daughters, Purva P. Bhandari and Neha P. Bhandari, who have actually helped me in typing this matter.

Contents

Foreword

Of all the subjects that are there in the medical curriculum, pharmacology can sometimes be abstract, dry, and theoretical. This makes the subject difficult to remember, and hence to reproduce during examinations.

Although there has been a huge growth in the electronic resources and some excellent books have been written, there remains a critical need for a book on the current competency-based medical education (CBME) syllabus that can be referred to. This *Textbook of Pharmacology* fills this gap. It is highly recommended for students.

It was for this reason that this project was undertaken, and I hope that it would be easily adopted as an additional reference material along with the standard textbooks.

I wish Dr Prasan R. Bhandari every success in his endeavor.

Dr Rajiv Yervadekar, MD, PhD
Dean and Faculty of Health & Biomedical Sciences
Symbiosis International University
Pune, Maharashtra

Preface

Competency-based medical education (CBME) is acquiring impetus throughout the world. Hence, the National Medical Commission (NMC) has designated the basic competencies mandatory of an Indian medical graduate and introduced a competency-based element on attitudes and communication in the syllabus. Extensive acceptance of a competency-based approach would indicate a paradigm shift in the present attitude to medical education.

The course in pharmacology is undergoing a sea change from stressing on animal experiments and dispensing pharmacy-based curriculum to an "applied" approach, wherein the importance is on how the student prescribes rationally, considering the numerous aspects of medicine and patient. Traditional pharmacology education has been censured for not grooming students for medical practice or teaching safe and rational use of medicines. The mention of these in the textbook is cursory.

Textbook of Pharmacology is based on the new CBME curriculum for the Indian medical graduate introduced by NMC in 2018. It comprises all the competencies required to develop skills in students as per the latest NMC recommendations and provide good healthcare to the growing needs of the nation and the world.

This book presents condensed and succinct descriptions of relevant and current information pertaining to pharmacology. It is not meant to be a substitute for the comprehensive presentation of information and difficult concepts found in standard textbooks of pharmacology.

The book's format has been designed with the students in mind. We have incorporated numerous illustrations, figures, and tables, in tune with the proverb "one picture is worth a thousand words," to summarize a variety of aspects.

Multiple choice question of case-based learning types have been included at the end of most chapters, which will be of benefit in better understanding of clinical scenarios.

I am eager to receive feedback and want to hear what you like about the book, and what could be improved. Please share your feedback by email at prasangeeta2012@gmail.com.

I am grateful to my students and colleagues who have taught most of what I know about teaching.

Wishing "All the Best" to the students for their examinations.

God bless all.

Prasan R. Bhandari, MBBS, MD

Acknowledgments

I thank the management of Symbiosis Medical College for Women, Pune for their support, especially:

- Dr S.B. Mujumdar (Padmashree and Padmabhushan, Founder and President and Chancellor of Symbiosis International University)
- Dr Vidya Yervadekar (Pro Chancellor, Symbiosis International University)
- Dr Rajiv Yervadekar (Dean, Faculty of Health & Biomedical Sciences of Symbiosis International University)
- Dr Vijaya Sagar (Dean, Symbiosis Medical College for Women)
- Dr Vijay Natrajan (CEO, Symbiosis University Hospital & Research Centre)
- Dr Mohan Jadhav (Medical Superintendent, Symbiosis University Hospital & Research Centre), for their support.

My sincere thanks to Dr Shraddha Yadav, Dr Ramanand Patil, Dr Viraj Shinde, Madhura Bhosale, Prachitee Borkar, and Akanksha Mate, from the Department of Pharmacology at Symbiosis Medical College for Women, Pune for helping me in editing the book.

I would like to take this opportunity to thank my family members, relatives, friends, and the departmental staff members for their active support, suggestions, and solutions. Additionally, my sincere thanks to the entire publication team at Thieme for providing me an opportunity to author this book.

Prasan R. Bhandari, MBBS, MD

Contributors

Ajay Prakash, PhD
Assistant Professor
Department of Pharmacology
Post Graduate Institute of Medical Education & Research
Chandigarh

Alka Bansal, MBBS, MD (Pharmacology)
Professor
Department of Pharmacology
Sawai Man Singh Medical College
Jaipur, Rajasthan

Amit Khurana, PhD (Pharmacology and Toxicology)
Department of Veterinary Pharmacology and Toxicology
P.V. Narsimha Rao Telangana Veterinary University
Rajendranagar, Hyderabad, Telangana

Amit Khurana, PhD
Research Scientist
Institute of Molecular Pathobiochemistry, Experimental Gene Therapy and Clinical Chemistry
RWTH Aachen University Hospital
Aachen, Germany

Amit Singh, MD, PhD
Professor and Head
Department of Pharmacology
Institute of Medical Sciences
Banaras Hindu University
Varanasi, Uttar Pradesh

A. Meenakumari, MBBS, MD (Pharmacology)
Professor of Pharmacology
Department of Pharmacology
Katuri Medical College
Guntur, Andhra Pradesh

Amrita Sil, MD (Pharmacology)
Associate Professor
Department of Pharmacology
Rampurhat Government Medical College
Rampurhat, Birbhum, West Bengal

Anuja Jha, MD (Pharmacology)
Assistant Professor
Department of Pharmacology
Sri Aurobindo Medical College & PG institute
Ujjain, Madhya Pradesh

Anupam Raja, PhD
Senior Research Fellow
Department of Pharmacology
Post Graduate Institute of Medical Education & Research
Chandigarh

Areeg Anwer Ali Shamsher, PhD (Pharmacology)
Professor
Department of Clinical Pharmacy and Pharmacology
RAK College of Pharmaceutical Sciences
RAK Medical and Health Sciences University
Ras Al Khaimah, United Arab Emirates

Arpita Shrivastav, PhD
Assistant Professor
Department of Pharmacology & Toxicology
College of Veterinary Science & Animal Husbandry
Rewa, Madhya Pradesh

Arshiya Sehgal, MD (Pharmacology)
Junior Resident
Department of Pharmacology
Government Medical College
Patiala, Punjab

Arulmozhi S., M Pharm, PhD (Pharmacology)
Assistant Professor and Head
Department of Pharmacology
Poona College of Pharmacy
Bharati Vidyapeeth
Pune, Maharashtra

Arunachalam Muthuraman, M Pharm, PhD
Associate Professor
Pharmacology Unit, Faculty of Pharmacy
Asian Institute of Medicine, Science and Technology
Bedong, Kedah Darul Aman, Malaysia

Asha B., MD (Pharmacology)
Additional Professor
Department of Pharmacology
Sri Devaraj Urs Medical College
Sri Devaraj Urs Academy of Higher Education and Research
Kolar, Karnataka

Aswinprakash Subramanian, MSc
Associate Professor in Medical Anatomy
Faculty of Medicine
Asian Institute of Medicine, Science and Technology
Bedong, Kedah Darul Aman, Malaysia

Awanish Mishra, PhD
Assistant Professor
Department of Pharmacology and Toxicology
National Institute of Pharmaceutical Education and Research
Guwahati, Assam

B. Dinesh Kumar, PhD
Senior Principal Scientist
Drug Toxicology Research Centre
ICMR-National Institute of Nutrition
Hyderabad, Telangana

Bhoomendra A. Bhongade, M Pharm, PhD (Pharmacology)
Professor
Department of Pharmaceutical Chemistry
RAK College of Pharmaceutical Sciences
RAK Medical and Health Sciences University
Ras Al Khaimah, United Arab Emirates

Bikash Medhi, MBBS, MD, MAMS, FIMSA
Professor
Department of Pharmacology
Postgraduate Institute of Medical Education and Research
Chandigarh

Biplab Sikdar, MSc
Research Scholar
Department of Pharmacology and Toxicology
National Institute of Pharmaceutical Education and Research
Raebareli, Lucknow, Uttar Pradesh

Bushra Hasan Khan, MD (Pharmacology)
Associate Professor
Department of Pharmacology
FH Medical College
Agra, Uttar Pradesh

Chandra Das, MBBS, MD, DM
Consultant Cardiologist
Rahman Hospital
Guwahati, Assam

C. S. Suthakaran, MD (Pharmacology)
Professor
Department of Pharmacology
Saveetha Medical College & Hospital
Saveetha Nagar Thandalam
Chennai, Tamil Nadu

D.H. Nandal, MBBS, MD (Pharmacology)
Professor and Head
Department of Pharmacology
Biratpur Medical College
Biratnagar, Nepal

Dipti Ramesh Sonawane, MBBS, MD, DNB (Pharmacology)
Assistant Professor
Department of Pharmacology
Vilasrao Deshmukh Government Medical College, Latur
Nashik, Maharashtra

D. Thamizh Vani, MD
Assistant professor
Thiruvannamalai Medical college
The Tamil Nadu Dr. M.G.R. Medical University
Thiruvannamalai, Tamil Nadu

Farhana Dutta Majumder, MD (Pharmacology)
Professor
Sree Balaji Medical College and Hospital
Bharath Institute of Higher Education and Research
Chennai, Tamil Nadu

Farhana Rahman, MBBS, MD (Pharmacology)
Professor
Department of Pharmacology
Sree Balaji Medical College and Hospital
Chennai, Tamil Nadu

Harish Kumar, PhD
Senior demonstrator,
Department of Pharmacology
Post Graduate Institute of Medical Education & Research
Chandigarh

Harpinder Kaur, MS (Pharmacology and Toxicology)
Senior Research Fellow
Department of Pharmacology
Postgraduate Institute of Medical Education and Research
Chandigarh

Harvinder Singh, PhD
Research Scholar
Department of Pharmacology
Post Graduate Institute of Medical Education & Research
Chandigarh

Iswar Hazarika, PhD
Assistant Professor
Department of Pharmacology
Girijananda Chowdhury Institute of Pharmaceutical Sciences
Guwahati, Assam

Jagadeesh Dhamodharan, MSc
Associate Professor in Medical Anatomy
Faculty of Medicine
Asian Institute of Medicine, Science and Technology
Bedong, Kedah Darul Aman, Malaysia

Jameel Ahmad, MD (Pharmacology), DCH
Associate Professor
Department of Pharmacology
J.N. Medical College
AMU, Aligarh, Uttar Pradesh

Janakidevi C.H., MBBS, MD
Assistant Professor
Department of Pharmacology
Sri Muthukumaran Medical college Hospital & Research Institute
Chennai, Tami Nadu

Jitendra H. Vaghela, MBBS, MD (Pharmacology)
Assistant Professor
Department of Pharmacology
NAMO Medical Education & Research Institute
Silvassa, Dadra and Nagar Haveli

Jitupam Baishya, DM (Neurology)
Assistant Professor of Neurology
Post Graduate Institute of Medical Education & Research
Chandigarh

Kala Kumar Bharani, MVSc, PhD (Pharmacology and Toxicology)
Professor and Head
Department of Veterinary Pharmacology and Toxicology
P.V. Narsimha Rao Telangana Veterinary University
Rajendranagar, Hyderabad, Telangana

Kamlesh M. Palandurkar, MBBS, MD (Biochemistry), DNB, MNAMS
Associate Professor
Department of Biochemistry
Hyderabad, Telangana
Institute of Medical Sciences
Banaras Hindu University
Varanasi, Uttar Pradesh

Kiran Rajendra Giri, MBBS, MD (Pharmacology)
Associate Professor
Department of Pharmacology
Institute of Medical Sciences, Banaras Hindu University
Varanasi, Uttar Pradesh

Leeela Talluri, MSc, MS (Pharmacology), MSc (Clinical Research)
Medical Writing Manager
Hetero Group of Pharma companies

Madhura Bhosale, MSc
Assistant Professor
Symbiosis Medical College for Women
Pune, Maharashtra

Manisha Prajapat, PhD
Research Scholar
Post Graduate Institute of Medical Education & Research
Chandigarh

Manju Agrawal, MD (Pharmacology)
Assistant Professor
Pt. Jawahar Lal Nehru Memorial Medical College
Raipur, Chhattisgarh

Manjunath G.N., MD (Pharmacology)
Professor and Head of Pharmacology
Sri Siddhartha Medical College
Tumakuru, Karnataka

Mayank Kulshreshtha, PhD
Sr. Assistant Professor
Department of Pharmacology
School of Pharmacy, Babu Banarasi Das University
Lucknow, Uttar Pradesh

M. Vijay Kumar, M Pharm, PhD
Department of Pharmacology
Nitte Gulabi Shetty Memorial Institute of Pharmaceutical Sciences
Deralakatte, Mangaluru, Karmataka

Narendrababu Kondapalli, PhD (Biochemistry)
Research Associate
Department of Microbiology and Immunology
ICMR-National Institute of Nutrition
Hyderabad, Telangana

Neeraj Kumar Fuloria, PhD
Senior Associate Professor
Faculty of Pharmacy & Centre of Excellence for Biomaterials Engineering
Asian Institute of Medicine, Science and Technology
Bedong, Kedah, Malaysia

Neeraj Shrivastava, PhD
Assistant Professor
Department of Microbiology
College of Veterinary Science & Animal Husbandry
Rewa, Madhya Pradesh

Nilofer Sayed, BAMS, MS (Pharmacology and Toxicology)
PhD Scholar
Department of Pharmacy
Pravara Rural Education Society's College of Pharmacy
Shreemati Nathibai Damodar Thackersey Women's University
Nashik, Maharashtra;
Department of Veterinary Pharmacology and Toxicology
P.V. Narsimha Rao Telangana Veterinary University
Rajendranagar, Hyderabad, Telangana

Nishigandha Suresh Jadhav, MBBS, MD (Pharmacology)
Ex-Post Graduate Student
Vilasrao Deshmukh Government Medical Institute of Sciences
Latur, Maharashtra

Nishita H. Darji, MBBS, MD (Pharmacology), PGDHHM
Junior lecturer
Department of Pharmacology
Smt. NHL Municipal Medical College
Ahmedabad, Gujarat

Nishtha Khatri, MD (Pharmacology)
JR-3, Department of Pharmacology & Therapeutics
Seth Gordhandas Sunderdas Medical College and the King
Edward Memorial Hospital
Mumbai, Maharashtra

Niti Mittal, MD, DM (Clinical Pharmacology)
Assistant Professor
Department of Pharmacology
Pandit Bhagwat Dayal Sharma Post Graduate Institute of
Medical Sciences
Rohtak, Haryana

Panini Patankar, MBBS, MD
JR-3, Department of Pharmacology & Therapeutics
Seth Gordhandas Sunderdas Medical College and the King
Edward Memorial Hospital
Mumbai, Maharashtra

Phulen Sarma, MBBS, MD, DM
Scientist
Department of Pharmacology
Postgraduate Institute of Medical Education and Research,
Chandigarh

Prachitee Borkar, MSc
Assistant Professor
Symbiosis Medical College for Women
Pune, Maharashtra

Prasan R. Bhandari, MBBS, MD
Professor and Head
Department of Pharmacology
Symbiosis Medical College for Women
Pune, Maharashtra

Prerna Singh, MBBS
Junior Resident
Department of Pharmacology
Jawaharlal Nehru Medical College
Aligarh Muslim University
Aligarh, Uttar Pradesh

Prince Allawadhi, M Pharm
PhD Scholar
Department of Biotechnology
Indian Institute of Technology Roorkee
Roorkee, Uttarakhand;
Department of Veterinary Pharmacology and Toxicology,
P.V. Narsimha Rao Telangana Veterinary University
Rajendranagar, Hyderabad, Telangana

R. Srinivasa Rao, MD (Ayurveda), PG Diploma in Clinical research, IIMBx Business Management MicroMasters Programme
General Manager - Clinical Trial Operations
Jeevan Scientific Technology Limited
Hyderabad, Telangana

Rahul Kumar, MD
Professor (J. Gr.)
Department of Pharmacology
King George's Medical University
Lucknow, Uttar Pradesh

Rajaneesh Kumar Chaudhary, M Tech
Assistant Professor
Amity Institute of Pharmacy
Amity University;
Research Scholar
School of Pharmacy
Babu Banarasi Das University
Lucknow, Uttar Pradesh

Rajendra S. Bhambar, PhD, MBA
Professor
Department of Pharmacognosy
Mahatma Gandhi Vidyamandir's Pharmacy College
Nashik, Maharashtra

Ramanand Patil, MD (Pharmacology)
Associate Professor
Department of Pharmacology
Symbiosis Medical College for Women
Pune, Maharashtra

Rashmi Bhaskarrao Kharde, MBBS, MD (Pharmacology)
Assistant Professor
Department of Pharmacology
Rural Medical College
Loni, Maharashtra

Reena Rajendra Giri, MBBS, MD (Pharmacology)
Associate Professor
Department of Pharmacology
Government Medical College
Akola, Maharashtra

R.S. Ray, M Pharm, PhD (Pharmacology)
Scientific Assistant
Indian Pharmacopoeia Commission
Ministry of Health and Family Welfare
Government of India
Raj Nagar, Ghaziabad, Uttar Pradesh

Rupali A. Patil, M Pharm, PhD
Associate Professor
Department of Pharmacology
GES's Sir Dr. M. S. Gosavi College of Pharmaceutical Education & Research
Nashik, Maharashtra

Sachin Karkale, MS (Pharmacology and Toxicology)
Toxicologist
Vivo Biotech Ltd.
Siddipet, Telangana;
Department of Pharmacology and Toxicology
College of Veterinary Science
P.V. Narsimha Rao Telangana Veterinary University
Rajendranagar, Hyderabad, Telangana

Sachin Parab, MBBS, PDCR
Consultant Pharmaceutical Physician
Ex- Abbott
Mumbai, Maharashtra

Saieswari Natesan, M Pharm
Executive
Enzene Biosciences Ltd.
Pune, Maharashtra

Sandeep Prakash Narwane, MBBS, MD (Pharmacology)
Professor
Department of Pharmacology
Dr. BVP Rural Medical College
Loni, Maharashtra

Sankha Shubhra Chakrabarti, MD
Associate Professor
Department of Geriatric Medicine
Institute of Medical Sciences
Banaras Hindu University
Varanasi, Uttar Pradesh

Sapna D. Desai, M Pharm, PhD
Associate Professor and Head
Department of Pharmacology
Pioneer Pharmacy Degree College
Vadodara, Gujarat

Satish Eknath Bahekar, MBBS, MD (Pharmacology)
Assistant Professor
Department of Pharmacology
Government Medical College
Aurangabad, Maharashtra

Shailesh Bhosle, MS (Pharm)
Research Scholar
Department of Pharmacology and Toxicology
National Institute of Pharmaceutical Education and Research
Raebareli, Lucknow, Uttar Pradesh

Shantanu R. Joshi, PhD Scholar
Department of Clinical Pharmacology
Seth Gordhandas Sunderdas Medical College and the King Edward Memorial Hospital
Mumbai, Maharashtra

Shardendu Kumar Mishra, PhD (Pharmacology and Toxicology)
Associate Professor
Department of Pharmacology
Ram-Eesh Institute of Vocational & Technical Education
Greater Noida, Uttar Pradesh

Sheshidhar G. Bannale, MBBS, MD (Pharmacology)
Professor
Department of Pharmacology
S Nijalingappa Medical College Bagalkot
Karnataka

Shikha Jaiswal Shivhare, MBBS, MD (Pharmacology)
Assistant Professor
Department of Pharmacology
Pt. Jawahar Lal Nehru Memorial Medical College
Raipur, Chhattisgarh

Shivam Yadav, M Pharm
Assistant Professor
Department of Pharmacognosy
S.N.A. Institute of Pharmacy
Lucknow, Uttar Pradesh

Shivkanya Fuloria
Associate Professor
Faculty of Pharmacy & Centre of Excellence for Biomaterials Engineering
Asian Institute of Medicine, Science and Technology
Bedong, Kedah, Malaysia

Shraddha M. Pore, MD (Pharmacology)
Professor & Head
Department of Pharmacology
Government Medical College And Hospital Miraj
Sangli, Maharashtra

Shraddha Yadav, MD (Pharmacology)
Associate Professor
Symbiosis Medical college for Women
Pune, Maharashtra

Shrikant V. Joshi, M, Pharm, PhD
Associate Professor
Maliba Pharmacy College
Uka Tarsadia University
Surat, Gujarat

Shruti Chandram, MBBS, MD (Pharmacology)
Assistant Professor
Department of Pharmacology
MGM Medical College
Aurangabad, Maharashtra

Shubhadeep Sinha, MD (Pharmacology)
Senior Vice President & Medical Director
Hetero Group of Pharma companies
Hyderabad, Telangana

Shubhangi H. Pawar, M Pharm
Assistant Professor
Department of Pharmacology
Mahatma Gandhi Vidyamandir's Pharmacy College
Nashik, Maharashtra

Shweta Sinha, PhD
Post-doctoral Research Associate
Department of Medical Parasitology
Post Graduate Institute of Medical Education & Research
Chandigarh

Snehal Lonare, MVSc
PhD Scholar
Department of Pharmacology and Toxicology
Guru Angad Dev Veterinary And Animal Sciences University
Ludhiana, Punjab

Sonali Karekar, MD (Pharmacology)
Associate Medical Advisor
Internal Medicine
Pfizer Ltd.;
Department of Pharmacology & Therapeutics
Seth Gordhandas Sunderdas Medical College and the King Edward Memorial Hospital
Mumbai, Maharashtra

Sri. H. Thakkalapally, PhD
Research Assistant
Department of Pharmacology
St John's University
New York, USA

Srinivasa Reddy Yathapu
Drug Toxicology Research Centre
ICMR-National Institute of Nutrition
Hyderabad, Telangana

Suhani V. Patel MBBS, MD (Pharmacology)
Clinical Researcher
SickKids - The Hospital for Sick Children
Toronto, Canada

Suneha Sikha, M Pharm (Pharmacology)
Drug Safety Associate
Bioclinica
Hyderabad, Telangana

Sunil V. Amrutkar, PhD
Professor
GES's Sir Dr. M. S. Gosavi College of Pharmaceutical Education & Research
Nashik, Maharashtra

Swetza Singh, PhD
Assistant Professor
Department of Pharmacology
School of Pharmacy, Babu Banarasi Das University
Lucknow, Uttar Pradesh

Swamy R.M., MD (Pharmacology)
Professor in Pharmacology
Sri Siddhartha Medical College
Tumakuru, Karnataka

Syed Ayaz Ali, M Pharm (Pharmacology)
Associate Professor
Department of Pharmacology
Y.B. Chavan College of Pharmacy
Aurangabad, Maharasthra

Tejus A, MBBS, MD (Pharmacology)
Associate Professor
Department of Pharmacology
Army College of Medical Sciences
Delhi Cantt, Delhi

Tithishri Kundu, MBBS, MD
Senior Resident
Department of Pharmacology
Bankura Sammilani Medical College
Bankura, West Bengal

T. Smitha, M Pharm
Assistant Professor
Jayamukhi College of Pharmacy
Affiliated to Kakatiya University
Narsampet, Telangana

Tuhin Kanti Biswas, MD, PhD
Assistant professor
J. B. Roy State Ayurvedic Medical College and Hospital
Kolkata, West Bengal

Upinder Kaur, MD
Assistant Professor
Department of Pharmacology
Institute of Medical Sciences
Banaras Hindu University
Varanasi, Uttar Pradesh

Vaishali Undale, M Pharm, PhD (Pharmacology)
Head of the Department
Department of Pharmacology
Dr. D.Y. Patil Institute of Pharmaceutical Sciences and Research
Pune, Maharashtra

S. Vasudeva Murthy, PhD
Professor and Head
Department of Pharmacology
Jayamukhi College of Pharmacy
Arshanapally, Chennaraopet, Telangana

Veena R.M., MBBS, MD (Pharmacology)
Associate Professor
Department of Pharmacology
BGS Global Institute of Medical Sciences
Bengaluru, Karnataka

Vetriselvan Subramaniyan, Ph.D., Cert. Health Res (CHRF)
Deputy Dean (Undergraduate)
Department of Pharmacology
Faculty of Medicine, Bioscience and Nursing
MAHSA University
Bandar Saujana Putra, Jenjarom, Selangor, Malaysia

Vijay Kumar Sehgal, MD (Pharmacology)
Professor & HOD
Department of Pharmacology
Government Medical College
Patiala, Punjab

Vijayakumar A.E., MD (Pharmacology)
Assistant Professor
Department of Pharmacology
ESIC Medical College and PGIMSR
Chennai, Tamil Nadu

Vinita Awasthi, MD
Student
Department of Pharmacology
King George's Medical University
Lucknow, Uttar Pradesh

Viraj A Shinde, MD (Pharmacology)
Assistant Professor
Department of Pharmacology
Symbiosis Medical College for Women
Lavale, Pune, Maharashtra

Vishalkumar K. Vadgama, MD (Pharmacology)
Assistant Professor
Department of Pharmacology
Government Medical College
Bhavnagar, Gujarat

Vishal Munjajirao Ubale, MBBS, MD
Assistant Professor
Department of Pharmacology
Government Medical Collage
Nagpur, Maharashtra

Vivek Jain, M Pharm, PhD (Pharmacology)
Assistant Professor
Department of Pharmaceutical Sciences
Mohanlal Sukhadia University
Udaipur, Rajasthan

Yogesh A. Kulkarni, PhD
Associate Dean
Pharmaceutical Sciences
Shobhaben Pratapbhai Patel School of Pharmacy & Technology Management
SVKM's NMIMS
Mumbai, Maharashtra

Competency Mapping Chart

Competency Code	Competency: The student should be able to	Page No.
Topic: Pharmacology		
PH1.1	Define and describe the principles of pharmacology and Pharmacotherapeutics.	2
PH1.2	Describe the basis of evidence-based medicine and therapeutic drug monitoring.	12, 13, 14
PH1.3	Enumerate and identify drug formulations and drug delivery systems.	7, 792
PH1.4	Describe absorption, distribution, metabolism,and excretion of drugs.	8-10, 11-13
PH1.5	Describe general principles of mechanism of drug action.	17, 18
PH1.6	Describe principles of pharmacovigilance and ADR reporting systems.	43-44
PH1.7	Define, identify, and describe the management of adverse drug reactions (ADRs).	43
PH1.8	Identify and describe the management of drug interactions.	37
PH1.9	Describe nomenclature of drugs, i.e., generic and branded drugs.	2
PH1.10	Describe parts of a correct, complete, and legible generic prescription. Identify errors in prescription and correct appropriately.	83
PH1.11	Describe various routes of drug administration, e.g., oral, subcutaneous, intravenous, intramuscular, sublingual.	792
PH1.12	Calculate the dosage of drugs using appropriate formulae for an individual patient, including children, elderly, and patient with renal dysfunction.	88
PH1.13	Describe mechanism of action, types, doses, side effects,indications, and contraindications of adrenergic and antiadrenergic drugs.	114, 131, 139
PH1.14	Describe mechanism of action, types, doses, side effects,indications, and contraindications of cholinergic and anticholinergic drugs.	104, 119
PH1.15	Describe mechanism/s of action, types, doses, side effects, indications, and contraindications of skeletal muscle relaxants.	123
PH1.16	Describe mechanism/s of action, types, doses, side effects, indications, and contraindications of the drugs that act by modulating autacoids, including: antihistaminics, 5-HT modulating drugs, nonsteroidal anti-inflammatory drugs (NSAIDs), drugs for gout, antirheumatic drugs, and drugs for migraine	360, 370, 380, 386, 399, 408
PH1.17	Describe the mechanism/s of action, types, doses, side effects, indications, and contraindications of local anesthetics	214, 215
PH1.18	Describe the mechanism/s of action, types, doses, side effects, indications, and contraindications of general anesthetics and preanesthetic medications	238
PH1.19	Describe the mechanism/s of action, types, doses, side effects,indications, and contraindications of the drugs that act on the central nervous system (including anxiolytics, sedatives and hypnotics, antipsychotic, antidepressant drugs, antimanic agents, opioid agonists and antagonists, drugs used for neurodegenerative disorders, and antiepileptics drugs)	267, 288, 301, 312, 327, 342, 354
PH1.20	Describe the effects of acute and chronic ethanol intake	278, 281–283
PH1.21	Describe the symptoms and management of methanol and ethanol poisonings	283–284
PH1.22	Describe drugs of abuse (dependence, addiction, stimulants,depressants, psychedelics, drugs used for criminal offences)	316
PH1.23	Describe the process and mechanism of drug deaddiction	41, 42, 283, 316

Competency Code	Competency: The student should be able to	Page No.
PH1.24	Describe the mechanism/s of action, types, doses, side effects,indications, and contraindications of the drugs affecting renal systems including diuretics, antidiuretics (vasopressin), and analogues	156, 157, 188, 226, 659
PH1.25	Describe the mechanism/s of action, types, doses, side effects, indications, and contraindications of the drugs acting on blood, such as anticoagulants, antiplatelets, fibrinolytics, and plasma expanders	206, 444, 470–473
PH1.26	Describe mechanisms of action, types, doses, side effects,indications, and contraindications of the drugs modulating the renin, angiotensin, and aldosterone system	148
PH1.27	Describe the mechanisms of action, types, doses, side effects, indications, and contraindications of antihypertensive drugs and drugs used in shock	148, 187, 204
PH1.28	Describe the mechanisms of action, types, doses, side effects, indications, and contraindications of the drugs used in ischemic heart disease (stable and unstable angina and myocardial infarction) and peripheral vascular disease	167, 175
PH1.29	Describe the mechanisms of action, types, doses, side effects, indications, and contraindications of the drugs used in congestive heart failure	155
PH1.30	Describe the mechanisms of action, types, doses, side effects, indications, and contraindications of the antiarrhythmics	210
PH1.31	Describe the mechanisms of action, types, doses, side effects, indications, and contraindications of the drugs used in the management of dyslipidemias	176, 178, 179, 181, 461
PH1.32	Describe the mechanism/s of action, types, doses, side effects, indications, and contraindications of drugs used in bronchial asthma and chronic obstructive pulmonary disease	422
PH1.33	Describe the mechanism of action, types, doses, side effects, indications, and contraindications of the drugs used in cough (antitussives, expectorants/mucolytics)	431
PH1.34	Describe the mechanism/s of action, types, doses, side effects, indications, and contraindications of the drugs used in the following: 1. Acidpeptic disease and gastroesophageal reflux disease 2. Antiemetics and prokinetics 3. Antidiarrheals 4. Laxatives 5. Inflammatory bowel disease 6. Irritable bowel disorders and biliary and pancreatic diseases	475, 485, 493, 497, 499, 500
PH1.35	Describe the mechanism/s of action, types, doses, side effects, indications, and contraindications of drugs used in hematological disorders such as: 1. Drugs used in anemias 2. Colony-stimulating factors	438
PH1.36	Describe the mechanism of action, types, doses, side effects, indications, and contraindications of drugs used in endocrine disorders (diabetes mellitus, thyroid disorders, and osteoporosis)	667, 695, 725, 731
PH1.37	Describe the mechanisms of action, types, doses, side effects, indications, and contraindications of the drugs used as sex hormones, their analogues, and anterior pituitary hormones	648, 675, 684
PH1.38	Describe the mechanism of action, types, doses, side effects, indications, and contraindications of corticosteroids	710
PH1.39	Describe mechanism of action, types, doses, side effects,indications, and contraindications of drugs used for contraception	675

Competency Code	Competency: The student should be able to	Page No.
PH1.40	Describe mechanism of action, types, doses, side effects,indications, and contraindications of: 1. Drugs used in the treatment of infertility 2. Drugs used in erectile dysfunction	60
PH1.41	Describe the mechanisms of action, types, doses, side effects,indications, and contraindications of uterine relaxants and stimulants	733
PH1.42	Describe general principles of chemotherapy	504
PH1.43	Describe and discuss the rational use of antimicrobials including antibiotic stewardship program	636
PH1.44	Describe the first-line antitubercular drugs, their mechanisms of action, side effects, and doses	570
PH1.45	Describe the drugs used in multidrug-resistant and extensively drug-resistant tuberculosis	570
PH1.46	Describe the mechanisms of action, types, doses, side effects, indications, and contraindications of antileprotic drugs	579
PH1.47	Describe the mechanisms of action, types, doses, side effects, indications, and contraindications of the drugs used in malaria, kala-azar, amebiasis, and intestinal helminthiasis	95, 605, 618
PH1.48	Describe the mechanisms of action, types, doses, side effects, indications, and contraindications of the drugs used in urinary tract infection/sexually transmitted diseases and viral diseases including HIV	560, 567
PH1.49	Describe mechanism of action, classes, side effects, indications, and contraindications of anticancer drugs	627
PH1.50	Describe mechanisms of action, types, doses, side effects,indications, and contraindications of immunomodulators and management of organ transplant rejection	409, 410, 752
PH1.51	Describe occupational and environmental pesticides, food adulterants, pollutants, and insect repellents	45
PH1.52	Describe management of common poisoning, insecticides,common sting, and bites	51
PH1.53	Describe heavy metal poisoning and chelating agents	742
PH1.54	Describe vaccines and their uses	91, 764
PH1.55	Describe and discuss national health programs including immunization, tuberculosis, leprosy, malaria, HIV, filaria, kala-azar, diarrheal diseases, anemia and nutritional disorders, blindness, noncommunicable diseases, cancer, and iodine deficiency	91
PH1.56	Describe basic aspects of geriatric and pediatric pharmacology	87
PH1.57	Describe drugs used in skin disorders	792
PH1.58	Describe drugs used in ocular disorders	143, 813
PH1.59	Describe and discuss the following: essential medicines, fixed-dose combinations, over-the-counter drugs, herbal medicines	15, 837
PH1.60	Describe and discuss pharmacogenomics and pharmacoeconomics	66
PH1.61	Describe and discuss dietary supplements and nutraceuticals	76
PH1.62	Describe and discuss antiseptics and disinfectants	806
PH1.63	Describe drug regulations, acts, and other legal aspects	79
PH1.64	Describe overview of drug development, phases of clinical trials, and good clinical practice	63

Competency Code	Competency: The student should be able to	Page No.
Skills: Clinical Pharmacy		
PH2.1	Demonstrate understanding of the use of various dosage forms (oral/local/parenteral; solid/liquid)	Practical
PH2.2	Prepare oral rehydration solution from ORS packet and explain its use	Practical
PH2.3	Demonstrate the appropriate setting up of an intravenous drip in a simulated environment	Practical
PH2.4	Demonstrate the correct method of calculation of drug dosage in patients including those used in special situations	Practical
Skills: Clinical Pharmacology		
PH3.1	Write a rational, correct, and legible generic prescription for a given condition and communicate the same to the patient	Practical
PH3.2	Perform and interpret a critical appraisal (audit) of a given prescription	Practical
PH3.3	Perform a critical evaluation of the drug promotional literature	Practical
PH3.4	To recognize and report an adverse drug reaction	Practical
PH3.5	To prepare and explain a list of P-drugs for a given case/condition	Practical
PH3.6	Demonstrate how to optimize interaction with pharmaceutical representative to get authentic information on drugs	Practical
PH3.7	Prepare a list of essential medicines for a healthcare facility	Practical
PH3.8	Communicate effectively with a patient on the proper use of prescribed medication	Practical
Skills: Experimental Pharmacology		
PH4.1	Administer drugs through various routes in a simulated environment using mannequins	Practical
PH4.2	Demonstrate the effects of drugs on blood pressure (vasopressor and vasodepressors with appropriate blockers) using computer-aided learning	Practical
Communication: Pharmacology		
PH5.1	Communicate with the patient with empathy and ethics on all aspects of drug use	Practical
PH5.2	Communicate with the patient regarding optimal use of:(1) drug therapy, (2) devices, and (3) storage of medicines	Practical
PH5.3	Motivate patients with chronic diseases to adhere to the prescribed management by the health care provider	Practical
PH5.4	Explain to the patient the relationship between cost of treatment and patient compliance	Practical
PH5.5	Demonstrate an understanding of the caution in prescribing drugs likely to produce dependence and recommend the line of management	Practical
PH5.6	Demonstrate ability to educate public and patients about various aspects of drug use including drug dependence and over-the-counter drugs	Practical
PH5.7	Demonstrate an understanding of the legal and ethical aspects of prescribing drugs	Practical
Integration		
Physiology		
PY3.5	Discuss the action of neuromuscular-blocking agents	124
Microbiology		
MI1.6	Describe the mechanisms of drug resistance, methods of antimicrobial susceptibility testing, and monitoring of antimicrobial therapy	507
MI3.3	Describe the enteric fever pathogens and discuss the evolution of the clinical course and the laboratory diagnosis of the diseases caused by them	768

Competency Code	Competency: The student should be able to	Page No.
Community Medicine		
CM3.8	Describe the mode of action and application cycle of commonly used insecticides and rodenticides	46
CM19.1	Define and describe the concept of Essential Medicines List (EML)	837
Forensic Medicine and Toxicology		
FM4.25	Clinical research and ethics: discuss human experimentation including clinical trials	63
FM9.1	Describe general principles and basic methodologies in treatment of poisoning: decontamination, supportive therapy, antidotetherapy, procedures of enhanced elimination with regard to caustics,inorganic (sulfuric, nitric, and hydrochloric acid) and organic (carbolic acid [phenol] andoxalic and acetylsalicylic acids)	43, 51
FM9.2	Describe general principles and basic methodologies in treatment of poisoning: decontamination, supportive therapy, antidotetherapy, procedures of enhanced elimination with regard to phosphorus, iodine, and barium	43, 51
FM9.3	Describe general principles and basic methodologies in treatment of poisoning: decontamination, supportive therapy, antidotetherapy, procedures of enhanced elimination with regard to arsenic, lead, mercury, copper, iron, cadmium, and thallium	58, 742
FM9.4	Describe general principles and basic methodologies in treatment of poisoning: decontamination, supportive therapy, antidote therapy, procedures of enhanced elimination with regard to ethanol, methanol, and ethylene glycol	283
FM9.5	Describe general principles and basic methodologies in treatment of poisoning: decontamination, supportive therapy, antidote therapy, procedures of enhanced elimination with regard to organophosphates, carbamates, organochlorines, pyrethroids, paraquat, aluminum, and zinc phosphide	46, 60, 117
FM9.6	Describe general principles and basic methodologies in treatment of poisoning: decontamination, supportive therapy, antidote therapy, procedures of enhanced elimination with regard to ammonia, carbon monoxide, hydrogen cyanide and derivatives, methyl isocyanate, and tear (riot control) gases	45
FM10.1	Describe general principles and basic methodologies in treatment of poisoning: decontamination, supportive therapy, antidotetherapy, procedures of enhanced elimination with regard to: 1. Antipyretics: paracetamol, salicylates 2. Anti-infectives (common antibiotics—an overview) 3. Neuropsychotoxicology barbiturates, benzodiazepines,phenytoin, lithium, haloperidol, neuroleptics, tricyclics 4. Narcotic analgesics, anesthetics, and muscle relaxants 5. Cardiovascular toxicology: cardiotoxic plants—oleander, odollam, aconite, digitalis 6. Gastrointestinal and endocrinal drugs: insulin	43, 51
Dermatology, Venereology, and Leprosy		
DR5.3	Enumerate and describe the pharmacology, administration, and adverse reaction of pharmacotherapies for scabies	794
DR7.3	Describe the pharmacology and action of antifungal (systemic and topical) agents. Enumerate side effects of antifungal therapy	583
DR8.7	Enumerate the indications and describe the pharmacology,administration, and adverse reaction of pharmacotherapies for common viral illnesses of the skin	793
DR9.4	Enumerate, describe, and identify lepra reactions and supportive measures and therapy of lepra reactions	579

Competency Code	Competency: The student should be able to	Page No.
DR9.5	Enumerate the indications and describe the pharmacology,administration, and adverse reaction of pharmacotherapies for various classes of leprosy based on national guidelines	94, 579
DR10.8	Enumerate the indications and describe the pharmacology,indications, and adverse reactions of drugs used in the nonsyphilitic sexually transmitted diseases (chancroid, donovanosis, and lymphogranuloma venereum)	568
DR14.5	Enumerate the indications and describe the pharmacology, indications, and adverse reactions of drugs used in urticaria and angioedema	365
DR15.3	Enumerate the indications and describe the pharmacology, indications, and adverse reactions of topical and systemic drugs used in the treatment of pyoderma	792
Anesthesiology		
AS3.6	Choose and write a prescription for appropriate premedications for patients undergoing surgery	251
AS4.1	Describe and discuss the pharmacology of drugs used in induction and maintenance of general anesthesia (including intravenous and inhalation induction agents, opiate and nonopiate analgesics, depolarizing and nondepolarizing muscle relaxants, anticholinesterases)	238
AS4.3	Observe and describe the principles and the practical aspects of induction and maintenance of anesthesia	240
AS5.4	Observe and describe the pharmacology and correct use of commonly used drugs and adjuvant agents in regional anesthesia	249
AS8.3	Describe the pharmacology and use of drugs in the management of pain	354, 400
AS8.4	Describe the principles of pain management in palliative care	354
AS8.5	Describe the principles of pain management in the terminally ill	354
Psychiatry		
PS4.4	Describe the treatment of alcohol and substance abuse disorders including behavioral and pharmacologic therapy	281
PS4.6	Enumerate and describe the pharmacologic basis and side effects of drugs used in alcohol and substance abuse	278, 316
PS5.5	Enumerate and describe the pharmacologic basis and side effects of drugs used in schizophrenia	343
PS6.4	Describe the treatment of depression including behavioral and pharmacologic therapy	327
PS6.6	Enumerate and describe the pharmacologic basis and side effects of drugs used in depression	327
PS8.4	Describe the treatment of anxiety disorders including behavioral and pharmacologic therapy	268
PS8.6	Enumerate and describe the pharmacologic basis and side effects of drugs used in anxiety disorders	268, 338
PS10.4	Describe the treatment of somatoform disorders including behavioral, psychosocial and pharmacologic therapy	329
PS10.6	Enumerate and describe the pharmacologic basis and side effects of drugs used in somatoform, dissociative, and conversion disorders	329
PS11.4	Describe the treatment of personality disorders including behavioral, psychosocial, and pharmacologic therapy	329

Competency Code	Competency: The student should be able to	Page No.
PS11.6	Enumerate and describe the pharmacologic basis and side effects of drugs used in personality disorders	329
PS12.4	Describe the treatment of psychosomatic disorders including behavioral, psychosocial, and pharmacologic therapy	329
PS12.6	Enumerate and describe the pharmacologic basis and side effects of drugs used in psychosomatic disorders	329
PS13.4	Describe the treatment of psychosexual and gender identity disorders including behavioral, psychosocial, and pharmacologic therapy	329
PS18.1	Enumerate the indications and describe the pharmacology, dose, and side effects of commonly used drugs in psychiatric disorders	329
General Medicine		
IM1.24	Describe and discuss the pharmacology of drugs including indications and contraindications in the management of heart failure including diuretics, angiotensin-converting enzyme inhibitors, beta blockers, aldosterone antagonists, and cardiac glycosides	148, 155
IM1.27	Describe and discuss the role of penicillin prophylaxis in the prevention of rheumatic heart disease	513
IM1.30	Administer an intramuscular injection with an appropriate explanation to the patient	5
IM2.15	Discuss and describe the medications used in patients with an acute coronary syndrome based on the clinical presentation	167, 175
IM2.18	Discuss and describe the indications, formulations, doses, side effects, and monitoring for drugs used in the management of dyslipidemia	461
IM2.20	Discuss and describe the assessment and relief of pain in acute coronary syndromes	167, 175
IM2.23	Describe and discuss the indications for nitrates, antiplatelet agents, GP IIb–IIIa inhibitors, beta blockers, angiotensin-converting enzyme inhibitors, etc., in the management of coronary syndromes	167, 175
IM3.12	Select, describe, and prescribe, based on the most likely etiology, an appropriate empirical antimicrobial based on the pharmacology and antimicrobial spectrum	504
IM3.13	Select, describe, and prescribe, based on culture and sensitivity, appropriate empaling antimicrobial based on the pharmacology and antimicrobial spectrum	504
IM4.22	Describe and discuss the pharmacology, indications, adverse reactions, and interactions of antimalarial drugs and basis of resistance	605
IM4.23	Prescribe drugs for malaria based on the species identified,prevalence of drug resistance, and national programs	605
IM4.26	Counsel the patient on malarial prevention	605
IM5.7	Enumerate and describe the causes and pathophysiology of drug-induced liver injury	42
IM5.7	Describe and discuss the management of hepatitis, cirrhosis, portal hypertension, ascites spontaneous, bacterial peritonitis, and hepatic encephalopathy	55
IM6.13	Describe and enumerate the indications and side effects of drugs for bacterial, viral, and other types of diarrheas	493
IM6.17	Discuss and describe the principles of highly active antiretroviral therapy (HAART), the classes of antiretrovirals used, adverse reactions, and interactions	598
IM6.18	Discuss and describe the principles and regimens used in postexposure prophylaxis	598

Competency Code	Competency: The student should be able to	Page No.
IM7.21	Select, prescribe, and communicate appropriate medications for relief of joint pain	400
IM7.22	Select, prescribe, and communicate preventive therapy for crystalline arthropathies	408
IM7.23	Select, prescribe, and communicate treatment option for systemic rheumatologic conditions	408
IM7.24	Describe the basis for biologic and disease-modifying therapy in rheumatologic diseases	408
IM8.14	Develop an appropriate treatment plan for essential hypertension	187
IM8.15	Recognize, prioritize, and manage hypertensive emergencies	187
IM9.14	Prescribe replacement therapy with iron, B_{12}, folate	439
IM9.15	Describe the national programs for anemia prevention	99
IM10.25	Identify and describe the priorities in the management of acute renal failure including diet, volume management, alteration in doses of drugs, monitoring, and indications for dialysis	88
IM11.16	Discuss and describe the pharmacologic therapies for diabetes, their indications, contraindications, adverse reactions, and interactions	698
IM11.18	Describe and discuss the pharmacology, indications, adverse reactions, and interactions of drugs used in the prevention and treatment of target organ damage and complications of type II diabetes including neuropathy, nephropathy, retinopathy,hypertension, dyslipidemia, and cardiovascular disease	698
IM11.19	Demonstrate and counsel patients on the correct technique to administer insulin	698
IM12.13	Describe the pharmacology, indications, adverse reaction, and interactions of thyroxine and antithyroid drugs	667
IM12.14	Write and communicate to the patient appropriately a prescription for thyroxine based on age, sex, and clinical and biochemical status	667
IM12.15	Describe and discuss the indications of thionamide therapy, radioiodine therapy, and general surgery in the management of thyrotoxicosis	667
IM13.17	Describe and enumerate the indications, use, and side effects of narcotics in pain alleviation in patients with cancer	357, 627
IM14.13	Describe and enumerate the indications, pharmacology, and side effects of pharmacotherapy for obesity	137, 177
IM15.14	Describe and enumerate the indications, pharmacology, and side effects of pharmacotherapy of pressors used in the treatment of upper gastrointestinal bleed	136, 232
IM15.15	Describe and enumerate the indications, pharmacology, and side effects of pharmacotherapy of acid peptic disease including *Helicobacter pylori*	476
IM16.13	Describe and enumerate the indications, pharmacology, and side effects of pharmacotherapy for parasitic causes of diarrhea	618
IM16.16	Describe and enumerate the indications, pharmacology, and side effects of pharmacotherapy including immunotherapy	493, 500
IM17.11	Describe the indications, pharmacology, dose, and side effects of abortive therapy in migraine	380
IM17.12	Describe the indications, pharmacology, dose, and side effects of prophylactic therapy in migraine	380
IM17.13	Describe the pharmacology, dose, adverse reactions, and regimens of drugs used in the treatment of bacterial, tubercular, and viral meningitis	512, 513, 539, 575

Competency Code	Competency: The student should be able to	Page No.
IM17.14	Counsel patients with migraine on lifestyle changes and need for prophylactic therapy	380
IM19.8	Discuss and describe the pharmacology, dose, side effects, and interactions used in the drug therapy of Parkinson's syndrome	301
IM20.7	Enumerate the indications and describe the pharmacology, dose, adverse reactions, and hypersensitivity reactions of anti–snake venom	61
IM20.8	Describe the diagnosis, initial approach, stabilization, and therapy of scorpion envenomation	51, 60
IM20.9	Describe the diagnosis, initial approach, stabilization, and therapy of bee sting allergy	51
IM21.1	Describe the initial approach to the stabilization of the patient who presents with poisoning	43, 51
IM21.2	Enumerate the common plant poisons seen in your area and describe their toxicology, clinical features, prognosis, and specific approach to detoxification	43, 51
IM21.3	Enumerate the common corrosives used in your area and describe their toxicology, clinical features, prognosis, and approach to therapy	43, 51
IM21.4	Enumerate the commonly observed drug overdose in your area and describe their toxicology, clinical features, prognosis, and approach to therapy	43, 51
IM21.5	Observe and describe the functions and role of a poison center in suspected poisoning	51
IM22.3	Describe the approach to the management of hypercalcemia	727
Pediatrics		
PE13.5	Propose a management plan for Fe-deficiency anemia	100, 439
PE13.6	Discuss the National Anaemia Control Program and its recommendations	100
PE14.1	Discuss the risk factors, clinical features, diagnosis, and management of lead poisoning	742
PE14.3	Discuss the risk factors, clinical features, diagnosis, and management of organophosphorus poisoning	60, 117
PE14.4	Discuss the risk factors, clinical features, diagnosis, and management of paracetamol poisoning	404
PE24.5	Discuss the role of antibiotics, antispasmodics, antisecretory drugs, probiotics, and antiemetics in acute diarrheal diseases	493
PE24.8	Discuss the causes, clinical presentation, and management of dysentery in children	493
PE34.3	Discuss the various regimens for management of tuberculosis as per national guidelines	570, 574
PE34.4	Discuss the preventive strategies adopted and the objectives and outcome of the National Tuberculosis Control Program	93
General Surgery		
SU13.2	Discuss the principles of immunosuppressive therapy. Enumerate indications and describe surgical principles and management of organ transplantation	719, 759
Physical Medicine and Rehabilitation		
PM3.5	Enumerate the indications and describe the therapies for spasticity including medications, serial casts, nerve blocks, and botulinum toxin injections	263

Competency Code	Competency: The student should be able to	Page No.
Respiratory Medicine		
CT1.4	Describe the epidemiology, the predisposing factors, and microbial and therapeutic factors that determine resistance to drugs	507
CT1.14	Describe and discuss the pharmacology of various antituberculous agents, their indications, contraindications, interactions, and adverse reactions	570
CT1.15	Prescribe an appropriate antituberculosis regimen based on the location of disease, smear positivity and negativity, and comorbidities based on current national guidelines including directly observed tuberculosis therapy (DOTS)	570
CT2.16	Discuss and describe therapies for obstructive airway disease including bronchodilators, leukotriene inhibitors, mast cell stabilizers, theophylline, inhaled and systemic steroids, oxygen, and immunotherapy	422

Part I

General Pharmacology

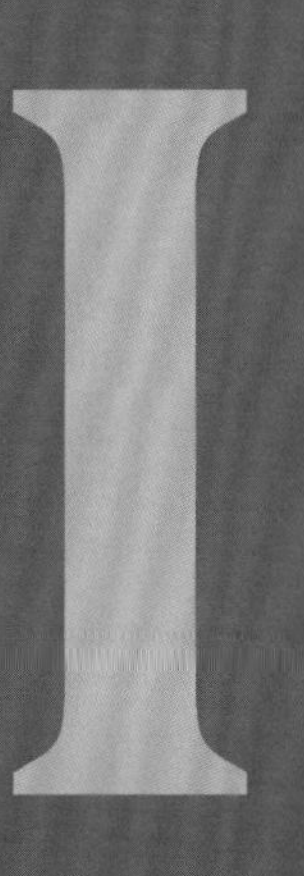

Chapter 1 Definitions and Sources of Drugs

Madhura Bhosale and Prachitee Borkar

Learning Objectives

- Common terms.
- Drug nomenclature.

Pharmacology (PH1.1)

Pharmacology is a science that deals with the effects of drugs on the living system. Widely, it encompasses all aspects of knowledge about drugs; however, medical pharmacology, which is relevant, is defined as the science of substances used to prevent, diagnose, and treat disease.

The World Health Organization (WHO) defines drug as any substance or product that is used or intended to be used, in order to modify or explore the physiological system or pathological states for the benefit of a recipient.

The two main divisions of pharmacology are as follows:

- **Pharmacokinetics:** It is the movement of drug within the body, which includes the processes of absorption (A) distribution (D), metabolism (M), and excretion (E). It also means "what body does to the drug."
- **Pharmacodynamics:** It is the study of drugs, their mechanism of action, pharmacological actions, and their adverse effects. It also means "what drug does to body."

Common Terms

Pharmacy: It is the science that deals with preparation, preservation, standardization, compounding, dispensing, and proper utilization of drugs.

Therapeutics: It is concerned with the treatment of diseases.

Toxicology: It is the study of poisons, their actions, detection, prevention, and treatment of poisoning.

Chemotherapy: It deals with treatment of infectious diseases/cancer.

Clinical pharmacology: It is the study of drug in man, both healthy volunteers and patients. It includes evaluation of pharmacokinetics and pharmacodynamics data, safety, efficacy, and adverse effects of a drug by comparative clinical trials.

Essential drugs: These are those drugs that satisfy the health care needs of majority of the population. They should be available at all times in adequate amounts and in appropriate dosage forms (WHO).

Orphan drug: The drugs used for diagnosis, treatment, or prevention of rare diseases.

Drug Nomenclature (PH1.9)

Chemical name: It describes the chemical composition of a drug, for example, acetylsalicylic acid. They are not suitable for use in prescribing.

Nonproprietary/generic name: It is the name assigned by a scientific authority, for example, the United States Adopted Name (USAN) Council and the British Approved Name (BAN). It is the same all over world, for example, aspirin.

Proprietary name (brand name): It is the name assigned by the manufacturer and is the property/trademark of the manufacturer, for example, Disprin. Often brand name is memorable, appealing, and indicative of drug use, for example, Asmanil (generic name Salbutamol), indicating its use in asthma. However, a drug may have different brand names; also, the same manufacturer can assign the same drug different brand names in different countries.

Sources of Drugs

There are various sources of drugs.

Natural

Drugs can be obtained from plants, animals, microorganisms, and recombinant deoxyribonucleic acid (DNA) technology.

- *Plants:* Plant products are being used in treatment since centuries. Based on their chemical composition, they can be divided into following categories:
  - Alkaloids: These are alkaline nitrogenous bases, having potent activity, for example, morphine, atropine, and quinine.
  - Glycosides: These are compounds with heterocyclic nonsugar moiety linked to a sugar moiety through ether linkage, for example, digoxin and digitoxin.
  - Oils: These are viscous liquids insoluble in water, for example, castor oil is a purgative, clove oil is used as an analgesic in dental pain, and *Nilgiri* oil is used as a counterirritant.
- *Animals: These are mainly organ extracts, for example, insulin and thyroxine.*
- *Minerals: Some minerals are used as medicinal substances, for example, ferrous sulfate and magnesium sulfate.*
- *Microorganisms: Most antibiotics are obtained from fungi, bacteria, for example, penicillin and streptomycin.*
- *Genetic engineering (recombinant DNA technology):* Several drugs are produced by recombinant DNA technology, for example, human insulin and hepatitis B vaccine.

Synthetic

Synthetic drugs form the largest source of medicines. Synthetic drugs are pure and designed to target specific macromolecules, for example, angiotensin-converting enzyme (ACE) inhibitors and thiazides. On the other hand, semisynthetic drugs are chemically modified natural products that are highly selective than their natural counterparts, for example, atropine substitutes.

Multiple Choice Questions

1. Which of the following is/are drug(s) obtained from natural sources?

A. Angiotensin-converting enzyme (ACE) inhibitors.
B. Thiazides.
C. Morphine.
D. Methamphetamine.

Answer: B

Alkaloids are alkaline nitrogenous bases, having potent activity, for example, morphine, atropine, and quinine. Drugs can be obtained from plants, animals, microorganisms, and recombinant deoxyribonucleic acid (DNA) technology. Morphine is an opiate alkaloid isolated from the plant *Papaver somniferum*.

2. "Essential drugs" are:

A. Life-saving drugs.
B. Drugs that meet the priority health care needs of the population.
C. Drugs that must be present in the emergency bag of a doctor.
D. Drugs that are listed in the pharmacopeia of a country.

Answer: B

The WHO has defined essential medicines (drugs) as "those that satisfy the priority health care needs of the population. They are selected with due regard to public health relevance, evidence on efficacy and safety, and comparative cost effectiveness."

3. An "orphan drug" is:

A. A very cheap drug.
B. A drug that has no therapeutic use.
C. A drug needed for treatment or prevention of a rare disease.
D. A drug that acts on orphan in receptors.

Answer: C

These are drugs or biological products for diagnosis/treatment/ prevention of a rare disease or condition, or a more common disease (endemic only in resource-poor countries) for which there is no reasonable expectation that the cost of developing and marketing it will be recovered from the sales of that drug.

Chapter 2 Routes of Drug Administration

Madhura Bhosale and Prachitee Borkar

PH1.3: Enumerate and identify drug formulations and drug delivery systems.

PH1.11: Describe various routes of drug administration, e.g., oral, SC, IV, IM, SL.

Learning Objectives

- Local route.
- Systemic route.

Introduction

It becomes more than important to know the numerous principles and modes of drug administration, as they are clinically pertinent in therapeutics, and help in evading any possible injury to patients getting these drugs. Although there are numerous principles of drug administration, the five significant ones are as follows: the right patient, the right drug, the right dose, the right time, and the right route of administration. Modes or routes of drug administration differ from the extensively administered oral route to parenteral and inhalational routes. There are also some specialized routes and modes of drug delivery, for example, the liposomal delivery, prodrug delivery, and others. Each of these routes of administration has its own advantages and disadvantages, which must be considered and compared to each other before selecting the same. This chapter deals with the key principles and routes or modes of drug administration.

Factors determining route of administration are as follows:

1. Drug characteristics like state of drug (solid/liquid/gas), and other properties of drug such as its solubility, stability, pH, and irritancy.
2. Clinical scenarios such as emergency or regular treatment.
3. Patient conditions like unconscious state, or if patient is experiencing diarrhea or vomiting.
4. Age.
5. Comorbid diseases.
6. Patient/doctor choice.
7. Rate and extent of absorption of the drug from different routes.
8. Effect of digestive enzymes and first-pass metabolism on the drug.

Routes of drug administration can be divided broadly into two categories: local and systemic (**Fig. 2.1**). Systemic route includes enteral route which further comprises oral and rectal (drug is directly administered into the gastrointestinal tract [GIT]), whereas parenteral route comprises sublingual (under the tongue), inhalation (into bronchi) and injection. Further, injection includes intravenous (IV, into the vein), intramuscular (IM, into the muscle), and subcutaneous (SC, under the skin).

Local Route

It is one of the simplest routes of drug administration, wherein the drug can be given at the desired site of action. Systemic absorption of drugs is minimal, hence systemic side effects can be avoided. Following are some of the local routes:

Topical

The drugs applied to skin/mucous membrane for local actions. A few examples are as follows:

- Oral cavity—Drugs can be delivered only to oral mucosa in the form of lozenges or rinse, for example, clotrimazole troche for oral conditions.
- GIT—Nonabsorbable drug can be used to have local effect only, for example, neomycin for gut sterilization before surgery.
- Rectum and anal canal—Drug in liquid/solid form is used through this route for various actions.
  - Evacuant enema: Through this route, drugs are used for bowel evacuation, for example, soap water enema. Soap acts as lubricant and water stimulates the rectum.
  - Retention enema, for example, methylprednisolone in ulcerative colitis.

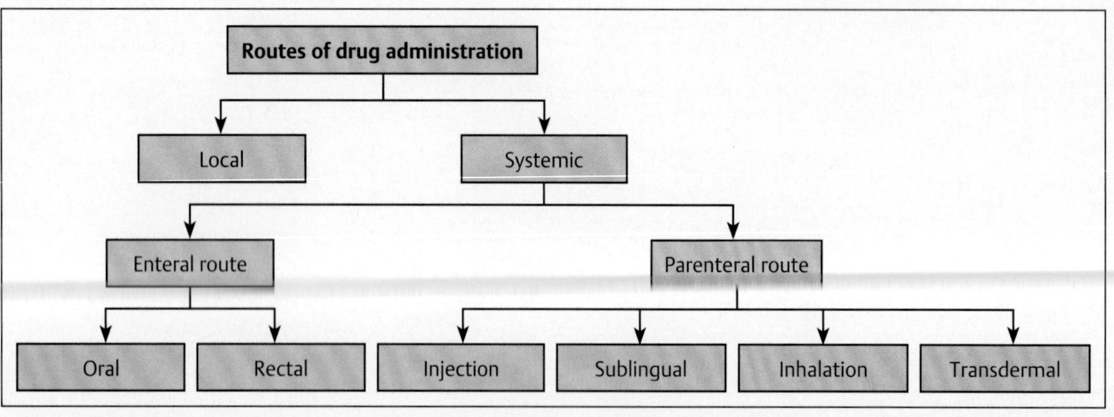

Fig. 2.1 Routes of drug administration.

- Suppository solid dosage form drug is inserted in rectum, for example, bisacodyl for bowel evacuation.
- Eye, ear, and nose—Drugs can be delivered to nasal mucosa, eyes, or ear canal in the form of drops, ointments, and sprays. This route can be employed for allergic/infective conditions of these organs.
- Bronchi (inhalational)—This route of drug administration is used for conditions like bronchial asthma and chronic obstructive pulmonary disorder (COPD), wherein drug is absorbed by bronchial mucosa through inhalation, for example, salbutamol.
- Vagina—Drugs can be applied/inserted in the form of tablet, cream, or pessary to vagina. This route is mainly used for vaginal candidiasis.
- Urethra—Medication in the form of solution/jellies can be applied to urethra, for example, lignocaine.

Deeper Areas

These are, for example, intra-articular tissue or retrobulbar region. They can be reached by using syringe and needle. However, in order to reduce systemic absorption of drug, only slowly absorbed drugs should be used, for example, lidocaine for local anesthesia can be given as intrathecal injection. Also, hydrocortisone acetate is given as an intra-articular injection.

Systemic Route

Through this route, drug reaches the blood, is distributed across the body, and produces systemic effects. Broadly, this route can be divided into enteral, parenteral, and specialized drug delivery.

Enteral Route

This route includes oral and rectal.

Oral

This is the most common and accepted route of drug administration. Following oral administration, drug reaches the systemic circulation and is widely distributed across all tissues. Oral route has advantages of being safe, painless, and convenient for repeat and long-term use. Moreover, through this route, drug can be self-administered and does not require professional assistance. However, oral route has few limitations like slow onset of action, and thus cannot be given in emergencies, unpalatable/irritant drugs (e.g., chloramphenicol), unabsorbable drugs (e.g., neomycin), drugs with high first-pass metabolism (e.g., lignocaine), medications destroyed by digestive juices (e.g., insulin). Other drawbacks included are they cannot be given in unconscious/uncooperative/unreliable patients and those having vomiting and diarrhea. Many dosage forms are available for oral administration; for example, solid forms like tablets, capsules, and liquid preparations such as syrups, elixirs, and suspensions. Tablets are made by compressing powdered drug along with binding agents and excipients, whereas capsules contain shell of gelatin, which is a tasteless natural substance. Two types of capsules are available—hard gelatin capsule (contain drug in solid form) and soft gelatin capsule (drug as an oily liquid form). In case of pediatric patients, swallowing of tablets/capsules is often problematic; in such cases, oral liquid preparations can be used.

Some of the abovementioned limitations of this route can be overcome by enteric coating of tablets and/or sustained/controlled release formulation. Enteric coating of tablets is done by cellulose and acetate. This has advantages like it prevents gastric irritation, protects drug from gastric acid, and retards drug absorption, thus increasing its duration of action. On the other hand, sustained/controlled release formulations have different coatings which dissolve at different time intervals. Advantages of this formulation are increase in duration of action, thus decreasing dosing frequency and increasing patient compliance, for example, sustained release nifedipine.

Sublingual

Drug which is lipid soluble is kept under the tongue or crushed and applied to buccal mucosa. Drug is absorbed into veins surrounding oral mucosa; later, it enters superior vena cava and heart and eventually reaches systemic circulation, for example, buprenorphine and nitroglycerin (used to terminate anginal attack). Advantages of this route is that drugs with high first-pass liver metabolism are readily available in systemic circulation when given by this route. Other advantages include rapid onset of action, drug can be self-administered, and action can be terminated by spitting out tablet. Limitations of this route is that it is irritant, lipid insoluble, and unpalatable; hence, it cannot be given. Additionally, it cannot be used in children.

Rectal

This route can be used for systemic effects apart from local effects. Drugs are absorbed by hemorrhoidal veins, and to some extent, they bypass liver metabolism. This route possesses certain advantages like irritant/unpleasant drug can be administered through this route. It can be used as suppository as well as in uncooperative/recurrent vomiting patients. Nevertheless, it has limitations like being embarrassing to patients, having erratic drug absorption, and leading to rectal inflammation in case of irritant drugs, for example, diazepam for febrile convulsions in children.

Parenteral Route (IM1.30)

This is route of drug administration other than the enteral route. It includes drugs administered by injection, inhalation, and transdermal route. It has advantages like rapid onset, thus can be used in emergency; also, it can be used in uncooperative patients and patients with vomiting/diarrhea. This route is suitable for irritant drugs, drugs with high first-pass metabolism, orally nonabsorbable drugs, and medication destroyed by digestive juices. Disadvantages of this route are that it is expensive and not easy for self-administration.

Inhalation

Volatile liquids and gases are administered by this route, for example, general anesthetics. Inhaled drug is absorbed through vast surface of alveoli; hence action is rapid.

Moreover, when drug administration is stopped, remaining drug in alveoli will be expelled quickly. Hence, termination of drug action as well as moment-to-moment drug regulation can be achieved through this route. However, irritant drugs can cause increased respiratory secretion and bronchospasm.

Transdermal Route (Adhesive Patches)

Patches deliver drug into circulation for systemic effects. Patches have multilayers like backing film, drug reservoir, rate controlling micropore membrane, and adhesive layer with priming dose, for example, scopolamine for motion sickness, nitroglycerin for angina, estrogen for hormone replacement therapy (HRT), and fentanyl for analgesia. Few advantages of this route include self-administration, good-patient compliance, prolonged action, minimal side effects, and constant plasma concentrations of drug. However, this route has drawbacks like being expensive, local irritation (itching, dermatitis), and patch may fall without being noticed.

Injection (Fig. 2.2)

Intradermal

Drug is injected into dermal layer of skin, for example, bacillus Calmette–Guerin (BCG) vaccination and drug sensitivity testing.

Subcutaneous (SC)

Drug is injected into SC tissue which has nerve supply but less vascular supply, for example, insulin and adrenaline. Self-administration is also possible; depot preparations for prolonged action can be used, for example, norplant for contraception. This route is unsuitable for irritant drugs as well as has slow onset, thus cannot be used in emergency.

Intramuscular (IM)

Drug is injected into large muscles, deltoid, gluteus maximum, and lateral aspect of thigh in children. With this route, rapid onset of action can be achieved compared to oral route; also, depot preparations (used to prolong drug action), mild irritants, soluble substances, and suspensions can be given. Nonetheless, IM route requires aseptic condition, administration by professionals, can be painful, and may lead to abscess and local tissue injury.

Intravenous (IV)

Direct injection of drug into vein. Drug can be given as bolus administration as well as slow IV infusion. Bolus administration is single, large dose rapidly/slowly injected as single unit, for example, furosemide, whereas slow IV injection involves addition of drug into a bottle containing dextrose/saline, for example, dopamine infusion in cardiogenic shock. With this route, 100% bioavailability and rapid onset of action can be achieved; hence it is suitable for emergencies. For example, when sedative drug midazolam is IV administered, sedation occurs in 2 to 4 minutes. Moreover, large volumes of fluids, for example, dextrose and highly irritant drugs, for example, anticancer drugs can be given through this route. Constant plasma concentration can be maintained using this route of administration. However, once drug is injected, drug action cannot be terminated. Administration of drug through this route can cause local irritation, thrombophlebitis, and necrosis.

Requirement of strict aseptic conditions and impossibility of self-administration are its other drawbacks. Also, depot preparations cannot be given. Caution in the form of ensuring tip of needle is in vein as well as slow administration of drug should be exercised while giving drugs through IV route.

Intra-arterial

This route is used when localized effect of a drug in a particular tissue or organ is desired. For example, in the treatment of renal tumor or head/neck cancer, drug is injected into renal artery or carotid artery, respectively.

Intrathecal

Injection of drug into subarachnoid space (into cerebrospinal fluid [CSF]). This route can be used as a method for direct delivery of a drug into central nervous system (CNS), for example, spinal anesthesia (lignocaine) and antibiotics (in meningitis).

Epidural Injection

This is injection into epidural space, which is area outside dura mater. It is different from intrathecal as drug is not

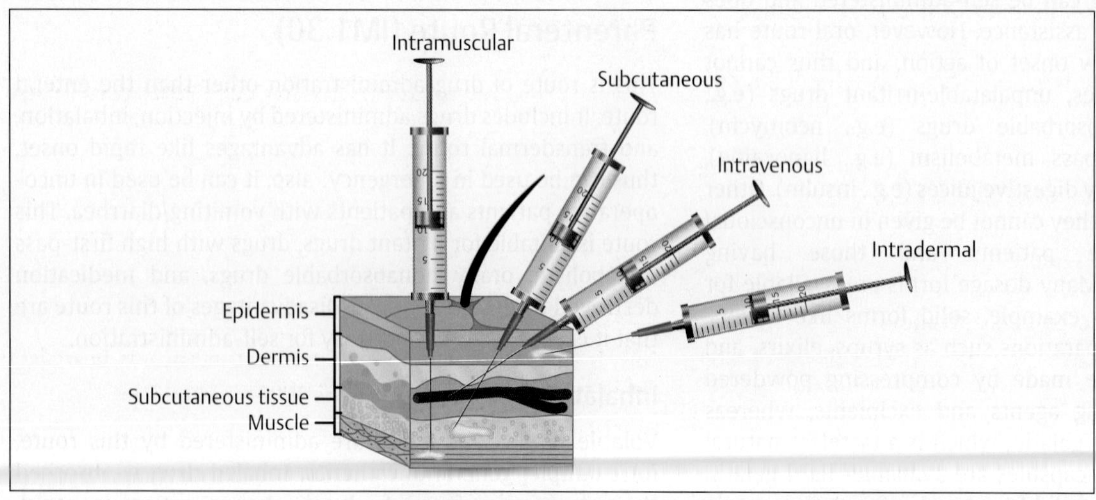

Fig. 2.2 Types of injection.

directly administered into CSF. Local anesthetic drugs are given by this route to provide analgesia during childbirth.

Intra-articular

Drug is injected into joint space, for example, hydrocortisone for rheumatoid arthritis. This route requires aseptic condition and can cause damage to cartilage on repeated use.

Specialized Drug Delivery (PH1.3)

Ocusert

Drug is kept beneath lower eyelid, for example, pilocarpine in glaucoma. Major advantage is single application releases drug for 1 week.

Progestasert

It is intrauterine contraceptive device which releases progesterone for 1 year.

Liposomes

Drug incorporated in minute phospholipid vesicles, for example, liposomal amphotericin for fungal infection.

Monoclonal Antibiotics

These are immunoglobulins which react with specific antigen. These can be used for targeted delivery, for example, anticancer drugs.

Multiple Choice Questions

1. Drug administered through the following route is most likely to be subjected to first-pass metabolism:

A. Oral.
B. Sublingual.
C. Subcutaneous.
D. Rectal.

Answer: A

Total drug absorbed orally is subjected to first-pass metabolism in the intestinal wall and liver, while approximately half of that absorbed from the rectum passes through the liver. Drug entering from any systemic route is exposed to first-pass metabolism in the lungs, but its extent is minor for most drugs.

2. Transdermal drug delivery systems offer the following advantages, except:

A. They produce high peak plasma concentration of the drug.
B. They produce smooth and nonfluctuating plasma concentration of the drug.
C. They minimize interindividual variations in the achieved plasma drug concentration.
D. They avoid hepatic first-pass metabolism of the drug.

Answer: A

The micropore membrane is such that the rate of drug delivery to skin surface is less than the slowest rate of absorption from the skin. As such, the drug is delivered at a constant and predictable rate irrespective of site of application. They provide smooth plasma concentrations of the drug without fluctuations.

3. In addition to slow intravenous infusion, which of the following routes of administration allows for titration of the dose of a drug with the response?

A. Sublingual.
B. Transdermal.
C. Inhalational.
D. Nasal insufflation.

Answer: C

When administration is discontinued, the drug diffuses back and is rapidly eliminated in the expired air. Thus, controlled administration is possible with moment-to-moment adjustment.

4. Which of the following drugs is administered by intranasal spray/application for systemic action?

A. Phenylephrine.
B. Desmopressin.
C. Azelastine.
D. Beclomethasone dipropionate.

Answer: B

Certain drugs, such as GnRH agonists and desmopressin applied as a spray or nebulized solution, have been used by this route. Desmopressin is the preparation of choice for all V2 receptor-related indications. The intranasal route is preferred.

5. Compared to subcutaneous injection, the intramuscular injection of drugs:

A. Is more painful.
B. Produces faster response.
C. Is unsuitable for depot preparations.
D. Carries greater risk of anaphylactic reaction.

Answer: B

The muscle is more vascular (absorption of drugs in aqueous solution is faster).

6. Select the route of administration that carries the highest risk of adversely affecting vital functions:

A. Intra-arterial injection.
B. Intrathecal injection.
C. Intravenous injection.
D. Intramuscular injection.

Answer: C

This is the most risky route, as vital organs such as heart and brain get exposed to high concentrations of the drug.

Chapter 3 Pharmacokinetics

Ramanand Patil

PH1.4: Describe absorption, distribution, metabolism, and excretion of drugs.

Learning Objectives

- Absorption of a drug.
- Distribution of a drug.
- Drug metabolism.
- Drug excretion.
- Pharmacokinetic parameters.

Introduction

The term *pharmacokinetics* (PK) is derived from two words, *pharmacon* (drug) and *kinesis* (movement). Simply, it deals with "what the body does to the drug." It includes absorption (A), distribution (D), metabolism (M), and excretion (E) of the drug. ADME involves passage of the drugs across various biological membranes in the body (**Fig. 3.1**). Each biological membrane has a lipid bilayer.

Drugs cross biological membranes via the following mechanisms:

- *Simple or passive diffusion:* It is a bidirectional process. Drug molecules move from a higher concentration region to a lower concentration region till equilibrium is achieved. The diffusion rate is directly proportional to the concentration gradient across membrane. Lipid-soluble (nonionized) drugs are passively transported (without energy), crossing the biological membranes to the other side.
- *Filtration:* It depends on the size and weight of the drug molecule. If drug molecules are smaller than the pores, they are easily filtered through the membrane.
- *Specialized transport:*
  - Active transport: It requires energy. Drug moves from a region of lower concentration to a region of higher concentration against the chemical or electrical gradient, for example, transport of choline to cholinergic neurons against the concentration gradient.
  - Facilitated diffusion: It does not require energy for transport. It is a carrier-mediated transport. In facilitated diffusion, the drug attaches to a carrier on the membrane, facilitating its diffusion across the membrane. In contrast to active transport, here, the drug moves from a higher concentration region to a lower concentration region, for example, absorption of vitamin B12 from gastrointestinal tract (GIT) and transport of amino acids in brain.

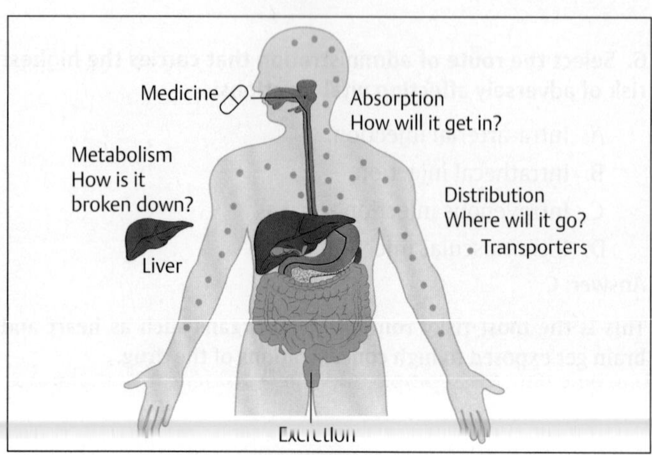

Fig. 3.1 Principles of pharmacokinetics.

Absorption of a Drug (PH1.4)

The process by which drug is transported from the site of administration to the blood circulation is known as absorption. Factors modifying drug absorption are mentioned in **Box 3.1**.

Physical State

Liquids are absorbed better compared to solids.

Particle Size

Drugs with smaller particle size are better absorbed, for example, microfine griseofulvin. Anthelmintic drugs have a larger particle size; hence, they are poorly absorbed and act better on gut helminths.

Disintegration Time

It is the time required by the tablet or capsule to disintegrate (break) into fine drug granules. Drugs having faster disintegration time demonstrate better absorption.

Dissolution Time

It is the time required for the drug to dissolve into solution. Drugs having faster dissolution time show better absorption.

Box 3.1 Factors modifying drug absorption

- Physical state
- Particle size
- Disintegration time
- Dissolution time
- Formulation
- Lipid solubility
- pH and ionization
- Area and vascularity of absorbing surface
- GI motility
- Presence of food
- GI diseases
- Metabolism

Formulation

Drug formulations affect drug absorption. Inert substances such as lactose and starch used in drugs may interfere with drug absorption.

Lipid Solubility

Lipid-soluble drugs penetrate the cell faster and better at cell surface and easily dissolve in phospholipids of cell membrane.

pH and Ionization

The degree of ionization of drugs depends on the pH level of the medium. Unionized form of lipid-soluble drugs is better absorbed compared to ionized drugs, which are poorly absorbed. Acidic drugs will remain unionized in the acidic medium of the stomach (e.g., aspirin, barbiturates) and basic drugs will remain unionized in the alkaline medium of the intestines (e.g., pethidine, ephedrine), and both unionized forms of drug are rapidly absorbed. Strong electrolytes are completely ionized at acidic and alkaline pH (e.g., heparin, streptomycin); hence, they are poorly absorbed. However, most drugs are weak electrolytes and they exist in both ionized and unionized forms.

Area and Vascularity of Absorbing Surface

Drugs are better absorbed from surfaces having larger area and more vascularity. As the small intestine has larger surface area than the stomach, drugs are better absorbed in the small intestine.

Gastrointestinal Motility

The faster the gastric emptying time (GET), the faster the drug reaches the intestine and rapid absorption occurs. Faster motility causes reduced drug absorption, as in diarrhea, due to less contact time with intestinal surface for absorption of the drug.

Presence of Food

The presence of food alters the GET and dilutes the drug. It slows down the absorption of the drug, and the complex of food and drug is incompletely absorbed, for example, tetracyclines chelate calcium.

Gastrointestinal (GI) Diseases

GI diseases such as malabsorption syndrome and achlorhydria reduce the absorption of drug. In achlorhydria, absorption of acidic drugs is reduced, for example, ketoconazole.

Metabolism

Most of the drugs are metabolized and inactivated during first-pass metabolism in the GIT or in the liver (e.g., nitroglycerine [NTG)], insulin); hence, such drugs are given either in high dose or parenterally.

First-Pass Metabolism (Presystemic Metabolism)

Metabolism of most of the orally administered drug occurs during its passage from the site of absorption to the systemic circulation either in the GIT wall or in the liver. It could be partial or total metabolism. Those drugs with partial first-pass metabolism require higher dose (e.g., propranolol, NTG) and those drugs with total first-pass metabolism require change of route of drug administration (e.g., insulin, isoprenaline).

Absorption from Parenteral Route

- Intravenous (IV) route: Drugs are directly given into the vein. This route produces a very rapid action with smaller doses.
- Intramuscular (IM) route: In this route, drug molecules are initially dissolved in the tissue fluid and then absorbed. Since muscles are highly vascular, fast absorption of drugs occurs. Lipid-soluble drugs are absorbed faster by IM route.
- Subcutaneous (SC) route: This route has a slow but steady absorption of drug with sustained and uniform action.
- Inhalation route: This route produces rapid effects. Lipid-soluble drugs are rapidly absorbed from pulmonary epithelium and produce rapid effects.
- Topical route: Drug absorption is slow via topical route because multiple epidermal layers are present; however, easy absorption occurs through the mucous membrane. Drugs having high-lipid solubility are absorbed from intact skin, for example, NTG.

Bioavailability

Bioavailability (BA) is a fraction or percentage of an active drug that reaches the systemic circulation following the administration. Large variations in BA of the drugs may lead to therapeutic failure or toxicity.

BA of drugs from different routes are as follows: IV, 100%; transdermal, 80 to 100%; IM/SC/sublingual, more than 75%; oral, 30 to 100% (lower because of the first-pass metabolism); and rectal, 30 to 100%.

Bioavailability (F) is calculated by,

$$F = \frac{\text{Area under the curve (AUC) (oral)} \times 100}{\text{AUC (IV)}}$$

To measure BA, the drug is administered by IV route, and plasma concentration is measured at hourly interval, and then plotted against timer. Similarly, for oral dosage of same dose, the plasma concentration–time graph is obtained, and then AUC is measured (**Fig. 3.2**).

Factors modifying bioavailability are similar to the factors modifying drug absorption.

Bioequivalence

Bioequivalence is a comparison of BA of different formulations of the same amount of drug. Oral formulations containing the same amount of drug from different manufacturers or different batches from the same manufacturer may

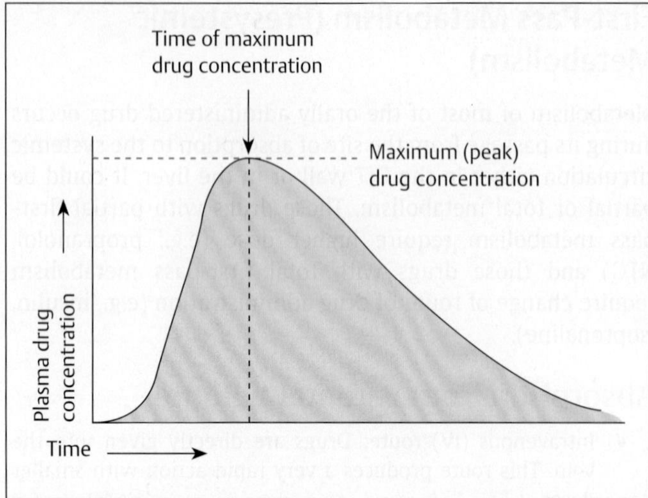

Fig. 3.2 Area under the curve (AUC).

have different plasma concentration and could become nonbioequivalent. Differences in bioequivalence may be due to difference in disintegration and/or dissolution rate. Nonbioequivalence or bioequivalence may lead to therapeutic failure or toxicity of the drug, such as drugs with low safety margin (digoxin, anticoagulants).

Distribution of a Drug

After absorption through the systemic circulation, the drug is distributed to different tissues. Through this process, the drug crosses many barriers to reach the site of action. It also involves the same process of absorption such as filtration, diffusion, and specialized transport.

Factors determining distribution are lipid solubility, ionization, vascularity, and binding to plasma and cellular proteins.

Plasma Protein Binding

In the blood, acidic drugs are bound to albumin, basic drugs are bound to α-acid glycoprotein, and free drug is available for action, metabolism, and excretion. Protein-bound drug acts as a reservoir drug. Plasma protein binding (PPB) is variable for every drug such as 0% for lithium and ethosuximide and 99% for warfarin.

Clinical significance of PPB:

- Only the free fraction of drug is available for action, metabolism, and excretion, and when the concentration of the free fraction of drug decreases, bound drug is released.
- Protein-bound drug serves as a reservoir (store) drug.
- PPB increases the drug's half-life ($t_{½}$) and also its duration of action.
- Plasma-bound drugs are not metabolized or excreted, and hence highly plasma-bound drugs are generally long-acting.
- When binding site is same for many drugs, they compete for that; therefore, a drug having higher affinity for same binding site displaces another drug with low affinity. This may result in drug interactions. Warfarin is 99% plasma-bound and 1% free in blood. When warfarin is coadministered with indomethacin, indomethacin displaces warfarin from binding site and reduces warfarin PPB to 95%, and 5% warfarin is free. This results in fivefold increase in the warfarin concentration and therefore the toxicity of warfarin (bleeding) increases. However, there is also a simultaneous increase in metabolism and excretion of warfarin, which decrease toxicity.
- When a drug is administered repeatedly for shorter duration, saturation of binding sites occurs; thereafter, there is increase in free drug concentration.
- Diseases such as chronic renal failure, chronic hepatic dysfunction, and anemia cause hypoalbuminemia. This decreases the concentration of plasma-bound drugs and careful administration of highly protein-bound drugs is needed.
- In drug poisoning, highly bound drugs cannot be removed by hemodialysis easily.

Tissue Binding

Certain drugs, because of their special affinity for some tissues, bind to them. Due to this binding, there is a delay in excretion and metabolism of these drugs, which results in increase in their duration of action (e.g., lipid-soluble drugs binding to adipose tissue). Tissue binding also serves as a drug reservoir (store).

Redistribution

Drugs with high lipid solubility are redistributed, for example, they are initially distributed to highly vascular organs (brain, heart, and kidney) and later redistributed to less vascular organs (muscle, fat), which terminates their action (e.g., thiopentone).

Blood–Brain Barrier

Endothelial cells of brain capillaries are joined by a continuous tight intercellular junction, instead of pores and capillaries, covered by glial cells. Together, they constitute the blood–brain barrier (BBB).

Only unionized lipid-soluble drugs can cross the BBB (e.g., barbiturates, diazepam, volatile anesthetics). During inflammation, such as in meningitis, the permeability of the BBB increases (e.g., penetration of penicillin during meningitis). Some areas in brain have weak barrier such as chemoreceptor trigger zone (CTZ), posterior pituitary, and parts of hypothalamus. As the pH level of cerebrospinal fluid (CSF) is 7.35, the concentration of weakly basic drugs in CSF is more than that of acidic drugs.

Placental Barrier

Unionized lipid-soluble drugs can cross the placental barrier more than lipid-insoluble drugs, which results in increased fetal adverse effects. Lipid-soluble drugs having 200- to 500-Da molecular weight have the ability to cross the placental barrier easily than drugs with more than 1,000-Da molecular weight, which hardly cross it (e.g., anesthetics, alcohol easily crosses placental barrier, whereas d-tubocurarine [d-TC] and insulin do not cross it).

Volume of Distribution (V_d)

The volume of distribution is the volume into which the total amount of a given drug in the body appears to be distributed.

The volume of distribution (V_d) is calculated by the following formula:

$$V_d = \frac{\text{Amount of drug in the body}}{\text{Plasma concentration}}$$

Therefore, if the dose of drug is 500 mg and its plasma concentration is 10 mg/L, then V_d is 50 L. Highly plasma protein–bound drugs have small V_d (e.g., aspirin, phenylbutazone) and low plasma protein–bound drugs have large V_d (e.g., pethidine). The volume of distribution (V_d) is important in cases of drug poisoning. Drugs that have large V_d are not easily removed by hemodialysis because of wide distribution. Changes occur in volume of distribution (V_d) in disease states due to alteration in tissue permeability and protein binding. Those drugs that have a low V_d have a large V_d in patients with edema or ascites (e.g., aminoglycosides).

Factors Determining Distribution

- Physicochemical properties of the drug: Unionized lipid-soluble drugs are widely distributed (e.g., lignocaine, propranolol), while ionized drugs are confined to the intravascular compartment (e.g., heparin).
- PPB: Drugs with high PPB have low V_d and those with low PPB have high V_d.
- Tissue storage: Certain drugs are sequestered in certain tissue, such as digoxin (V_d of 66 L/kg) in the heart.
- Diseases: Diseases such as congestive cardiac failure and uremia can alter the V_d of the drug. Diseases can increase V_d due to increase in extracellular fluid volume or can decrease V_d due to decrease in tissue perfusion.
- Fat: Highly lipid-soluble drugs get distributed in adipose tissue; therefore, they have a high V_d, as fat acts as a reservoir of drug.

Drugs Metabolism (Biotransformation) (PH1.4)

Biotransformation (metabolism) is defined as the chemical alteration of drug in living organism. Lipid-soluble unionized drugs are converted to water-soluble ionized drugs, as the latter are not reabsorbed by kidneys and excreted from body. Highly polar ionized parent molecule may not get metabolized and is excreted as it is. Drug metabolism occurs at the liver (primary site), GIT, kidneys, lungs, blood, skin, placenta, etc.

Consequences of Metabolism of Drug

- Active drug to inactive metabolite: it is the most common (phenobarbitone to hydroxyphenobarbital and phenytoin to p-hydroxyphenytoin).
- Active drug to active metabolite (codeine to morphine and diazepam to oxazepam).
- Inactive drug to active metabolite (prodrug) (L-dopa to dopamine and prednisone to prednisolone).
- Active drug to toxic metabolite (paracetamol to N-acetyl-p-benzoquinoneimine [NAPQI]).

Pathways of Drug Metabolism

- Phase I or nonsynthetic: oxidation, reduction, and hydrolysis.
- Phase II or synthetic: conjugation reactions.

Phase I (Nonsynthetic Reactions)

Oxidation

Oxidation is the most common and important reaction. In oxidation, addition of O_2 and/or removal of hydrogen occurs (phenytoin, phenobarbitone, propranolol).

Reduction

In reduction, removal of O_2 or addition of hydrogen occurs in contrast to oxidation (chloramphenicol, methadone).

Hydrolysis

In hydrolysis, compounds are broken down by addition of water. It is common among esters and amides (esters: procaine, succinylcholine; amides: lignocaine, procainamide). At the end of phase I, nonsynthetic reactions metabolite may be inactive or active.

Phase II (Synthetic Reactions)

Phase II consists of conjugation reactions. In phase I, if a metabolite is polar, it is excreted by kidneys. However, many metabolites are still lipophilic and they are reabsorbed and undergo subsequent conjugation reaction with endogenous substrates such as glucuronic acid, sulfuric acid, acetic acid, and amino acid (**Table 3.1**). These conjugates are inactive, polar, and water soluble. Not all drugs undergo phase I and then phase II reactions—some drugs such as isoniazid/isonicotinic acid hydrazide (INH) undergo phase II reaction first and then phase I reaction.

Enzymes for Drug Metabolism

Microsomal Enzymes

These enzymes are mainly present in endoplasmic reticulum and catalyze most of phase I as well as phase II glucuronide conjugation reactions. Examples include cytochrome P450 and glucuronyl transferase. They are inducible enzymes.

Table 3.1 Reactions and examples of phase II metabolic reactions

Reactions	Examples
Glucuronide conjugation	Paracetamol, morphine
Acetylation	INH, dapsone, sulfonamides
Glycine conjugation	Salicylic acid
Sulfate conjugation	Sex steroids
Glutathione conjugation	Paracetamol
Methylation	Adrenaline, dopamine

Nonmicrosomal Enzymes

These enzymes are mainly present in cytoplasm, plasma, and mitochondria of liver cells and catalyze all phase II reactions (except glucuronide conjugation). They are mostly involved in reduction and hydrolysis reactions. They are noninducible enzymes.

Enzyme Induction

Repeated administration of drugs stimulates or induces synthesis of microsomal enzymes. It is a slow process and can take around 2 to 3 weeks. Some examples of drugs that undergo enzyme induction are rifampicin, phenytoin, phenobarbitone, carbamazepine, and griseofulvin.

Clinical Importance of Enzyme Induction

- It hastens metabolism and thus reduces duration and efficacy of drug action, leading to therapeutic failure, for example, rifampicin inducing oral contraceptive (OC) pills, which, in turn, leads to contraceptive failure.
- Autoinduction can lead to drug tolerance (carbamazepine).
- Due to increased production of toxic metabolites during enzyme induction, drug toxicity can occur, for example, hepatotoxicity can occur due to paracetamol in alcoholics.
- Osteomalacia can occur due to increased metabolism of vitamin D by phenytoin.
- Overproduction of porphobilinogen can lead to porphyria.
- Consumption of enzyme inducers such as cabbage and spinach can lead to rapid elimination of drugs.
- Enzyme induction also have benefits; for example, phenobarbitone given to neonatal patients with jaundice can induce glucuronyl transferase, leading to increased metabolism of bilirubin and thus decreasing bilirubin levels.

Enzyme Inhibition

Enzyme inhibitors are defined as drugs that inhibit the activity of metabolizing enzymes. Unlike enzyme induction, it is a rapid process. Some of the examples of enzyme inhibitors are erythromycin, ketoconazole, cimetidine, chloramphenicol, and ciprofloxacin. This may lead to increased effects, for example, warfarin when given with enzyme inhibitors causes increased bleeding.

Factors Modifying Drug Metabolism

- *Age:* Neonates and elderly patients have low-metabolizing capacity, which may lead to increased toxicity–for example, gray-baby syndrome in neonates due to decreased glucuronyl transferase, and increased toxicity of propranolol and lignocaine in the elderly.
- *Diet:* Protein deficiency may reduce the drug metabolism and protein-rich food increases the metabolism (theophylline and caffeine). Food rich in carbohydrate reduces metabolism.
- *Diseases:* Diseases of liver (e.g., cirrhosis) reduce the metabolism of drugs and increase the duration of action of drugs (e.g., diazepam).
- *Pharmacogenetics:* It is the study of genetically determined variations in drug responses. Genetic defect may alter drug response. Some examples of genetic variation are:
  - INH slow acetylators increase in peripheral neuritis and INH fast acetylators require a larger dose.
  - Succinylcholine (SCh): It is a depolarizing skeletal muscle relaxant, metabolized in 3 to 6 minutes by plasma pseudocholinesterase. Persons having abnormal or atypical pseudocholinesterase metabolize SCh very slowly, which can lead to respiratory paralysis and apnea.
  - Glucose-6-phosphate dehydrogenase (G6PD) (maintains RBCs' integrity) deficiency may lead to hemolysis in a patient who is exposed to primaquine, sulfonamides, dapsone, salicylates, etc.

Prodrug

It is an inactive drug that metabolizes to active drug. Advantages of prodrug are as follows:

- It increases the bioavailability of the drug; for example, in parkinsonism, there is a deficiency of dopamine in the brain and dopamine cannot cross the BBB, but a prodrug of dopamine, L-dopa, crosses the BBB and is then converted to dopamine.
- It increases the duration of action; for example, phenothiazine has a short duration of action, but when it is esterified as fluphenazine, the duration of action is increased.
- It enhances taste, for example, clindamycin is bitter, but clindamycin palmitate has better taste.
- Site-specific drug is delivered; for example, methanamine is converted to active formaldehyde in acidic pH of urine and acts as urinary antiseptic.

Drug Excretion (PH1.4)

Drug excretion is the removal of drug and its metabolite from the body. Major routes of excretion are the kidney, lungs, bile, and feces, and minor routes of excretion are sweat, saliva, and milk.

Kidney

The processes involved in drug excretion through the kidney include glomerular filtration, active tubular secretion, and passive tubular reabsorption. Glomerular filtration and tubular secretion facilitate excretion, while tubular reabsorption decreases drug excretion.

Glomerular Filtration (PH1.2)

Drugs with smaller molecular weight are easily filtered compared to those with larger molecular weight. The extent of glomerular filtration is directly proportional to glomerular filtration rate and the fraction of unbound or free drug in plasma.

Passive Tubular Reabsorption

It depends on the pH of renal tubular fluid and the degree of ionization. Strong acids and basic drugs remain ionized at any urinary pH and hence are excreted. Weakly acidic drugs (e.g., salicylates, barbiturates) are unionized at acidic pH of urine and are reabsorbed, but by making urinary pH alkaline with sodium bicarbonate, they become ionized and are easily excreted. Similarly, weakly basic drugs (e.g., morphine, amphetamine) remain unionized in alkaline urine and are reabsorbed, but by making urine acidic with vitamin C (ascorbic acid), they become ionized and are easily excreted. The principle of making urine acidic or alkaline is employed for excretion of basic or acidic poisons from the kidneys.

Active Tubular Secretion

This process of drug excretion is a carrier-mediated active transport that requires energy and is unaffected by changes in urinary pH and protein binding. The carrier system is nonselective and there is competition between drugs with similar physicochemical properties for carrier system, for example, probenecid competitively inhibits tubular secretion of penicillin and cephalosporin and increases the duration of action/plasma concentration/efficacy of penicillin/cephalosporin.

Lungs

Alcohol and volatile general anesthetics (e.g., ether, halothane) are partially excreted.

Feces

Drugs that are not completely absorbed through the gut are excreted through feces (purgatives).

Bile

Drugs that are excreted from the bile get reabsorbed in the intestine and are again re-excreted from the bile repeatedly, a process known as enterohepatic circulation. This process increases the BA and duration of drug action (e.g., erythromycin, phenolphthalein).

Skin

Metals such as arsenic and mercury are excreted through the skin in smaller amounts.

Saliva

Drugs such as lithium, potassium iodide, phenytoin, and metronidazole are excreted in the saliva. This process of excretion is used for monitoring lithium therapy.

Milk

During lactation, certain drugs are secreted in milk. As milk is acidic, basic drugs (e.g., tetracycline, chloramphenicol, morphine, diazepam) are excreted easily. This can affect the suckling infant—for example, tetracyclines secreted in milk chelates developing teeth and bones in suckling infant.

Pharmacokinetic Parameters

Plasma Half-Life ($t½$)

It is defined as the time required for the plasma concentration of the drug to become half, that is, 50% of its original value. It determines the duration of action and dosage frequency and also estimates the time required for plasma to reach concentration at steady state (PSS). After repeated administration, drug requires approximately 4 to 5 $t_{½}$ to reach steady-state concentration and is almost completely eliminated in 4 to 5 $t_{½}$ after single administration (**Fig. 3.3**).

Clearance

Clearance (CL) is a fraction of the volume of distribution from which drug is removed in unit time.

$$\text{CL} = \frac{\text{Rate of elimination}}{\text{Plasma concentration of drug}}$$

First-Order Kinetics

A constant fraction of drug in the body is eliminated per unit time, and the rate of drug elimination is directly proportional to its plasma concentration. In first-order kinetics, half-life ($t_{½}$) remains constant. Majority of drugs are eliminated through first-order kinetics (**Fig. 3.4a**).

Zero-Order Kinetics

In zero-order kinetics, a constant amount or a fixed quantity of drug is eliminated per unit time, and the rate of drug elimination is independent of its plasma concentration. In this kinetics, half-life ($t_{½}$) is never constant. Examples of drugs following this kinetics are alcohol, aspirin, phenytoin, and heparin (**Fig. 3.4b**).

Mixed-Order Kinetics (Michaelis–Menten Kinetics or Saturation Kinetics) (PH1.2)

It depends on the dose. At low doses, the elimination kinetics is of first order, but as the dose increases, the elimination processes get saturated and the kinetics changes to zero order. Some drugs following this kinetics are phenytoin, higher doses of aspirin, warfarin, and digoxin. The plasma concentration of such drugs needs to be monitored because

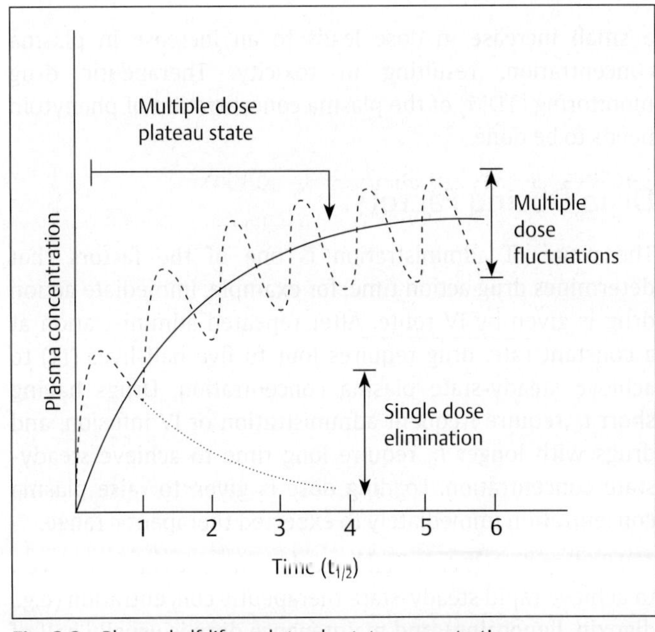

Fig. 3.3 Plasma half-life and steady-state concentration.

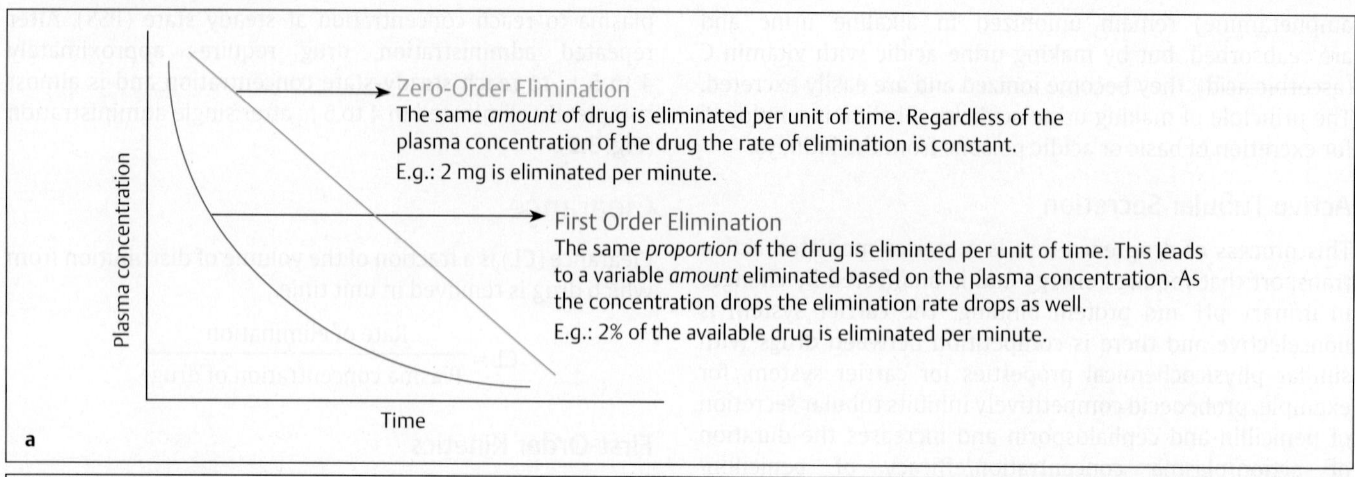

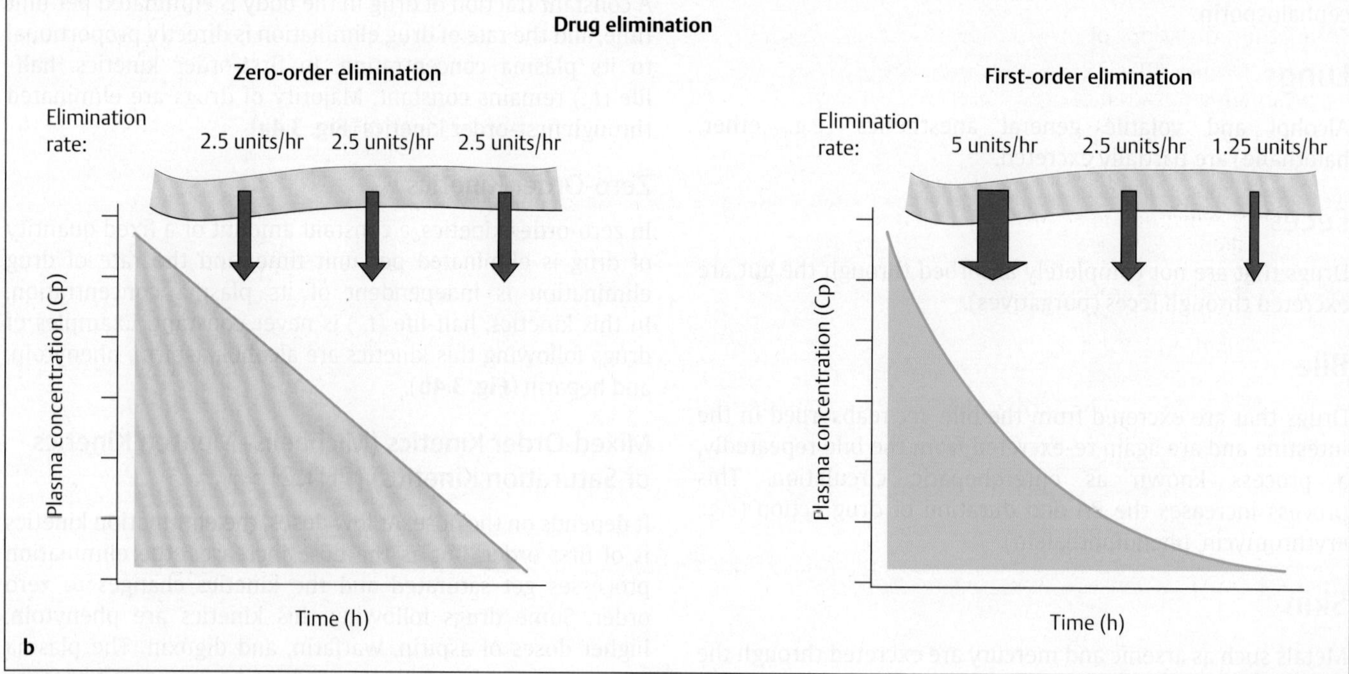

Fig. 3.4 **(a)** Zero-order and **(b)** first-order kinetics.

a small increase in dose leads to an increase in plasma concentration, resulting in toxicity. Therapeutic drug monitoring (TDM) of the plasma concentration of phenytoin needs to be done.

Drug Dosing Factors

The route of administration is one of the factors that determines drug action time, for example, immediate action drug is given by IV route. After repeated administration at a constant rate, drug requires four to five half-lives ($t_{½}$) to achieve steady-state plasma concentration. Drugs having short $t_{½}$ require frequent administration or IV infusion, and drugs with longer $t_{½}$ require long time to achieve steady-state concentration. Loading dose is given to raise plasma concentration immediately to expected therapeutic range.

Loading dose is an initial large dose or series of doses given to achieve rapid steady-state therapeutic concentration (e.g., digoxin, lignocaine), and maintenance dose is usually half of loading dose administered at every half-life of the drug.

Therapeutic Drug Monitoring (PH1.2)

It is a measurement of the plasma concentration of a drug to monitor drug therapy. TDM is useful for the following cases:

- Drugs having narrow therapeutic index (e.g., phenytoin, digoxin, lithium, aminoglycosides).
- In renal failure patients (aminoglycosides).
- To ascertain BA.
- For checking compliance of patients.
- For drugs having wide interindividual variations.
- For nonresponsive patients.
- To treat drug poisoning.

TDM is not useful for the following cases:

- When clinical and biochemical parameters are available to monitor drug effects such as blood pressure, blood sugar, and prothrombin time.
- Drugs with tolerance such as opioids.
- Hit-and-run drugs whose effect persist longer than the drug itself, for example, proton pump inhibitors such as omeprazole.

Fixed-Dose Combination (PH1.59)

It is a combination of two or more drugs in a single formulation, such as sulfamethoxazole and trimethoprim (cotrimoxazole) as antibiotic, levodopa and carbidopa for parkinsonism, estrogen and progesterone as OC, and amoxicillin and clavulanic acid (co-amoxiclav) as antibiotic.

Advantages of fixed-dose combination are increased patient compliance, synergism, increased efficacy, lower side effects, lower cost, and lower drug resistance. Disadvantages include inflexible fixed dose, different pharmacokinetics of drugs, increased side effects, and ignorance of contents by physician and/or patient.

Methods of Prolonging Drug Action

Prolonging duration of drug action reduces the dosing frequency and increases patient compliance. Methods used for prolonging duration of drug action are as follows:

- Oral drugs by enteric coating (e.g., erythromycin) or sustained-release (SR) preparations (e.g., diclofenac). SR diclofenac tablet acts for 24 hours compared to diclofenac tablet, which acts for 12 hours.
- Parenteral drugs:
  - By reducing vascularity of absorbing surface: Adding an adrenaline (vasoconstrictor) to local anesthetics (LA) delays removal of LA from site, increases duration of action, decreases systemic absorption (reduces toxicity of LA), and decreases local bleeding (improves operative field). Adrenaline–LA combination should not be used on end arteries (fingers, toes, ears, nose, penis). This combination delays wound healing due to reduced tissue blood supply. Adrenaline should not be used in cardiovascular diseases such as hypertension, cardiac failure, ischemic heart diseases, and arrhythmias.
  - By decreasing solubility: By combining drug with water, insoluble agent such as penicillin G has 4 to 6 hours' duration of action only, while procaine penicillin has 12 to 24 hours' duration of action and benzathine penicillin has 3 to 4 weeks' duration of action.
  - By injecting drug in oily solution such as depot progestin (depot medroxyprogesterone acetate).
  - Pellet implantation such as Norplant implantation.
  - Ocusert, Progestasert, transdermal patch.
  - By increasing PPB, for example, sulfadiazine is less protein bound and has 6 hours of duration of action, while sulfadoxine is highly protein bound and has 7 days of duration of action.
  - By decreasing metabolism—for example, anticholinesterases (physostigmine, neostigmine) increase duration of action of ACh by inhibiting cholinesterases.
  - By decreasing renal excretion—for example, probenecid decreases excretion and increases duration of action of penicillin/cephalosporin.

Multiple Choice Questions

1. A 56-year-old male patient with presumed staphylococcal sepsis is admitted in the intensive care unit and is empirically given intravenous (IV) vancomycin to avoid problems with possible resistance while waiting for the culture results to come back. His creatinine level is 4.1, which is indicative of acute renal failure. Vancomycin is excreted by the renal route. What actions need to be taken with regard to adjustments of the prescribed medication?

A. Change the drug to an oral route.
B. Restriction of water intake.
C. No changes in current treatment.
D. Vancomycin dose will need to be reduced.

Answer: D

As vancomycin is excreted by the renal route, functional status of the kidney needs to be considered while prescribing because it may produce undesirable toxic side effects due to accumulation.

2. A 42-year-old patient on an antidepressant drug visited the psychiatrist to change the antidepressant drug, as he felt his current drug is not helping. Due to this, he started drinking heavily. The psychiatrist wanted to try imipramine, but before prescribing it, he ordered a hepatic function panel, as this drug undergoes an extensive first-pass effect and the patient has a recent history of alcohol use. What is the rationale behind the doctor's decision?

A. Hepatic function panel results may reveal a particular susceptibility to the drug.
B. Imipramine bioavailability increases.
C. Drugs with a high first-pass metabolism achieve high systemic concentrations in hepatic dysfunction.
D. The drug is more rapidly metabolized by the liver when hepatic aminotransferase level increases.

Answer: C

In hepatic dysfunction, drug levels may reach higher systemic concentrations.

3. A 52-year-old highly paid employee was recently fired from his job due to the COVID-19 pandemic. He started a new job but was not happy with it. Due to frustration, he decided to commit suicide and ingested a jarful of phenobarbital (antiseizure drug). Subsequently, he developed diminished breathing, lower body temperature, and skin reddening and is brought to the hospital. He is diagnosed with barbiturate overdose and is given bicarbonate to alkalinize urine. How are the toxic effects of phenobarbital overcome by making urine alkaline with bicarbonate?

A. Alkalinization of urine with bicarbonate increases glomerular filtration.
B. Alkalinization of urine with bicarbonate decreases proximal tubular secretion.
C. Alkalinization of urine with bicarbonate decreases untoward side effects.
D. Alkalinization of urine with bicarbonate decreases distal tubular reabsorption.

Answer: D

Alterations of the pH of urine affect renal distal tubular reabsorption of drugs by ion trapping as well as the ionization of weak acids and bases. Phenobarbital is a weak acid, and increasing the urinary pH will increase the ionized form and trap it in the ultrafiltrate because charged molecules cannot be reabsorbed back across membranes in the tubule into the plasma. This results in increase in elimination of the phenobarbital in the urine.

4. A 16-year-old patient has three tonic-clonic seizures within 8 days and was diagnosed with epilepsy. He is started on phenytoin. Initially, loading dose is given to achieve proper drug concentrations in plasma, followed by maintenance doses. As phenytoin has narrow therapeutic window, its blood level needs to undergo therapeutic drug monitoring (TDM) to adjust the maintenance dose as needed. The rationale behind this regimen of phenytoin is:

A. To achieve the desired plasma concentration rapidly, a loading dose is given.
B. Steady-state concentration will be achieved with three half-lives if the drug is administered at a maintenance dose rate.
C. Maintenance dose rate usually does not equal the elimination rate.
D. Loading dose of the drug does not depend on the volume of distribution, and maintenance dose rate does not depend on clearance of the drug.

Answer: A

In some conditions, for example, to prevent further seizures, a loading dose is given in sufficient dose to achieve the desired effect quickly.

5. When a 50-mg X tablet is administered for every 24 hours, it will achieve an average steady-state plasma concentration of 8 mg/L. What will be the resulting average plasma concentration after five half-lives if regimen changed to 25-mg tablet every 12 hours?

A. 3 mg/L.
B. 8 mg/L.
C. 6 mg/L.
D. 10 mg/L.

Answer: B

A 50-mg tablet every 24 hours is the same dose rate as 25-mg tablet every 12 hours and the average plasma concentration will remain the same.

6. To achieve a steady-state plasma concentration of 5 μg/L, a calculated oral maintenance dose of drug is administered to a patient, but after dosing steady-state, the average plasma concentration of drug is 10 μg/L. This is due to decrease in which of the following?

A. Bioavailability.
B. Volume of distribution.
C. Half-life.
D. Clearance.

Answer: D

A decrease in clearance will increase the plasma drug concentration.

7. Morphine 10 mg is administered orally for severe cancer pain, but a plasma concentration of only 30% of intravenous administration is achieved of the same dose. The amount of active drug in the body is reduced after administration but before entering the systemic circulation due to which of the following?

A. Excretion.
B. First-order elimination.
C. Metabolism.
D. First-pass effect.

Answer: D

In first-pass effect, the drug is eliminated before it enters into the systemic circulation on its passage through the portal circulation and the liver.

8. Therapeutic drug monitoring (TDM), a measurement of the plasma concentration of drug to monitor drug therapy, is not used for:

A. Drugs having narrow therapeutic index.
B. For checking compliance of patients.
C. To treat drug poisoning.
D. When clinical and biochemical parameters, such as blood pressure, blood sugar, and prothrombin time, are available to monitor drug effects.

Answer: D

TDM is not required when clinical and biochemical parameters are available.

9. In a 40-year-old patient, an adrenaline is added to local anesthetics (LA). What is the rationale behind it?

A. Adrenaline delays removal of LA from site.
B. Adrenaline decreases duration of action.
C. It increases systemic absorption.
D. It increases local bleeding.

Answer: A

By adding an adrenaline, which is a vasoconstrictor, to LA, it delays removal of LA from site.

10. Pharmacokinetics (PK) involves passage of the drugs across various biological membranes in the body. Each biological membrane has a lipid bilayer. How do you differentiate active transport from facilitated transport?

A. It is not a carrier-mediated transport.
B. Drug moves from a lower concentration region to a higher concentration region against the chemical or electrical gradient.
C. It requires energy for transport.
D. All of the above.

Answer: D

It requires energy. Drug moves from a lower concentration region to a higher concentration region against the chemical or electrical gradient, e.g., transport of choline to cholinergic neurons against the concentration gradient.

Chapter 4 Pharmacodynamics

Shraddha Yadav and Prasan R. Bhandari

PH1.5: Describe the general principles of mechanism of drug action.

Learning Objectives

- Principles of drug action.
- Site of drug action.
- Mechanism of drug action.
- Dose–response relationship.
- Quantitative aspect of drug action.
- Drug antagonism.
- Assessment of safety of drugs/therapeutic index/ therapeutic window.

Introduction

Pharmacology is the study that deals with biological and therapeutic effects of drugs. It is all about what a drug does to the body and how it does it. In simple terms, pharmacodynamics is about "what a drug does to the body." It explains the whole action–effect sequence and the dose–effect relationship.

Many a times, the terms *action* and *effect* are used synonymously, but actually they are distinct. The response produced by a drug is called its effect; it can be measured and thus quantified. How/where this effect is produced is called action and action can be identified. For example, increased force of contraction and increased cardiac output produced by administration of dobutamine are its effect, which occur due to its action of stimulation of β receptors. Thus, it can be concluded that action is drug–cell interaction and effect is subsequent event that occurs after action.

Principles of Drug Action (PH1.5)

Most of the drugs other than gene-based drugs do not produce new function to any biological system. They only change the speed of the proceeding activity. These alterations, however, can have a prominent medicinal or toxicological influence. The classification of various types of drug action is as follows.

Stimulation

This involves increase in activity of a particular physiological system or a selective tissue or cells, for example, adrenaline increases heart rate and pilocarpine activates salivary glands.

Depression

It involves decrease in activity of a particular physiological system or a selective tissue or cells, for example, benzodiazepines inhibit the central nervous system (CNS), quinidine decreases heart rate, and omeprazole reduces gastric acid secretion.

Replacement of Endogenous Substance

Numerous diseases occur due to deficiency of hormones or vitamins or minerals and hence the substance that is deficient needs to be replaced, for example, insulin in diabetes mellitus and vitamin C in scurvy.

Alteration of Immune Status

Autoimmune diseases occur due to overactivity of the immune system. Thus, immunosuppressants such as corticosteroids are used to reduce the overactive immune system. Immunity also can be activated by using vaccines and antisera, for example, polio vaccine and antisera (for snake poisoning).

Cytotoxic Action

Selective cytotoxic effect on invading microbes such as bacteria, parasite, and virus or on cancer cells, by reducing them without significantly affecting the host cells, is used for treatment of various diseases. Examples include penicillin, chloroquine, zidovudine, and cyclophosphamide.

Irritation

It is a nonspecific phenomenon and may occur in any living tissues or organism. Sometimes, irritating agents such as methyl salicylate and capsaicin are applied locally to relieve pain arising due to deeper structure, known as the counterirritant effect. Irritants also cause vasodilation and block the pain impulse from deeper structures by stimulation of sensory nerve endings in the skin as a result of irritation.

Site of Drug Action

Locally

At the site where drug is applied.

Systemically

Extracellular

For example, antacids, which are used to neutralize the gastric acid, and osmotic purgatives.

Cellular

For example, effect of adrenaline on the heart and blood vessels, and inhibition of enzyme Na^+/K^+-ATPase by digoxin.

Intracellular

For example, rifampicin inhibits the synthesis of nucleic acid.

Mechanism of Drug Action (PH1.5)

The concept of a chemical interaction between drug and tissue, resulting in drug action, was suggested by Paul Ehrlich. Most drugs exhibit their action by interaction with a distinct target biomolecule, generally a protein. This bestows selectivity of action to the drug. Functional proteins that are targets of drug action can be grouped into four major categories, namely, enzymes, ion channels, transporters, and receptors. However, a few drugs do act on other proteins (e.g., colchicine, vinca alkaloids, taxanes bind to the structural protein tubulin) or on nucleic acids (alkylating agents). The knowledge of mechanism of action is important due to the following reasons:

1. It serves as significant basis for proper use of drugs.
2. It forms the basis for developing a new or improved drug that has the anticipated actions and minimizes the untoward effects.

There are four major types of regulatory proteins that are the primary target for various drugs (**Fig. 4.1**). These are as follows:

1. Enzymes.
2. Ion channels.
3. Carrier molecules/membrane transporters.
4. Receptors.

Only few drugs have effects due to their simple physical or chemical property; examples are:

- Physical mass: ispaghula (bulk laxatives).
- Physical form, opacity: petroleum jelly, dimethicone.
- Absorption of UV rays: para-aminobenzoic acid.
- Adsorptive property: activated charcoal.
- Osmotic activity: magnesium sulfate, mannitol.
- Radioactivity: radioisotopes such as I^{131}.
- Chemical neutralization of gastric HCl: antacids.
- Oxidizing property: potassium permanganate.
- Chelation of heavy metals: chelating agents (dimercaprol, ethylenediamine tetraacetic acid [EDTA]).
- Sequestration of bile acids and cholesterol in the gut: cholestyramine.

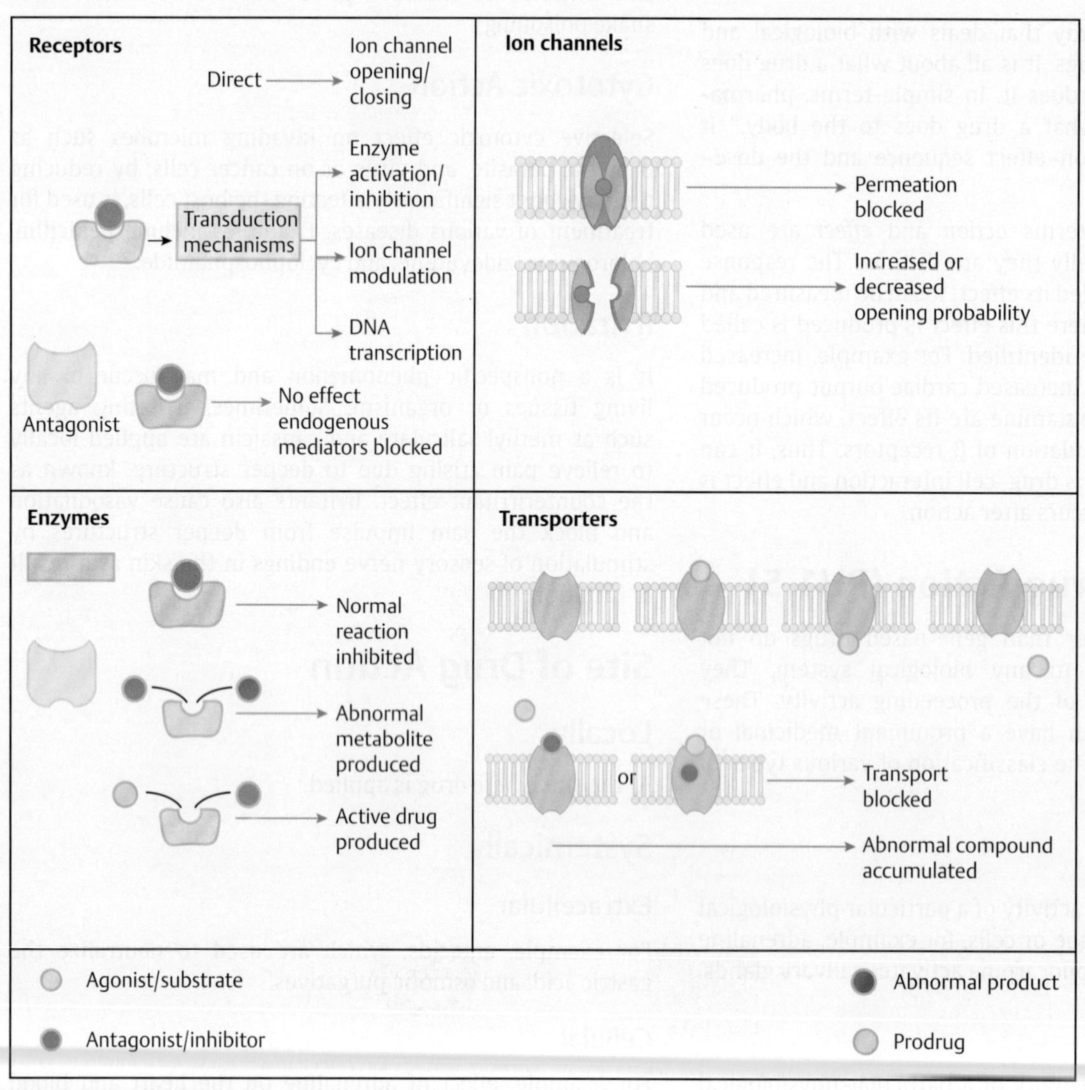

Fig. 4.1 Four primary targets for various drugs.

Enzymes

Enzymes are vital in carrying out majority of biological reactions. Drugs can alter enzymatic reactions. They can alter the rate of such reactions.

Enzyme Stimulation

Enzyme stimulation is a natural physiological process. For example, pyridoxine, being a cofactor, enhances the activity of decarboxylase. Enzymes are activated via receptors and second messengers, such as adrenaline activates hepatic glycogen phosphorylase via β receptors and cyclic adenosine monophosphate (cAMP). In enzyme stimulation, the affinity of enzyme for substrate is increased (k_m reduced).

Enzyme activity is also increased through enzyme induction causing various drug interactions, but enzyme induction is not the same as enzyme stimulation, as the affinity of the enzyme does not change (k_m is constant). In enzyme induction, synthesis of the enzyme protein is increased and thus there is apparent increase in enzyme activity.

Enzyme Inhibition

Many drugs act by targeting important enzymes. Inhibition of enzymes is an important mechanism of action for many drugs (**Fig. 4.2**). Enzyme inhibition may be nonspecific by changing the structure of enzyme, that is, denature the protein or enzyme. But such chemicals are not useful for systemic therapeutic purpose. Examples of nonspecific enzyme inhibitors include strong acids and alkalis, phenol, and formaldehyde. Many drugs used clinically inhibit a specific enzyme. Such drugs are useful for therapeutic purpose. The specific enzyme inhibition may be competitive or noncompetitive. The enzyme inhibitors are highly effective drugs depending on the blockade of subsequent process. For example, the synthesis of uric acid involves xanthine oxidase enzyme. Allopurinol is a drug that inhibits xanthine oxidase enzyme, thus preventing the further synthesis of uric acid, and serves as an important drug in the treatment of chronic gout and hyperuricemia.

Similarly, thromboxane A_2 is an enzyme involved in platelet aggregation. Aspirin in low dose inhibits thromboxane A_2 and hence is widely used as antiplatelet drug.

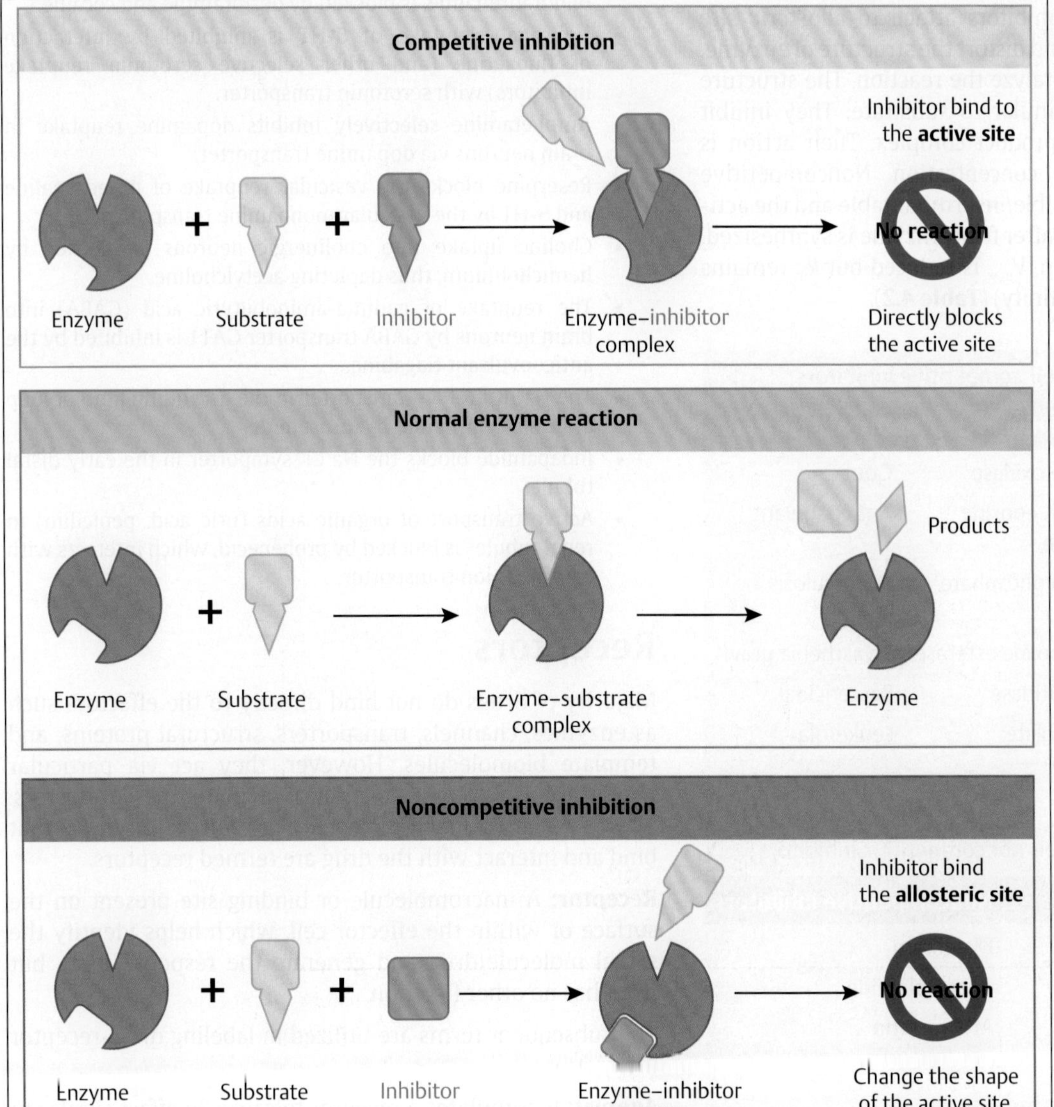

Fig. 4.2 Normal reaction: competitive and noncompetitive inhibition.

Competitive Inhibition

The competitive enzyme inhibitors prevent the formation of enzyme–substrate complex due to similar shape. The drug in such case is a structural analogue of enzyme and competes for enzyme. The inhibition depends on relative concentration of substrate and inhibitor, as they compete for active site of enzyme. Hence, it is usually temporary or equilibrium type/surmountable. In competitive inhibition, V_{max} remains unchanged but K_m is increased (reduced affinity), thus achieving a new equilibrium in presence of inhibitor drug, that is, higher substrate concentration is necessary and thus higher amount of the substrate will displace the inhibitor drug, achieving the previous rate as observed initially without the enzyme inhibitor. For example, physostigmine competes with acetylcholine for cholinesterase enzyme (**Table 4.1**). However, enzyme inhibition may be irreversible (nonequilibrium) type, where V_{max} is reduced and K_m is increased, for example, methotrexate (strong inhibitor of dihydrofolate reductase [DHFR]; affinity 50,000 times). In such case, the enzyme inhibitor cannot be displaced with increase in concentration of the substrate.

Noncompetitive Inhibition

Noncompetitive enzyme inhibitors attach to allosteric site (different from active site) and distort the structure of enzyme, thus making it unable to catalyze the reaction. The structure of the drug may not be similar to substrate. They inhibit the formation of enzyme–product complex. Their action is not affected by substrate concentration. Noncompetitive inhibition is usually irreversible/insurmountable and the activity of enzyme returns only after fresh enzyme is synthesized. In noncompetitive inhibition, V_{max} is reduced but k_m remains unchanged (no change in affinity) (**Table 4.2**).

Table 4.1 Enzymes and their competitive inhibitors

Inhibitor (drug)	Enzyme inhibited	Disease treated
Allopurinol	Xanthine oxidase	Gout
Dicumarol	Vitamin K epoxide reductase	Anticoagulant
Isonicotinic acid hydrazide (INH)	Pyridoxal phosphate	Tuberculosis
Neostigmine	Acetyl choline esterase	Myasthenia gravis
Penicillin	Transpeptidase	Bactericidal
Methotrexate	Dihydrofolate reductase	Leukemia

Table 4.2 Enzymes and their noncompetitive inhibitors

Enzymes	Noncompetitive inhibitors
Aldehyde dehydrogenase	Disulfiram
Carbonic anhydrase	Acetazolamide
HMG-CoA (β-Hydroxy β-methylglutaryl-CoA) reductase	Atorvastatin
H^+/K^+-ATPase	Omeprazole

Ion Channels

These are proteins that act as ion selective channels, are involved in transmembrane signaling, and regulate intracellular ionic composition. They are a common target for drug action (**Fig. 4.1**). Many of these ion channels are activated by particular signal molecules either directly or through some other proteins, and thus are receptors. These ions channels can be of following types:

1. Ligand-gated channels.
2. G-protein regulated channels.
3. Voltage-gated channels.

Transporters

Several molecules are shifted through membranes by binding to distinct transporters (carriers), which either enable diffusion in the direction of the concentration gradient or drive the metabolite/ion against the concentration gradient using metabolic energy. Many drugs act by directly interacting with the transporter proteins to impede the occurring physiological transport of the metabolite/ion. For example:

- Norepinephrine transporter, which is involved in reuptake of noradrenaline, is blocked by desipramine and cocaine.
- Neuronal reuptake of 5-HT is inhibited by interaction of fluoxetine (and other selective serotonin reuptake inhibitors) with serotonin transporter.
- Amphetamine selectively inhibits dopamine reuptake in brain neurons via dopamine transporter.
- Reserpine blocks the vesicular reuptake of noradrenaline and 5-HT by the vesicular monoamine transporter 2.
- Choline uptake into cholinergic neurons is blocked by hemicholinium, thus depleting acetylcholine.
- The reuptake of gamma-aminobutyric acid (GABA) into brain neurons by GABA transporter GAT1 is inhibited by the anticonvulsant tiagabine.
- The $Na^+/K^+/2Cl^-$ cotransporter in the ascending limb of loop of Henle is inhibited by furosemide.
- Indapamide blocks the Na^+Cl^- symporter in the early distal tubule.
- Active transport of organic acids (uric acid, penicillin) in renal tubules is blocked by probenecid, which interacts with organic anion transporter.

Receptors

Majority of drugs do not bind directly to the effectors such as enzymes, channels, transporters, structural proteins, and template biomolecules. However, they act via particular regulatory macromolecules that regulate these effectors. These regulatory macromolecules, or the sites on them, that bind and interact with the drug are termed receptors.

Receptor: A macromolecule or binding site present on the surface or within the effector cell, which helps identify the signal molecule/drug and generate the response to it, but itself has no other function.

The subsequent terms are utilized in labeling drug–receptor interaction:

Agonist: It stimulates a receptor to cause an effect similar to that of the physiological signal molecule.

Partial agonist: It stimulates a receptor leading to a submaximal effect; however, it antagonizes the action of a full agonist.

Inverse agonist: An agent that activates a receptor to produce an effect in the opposite direction to that of the agonist.

Antagonist: It blocks the action of an agonist on a receptor or the subsequent response; however, it does not possess any effect of its own.

Ligand (Latin: ligare—to bind): Any molecule that binds specifically to particular receptors or sites. It merely suggests affinity or ability to bind without regard to functional change: agonists and competitive antagonists are both ligands of the same receptor.

Receptor Occupation Theory

While learning quantitative characteristics of drug action, Clark (1937) proposed a theory of drug action on the basis of occupation of receptors by specific drugs. According to this theory, the speed of a cellular function can be controlled by interaction of these receptors with drugs that are small molecular ligands. He suggested that the interaction among the drug (D) and receptor (R) is controlled by the law of mass action, and the effect (E) will be a direct function of the drug–receptor complex (DR) formed:

$$D + R \underset{K_2}{\overset{K_1}{\rightleftharpoons}} DR \longrightarrow E \quad \text{...(1)}$$

Further, it has been understood that occupation of the receptor is necessary but it is not itself enough to produce a response; the agonist should also be capable of inducing a conformational change in the receptor. The ability of the drug to bind with the receptor is labeled as affinity, and the ability to develop a functional change in the receptor is labeled as intrinsic activity (IA) or efficacy. Affinity and IA are independent properties. Competitive antagonists occupy the receptor; however, they do not activate it. Additionally, some drugs are partial agonists that occupy and start the receptor at submaximal level. An all-or-none action is not necessary at the receptor. A theoretical quantity (S) representing intensity of stimulus imparted to the cell was interposed in the Clark equation:

$$D + R \underset{K_2}{\overset{K_1}{\rightleftharpoons}} DR \Longrightarrow S \longrightarrow E \quad \text{...(2)}$$

Depending on the agonist, DR might produce a stronger or weaker S, perhaps as a function of the conformational change got about by the agonist in the receptor. Hence:

1. **Agonists** possess both affinity and maximal IA (i.e., IA = 1), for example, histamine, adrenaline, and morphine.
2. **Partial agonists** possess affinity and submaximal IA (i.e., IA between 0 and 1), for example, pentazocine (on μ-opioid receptor) and dichloroisoproterenol (on β-adrenergic receptor).
3. **Competitive antagonists** possess affinity but no IA (i.e., IA = 0), for example, atropine, propranolol, naloxone, and chlorpheniramine.
4. **Inverse agonists** possess affinity but IA with a minus sign (i.e., IA between 0 and −1), for example, DMCM (methyl-6, 7-dimethoxy-4-ethyl-beta-carboline-3-carboxylate) (on benzodiazepine receptor) and chlorpheniramine (on H_1 histamine receptor).

It has been established that several agonists could produce maximum response in spite of occupying less than 1% of the available receptors. A large receptor backup is available in such a case, or a number of spare receptors are present.

Nature of Receptors

Regulatory macromolecules, generally proteins, or nucleic acids could likewise function as receptors. Huge number of receptor proteins have been isolated, refined, and cloned and their major amino acid (AA) sequence has been done.

Molecular cloning has played an important role in discovering the receptor protein and in studying its structure and properties, as well as in subclassifying receptors. The cell surface receptors, besides their coupling and effector proteins, are regarded to be moving in an ocean of membrane lipids—the bending, alignment, and structure of the system being calculated by relations between the lipophilic and hydrophilic domains of the peptide chains with solvent molecules. Nonpolar fragments of the AA chain entomb inside the membrane, whereas polar groups emerge in the aqueous medium. In such a precisely well-adjusted system, it is easy to imagine that a minute molecular ligand binding to one site in the receptor molecule might upset the balance (by altering distribution of charges, etc.) and generate a conformational modification at distant sites. Each of the four main families of receptors possesses a distinct common structural motif; however, the specific receptors vary in the AA sequencing, length of intra/extracellular loops, etc. Majority of receptor molecules are comprised of numerous dissimilar subunits (heteropolymeric), and agonist binding has been revealed to generate alterations in their quaternary configuration or relative arrangement of the subunits, for example, on stimulation, the subunits of nicotinic receptor split up, unlocking a centrally situated cation channel. Several drugs act upon physiological receptors that facilitate reactions to hormones, transmitters, autacoids, and additional endogenous signal molecules—examples include adrenergic, cholinergic, histaminergic, steroid, leukotriene, insulin, and other such receptors. Furthermore, presently certain truly drug receptors have been labeled for which there are no identified physiological ligands, for examples, benzodiazepine receptor and sulfonylurea receptor. Receptors for which no endogenous mediator or ligand is known have been termed “orphan receptors.”

Receptor Classification

The basis of receptor classification can be on the effect of a particular drug, ligand binding to receptor, molecular cloning, or biochemical pathway analysis in response to activation.

Depending on molecular configuration and type of transduction system, there are four types of receptors (**Fig. 4.3**).

1. Ligand-gated ion channel (ionotropic receptor).
2. G-protein-coupled receptor (GPCR) (metabotropic receptor).
3. Enzyme/kinase-linked receptor.

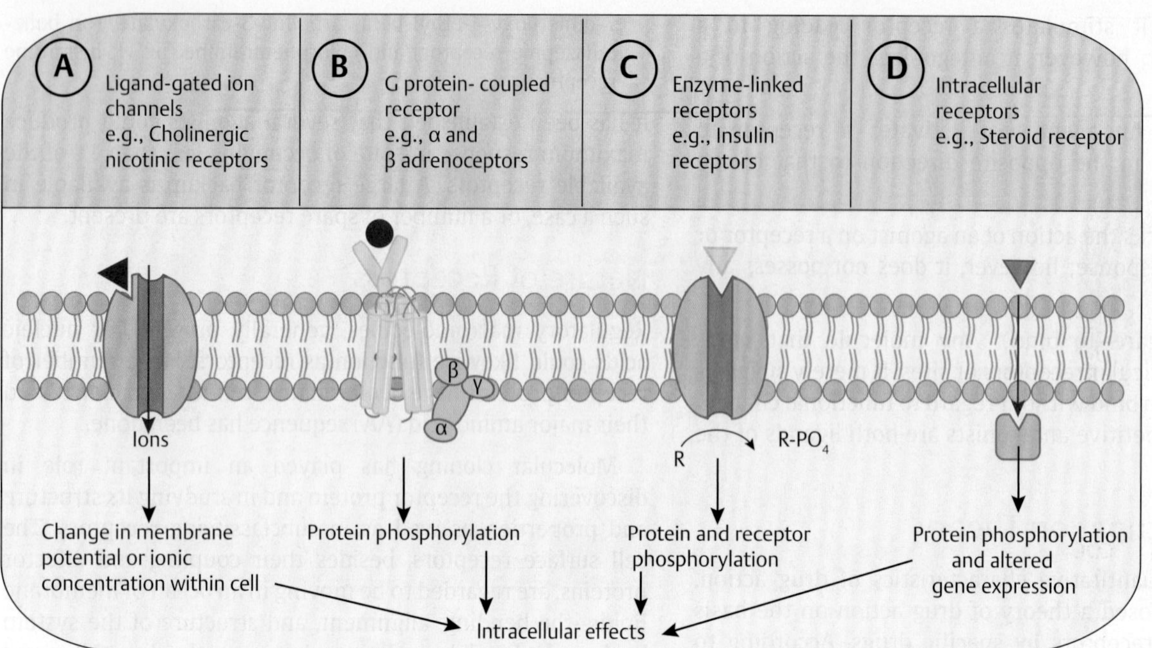

Fig. 4.3 Four major types of receptors.

4. Receptor linked to gene transcription (nuclear/cytoplasmic receptors).

Receptor Subtypes

The understanding of various types as well as subtypes of receptors for signal molecules has been pivotal in the advance of targeted and more selective drugs. Even during the development of receptor pharmacology, it was witnessed that actions of acetylcholine may be assembled into "muscarinic" and "nicotinic" subject to whether they represented muscarine or nicotine alkaloids. Therefore, these were facilitated by two types of cholinergic receptors, namely, muscarinic (M) and nicotinic (N). This idea was reinforced by the discovery that muscarinic actions were inhibited by atropine; likewise, nicotinic actions were suppressed by curare. In a revolutionary study, Ahlquist (1948) separated adrenergic receptors into "α" and "β" depending on two distinct rank order of potencies of adrenergic agonists. These receptors presently have been further subdivided into (M_1, M_2, M_3, M_4, and M_5), (NM, NN) (α_1, α_2) (β_1, β_2, β_3). Numerous subtypes of receptors for almost all transmitters, such as autacoids and hormones, are currently identified and have carved the way for various clinically improved drugs. In several cases, receptor classification has added to complete account for variances witnessed in the actions of closely interrelated drugs.

Receptors are involved in two essential functions, the first being acknowledgment of the particular ligand molecule and the second being transduction of the signal into a response. Hence, the receptor molecule possesses a ligand-binding domain (spatially and energetically appropriate for attaching the particular ligand) and an effector domain that goes through a functional conformational change. These domains have truly been recognized in certain receptors these days. The modification in the receptor molecule is interpreted into the response. The serial relationship among drug action, transducer, and drug effect can be understood.

Transducer Mechanisms

Significant progress has been made in understanding the mechanisms of transducer. It has been established to be extremely intricate activities, which indicate the amplification and incorporation of synchronously received extracellular and intracellular signals at each step. Since only a limited number of transducer pathways are common to a large number of receptors, the cell is capable of making a combined response reproducing the sum total of various signal input. The transducer mechanisms are clustered into four main classes. Receptors clustered in one class could also possess significant structural homology and fit to one superfamily of receptors.

G Protein–Coupled Receptors

GPCRs are the commonest single class of target for therapeutic drugs. The GCPR family involves many receptors such as muscarinic, acetylcholine receptors (AChRs), adrenoreceptors, dopamine receptors, and 5-HT (serotonin) receptors. For majority of them, studies have discovered an array of subtypes.

Many of the neurotransmitters can interact with both GPCRs and ligand-gated channels, thus permitting the same transmitter to yield fast and slow effects through ligand-gated and GPCRs, respectively.

Molecular Structure

In 1986, β_2 adrenoreceptor, a GPCR, was cloned. Subsequently, rapid developments in molecular biology led to AA sequencing of GPCRs along with study of the three-dimensional structure of these receptors in detail. Now, with the help of computational molecular docking and nuclear magnetic resonance methods, the ligand binding and conformational change associated with activation of these have also been studied. From such studies, a more in-depth understanding of mechanism of stimulation of GPCRs and

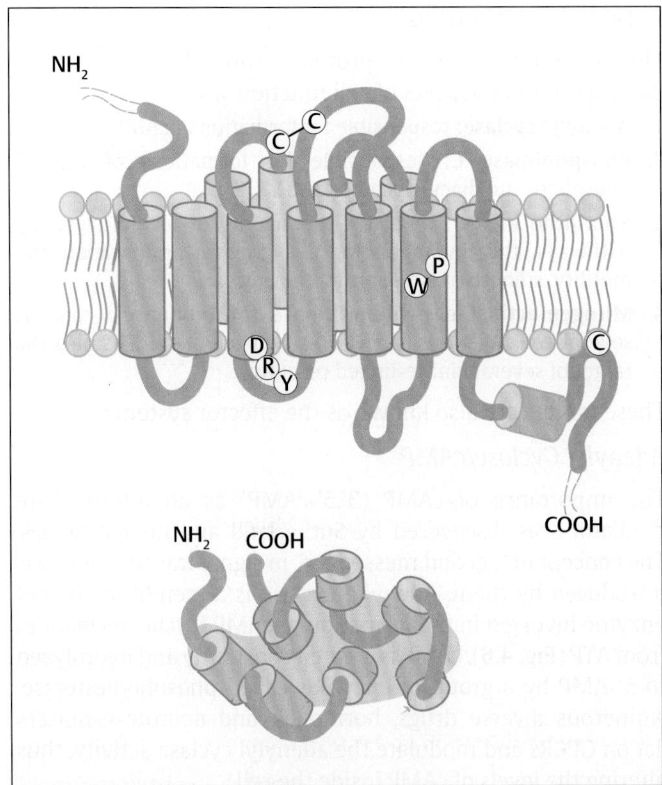

Fig. 4.4 Schematic molecular structure of G protein–coupled receptor.

factors responsible for the agonist efficacy is coming up. This, in turn, will be echoed in having a better approach to designing new GPCRs drugs/ligands.

GPCRs comprise a single polypeptide chain, with AA residues in the range of 35 to 1,100 residues. Their distinctive structure consists of seven transmembrane α-helices, with an extracellular N-terminal domain of varying length and an intracellular C-terminus; the agonist binding site is located in between the helices on the extracellular face, while another recognition site formed by cytosolic segments binds the coupling G protein. These G proteins drift in the membrane with their exposed domain lying in the cytosol (**Fig. 4.4**).

G Proteins and Their Roles

G proteins are membrane proteins whose primary role is to respond to GPCR activation and convey the message inside the cell to the effector systems, which produce a cellular response (**Fig. 4.5**). They are essentially middle management in the process. They are termed *G proteins* due of their interaction with guanine nucleotides, guanosine triphosphate (GTP), and guanosine diphosphate (GDP).

These G proteins contain three subunits, α, β, and γ, where the α subunit possesses the GTPase activity. During the resting phase, the G proteins exist in an αβγ trimer; these may or may not be necessarily coupled with the receptor. In the inactive condition, GDP is attached to the α subunit

Ligand
α β γ GDP
ON
GTP GDP
α GTP
β γ
OFF
RGS
Pi
α β γ GDP
Downstream signaling
PLCβ, PI3K, ion channel
Desensitization and apoptosis

$α_s$ | $α_i$ | $α_q$ | $α_{12}$

Activation of adenylyl cyclase (cytosolic cAMP) Activation of PKA ↓ **Cell growth and motility**

Inactivation of adenylyl cyclase (cytosolic cAMP) ↓ **Cell motility**

Activation of PLC (intracellular Ca^{2+}) Activation of PKC ↓ **Cell proliferation**

Strong activation of Rho GTPase ↓ **Cancer progression and metastasis**

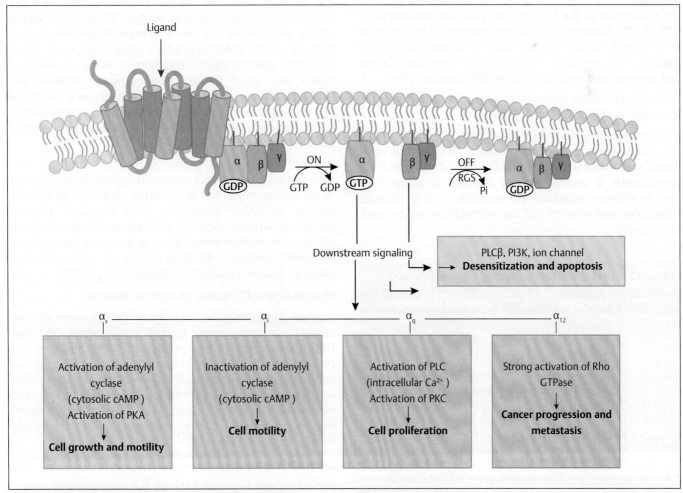

Fig. 4.5 Schematic representation and function of G protein.

at the visible domain; stimulation through the receptor causes displacement of GDP by GTP. The actuated α subunit transporting GTP separates from the other two subunits and modulates the effector. In some cases, the βγ subunit is the activator species. Activation of the effector is ended when the bound GTP molecule is hydrolyzed, which lets the α subunit to combine with the βγ.

Agonist activates GPCR, leading to minor changes in residues around the ligand-binding site; this, in turn, decodes to bigger rearrangements of the intracellular regions of the receptor. This leads to opening of a cavity on the intracellular side of the receptor into which the G protein can bind. This causes interaction of αβγ with receptor and it occurs within 50 ms due to high affinity. This results into dissociation of GDP, to be substituted with GTP (GDP–GTP exchange). This further leads to dissociation of G protein trimer, causing the release of α-GTP from βγ subunits. These are functioning forms of G-protein, which spread in the membrane and combine with several enzymes and ion channels, leading to stimulation of the target.

Connection of α and βγ subunits with target enzymes or channels could lead to modulation based on the concerned G protein. Activation of G protein leads to amplification, as a single agonist–receptor complex could stimulate numerous G protein molecules and all of these remain connected with their effector enzyme long enough to create several molecules of the product. The product is generally a second messenger and additional magnification follows prior to the production of the final cellular response. Hydrolysis of GTP to GDP happens through the inherent GTPase activity of α subunit, which further leads to termination of the signaling. The resulting α-GDP detaches from the effector and subsequently reunifies with βγ, finishing the cycle.

Four main classes of G protein that are pharmacologically important are G_s, G_i, G_o, and G_q (**Table 4.3**).

G proteins exhibit specificity as regards both receptors and effectors with which they couple. They have distinct identification domains in their configuration complementary to particular G protein–binding domains in receptor as well as effector molecules. For example, G_s & G_i produce stimulation and inhibition of the adenylyl cyclase enzyme, respectively.

Table 4.3 The main G protein types and their functions

G protein	Receptors	Signaling pathway
G_s	β-adrenergic receptors, glucagon, histamine, serotonin	Increase adenylyl cyclase cAMP Excitatory effects
G_i	α_2-adrenergic receptors, mAChR, opioid, serotonin	Decrease adenylyl cyclase cAMP Cardiac K^+ channel open-decrease heart rate
G_q	mAChR, serotonin 5-HT_{1C}	PLC-IP_3, DAG Increase cytoplasmic Ca

Abbreviations: cAMP, cyclic adenosine monophosphate; DAG, diacylglycerol; mAChR, muscarinic acetylcholine receptors; PLC-IP3, phospholipase C-inositol triphosphate.

Targets for G Proteins

The main targets for G proteins, through which GPCRs control different aspects of cell function, are:

1. **Adenylyl cyclase**: responsible for formation of cAMP.
2. **Phospholipase C**: responsible for formations of inositol phosphate and diacylglycerol (DAG).
3. **RhoA/Rho kinase**: regulates the activity of several signaling pathways, thereby regulating cell growth, proliferation and motility, smooth muscle contraction, etc.
4. **Mitogen-activated protein kinase (MAP kinase)**: controls several cell functions, such as cell division, and it is also the target of several kinase-linked receptors.

These targets are also known as the effector systems.

Adenylyl Cyclase/cAMP

The importance of cAMP (3′,5′-cAMP) as an intermediate mediator was discovered by Sutherland and his colleagues. The concept of "second messenger" in signal transduction was introduced by them. Adenylyl cyclase is a membrane-bound enzyme involved in the formation of cAMP (cyclic nucleotide) from ATP (**Fig. 4.6**). cAMP is created constantly and hydrolyzed to 5′-AMP by a group of enzymes called phosphodiesterase. Numerous diverse drugs, hormones, and neurotransmitters act on GPCRs and modulate the adenylyl cyclase activity, thus altering the levels of cAMP inside the cell.

cAMP controls many facets of cell functions such as enzymes involved in energy metabolism, cell division and cell differentiation, ion transport, ion channels, and the contractile proteins in smooth muscle. These wide-ranging effects are carried out by activation of protein kinases through cAMP. cAMP-dependent protein kinase A is an important protein kinase. This protein kinase A phosphorylates and alters the function of many enzymes, ion channels, transporters, transcription factors, and structural proteins. Further, it leads to effects such as increased contractility/impulse generation of the heart, relaxation of smooth muscle, glycogenolysis, and lipolysis.

cAMP also opens a particular type of membrane Ca^{2+} channel, known as cyclic nucleotide–gated channel found in the kidney, heart, and brain. Other mediators for cellular actions of cAMP comprise: cAMP-regulated guanine nucleotide exchange factors, cAMP response element binding protein, the transcription factor, and certain transporters. Responses contrary to the those mentioned are formed when adenylyl cyclase is blocked via inhibitory G_i protein.

Phospholipase C/Inositol Phosphate System

Enzyme phospholipase C catalyzes development of two intracellular messengers, inositol triphosphate (IP_3) and DAG from membrane phospholipids. The IP_3 augment free cytosolic Ca^{2+} by releasing calcium from intracellular stores, and this surge in intracellular calcium initiates many events such as contraction, secretion, enzyme activation, and membrane hyperpolarization. DAG activates protein kinase C that phosphorylates a variety of proteins and regulates many cellular functions (**Fig. 4.7**).

Channel Regulation

The stimulated G proteins (G_s, G_i, G_o) could likewise modulate ionic channels, particularly for Ca^{2+} and K^+, lacking the

One signal molecule
Adenylyl cyclase
GPCR
G protein
ATP
cAMP
Protein kinase A
Phosphorylated protein
Cell response

1. Signal molecule binds to G protein-coupled receptor (GPCR), which activates the G protein.
2. G protein turns on adenylyl cyclase, an ampilfier enzyme.
3. Adenylyl cyclase converts ATP to cyclic AMP.
4. cAMP activates protein kinase A.
5. Protein kinase A phosphorylates other proteins, leading ultimately to a cellular response.

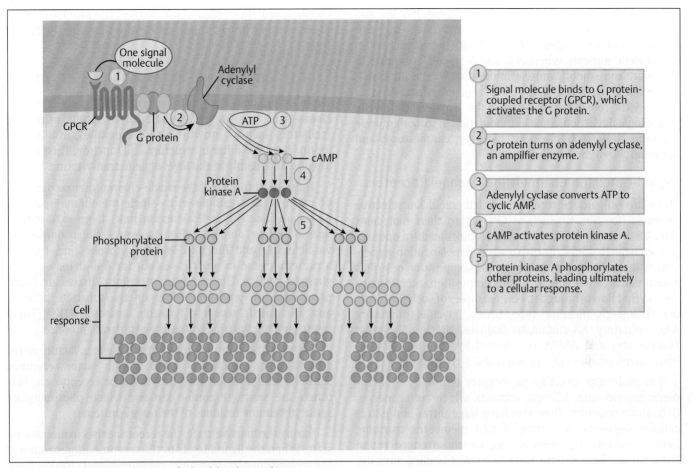

Fig. 4.6 Schematic representation of adenylyl cyclase pathway.

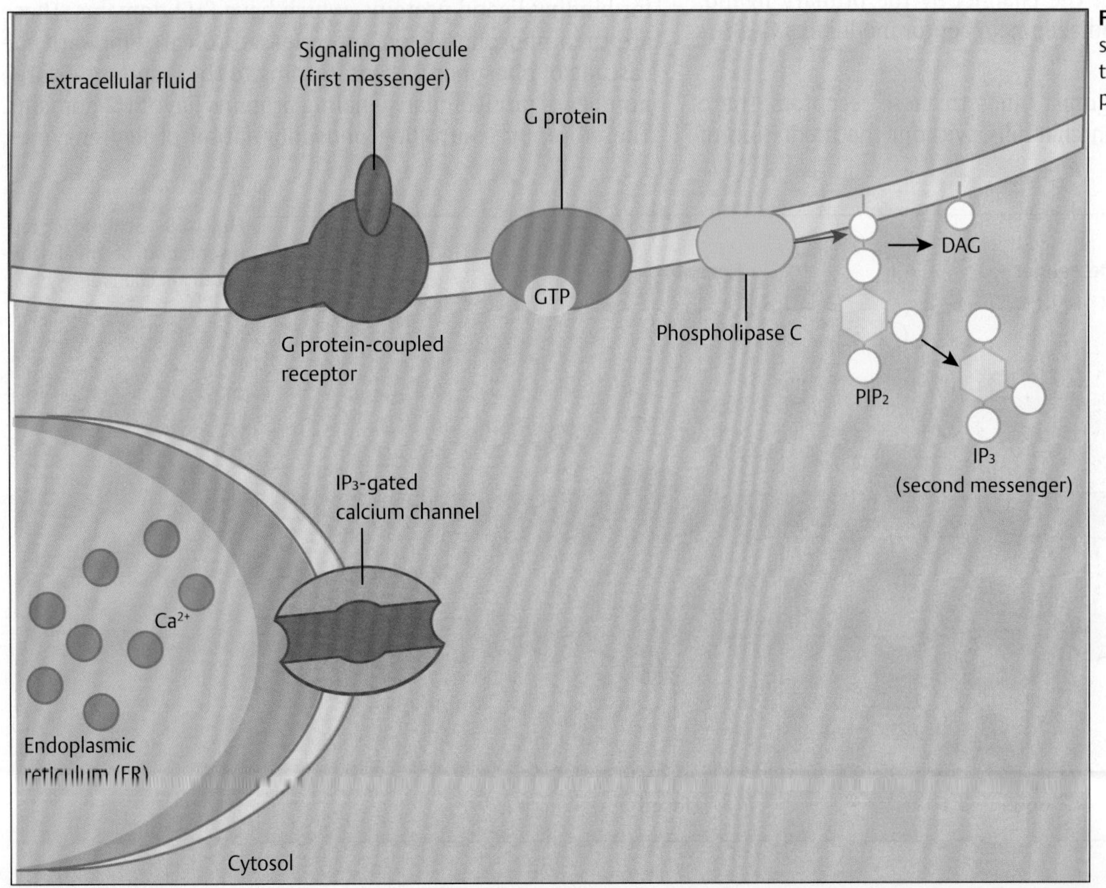

Fig. 4.7 Schematic representation of signal transduction of GPCR through phospholipase C.

involvement of second messengers such as cAMP or IP_3, and thus generate depolarization/hyperpolarization/changes in intracellular Ca^{2+}. G_s opens the Ca^{2+} channels in myocardium and skeletal muscles, whereas G_i and G_o open K^+ channels in the heart and smooth muscle in addition to the inhibition of neuronal Ca^{2+} channels. Direct channel regulation is typically the role of the βγ dimer of the separated G protein. Physiological reactions such as modulation in smooth muscle relaxation, transmitter release, inotropy, chronotropy, and neuronal activity will ensue.

Ligand-Gated Ion Channels/Ion Channel Receptors

These are cell surface receptors, which enfold ion selective channels (for Na^+, K^+, Ca^{2+}, or Cl^-) within their molecules (**Fig. 4.8**). Agonist binding to such receptors leads to opening of the channel, which, in turn, causes depolarization/hyperpolarization/changes in cytosolic ionic composition or brings about a change in cytosolic ionic composition, according to the ion that flows through it. Few examples of such receptors are cholinergic nicotinic type, $GABA_A$, glycine (inhibitory AA), excitatory AA-glutamate (kainate, NMDA [N-methyl D-aspartate] and AMPA [α-amino-3-hydroxy-5-methyl-4-isoxazolepropionic acid receptor]) and 5-HT_3 receptors.

The molecular structure of receptor is usually a pentameric protein with different subunits, which are termed α, β, δ, and γ subunits. They also have large intra- and extracellular segments, consisting of four membrane-spanning helical domains. The subunits are mostly arranged round the channel like a rosette and the agonist binding sites are on the α subunits. Certain ligand-gated ion channels also have secondary ligands, which bind to an allosteric site and modulate the gating of the channel by the primary ligand, for example, the benzodiazepine receptor modulates $GABA_A$-gated Cl^- channel.

Hence, when the agonist binds to these receptors, there is direct opening of ion channels, without the mediation of coupling protein or second messenger. The onset and offset of responses through this class of receptors are the fastest (in ms).

Transmembrane Enzyme-Linked Receptors

These membrane receptors, unlike the ligand-gated ion channels and GPCRs, are activated by a variety of protein mediators such as growth factors, cytokines, insulin, and leptin. They also differ in structure and function. Their effects are directed mainly at the level of gene transcription.

These receptors are large single-chain proteins consisting of up to 1,000 residues with single-membrane spanning helical region. This helical region links large extracellular ligand-binding domain with the intracellular domain of variable size and function. At the cytosolic side, there is a protein kinase in most cases but for few it may also be guanylyl cyclase. The commonest protein kinases are called phosphorylate tyrosine residues on the substrate proteins and are called "receptor tyrosine kinases" (RTKs). These phosphorylate tyrosine residues on substrate proteins.

Examples are insulin, epidermal growth factor, nerve growth factor, and many other growth factor receptors. However, the transforming growth factor receptor and few others are serine/threonine kinases, which phosphorylate serine/threonine residues of the target proteins.

During the inactive state, the receptor exists in monomeric state. When the ligand binds to the receptor, dimerization of the receptor occurs, leading to conformational changes. This, in turn, activates the kinase to autophosphorylate tyrosine residues on each other. This further increases their affinity for binding ligand proteins, which have SH2 domains. These are then phosphorylated and released to carry forward the cascade of phosphorylations, leading to the response. A large number of intracellular signaling proteins have SH2 domains. Therefore, by controlling phosphorylation of key enzymes,

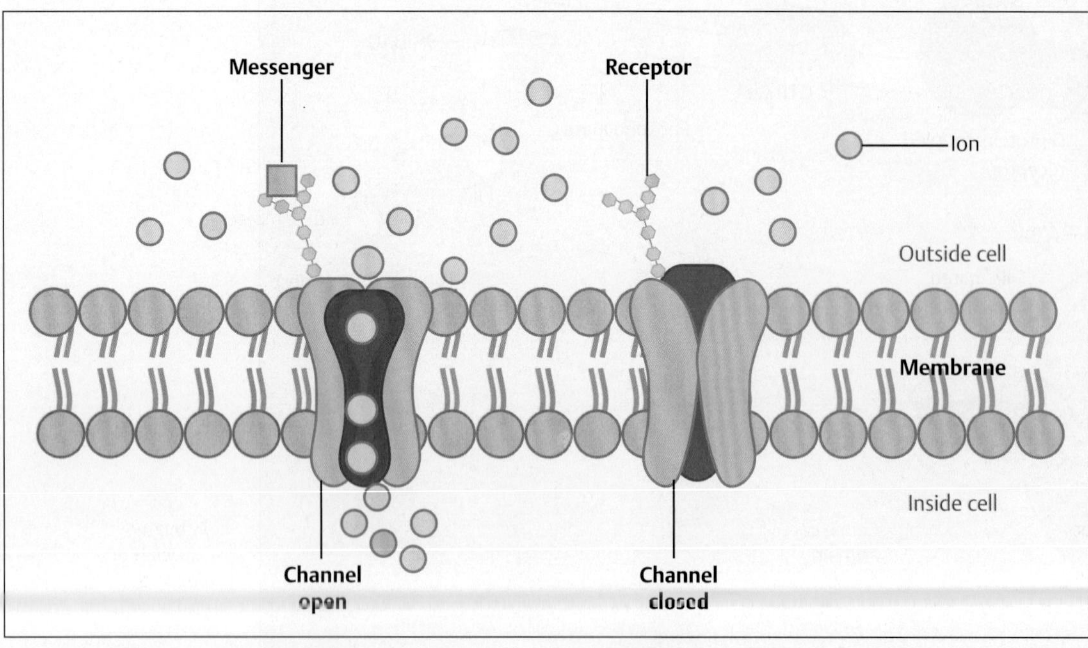

Fig. 4.8 Schematic representation of the ligand-gated ion channel.

ion channels, transporters, etc., the RTKs are able to regulate diverse cellular functions including metabolic reactions, cell growth, and differentiation. One such SH2 domain enzyme is phospholipase C, which is activated by certain RTKs, and generates IP_3 and DAG as second messengers for response effectuation. The dimerization of these receptors also promotes receptor internalization, degradation in lysosomes, and downregulation when required.

Instead of protein kinase, the enzyme can be guanylyl cyclase, as in the case of atrial natriuretic peptide. Agonist activation of these receptor generates cGMP in the cytosol as a second messenger, which in turn activates cGMP-dependent protein kinase and alters cellular activity.

These receptors have key role in regulating the cell division, intermediary metabolism, growth, differentiation, inflammation, tissue repair, apoptosis, and immune response (**Fig. 4.9**).

Transmembrane JAK-STAT Binding Receptors

These receptors diverge from RTKs in not having any intrinsic catalytic domain, that is, the receptors lack intrinsic protein kinase activity. Ligand induces dimerization, leading to a conformational change, which leads to increased affinity for a cytosolic tyrosine protein kinase JAK (Janus kinase). On binding, JAK is activated and phosphorylates tyrosine residues of the receptor, which in turn binds to another free-moving protein STAT (signal transducer and activator of transcription). This is also phosphorylated by JAK. Pairs of phosphorylated STAT dimerize and translocate to the nucleus to regulate gene transcription, resulting in a biological response. Many cytokines, growth hormone, prolactin, interferons, etc., act through this type of receptor.

Receptors Involved in Regulating Gene Expression (Transcription Factors and Nuclear Receptors)

This class of receptors are unique, as they are intracellular (cytoplasmic or nuclear) soluble proteins distinct from other classes of receptors. They respond to lipid-soluble chemical messengers, which penetrate the cell. These receptor proteins are specific for each hormone/regulator, and are fundamentally capable of binding to specific genes. However, proteins such as HSP-90 prevent them from adopting the configuration needed for binding to DNA. When the hormone binds at the carboxy terminus of the receptor, the restricting proteins (HSP-90, etc.) are released, and receptor dimerizes. Subsequently, the DNA-binding regulatory segment located in the middle of the molecule folds into the requisite configuration. Then, the ligand receptor dimer moves to the nucleus and binds to other coactivator/co-repressor proteins, which have a modulatory influence on its ability to alter gene function. The whole complex is then attached to hormone response element (specific DNA sequence) of the target gene, and modulates their expression so as to synthesis or repress the specific mRNA on the template of the gene. This mRNA subsequently moves to the ribosomes and shows the way to synthesis of specific proteins that control activity of target cells (**Fig. 4.10**).

All the steroidal hormones such as glucocorticoids, mineralocorticoids, androgens, estrogens, progesterone, thyroxine, vitamin D, and vitamin A are examples of receptors regulating gene expression; thus, they function in the manner described earlier. Various steroidal hormones affect different target cells and yield diverse effects. This occurs due to the fact that each hormone binds to its own receptor, which in turn leads to synthesis of specific proteins in an exclusive pattern. The specificity of the receptor for the hormone is determined by the hormone-binding domain, whereas the DNA-binding/N-terminus domain functions to determine the specificity of the gene that will be activated or repressed. Different ligands of same nuclear receptor have been found to induce ligand-specific conformations of the receptor, so that different combinations of co-activators and co-repressors may be bound in different target tissues, for example, selective estrogen receptor modulators (SERMs).

Nuclear receptors have been found to have different ligands. They have been found to bring about ligand-specific conformations of the receptor. This may also involve different combinations of co-activators and co-repressors bound in different target tissues, for example, SERMs. Tamoxifen and raloxifene have different patterns of action on various estrogenic target organs.

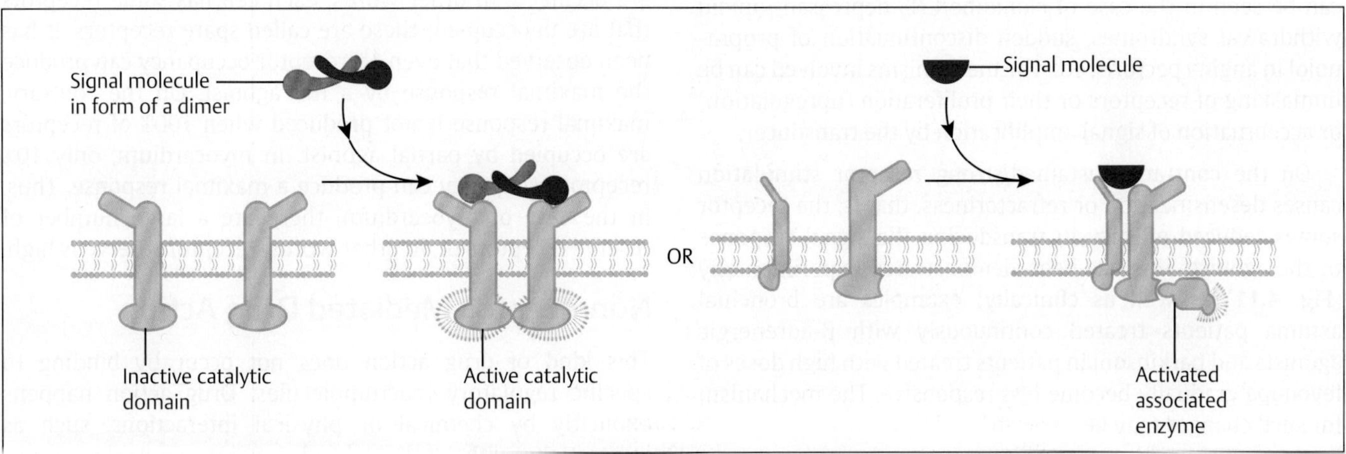

Fig. 4.9 Schematic representation of transduction of enzyme-linked receptor.

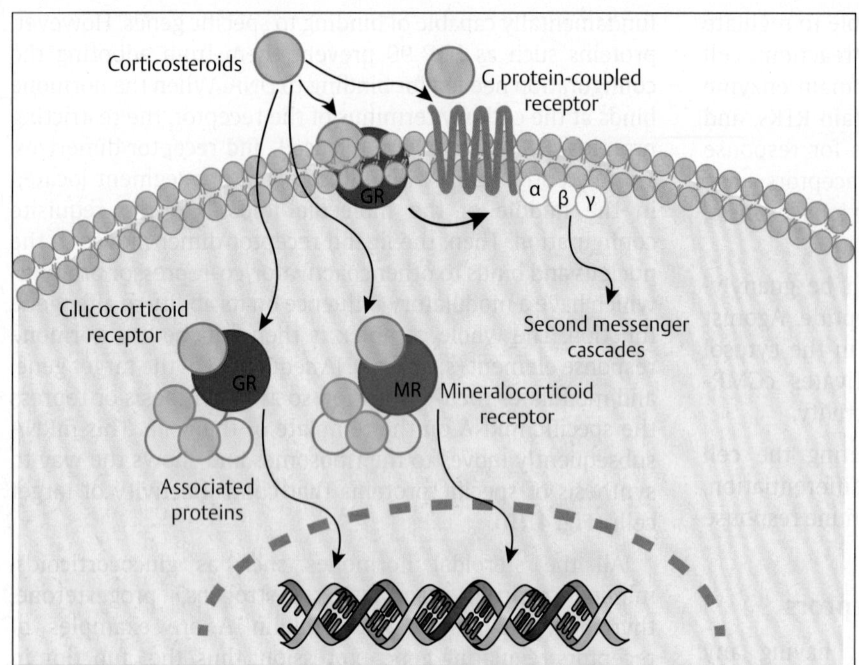

Fig. 4.10 Schematic representation of intracellular (glucocorticoid) receptor.

This transduction mechanism is slowest in the time course of action; it takes hours to manifest, as adequate quantity of effector protein will have to be produced before the response occurs. The effects generally occur after the hormone or signal has been eliminated as majority of the effector proteins have slow turnover.

Regulation of Receptors

Receptors are always in a dynamic state. Their concentration as well as efficacy to elicit a response is modulated by the level of ongoing activity feedback from their own signal output and other pathophysiological influences, for example, estrogens increase the density of oxytocin receptors on the myometrium. There is a progressive increase in sensitivity of the uterus to the contractile action of oxytocin during the third trimester of pregnancy, especially near term. If there occurs a prolonged deprivation of agonist either by denervation or by continued use of antagonist or drug that reduces input, it results in supersensitivity of receptor as well as the effector system to the agonist. The clinical relevance of this can be seen in the case of clonidine/CNS depressant/opioid withdrawal syndromes, sudden discontinuation of propranolol in angina pectoris, etc. The mechanisms involved can be unmasking of receptors or their proliferation (upregulation) or accentuation of signal amplification by the transducer.

On the contrary, sustained/strong receptor stimulation causes desensitization or refractoriness, that is, the receptor shows reduced efficacy in transducing the signal response to the agonist. This has been demonstrated experimentally (**Fig. 4.11**) as well as clinically; examples are bronchial asthma patients treated continuously with β-adrenergic agonists and parkinsonian patients treated with high doses of levodopa gradually become less responsive. The mechanism for such changes may be:

1. Internalization of receptor, masking, or impaired coupling of the transducer to the receptor. In such cases, the refractoriness progresses as well as disappears quickly.
2. Reduced synthesis/augmented destruction of the receptor (downregulation). In these conditions, refractoriness develops gradually over weeks or months and regresses slowly. Tyrosine kinase receptors as well as GPCRs are known to exhibit such kind of downregulation. The transducer and effector proteins are too up- or downregulated.

Functions of Receptors

1. Propagation of signal in an effector cell from extracellular to intracellular compartment when molecular entity conveying the signal cannot infiltrate the cell membrane itself.
2. To strengthen the signal.
3. To assimilate a variety of extracellular and intracellular regulatory signals.
4. To adjust to short-term and long-term changes in the regulatory environment and maintain homeostasis.

Spare Receptors (Reserve Receptors)

Drugs act on receptors to produce response. For maximal response by agonist, it is not necessary that all receptors are occupied. In other words, each cell has some receptors that are unoccupied; these are called spare receptors. It has been observed that even 1% receptor occupancy can produce the maximal response by a full agonist. On the contrary, maximal response is not produced when 100% of receptors are occupied by partial agonist. In myocardium, only 10% receptor occupancy can produce a maximal response. Thus, in the case of myocardium, there are a large number of reserve receptors or, in other words, receptor reserve is high.

Nonreceptor-Mediated Drug Action

This kind of drug action does not occur by binding to specific regulatory macromolecules. Drug action happens explicitly by chemical or physical interactions, such as interactions with small molecules or ions as in the case of antacids, chelating agents, cholestyramine, etc. In addition, drugs such as alkylating agents that bond covalently with

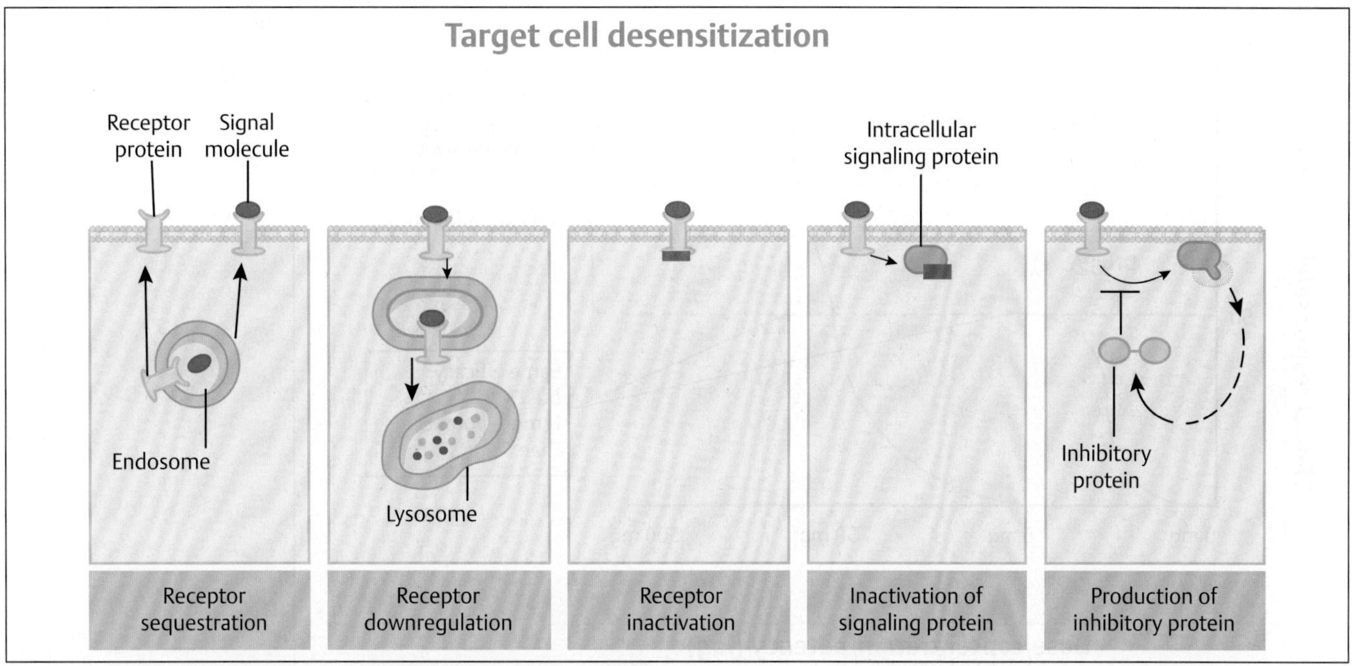

Fig. 4.11 Schematic representation of phenomenon of desensitization.

numerous critical biomolecules, such as nucleic acids, show cytotoxic activity, which is beneficial in the treatment of cancer. Additional significant class of drugs includes the antimetabolites (purine/pyrimidine analogues) leading to creation of nonfunctional or dysfunctional cellular constituents which exert antiviral, antineoplastic, and immunosuppressant activity.

Dose–Response Relationship

Once a drug is given systemically, the dose–response relationship has two constituents:

1. Plasma concentration–response relationship.
2. Dose–plasma concentration relationship.

Pharmacokinetic considerations determine the dose–plasma concentration relationship, whereas pharmacodynamic considerations determine the plasma concentration–response relationship, which is studied easily in vitro.

Usually, the strength of the response rises with increase in dose, more specifically the concentration of the drug at the receptor. However, at higher doses, the increase in response gradually becomes less noticeable and the dose–response curve (DRC) is a rectangular hyperbola (**Fig. 4.12**). Such response occurs since the drug–receptor interaction observes law of mass action, which is described by the following equation and is applicable to interaction between any two molecules having a given affinity for each other:

$$E = \frac{E_{max} \times [D]}{K_D + [D]},$$

where:

E is the witnessed effect at a dose [*D*] of the drug,

E_{max} is the maximal response,

K_D is the dissociation constant of the drug–receptor complex, that is, the degree of affinity between the two, and is equivalent to the dose of the drug at which half-maximal response is observed.

In case the dose is plotted on logarithmic scale, the curve turns out to be sigmoid and a linear relationship between the log of dose and the response is realized in the intermediate (30–70% response) zone as is expected from the equation. Other benefits of plotting log DRCs are:

1. A wide range of drug doses can be exhibited on a chart.
2. Assessment between agonists and study of antagonist become easier.

The log DRC could be described by its shape (slope and maxima) and position on the dose axis.

Drug Potency and Efficacy

Drug potency is the amount (dose) of drug required to produce a certain response. It is a quantitative parameter. When two drugs have similar effect, then the drug that produces similar response in lower dose is more potent, that is, its ED_{50} is less. In other words, dose required is higher for drugs with lower potency and vice versa. If we refer to DRC, the position of the DRC on dose axis is the drug potency. A DRC sited toward right depicts low potency. Relative potency is often a useful tool as compared to absolute potency. The relative potency is defined by comparing the dose (concentration) of the two agonists at which they produce half-maximal response (EC_{50}). For example, 10 mg of morphine is equal to 100 mg of pethidine as analgesic; here, morphine is 10 times more potent than pethidine as analgesic. Nevertheless, higher potency does not indicate clinical superiority unless the potency for therapeutic effect is selectively increased over potency for adverse effects. Drug potency is one of the factors considered in choosing the dose of the drug (**Fig. 4.12**).

Drug efficacy denotes the maximum response that could be exhibited by a drug, for example, morphine produces

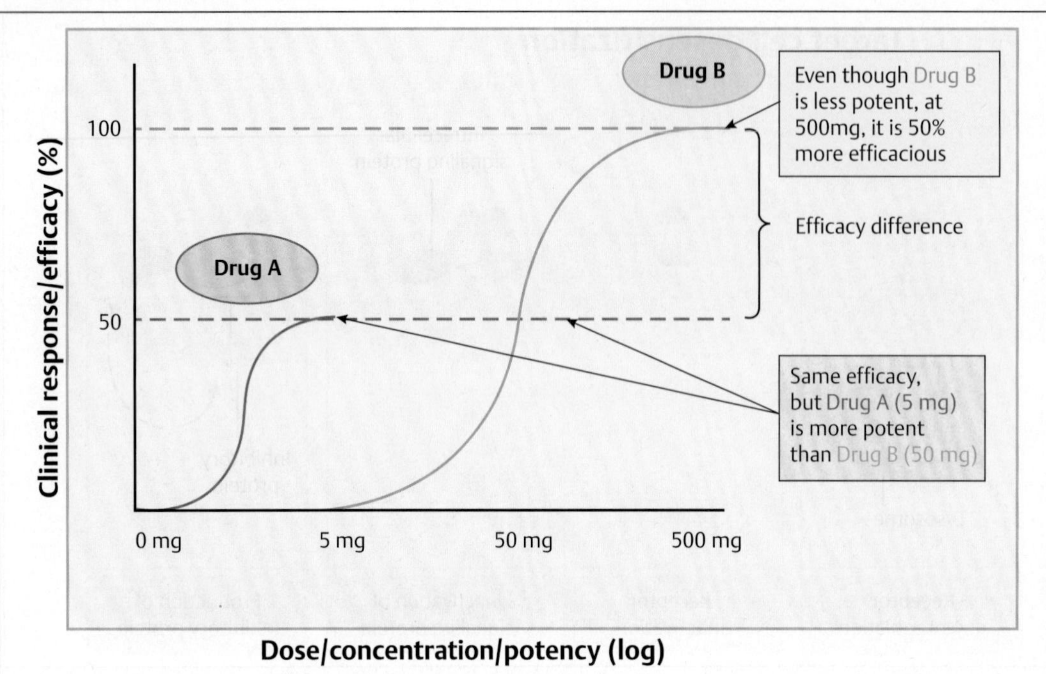

Fig. 4.12 Graphical representation of drug potency and drug efficacy.

higher degree of analgesia, which cannot be obtained by any dose of aspirin. Thus, morphine has higher efficacy than aspirin. While selecting a drug for treatment, efficacy is an important parameter involved. It is a qualitative parameter. *Drug potency* and *drug efficacy* are the terms that are utilized interchangeably; however, these are not the same. They emphasize dissimilar characteristics of the drug. The two can differ individually:

1. Aspirin has lower potency and lower efficacy when compared to morphine.
2. Pethidine has lower potency but equal efficacy as that of morphine.
3. Furosemide has lower potency but more efficacy than metolazone as a diuretic.
4. Diazepam is relatively more potent, yet less efficacious than pentobarbitone.

The type of drug determines whether higher efficacy or lower efficacy can be clinically beneficial. For example, higher efficacy of furosemide confers its utility in mobilizing edema fluid and in renal failure, whereas in the case of diazepam lower efficacy confers safety in overdose.

The slope of DRC is also an important parameter to be considered. A sharp slope shows that the moderate escalation in dose can distinctly increase the response. This means that the dose needs to be individualized. Conversely, a flat DRC indicates that slight escalation in response can follow over a wide range of doses; thus, standard doses could be administered to most patients. Hydralazine exhibits steep DRC, whereas hydrochlorothiazide has flat DRC for their antihypertensive effect (**Fig. 4.13**).

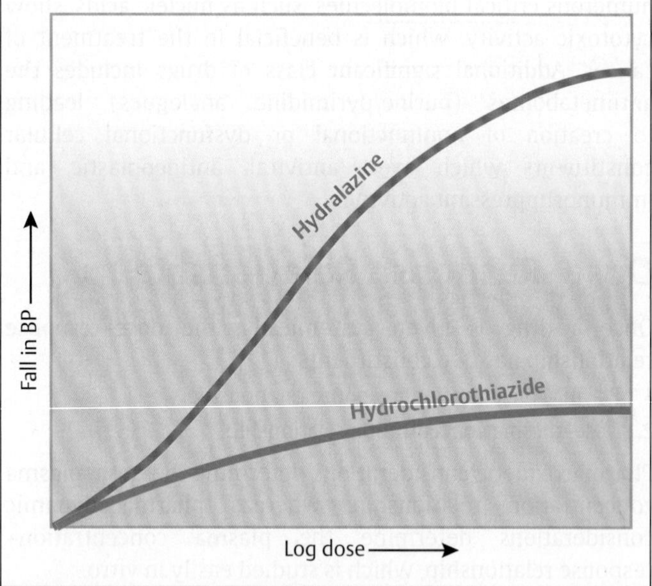

Fig. 4.13 Comparative efficacy of two diuretic drugs.

Therapeutic Efficacy

Therapeutic efficacy is articulated as follows:

1. Amount of benefit produced by the drug (in recommended dose range), that is, graded DRC relationship. For example, the extent of help in parkinsonian symptoms produced by levodopa–carbidopa is much more than that produced by the drug trihexyphenidyl: thus, levodopa–carbidopa has higher therapeutic efficacy than trihexyphenidyl.
2. Success rate for attaining a defined therapeutic end point, that is, quantal dose–response relationship. For example, an antibiotic that cures 95% cases of gonorrhea is a more efficacious drug than the one that cures 75% of patients. Similarly, a more effective antiepileptic drug would be capable of making a greater proportion of epileptic patients completely seizure-free as compared to another drug.

Drug Selectivity

Drugs occasionally produce single action but most of the time a drug produces different effects. The DRCs of different effects may be different. The distance between the DRCs of a drug for diverse effects is an extent of its selectivity. For example, DRCs of isoprenaline for bronchodilation and cardiac stimulation are fairly comparable but distant in the case of salbutamol. Thus, salbutamol is a more selective bronchodilator.

Quantitative Aspect of Drug Action

Quantitative feature of drug is significant as it helps us to make choice on its mode of use. **Dose–response (effect)** or **concentration–response (effect)** is more important in this aspect.

Dose–Response Relationship

There are two types of drug response: graded response and quantal response.

Graded Response

In graded response, the degree of response changes as per concentration, that is, response is more at higher concentration. The response of a drug on any parameter can be measured with dose increment, for example, effect of drug on blood pressure, blood glucose, or contraction or relaxation of muscles, etc. Graded response can be studied in vitro as well as in vivo, but in vitro studies are preferred because, in the case of in vivo, the system is complicated by various factors that can modify the response, while in in vitro it is not so. The response increases with increase in concentration of agonist till it reaches the maximum response. The concentration–response curve, when plotted, is a hyperbola. The log dose (concentration)–response curve is sigmoidal and the middle portion (precisely 30–70% response) is linear and thus suitable for various calculations and conclusions (**Fig. 4.14**).

1. Since the middle portion is linear, it shows that the response is directly proportional to log concentration within a range of doses.
2. The effective dose (ED) or effective concentration (EC) can be determined, such as ED_{50} (median effective dose) and ED_{100} or ED_{max} (maximum effective dose).

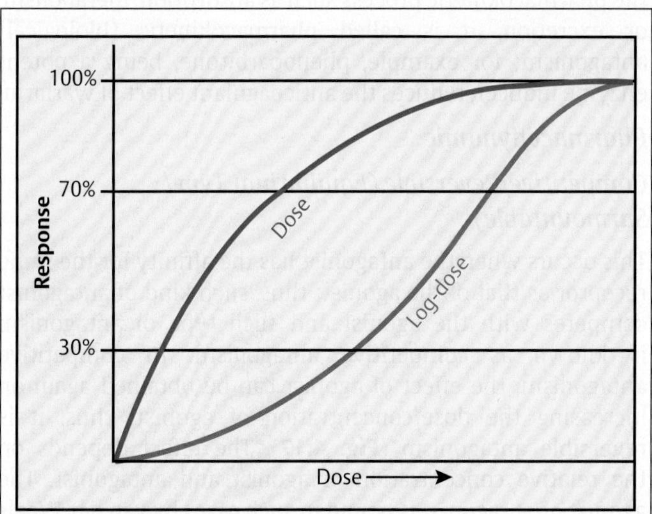

Fig. 4.14 Graded dose–response curve.

Quantal Response

In such kind of response, all-or-none law exists, that is, response is either produced or not produced—for example, anticonvulsant actions of drugs in which drug produces either anticonvulsant action or no action but there is no response in between (**Fig. 4.15**). Usually, intact animal is used to study the quantal response. In this kind of response, also the log dose curve is sigmoidal. It can be used to determine the lethal dose during acute toxicity study, that is, LD_{50}.

Drug Antagonism

Definitions

1. **Ligand (Latin: ligare—to bind):** It is a molecule that combines specifically to a particular site or receptor, that is, ligand can be either agonist or antagonist.
2. **Affinity:** It refers to the ability of a drug to bind to its receptor, that is, the ability to form drug–receptor complex.
3. **IA or efficacy:** If the drug–receptor complex formed due to affinity produces a pharmacological response, it is called its IA or efficacy.

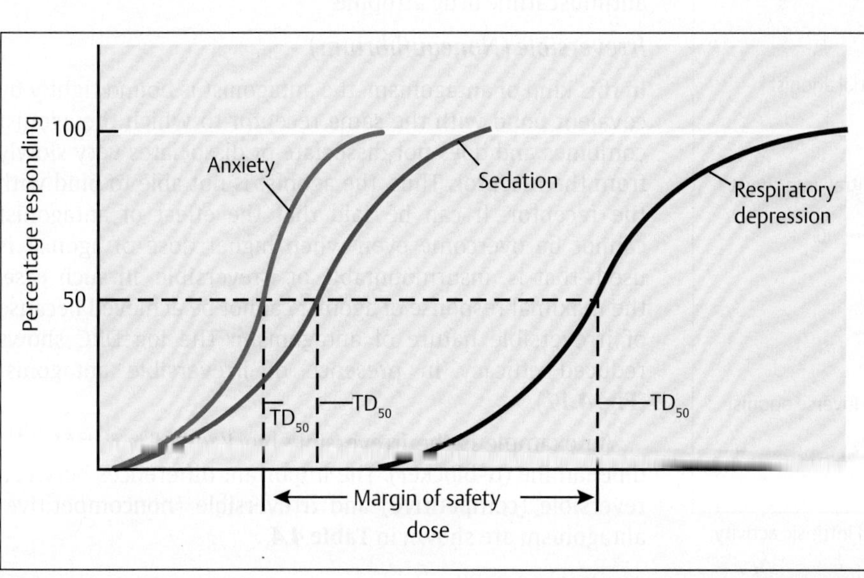

Fig. 4.15 Schematic representation of quantal dose–response curve after administration of different doses of sedative hypnotic.

On the basis of affinity and IA, drugs can be categorized as follows (**Fig. 4.16**):

1. **Affinity + IA = agonist:** A drug that has affinity as well as IA/efficacy is known as agonist. For example, salbutamol is agonist to β_2-receptor.
2. **Affinity + no IA = antagonist:** A drug having affinity but no IA is known as antagonist. For example, atenolol is antagonist at β_1-receptor.
3. **Affinity + submaximal IA = partial agonist:** A drug having affinity for a receptor but submaximal IA or efficacy is called partial agonist. For example, buprenorphine is partial agonist at μ-opioid receptors. Partial agonist antagonizes the action of full agonist and, in absence of full agonist, produces some agonistic action but they do not produce maximal response even at higher concentration.
4. **Affinity + negative IA = reverse agonist/inverse agonist:** A drug having affinity for a receptor but producing action opposite to that of full agonist. For example, β-carbolines have affinity of benzodiazepines receptor but produce anxiety, arousal, and increased skeletal muscle tone. These are actions opposite to benzodiazepines.
5. **Agonist–antagonist:** There are multiple opioid receptors, and some drugs act as agonist at some receptor and as antagonist at other receptors. Such molecules are called agonist–antagonist. For example, pentazocine is antagonist at μ-receptor but agonist at ⱪ-receptor.
6. **Receptor selectivity:** If a drug produces any of the above-mentioned action only at one receptor, it is called selective agonist or selective antagonist. For example:
   a. Salbutamol is a β_2-receptor selective agonist, while isoprenaline is nonselective agonist at β-receptor, that is, at both β_1- and β_2-receptor.
   b. Atenolol is β_1-receptor selective antagonist, while propranolol is nonselective antagonist at β-receptor, that is, it is antagonist at both β_1- and β_2-receptor.
7. **Absolute and relative selectivity:** Selectivity can be absolute or relative. For example, salbutamol is β_2-receptor selective agonist in usual therapeutic doses but at higher doses it also stimulates β_1-receptor. This indicates that selectivity is lost at higher dose and this is known as relative selectivity for β_2-receptor. Conversely, whatever high dose of salbutamol is used, it will not stimulate α-receptors; thus, selectivity of salbutamol for β-receptor is absolute.

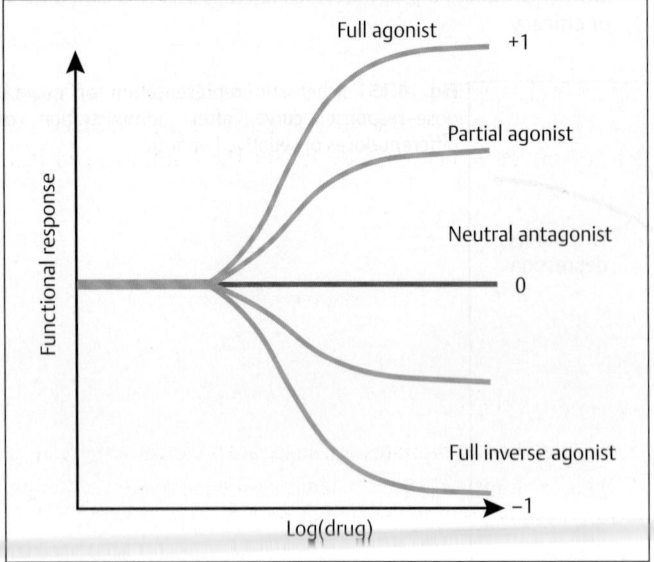

Fig. 4.16 Drug categories on the basis of affinity and intrinsic activity.

Antagonism

Chemical

In this type, the action of a drug reduces or inhibits a chemical reaction; for example, antacids neutralize the gastric acid and thus are used for peptic ulcer treatment.

Physiological/Functional

In such type of antagonism, a drug, which is receptor agonist, reverses the action of another drug on the same physiological system but on different receptors. This phenomenon is known as physiological antagonism. For example, adrenaline overcomes the effect of acetylcholine on the heart. Similarly, adrenaline overcomes the effect of histamine in anaphylactic shock by acting on different receptors.

Pharmacological

Pharmacokinetic

When a drug reduces the effect of another drug by altering the pharmacokinetic process such as absorption, metabolism, or excretion, it is called pharmacokinetic (biological) antagonism; for example, phenobarbitone, being a potent enzyme inducer, reduces the anticoagulant effect of warfarin.

Pharmacodynamic

Competitive/Reversible (Equilibrium Type/ Surmountable)

This occurs when the antagonist has the affinity for the same receptor as that of the agonist; thus, such kind of antagonist competes with the agonist and such type of antagonism is known as competitive antagonism. In competitive antagonism, the effect of agonist can be obtained again on increasing the dose/concentration of agonist; thus, it is reversible antagonism (**Fig. 4.17**). The effect depends on the relative concentration of agonist and antagonist. The agonist or antagonist is bound in such cases by van der Waals or hydrogen bond, for example, α-blocker (prazosin) and antimuscarinic drug atropine.

Irreversible (Nonequilibrium)

In this kind of antagonism, the antagonist is bound tightly by covalent bond with the same receptor to which the agonist combines and does not dissociate or dissociates very slowly from the receptor. Thus, the agonist is not able to bind with the receptor. It can be said that the effect of antagonist cannot be overcome even when higher dose of agonist is used—that is, insurmountable or irreversible. In such case, the maximal response of agonist cannot be achieved because of irreversible nature of antagonism. The log DRC shows reduced efficacy in presence of irreversible antagonist (**Fig. 4.17**).

An example is the irreversible blockade of α-receptor by dibenamine (α-blocker). The important differences between reversible (competitive) and irreversible (noncompetitive) antagonism are shown in **Table 4.4**.

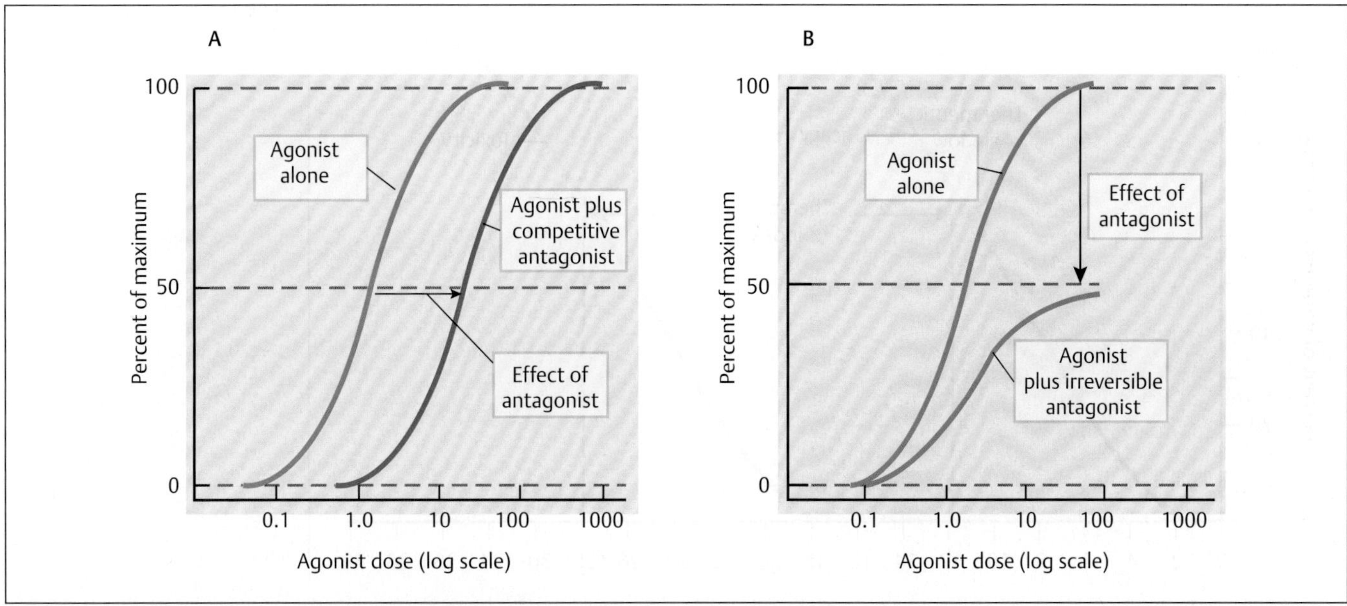

Fig. 4.17 Log dose–response curve for competitive antagonism.

Table 4.4 Differences between reversible (competitive) and irreversible (noncompetitive) antagonism

Competitive	Noncompetitive
Binds to same receptor	Binds to other site
Resembles chemically	No resemblance
Parallel right shift of DRC in increasing dose of agonist	Maximal response is suppressed
Intensity depends on the concentration of agonist and antagonist	Depends only on concentration of antagonist
Example: ACh and atropine, morphine, and naloxone	Diazepam, bicuculline

Abbreviations: ACh, acetylcholine; DCR, dose–response curve.

Noncompetitive

Often, the term *irreversible* is interchangeably used with *noncompetitive*. However, it must be clarified that noncompetitive is not a receptor antagonism. In noncompetitive antagonism, the response of the agonist is blocked by the antagonist by acting at a different site and not on the receptor of the agonist.

Clinical Relevance of Drug Antagonism

1. Treatment of certain conditions and poisoning, for example:
   a. Use of antacids for peptic ulcer (chemical antagonism).
   b. Use of adrenaline for anaphylactic shock (physiological antagonism).
   c. Poisoning, for example, use of naloxone for opioid poisoning, atropine for organophosphorus (competitive antagonism).
2. To overcome or reduce the adverse effect of a drug, for example, use of benzhexol with trifluoperazine reduces the extrapyramidal side effect of trifluoperazine (competitive antagonism).
3. To assess the efficacy of a drug in presence of other drug or when two drugs are used simultaneously, for example, bacteriostatic drug (e.g., tetracycline) reduces efficacy of bactericidal (penicillin) when used together.

Assessment of Safety of Drugs/ Therapeutic Index

On the basis of animal data of lethal dose and effective dose, the therapeutic index is calculated as follows (**Fig. 4.18**).

$$\text{Therapeutic index} = LD_{50}/ED_{50}.$$

Here, LD_{50} is the dose of a drug that kills 50% of animals used in a study and ED_{50} is the dose of a drug that produced the desired effect or response in 50% of the animals used in a study.

Significance of Therapeutic Index

1. Therapeutic index is an indicator of safety margin of a drug. For example, if there are two drugs A and B with therapeutic index of 10 and 20, respectively, it means drug B is much safer than drug A. Therapeutic index of benzodiazepines is around 100, while that of barbiturates is 8 to 10 and thus benzodiazepines are safer than barbiturates and hence are preferred as hypnotics.
2. High therapeutic index indicates wide safety margin. Appropriate precautions should be taken while using a drug with narrow safety margin as slight increase in dose may lead to toxicity.

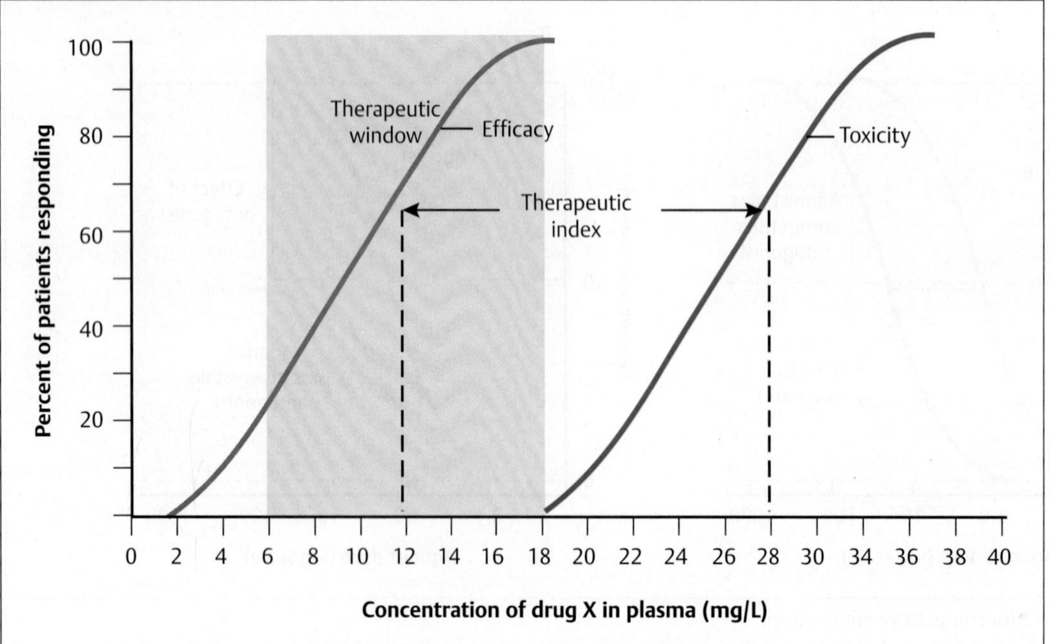

Fig. 4.18 Therapeutic index.

Limitations

LD_{50} is not a good indicator of toxicity in therapeutic settings as it is the extrapolation of animal data to clinical condition. Idiosyncratic and allergic reactions, toxicity due to associated condition, or effect of drug on pregnancy cannot be predicted on the basis of therapeutic index.

Drugs with High Therapeutic Index

Majority of drugs have high therapeutic index and their DRC is not steep. Examples are penicillin G, ampicillin, amoxycillin, aspirin, benzodiazepines (diazepam), atenolol, and atropine.

Drugs with Low Therapeutic Index

Drugs that have low therapeutic index have a steep DRC. Examples are theophylline, barbiturates, lithium, digoxin, phenytoin, gentamicin, and cytotoxic drugs.

Therapeutic Window

It is the range of plasma concentration of the drug that produces therapeutic effect in majority of patients. It is the range of doses of a drug between the dose that produce minimal therapeutic effect at one end and the dose that produce maximum adverse effect.

Therapeutic Window Phenomenon

This phenomenon is observed with certain drugs, for example, tricyclic antidepressants, clonidine, and glipizide. In this phenomenon, therapeutic effect of the drug is detected within narrow range of plasma concentration. Thus, below and above that plasma concentration the therapeutic effect is suboptimal, reduced, or lost (**Fig. 4.19**).

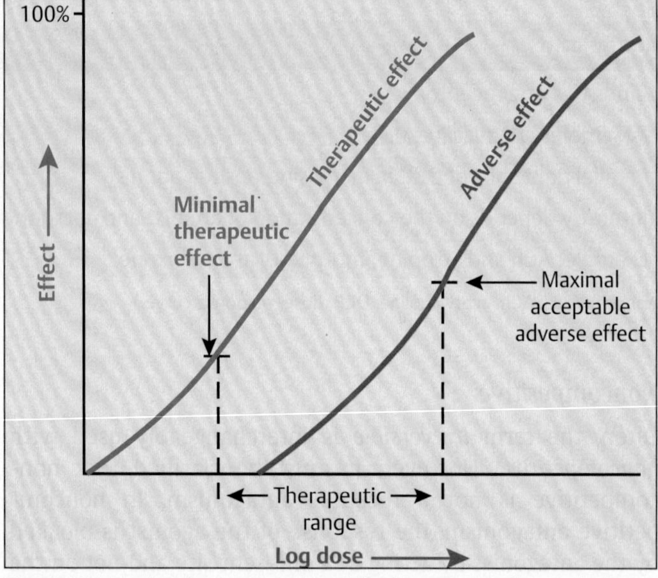

Fig. 4.19 Graphical representation of the therapeutic effect and adverse effect on log dose curve.

In clinical setup, the therapeutic index may be calculated as follows:

Clinical therapeutic index = Maximum tolerated doses/ Minimum dose for clinical response.

Risk–Benefit Ratio

At times it is difficult to decide whether to use the drug for its therapeutic effect or not due to a drug's narrow safety margin. In such cases, the benefit versus risk should be calculated and if benefit outweighs the risk, the drug can be used. For making such kind of decisions pharmaco-epidemiological data should be considered.

Multiple Choice Questions

1. All of the following agents act by intracellular receptors, except:

A. Thyroid hormones.
B. Vitamin D.
C. Insulin.
D. Steroids.

Answer: C

Transmembrane enzyme-linked receptors. These membrane receptors, unlike the ligand-gated ion channels and GPCRs, are activated by a variety of protein mediators such as growth factors, cytokines, insulin, and leptin.

2. Which of the following statement is true regarding inverse agonist?

A. Binds to the receptor and causes intended action.
B. Binds to the receptor and causes opposite action.
C. Binds to the receptor and causes no action.
D. Binds to the receptor and causes submaximal action.

Answer: B

Inverse agonist is a drug having affinity for a receptor but producing action opposite to that of full agonist. For example, β-carbolines have affinity of benzodiazepines receptor but produce anxiety, arousal, and increased skeletal muscle tone. These are actions opposite to benzodiazepines.

3. Which of the following is an ionotropic receptor?

A. Muscarinic cholinergic receptor.
B. Nicotinic cholinergic receptor.
C. Glucocorticoid receptor.
D. Insulin receptor.

Answer: B

Ligand-gated ion channels/ion channel receptors. These are cell surface receptors, which enfold ion selective channels (for Na^+, K^+, $Ca2^+$, or Cl^-) within their molecules (Fig. 4.8). Agonist binding to such receptors leads to opening of the channel, which, in turn, causes depolarization/hyperpolarization/changes in cytosolic ionic composition or brings about a change in cytosolic ionic composition, according to the ion that flows through it. Few examples of such receptors are cholinergic nicotinic type, GABAA, glycine (inhibitory AA), excitatory AA-glutamate (kainate, NMDA, and AMPA) and 5-HT3 receptors.

4. Which of the following does not act as second messenger?

A. Cyclic AMP.
B. Inositol trisphosphate.
C. Diacylglycerol.
D. G proteins.

Answer: D

G proteins are membrane proteins whose primary role is to respond to GPCR activation and convey the message inside the cell to the effector systems, which produce a cellular response (Fig. 4.5). They are essentially middle management in the process.

5. A 56-year-old man with heart failure is to be treated with a diuretic drug. Drugs A and B have same mechanism of action. Drug A in dose of 50 mg produces the same magnitude of diuresis as 500 mg of drug B. This means that:

A. Drug B is less efficacious than drug A.
B. Drug A is more potent than drug B.
C. Drug A is a safer drug than drug B.
D. Drug A will have shorter duration of action than drug B.

Answer: B

The drug producing the same response at lower dose is more potent. In this case, drug A is 10 times more potent than drug B.

6. Which of the following has cytoplasmic receptor?

A. Epinephrine.
B. Insulin.
C. FSH.
D. Cortisol.

Answer: D

Receptors involved in regulating gene expression (transcription factors and nuclear receptors). This class of receptors are unique, as they are intracellular (cytoplasmic or nuclear) soluble proteins distinct from other classes of receptors.

All the steroidal hormones such as glucocorticoids, mineralocorticoids, androgens, estrogens, progesterone, thyroxine, vitamin D, and vitamin A are examples of receptors regulating gene expression.

7. G protein–coupled receptor is:

A. Metabotropic receptors.
B. Ionic receptors.
C. Kinase-linked receptors.
D. Nuclear receptors.

Answer: A

A metabotropic receptor is a type of membrane receptor that initiates a number of metabolic steps to modulate cell activity.

8. Which of the following is true for agonist?

A. Affinity with intrinsic activity is 1.
B. Affinity with intrinsic activity is 0.
C. Affinity with intrinsic activity is-1.
D. None.

Answer: A

Agonist stimulates a receptor to cause an effect similar to that of the physiological signal molecule.

9. Which of the following plasma membrane receptors activate signaling pathways usually by forming molecular dimers that result in protein phosphorylation reactions upon binding of their specific ligand?

A. Steroid hormone receptors.
B. Receptor tyrosine kinases.
C. Ligand-gated ion channels.
D. G protein-coupled receptors.

Answer: B

During the inactive state, the receptor exists in monomeric state. When the ligand binds to the receptor, dimerization of the receptor occurs, leading to conformational changes. This, in turn, activates the kinase to autophosphorylate tyrosine residues on each other.

10. Which of the following most accurately describes the transmembrane signaling process involved in the steroid hormone action?

A. Action on a membrane spanning tyrosine kinase.

B. Action of a G protein, which activates or inhibits adenylyl cyclase.

C. Diffusion across the membrane and binding to an intracellular receptor.

D. Opening of transmembrane ion channels.

Answer: C

Steroid hormones are lipid soluble and act on cytoplasmic receptors after crossing the plasma membrane.

Drug Interactions

Mayank Kulshreshtha, Shivam Yadav, and Prasan R. Bhandari

PH1.8: Identify and describe the management of drug interactions.

Learning Objectives

- Classification of drug interactions.
- Drug–food interactions.
- Drug–herb interaction.

Introduction

A drug interaction can be defined as a variation of response of one drug caused by another when they are given concurrently or in rapid sequence. The variation is generally quantitative, that is, the response could be either enhanced or reduced in strength; however, occasionally, it could be qualitative, that is, an atypical or a diverse kind of response is seen. The likelihood of drug interaction happens when a patient simultaneously takes more than one drug, and the probabilities grows with the quantity of drugs taken.

Various medical/dental situations are managed with a combination of drugs. The constituents of the combination are so carefully chosen that they supplement each other's effects; for example, an antibiotic is combined with an analgesic to manage a sore infective condition; adrenaline is added to lignocaine for dental anesthesia; mixed aerobic–anaerobic bacterial infections, comprising various orodental infections, are managed by a combination of antimicrobials. In addition, frequently, several drugs are utilized to manage a patient who is enduring from multiple diseases simultaneously. The probabilities of inadvertent/adverse drug interactions are higher in this condition, since a variety of diverse medications could be dispensed to a patient depending on his/her diseases/symptoms. The seriousness of drug interactions in maximum number of situations is extremely unpredictable.

Significantly, a large percentage of patients are old and are expected to be getting one or numerous drugs for their prolonged disorders such as hypertension, diabetes, and arthritis. The clinician could inadvertently recommend medications that could possibly interact with the existing ones consumed by the patient, causing serious complications. Hence, it is necessary that the physician take a thorough medical and drug history of the patient and document all the drugs the patient is presently consuming.

The number of possible drug–drug interactions is extensive and still rising. Hence, it is quite difficult to recognize and recollect all of these. However, the clinically relevant and significant and frequent drug interactions are comparatively limited.

These are summarized in **Table 5.1**. Some of these can be recognized, which are more common in clinical situations. Hence, attention should be paid while the patient is being administered one or more of such medications.

Drugs most likely to be involved in clinically important drug interactions are as follows:

- Highly protein bound drugs—nonsteroidal anti-inflammatory drugs (NSAIDs), warfarin, sulfonylureas.
- Drugs with narrow therapeutic index (thus narrow safety margin)—aminoglycoside antibiotics, digoxin, lithium.
- Drugs impacting strictly regulated body functions—antihypertensives, antidiabetics, anticoagulants.
- Drugs undergoing metabolism by saturation kinetics—phenytoin, theophylline.

Classification of Drug Interactions

Drug interactions can generally be classified as pharmacokinetic and pharmacodynamic interactions. In some situations, however, the mechanisms are complicated and could not be easily recognized. Some drug interactions occur even externally (in vitro) when drug solutions are mixed prior to their administration.

Table 5.1 Some selected herb–drug interactions

Herb	Common use	May interact with	Potential effect
Aloe vera	Laxative	Cardiac glycosides, thiazide diuretics	Can cause electrolyte imbalance and hypokalemia
Garlic	Hyperlipidemia	Anticoagulants, antiplatelet agents	Inhibits platelet aggregation; additive anticoagulant, antiplatelet effects
Ginger	Motion sickness, nausea, arthritis	Anticoagulants, antiplatelet agents	Inhibits thromboxane synthetase; may have additive anticoagulant, antiplatelet effects
Karela (bitter gourd)	Diabetes mellitus	Hypoglycemic drugs	Potentiates drug effect
Turmeric	Dyspepsia	Antiplatelet agents	Herb contains curcumin; may potentiate antiplatelet activity

In Vitro Drug Interactions

Some medications react with one other and become inactivated if they are mixed prior to their administration. During real-life situations, it can happen when parenteral medications are mixed in the same syringe or infusion bottle. Certain examples include:

- Penicillin G or ampicillin + aminoglycosides.
- Thiopentone sodium + succinylcholine/morphine.
- Heparin + penicillin/gentamicin/hydrocortisone.
- Noradrenaline + sodium bicarbonate solution.

Hence, it is recommended to refrain from mixing any two or more injectable drugs prior to their administration.

In Vivo Drug Interactions

Pharmacokinetic Interactions

These drug interactions change the concentration of the medication at its site of action (and thus its strength of response) by disturbing its absorption, distribution, metabolism, or excretion. This could be due to alteration of absorption or first-pass metabolism, displacement of plasma protein–bound drug, or modification of drug binding to tissues, thus changing its volume of distribution and clearance, inhibition/induction of metabolism, or modification of excretion.

Absorption Level Interactions

Absorption of an orally given medication can be altered by other simultaneously administered drugs. This occurs because of the development of insoluble and poorly absorbed complexes in the gastrointestinal (GI) lumen, for example, tetracyclines and calcium/iron salts, antacids, or sucralfate. For example, phenytoin absorption is also reduced by sucralfate. These could be decreased by giving the two drugs 2 to 3 hours apart, with the aim that these agents do not react in the gastric lumen. Antimicrobial agents such as ampicillin, tetracyclines, and cotrimoxazole significantly decrease the gastrointestinal commensal bacterial flora, which generally deconjugates oral contraceptive steroids secreted in the intestine and results in their enterohepatic circulation. Quite a lot of cases of contraceptive failure have occurred because of the simultaneous administration of these antibiotics because of a reduced levels of contraceptive blood levels. Modification of gastrointestinal motility by anticholinergic drugs (e.g., atropinic drugs, tricyclic antidepressants, opioids) and prokinetic drugs (e.g., metoclopramide or cisapride) could likewise alter drug absorption.

Distribution Level Interactions

These are generally because of displacement of one drug from its binding sites on plasma proteins by another drug. Highly plasma protein–bound medications, which have a generally less volume of distribution, for example, warfarin (oral anticoagulant), sulfonylureas, NSAIDs, and antiepileptics, are specifically vulnerable to develop these drug interactions. Displacement of the plasma protein–bound drug will result in an elevated blood levels of the free and active form of the drug, consequently causing toxicity. However, these are typically of a short duration, since the free form quickly gets distributed, metabolized, and excreted; therefore, its steady-state level is only slightly increased. The clinical significance of such drug interactions is usually important only when displacement spreads to tissue-binding sites along with inhibition of metabolism and/or excretion. For example, quinidine has been demonstrated to decrease the binding of digoxin to tissue proteins and also its renal and biliary elimination, causing approximately doubling of digoxin blood levels and toxicity.

Metabolism Level Interactions

Some drugs increase or decrease the extent of metabolism of other drugs. These drugs could therefore alter the bioavailability (if the drug exhibits a high first-pass metabolism in liver) and the plasma half-life of the drug (if the drug is chiefly eliminated by metabolism). Inhibition of drug metabolism could be because of competition for the same cytochrome P450 (CYP) isoenzyme or cofactor, and achieves clinical relevance primarily for drugs that are metabolized by saturation kinetics. Antifungals such as ketoconazole, macrolide antibiotics such as erythromycin and cimetidine, and proton-pump inhibitors such as omeprazole, chloramphenicol, ciprofloxacin, and metronidazole are certain drugs that are potent enzyme inhibitors. Since lignocaine metabolism is related to hepatic blood flow, propranolol has demonstrated an increase in its plasma half-life by decreasing hepatic blood flow.

Certain drugs are microsomal enzyme inducers, and they increase the metabolism of numerous drugs (including their own). Induction occurs because of gene-mediated enhanced synthesis of some CYP isoenzymes; it happens in 1 to 2 weeks after the consumption of these drugs and causes a maximal effect (whereas enzyme inhibition develops quickly) and reverts to normal slowly over a period of 1 to 3 weeks following stoppage of the enzyme inducer. Rifampicin, phenytoin, barbiturates, carbamazepine, cigarette smoking, chronic alcoholism, and certain pollutants are examples of potent microsomal enzyme inducers. Cases of failure of antibiotic treatment have happened in patients treated with chronic enzyme inducer therapy. Contraceptive failure and loss of efficacy of several drugs have occurred because of enzyme induction. However, the toxic dose of paracetamol is lesser in chronic alcoholics and in those consuming enzyme inducers, since one of the metabolites of paracetamol is responsible for its overdose hepatotoxicity.

Excretion Level Interaction

These are significant especially in drugs actively secreted by tubular transport mechanisms, for example, probenecid inhibits tubular secretion of penicillins and cephalosporins and prolongs their plasma $t_{½}$. This is mostly used in the single-dose treatment of gonorrhea. Aspirin inhibits the uricosuric action of probenecid and reduces the tubular secretion of methotrexate. Alteration in urinary pH could also alter excretion of weakly acidic or weakly basic drugs. This feature has been used in poisoning therapy. Diuretics, tetracyclines, angiotensin-converting enzyme (ACE) inhibitors, and some NSAIDs could increase the plasma concentration of lithium by increasing its tubular reabsorption.

Pharmacodynamic Level Interactions

These drug interactions occur due to alteration of the effects of one drug at the target site by another drug independent of a variation in its plasma levels. Consequently, a heightened response (synergism), a reduced response (antagonism), or a bizarre response takes place. The occurrences of synergism and antagonism are intentionally used in the treatment of certain situations. Certain examples include:

- Extreme reduction in blood pressure (BP) because of simultaneous therapy with vasodilators, ACE inhibitors, high-ceiling diuretics (furosemide), α1 blockers, and cardiac depressants.
- Increased drowsiness, respiratory depression, and motor incoordination because of simultaneous treatment with benzodiazepine (diazepam), a sedating antihistaminic (promethazine), a neuroleptic (chlorpromazine), an opioid (morphine), or consumption of alcoholic beverage.
- Increase in the prothrombin time consequently increased bleeding due to the therapy of ceftriaxone or cefoperazone with oral anticoagulants such as warfarin.
- Increased chances of ototoxicity because of concurrent use of aminoglycoside antibiotic (e.g., gentamicin) with high-ceiling diuretics (e.g., furosemide).
- Antagonism of bactericidal action of β-lactam antibiotic by combining it with a bacteriostatic drug such as tetracycline, erythromycin, or clindamycin.
- Antagonism of antibacterial effects of macrolides such as erythromycin, clindamycin, and chloramphenicol because of their interference with each other's binding to the bacterial 50S ribosome.
- NSAIDs reducing the antihypertensive effect of ACE inhibitors/β-blockers/diuretics by inhibition of renal prostaglandin (PG) synthesis.
- Inhibition of the antiparkinsonian effects of levodopa due to the neuroleptics and metoclopramide, which possess antidopaminergic action.

However, not all patients consuming multiple drugs simultaneously develop adverse reactions. Nevertheless, caution is recommended to prevent any dire consequences in all situations where interactions are likely. Basically, two drugs having the possibility to interact do not certainly contraindicate their simultaneous use. In several clinical situations, familiarity of the character, type, and mechanism of the probable interaction can allow their simultaneous administration as long as suitable dose modifications are done or additional remedial actions are taken. Yet, it is a helpful practice to think of the chances of drug interaction whenever two or more drugs are administered to a patient, or any medication is supplemented to what the patient is already consuming.

Beneficial Drug Interactions

Many drug interactions are beneficial and intentionally utilized in therapeutics, for example, the synergistic action of ACE inhibitors + diuretics to manage high BP, sulfamethoxazole + trimethoprim to tackle bacterial infection, or furosemide + amiloride to avoid hypokalemia. These are well-established drug interactions and do not lead to any harm to the patient.

Drug groups frequently implicated in drug interactions include antidiabetics, antihypertensives, antianginal drugs, antiarthritic drugs, antiepileptic drugs, oral contraceptives, anticoagulants, psychopharmacological agents, antiulcer drugs, corticosteroids, and antitubercular drugs.

Drug–Food Interactions

The relationships and interactions between foods, the nutrients they contain, and drugs are increasingly acknowledged. Some foods and specific nutrients in foods, if consumed simultaneously with certain medications, could alter the therapeutic efficacy of the drugs. Additionally, the therapeutic efficacy of several medications is contingent on the nutritional status of the patient. Drug–food interactions can occur with both prescription and over-the-counter medicines, including antacids, vitamins, and iron pills. Foods having active substances that interact with some drugs can result in unexpected or adverse effects. Some of the examples are discussed in the following sections.

Food

Dietary fiber also alters drug absorption. Pectin and other soluble fibers retard the absorption of acetaminophen. Bran and other insoluble fibers have a similar effect on digoxin. Large amounts of broccoli, spinach, and other green leafy vegetables with high levels of vitamin K, which promotes the formation of blood clots, can antagonize the effects of heparin, warfarin, and other drugs given to prevent clotting.

Dietary Supplements

Dietary supplements are products that contain a vitamin, mineral, herb, or amino acid and that are meant as a supplement to the normal diet. Supplements are controlled as foods and not as drugs; hence, they are not evaluated as carefully. However, they may interact with prescription or over-the-counter drugs. People who consume dietary supplements must apprise their treating physician, so that interactions could be prevented. Some dietary components increase the risk of side effects. Theophylline, used to treat asthma, contains xanthine, which is also present in tea, coffee, chocolate, and other sources of caffeine. Ingesting high quantities of these substances while consuming theophylline enhances the chances of drug toxicity.

Drug–Herb Interaction

Plants have been continuously used as a significant source of medicine. These could be used by natives in folk medicine. Any pharmacological alteration can occur because of herbal substances. A herb can alter the actions of concurrently administered drugs. These could be desirable, adverse, or harmful effects. Interactions between herbs and drugs may increase or decrease the pharmacological or toxicological effects of either component. Herbal medicines are abundant: the lack of information of adverse events and interactions perhaps reveals a combination of underreporting and the benign character of most herbs used.

Multiple Choice Questions

1. High plasma protein binding:

A. Increases volume of distribution of the drug.

B. Facilitates glomerular filtration of the drug.

C. Increases drug interactions and toxicity.

D. Generally makes the drug short-acting.

Answer: C

Distribution-level interactions are generally because of displacement of one drug from its binding sites on plasma proteins by another drug. Highly plasma protein–bound medications, which have a generally less volume of distribution, for example, warfarin (oral anticoagulant), sulfonylureas, NSAIDs, and antiepileptics, are specifically vulnerable to develop these drug interactions. Displacement of the plasma protein–bound drug will result in an elevated blood levels of the free and active form of the drug, consequently causing toxicity.

2. Beneficial drug interactions include all of the following EXCEPT:

A. ACE inhibitors + diuretics.

B. Sulfamethoxazole + trimethoprim.

C. Furosemide + amiloride.

D. NSAIDs + ACE inhibitors.

Answer: D

Many drug interactions are beneficial and intentionally utilized in therapeutics, for example, the synergistic action of ACE inhibitors + diuretics to manage high BP, sulfamethoxazole + trimethoprim to tackle bacterial infection, or furosemide + amiloride to avoid hypokalemia. These are well-established drug interactions and do not lead to any harm to the patient.

3. All of the following are in vitro drug interactions EXCEPT:

A. Penicillin G or ampicillin + aminoglycosides.

B. Thiopentone sodium + succinylcholine/morphine.

C. Heparin + penicillin/gentamicin/hydrocortisone.

D. Phenytoin + theophylline solution.

Answer: D

Some medications react with one another and become inactivated if they are mixed prior to their administration. During real-life situations, it can happen when parenteral medications are mixed in the same syringe or infusion bottle. Some examples include: penicillin G or ampicillin + aminoglycosides, thiopentone sodium + succinylcholine/morphine, heparin + penicillin/gentamicin/hydrocortisone, and noradrenaline + sodium bicarbonate solution. Hence, it is recommended to refrain from mixing any two or more injectable drugs prior to their administration.

4. Which of the following drugs is an enzyme inducer?

A. Ketoconazole.

B. Macrolide antibiotics.

C. Rifampicin.

D. Cimetidine.

Answer: C

Certain drugs are microsomal enzyme inducers, and they increase the metabolism of numerous drugs (including their own). Rifampicin, phenytoin, barbiturates, carbamazepine, cigarette smoking, chronic alcoholism, and certain pollutants are examples of potent microsomal enzyme inducers.

5. Which of the following drug's toxicity could be increased by consumption of tea, coffee, or chocolate?

A. Rifampicin.

B. Theophylline.

C. Phenytoin.

D. Barbiturates.

Answer: B

Some dietary components increase the risk of side effects. Theophylline, used to treat asthma, contains xanthine, which is also present in tea, coffee, chocolate, and other sources of caffeine. Ingesting high quantities of these substances while consuming theophylline enhances the chances of drug toxicity.

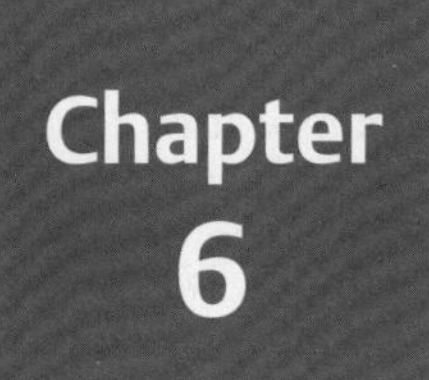

Adverse Drug Reactions and Its Monitoring and Pharmacovigilance

Viraj A. Shinde and Ramanand Patil

PH1.6: Describe the principles of pharmacovigilance and adverse drug reaction reporting systems.

PH1.7: Define, identify, and describe the management of adverse drug reactions (ADR)

Learning Objectives

- Types of adverse drug reactions.
- Pharmacovigilance.

Introduction

Adverse drug reaction is defined as any undesirable or unwanted effect due to drug administration, which requires treatment or reduction in dose or indicates watchfulness for later use of the same drug.

Types of Adverse Drug Reactions

There are two types of drug reactions, dose-related and non–dose-related.

Dose-Related

Dose-related adverse drug reactions are most common and predictable.

Side Effects

These are adverse drug reactions seen with therapeutic doses, for example, atropine causing dryness of mouth. Side effects can be beneficial in some situations and may be problematic in other situations. For example, dryness of mouth can be beneficial when atropine is administered as preanesthetic medication, while it can be problematic in patients suffering from intestinal colic. Side effects of some drugs may be used to design drugs, for example, sulfonamides have side effects like hypoglycemia and acidosis. This finding led to development of sulfonylureas as a hypoglycemic agent and acetazolamide as a carbonic anhydrase inhibitor.

Toxic Effects

These are the effects seen due to overdosing or chronic use. Excessive dose could also be absolute (accidental, homicidal, suicidal) or relative (standard dose of gentamicin in case of renal failure). Examples include nephrotoxicity seen with aminoglycosides and bleeding due to anticoagulants.

Non–Dose-Related

Hypersensitivity Reactions (Drug Allergy)

These reactions are not related to the pharmacodynamic profile of a drug. These can occur even at low doses. The antigen–antibody (Ag–Ab) reaction results in release of various mediators. These reactions are classified on the basis of immunological mechanism mediating the reaction. Type I, II, and III are humoral (Ab)-mediated, while type IV is cellular (delayed hypersensitivity)-mediated.

Type I Hypersensitivity (Immediate, Anaphylactic) Reactions

Type I hypersensitivity reactions occur rapidly and immediately. Manifestations of type I hypersensitivity reactions are itching, urticaria, hay fever, asthma, or even anaphylactic shock. Immunoglobulin E (IgE) mediates acute allergic reaction to drugs (penicillin, aspirin, etc.). When re-exposure to same drug occurs, there is an Ag—Ab reaction on mast cell surface.

There is release of mediators such as histamine, 5-hydroxytryptamine (5-HT), prostaglandins (PG), leukotrines (LTs), and platelet-activating factor (PAF), leading to hypotension, bronchoconstriction, angioedema, and urticaria. As type I hypersensitivity reaction is a medical emergency, prompt treatment becomes necessary. It consists of injecting intravenously (IV) 100 to 200 mL of adrenaline, 100 to 200 mL of IV administered hydrocortisone, and IV fluids. Adrenaline is the drug of choice.

Type II Hypersensitivity (Cytotoxic) Reactions

In the presence of complement, antibody reacts, which destroys cell-bound antigen. IgG and IgM antibodies react with cell-bound antigen. This results in activation of complement and destruction of cells, such as blood transfusion reaction, hemolytic anemia due to quinine, and cephalosporins.

Type III Hypersensitivity (Immune Complex–Mediated, Retarded, Arthus) Reactions (PH1.23)

The antibody that is mainly involved in type III hypersensitivity is IgG. The Ag–Ab complex formed to fix complement. The Ag–Ab complex is deposited on vascular endothelium. This results in destructive inflammatory response. Examples include serum sickness (fever, urticaria, joint pain, lymphadenopathy) due to penicillins and sulfonamides, acute interstitial nephritis with nonsteroidal anti-inflammatory drugs (NSAIDs), and Stevens–Johnson syndrome due to sulfonamides.

Type IV Hypersensitivity (Cell-Mediated/Delayed) Reactions

T-lymphocytes cause type IV hypersensitivity reaction. Local inflammation results from re-exposure to antigen. Secondary cellular response, which is seen 48 to 72 hours after exposure to antigen, is said to be delayed. Examples include contact dermatitis due to local anesthesia (LA).

Type II, III, and IV are treated with corticosteroids.

Idiosyncrasy

It is an abnormal response to a drug which is genetically determined. Examples include apnea due to succinyl, chloramphenicol-induced aplastic anemia, and hemolytic anemia due to primaquine.

Drug Dependence (PH1.23)

Drug dependence is defined as "a state, psychic and sometimes physical, resulting from the interaction between living organism and a drug, characterized by behavioral and other responses that always include a compulsion to take the drug on a continuous or periodic basis in order to experience its psychic effects and sometimes to avoid the discomfort of its absence." Examples include alcohol, barbiturates, amphetamines, and opioids.

Types of Drug Dependence

Psychological Dependence

Individuals with psychological dependence have an intense desire to continue taking the drug. They feel their well-being depends on the drug.

Physical Dependence

Repeated use of a drug produces physiological changes in the body. This makes continuous presence of the drug in the body necessary to maintain normal function.

Abrupt stoppage leads to "withdrawal syndrome." The effects produced by withdrawal syndrome are opposite to those of the abused drug.

Treatment

Treatment of dependence consists of hospitalization. Abrupt stoppage of agents such as alcohol, central nervous system (CNS) depressants, antiepileptics, clonidine, and nitrates results in withdrawal syndrome. The cessation of therapy should be gradual in such a scenario, with small decrease in dose. In some cases, treatment consists of replacing drug with substitution therapy, for example, methadone or buprenorphine for morphine addicts, while in other cases it could be aversion therapy such as disulfiram for alcohol withdrawal or blockade therapy such as naltrexone for opioid dependence. General measures for deaddiction include nutrition, family support, and rehabilitation.

Iatrogenic Diseases

The meaning of "iatros" is physician. Iatrogenic means physician-induced disease due to drug therapy. Examples include NSAID-induced peptic ulcer and metoclopramide-induced parkinsonism.

Carcinogenicity and Mutagenicity

The ability of drug to cause cancer is known as carcinogenicity. The ability of drug to produce abnormal genetic materials in the cell is known as mutagenicity. Reactive intermediates which are produced due to oxidation of the drug may result in harmful effect on genes and may cause structural changes in the chromosomes. Examples include anticancer drugs and estrogens.

Photosensitivity Reactions

These are drug-induced cutaneous reactions that follow after exposure to ultraviolet radiation. Examples include doxycycline, demeclocycline, and dapsone.

Hepatotoxic Reactions (IM5.7)

These occur when drugs cause impairment of liver function. Examples include antituberculosis drugs (isonicotinic acid hydrazide [INH], rifampicin, pyrazinamide), paracetamol, and halothane.

Nephrotoxic Reactions

Reactions are termed as nephrotoxic reaction when the drugs used cause damage to kidneys—for example, aminoglycosides (streptomycin, gentamicin), amphotericin B, cisplatin, cyclosporine, and heavy metals.

Ototoxic Reactions

These are defined as reactions that cause ototoxicity and impairment of hearing due to intake of some drugs, for example, aminoglycosides, loop diuretics (frusemide), and cisplatin.

Ocular Reactions

Some drugs may cause impairment of vision, for example, ethambutol, chloroquine, and glucocorticoids.

Teratogenicity

The ability of drug to cause fetal abnormalities when administered to pregnant woman is known as teratogenicity. "Teratos" is a Greek word which means monster. Examples include thalidomide (sedative drug) causing phocomelia (babies with seal limbs), tetracyclines causing yellowish discoloration of teeth, and antithyroid drugs causing fetal goiter. The abnormalities produced depends on the stage of pregnancy. The period from conception till 16 days is usually resistant. If a fetus is affected during this period, it causes abortion. The period of organogenesis (17–55 days) is the most vulnerable period. If a fetus is affected during this period, it leads to major physical abnormalities. The fetal period 56 days onward is the period of growth and development. Developmental and functional abnormalities result if the fetus is affected during this period. The general rule is to avoid drugs during the first trimester of pregnancy.

Poisoning (FM9.1, FM9.2, FM10.1)

A substance that threatens life by severely affecting one or more vital functions is known as poison. Any drug may cause poisoning, for example, barbiturates, morphine, and salicylate.

General Principles of Treatment

Antidote (PH1.7, IM21.1, IM21.2, IM21.3, IM21.4)

Activated charcoal may be used to decrease the absorption of a poison from the alimentary canal. Most of the drugs and poisons are adsorbed by activated charcoal but alkalis, arsenic, lithium carbonate, cyanide, mineral acids, and ferrous sulfate are not adsorbed. Universal antidote, which consists of two parts of powdered charcoal with one part of tannic acid and one part of magnesium oxide, may be used if activated charcoal is not available. Specific antidotes for the respective drug poisoning are mentioned in **Table 6.1**.

Breathing Should Be Assessed

If it is insufficient, mechanical ventilation may be given to the patient. Airway should be cleared of secretions and vomitus by inserting endotracheal tube, and secretions should be regularly aspirated.

Circulation Should Be Maintained

Blood pressure and pulse should be checked. IV line should be started.

Table 6.1 Specific antidotes

Drug toxicity	Antidote
Paracetamol	N-acetylcysteine
Theophylline	Propranolol
Mercury, arsenic, and copper	British anti-Lewisite (BAL)
Benzodiazepines	Flumazenil
Atropine and other antimuscarinics	Physostigmine
Organophosphate compounds	Atropine; pralidoxime
Carbon monoxide	Oxygen
Cyanide	Dicobalt edetate; amyl nitrite followed by sodium nitrite, then sodium thiosulfate
Warfarin	Vitamin K_1
Methyl alcohol and ethylene glycol	Ethyl alcohol
Beta-adrenergic stimulants	Propranolol
Lead	Calcium disodium edetate; dimercaptosuccinic acid
Nitrites	Methylene blue
Opioids	Naloxone

Diuretics

This promotes elimination of poison that is absorbed. IV mannitol or furosemide can be used. Alkalinization of urine with sodium bicarbonate will fasten the elimination of acidic poisons (e.g., salicylic acid, barbituric acid), while acidification of urine with ascorbic acid will fasten elimination of basic poisons (e.g., amphetamines).

Dialysis

It is indicated in severe poisoning. It is suitable only for drugs that are not highly protein-bound and for drugs with low volume of distribution, for example, aspirin, methanol, and lithium.

Electrolyte Balance

It should be maintained by checking serum electrolyte level.

Fluid Balance

This should be maintained.

Gastric Lavage

It is done with normal saline. It removes the unabsorbed portion of drug. If the patient is unconscious, endotracheal intubation should be done before gastric lavage. After gastric lavage, add activated charcoal to the stomach. Activated charcoal adsorbs drugs and poisons (by physical antagonism).

Hospitalization

This step precedes all the above-mentioned steps.

Immediate Symptomatic Treatment

It consists of IV diazepam for seizure and external cooling for hyperpyrexia.

Pharmacovigilance (PH1.6)

Pharmacovigilance is the study of safety of marketed drugs under the practical conditions of clinical use in large communities. It is concerned with the development of science and regulation in the area of drug safety. It aims at the detection, assessment, and prevention of adverse effects and other problems related to the use of medicines.

Importance of Pharmacovigilance

Thalidomide Tragedy (1961–1962)

This was the greatest of all drug disasters. Thalidomide had been introduced and welcomed as a safe and effective hypnotic and antiemetic. It rapidly became popular for the treatment of nausea and vomiting in early pregnancy. Tragically, the drug proved to be a potent human teratogen that caused major birth defects in an estimated 10,000 children. Phocomelia was the characteristic feature.

Other Historic Violations

- Elixir sulfanilamide was an improperly prepared sulfanilamide medicine that caused mass poisoning in the United States in 1937. It caused the death of more than 100 people.

The public outcry caused by this incident and other similar disasters led to the passing of the 1938 Federal Food, Drug, and Cosmetic Act.

- The thalidomide disaster led, in Europe and elsewhere, to the establishment of the drug regulatory mechanisms of today.
- These mechanisms require that new drugs shall be licensed by well-established regulatory authorities before being introduced into clinical use.

Glossary of Terms

- *Adverse event:* Any untoward medical occurrence that may present during treatment with a pharmaceutical product, but that does not necessarily have a causal relationship with the treatment.
- *Adverse reaction:* The World Health Organization (WHO) technical report—a response to a drug, which is noxious and unintended, and which occurs at doses normally used in humans for the prophylaxis, diagnosis, or therapy of disease or for the modification of physiological function.
- *Expected:* As opposed to "unexpected," an event that is noted in the investigator brochure or labeling (package insert or summary of product characteristics).
- *Unexpected adverse reaction*: The nature or severity of which is not consistent with the domestic labeling or market authorization, or expected from characteristics of the drug.
- *Signal:* Reported information on possible causal relationship between an adverse event and a drug, with the relationship being unknown or incompletely documented previously. Usually, more than one single report is required to generate a signal, depending on the seriousness of the event and quality of information.
- *Data mining:* It is used to describe various automated or semiautomated techniques to generate signals from existing databases.

Methodologies in Pharmacovigilance (PH1.6)

The various methods used for pharmacovigilance are passive surveillance, stimulated surveillance, active surveillance, and comparative observational studies. Passive surveillance consists of methods such as spontaneous reporting, case reports, and case series. Comparative observational studies consist of studies such as cross-sectional, case–control, and cohort studies.

Important Organizations Involved in Pharmacovigilance

- The Food and Drug Administration (FDA or USFDA) is an organization of the United States Department of Health and Human Services.
- The European Medicines Agency (EMEA) is a decentralized body of the European Union located in London.
- The Ministry of Health, Labor and Welfare (MHLW), Japan.
- The Central Drugs Standard Control Organization (CDSCO): The Government of India with the assistance of the World Bank has initiated the national pharmacovigilance program. The pharmacovigilance program is coordinated by CDSCO under the aegis of the Ministry of Health & Family Welfare, DGHS, New Delhi.

Uppsala Monitoring Center

Vigibase: The Uppsala monitoring center ([UMC] on behalf of WHO) has over 3 million adverse event case reports from over 75 countries. The data are supplied by national health authorities. Most of the data are from the United States and supplied by the FDA. The UMC does not review or assess the individual cases put into database, but it does pharmacovigilance analyses and signaling.

Multiple Choice Questions

1. Type B (unpredictable) adverse drug reaction is:

A. Side effect.
B. Toxic effect.
C. Idiosyncrasy.
D. Physical dependence.

Answer: C

Idiosyncrasy is uncommon, not dose-related, and generally more serious, and requires withdrawal of the drug.

2. An unwanted effect of a drug that is seen with therapeutic doses is:

A. Side effect.
B. Toxic effect.
C. Allergic reaction.
D. Idiosyncrasy.

Answer: A

Side effects are unwanted, unavoidable pharmacodynamic effects that are seen with therapeutic doses.

3. In a case of anaphylactic shock, which of the following is the route of choice for administration of adrenaline?

A. Intracardiac.
B. Intravenous.
C. Intramuscular.
D. Subcutaneous.

Answer: C

Life-saving measure in anaphylactic shock is intramuscular adrenaline hydrochloride.

Chapter 7

Occupational and Environmental Pesticides, Food Adulterants, and Insect Repellents

Manjunath G.N. and Swamy R.M.

PH1.51: Describe occupational and environmental pesticides, food adulterants, pollutants, and insect repellents.

Learning Objectives

- Environmental toxins.
- Solvents.
- Pesticides.
- Food adulteration.
- Insect repellents.

Glossary of Terms

1. *Environment:* It is the complex changes in the ecosystem, which is a result of changes in the soil, living things, and climate.
2. *Toxicology:* It is a scientific discipline, overlapping with biology, chemistry, pharmacology, and medicine, that involves the study of the adverse effects of chemical substances on living organisms and the practice of diagnosing and treating exposures to toxins and toxicants.
3. *Hazard:* Any agent, either natural or human-induced, that is known to produce damage to the susceptible target and its surrounding environment.
4. *Risk:* The possibility of developing damage or derangement to the host, following exposure to certain agents.
5. *Threshold limit value (TLV):* TLV of a chemical substance is believed to be a level to which a worker can be exposed day after day for a working lifetime without adverse effects.

Environmental Toxins

They are chemicals that can cause cancer and alter the endocrine system, leading to disruption of biological system and, further, to ill health of humans. It can be natural or human-made.

Air Pollutants (FM9.6)

These are pollutants that are widely distributed across the country; they are regulated and used as air quality indicators. Air pollutants include carbon monoxide, nitrogen dioxide, sulfur dioxide, ozone, hydrocarbons, pesticides/insecticides, and halogenated biphenyl compounds.

Carbon Monoxide (CO)

It is a tasteless and odorless gas present in the air and is invisible and poorly detected by humans. The permissible limit of CO in the air without producing any harm is 0.2 parts per million (ppm).

The main sources of carbon monoxide are from exhaust of motor vehicles, forest fire, and steel industries. Smoke from tobacco is one of the main indoor sources of carbon monoxide. Concentrations above 10% are found to be deadly and require administration of pure oxygen for at least 24 hours.

CO can damage vital organs such as the heart and brain due to reduction in oxygen-carrying capacity of the organs. Concentrations of CO above 40% bound to hemoglobin can be lethal, whereas a small increase in the level of CO can produce lack of concentration, clumsy feeling, and fatigue. Fetuses and those belonging to the pediatric age group are particularly at risk.

Treatment

Exposed person should be immediately shifted to fresh air. The patient should be shifted to emergency medical facility if he/she develops signs and symptoms of carbon monoxide poisoning, that is, nausea, dizziness, headache, shortness of breath, confusion, and weakness.

Pure Oxygen Therapy

Pure oxygen is supplied through face mask and ventilator support in patients with difficulty in breathing. In cases of severe poisoning, hyperbaric oxygen therapy is recommended to protect the heart and brain. This accelerates the replacement of carbon monoxide with oxygen. It is also given to pregnant women to prevent fetal damage.

Preventive Measures

- Maintenance of fuel quality standards.
- Using alternative fuels as much as possible.
- Stringent vehicle emission standards.

Sulfur Dioxide

It is a colorless gas with suffocating odor. It may explode when heated but is not inflammable. It is highly toxic and fatal when inhaled, as it releases sulfate particles and sulfuric and sulfurous acid.

The main source of sulfur dioxide is industrial processes—materials generated out of coal, oil, or gas in the production of electricity, processing of mineral ores containing sulfur, and fossil fuel burning. It is also present in motor vehicle emissions.

Sulfur dioxide, when inhaled, irritates the nasopharynx and airways, leading to cough, breathlessness, and wheeze within 10 to 15 minutes.

Treatment

There is no specific antidote, and only symptomatic treatment is sufficient.

Nitrogen Dioxide

It is another nasty gas formed naturally in the atmosphere following lightning. Other sources include soil, water, and plants. This contributes to the development of photochemical smog, which has deleterious effects on human health.

The burning of fossil fuels (coal, gas, and oil) is the chief source of nitrogen dioxide. Motor vehicle exhaust contributes about 80% of nitrogen dioxide in cities. Other sources are refineries of petrol and metal, coal-fired power electricity generation stations, food processing units, and other manufacturing industries.

The main problems of inhaling are the inflammation of epithelial lining and increased chances of infections of lung. The symptoms are wheezing, cough, colds, flu, and bronchitis. Asthmatic children and elderly people with cardiac problems are at higher risk.

Treatment

There is no specific antidote. Patients who have developed symptoms and signs of hypoxia or those with methemoglobin levels > 30% should be given methylene blue 1 to 2 mg/kg bodyweight intravenously (IV) slowly. This dose may be repeated after 1 hour. Clinical response is seen within half an hour. It is not required if only cyanosis is observed, and it is not effective in G6PD-deficient patients. Initial dose should not exceed 7 mg/kg. (Doses greater than 15 mg/kg may cause hemolysis.) Side effects include nausea, vomiting, abdominal pain, chest pain, dizziness, excessive sweating, and difficulty in urination.

Exchange transfusion is the treatment of choice in those with severe poisoning who have stopped responding to methylene blue. Steroids, when started immediately, can prevent the patient ending up in bronchiolitis obliterans. It should be continued for 8 weeks and tapered gradually.

Preventive Measures

- Mandatory emission tests for vehicles, and improving the national fuel quality through regulation.
- Reduction in diesel vehicles and its consumption.

Ozone

Ozone is formed when heat and sunlight react chemically with nitrogen oxides and volatile organic compounds or hydrocarbons at the ground level or high in the atmosphere.

The sources for this reaction come from the exhaust of motor vehicles, aviation, oil refineries, printing, petrochemicals, and forest fires. The safe limit of ozone in the ground-level atmosphere is around 0.04 ppm.

Ozone can irritate the lining of the nose, airways, and lungs. Pain is observed initially in the eyes, nose, and throat. Later on, earache and cough develop, followed by chest pain. It reduces athletic performance and causes exacerbation of asthma.

Preventive Measures

- Emission quality and fuel quality standards need to be maintained.
- Forecasting of pollution should be done effectively.

Hydrocarbons

Hydrocarbons are organic compounds that consist of hydrogen and carbon atoms and form more complex compounds such as cyclohexane. Methane, ethane, butane, pentane, propane, and hexane are some common hydrocarbons that are present in crude oils such as petroleum and natural gas. These are used in lanterns, lighters, grills, internal combustion units, engine lubricants, and greases. Also, these compounds are used in highway construction and roofing.

They produce the greenhouse effect and deplete ozone layer when exposed to sunlight and/or nitrogen oxides. As a result of this, photosynthetic ability of plants is reduced, increasing the risk of cancer and respiratory illness. Oil spills can destroy marine plant life.

Prevention and Treatment

The first would be through biofiltration using microorganisms to degrade organic and inorganic substances. The second way is by using vapor combustion unit or flare and lastly carbon adsorbed can be used to dispose of hydrocarbons.

Air Toxics

These are the pollutants present in low concentrations in air, in the form of gas, aerosol, or particulate form, that can produce harmful effects on living beings due to its toxicity. The common sources are emissions from industries, motor vehicles, and solid fuel combustion. Other sources are paints and adhesives in new buildings.

Biological Pollutants (CM3.8)

They are airborne microbiological contamination that can affect the quality of indoor environment, such as molds, the skin shedding of animals and humans, and dropping of cockroaches.

Solvents (FM9.5)

They are organic liquids, such as acetone, petroleum spirits, hexane, methanol, and white spirit, that are used to dissolve or dilute other substances or materials.

The most common places where solvents are used are in paints, varnishes, cleaning products, adhesives, resins, lacquers, degreasing materials, pesticides, paint removers, inks and ink removers, and toiletries.

Effects of Solvents

- These substances produce vapors that are harmful when inhaled. Deliberate breathing (sniffing) can be lethal.
- Skin contact causes dermatitis. Eye contact can result in redness and irritation.
- They can be ingested by consuming contaminated food and drink. There are cases of accidental consumption from old unlabeled containers.

Precautions

- *Preventing exposure:* Use of water-based formulation can reduce the harmful effects.
- *Control exposure:* Work area should be well-ventilated with doors and windows open and with mechanical ventilation. Brush instead of spray should be used with solvent-based products. Store solvents in properly labelled containers and dispose in spillage-proof closed containers. Train the employees on handling and use of solvents. Provide workers with safety data sheets.
- *Fire:* Smoking near solvents can produce fire explosion and hence "no smoking" and "no naked flame" signs are mandatory boards near solvent storages. Compulsory use of personal protective equipment is advised.
- *Hygiene:* Facilities should be provided for washing, and it is recommended to wash before eating, drinking, smoking, and using toilet. Separate changing rooms should be provided.
- *First aid:* Move the person to fresh air, and heavily contaminated clothing should be removed immediately. Any solvent splashes on the skin or eye are to be washed with water immediately for a minimum of 8 minutes. Any open wound should be covered with appropriate dressing. If it is severe, the patient should be shifted to the hospital.

Pesticides

Pesticides are a complex mixture of substances used to kill, eliminate, or repel insects, weeds, rodents, fungi, or other organisms. Although exposure to pesticides causes hazardous genetic effects, they are still being used in agriculture. Despite their benefit in increasing crop yield and reduction in postharvest losses in agriculture, their extensive use results in the accumulation of pesticide in food residue, soil, runoff water, etc.

Types

There are different types of pesticides, and exposure depends on the class of organisms designed to control (weedicide, fungicide, rodenticide, and herbicide) or on the chemical structure (organochlorine, organophosphates, carbamates, chlorinated hydrocarbons, and dipyridyls).

Mechanism of Action

These substances produce reactive oxidative species, which are free radicals. Long term exposure can cause harm to human health by damaging DNA, resulting in disturbance in various organs systems of the body. Herbicides such as phenylamides inhibit RNA synthesis, resulting in impaired protein synthesis and thus affecting the enzymatic function.

WHO Toxicity Classification

- *CLASS 1a:* extremely hazardous (red color code).
- *CLASS 1b:* highly hazardous (red color code).
- *CLASS 2:* moderately hazardous (yellow color code).
- *CLASS 3:* slightly hazardous (blue color code).
- *CLASS U:* unlikely to be hazardous (green color code).

Health Effects

The acute effects are headache and nausea, while the more serious and long-term effects include carcinogenesis, cardiac diseases, immunotoxicity, teratogenicity, reproductive disorders, neurological disorders and other disorders such as diabetes, chronic respiratory diseases, chronic nephropathies, autoimmune diseases, hyperglycemia/diabetes, and many other disorders.

Biomonitoring

Biomonitoring is the direct assessment of a pesticide, its metabolite, or its product in the biological sample such as blood or urine. Moreover, serum, plasma, amniotic fluid, breast milk, and hair can be used. Blood is considered to be the most reliable source for the estimation of parent pesticide, whereas urine can be used to measure the metabolites of a pesticide by chromatography. In blood, measurement is to be done within 24 hours of exposure, because pesticides get metabolized and eliminated through urine. Apart from these, various cytogenetic markers such as micronuclei tests and comet assays are also used to estimate the DNA damage.

Prevention

Decrease exposure: Avoiding contact as much as possible, self-protection, using less pesticides, and using safe and less toxic pesticides.

- Personal protection such as hat, mask, long-sleeved shirts, trousers, rubber gloves, rubber boots, and waterproof apron.
- Protecting others by spraying at the end of the day, avoiding spraying in strong winds, and not allowing anyone in or near the fields for some hours after spraying pesticides.
- Personal hygiene by washing hands with soap and water before entering the house for eating, drinking, or smoking. Removing the pesticide-contaminated dress before entering the house/taking bath/showering separately, and washing the protective clothes; not mixing the contaminated clothes with regular clothes. Keeping the pesticides out of reach of children. Proper disposing of pesticide container.

Food Adulteration

It is the process of adding or mixing substandard, harmful, useless, or unnecessary substances in foods to increase its sale or profit. Debasing or making a substance impure by adding an inferior substance, with the motive of increasing the quantity, is called adulteration, and the inferior substance being added is known as an adulterant.

Types of Adulteration

Physical Contamination

Substances commonly used include sand, gritty matter, soap stone, common salt, coriander powder, chili powder, sawdust, rice bran (flour), refined flour (*maida*), gram flour (*besan*), spices, and washing soda. Mustard seeds are adulterated with argemone seeds; lovely silver leaves are used to decorate sweetmeats and *burfi*. Pan is adulterated with aluminum leaf or foil.

Chemical Contamination

Chemicals can affect the quality and disguise the deterioration, which is potentially very harmful to the human. For example, metanil yellow dye is added to starch-based material to color *besan* or gram flour and pulses; lead chromate is added to turmeric to color sweetmeats such as *laddoo*, *burfi*, *jalebi*, *dalmoot*, and *papad*; ultramarine blue is added for developing deep pink color (*gulabi*); melamine is added in toy painting, and it also increases the flavor of protein in infant milk.

Adulterants

The most common food products that are adulterated include spices, milk products, edible oil, beverage drinks, sweets, pulses, sugar, processed foods, and rice and cereal products such as flour, *maida*, and *sooji*.

- *Mineral poisons* are used to make confectionaries light-colored and also to make pickles and tea in fine green shades.
- *Alums* or cheaper and poor nutritious adulterants such as rice, potatoes, corn, beans, and rye are added to white bread. Chemicals such as carbonate and sulfate of lime, silicate of magnesia in the form of soapstone, white clay, carbonate of magnesia, bone dust, and bone ashes absorb more water and hence addition of these substances to flour increases its actual weight.
- *Milk adulteration:* By diluting with water, or mixing with soya milk, starch, groundnut milk, formalin, detergent, and wheat flour, the nutritional value of milk is reduced. This can also lead to cancer or acute renal failure.
- *Ghee* adulteration: *Ghee* essence is added in cheaper oils. Argemone oil, used for adulteration of *ghee* and butter, is highly toxic and produces a disease known as dropsy. Mashed potatoes, sweet potatoes, and other starches are also used.
- *Mustard seeds and oil:* Argemone seeds, argemone oil, and mineral oil are added. This can lead to epidemic dropsy, glaucoma, and cancer.
- *Sugar and salts:* Chalk powder, white sand, washing soda, plastic crystals, urea, *rava*/*sooji*, etc., are added. Chalk powder inhalation can cause respiratory problems, and washing soda can cause diarrhea, nausea, and vomiting.
- *Tea powder:* Used tea leaves are mixed with coal tar dyes, dye, or artificial color or iron filings. This can lead to cancer and tetanus.
- *Coffee:* Chicory powder, ground tamarind seeds, and date seeds are added, which can cause diarrhea, gastrointestinal disturbances, giddiness, and arthralgia. Ground coffee can be adulterated with maize, soybean, sugar, and acai seed. Other substances such as Sudan dye, aniline dye, and metanil are carcinogenic.
- *Turmeric and spices:* Lead chromate is added, which can produce anemia, paralysis, brain damage, and abortion.
- *Sweets:* Metal yellow in excess of safe limit can cause allergies, hepatic damage, infertility, anemia, carcinomas, and teratogenicity. Formalin, which is used to preserve food, can cause carcinomas, bronchial asthma, and skin diseases.
- *Vegetable oils and fats:* Mixing palm oil or cheaper edible oils such as rice bran with cooking oils.
- *Fish*: Mercury can be contaminating, leading to brain damage, paralysis, and death.
- *Food grains and other products: Kesari dal* is mixed with Bengal gram and *toor dal*, wheat and other food grains with ergot, asafetida with galbanum and colophony resin, aniline and metanil dye with turmeric, and brick powder and artificial colors with chili powder.

Food Additives

- To enhance and retain the quality of processed foods in terms of taste, flavor, and texture, certain chemical substances are added. They enhance the shelf life. These additives become adulterants if they exceed the prescribed limit, and can cause serious hazard to human health.
- Tartrazine, a synthetic color, is an azo dye primarily used as a food coloring agent. It can cause rashes, urticaria, rhinorrhea, and bronchial asthma. Artificial sweeteners such as saccharin and cyclamate can produce bladder cancer.
- Carcinoma of stomach and intestine can be caused by nitrates and nitrites used as preservatives in packaged meat.
- Monosodium glutamate, which is a food flavor enhancer, causes nausea and headache. Occasionally, it causes chest tightness and asthmatic attack. Brain damage can occur on long-term usage.
- Sodium metabisulfite and sulfur dioxide are used as preservatives for dry fruits, wines, and beers but can cause breathing and heart problems.

Insect Repellents

Insect repellents (IRs) are chemical substances that when sprayed in air can prevent insect bite by being suspended in the air at least about 1.5 inch above the skin. For example, oil of lemon eucalyptus and citronella are natural IRs, and (*N*, *N*-diethyl-3-methylbenzamide (DEET), picaridin, permethrin, and IR3535 are synthetic IRs.

Synthetic

- DEET can provide protection for short period after applying to the skin and clothing against blackflies, biting flies, fleas, and ticks. It repels rather than kills, and it is available as liquid, lotion, sprays, and impregnated material in the concentration range of 4 to 100%. Skin sensitivity develops on repeated use. In the case of children, the concentration is less than 6%. Protection time depends on the concentration.
- Picaridin, when compared to DEET, lacks chemical odor and is nongreasy and nondamaging to clothing and plastics. It produces noxious vapor to mosquitoes, flies, and ticks.

Picaridin 20% spray can protect against *Aedes*, *Anopheles*, and *Culex* mosquito species at least for 8 to 14 hours. It should be avoided in children younger than 2 years. No proven toxicities have been found in human and animal studies.

- Permethrin is an insecticide and repellent used especially on clothing, shoes, mosquito nets, and camping gear. Clothing treated with permethrin repels and kills ticks, mosquitoes, and other arthropods and also retains its effect even after repeated washing. Mosquito net impregnation can provide protection for 1 year. Nylon nets retain mosquitos for longer period than cotton nets. The benefits given by nets depend on biting habits of mosquito, the size and constitution of the nets, and its treatment with insecticides.
- IR3535 is basically a skin moisturizer that has shown greater effectiveness against black fly and sand fly bites. A 20% solution can protect against *Aedes* and *Culex* mosquitoes for 7 to 10 hours. However, it should be avoided in malaria-endemic areas. It produces eye irritation and can damage plastics and fabrics also.

Natural

- Citronella or lavender oil protects against mosquito bites for less than an hour. It is a potential dermal sensitizer available as lotion, oil, and solid wax. It is to be avoided in children younger than 2 years. Citronellol and geraniol are the active ingredients of oil of citronella. It is also a component of candles and flame pots. The duration of action is short, less than an hour in the concentration of 4.2%.
- Lemon eucalyptus oil is an extract from the leaves of the lemon eucalyptus tree, *Corymbia citriodora*. It is more long-lasting and effective than DEET in lower concentrations. It can also be used in malaria-endemic areas but has to be applied more frequently. It has less risk of allergic skin reactions, but should not to be used in children younger than 3 years.

Polyhalogenated Biphenyls

They are a group of compounds that are manufactured for commercial purposes, having congeners such as polychlorinated biphenyl and polybrominated biphenyls. They are extensively used in dielectric fluids, transformers, capacitors, vacuum pump, gas turbines, and hydraulic fluids. They are noninflammable. These compounds have a low-to-moderate acute toxicity in mammalian species and greater toxicity in invertebrates, but produces pronounced subacute and chronic toxicity. There is some variability between species with respect to toxicity.

Multiple Choice Questions

1. A patient was brought to the emergency room with symptoms of headache, fatigue, weakness, dizziness, restlessness, nervousness, nausea, diarrhea, soreness of joints, and irritation of skin, eye, and throat after exposure to pesticide. What could be the possible mechanism of action of these pesticides?

A. Inhibition of photosynthesis.
B. Inhibition of cholinesterase enzyme.
C. Inhibition of RNA function.
D. Inhibition of DNA function.

Answer: D

Pesticides tend to produce free-radical reactive oxidative species that damage the DNA on long-term exposure.

2. A 30-year-old patient was brought to the emergency room with history of consumption of a pesticide. The doctor wants to know the concentration and the type of agent consumed within 24 hours. Which sample can give you the estimation of parent pesticide?

A. Blood.
B. Urine.
C. Hair.
D. Stools.

Answer: A

Urine and stools contain the metabolites, not the parent pesticide, and accumulation of pesticides in the hair takes longer.

3. A 45-year-old female patient visited the medicine OPD with symptoms of headache, nausea, breathlessness, loose bowels, and bilateral pitting edema after consumption of mustard seeds on a daily basis. The mustard seeds were later found to be adulterated with argemone seeds. What is the probable diagnosis?

A. Tetanus.
B. Dropsy.
C. Diarrhea.
D. Respiratory problems.

Answer: B

Dropsy is a term used to indicate swelling in soft tissues due to the accumulation of excess water, and argemone seeds cause accumulation of water in soft tissues.

4. The most common additive in preserving beer, wine, and dry fruits is:

A. Cyclamate.
B. Monosodium glutamate.
C. Sulfur dioxide.
D. Picaridin.

Answer: C

Sulfur dioxide prevents reaction with oxygen, which prevents the food from browning.

5. Which chemical, when compared to DEET, is found to be nongreasy and nondamaging on clothes and plastics and is used as an insect repellent?

A. Lavender oil.
B. Picaridin.
C. Permethrin.
D. Oil of citronella.

Answer: B

Picaridin produces vapors noxious to mosquitoes, flies, and tics, and a 20% solution spray can protect against *Aedes, Anopheles,* and *Culex* mosquitoes.

6. DDT is a form of:

A. Insecticide.
B. Herbicide.
C. Preservative.
D. Repellent.

Answer: A

Insecticides are the substances used to kill insects.

7. Which of the following is true about carbon monoxide poisoning?

A. Concentration of CO above 10% is found to be deadly and requires administration of pure O_2 for over 24 hours.
B. It has more than 10 times the affinity of oxygen.
C. Seventy percent is not deadly.
D. Concentration above 10% is dangerous and needs observation.

Answer: A

CO concentration above 10% is lethal, and such cases not just need observation but also should be treated immediately with oxygen.

8. The treatment protocol for nitrogen dioxide includes all except:

A. Methylene blue.
B. Exchange transfusion.
C. Steroids.
D. Sodium nitrite.

Answer: D

For the treatment of poisoning by nitrogen dioxide, we use methylene blue (for patients with hypoxia) and exchange transfusion (for severe poisoning); also, the use of steroids will prevent the patient from getting bronchiolitis obliterans.

Chapter 8 Management of Common Poisonings, Insecticides, and Common Stings and Bites

Sri H. Thakkalapally

PH1.52: Management of common poisoning, insecticides, and common stings and bites

Learning Objectives

- Initial management of the poisoned patient.
- Treatments that enhance elimination.
- Antidotes.
- Management of specific poisonings.
- Poisonings from animal and insect bites.

Understanding General Aspects of Poisoning (PH1.7, FM9.1, FM9.2, FM10.1, IM20.8, IM20.9, IM21.1, IM21.2, IM21.3, IM21.4, IM21.5)

The fields of pharmacology and toxicology are rife with examples of substances that can elicit serious side effects or cause outright poisoning. Many substances that are deemed safe for use may cause serious adverse effects in overdoses, as paracetamol (LD_{50} > 2000 mg/kg) is fatal to adults in doses above 12 grams, while substances like botulinum toxin (LD_{50}: 0.00001 mg/kg), which are inherently toxic by nature, can be used to treat lateral canthal lines (crow's feet) in appropriate dosages. It is, therefore, logical to conclude that the dose determines whether a chemical acts as a poison.

We lose a significant portion of our population every year to poisonings. Just in the year 2012, at least 1.2 million deaths were recorded as a result of either deliberate or unintentional poisonings. Just organophosphates account for about 300,000 deaths per year. The cases of overall poisonings are well above this number, since many cases of poisoning are never reported to a poison center, as centers often do not exist, or the patient is unable to seek required medical help. This is often the case in middle- and low-income countries.

Not all poisoning cases lead to moribund conditions. Depending on the level of exposure, the effects could be mild, moderate, or severe. Depending upon the dosage of the poison substance and the length of exposure, a poisoning can either be acute or chronic (**Table 8.1**). When a patient is exposed to a one-time fatal dosage of a toxic compound, poisoning symptoms are precipitated within minutes after ingestion. The patient's condition deteriorates quickly; without appropriate medical care, irreversible damage occurs to the body, and in serious cases, death ensues. This kind of poisoning is acute in nature. Chronic poisonings, on the other hand, are slow to precipitate observable symptoms. The poisonous substance is introduced to the patient in such minute doses that it does not immediately cause noticeable harm. The human body can eliminate most such compounds over time, but with repeated exposure, the toxin deposits in the body accumulate and produce irreversible damage to the patient.

Even if the same substance causes acute and chronic poisoning cases, the clinical features of the poisonings differ significantly.

Arsenic, a naturally occurring heavy metal, can cause chronic poisoning when arsenic-contaminated ground water is consumed for a prolonged time period; acute poisoning is caused when pesticides or insecticides with inorganic arsenic is consumed either accidentally or with suicidal intent. While the poisoning substance in both cases is the same, the clinical features differ significantly.

A patient suffering from serious acute arsenic poisoning (100–300 mg) usually exhibits acute psychosis, excess salivation, cardiomyopathy, gastrointestinal (GI) distress, diffused skin rash, and seizures. Chronic arsenic poisoning, on the other hand, takes years to physically manifest in a patient. Clinical features vary among populations but usually they are as follows: hyperpigmentation, keratosis, recurrent bouts of diarrhea, behavioral changes, memory loss, and cancers.

Acute poisoning is a dynamic medical condition that can devolve quickly without appropriate medical attention and requires early management decisions to ensure an optimal outcome for the patient. Chronic poisonings, on the other

Table 8.1 Types of poisoning based on length of exposure to the poisoning agent

Category	Length of exposure
Acute	> 24 hours
Subacute	> 1 month
Subchronic	1–3 months
Chronic	> 3 months

hand, are not well understood. Not only do the symptoms vary widely, based on the population and geographical area, many symptoms are still being documented. Minamata disease, first documented in 1956, Japan, is still being studied to understand the toxidrome evolution of chronic mercury poisoning.

Because of such disparities, treatment strategies for acute and chronic poisoning differ significantly. This chapter, therefore, will exclusively cover the strategies to manage acute poisoning cases, which have well-developed research material.

Initial Management of the Poisoned Patient

The definitive way to identify the cause of acute poisoning in a patient is through laboratory diagnosis. However, acute poisoning is a dynamic condition that requires immediate care, and a patient in a critical condition can seldom afford the time. As a result, physicians tend to administer supportive care to address threats to basic life functions first. Supportive care provides a chance for the patient's condition to stabilize while giving more time to develop a tailored strategy.

Mild-to-moderate poisonings do not generally affect a patient's consciousness, but many moderate-to-severe overdoses can alter the mental status of the patient. If the admitted patient exhibits an altered state of consciousness or is in coma, 50% dextrose solution (50 mL) should be administered to treat hypoglycemia. Thiamine (100 mg intravenous [IV]/intramuscular [IM]) is usually administered ahead of dextrose to prevent the onset of Wernicke–Korsakoff syndrome, especially in people suffering from thiamine deficiency and alcoholics. Flumazenil may help reverse sedation in benzodiazepine poisonings if no other coingestant is involved.

Upon admission, threats to the airway, breathing, and circulation (ABC) of the patient should be assessed and managed first.

Airway

The priority for critically ill patients is to secure them a clear airway for aspiration. Any foreign materials or vomitus obstructing the passage should be cleared. In cases where a clear airway cannot be achieved, an endotracheal tube is inserted to aid breathing. If the patient is unconscious, care should be taken to avoid blockage of airway passage with tongue by placing the neck in a comfortable position, without flexion, or position them on their side to dislodge any obstruction by the tongue.

Breathing

After establishing a clear airway, the next step is to assess the respiratory functions. Death due to breathing difficulties is one of the common outcomes in cases of a drug overdose. There are three major breathing complications in poisoning cases: ventilatory failure, hypoxia, and bronchospasm.

Ventilatory Failure

The partial pressure of carbon dioxide (normal pCO_2 levels: 35–45 mm Hg) in arterial blood gases is a good indicator of the patient's ventilatory status. A patient with elevated levels of pCO_2 should receive ventilator assistance. Ventilatory failure occurs either due to muscular paralysis (neuromuscular blockers and nicotine overdoses) or respiratory depression (alcohol and opiate poisoning).

Hypoxia

Hypoxia is a common side effect of cyanide (CN) and carbon monoxide (CO) poisonings. Both cause cellular hypoxia, CO by disrupting hemoglobin's capacity to carry oxygen, and CN by interfering with a cell's oxygen utilization. Hypoxia can also be caused due to decreased oxygen in the environment or pulmonary edema. Hypoxia can be addressed by increasing the oxygen content of the inspired air through intubation and using a hyperbaric chamber.

Bronchospasm

If the bronchospasm is not caused by preexisting conditions like asthma, obstructions, or injuries, the patient can be treated with bronchodilators (ipratropium bromide). Beta-blockers are contraindicated in the management of bronchospasm, and bronchospasm caused by them can be treated with aminophylline (6 mg/kg one-time dose as IV over 30 minutes).

Circulation

Blood pressure, pulse rate, and pulse rhythm of a patient are good indicators of basic cardiovascular health. Cases that are suspected of poisoning by cardiotoxic agents should also have ECGs monitored for at least 6 to 8 hours after the ingestion. Poisoning can produce either or one or more of the following complications, depending on the pharmacologic mechanism of the toxic agent and condition of the patient.

Arrhythmias

Sympathomimetic drugs (cocaine and amphetamine), tricyclic antidepressants (TCAs), and sodium channel blockers overdoses can cause ventricular arrhythmias. Treatment options vary based on the toxin involved and the condition of the patient. A total of 1 to 2 mEq/kg dose of sodium bicarbonate in the form of an IV bolus can be administered to treat arrhythmias in patients suffering from an overdose of TCAs and sodium channel blockers.

Bradycardia

Calcium channel blockers (CCBs), TCAs, and organophosphates are some drug categories that can cause bradycardia in an overdose. Bradycardia is generally not treated in patients, as it could be the body's reflex mechanism to cope with toxin-induced hypertension.

Hypertension

Hypotension is usually treated with IV fluids and small doses of vasopressor drugs.

Prolonged QRS Interval

Serious overdose of TCAs and sodium channel blockers produce prolonged QRS interval. This is caused by interventricular conduction delay as a result of sodium channel blockade. As the QRS complex gets wider, the adverse events precipitated deteriorate from hypotension to seizures and then ventricular arrhythmias. In the above cases, sodium bicarbonate is administered as IV bolus (1–2 mEq/kg).

Treatments That Enhance Elimination

Decontamination

Toxic substances are usually introduced into body via one of the following routes: absorption through dermal or mucosal membranes, inhalation, ingestion, or parenteral. The goal of decontamination is to reduce further absorption of poison into the system. It is conducted by removing toxins from the skin if the poison is absorbed percutaneously, or from the digestive system if ingested orally. This process is usually undertaken alongside the initial management and evaluation of the patient.

Skin Decontamination

Poisons that are corrosive in nature and poisons like organophosphates that are absorbed through the dermis are the main targets of skin decontamination. These toxins can adhere onto clothes and skin, continuously entering the circulatory system for hours. To avoid further contamination, the clothing should be removed and double-bagged for poison analysis, and patient's skin should be thoroughly washed using soap and water.

Gastric Decontamination

The rationale of gastric decontamination is to remove the yet unabsorbed poison in the digestive tracts. Until recently, gastric decontamination procedures like emesis, gastric lavage, and cathartics were highly regarded and performed regularly. But recent studies indicate that these procedures' contribution to the change in the outcome of the patient is insignificant. At the same time, they can sometimes cause undue side effects. On the other hand, under right conditions, some of the procedures have proven to be potentially lifesaving. This is especially true in cases of poisonings involving ingestion of massive doses of a drug, sustained-release (SR) and enteric-coated drugs, or drugs that cannot be removed using activated charcoal.

Emetics and gastric lavage aim to cleanse the stomach of its toxic substances, while activated charcoal, cathartics, and whole bowel irrigation (WBI) are aimed at cleansing the intestines.

Emesis

Ipecac syrup is the most commonly used emetic in patients who have ingested poisons. The early studies focused on analyzing the dose–response relationship between ipecac and the medication or marker substances (e.g., barium) to prove its efficacy, but recent clinical studies focused on the understanding the contribution of emesis toward clinical outcome demonstrated a lack of significant effect on the patient outcome.

Gastric Lavage

This is a procedure in which the stomach contents are flushed out through an orogastric/nasogastric tube using lavage solution (generally, 0.9% saline solution). For decades, physicians performed gastric lavages to flush out remaining poison substance from the stomach. This procedure requires an experienced practitioner, and its usefulness is dependent upon the amount of poison left in the stomach and the time after ingestion. Gastric lavage is useful in cases where the patient has ingested massive amounts of drugs. This procedure is more effective if conducted within 1 hour of ingesting poison. It is contraindicated in patients with altered mental state and convulsing patients.

Cathartics

Lone use of cathartics is not recommended in gut decontamination. Usually, cathartics (sorbitol, magnesium citrate) are used in combination with activated charcoal. A cathartic is intended to accelerate the elimination of bowel contents along with the activated charcoal–poison complex. However, studies have shown that simultaneous administration actually decreases the efficacy of both agents and disrupts the adsorption capacity of activated charcoal. More recent position statements have declared that cathartics have no role in poison management. Even with activated charcoal, some studies indicated that cathartics make no significant difference in the patient outcome. As such, they are not endorsed for gut decontamination. If used, it is recommended to use them in cases where the poisonous substance cannot be adsorbed by activated charcoal, and in single dose, to avoid side effects.

Single-Dose Activated Charcoal

Activated charcoal is a highly porous form of carbon with a surface area of 950 to 2000 m^2/g, which is conducive for adsorption of substances with molecular weight in the range of 100 to 1000 Da. Despite this limitation, activated charcoal is used even if the poisonous substance is unknown, as it has few side effects compared to the benefits. Activated charcoal has an affinity with most medications like acetaminophen, CCBs, salicylates, TCAs, vitamin K antagonists, and alkaloids, but is contraindicated for corrosive substances like inorganic acids, surfactants, liquid hydrocarbons or in cases where the patient's respiratory tract is not protected, as it poses the risk of aspiration. The rationale behind the usage of activated charcoal is to eliminate further absorption of poison by adsorbing it. The effectiveness of activated charcoal in managing poison is dependent not only on the adsorptive properties of the poison but also on the time of ingestion. As the time of ingestion increases, the effectiveness of activated charcoal decreases. Theoretically, highest effect is shown when administered within an hour of poison ingestion.

Also, activated charcoal is not very effective in adsorbing SR/controlled release drugs or enteric-coated drugs. In the case of poisoning from such pharmaceutical preparations, WBI is recommended.

When used, a dosage of 25 to 50 grams of activated charcoal dissolved in water is administered to be ingested. Some studies suggest using 0.5 to 1 g/kg bodyweight for increased efficiency, especially in cases of overdose, where the excessive substance may form bezoars that can produce prolonged resorption long after ingestion to the detriment of the patient.

Whole Bowel Irrigation

This was originally designed to clean bowels before surgeries. It was only in the last three decades that WBI found use in poison management. It is mainly used to flush out overdose ingestions of SR and enteric-coated pharmaceuticals. It is also beneficial in cases where a patient has ingested significant amounts of iron, lithium, potassium tablets, or narcotic packets (in case of body packers while smuggling drugs). WBI is performed by enteral administration of saline or polyethylene solution until the effluent is clear, indicating an end point. Unfortunately, this does not translate to complete elimination of the poison unless the substance is radiopaque and can be quantified. As a result, there are currently no dose response studies on this procedure.

WBI is not routinely recommended due to its contraindications and side effects. It cannot be used in patients suffering from bouts of vomiting, GI hemorrhaging, bowel obstruction or perforation, or with an unprotected or compromised airway. WBI is only considered in situations where activated charcoal cannot be used due to its incompatibility with the poison or when more than 2 hours have passed from the time of ingestion.

Enhanced Elimination

In poison management, enhanced elimination procedures are rarely indicated, as most acute poisoning cases produce good outcomes with supportive care. They are, therefore, used in cases where supportive care does not yield desired results. Their usage also reduces the need for more invasive interventions. An important thing to note here is that the preferred method depends on the pharmacokinetic (toxicokinetic) properties of the poisonous substance. Some parameters in consideration are as follows: small volume of distribution, small molecular size, low protein binding, and slow endogenous elimination. Enhanced elimination methods are especially useful in management of toxic substances with long half-lives.

Multiple-Dose Activated Charcoal

Similar to single-dose activated charcoal, use of multiple-dose activated charcoal (MDAC) depends on the adsorptive properties of the toxin and its active metabolite. MDAC is recommended for poison substances that have a small volume of distribution and undergo either enterohepatic or enterogastric circulation. MDAC adsorbs the toxin in the window between its secretion into the intestine and reabsorption. Similar to single-dose activated charcoal, MDAC reduces the amount of toxin reabsorbed into the blood stream. By decreasing the amount of toxin in the intestinal lumen, it creates a concentration gradient across the intestinal wall, which then functions as a dialysis membrane.

Clinical trials on MDAC show that it exerts a significant effect on clearance of the following drugs: carbamazepine, theophylline, dapsone, phenobarbital, and quinine. It is however ineffective against phenytoin, according to a recent trial. MDAC is preferred method of elimination enhancement when applicable due to the minimally invasive nature of its procedure. A dose of 20 to 50 g or 0.5 to 1 g/kg is administered every 4 to 6 hours. MDAC is contraindicated in patients with GI obstruction.

Modification of Urine pH

Modification of urine pH enhances elimination of polar drugs like salicylates. Alkalization of urine can increase ionization/dissociation of weak acids and increase the fraction of drug excreted by urine, which is poorly resorbed across renal tubular epithelium. Urine alkalization is effective in salicylate overdose (quadrupled clearance), 2.4-dichlorophenoxyacetic acid and mecoprop poisonings, both of which are weak acids. It was also used for barbiturate poisoning but discontinued, since activated charcoal works more efficiently in this case.

The pH of the urine can also be modulated to acidification, in order to assist with the elimination of drugs with weak basic qualities like amphetamine and phencyclidine, but supportive care seems to precipitate sufficiently good outcomes for these poisonings.

Urine alkalization is done by administering an IV solution of sodium bicarbonate. Contraindications include hypokalemia and renal impairment.

Extracorporeal Procedures

Extracorporeal procedures involve filtering the toxin from blood once it is taken out of the body. Anticoagulants are used to prevent clotting. Filtered blood is reintroduced into the patients' body. These procedures are helpful in cases where expedited removal of toxin provides an opportunity to secure the condition of a critically ill patient unresponsive to other methods. Presence of acute kidney injury or electrolyte imbalances are not conducive for performing extracorporeal procedures. Due to the nature of these procedures, nephrologists play a critical role in their administration.

Hemodialysis

This procedure induces diffusion of targeted molecules from blood into the dialysate across a semipermeable membrane. Therefore, properties of the targeted molecule (size, low affinity to protein binding, water-soluble, and low-volume distribution) and dialysis factors determine the feasibility of administering this procedure.

For a molecule to be effectively removed under hemodialysis, it needs to have a molecular weight under 500 Da. Molecules around 300 Da are most effectively removed, but dialysis parameters can be adjusted to increase the efficiency to up to 500 Da. As a result, short-chain alcohols are good candidates for the usage of hemodialysis if the patient's condition cooperates.

Administration of hemodialysis is found to be highly effective in the treatment of poisonings caused by lithium, methanol, ethylene glycol, salicylates, valproate, carbamazepine, phenytoin, and metformin. This procedure can also correct fluid and electrolyte abnormalities simultaneously while removing the toxins.

Hemoperfusion

As the name indicates, this procedure involves passing the patient's blood over a column of adsorbent material that then adsorbs the toxin molecules. The adsorbent material used in this procedure is usually activated charcoal or resin. Using this procedure, molecules as heavy as 40,000 Da can be adsorbed onto the hemoperfusion cartridge. However, this procedure is more complex and expensive than hemodialysis, requiring continuous administration of heparin, which causes side effects including thrombocytopenia. Hemoperfusion precipitates the same effect as administering MDCA and is therefore rarely used for poison management.

Despite these drawbacks, this procedure is used to treat some poisonings due to its superiority over hemodialysis. Examples include paraquat, phenobarbital, and pentobarbital poisonings.

Hemofiltration

In this procedure, the heavier toxin molecules are separated from blood through convection. In hemodiafiltration, a variant of the procedure, both convection and diffusion are employed to segregate molecules. This procedure is used rarely due to lack of availability and paucity of studies exploring its use in poison management.

Peritoneal Dialysis

It uses peritoneum as a natural semipermeable membrane which filters the toxins. Although administration of this procedure is easier than hemodialysis and hemoperfusion, the effectiveness is very poor. This procedure is also very rarely used and is restricted to usage in infants and children and in cases where other procedures are unavailable. One main advantage of this procedure is the ability to maintain core temperature in hypothermic patients.

Plasmapheresis

Plasma exchange or plasmapheresis is an extracorporeal method where the patient's blood is passed through an apheresis machine, where the plasma is filtered and discarded, followed by reinfusion of plasma from a healthy donor.

These procedures are rarely, if ever, used in normal situations. They are mostly employed in poison management under the discretion of physician in situations where the commonly used procedures like hemodialysis are less effective or more deleterious.

Antidotes

One could assume that antidotes are the most effective way to treat poisonings, but studies have shown that timely supportive care provides comparable, if not better, clinical outcomes. This is because antidotes are limited by their availability, prescriber's understanding of the poison as well as the antidote, severity of the poisoning, costs, and their adverse effects.

An antidote counteracts a toxin primarily by one of the following methods: (i) It directly interacts with the toxin, as seen in chelation therapy and activated charcoal therapy. (ii) It interacts with the toxin's target receptor or enzyme. Ethanol and naloxone, antidotes for methanol and opioids respectively, act through this mechanism. (iii) The antidote affects the concentration of the toxic metabolite, for example, N-acetyl cysteine replenishes glutathione stores in the body, which conjugates to N-acetyl-p-benzoquinoneimine (NAPQI) and decreases toxicity. (iv) The antidote counteracts the harmful effects precipitated by the toxin. Atropine inhibits acetylcholine (ACh) binding at muscarinic receptors and impedes muscarinic activity of the organophosphates.

Many poisoned patients show good clinical outcomes with supportive care alone; as a result, usage of antidotes is reserved for situations where a patient is rapidly deteriorating despite receiving supportive care. Certain predictors like high levels of serum methanol, or marked QRS prolongation may warrant the use of an antidote to increase the patients' chance of survival. **Table 8.2** summarizes some of the important features of different antidotes.

Management of Specific Poisonings

Acetaminophen (IM5.7)

Paracetamol overdoses causes hepatotoxicity primarily through acetaminophen's (APAP) highly reactive intermediate NAPQI.

When taken in therapeutic doses, NAPQI is converted into nontoxic cysteine or mercapturic conjugates by glutathione (GSH) through CYP450 pathway in hepatic cells. But, in APAP overdoses, stores of GSH are exhausted and NAPQI is formed in excess, leaving it free to react with key target proteins, DNA, unsaturated lipids, and nucleophilic macromolecules, resulting in damage to liver cells and renal cells.

For adults, taking the drug in excess of 100 mg/kg body weight leads to hepatotoxicity and renal failure, and is potentially fatal when taken in excess of 12 grams. This effect is potentiated when APAP is consumed with alcohol by induction of CYP450 isoenzyme 2E1.

APAP overdose is usually asymptomatic, but in very high doses, the patient may demonstrate lactic acidosis. Without proper medical care, hepatoxicity and renal failure may set within 48 to 72 hours.

N-acetylcysteine (NAC) is an antidote that can replenish GSH and assists in neutralizing NAPQI. NAC is effective, free of adverse effects, and shows good results; hence, it is generally administered to a patient presenting with acute APAP poisoning to protect the liver from hepatotoxicity. NAC infusion is initiated with a loading dose of 200 mg/kg in the first 4 hours, followed by 100 mg/kg over the next 16 hours.

If the patient is admitted within first 2 hours of ingestion gastric lavage or activated charcoal may be used to reduce

Table 8.2 Summary of the important features of antidotes

Antidote	Indications	Dosage	Adverse reactions
Activated charcoal	Drug and poison overdoses	Loading dose: 25–100 g Repeat dose: 10–25 g every 2–4 hours	Constipation
Acetylcysteine	Paracetamol	Loading dose: 15 g over an hour Repeat dose: 5 g over 4 hours	Nausea, tachycardia, and others
Atropine	Organophosphates	2–5 mg	Dry mouth, blurred vision, and others
Antivenom	Snakes, scorpions, and other poisonous bites	Case-dependent	Rash, fever, body aches, and others
Calcium disodium edetate	Chromium, manganese, nickel, zinc	10–40 mg/kg/day	Nephrotoxicity
Deferoxamine	Iron	15 mg/hr, 6 g/day	Hypotension, allergic reaction
Digoxin specific antibodies	Digoxin	Serum digoxin (ng/mL) x body weight (kg)/100	Serum sickness, heart failure
Dimercaprol	Arsenic, copper, mercury, gold	2.5–3.5 mg/kg every 4 hours	Hypertension, nephrotoxicity, and others
Flumazenil	Benzodiazepines	Initial dose: 0.2 mg Repeat doses: 0.5 mg	Nausea, seizure, and others
Glucagon	Beta-blockers	Loading dose: 5–10 mg Maintenance dose: 1–5 mg/hr	Nausea, hyperglycemia
Naloxone	Opioids	0.8–2 mg, repeated 5 to 10 times	Withdrawal symptoms in case of opiate dependency
Sodium nitrite	Cyanide	300 mg	Methemoglobinemia
Physostigmine	Anticholinergic agents	0.5–2 mg	Bradycardia, bronchospasms, and others
Pralidoxime	Organophosphate insecticides	1 g over 30 minutes	Nausea, headache, and others
Protamine	Heparin	1–1.5 mg per 100 units of heparin	Anaphylactoid reactions

further absorption through gut. This might not be a viable option in patients who are unconscious; in such cases, many studies have shown the benefits of administering NAC as soon as the patient is presented with APAP poisoning to reduce hepatotoxicity. In cases of large overdoses where the lactic acidosis cannot be controlled with the help of fluid resuscitation and NAC, hemodialysis can prove efficient in eliminating most of the drug as APAP is moderately dialysable.

Once the necessary supportive measures are taken, the patient should be monitored for the next 24 hours. NAC can be discontinued once the level of paracetamol drops to normal level (< 10 mg/L).

Tricyclic Antidepressants

TCAs have a narrow therapeutic index and tend to show intoxication at comparatively smaller doses; consequently, they are now largely supplanted by selective serotonin reuptake inhibitors (SSRIs). They have, however, still retained a narrow range of uses, especially in treating depression resistant to other antidepressant classes.

TCA poisoning mainly produces three toxic syndromes: cardiotoxic effects, central nervous system (CNS) disturbances, and anticholinergic effects. Intensity of these toxidromes depends on the dose and the type of TCA ingested. Commonly, an overdose of > 20 mg/kg can quickly precipitate life-threatening cardiotoxicity.

If an admitted patient is suspected of TCA poisoning, ECG should be obtained, and any abnormalities should be immediately addressed. A QRS interval prolongation greater than 120 ms indicates severe TCA poisoning. Inquiries and investigations should be made to find the involvement of any coingestants like SSRIs and paracetamol.

TCAs do not have any known antidotes; therefore, primary management is carried out by providing appropriate supportive care. Due to TCAs' cardiotoxicity, ECG should be monitored in regular intervals for abnormalities. A prolonged QRS (> 100 minutes) is indicative of seizures, while QRS greater than 160 ms is associated with ventricular arrhythmia, which are treated by anticonvulsants and sodium bicarbonate (1–2 mEq/kg IV), respectively.

ABC should be properly managed. Detaining the absorption of the drug is considered beneficial and both single and MDCA have showed benefits if administered within 2 hours of ingestion. Gastric lavage might be useful in case of large-dose ingestions. Due to TCAs' high volume of distribution and high protein binding, extracorporeal methods are not very useful in enhancing the elimination of the drug.

Table 8.3 CNS and cardiovascular symptoms are caused in part due to anticholinergic effects of TCAs

Cardiovascular effects	CNS effects	Anticholinergic effects
Hypotension	Lethargy	Altered mental state
Vasodilation	Respiratory depression	Sinus tachycardia
Prolonged QRS complex	Seizures	Fever and altered mental state
Wide complex tachyarrhythmia	Coma	Dilated pupils, dry mouth, and dry skin

Abbreviations: CNS, central nervous system; TCA, tricyclic antidepressants.

Both flumazenil (benzodiazepine antagonist) and physostigmine (a cholinergic agent) are contraindicated in TCAs' poisoning management, as they exacerbate the seizures. **Table 8.3** shows treatment options considered for specific conditions elicited due to TCA toxicity.

In cases where a patient does not respond to standard management procedures, intravenous lipid emulsion and high dose of insulin should be considered. Before discharging, the patient's ECG should be monitored until normal for 12–24 hours.

Antidepressants, Selective Serotonin Reuptake Inhibitors

SSRIs are safer than TCAs and rarely precipitate life-threatening symptoms, only causing serious adverse events at doses 75 times the normal daily dose. At moderate overdoses, common symptoms of SSRI overdose are nausea, vomiting, drowsiness, tremors, and lethargy. Serotonin overdose symptoms are exacerbated when consumed with alcohol. Serotonin syndrome (symptoms: altered mental state, autonomic hyperactivity, and neuromuscular abnormalities) may develop in some cases. Supportive care and gut decontamination are common management strategies for SSRI overdose. Extracorporeal methods do not yield increased elimination of the drug due to its high volume of distribution. In most cases, symptoms resolve quickly after discontinuation of the serotonergic drugs.

Anticholinergic Poisoning

Anticholinergic poisoning can develop due to ingestion of high doses of drugs with anticholinergic properties (e.g., antihistamines and antipsychotics; **Box 8.1**), some plant parts (e.g., roots of *Atropa belladonna*), or mushrooms (e.g., *Amanita muscaria*). Anticholinergic drug overdose is rarely fatal. Patients usually exhibit flushing caused by vasodilation, anhydrosis, dry mucous membranes, mydriasis, altered mental state, fever caused by impaired thermoregulation, and urinary retention due to impaired bladder emptying. These symptoms are easily remembered by the mnemonic red as a beet, dry as a bone, blind as a bad, mad as a hatter, hot as hare, and full as a flask.

Anticholinergic drug overdose can be confused with sympathomimetic toxicity, in which case, absence of sweating indicates anticholinergic drug overdose.

The standard approach to treating anticholinergic overdose is by administering supportive care, in order to maintain the ABC of the patient. Cardiac activity should be continuously monitored. Single-dose charcoal can be administered if the ingestion occurred in an hour. However, it could be considered outside this window too, as anticholinergic drugs reduce gut motility. Enhanced elimination methods are ineffective in managing anticholinergic intoxication.

Box 8.1 A noncomprehensive list of some common anticholinergic agents

- Amitriptyline (TCAs)
- Atropine (Antimuscarinic agent)
- Benztropine (Anti-Parkinson drug)
- Diphenhydramine (Antihistamines)
- Dicyclomine (Antispasmodic)
- Oxybutynin (Antimuscarinic)
- Plants
  - *Atropa belladonna* (Deadly nightshade)
  - *Datura stramonium* (Jimsonweed)

If the patient displays agitation, benzodiazepines (BZDs) can be considered for treatment. IV fluids should be administered in case of hypotension, and cooling measures should be initiated in cases of significant hyperthermia. In cases of wide complex dysrhythmias, sodium bicarbonate IV preparation should be administered.

Physostigmine is an acetylcholinesterase inhibitor that is active in both CNS and peripheral nervous system (PNS) and is the recommended antidote in cases where both CNS and PNS are affected by the poisoning at a dose of 0.5 to 2 mg/kg.

Opioid Analgesic Drugs

Opioids are one of the most commonly misused drugs which effect multiple organ systems and lead to life-threatening repercussions. Opioid overdosing also tends to form bezoars in the gut, resulting in erratic drug absorption rates and leading to delayed advent of toxicity.

Classic symptoms of opioid overdose are respiratory depression, apnea or hypopnea, miosis, and stupor. Patients with apnea should be helped with their breathing by a pharmacologic agent or with the help of a mechanical stimulus. For patients with respiratory rate of less than 12 breaths per minute, respiratory assistance should be immediately provided.

Naloxone is one of the safest antidotes available and can be administered to treat opioid poisoning. It is a competitive opioid receptor antagonist and quickly reverses the signs of opioid intoxication. An initial dose of 0.4 mg is administered to the patient with gradual increase in the dosage every 2 minutes until 15 mg of dose is reached or until the respiratory depression is resolved.

Calcium Channel Blockers

CCBs or calcium antagonists are commonly prescribed for hypertension, arrhythmia, and angina, as they decrease cardiac inotropy, dromotropy, chronotropy, and vascular tone by blocking L-type calcium channels. Overdosing can happen with relatively small doses, generating hypotension, bradycardia, lethargy, syncope, hyperglycemia, lactic acidosis, seizures, and noncardiogenic pulmonary edema in the patient.

Overdosing of CCBs can cause a patients' condition to deteriorate rapidly. Initial management of a critically ill patient is focused on applying standard supportive care. Gastric lavage or activated charcoal is recommended within an hour of ingestion. CCBs have a high protein binding capacity; as a result, enhanced elimination procedures are not recommended.

Administration of an initial dose of 10 to 20 mL of 10% calcium chloride with three to four repeated boluses every 20 minutes can promote calcium influx and offset cardiac depression. Patients should be continuously monitored for signs of hypercalcemia and hypokalemia. Glucagon (bolus of 5–10 mg over 1–2 minutes) induces positive chronotropic and inotropic effects, resulting in increased heart rate.

Hyperinsulinemic euglycemia therapy (HIET) is a new therapy that is finding its place in the management of severe CCB toxicity. HIET corrects hypoinsulinemia caused by CCBs and reverses metabolic acidosis while increasing myocardial contractility. A starting dose of 0.5 to 1 U/kg insulin is IV administered, followed by 1 to 10 U/kg/hr continuous infusion. Glucose is administered concomitantly to maintain serum glucose levels.

Heavy Metals (FM9.3)

Human body has a low tolerance for heavy metals, and even the essential heavy metals cause toxicity when present above the threshold levels. At significant levels, they interfere with cell growth, development, cell division, signal transduction pathways, and electrolyte balance.

Chelation therapy is the primary treatment strategy for heavy metal poisoning. It uses chelators which are metals capable of donating a pair of electrons to form covalent bonds with heavy metals. The nontoxic complexes formed are then removed from the body through excretion. Chelation therapy is sometimes accompanied by antioxidant therapy to improve oxidative damage.

Chelation therapy is not risk-free and should be administered by an experienced medical practitioner.

Plasmapheresis or plasma exchange is an alternate treatment option for severe heavy metal intoxication. Some studies indicated it to be a viable option for inorganic mercury poisoning. Also, sauna therapy (inducing sweat) has shown increased amounts of heavy metals in sweat and can be considered as a concomitant supportive care to eliminate heavy metals.

Table 8.4 presents a noncomprehensive list of heavy metal toxicities and common chelating therapies. Heavy metal intoxication will be further discussed in detail in Chapter 81.

Carbon Monoxide

CO is an odorless and colorless gas and has 200 times greater affinity for hemoglobin than oxygen. Subsequently, CO poisoning, which happens when a person is exposed

Table 8.4 Heavy metal toxicities and common chelating therapies

Heavy metal	Clinical symptoms	Chelation therapy
Arsenic	Vomiting, abdominal pain, diarrhea, dark urine, dehydration	DMSA DMPS
Cadmium	Severe nausea and vomiting, abdominal pain, diarrhea, salivation	EDTA DMSA DMPS
Copper	Dizziness, headache, convulsions, lethargy, stupor, and coma	Penicillamine
Iron	Nausea, vomiting, abdominal pain, diarrhea, dehydration, and lethargy	DFO Deferiprone Deferasirox Clioquinol—can cross BBB
Lead	Anemia, abdominal pain, and headache. In serious cases, convulsions and coma	Sodium-calcium EDTA Succimer Dimercaprol (also known as BAL)
Mercury	Hypertension, tremors, changes in nerve response, insomnia, impaired cardiac, cognitive, and renal functions	DMSA—can cross BBB DMPS

Abbreviations: BAL, British anti Lewisite; BBB, blood–brain barrier; EDTA, ethylenediaminetetra-acetic acid; DFO, deferoxamine; DMPS, dimercaptopropanesulfonate; DMSA, dimercaptosuccinic acid.

to CO concentration above 1000 ppm, can cause cellular hypoxia by displacing oxygen in hemoglobin to form carboxyhemoglobin (HbCO) complex. The intensity of the poisoning is proportional to the length of exposure, and exposure to levels above 1200 ppm can be fatal.

CO poisoning affects mainly the brain and the heart, with majority of the patients reporting headache, dizziness, and nausea. In severe poisoning, the patient can show altered mental status, convulsions, arrhythmias, and slip into coma. The mechanism of effects precipitated by CO are not fully understood, but some studies report that it attacks mitochondrial electron transport chain.

Clinical diagnosis of CO toxicity requires HbCO measurement. Patients suspected of CO poisoning are administered 100% oxygen until symptoms are resolved. HbCO half-life decreases in about 20 to 30 minutes. 100% oxygen is administered at 2 to 3 atm in a hyperbaric chamber.

Amphetamines

Most amphetamine intoxications reported occur due to their illicit usage in the form of methamphetamine (speed), lysergic acid diethylamide (LSD), or methylene-dioxy-methamphetamine (ecstasy).

Due to their narrow therapeutic index, amphetamines can quickly precipitate adverse effects. Patients may present with paranoia, seizures, and arrhythmia among other peripheral manifestations and CNS effects.

Upon admission, patient should be immediately administered supportive care. Activated charcoal may be useful if the patient is conscious. Because of their high volume of distribution, amphetamines are suitable for enhanced elimination procedures. BZDs can be used to sedate and to treat seizures; hypertension is treated with a vasodilator and propranolol is used to correct tachyarrhythmias. Amphetamine intoxication rarely causes death, but the chances are higher when they are used alongside other stimulants.

Alcohols

Ethylene glycol and methanol poisoning can cause significant morbidity in patients due to their toxic metabolites produced by alcohol dehydrogenase (**Table 8.5**). Traditionally, ethanol therapy was used to treat methanol and ethylene glycol poisonings by administering ethanol to the patient, which would then compete for the enzyme. This procedure requires careful calculations and frequent monitoring of ethanol levels in the blood.

Short-chained alcohols are great candidates for hemodialysis, especially if the patient exhibits metabolic acidosis. Fomepizole (4-methyl pyrazole), a competitive inhibitor of alcohol dehydrogenase, can be given alongside hemodialysis. If given early, it can also obviate the need for hemodialysis. Simultaneous administration of sodium bicarbonate IV can enhance urinary clearance of less toxic metabolites.

Benzodiazepines

Most often, BZDs are well-tolerated and their poisoning alone does not produce any significant symptoms, but this tolerance decreases when they are consumed with other CNS depressants like ethanol. In such cases, the common symptoms are slurred speech, confusion, and incoordination. Respiratory depression is uncommon but should be addressed promptly if present.

Management strategy focuses primarily on supportive care, as enhanced elimination methods are ineffective. 0.1 to 0.2 mg initial dose of flumazenil can be considered if the poisoning is caused by BZD alone and the patient is a nonhabituated user.

Flumazenil is a BZD antagonist which acts on gamma-aminobutyric acid (GABA) receptor and can reverse some adverse effects of BZD poisoning. It may, however, cause uncontrollable seizures in patients with history of seizures. Therefore, supportive care is preferred. Flumazenil is to be administered only when absolutely sure that BZD is taken alone; otherwise, it can unmask the adverse effects of coingestants.

Cyanide

CN can enter the system via ingestion (NaCN, KCN) or inhalation (HCN) and reversibly bind to mitochondrial cytochrome oxidase a3 to cause intracellular hypoxia. The onset of symptoms occurs quickly, and the intensity depends on the level of exposure.

In early stages, cellular hypoxia causes headache, dizziness, and confusion, which can develop into hypotension, arrhythmias, seizures, and coma later.

Decontamination is an important step in CN toxicity. Clothing contaminated with fumes should be removed and skin in contact with CN should be washed with soap and water. Activated charcoal and hemodialysis are not very effective in managing the poison but hydroxycobalamine (5 g, IV) is an effective antidote for acute poisoning. Hydroxycobalamine forms cyanocobalamine with CN;

Table 8.5 Toxicity information on some common alcohol poisonings

Alcohol	Toxic levels	Toxic metabolite	Treatment
Ethanol	9–12 mL/kg	Formaldehyde	Fomepizole
Ethylene glycol	1–1.5 mL/kg	Glycolic acid	Hemodialysis, Fomepizole
Isopropyl alcohol	2–4 mL/kg	Isopropyl alcohol	Intravenous hydration
Methanol	> 0.1 mL/kg	Formic acid	Hemodialysis, Ethanol, Fomepizole

the complex is harmless and undergoes renal excretion. Alternatively, a CN antidote kit containing sodium nitrite and sodium thiosulfate may also be used.

Organophosphorus Compounds (FM9.5, PE14.3)

Organophosphorus (OP) compounds are mostly used as pesticides. Their use has been slowly declining in the last three decades due to their toxicity; however, they are still widely available in rural areas. They cause overstimulation of nicotinic and muscarinic receptor by inhibiting the breakdown of ACh. As a result, OP toxicity produces signs of weakness, muscular fasciculations, mydriasis, hypertension, and tachycardia through nicotinic receptor stimulation; muscarinic receptor stimulation produces vomiting, hypersecretion (defecation, urination, lacrimation, and salivation), miosis, and bronchospasms.

OPs can enter the system through dermal absorption, inhalation, and ingestion; therefore, decontamination procedures play an important role in treatment. Airway should be secured, and the patients' pulse oximetry and ECG should be monitored.

Activated charcoal may be helpful if administered within 1 to 2 hours of ingestion. Cathartics do not have a place in the management as the patient may already be suffering from diarrhea. Dialysis and other extracorporeal methods are not efficient due to OPs' large volume of distribution.

Multiple doses of atropine (initial dose of 0.5–3 mg IV) reverses muscarinic effects. In case of severe respiratory depression, pralidoxime (initial dose of 1–2 mg IV) should be administered. Pralidoxime is a cholinesterase reactivator and is given even after atropine administration is stopped, as it can slow down the adverse effects precipitated by the release of OP from fats.

Salicylates

Salicylates are over-the-counter (OTC) medications commonly used as analgesics and antipyretics. In overdoses, salicylate poisoning has a high mortality rate. In high doses, they cause metabolic disorders, hyperventilation, and respiratory alkalosis. Salicylates disrupt oxidative phosphorylation in mitochondria, which ultimately results in metabolic acidosis. Without any supportive care, salicylate poisoning leads to end organ damage and hemodynamic instability.

Activated charcoal and gastric lavage can help decrease the amount of salicylate absorbed. In severe poisoning, mechanical respiration might be required. Sodium bicarbonate IV administration (1–2 mEq/kg) can help with the correction of metabolic acidosis, and replenishment of body fluids and dextrose can help with hypoglycemia.

If acidosis persists, despite sodium bicarbonate administration, hemodialysis can enhance serum salicylate elimination.

Poisonings from Animal and Insect Bites

Threat of poisoning surrounds us not only from industrial chemicals, pharmaceuticals, and plant extracts but also from the thousands of poisonous insects and animals distributed around the planet. Understandably, the threat from these poisonous species has decreased since the advent of cities and towns, but cases of poisonous bites and stings are not uncommon.

Hymenoptera Stings

The order hymenoptera includes insects like bees, wasps and fire ants among 150,000 other insect species. While the venom from these insect stings is not lethal to humans, they are responsible for a significant amount of deaths caused due to anaphylaxis induced by envenomation.

The venom contains high-molecular weight proteins, which are responsible for the allergic reactions via systemic immunoglobulin E (IgE)-mediated histamine release, and low-molecular weight proteolytic enzymes which cause inflammatory reactions at the site of sting.

Hymenoptera stings usually cause immediate pain and local reaction and can last for hours. Without anaphylaxis, these stings resolve themselves in a couple of days. However, in cases of severe anaphylaxis, patients exhibit symptoms like urticaria, flushing, hypotension, compromised breathing ability, and angioedema.

On admission, patients exhibiting anaphylactic reactions should be assessed for their ABC. IV fluids should be administered along with epinephrine (0.3–0.5 mg IM), corticosteroids, and H1 and H2 antagonists to improve the allergic symptoms. Stings without systemic allergic reactions can be treated with analgesics and ice packs.

Before discharging, the patient should be warned of rebound anaphylaxis and serum sickness-like reactions, in case of which they should seek medical attention immediately.

Scorpion Stings (IM20.8)

Only 1.5% of all scorpion species' venom cause lethal harm to humans. Most stings sustained are painful but relatively harmless. The effects precipitated by the sting vary from one species to another and the age of the patient; young children and elderly are more vulnerable to the effects of a scorpion venom.

The Indian red scorpion, native to Indian subcontinent, carries lethal venom. Its envenomation can produce loss of consciousness, cardiotoxicity, acute pulmonary edema, convulsions, and multiorgan failure, followed by death within the first 24 hours. Early administration of prazosin (500 µg repeated every 3 hours), a postsynaptic alpha 1 blocker, can improve the clinical outcome.

Scorpion stings are usually diagnosed by patient's report that they saw a scorpion in the vicinity. The site of sting becomes red due to local inflammation and numbness, and weakness may also be observed. In mild cases of envenomation, application of analgesic at the sting site, followed by intermittent ice pack, is recommended. Young children should be kept under observation to avoid development of severe symptoms. In severe envenomation, antivenin (IV infusion of three vials in 50 mL of saline over 30 minutes) is administered along with supportive care. The patient should be closely monitored for any hypersensitivity to the antivenin.

Snake Bites (IM20.7)

As much as 10 to 15% of the 3,000 snake species are venomous. They are ubiquitous to every continent except Antarctica, and they are usually encountered by humans during outdoor activities in warm weather.

Depending on the snake species, its venom can be of one of the following categories: coagulant, cytoxin, hemotoxin, myotoxin, or nephrotoxin. King cobra, kraits, mamba, and coral snake bites are neurotoxic; viper and asp disrupt clotting system; and rattle snake bites produce myotoxic effects.

Diagnosing a snake bite requires proper identification of the snake. Information on its color pattern, unique features, and geographic area in which the patient sustained the bite are helpful in identifying the species. In prehospital setting, it is recommended that that the site of injury is immobilized and bandaged with an elastic band (without cutting off arterial blood flow), and rushed to an emergency center.

Mild cases of envenomation do not need administration of antivenom, but for moderate-to-severe envenomation, antivenins are the only effective treatment strategy. Once admitted, the bite is decontaminated using water and soap, followed by administration of broad-spectrum antibiotics if the patient exhibits signs of infection. The patient is then monitored closely for 12 to 14 hours to address any symptoms that may arise due to envenomation.

Generally, eight vials of antivenin (specific to the venom) is administered via IV, followed by a maintenance dose of four vials. It is recommended that the patients receiving antivenin should be pretreated with epinephrine to avoid hypersensitivity reactions.

Disposition of a Patient

All patients reporting severe toxicities should be kept in observation until they show a stabilized condition for more than 6 to 8 hours, but some poisonings may require a patient to be kept under observation longer. Special attention should be paid to cases involving SR preparations. If poisoning is caused as a result of suicidal intent or misuse of drugs, the patients is to be referred to appropriate counselling for further help. Patients and their family members should be informed about any possible delayed adverse events before discharging.

Ultimately, the decision of whether to discharge a patient depends on the discretion of a qualified medical practitioner, as effects of poisoning are unique to each case.

Multiple Choice Questions

1. A woman in mid-40s is admitted with tricyclic antidepressant (TCA) overdose. She is unconscious and the time of ingestion is estimated to be more than 4 hours. Her ECG reveals a widened QRS (174 ms). Which of the following treatment options should not be considered for this patient?

A. 2 mmol/kg sodium bicarbonate bolus.
B. Flumazenil (a benzodiazepine antagonist).
C. Phenobarbital (a barbiturate).
D. All the above.

Answer: B

Flumazenil is a benzodiazepine antagonist which exacerbates seizures in patients suffering from TCA overdose.

2. Which of the following parameters must be true for a drug to qualify for extracorporeal methods to enhance its elimination?

A. Low protein binding capacity.
B. High volume of distribution.
C. Low volume of distribution.
D. Large molecular size.
E. Small molecular size.

Answer: A, B, E

A drug needs to have low volume of distribution, low protein binding capacity, and small molecular size to qualify for extracorporeal procedures.

3. Ethanol and fomepizole are used as antidotes in both methanol and ethylene glycol poisonings. What is their target molecule?

A. Methanol and ethylene glycol.
B. Aldehyde dehydrogenase.
C. Alcohol dehydrogenase.
D. Formic acid and glycolic acid.

Answer: C

Ethanol and fomepizole competitively inhibit alcohol dehydrogenase enzyme and prevent the formation of toxic metabolites like formic acid, glycolic acid, and oxalic acid.

4. How should a scorpion sting be managed in clinical setting?

A. Antivenin.
B. Intravenous (IV) sodium bicarbonate.
C. Prazosin.
D. Nonsteroidal anti-inflammatory drugs (NSAIDs).

Answer: A, C, D

Antivenin and prazosin are prescribed for serious envenomation, while NSAIDs can help with the localized pain of the sting

5. A 64-year-old man accidentally ingested *Atropa belladonna* fruits on his hike. At the time of admission, the man was unconscious with signs of anticholinergic toxic syndrome. His medical history was normal with no known complications. Which of the following drugs can be used to treat this patient?

A. Physostigmine.
B. Flumazenil.
C. Fomepizole.
D. Pralidoxime.

Answer: A

Physostigmine reversibly inhibits anticholinesterase.

6. How can you prevent the formation of bezoars?

A. Emesis.
B. Administer sodium bicarbonate intravenously (IV).
C. Increase the dosage of activated charcoal.
D. Hemodialysis.

Answer: C

Increasing activated charcoal quantity will prevent the formation of bezoars by adsorbing the excess chemical.

7. Which of the following is used in the treatment of lead poisoning?

A. Dimercaprol.
B. Penicillamine.
C. Succimer.
D. Deferoxamine.

Answer: A, C

Dimercaprol is a dithiol that acts by forming a stable five-membered ring between its sulfhydryl groups and certain heavy metals, thereby neutralizing its toxicity and promoting its elimination. Dimercaprol is more efficacious when given soon after the metal exposure, because it is better at preventing enzyme inhibition rather than reactivating enzyme function.

Succimer is an organosulfur compound with two sulfhydryl groups that bind divalent metal ions such as lead, cadmium, mercury, and arsenic. Succimer does not significantly chelate essential metals such as zinc, copper, or iron, and its specificity, safety, and oral availability make it preferable to other chelating agents for treating lead poisoning such as Ca-EDTA, which must be given intravenously (IV), and dimercaprol (British anti-Lewisite [BAL]), which requires intramuscular (IM) administration.

8. Which of the following elimination methods are dispensable in the management of organophosphate poisoning?

A. Decontamination.
B. Activated charcoal.
C. Dialysis.
D. Airway management.

Answer: C

Organophosphates have a large volume of distribution, which is not conducive for dialysis.

9. Why is epinephrine administered to a patient who was subject to a snake bite?

A. To prevent anaphylactic reactions that may be caused by the proteins in venom.
B. To prevent any allergic reactions in case the person has asthma.
C. To prevent anaphylactic reactions that may be caused by antivenin.
D. There is no need to use epinephrine.

Answer: C

Generally, eight vials of antivenin (specific to the venom) is administered via IV, followed by a maintenance dose of four vials. It is recommended that the patients receiving antivenin should be pretreated with epinephrine to avoid hypersensitivity reactions.

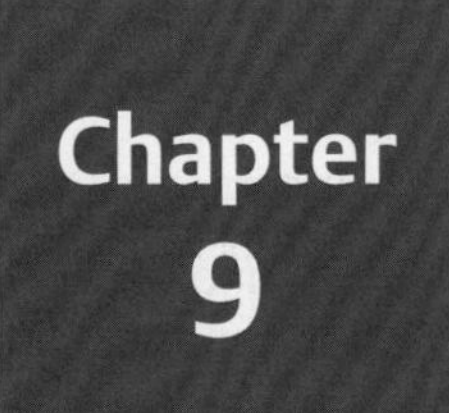

Chapter 9

New Drug Approval Process and Clinical Trials

Viraj A. Shinde

PH1.64: Describe overview of drug development, phases of clinical trials, and good clinical practice.

Learning Objective

- Overview of the drug approval process.

Introduction

The new drug application (NDA) procedure is supervised by the Food and Drugs Administration (FDA). Before endorsement, declaration of the ingredients and formulation, assay methods, manufacturing processes, and all animal and human testing centered on the twin properties of safety and efficacy of novel drug products is at the heart of the NDA process. Investigational new drug (IND) applications has to be filed by investigator before testing novel drugs in human beings. Center of Drug Evaluation and Research (CDER) underneath FDA is accountable for drugs and drug efficacy of all prescriptions and over-the-counter drug products before merchandising. The CDER is accountable for keeping a track of drug safety and securing early market endorsement. It also has power to retreat a drug from the market, which is posing high volume of health risk.

Overview of the Drug Approval Process

Preclinical testing and clinical testing are two segments of development process. Lead compound culling and animal testing of novel chemicals are two parts of preclinical testing. Administration of new chemicals to humans is clinical testing.

Drug Discovery and Lead Compound Selection

1. Lead compound, which must first be identified by researchers, is a chemical with potential therapeutic benefits. Sizeable number of chemicals are expeditiously screened by using numerous assay techniques for biological activity.
2. Biological testing of a sizeable array of disparate compounds from extant chemical athenaeum is known as random screening.
3. Targeted synthesis is more mechanism-based drug designing. One step involves focusing by the researchers in a targeted synthesis for drug intervention.
4. The boundless proficiency of disease state is essential, which is a more controlled path and expands the likelihood of successfully finding out the lead compound.
5. The lead compound is picked out by amalgamation of these discovery techniques.

Preclinical Testing

Pharmacological profile of a prospective compound is unfolded using experimentation on animals. The animals used for experimentation are rodents (guinea pig, mouse, rat, hamster, rabbit) and larger animals (cat, dog, monkey). Unfavorable compounds are removed at each step. Preclinical testing consists of the following:

1. Discovery testing done to establish biological activity in vivo.
2. Adequate quantities of high purity can be ensured by chemical synthesis and scaling up.
3. Formulation development and stability testing to characterize various chemical properties develop the initial drug delivery system and determine the stability of the compound.
4. Restricted toxicities of the lead agent can be ensured by animal safety testing.
5. The set of compound's characteristics such as mechanism of action in animal models, specificity of compound, duration of action, and serious adverse reaction are understood during discovery testing.
6. This phase is characterized by determination of physiochemical characteristics of the active compound and unfolding of the drug delivery system to be used in human testing.
7. The utmost suitable animal model to anticipate response in human being is often unknown.
8. To gain a complete knowledge of the potential toxicity, toxicity studies need to be performed in at least twin animal species, one non-rodents and another rodent.
9. Animals should be administered novel drug product by the very same route of administration for testing purpose, as is intended for human use.
10. The chemical synthesis, formulation development, and animal safety testing goes on simultaneously once discovery testing shows therapeutic promise.

Investigational New Drug (IND) Applications

Filing of IND application with the FDA and approval of FDA is necessary before new drug product is administered to human beings. All preclinical data related to animal testing and the locations and names of the investigators who are going to perform the planned clinical trials is a part of IND.

Clinical Trials (FM4.25)

Clinical trials involve the administration of a drug to human beings. Substantial monetary and time dedication is required by this segment of the drug development process. Phase 1, phase 2, phase 3, and phase 4 are four phases of human testing, each one with definite objectives. Good clinical practice (GCP) guidelines by an International Conference on Harmonization (ICH) has laid down standards for the design, conduct, monitoring, ethics, auditing, recording and analyzing data, and reporting of clinical trials. Ethical guidelines for conducting clinical trials in India are also framed by Indian Council of Medical Research (ICMR) in India.

Phase 1

Phase 1 clinical testing is characterized by the first series of experiments to be carried out in human beings. Twenty to thirty healthy human participants are generally chosen. In phase 1 of clinical trial, the beginning dose is by and large small. Normally, one-tenth of the bigger dose without any effect in animal models is chosen. Supplementary participants may be enrolled and administered bigger doses to decide the maximum tolerated dose with no significant side effect after initial treatment is completed. This phase is characterized by the evaluation of preliminary absorption, distribution, metabolism, and excretion (ADME) data of the parent drug and all its metabolites. Qualified clinical pharmacologists/trained physicians monitor this phase.

Phase 2

A change in center of attention of phase 2 clinical trial from safety to efficacy is seen. Individuals in a large number (100–300) engage in this phase, where most of the human beings suffer from targeted disease. This phase is additionally looked into to gather information regarding side effect from the new drug. Before starting this phase of trial clinical protocols have to be directed to the FDA to rectify the IND.

Phase 3

A careful assessment of the preclinical and clinical data is done in the analysis of the proposed phase 3 protocol, which is carried out by scientists. The proposed phase 3 trials have specific areas which are as follows: inclusion/exclusion criteria, dosing schedule, method and timing of data collection, duration of treatment and follow-up assessment, blinding of the drug product and plans to access compliance with the protocol, identification of primary outcome variables, and various ways to account for dropouts. It is the lengthiest and most compendious trials concerning efficacy and safety of new compounds. Notably, a huge volume of participants is chosen for testing (1,000–3,000 patients) who are stricken with the targeted disease. A comparison may be done between the new drug with the present therapeutic regimen or placebo. Before starting these phase 3 clinical trials, the ultimate marketed formulation of the drug product should be optimized. In this phase, a "new drug application" (NDA) is made to the licensing authority. The licensing authority may give marketing permission if it is satisfied with the results of the trial.

Phase 4

These trials are postapproval clinical trials planned for one among the several reasons. To further assess efficacy and side effects of a drug, the NDA committee may order phase 4 testing in a certain patient population. Auxiliary clinical trials may be performed by companies to more completely comprehend how their product stands in comparison to other commercially available therapeutic regimens. Rare/idiosyncratic adverse effects and unexpected drug interactions are detected in this phase. Adverse effects on chronic use of drug are also detected in this phase. These are done once the drug enters the market.

New Drug Application

The final obstacle prior to acceptance and merchandising is the NDA process. Highly explicit information is present in a NDA document. Side effects and efficacy of the drug therapy, constituents of drug products, elucidation of method and controls used in production of the active ingredients, the delivery system and its packing, and proposed labeling are the chief items that NDA includes. First assessment for completeness of NDA is done when the NDA is first submitted. The NDA is accepted for evaluation only if the document is acceptably complete. In a period of 60 days of the date of submission, the decision to accept the NDA is made. The FDA has 180 days from the date of submission of NDA to complete the scrutiny and give the decision of approval/nonapproval.

Postapproval Activities Safety Monitoring

The drug safety is constantly tracked once the NDA has been accepted and marketing of the drug product is started. Regular submission of reports of adverse events is mandatory to sponsors/company of the NDA. These are submitted quarterly for 3 years and then yearly for the new drugs. In case of serious adverse events, small labeling changes or inclusion of warning or precaution declaration may be required. The approval may stand withdrawn if serious safety concerns arise.

Changes to an Approved Product

The FDA must receive information regarding any changes that are done to an FDA-approved drug product, including constituent or constitution, chemical synthesis, production process, site, analytical methods, batch size, or labeling. The FDA should be notified through annual reports or supplemental new drug applications (SNDA), subject to type of revision and the influence of revision on the quality of drug product.

Multiple Choice Questions

1. In which phase of clinical trials, there is comparison of efficacy between the new and existing drugs?

A. Phase I.
B. Phase II.
C. Phase III.
D. Phase IV.

Answer: C

The aim of a phase III trial is to establish the value of the drug in relation to existing therapy.

2. Good clinical practice (GCP) is required in all, EXCEPT:

A. Preclinical phase.
B. Phase I trial.
C. Phase II studies.
D. Phase IV studies.

Answer: A

Preclinical testing does not require GCP guidelines as it is not part of the clinical phase.

3. Which of the following is true with respect to clinical trials of new drugs?

A. Phase I involves the study of a small number of normal volunteers by highly trained clinical pharmacologists.
B. Phase II involves the use of the new drug in a large number of patients (1,000–5,000) who have the disease to be treated.
C. Phase III involves the determination of the drug's therapeutic index by the cautious induction of toxicity.
D. Phase IV involves the detailed study of toxic effects that have been discovered in phase III.

Answer: A

Phase I trials involve small numbers of healthy volunteers usually meant to check for safety and pharmacokinetic profiles of the experimental drug.

4. In which of the following phases of clinical trials do healthy normal human volunteers participate?

A. Phase I.
B. Phase II.
C. Phase III.
D. Phase IV.

Answer: A

Phase I trials require healthy volunteers.

5. Postmarketing surveillance of a drug is also called:

A. Phase I trial.
B. Phase II trial.
C. Phase III trial.
D. Phase IV trial.

Answer: D

Phase IV trials involve postmarketing surveillance.

Chapter 10

Pharmacogenomics and Pharmacoeconomics

Manju Agrawal

PH1.60: Describe and discuss pharmacogenomics and pharmacoeconomics.

Learning Objectives

- Genetic polymorphism.
- Pharmacogenomic examples.
- Pharmacoeconomic analysis.
- Pharmacoeconomic calculations.

Pharmacogenomics

Pharmacogenomics is a branch of pharmacology that deals with the effect of a person's genetic makeup on the response to a drug. A number of factors influence drug response in an individual such as the age, body weight, disease, drug interactions, drug compliance, and genetic factors. Genetic factors are the most important factors for interindividual and intraindividual differences in drug response but least understood. This comparatively new field combines pharmacology (the science of drugs) and genomics (the study of genes and their functions) to develop effective, safe medications that will be personalized to a person's genetic makeup. The term pharmacogenetics and pharmacogenomics are used interchangeably, however, the two terms vary. Pharmacogenetics is the study of single gene influencing a drug response, while pharmacogenomics is the study of entire spectrum of genes (genome) influencing drugs response and **Table 10.1** illustrates the difference.

Heredity influences drug response, and this was first described in 1956 with the identification of glucose-6-phosphate dehydrogenase (G6PD) deficiency, leading to hemolytic reactions after ingestion of fava beans, and later on to certain therapeutic drugs like the antimalarial drug primaquine, sulfonamides, nitrofurantoin, and high-dose ascorbic acid. Friedrich Vogel first coined the term "pharmacogenetics" in 1959, when he defined it as the "study of the role of genetics in drug response." The completion of the human genome project in 2003 fuelled the discipline of pharmacogenomics by extensively cataloguing genetic variations in the DNA and developing more personalized drug therapies. Until then, drugs were prescribed with the idea that "one drug fits all." Advancement in technology to assess such variation and correlation with phenotypic data served as a foundation for implementing pharmacogenomics and developing more personalized drug therapies. The Clinical Pharmacogenetic Implementation Consortium (CPIC), and the US Food and Drugs Administration (FDA) regularly publish a series of guidelines for using genetic information in selecting drugs and dosing. The US National Institute of Health (NIH) funds a pharmacogenetic and pharmacogenomic knowledge base (PharmGKB), which is an online database website with downloadable content. Users can search and browse the knowledge base by genes, variants, drugs, diseases, and pathways and integrate the information toward personalized medicine.

Common terminology used in pharmacogenomics

- **Deoxyribonucleic acid (DNA):** The genetic code made up of nucleotides bases, two purine bases: Adenine (A), guanine (G), and two pyrimidine bases: thymine (T), and cytosine (C), always pair together as A-T and C-G in the two DNA strands to form a double helix.
- **Codon**: Three consecutive nucleotides form a codon, and each codon specifies an amino acid. There are 64 possible codons, three of which do not code for amino acids and the remaining 61 code for 20 amino acids, implying two or more codons code for the same amino acid.
- **Gene**: This is a series of codons that specify a particular protein.
- **Allele**: This is one or more alternative forms of a pair of genes that arise by mutation, appear at the same location on a particular chromosome, and control the same characteristic. Example: CYP2D6*3 is a variant allele for drug metabolizing enzyme CYP2D6.
- **Polymorphism/variant**: Variation in the DNA nucleotide sequence that occurs at a frequency of at least in 1% population.
- **Single nucleotide polymorphism (SNP)**: Base pair substitution that occurs in the coding region.

Table 10.1 Difference between pharmacogenetics and pharmacogenomics

Pharmacogenetics	Pharmacogenomics
The study of single gene influencing a single drug response. E.g., Influence of one gene coding for CYP2C9 on warfarin dose.	The study of entire spectrum of genes (genome) influencing drugs response. E.g., Influence of multiple genes coding for CYP2C9, VKORC1, and CYP4F2 on warfarin dose.

The goals of pharmacogenomics are as follows:

1. To optimize drug therapy—choose the right drug at the right dose for the right duration.
2. Reduce the risk of serious adverse responses or loss of response.
3. Reduce health care costs associated with hospitalizations and outpatient visits due to adverse drug responses and multiple drug prescriptions.

Types of Genetic Polymorphism

Genetic variation may affect either the drug pharmacokinetics or drug pharmacodynamics or both by affecting gene coding for the following:

a. Drug-metabolizing enzymes.
b. Drug transporters.
c. Drug targets.
d. Disease-associated genes.

Variation in drug-metabolizing enzymes and transporters usually alter the pharmacokinetics of a drug, while variation in drug targets and disease-associated genes often alter the pharmacodynamics of the drug. The most common type of variation is SNPs (**Fig. 10.1**), while less commonly seen variations are insertion and deletion (Indels), tandem repeats, frame shift mutation, defective splicing, aberrant splice site, premature stop codon polymorphism, and copy number variants.

Genotype analysis can be used to identify DNA changes in specific metabolizing enzymes that produce aberrant phenotypes. Genotyping is done using DNA extracted from white blood cells (WBCs) or buccal cells. It determines differences in genetic complement by comparing a DNA sequence to that of another sample or a reference sequence.

Polymorphism in Drug Metabolizing Enzymes

Polymorphism in drug metabolizing enzymes are the most documented examples of genetic variation affecting serum drug concentration and are important determinants of therapeutic drug response and adverse drug effects. The potential for a clinically significant event is aggravated if these enzymes metabolize drugs with narrow therapeutic index or are eliminated by zero order kinetics or if the number of therapeutic alternatives are limited. The enzymes exhibiting polymorphism in the phase 1 enzyme are cytochrome P450 (CYP) enzyme super family which metabolize over 75% of prescription drugs and phase II enzymes like N-acetyl transferase. Other enzymes exhibiting pharmacogenetic polymorphism are as follows: thiopurine S-methyltransferase (TPMT), pseudocholinesterase, glucose 6 phosphate dehydrogenase, etc. Standardized terminology for clinical pharmacogenetic test results, depending upon the functional status and phenotypes, have been laid down and include:

- Poor metabolizer (PM)—individuals with little or no functional enzyme activity.
- Intermediate metabolizer (IM)—individuals with decreased enzyme activity.
- Normal metabolizer (EM)—individuals with fully functional enzyme activity.
- Rapid or ultrarapid metabolizer (UM)—individuals with substantially increased enzyme activity.

SNPs alter drug response, resulting in either of the following:

- Loss of efficacy due to decrease in drug concentration: if the polymorphism involves enzyme for bioactivation of a prodrug as seen in poor metabolizers, or if the enzyme is responsible for metabolism of drug, as seen in rapid/ultrarapid metabolizer, necessitating increase in therapeutic dose.
- Increase in adverse effects due to increase in drug concentration: if the polymorphism results in extensive bioactivation of a prodrug, as seen in rapid/ultrarapid metabolizer, or decrease in metabolism, as seen in poor metabolizers, necessitating reduction in therapeutic dose.

Some examples of pharmacogenetic polymorphism in drug metabolizing enzymes.

Phase I Enzymes

- **CYP2D6:** This enzyme metabolizes a large number of drugs like tricyclic antidepressants, selective serotonin reuptake inhibitors, beta-blockers, and opioid analgesics, and displays a marked allelic heterogeneity best characterized among all CYP variants. The gene coding for CYP2D6 is highly polymorphic. Analgesic *codeine* is a prodrug, and CYP2D6-mediated activation to morphine is essential for its analgesic activity. Individuals with CYP2D6*2 variation, due to duplication and amplification, have increased enzyme activity, known as UM phenotype, resulting in rapid conversion of codeine to morphine. These patients are at higher risk of life-threatening respiratory depression or experience signs of overdose at therapeutic dose and should be prescribed codeine with caution.
- **CYP2C9:** This is a major enzyme metabolizing warfarin, phenytoin, valproic acid, and tolbutamide. The gene that encodes CYP2C9 is also highly polymorphic. Warfarin is a narrow therapeutic index drug and routine monitoring of the internationalized normal ratio (INR) is necessary. Individuals carrying any of the variant CYP2C9 *2 or *3 alleles exhibit reduced enzyme activity (PM), leading to reduced elimination of S-warfarin with consequences of significant increase in drug plasma concentration which, in turn, leads to higher incidence of bleeding.
- **CYP2C19:** Drugs including proton pump inhibitor, antidepressant, and antiplatelet drugs are metabolized by CYP2C19. CYP2C19*2 (due to aberrant splicing) and CYP2C19*3 (due to premature stop codon) result in inactive/nonfunctional enzymes and are termed PM phenotypes

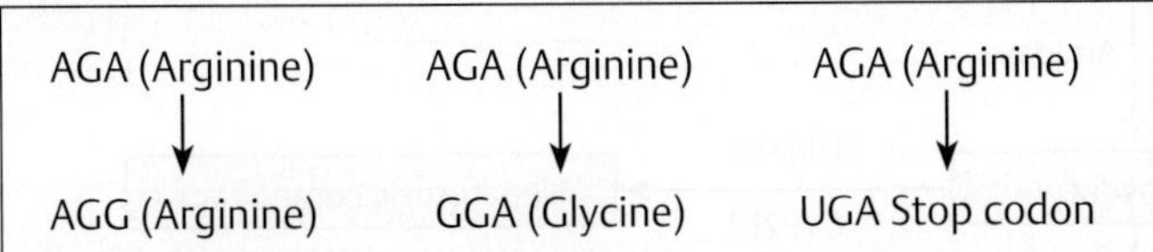

Fig. 10.1 SNP base-pair substitution: AGA codon codes for arginine, and substitution of adenine with guanine at third base results in codon AGG, which also codes for arginine; when similar substitution is at first base GGA glycine is formed, and when adenine is substituted for uridine at first base, a stop codon is formed.

which are more common among Asians. Omeprazole is inactivated by CYP2C19; individuals with these variants have decreased clearance, resulting in higher plasma concentration and hence higher cure rates in *H. pylori* eradication.

- Conversely, an antiplatelet agent *clopidogrel* is a prodrug that requires CYP2C19-mediated bioactivation. Individuals who carry two nonfunctional copies of the CYP2C19 variant (PM phenotype) have decreased active metabolites, resulting in reduced response to clopidogrel therapy. Such individuals who underwent percutaneous coronary intervention (PCI) for the treatment of acute coronary syndrome (ACS) are more prone to cardiovascular events and stent thrombosis and must be prescribed another agent.
- **CYP3A4:** This is usually not implicated in interindividual variability in drug metabolism, as it is highly inducible, and its activity is dominated by environmental factors.

Phase II Enzymes

- **N-acetyl transferase (NAT):** This acetylates isoniazid used in the treatment of tuberculosis and exists in two isoforms, NAT1 and NAT2 (**Fig. 10.2**). Polymorphism in NAT2 enzyme results in fast and slow acetylator phenotypes and modulates isoniazid toxicity. Fast acetylators will rapidly acetylate acetyl hydrazine to nontoxic metabolite, while in slow acetylators, acetyl hydrazine will not be acetylated but will be oxidized to a hepatotoxic metabolite.

Other Enzymes

- **Butyl cholinesterase** (also known as plasma cholinesterase/pseudocholinesterase): This rapidly hydrolyses succinylcholine, a depolarizing neuromuscular blocking agent. Individuals carrying the variant/atypical enzyme either have reduced affinity of the enzyme for the substrate or have reduced amount of normal enzyme. In these individuals, the drug persists in the blood and predisposes them to risk of prolonged apnea called succinyl apnea. In such patients, a 5- to 10-mg test dose of succinylcholine could be given to assess sensitivity to succinylcholine, or neuromuscular blockade could be induced by injecting a 1-mg/mL solution of succinyl choline slow intravenous (IV) infusion. Apnea or prolonged muscle paralysis should be treated with controlled respiration.

Polymorphism Affecting Drug Transport Genes

Several proteins facilitate drug transport, and polymorphism in organic anion transporter (OAT) has been recognized as clinically important. OAT encoded by SLC01B1 regulates uptake of hypolipidemic drug simvastatin (HMG-CoA reductase inhibitor) into the liver. Reduced function SLC01B1*5 allele due to amino acid substitution impairs simvastatin clearance and is associated with drug-induced myopathy, which requires lowering the dose or alternate statin.

Polymorphism in Drug Target Genes

Genetic polymorphism occurs in drug target proteins, which include enzymes, ion channels, receptors, and intracellular signaling proteins, and affects the pharmacodynamics of the drug.

- Polymorphism involving vitamin K epoxide reductase complex subunit 1 (VKORC1) encoded by VKORC1 gene affect the enzyme vitamin K oxidoreductase, a target for warfarin (a vitamin K antagonist). Warfarin, an anticoagulant, acts by inhibiting the synthesis of vitamin K-dependent clotting factors by inhibiting VKORC1 enzyme complex. SNP in the VKORC1 leads to lesser functional copies of the rate-limiting enzyme, requiring reduction in warfarin dosage (**Fig. 10.3**).
- Glucose 6 phosphate dehydrogenase (G6PD) deficiency exposes the red blood cells (RBCs) to the damaging effects of reactive oxygen species and leads to hemolytic reactions on account of exposure to certain drugs like antimalarial primaquine, sulfonamides, and nitrofurans. G6PD deficiency is defined as enzyme activity less than 60% of the enzyme activity. The frequency of G6PD deficiency is approximately 8% in malaria endemic zones. Quantitative tests in whole blood to determine G6PD status for high-dose primaquine is recommended.

Disease Associated Genes and Its Influence on Drug Behavior

The human leukocyte antigen (HLA) gene is associated with grave and occasionally lethal dermatologic reactions, like toxic epidermal necrolysis (TEN) and Stevens–Johnson syndrome (SJS), with carbamazepine and phenytoin, commonly prescribed antileptic drugs. Patients should be tested for the presence of HLA-B*15:02 before starting carbamazepine, and those who are positive, should be prescribed an alternative agent.

Similarly, use of abacavir, an antiretroviral agent has been associated with serious and sometimes fatal hypersensitivity reactions in patients who carry the HLA-B*57:01 allele.

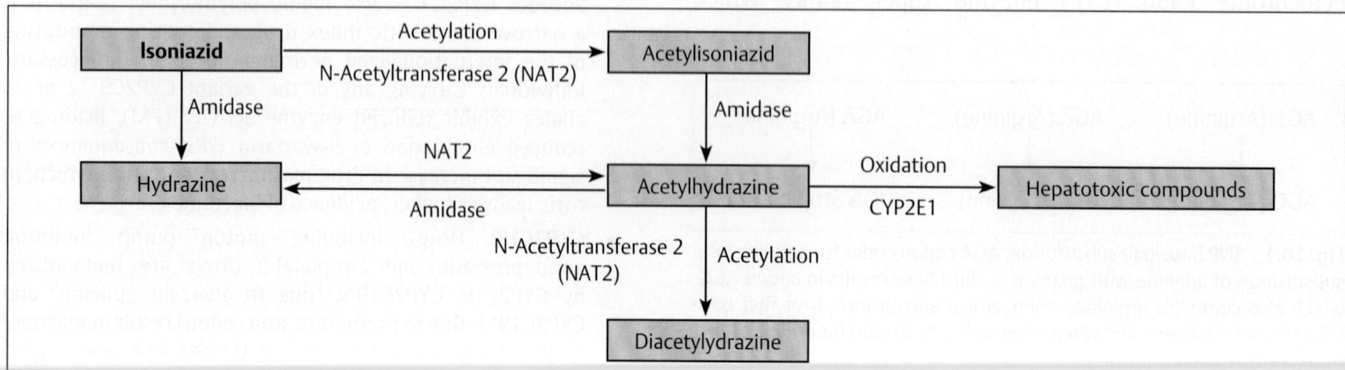

Fig. 10.2 Schematic diagram of the biotransformation of isoniazid.

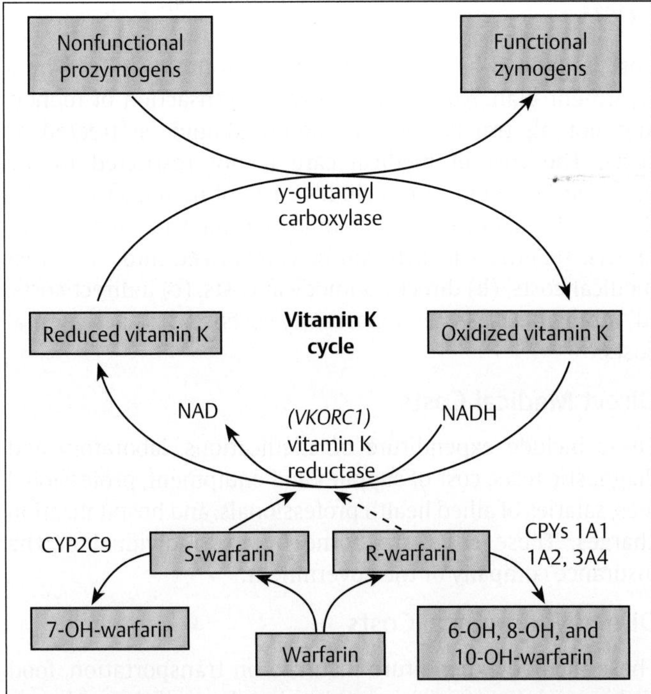

Fig. 10.3 Schematic diagram showing mechanism of action of warfarin.

Human epidermal growth factor receptor 2 (HER2) is overexpressed in 20% of metastatic breast cancers and is associated with aggressive cancer growth and poor survival. Trastuzumab, an anticancer drug, blocked HER2-mediated tumor growth and showed improvement in survival. HER2 testing is mandatory to identify patient who will respond to trastuzumab.

Epidermal growth factor receptor (EGFR) overexpression in head and neck, colon and rectal carcinoma is associated with poor prognosis. Patients with colorectal carcinoma carrying activating K-Ras gene mutation do not benefit from anti-EGRF therapy with cetuximab and panitumumab.

Pharmacogenomic Biomarkers in Drug Labeling

Drug labels are regularly updated to include pharmacogenetic information. A total of 261 drugs and 362 drug biomarkers pairs have been identified by FDA. The labeling includes specific actions to be taken, based on the biomarker information for some drugs, and the table can be accessed from the website– https://www.fda.gov/drugs/science-and-research-drugs/table-pharmacogenomic-biomarkers-drug-labeling. Information about genetic polymorphism and implicated drugs can also be accessed from *pharmgkb.org*, which provides information about clinical guidelines and drug labels concerning drugs and pharmacogenomic variations.

Challenges in Pharmacogenomic Implementation

The increasing understanding of pharmacogenomics will help clinicians to predict the drug therapy outcomes, based on the patient's genotype. Challenges in implementing pharmacogenomics in clinical practice are as follows:

- Clinician's knowledge about genetic determinants of drug response.
- Availability of biomarker testing.
- Multiple genes are likely to be involved in certain drug behaviors, making it very complex to identify the biomarkers.
- Pharmacoeconomics of biomarkers testing.

Application of Pharmacogenomics to Disease Management and Drug Development

Predicting a drug response prior to initiating a drug therapy does limit treatment options, but application of pharmacogenomics has its advantages:

- It eliminates the trial and error approach to drug prescription and consequent adverse drug reactions, for example, use of abacavir in HIV infection.
- It allows a clinician to avoid certain medications or modulate the dose if pharmacogenetic variability predisposes to adverse effects, for example, warfarin and clopidogrel dose modification for desired effect.
- It decreases the overall cost of health care by reducing the cost of managing the adverse reaction associated with polymorphism.
- It helps in development of new drugs, for example, imatinib, a selective tyrosine kinase inhibitor, was created for treatment of chronic myeloid leukemia that are Philadelphia chromosome positive.
- It promotes development of new drugs, focusing on treating genetically determined rare disease.

Ethical Issues

The "genetic information nondiscrimination law" prohibits health insurance companies and employers from discriminating against individuals based on genetic information.

Although pharmacogenomics is in its infancy with multiple challenges, understanding the genetic basis of variability in drug response to medication and accordingly modification of the prescription will become a necessary trend in drug and dose selection in the coming future.

Pharmacoeconomics

Health care around the globe has made great progress in the past few decades coupled with the impressive advancement in technology and understanding of human disease and treatment options. Every clinician is responsible for providing high-quality care which is most economical to the patient, but in this pursuit, she or he may not be able to provide the best treatment. Health care researchers from various disciplines have developed methods for the evaluation of the economic effects on treatment modalities. Pharmacoeconomics is the evolving discipline of health economics, which is dedicated to the study of how different treatment modalities influence the consumption of resources in monetary terms. Pharmacoeconomics is defined as "the description and analysis of the cost of drug therapy to health care system and society."

Genesis of Pharmacoeconomics (PH1.2)

In 1978, McGham, Rowland, and Bootman from the University of Minnesota introduced the concept of cost benefit and cost effectiveness analysis. The term, pharmacoeconomic, was first used in 1986 by Ray Townsend in a public forum as the description and analysis of the cost of drug therapy to health system and society. Health economic studies at that time were largely used to guide government policies dealing with reimbursement for health care services or drugs and health policy issues. At the same time, evidence-based medicine gained momentum, and therapeutic options had to be analyzed both therapeutically and economically. Pharmaceutical companies in various countries had to submit an economic study on the implications of introducing new drugs for the government to consider placing the drug on the formulary for government reimbursement. This trend soon followed for all new drugs and treatment modalities in all countries, and the discipline of pharmacoeconomic became recognized.

Goals of Pharmacoeconomics

Pharmacoeconomics addresses the economic, clinical, and humanistic aspects of health care interventions. The goals of pharmacoeconomic evaluation are:

1. To identify, measure, and compare the costs, risks, and benefits of drug therapy or treatment modality to health care system and society.
2. To determine which alternative treatment provides the best health outcome for the resources invested for an individual patient.
3. To effectively manage the hospital formulary.
4. To design economically viable health programs.
5. To formulate health insurance policy guidelines.
6. To guide new drug development.
7. To regulate drug pricing.
8. To efficiently allocate budget in health care systems.

The need for pharmacoeconomic analysis has increased over the last few decades due to increase in health care spending as a result of improved life expectancy, better technology, greater expectations, increased standards of living, and an increased demand in quality of health care. Increasing health expenditure has forced clinicians to find the best therapy at the lowest price. Availability of numerous drug options and well-informed patients also generate the need for economic assessment of health care costs.

Pharmacoeconomic Evaluation

The three dimensions of health economic evaluation are as follows:

1. Costs.
2. Consequences (benefits).
3. Perspective.

Costs

Cost is defined as the value of the resources utilized by a treatment plan. Not all costs involve transaction of money, and not all transactions of money should be treated as costs. The cost of medical care is not restricted to the purchase price but also includes costs of manufacturing the drugs, administration, and monitoring for and treating side effects. Health care costs can be categorized into: (a) direct medical costs, (b) direct nonmedical costs, (c) indirect costs, (d) intangible costs, (e) opportunity costs, and (f) incremental costs.

Direct Medical Costs

These include expenditure on medications, laboratory and diagnostic tests, cost of supplies and equipment, professional fees, salaries of allied health professionals, and hospitalization charges. These costs are borne by the individual or the insurance company or the government.

Direct Nonmedical Costs

These include expenditure incurred on transportation, food and special diets, special clothing, hotel stay if the patient is going to a distant location, home aides, and modification of homes to accommodate an ill individual—like making a ramp for wheel chair accessibility or bar handles for support. These costs are usually paid as out-of-pocket expenses and not reimbursed.

Indirect Costs

These represent the nonmedical cost of morbidity and mortality and include loss of earnings or income forgone due to premature death. It varies between individuals, depending on the duration and type of illness and the patient's earning capacity.

Intangible Costs

These are the cost of pain, grief, suffering, and inconvenience. They are difficult to measure in monetary terms and are often omitted in clinical economics research.

Opportunity Costs

These signify the monetary advantage skipped when choosing one treatment in place of an alternative treatment.

Incremental Costs

These are the extra costs required to avail an extra unit of benefit and are expressed as incremental cost effectiveness (ICER) ratio.

Consequences

Consequences or benefits are an important component for pharmacoeconomic evaluation and are categorized as economic, clinical, and humanistic outcomes; and they may be either positive, negative, or intermediate final outcome. A proposed model for outcomes evaluations is the ECHO model

Economic outcomes are the direct, indirect, and intangible costs of a treatment coordinated to the outcomes of an alternative treatment.

Clinical consequences are the medical situations happening as a result of disease or treatment.

Humanistic consequences are the result of treatment on patient's quality of life, which is measured by physical functioning, social functioning, well-being, and satisfaction. It is the indirect cost linked with the period lost from work.

Positive outcome means improved health manifested as life years gained after treatment and improved health related quality of life. Negative outcome is manifested either as treatment failure, drug resistance, adverse drug reaction, toxicity, or death.

Perspective

Costs and consequences can be calculated with regard to the patient's, the payer's, the provider's, and the society's point of view (perspective). Cost of medical care may not be solely borne by the patient who benefits from the treatment, so economic evaluation should be made taking into account all perspectives. Patient perspective is of utmost importance.

Patient's Perspective

This is what the patient pays for the therapeutic product or services and consequences are the clinical effects of a treatment option which could be either helpful or undesirable.

Payers

It comprises the insurance establishments, employers, or the government, and from their viewpoint, cost is the "reimbursement" done by them.

Providers

These are the hospitals, clinics laboratories, pharmacy, etc., and from their outlook, direct costs comprise cost of medicines, hospitalization, laboratory investigations, consultation fees, or salary of health care professionals.

Societal Perspective

It includes all the direct and indirect costs and consequences to the society and is the broadest of all. The cost and outcome also differ, depending on the perspective and across different interventions; therefore, it is important for economic analyses to adopt a societal perspective.

Methods of Pharmacoeconomic Evaluation

Pharmacoeconomic evaluation aims to identify, measure, value, and compare the cost and consequences of the treatment options **(Fig. 10.4)**.

Four types of economic evaluation used are:

a. Cost-minimization analysis (CMA).
b. Cost-benefit analysis (CBA).
c. Cost-effectiveness analysis (CEA).
d. Cost-utility analysis (CUA).

All analyses measure cost in monetary terms, but measure outcome in different humanistic terms. Comparing the cost and consequences or outcome of two treatment options are necessary for economic evaluation.

Cost of illness or burden of illness is calculated by adding the overall cost of a particular illness in a given area. It helps in estimation of financial burden of disease. This evaluation is helpful to measure the cost of prevention and treatment options against the illness cost and not for comparing treatment alternatives. Example: cost or burden of schizophrenia, diabetes, or peptic ulcer.

Cost-Minimization Analysis (CMA)

It determines the least expensive among the available treatment options which are therapeutically same in monetary terms. This method is frequently used when approving new drugs and comparing it with existing therapeutic options, comparing two brands of the same drug or comparing branded and generic drugs.

Example: Cost-minimization analysis (CMA):

1. Cost of branded amoxicillin—clavulanic acid tablet is Rs. 25 per tablet.
2. Cost of generic amoxicillin—clavulanic acid tablet is Rs. 15 per tablet.
3. Cost of therapy of a dosing schedule of one tablet twice daily for 5 days.
4. Cost for branded tablet is = 25 × 2 × 5 = Rs. 250.
   Cost for generic tablet is = 15 × 2 × 5 = Rs. 150.
5. The generic formulation is less expensive (economical) and preferred.

Cost-Benefit Analysis (CBA)

It measures and compares the expenses and benefits of treatment options or programs. Both prices and benefits are measured in monetary terms. Investment in any intervention must be undertaken only if benefits exceed the costs and is expressed as benefit to cost ratio. This ratio must be >1 to

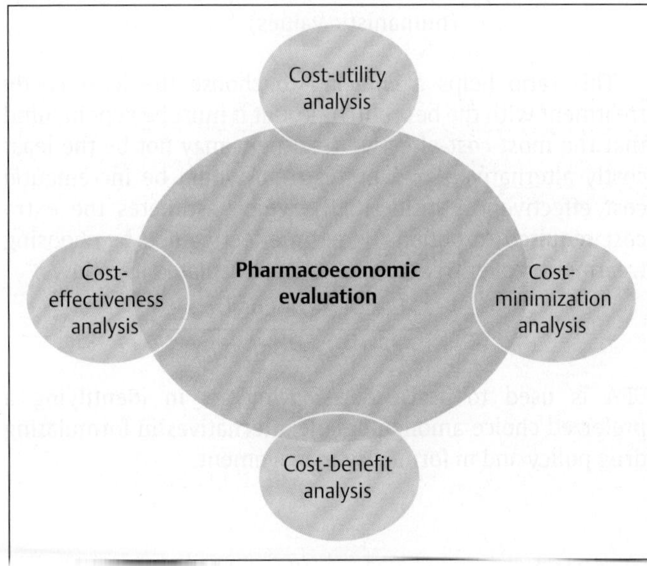

Fig. 10.4 Methods of pharmacoeconomic evaluation.

be of benefit, if it is = 1, the benefit is same as cost, and if it is <1 the cost outweighs the benefit and investment in this is not economical. CBA is used to (i) decide the most beneficial treatment/program from the existing alternatives which can be either surgical or medical and (ii) justify the value of an existing treatment/health program in comparison to the new one or vice versa for the patient or society when the resources are limited. The difficulty with this method of evaluation is that the researcher has to express both costs and outcomes in monetary terms. Values for years of life lost or years of life gained cannot be expressed in terms of currency. Moreover, indirect costs and intangible costs are difficult to estimate and not taken into account here. It is the least used method of evaluation.

Example: Cost-benefit analysis (CBA)

Cost for treatment A is Rs. 100 and value of benefit (outcome) of treatment is Rs. 1000.

Benefit to cost ratio is = benefit ÷ cost = Rs. 1000 ÷ Rs. 100 = 10.

Cost of treatment B is Rs. 200 and value of benefit (outcome) of treatment is Rs. 1000.

Benefit to cost ratio = Rs. 1000 ÷ Rs. 200 is = 5.

Treatment A is more beneficial compared to treatment B.

Cost-Effectiveness Analysis (CEA)

It is a more commonly applied form of economic analysis. It compares health schemes or treatment options with dissimilar efficacy and safety outcomes. It does not compare two totally different types of treatment options with different outcomes like surgical compared to medical treatment or prophylaxis compared to therapeutic. Cost is measured in financial terms, and outcome is measured in clinical terms like lives saved, disease cured, complication prevented or increased life expectancy. It is also expressed as ratio—average cost-effectiveness ratio (ACER).

$$\text{ACER} = \frac{\text{Total health care cost in rupees}}{\text{Clinical outcome NOT in rupees (humanistic values)}}$$

This ratio helps a clinician to choose the least costly treatment with the best outcome. But it must be kept in mind that the most cost-effective treatment may not be the least costly alternative. So, a better ratio would be incremental cost effectiveness ratio (ICER), which estimates the extra cost required to obtain the extra effect gained by choosing treatment B over treatment A and is calculated as follows:

$$\text{ICER} = \frac{Cost\ A\ (rs) - CostB\ (rs)}{Effect\ A\ (\%) - Effect\ B\ (\%)}$$

CEA is used to assist decision-makers in identifying a preferred choice among possible alternatives in formulating drug policy and in formulary management.

Example: Cost-effectiveness analysis (CEA)

New intervention A costs Rs. 100 and is assigned an effectiveness value of 0.9 (90%).

Existing intervention B costs Rs. 1000 and is assigned an effectiveness value of 0.8 (80%).

Incremental cost = Cost A (Rs.) – Cost B (Rs.)
= Rs. 100 – Rs. 1000 = – Rs. 900.

Incremental effectiveness = Effect A (%) – Effect B (%)
= 0.9 – 0.8 = 0.1.

ICER = – Rs. 900/0.1 = – Rs. 9000.

Each unit of effectiveness saves Rs. 9000 with the new intervention strategy.

Cost-Utility Analysis (CUA)

This is a method to compare therapy cost or health care program cost in monetary terms and result in patient's quality of life. It is measured as treatment cost in rupees per quality adjusted life year (QALY) gained. QALY is a measure which includes both the quantity and quality of life to assess the value of medical treatment, and one QALY is equal to one year of good health. CUA is used to compare two different drugs or procedures whose benefits may be different. This analysis is used less frequently as calculating QALY is highly subjective.

Example: Cost-utility analysis (CUA)

If a patient diagnosed as prostate cancer is found to have 70% quality of life, then

1 year of life with prostate cancer is equivalent to 0.70 years of life with perfect health which is = 0.70 QALYs.

If the patient improves to 90% after treatment A with Rs. 50,000 as annual cost of treatment, then 1 year of life after treatment is equivalent to 0.90 years of life in perfect health which is = 0.90 QALYs.

The treatment A benefit = (0.90 – 0.70) QALYs = 0.20 QALYs of life.

Another treatment B costs Rs. 60,000 annually and brings an improvement to 95%, then

1 year of life after treatment B is equivalent to 0.95 years of life in perfect health.

The treatment B benefit is 0.25 years of life = 0.25 QALYs.

Cost utility ratio of treatment A = Rs. 50,000/0.20 QALY
= Rs. 250,000/QALY.

Cost utility ratio of treatment B = Rs 60,000/0.25 QALY
= Rs. 240,000/QALY.

Although treatment B appears costly but in terms of cost per QALY gained, it is more economic.

Types of Pharmacoeconomic Studies

Three types of pharmacoeconomic studies are used, as no single type of study provides complete information, so specific studies are undertaken to address economic concerns from specific perspective. Pharmacoeconomic studies are increasingly being used to help determine the effects of new intervention before they are brought to the market and designed to meet the information needs of health care purchasers and regulatory authorities.

Prospective Studies

These are usually comparative multicentric studies, which yield organization-specific data and also used to assess effectiveness. The limitation of this type of study is that it is time-intense, expensive, difficult to regulate and randomize, and also has the possibility for patient selection bias.

Retrospective Studies

This uses published literature, comparing treatment users and nonusers who are followed from certain point in the past to the present. They are quick, inexpensive, and in the form of randomized control trials. The limitation is that it is problematic to oversimplify the results and might not be proportional due to variation in quality of the trial.

Model Studies

They employ data analysis to predict clinical outcomes in future. It uses a scientific approach and is both quantitative and prescriptive to choose the best treatment option. A prescriptive model is one which is used by decision-maker and is in accordance with the specific situation and needs of the decision maker. Using an economic model can aid the physician to forecast the influence of medication-use choices on a patient, organization, or health care system. It is a quick, relatively inexpensive evaluation method which bridges efficacy and effectiveness but is dependent on assumptions, and therefore decision-makers are reluctant to accept results.

Applied Pharmacoeconomics

Pharmacoeconomics values being utilized to evaluate the cost of pharmaceutical product or other intervention in real practice settings is known as applied pharmacoeconomics. Pharmacoeconomic data is used by clinicians, health systems, health insurers, policy-makers, pharmaceutical industry, health technology assessment agencies, and even patients. It is used in:

1. Therapeutic decision-making: Pharmacoeconomic information assists health care professionals, and hospitals, in making important decisions as to which therapy should be chosen. The goal is to deliver quality patient care by balancing economic, humanistic, and clinical outcomes and taking the emphasis away from "what's the cheapest?"
2. Formulary management of hospitals, so as to include all essential drugs and medical devices which are cost-effective.
3. Reimbursement policy: Government needs a pharmacoeconomic data at the time of registration of pharmaceutical product to be eligible for reimbursement.
4. Pricing for pharmaceutical products and medical devices, so that they do not profit beyond reasonability.
5. Health program evaluation, so that necessary amendments can be made.
6. Drug policy decision and treatment guidelines, so that wasteful or unwanted prescriptions are avoided.
7. Approval of new drugs.

Pharmacoeconomics and Drug Development

For the development of a new drug, a large amount of money, human resources, and technology is needed, along with good manufacturing practices, so that it can be used safely in the general population. Drug development undergoes these four different steps before it is available in the market:

- **Choosing discovery and development projects:** Pharmacoeconomic studies help a company to ascertain if the proposed new drug will generate profit or not, and if the cost of manufacturing is more than the revenue it will generate, it may abandon the project before starting it.
- **Anticipating drug price:** A company's new drug candidate takes a long period before entering the market, and a big amount of money is spent in clinical trials and drug approval. So, the companies anticipate price based on expenditure till approval, the revenue it will generate depending on the incidence and prevalence of the disease, and number competitor drugs in the market taking inflation into consideration.
- **Raising finances:** A company calculates the maximum price and the amount of drug that can be sold at that price and generate finances according to the development costs.
- **Negotiating with health care payers for reimbursement:** The company must conduct pharmacoeconomic study to ascertain the cost and benefits of the new drug, so that it can be reimbursed by the stakeholders.

Healthcare and Pharmacoeconomics in India

India is the largest provider of generic drugs globally. Indian pharmaceutical sector and medical device market is growing exponentially, and it is among the leading countries in terms of medicine expenditure.

Although India is a producer of high-quality drug at low cost, only one-third of its population has access to essential medicines. Limited numbers of people are covered by health insurance in India. Only 10% of the total population has insurance through private health financing schemes. As of 2020, more than 68.86% of the Indian population lives in villages and depend heavily on the government-funded hospitals for procuring health care. Thrust on rural health programs, speedy introduction of generic drugs into the market, and availability of lifesaving drugs at economic prices has remained in focus to bring down cost of treatment

There is a lack of awareness about the concepts and methods for conducting pharmacoeconomic valuations in India, as we do not have policies or guidelines for it. There are few practitioners of health economic analyses at academic and research institutes in India. The first pharmacoeconomic guidelines of India have been formulated and presented to the stakeholders, which has helped in the drug price control, and soon other fields will incorporate these guidelines for ensuring economical health care.

Conclusion

There are multiple challenges in use of pharmacoeconomics, as this branch is in its infancy and there is insufficient training and shortage of health economists along with lack of established guidelines regarding its application in our country. Implementing pharmacoeconomics requires robust training of all the stakeholders in the health sector. Health economics play an increasingly important role of providing insights into comparing the costs and benefits of medical care.

Multiple Choice Questions

1. A 40-year-old businessman was diagnosed with gastroesophageal reflux disease (GERD) and was prescribed metoclopramide (metabolized by CYP2D6) by the gastroenterologist. On eliciting past history, patient informed that he was sensitive to codeine and had difficulty in breathing when it was prescribed for pain relief sometimes back. How will the patient respond to metoclopramide therapy?

A. Will experience extra pyramidal symptoms in one dose.
B. Will not respond to metoclopramide.
C. Will respond very well to a single dose.
D. Will have poor response to metoclopramide.

Answer: D

Metoclopramide is metabolized by CYP2D6 but to inactive product. Moreover, other CYPs, namely, 1A2, 2C9, 2C19, and 3A4, also metabolize metoclopramide. The past history of difficulty in breathing with codeine suggests that the patient is rapid/ultrarapid metabolizer (UM) due to CYP2D6 polymorphism. The patient seems to be a rapid metabolizer, so the drug will be metabolized earlier, and he will show poor response to metoclopramide. If the patient was a slow metabolizer, then there was a possibility of decreased metoclopramide metabolism, leading to increased drug concentration and risk of extra pyramidal side effects.

2. A 50-year-old man with colon cancer was prescribed moderate dose irinotecan intravenously (IV) once in 2 weeks treatment as a single agent. One day before the second dose, patient experienced diarrhea and fever. On measuring the plasma concentration of SN-38, an irinotecan bioactivation product, it was found to be two-fold higher than expected. Identify the cause of increased drug plasma concentration.

A. Homozygous for the reduced function UGT1A1*28 allele.
B. Heterozygous for the increased function UGT1A1*28 allele.
C. Side effects unrelated to drug concentration.
D. Amoebiasis.

Answer: A

Raised SN-38 (bioactive irinotecan) is due to the fact that the patient may be homozygous for the reduced function UGT1A1*28 allele. Irinotecan is a prodrug which is hydrolyzed by carboxylesterase to the active drug SN-38 responsible for therapeutic action as well as dose-limiting gastrointestinal and bone marrow toxicities. Mutation in UGT1A1 gene results in polymorphic alleles UGT1A1*28, which has reduced enzymatic activity. Carriers of UGT1A1*28 variant cannot metabolize the active drug SN-38 and consequently are at higher risk of diarrhea and febrile neutropenia.

3. A young truck driver is diagnosed with HIV and is prescribed abacavir containing triple drug regimen. What test the doctor must advise before staring abacavir?

A. HLA-B 27 polymorphism.
B. CYP2D6 polymorphism.
C. HLA-B*5701.
D. TPMT deficiency.

Answer: C

The doctor must advise genotype screening for HLA-B*5701 allele as occasionally hypersensitivity reactions have been reported in patients who carry this allele. The results for this genotyping are either positive or negative and not intermediate type. HLA-B*5701 positive individuals are at a greater risk of hypersensitivity reactions, with the involvement of several organs. It is an inflammatory immune reaction characterized by fever, rash, diarrhea, arthralgia, and myalgia. It is not related to metabolism of the drug and appears within the first 4 weeks of start of abacavir, necessitating drug withdrawal. Abacavir is not recommended in patients with preceding history of hypersensitivity to the drug as it lasts for a lifetime. Such patients may be prescribed tenofovir lamivudine efavirenz combination. HLAb27 is associated with ankylosing spondylitis, CYP2D6 polymorphism affects metoclopramide therapy, and TPMT deficiency affects mercaptopurine metabolism.

4. A 45-year-old company executive comes with complaints of recurrent pain in the epigastrium and is diagnosed as suffering from peptic ulcer and was prescribed PPI-based anti *H. pylori* regimen. On eliciting previous history of drug allergy or disease, the patient informed us that he had undergone angioplasty and was prescribed clopidogrel which was ineffective and was later changed to prasugrel which he is still taking. What will be his response to PPI-based anti *H. pylori* regimen?

A. No cure.
B. 50% cure rate.
C. 100% cure rate.
D. Increased side effects.

Answer: C

Past history of clopidogrel unresponsiveness and replacement by prasugrel suggests poor metabolizer (PM) phenotype of CYP2C19. PPI like omeprazole and lansoprazole are metabolized

to inactive product by CYP2C19; individuals inheriting PM variants have decreased drug clearance, resulting in higher plasma concentration and hence higher cure rates in ***H. pylori*** eradication. The cure rate after dual (omeprazole and amoxicillin) therapy was 100% in homozygous PMs compared with 60% in heterozygous PMs and 29% in homozygous wild type genotypes.

5. A pharmaceutical company presents a new drug A to treat influenza for approval to the regulating authority with the following information: There is already an existing drug B for the management. As a health economist which ratio you will calculate?

Details about both drugs: Cost of new drug A for 100 patients = Rs. 200,000.

Number of lives saved per 100 patients = 80.
Cost of existing drug B for 100 patients = Rs. 100,000.
Number of lives saved per 100 patients = 70.

A. Average cost effectiveness ratio (ACER).
B. Incremental cost effectiveness ratio (ICER).
C. Both ACER and ICER.
D. Cost-utility analysis (CUA).

Answer: C

As a health economist, I will calculate the ACER and ICER.

ACER for drug A = health care cost in rupees/clinical outcome in lives saved

= Rs. 200,000/80 lives saved.

= Rs. 2,500/life saved.

ACER for drug B = health care cost in rupees/clinical outcome in lives saved

= Rs. 100,000/70 lives saved.

= Rs. 1428.57/life saved.

$$\text{ICER} = \frac{\text{Cost A (Rs)} - \text{Cost B (Rs)}}{\text{Effect A (\%)} - \text{Effect B (\%)}}$$

$$= \frac{\text{Rs. } 200{,}000 - \text{Rs. } 100{,}000}{(80 - 70) \text{ lives saved}}$$

$$= \frac{\text{Rs. } 100{,}000}{10 \text{ lives saved}}$$

ICER for new drug A is = Rs. 10,000 per life saved.

The new drug A is costly as the cost of saving one life is Rs. 2,500 compared to drug B which costs only Rs. 1,428 to save one life.

There is an incremental cost of Rs. 10,000 per life saved if drug A is used. In monetary terms, it may look logical to save this amount, but in humanistic values, it costs only Rs. 10,000 per life saved, and therefore drug A must be approved.

Chapter 11 Dietary Supplements and Nutraceuticals

Prasan R. Bhandari

PH1.61: Describe and discuss dietary supplements and nutraceuticals.

Learning Objectives

- Polyphenols (flavones).
- Fish oils and polyunsaturated fatty acids.
- Glucosamine sulfate and chondroitin sulfate.
- Coenzyme Q10.

Introduction

The Greek physician Hippocrates, known as the "father of medicine," said "let thy food be thy medicine, and the medicine be thy food." The philosophy behind this is: "focus on prevention."

The term nutraceuticals, obtained from the combination of "nutrition" and "pharmaceutical," was coined by Stephen De Felice in 1989 to label "a food or part of a food which offers medical or health advantages, comprising prevention and treatment of disease." "Nutraceuticals" often contain modified/unmodified whole food, plant extracts alone or in combination, semipurified and purified phytochemicals, or a combination of different phytochemicals. On the other hand, nutritional supplements are nutritional compounds that supplement one's diet by increasing one's total daily intake. These group of agents fade the line between food and drugs.

Nearly two-thirds of the world's 6.1 billion people rely on the healing power of plant-based materials for many reasons—availability, affordability, safety or their belief in traditional affordability, or belief in traditional cures. Medical benefits of food have been explored for thousands of years. Modern nutraceutical industry began to develop during the 1980s. They have astronomical profit margins and are being commercialized by the food, pharmaceutical, herbal medicine, and dietary supplement industries.

Dietary Supplement

Dietary supplement is a general term that comprises an assorted class of manufactured products that are taken orally to assist in maintaining good health and enhancing the beneficial value of diet. These are neither medications and nor are these supplements to be considered as alternatives to food. Dietary supplements are not governed by the same process like medicines, and manufacturers need not document their efficacy prior to obtaining the marketing permission. As per law, dietary supplements are not permitted to claim to cure or treat a disease. Thousands of dietary supplements are present in the market in a different formulations, for example, tablets, capsules, bulk powders, energy bars, drinks, etc. They are sold by chemists, grocery stores, gymnasiums, as well as online.

The dietary supplements offer nutrients either extracted from food sources or manufactured synthetically. They could likewise include ingredients not documented to be vital for life; however, they are stated to possess helpful health effects. Additionally, no dose-response studies or toxicity studies are usually carried out for dietary supplements. Majority of the population having a normal balanced diet may not need them; however, malnourished persons, elderly people, cancer/AIDS-related cachexia patients, etc. could benefit from these agents.

Both of these groups are conventionally highly priced as compared to normal food; however, they are consumed due to the acceptance that these agents are concentrated foods packed with energy. Nevertheless, most of these supplements are rarely standardized and statements made regarding these are generally not well-verified.

These agents could be single or multiple ingredient products and could include herbs, proteins, vitamins, minerals, amino acids, herbs, and other specialty ingredients like antioxidants, polyphenols (flavones), glucosamine, chondroitin sulfate fish oils, polyunsaturated fatty acids (PUFAs), diacerein, dietary fiber, etc.

Other nomenclatures for dietary supplements:

- Natural health product in Canada.
- Dietary supplement in the US.
- Food for special health use (FOSHU) in Japan.
- Biologically active food supplements in Russia.
- Complementary medicine in Australia.
- Food supplements in the European Union (EU).
- Foods for special dietary use in India.

Polyphenols (Flavones)

Polyphenols are secondary metabolites of plants which are generally found in fruits, vegetables, cereals, and beverages made from plants. They are thought to be formed to defend plant cells from photosynthetic stress and reactive oxygen species (ROS). The most significant polyphenols in foods are flavones, flavonoids, and phenolic acids. Dietary polyphenols possess antioxidant, anti-inflammatory, anticarcinogenic, antiatherogenic, and other properties. Some polyphenols have demonstrated to be more effective antioxidants than vitamins E and C. They are protective against hypertension, other cardiovascular diseases, diabetes, neurodegenerative diseases and cancer, etc.

Curcumin is a polyphenol present in turmeric, the yellow spice widely used in Indian cooking. It possesses anti-inflammatory, antioxidant, and anticarcinogenic properties. Turmeric has been expansively used in traditional medicine and as a household remedy for traumatic swelling, promoting wound healing, treating sore throats, etc.

Tea too is an abundant source of polyphenol, especially catechins. Consumed as black tea or green tea, it is alleged to have cancer-thwarting property for skin, esophagus, stomach, pancreas, colon, lungs, and breasts. It is also stated to reduce lipid levels and risk of cardiovascular disease.

Red wine is claimed to reduce the incidence of coronary artery disease (CAD). The benefit has been credited to the existence of numerous polyphenols. Red wines have demonstrated to decrease the production of endothelin-1 which promotes atherogenesis.

Besides all of these, numerous legumes, particularly soybean, vegetables like broccoli and red pepper, and spices contain polyphenols and are considered good for health.

Fish Oils and Polyunsaturated Fatty Acids

Polyunsaturated fatty acids (PUFAs) are essential fatty acids (FAs) that have to be obtained from diet, as these cannot be synthesized inside the body. The omega-3 FAs (ω-3 FAs) are a class of essential PUFAs. The main ω-3 FAs are α-linoleic acid (ALA), eicosapentaenoic acid (EPA), and docosahexaenoic acid (DHA). EPA and DHA are obtained primarily in fatty fishes, for example, salmon, herring, halibut, mackerel, and tuna and in fish oils. These can likewise be synthesized from ALA, whose primary sources are flax seeds, soybeans, canola oil, and nuts like walnut.

A variety of health benefits have been attributed to fish oils and ω-3 FAs, notably decreased risk of sudden cardiac death and CAD. They reduce blood lipids, especially low-density cholesterol (LDL)-cholesterol (LDL-Ch) and exert antiarrhythmic and antithrombotic effects.

Glucosamine Sulfate and Chondroitin Sulfate

Glucosamine

It is an amino sugar constituent of glycosaminoglycans and proteoglycans which together constitute collagen and cartilage. It is claimed to enhance the body levels of glucosamine and hasten reconstruction of injured cartilage. It is sourced from crustaceans (crabs and prawns). It is also frequently combined with chondroitin sulfate for osteoarthritis (OA) to alleviate joint pain and slow/halt cartilage damage. Although some patients get short-term symptomatic relief, controlled trials suggest that long-term therapy is ineffective in relieving OA pain and in reversing cartilage damage.

Chondroitin Sulfate

It is a sulfated glycosaminoglycan including 100 or more alternating sugar moieties. Attached to proteins as part of proteoglycan, chondroitin sulfate is a constituent of cartilage and bone. Commercially, it is manufactured from animal cartilage. It is thought to aid cartilage hold water, augment shock absorbing property of collagen, and prevent/reverse cartilage loss when combined with glucosamine, although the definite benefits, if any, are contentious.

Side effects like abdominal pain, dyspepsia, constipation, or diarrhea are minimal. It is contraindicated in subjects with shellfish allergy.

Coenzyme Q10

Coenzyme Q10 (CoQ10) or ubiquinone is a natural antioxidant existing in the mitochondria of many organs like skeletal muscle, heart, liver, etc. It is also obtainable from meat, fish, seafood, and vegetable oils. It functions as a cofactor in the electron transport chain and in synthesis of ATP. Since it is an antioxidant, it thwarts generation of free radicals and alterations of lipids, proteins and DNA. CoQ10 defends cells from damage. Ageing and certain medical disorders are related to reduced CoQ10 levels; however, benefits of CoQ10 supplementation in these situations are likewise not confirmed. However, most healthy people have sufficient CoQ10 in the body, and the value of supplementing more is controversial.

CoQ10 is believed to allay fatigue, enhance energy, and increase immunity. It is also stated to slow the advance of Parkinson's disease, Alzheimer's disease, and periodontal disease. The following conditions, albeit controversially, are said to benefit: ischemic heart disease, hypertension, muscle aches, statin-induced myopathy, heart failure, and radiation injury. It is generally well-tolerated; side effects comprise nausea, heart burn, anorexia, and diarrhea, which are mild in severity and infrequent. It can reduce the anticoagulant activity of warfarin; simultaneous use is avoided.

Diacerein

It is a diacetylated derivative of rhein, an anthraquinone purgative obtained from rhubarb. Diacerein has been consumed for osteoarthritis in certain European and Asian countries since 1994, however, it was approved by the US Food and Drugs Administration (FDA) only in 2008. It is believed to be chondroprotective in nature, which acts by inhibiting synthesis of IL-1β which, in turn, is instrumental in cartilage breakdown. It also enhances synthesis of TGFβ, which activates chondrocyte production. Diacerein, likewise, slows superoxide production, chemotaxis, and phagocytic action of neutrophils. It acts slowly to relieve pain of OA, taking one month or more. In clinical trials and meta-analysis, diacerein has been demonstrated to possess actions similar to nonsteroidal anti-inflammatory drugs (NSAIDs) for OA after 1-month therapy. Pain relief continued for few months even following the stoppage of the medicine. The common side effect includes diarrhea, which restricts its use. Mild skin rashes are also common, and it has the potential to cause hepatobiliary disorders.

Multiple Choice Questions

1. Curcumin is a polyphenol present in:

A. Grapes.

B. Coenzyme Q10.

C. Chondroitin.

D. Turmeric.

Answer: D

Curcumin is a polyphenol present in turmeric, the yellow spice widely used in Indian cooking. It possesses anti-inflammatory, antioxidant, and anticarcinogenic properties. Turmeric has been expansively used in traditional medicine and as a household remedy for traumatic swelling, promoting wound healing, treating sore throats, etc.

2. The following are features of glucosamine EXCEPT:

A. It is an amino sugar constituent of glycosaminoglycans and proteoglycans, which together constitute collagen.

B. It is claimed to hasten reconstruction of injured cartilage.

C. It is sourced from crustaceans (crabs and prawns).

D. It is a sulfated glycosaminoglycan.

Answer: D

It is an amino sugar constituent of glycosaminoglycans and proteoglycans, which together constitute collagen and cartilage. It is claimed to enhance the body levels of glucosamine and hasten reconstruction of injured cartilage. It is sourced from crustaceans (crabs and prawns). It is also frequently combined with chondroitin sulfate for osteoarthritis (OA) to alleviate joint pain and slow down/halt cartilage damage. Although some patients get short-term symptomatic relief, controlled trials suggest that long-term therapy is ineffective in relieving OA pain and in reversing cartilage damage. Chondroitin sulfate is a sulfated glycosaminoglycan.

3. The following are features of PUFA, EXCEPT:

A. Omega-3 FAs (ω-3 FAs) are a class of essential PUFAs.

B. They are essential fatty acids (FAs) that are synthesized inside the body.

C. The main ω-3 FAs are α-linoleic acid (ALA), eicosapentaenoic acid (EPA), and docosahexaenoic acid (DHA).

D. EPA and DHA are obtained primarily in fatty fishes.

Answer: B

Polyunsaturated fatty acids (PUFAs) are essential fatty acids (FAs) that have to be obtained from diet, as these cannot be synthesized inside the body.

4. Which of the following about coenzyme Q10 is true?

A. It is widely used in Indian cooking.

B. It is also called ubiquinone.

C. It is sourced from crustaceans (crabs and prawns).

D. It is an amino sugar.

Answer: C

Coenzyme Q10 (CoQ10) or ubiquinone is a natural antioxidant existing in the mitochondria of many organs such as the skeletal muscle, heart, and liver. It is also obtainable from meat, fish, seafood, and vegetable oils. It functions as a cofactor in the electron transport chain and in synthesis of ATP. Since it is an antioxidant, it thwarts generation of free radicals and alterations of lipids, proteins, and DNA. CoQ10 defends cells from damage. Ageing and certain medical disorders are related to reduced CoQ10 levels; however, benefits of CoQ10 supplementation in these situations are likewise not confirmed.

5. The following are features of diacerein, EXCEPT:

A. It is a diacetylated derivative of rhein.

B. It is an anthraquinone purgative obtained from rhubarb.

C. It has been consumed for osteoarthritis in European and Asian countries.

D. It is stated to reduce lipid levels and risk of cardiovascular disease.

Answer: D

It is a diacetylated derivative of rhein, an anthraquinone purgative obtained from rhubarb. Diacerein has been consumed for osteoarthritis in certain European and Asian countries since 1994. Red wine is claimed to reduce the incidence of coronary artery disease (CAD).

Drug Regulations, Acts, and Other Legal Aspects

Sachin Parab and Prasan R. Bhandar

PH1.63: Describe drug regulations, acts, and other legal aspects.

Learning Objectives

- Drugs regulatory system in India.
- Schedules under the drugs and cosmetics rules.

Drugs Regulatory System in India

Drug Regulatory Authority

The drug regulatory authority (DRA) is the agency that creates and executes most of the legislation and regulations on pharmaceuticals. Its primary role is to safeguard the quality, safety, and efficacy of drugs as well as the correctness of product information. This is accomplished by formulating some rules so that the manufacture, procurement, import, export, distribution, supply and sale of drugs, product promotion and advertising, and clinical trials are carried out as per stated criteria.

The primary legislation that controls manufacture import, distribution, and sale of drugs and cosmetics in India is the "Drugs and Cosmetics Act, 1940" (D&C Act)–and its subordinate legislation, the "Drugs and Cosmetics Rules, 1945" (D&C Rules). The act and rules pertain to all classes of medicines, for example, allopathic (modern medicine), Ayurvedic, Siddha, Unani, and homeopathic, whether manufactured in India or imported, and possess nationwide applicability.

Functions of Regulatory Authority

These include the following:

1. Product registration (drug evaluation and authorization, and monitoring of drug efficacy and safety).
2. Regulation of drug manufacturing, importation, and distribution.
3. Regulation and control of drug promotion and information.
4. Adverse drug reaction monitoring.
5. Licensing of premises, persons, and practices.
6. The main goal of drug regulation is to guarantee safety, efficacy, and quality of drugs.

Medical Regulatory Structure in India

These comprise the following:

1. Ministry of Health and Family Welfare (MHFW).
2. National drug authority.
3. State-level authority.
4. Central Drugs Standard Control Organisation (CDSCO)

Regulatory influence on the quality, safety, and efficacy of drugs in the country is implemented by a central legislation termed the Drugs and Cosmetics Act, 1940, and the rules made thereunder. The state governments allot licensing of manufacturing and sales sites, while the central government permits imports and permissions for marketing of new drugs in the country and for conduct of clinical trials. The MHFW is an Indian government ministry responsible for health policy in India. It is likewise accountable for all government programs concerning family planning in India. The ministry consists of two departments, namely, the Department of Health and Family Welfare and the Department of Health Research (DHR).

Department of Health

This department is responsible for the implementation of the 13 national health programs. It also includes the Medical Council of India, Food Safety and Standards Authority of India, and the CDSCO.

Department of Welfare

This includes the Central Drug Research Institute (CDRI), Lucknow, and the Indian Council of Medical Research (ICMR), New Delhi. The DHR has a scheme to provide advanced training in India and abroad to medical and health research personnel in cutting-edge research areas concerning medicine and health to create trained human resource for carrying out research activities.

CDSCO

It is the national regulatory body for Indian pharmaceuticals and medical devices. Within CDSCO, DCGI (Drug Controller General of India) controls pharmaceutical and medical devices under the scope of MHFW.

Functions of CDSCO

These include:

1. To protect and promote public health.
2. To safeguard and enhance the public health by assuring the safety, efficacy, and quality of the drugs, cosmetics, and medical devices.
3. Regulatory control over import, manufacturing, sale, and distribution of drugs.
4. Approval of certain drugs and clinical trials.

5. Meetings of the Drug Consultative Committee (DCC) and the Drug Technical Advisory Board (DTAB).
6. Approval for licenses as Central License Approving Authority.
7. Coordination with activities of state drug control organization.
8. DCGI:
   a. He/she is responsible for approval of new drugs, medical devices, and clinical trials to be conducted in India.
   b. He/she is appointed by the central government.
   c. The DCGI is advised by the DTAB.

Labeling of Medicines and Patient Information

The Rule 96 (Manner of Labelling) of the D&C Rules mandates that the following minimum information must be put on the label of all modern system medicines:

1. Proper (generic) name and trade (brand) name of the drug, if any, should be printed in the same font but proper (generic) name must be at least two font sizes larger than the brand or trade name.
2. Net contents and content of the active ingredients.
3. Name and address of the manufacturer along with manufacturing license number.
4. Distinctive batch number, date of manufacture, and expiry date.
5. Maximum retail price (MRP) inclusive of all taxes.

Schedules under the Drugs and Cosmetics Rules

The D&C Rules comprise numerous schedules to assist the rules. However, only a limited schedules are related to modern medicine drugs.

- Schedule A: Comprises specimens of prescribed forms for preparing different applications, allotting certificates, permits, licenses, etc.
- Schedule B: Recommends fees for tests/analysis by the central or state drugs laboratories.
- Schedule C: Is concerned with biological and special products, for example, sera, vaccines, toxins, antitoxins, insulin, etc.
- Schedule D: Explains exceptions concerning import of substances not for medicinal use or those used both as food and drugs.
- Schedule F: Specifies prerequisites for functioning of blood banks.
- Schedule G: Lists drugs that shall bear the label: "Schedule G prescription drug–caution: It is dangerous to take this preparation except under medical supervision." This schedule contains some anticancer, diuretic, antiepileptic, antidiuretic, and many antihistaminic drugs.
- Schedule H: These are prescription drugs, which should be labeled: "Schedule H prescription drug–caution: Not to be sold by retail without the prescription of a Registered Medical Practitioner." Most of the drugs are listed under this schedule.
- Schedule I: Omitted.
- Schedule J: Diseases and ailments (e.g., AIDS, baldness, gangrene, glaucoma, etc.) for which no drug may purport or claim to prevent or cure are listed in this schedule.
- Schedule K: It states conditions for grant of exemption from the provisions of Chapter IV of D&C Act. This comprises medicines listed as "Household remedies," for example, aspirin, paracetamol, pain balms, antacids, ointment for burns, etc., and provides that these can be sold from nondrug-licensed stores in villages whose population is less than 1,000 and in some other conditions.
- Schedule L: It mentions good laboratory practices (GLP) and prerequisites of sites and equipment for testing laboratories.
- Schedule M: It states good manufacturing practices (GMP) and requirements of premises, plant, and equipment for pharmaceutical products.
- Schedule N: It mentions the minimum equipment for running a pharmacy.
- Schedule O: It lists standards for disinfectant fluids.
- Schedule P: It lists maximum "life period" (expiry) of drugs and formulations in months under specified conditions of storage. The preparation is expected to retain the labeled potency till the expiry date.
- Schedule Q: Mentions about dyes, colors, and pigments allowed for use in cosmetics and soaps.
- Schedule R: Lists standards for single-use latex condoms and other mechanical contraceptives.
- Schedule S: Mentions standards for cosmetics.
- Schedule T: It states GMP for Ayurvedic, Siddha, and Unani medicines.
- Schedule U and U1: Mentions about particulars to be shown in manufacturing records.
- Schedule V: It enlists standards for patent and proprietary medicines.
- Schedule X: It mentions about certain drugs that are covered under the Narcotic Drugs and Psychotropic Substances Act, 1985, and those needing special license for manufacture and sale. These drugs must bear the label: "Schedule X prescription drug–warning: To be sold by retail on the prescription of a registered medical practitioner only." The label should be marked with the symbol XRx in red.
- Schedule Y: It describes requirements and protocols for permission to conduct clinical trials, and for import and/or manufacture of new drugs for sale.

Drugs (Magic Remedies) Objectionable Advertisement Act, 1954, and Rules, 1955

This act, and the rules under it, regulates the advertisements for some classes of drugs, so that overstated declarations made through the advertisements are not able to influence people and thereby avert them from indulging in self-medication. It forbids incorrect or deceptive advertisements that clearly or subtly produce incorrect imprints regarding the genuine capability/character of the drug, or compose incorrect declarations or else confusing in any specific way. There is likewise a register of diseases/ailments for which no advertisement professing prevention or cure is allowed (Schedule J).

Sale of Drugs

In India, buying and selling of modern medicine (allopathic) drugs is controlled by a licensing system, via the central authority or by state drug control authorities. Manufacture, storage, and sale of drugs without a valid license is an offense. Drug products must only be sold through licensed stores. Distance-selling or teleshopping of nonprescription medicines is not allowed.

Drugs (Prices Control) Order 1995 (DPCO)

This order regulates prices of certain drugs under the framework of Section 3 of the Essential Commodities Act 1955 (ECA). The Ministry of Chemicals and Fertilizers, Government of India, executes the DPCO through the National Pharmaceutical Pricing Authority (NPPA). The NPPA brings out a classification and list of price-controlled products along with their maximum prices. It also specifies the methods of price fixation and price revision. The manufacturer is not permitted to raise the retail price of these scheduled drugs without the sanction of NPPA. Certain vitamins and supplements, along with some nonscheduled drugs (e.g., aspirin), also come under price control through DPCO. For nonscheduled drugs, the manufacturer is permitted to fix the retail price, subject to a maximum increase of 10% on the prevailing price over a 12-month period. However, Ayurvedic and Unani drugs do not come under the purview of NPPA.

Trade Names

Trade (brand) names are controlled by the Trade and Merchandise Marks Act (TMMA). It offers for registration of trademarks for 7 years at a time, and could be renewed at comparable intervals. For any item, the trademark applied for should not already be registered or applied to be registered in India, and should not be objectionable from a social or religious point of view. However, a foreign trademark can be used in India without any restriction.

Multiple Choice Questions

1. As per the "Drugs and Cosmetics Act," prescription drugs are included in:

A. Schedule C.
B. Schedule H.
C. Schedule P.
D. Schedule X.

Answer: B

As per drug rules, majority of drugs, including all antibiotics, must be sold in retail only against a prescription issued to a patient by a registered medical practitioner. These are called "prescription drugs," and in India they have been placed in Schedule H of the Drugs and Cosmetic Rules (1945), as amended from time to time.

2. The warning "To be sold by retail by the prescription of a Registered Medical Practitioner Only" shall appear on the label of:

A. Schedule H drug.
B. Schedule X drug.
C. Schedule M drug and Schedule X drug.
D. Schedule G drug.

Answer: A

These are prescription drugs, which should be labeled: "Schedule H prescription drug–caution: Not to be sold by retail without the prescription of a Registered Medical Practitioner." Most of the drugs are listed under this schedule.

3. Which of the following is prescribed by Schedule F of the Drugs and Cosmetics Rules, 1945?

A. Requirements for the functioning and operation of a blood bank.
B. Standards for surgical dressings.
C. List of drugs to be prescribed.
D. Standards for disinfectant fluids.

Answer: A

Schedule F specifies prerequisites for functioning of blood banks.

4. Which of the following schedules of Drugs and Cosmetic Rules 1945 deals with objectionable advertisements?

A. Schedule F.
B. Schedule H.
C. Schedule J.
D. Schedule C.

Answer: C

Diseases and ailments (e.g., AIDS, baldness, gangrene, glaucoma, etc.) for which no drug may purport or claim to prevent or cure are listed in this schedule. A register of diseases/ailments for which no advertisement professing prevention or cure is allowed is mentioned in Schedule J.

Chapter 13 Prescription Writing

Prachitee Borkar and Viraj A. Shinde

PH1.10: Describe parts of a correct, complete, and legible generic prescription. Identify errors in prescription and correct appropriately.

Learning Objectives

- Prescription.
- P-Drug.

Prescription

It is a written order by a registered medical practitioner to a pharmacist to dispense mentioned drug/device/medicine in the stated dose, formulation, and quantity for a particular patient. There are five "R's" that govern prescription writing: right drug, right patient, right dose, right route, right time intervals.

Who Can Prescribe?

A doctor/nurse practitioner who holds qualifications duly recognized by the Medical Council of India/National Medical Commission (MCI/NMC) and is registered with MCI/state medical council can prescribe allopathic/modern medicines.

Parts of Prescription

Prescription contains the following parts:

1. Superscription.
2. Inscription.
3. Subscription.
4. Signa.
5. Name and signature, and registration number of the prescriber.

Fig. 13.1 depicts a model of prescription and its parts.

Superscription

It should contain the following details:

1. Name, qualifications, address, and contact number of the prescriber. Mostly, these details are printed on the letterhead.
2. Date on which prescription was written.
3. Name, age, gender, weight (in kg), and address of the patient.
4. Conclusive or interim diagnosis.
5. R_x is written just above names of drugs. It is an abbreviation for the Latin word "recipere" meaning "take." This symbol stands as an instruction to pharmacist because during earlier times medicines were compounded by pharmacist and dispensed. This practice is largely replaced due to availability of ready-made formulations; nevertheless, the use of the symbol R_x is mandatory.

Inscription

It is the body of prescription. It consists of name, dosage form (such as tablet, capsule, ampoule, vial), and strength of the drug. In India, it is mandatory to write generic name of the drug and not brand name in the prescription. Also, written name should be legible and preferably in capital letters. The strength of the drug should be carefully written

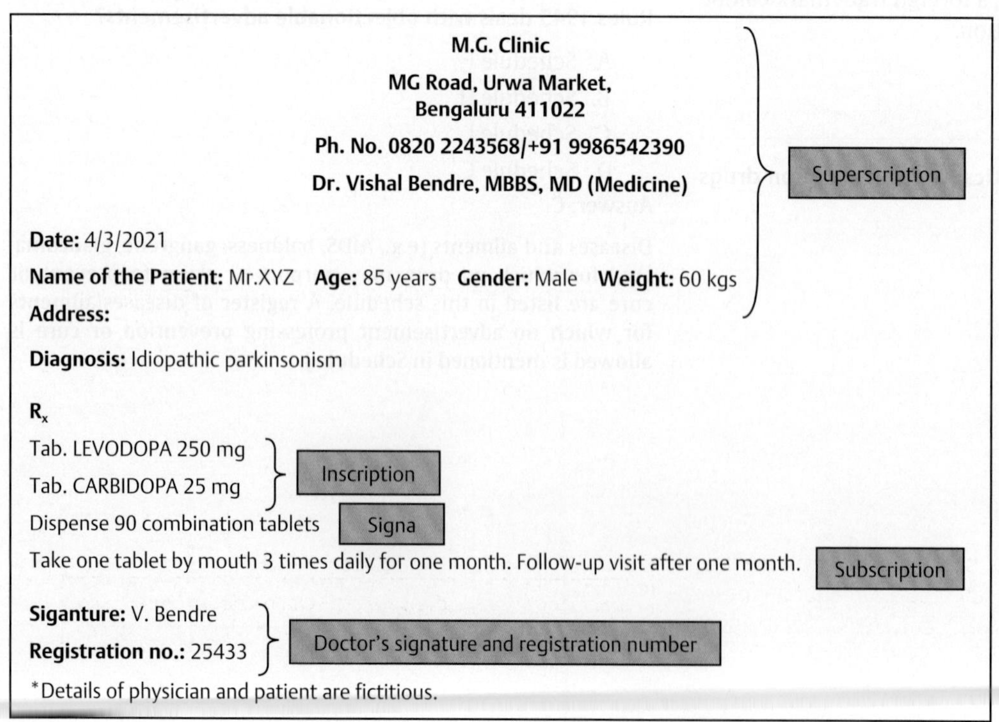

M.G. Clinic
MG Road, Urwa Market,
Bengaluru 411022
Ph. No. 0820 2243568/+91 9986542390
Dr. Vishal Bendre, MBBS, MD (Medicine)

Date: 4/3/2021
Name of the Patient: Mr.XYZ **Age:** 85 years **Gender:** Male **Weight:** 60 kgs
Address:
Diagnosis: Idiopathic parkinsonism

R_x

Tab. LEVODOPA 250 mg
Tab. CARBIDOPA 25 mg
Dispense 90 combination tablets
Take one tablet by mouth 3 times daily for one month. Follow-up visit after one month.

Siganture: V. Bendre
Registration no.: 25433

*Details of physician and patient are fictitious.

Fig. 13.1 Model of prescription and its parts.

and abbreviations/symbols, such as U for units and μg for microgram, should be avoided. When strength of the drug involves decimals, trailing "zero" must be mentioned (e.g., 0.75 mg and not .75 mg). Abbreviations of drugs (e.g., GTN for glyceryl trinitrate or Mtx for methotrexate) should not be used.

Subscription

This part includes instruction to pharmacist and is about quantity of medicine (e.g., 20 tablets/capsules) to be dispensed. It should be clearly stated and must not exceed patient's requirement, as excessive medicine can cause harm if used inappropriately. The physician should also state whether prescription can be refilled. This is mandatory for the controlled substances.

Signa

In Latin, the word "signa" means label. This part consists of instructions to the patient regarding how to take the drug as well as when to follow-up. For example, "take one tablet orally 2 times a day for 7 days." Abbreviations such as TDS and BD should not be used.

Doctor's Signature and Registration Number

This section contains signature of the registered medical practitioner along with his/her registration number. Signature validates prescription, and pharmacists should not dispense medicine in case signature of the physician is missing.

Electronic Prescribing (e-Prescribing)

In this, patient details and other data involving diagnosis of the patient, test results, drug name along with dose, frequency, and duration of treatment are entered into the electronic system, which is further connected to the drug database. Drug databases can ensure that the right drug is administered to the right patient in the right dose. However, physicians must not solely rely on the system and should refer authentic text if required. Advantages of e-prescribing are that errors due to illegible handwriting are avoided and errors due to incorrect drug and dose are minimized. Databases can also point out details such as potential drug interactions and other problems related to therapy.

Rational Prescribing

It is a comprehensive process consisting of series of steps, from establishing a diagnosis to follow-up. As described earlier, rational prescribing involves the use of right drug in the right patient for the right indication at the right dose by the right route (**Fig. 13.2**).

While selecting a specific drug, series of drug- and patient-related factors need to be taken into considerations. Drug-related factors are efficacy, safety, pharmacokinetics, pharmacodynamics, evidence-based, and cost-effectiveness. Patient-related factors are age, sex, comorbid conditions, potential drug interactions (if patient is on other drugs), and genetics.

Adequate and relevant information/instructions must be provided by the prescriber to the patient. It consists of the following.

Effects of the Drug

The physician should explain whether the patient can expect just symptomatic relief or cure of the disease, as well as how long it will take to have those effects and what happens if the drug is not taken.

Adverse Effects of the Drug

There is no consensus among physicians on whether or not to disclose all adverse effects to the patient. Elaboration of all possible side effects may reduce patient compliance, while not informing common ones may upset uninformed patient.

Instructions

The patient must be instructed on how and when drug must be taken. Moreover, duration of treatment and special instructions about diet and exercise to be followed must be made known to the patient. The patient must also be told when to come for follow-up visit and laboratory tests (if any) he/she must perform prior to visit (e.g., glucose level for antidiabetic drugs).

Precautions

The patient should be told if there are any precautions he or she must take while on medication (e.g., handling of heavy machinery while on conventional antihistaminic).

Prescribing Errors (PH1.10)

Prescription errors can be broadly divided into

1. Errors of omission.
2. Errors due to poor prescription writing.
3. Errors due to prescribing an inappropriate drug.

Table 13.1 describes the above-mentioned errors and steps to be taken to avoid those.

P-Drug

P-drugs (or personal drugs) are a short list of drugs that a physician has decided to prescribe frequently for the

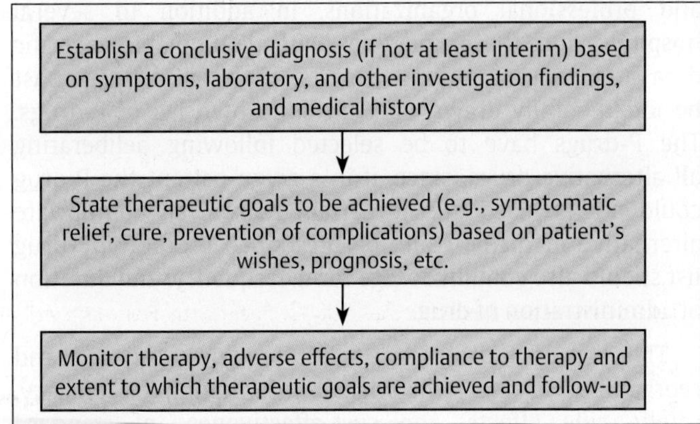

Fig. 13.2 Process of rational prescribing.

Table 13.1 Prescription errors and steps taken to avoid them (PH1.10)

Prescription errors	Steps to be taken to avoid errors
Errors of omission	
Incomplete and omission of certain details such as patient/physician's information or diagnosis, duration of treatment, refill instructions, instructions to patient, etc.	Use of printed proforma for prescription
	Proofreading of prescription
	Use of e-prescription
Errors due to poor prescription writing	
Illegible handwriting can lead to dispensing errors in case of "look-alike and sound-alike drugs"	Write in capital letters and prescribe using generic names
Use of abbreviations such as U, OD, BD, S.O.S, HS, etc., for instructions to the patient or for the drug such as GTN for glyceryl trinitrate or Mtx for methotrexate	Do not use abbreviations
Use of decimal point without trailing zero, e.g., 0.1 mg	Trailing zero must be mentioned when strength of the dose is in decimals, e.g., 0.1 mg
Errors due to prescribing of an inappropriate drug	
Failure to recognize potential drug interactions, contraindications, medical history, or drugs patient is already on	Critical evaluation of case before prescribing. Using authentic references when in doubt

diseases/disorders that he/she treats regularly. Because of frequent prescribing and noticing the beneficial and adverse effects of these P-drugs, the clinician becomes accustomed with them, and achieves expertise and faith in their use. Although thousands of drugs are registered in any country, and likewise essential drugs lists (WHO or National) include around 400 drugs, a clinician usually does not utilize more than 40 to 60 drugs on a frequent basis. These drugs could be deemed to be his/her P-drugs. The word "P-drug" includes the nonproprietary name of the drug, in addition to its dosage form, schedule, and treatment duration for specific diseases.

Instead of choosing these personal drugs arbitrarily or replicating from essential drug lists or from other senior physicians, it is necessary for any physician to wisely assemble his/her own P-drug list. P-drugs regularly differ from physician to physician and from nation to nation due to varying availability and prices of drugs, range of diseases/conditions confronted, distinct approaches, and understanding of accessible information. Standard treatment guidelines for several regular diseases/disorders have been established by the WHO, national health programs, and professional organizations, in addition to several hospitals. Since these guidelines depend on reliable scientific data and consent among experts, these guidelines must be judgmentally drawn upon in one's own list of P-drugs. The P-drugs have to be selected following deliberating all alternative drugs, since, if in a given patient the P-drug could not be used due to certain reason, an appropriate alternative medicine could be prescribed promptly. P-drug list should also contain dosage form, frequency, and duration of administration of drug.

The list of P-drugs must be frequently revised and reorganized as and when latest information on efficacy, safety, side effects, and cost-effectiveness of standard and new drugs list is made accessible. In this setting, the physician must be capable of judgmentally evaluating new and occasionally differing evidence.

There are four objectives that specify why a P-drug must on no occasion be the one that has been recommended or proposed by clinical instructors, senior classmates, or sales representatives:

1. The most recent and the costliest drug is not certainly the best, most safe, or the most cost-effective.
2. By preparing individual set of personal drugs, one can pick up to manage pharmacological principles and medicine-related information in a successful way.
3. By making individual own list of personal drugs, individual can prescribe substitutes when he or she is unable to prescribe personal drug.
4. The physician has the ultimate responsibility for patient's welfare, which the physician cannot authorize on to others.

Although expert opinion and consensus guidelines could be taken into consideration by clinicians, they should regularly think for themselves.

Example for choosing a P-drug for acute amebic dysentery:

A 60-year-old male patient has signs and symptoms comprising bloody, mucoid stools and abdominal pain. There is no history of alcoholism. The diagnosis made by you is of a case of acute amebic dysentery. Select a suitable drug and state its dosage schedule and duration of therapy.

Answer:

The steps involved in selecting a P-drug can be divided into five steps:

1. Define the diagnosis.
2. Specify the therapeutic objective.
3. Make an inventory of effective groups of drugs.
4. Choose an effective group according to criteria.
5. Choose a P-drug.

Step 1: Define the Diagnosis

The ingestion of amebic cysts of *Entamoeba histolytica* in the form of polluted food or water leads to development of protozoal infection known as amebiasis. In the gastrointestinal tract, cysts undergo changes to produce trophozoites. The trophozoites survive on the surface of colonic mucosa or invade it. The cysts are commensals on the mucosal epithelium. The spread of amebiasis is assisted by passing of cysts into the fecal matter (luminal cycle). The cysts invade the mucosa and produce amebic ulcers; this results in either amebic dysentery or chronic amebic dysentery. Acute amebic dysentery is characterized by blood as well as mucus in stools. Chronic intestinal amebiasis is characterized by nonspecific abdominal pain and ameboma. In certain situation, trophozoites could likewise invade extraintestinal tissues, chiefly hepatic tissues and infrequently the brain, where they lead to amebic abscess and systemic disease. Asymptomatic carriers are patients who harbor the parasites without any symptoms; however, their stool is positive for cysts. Asymptomatic carriers can transmit disease to other healthy individuals.

Step 2: Specify the Therapeutic Objective

Amebiasis is transmitted by the fecal–oral route and hence inadequate hygiene has an important part in the dissemination of the disease; refraining from consuming contaminated water and food along with adequate sanitation can assists in interruption of transmission of the disease. However, in the above-mentioned situation, only drug treatment would be discussed. The specific therapeutic objectives consist of treatment of the signs and symptoms, and eliminating the disease and averting transmission of the amebiasis and additional complications.

Step 3: Make an Inventory of Effective Groups of Drugs

Efficacy is the foremost basis for any class of drugs. In the following example, the drugs should possess antiamebic property. The five classes of drugs with antiamebic properties are as follows:

1. Nitroimidazoles (metronidazole, secnidazole, tinidazole, ornidazole, satranidazole).
2. Alkaloids (dehydroemetine, emetine).
3. Amide (diloxanide furoate).
4. 8-Hydroxyquinolines (diiodohydroxyquin, iodochlorhydroxyquin).
5. Antibiotics (tetracyclines and paromomycin).

Step 4: Choose an Effective Group According to Criteria

An effective group should be chosen based on the criteria of efficacy, safety, suitability, and cost of treatment.

Efficacy

The drug should have a rapid onset of action (the therapeutic objective). While selecting a drug, both pharmacodynamics and pharmacokinetics should be considered for a specific condition. Among the five classes of drugs, nitroimidazoles and alkaloids are highly efficacious for acute amebic dysentery, and the other classes of drugs have a lesser efficacy. With a single dose of metronidazole 500 mg, mean effective concentration for most vulnerable protozoa is achieved within 0.25 to 4 hours.

Safety

Majority of antiamebic drugs have side effects. The alkaloids are very toxic medications, whereas there is a higher probability of adverse effects with antibiotic class in contrast to the nitroimidazole class.

Suitability

This is usually related to the individual patient; hence, it is not considered while compiling a list of P-drugs. In this example, oral nitroimidazoles should be preferred since alkaloids are administered by the parenteral route.

Cost of Treatment

There is a larger relation of cost with individual drug products than with drug class. The first choice for this case is nitroimidazole group.

Step 5: Choose a P-Drug

Choose an active substance and a dosage form.

Very little difference exists in efficacy and safety of the five drugs in the nitroimidazole group. With regard to suitability, the five drugs barely differ in contraindications and probable drug interactions. Satranidazole is known to have higher tolerability (no nausea, vomiting, or metallic taste) and absence of neurological and disulfiramlike reactions as compared to other drugs in this class. However, cost is also to be taken into consideration while choosing P-drug. This advocates that the final selection depends on the price. In this example, metronidazole is the most cost-effective active drug. Following metronidazole, a luminal amebicide should be prescribed to avoid carrier state (diloxanide furoate is the rational choice for this).

Standard dosage schedule is chosen: for acute intestinal amebiasis, metronidazole 400 mg thrice a day is adequate. Standard duration of treatment is chosen: duration of treatment for acute intestinal amebiasis is usually 5 to 7 days with 400 mg metronidazole.

In this example, metronidazole given orally must be the P-drug chosen (it should be drug on one's own personal formulary), that is, tablet metronidazole 400 mg three times a day for 5 days followed by tablet diloxanide furoate 500 mg three times a day for 10 days.

Multiple Choice Questions

1. Which of the following is/are part(s) of prescription?

A. Subscription.
B. Inscription.
C. Superscription.
D. All of the above.

Answer: D

Prescription contains the following parts: superscription, inscription, subscription, signa, name and signature, and registration number of the prescriber. Fig. 13.1 depicts a model of prescription and its parts.

2. Drug name in prescription must be written as:

A. Brand name of the drug using capital letters.
B. Brand name of the drug using small letters.
C. Generic name of the drug using capital letters.
D. Generic name of the drug using small letters.

Answer: C

In India, it is mandatory to write the generic name of the drug and not the brand name in the prescription. Also, the written name should be legible and preferably in capital letters. The strength of the drug should be carefully written and abbreviations/symbols, such as U for units and μg for microgram, should be avoided.

3. Signa part of prescription contains:

A. Signature of the prescriber.
B. Instructions to the patient regarding how to take the drug.
C. Registration number of the physician.
D. Dose of the drug.

Answer: B

In Latin, the word "signa" means label. This part consists of instructions to the patient regarding how to take the drug as well as when to follow up–e.g., "take one tablet orally 2 times a day for 7 days."

4. P-drug is defined as:

A. Short list of drugs that a physician has decided to prescribe frequently for the diseases/disorders that he/she treats regularly.
B. Any substance or product that is used or intended to be used to modify or explore physiological systems or pathological states for the benefit of recipient.
C. Drugs that satisfy health care needs of the population.
D. Drugs or biological products for diagnosis/treatment/prevention of a rare disease or condition.

Answer: A

P-drugs (or personal drugs) are a short list of drugs that a physician has decided to prescribe frequently for the diseases/disorders that he/she treats regularly. Because of frequent prescribing and noticing the beneficial and adverse effects of these P-drugs, the clinician becomes accustomed with them, and achieves expertise and faith in their use. The word "P-drug" includes the nonproprietary name of the drug, in addition to its dosage form, schedule, and treatment duration for specific diseases.

5. Which of the following is/are step(s) involved in selecting a P-drug?

A. Define the diagnosis.
B. Make an inventory of effective groups of drugs.
C. Choose a P-drug.
D. All of the above.

Answer: D

The steps involved in selecting a P-drug can be divided into five steps: define the diagnosis, specify the therapeutic objective, make an inventory of effective groups of drugs, choose an effective group according to criteria, and choose a P-drug.

Chapter 14

Basic Aspects of Geriatric and Pediatric Pharmacology

M. Vijay Kumar

PH1.12: Calculate the dosage of drugs using appropriate formulae for an individual patient, including children, elderly, and patients with renal dysfunction.

PH1.56: Describe basic aspects of geriatric and pediatric pharmacology.

Learning Objectives

- Geriatric pharmacology.
- Pediatric pharmacology.

Geriatric Pharmacology

Pharmacology is the branch of science that deals with the study of action of drugs. Recent advances in pharmacology have divided pharmacology into various specialized terms, under which one of the broader areas of study is geriatric pharmacology.

Drug–Body Interactions

Basically, pharmacology of drugs is dealt under two heads. What the drug does to the body is called pharmacodynamics. What the body does to the drug is called pharmacokinetics. Pharmacokinetic properties play a major role in the action of the drug. If it has to be dealt with in detail, pharmacokinetic properties can be studied under four main heads of absorption, distribution, metabolism, and excretion (ADME).

The regulatory authority defined those older than 65 years as people of extremely diverse group. Some of the geriatric patients have various comorbidities, which considerably implicate functional significance.

Geriatric pharmacotherapy is a very important aspect in modern medicine. Life expectancy is increasing, extensive research is taking place to explore drugs, and polypharmacy is the newer approach for symptomatic treatments of elderly patients. There is an increasing spike in preventive goals in elderly patients to increase the life expectancy. The researchers are in line with these points, because in the coming days, older patients will experience more weakness and fatigue with multimorbidities.

Old people usually have multimorbidities and are treated with four to five or more medicines. Among elderly individuals, the pharmacokinetics and pharmacodynamics of most of the drugs are altered. In this condition, the usage of drug regimens with a group of drugs in compliance with pharmacotherapy will be a challenge. Thus, the safe and effective use of medicines is the greatest challenge.

Proper prescription and follow-up of the same are essential in older patients. The systematic prescribing will lead to proper analysis of the benefits and harmful effects of the drugs; moreover, life expectancy and health will be taken into consideration. The existing prescribing guidelines may not be applicable fully to the older patients. Multiple medication may be advisable even though it is available in combination, as the combination dosage forms may be harmful, and the most important thing is most of the drug registries' studies are conducted without taking the vulnerable old patients into consideration. In spite of this, most the drugs individually or in combination are included in the pharmacotherapy of older patients. This clearly indicates that the prescriber does not have definite information regarding the best prescription for older patients.

Older patients with additional risk factors, such as advanced age, polypharmacy practice, multimorbidities, renal failure, and cognitive impairment, are at high risk of adverse drug reactions, which can result in hospital admission or even death. Thus, prescribing for older patients is challenging, because of its complexity not only for doctors but also for other paramedical staff.

The successful treatment of older people can be attained by following these golden rules:

1. Prescription strategy and therapeutic approach to ageing on the action of drugs.
2. Effect of ageing on the drug.
3. Considering the pharmacological aspects for the management of diseases in old age.

How Age Affects Pharmacokinetic Properties

As the age increases, there are several parameters that will get altered in the body. The major one is change in body weight; along with this, there are other changes that affect pharmacokinetics, mainly volume of distribution and renal clearance. All pharmacokinetic parameters are affected by aging. Remarkable alterations are seen in pharmacokinetic parameters such as distribution, metabolism, and excretion, but change in absorption is clinically negligible.

Drug Absorption

Absorption of orally administered drug is directly influenced by gastrointestinal tract (GIT), as it alters with age. Absorption rate of the orally administered medicine is altered due to the age-related variation in GIT. Drug interaction with food and other drugs, as well as comorbidities affecting GI system, must be considered. Most studies revealed the effect of ageing on drug absorption with mixed and conflicted results, with the definite conclusion that the effect is not generalized, that is, all drugs may not have a similar effect on the pharmacokinetic properties, but few drugs such as levodopa, which is absorbed by active transport, may have increased absorption. However, some of the studies revealed that drugs that follow passive diffusion will have a low-grade evidence for age-related changes. Bioavailability of the drug has an influence on age-related physiological changes, as most of the drugs are passively absorbed. As we understand the importance of pharmacokinetics, it is necessary that, as a generalized approach, one should have the patients' overall counselling, which includes age, disease state, coexistent medications, etc. Based on these factors, pharmacotherapy has to be followed.

Distribution

Distribution simply refers to where the absorbed drug enters into the bloodstream to reach the target sites. One aspect of drug distribution which is a very important pharmacokinetic parameter is the volume of distribution (V_d), which varies with age. Technically, in the distribution phase, the absorbed drug travels and reaches different parts of the tissue or the site of action. The total body may increase by total body water and lean body mass under the influence of V_d. There are various factors that affect individually the rate of distribution such as volume of blood, flow rate, protein binding, and composition of body. Almost all these factors affect V_d individually over the course of the ageing process.

The distribution of drugs differs among elderly people. The changes that take place in their body may exhibit variation in bringing the drug to the active site. It has been reported that with age, alteration in protein binding and decrease and increase of serum albumin and alpha-1-acid glycoprotein, respectively, lead to decreased tissue perfusion.

Metabolism

The liver is the largest organ in the human body where drug metabolism takes place. The important metabolic pathways, phase I and phase II, are carried out in the liver. These pathways convert xenobiotic of the various synthesized protein substrates into another form by liver. Drugs and other chemical substances are converted into hydrophilic forms, which can be easily eliminated from the body, and it is responsible for detoxification process, where the harmful substances extracted from the drugs are excreted at the earliest after converting to water-soluble substrates. Metabolism of drug in hepatocytes depends on various parameters such as protein binding, liver perfusion, capacity, and enzymatic activity of drug metabolism. It has been reported in a recent study that geriatric patient will have reduced blood flow to hepatocyte (40%) and reduced mass of liver (30%). Since blood flow and liver health play a major role in metabolism in the older patients, metabolism is affected as their age prolongs. No perfect formula has been established for the capacity of liver function, where the prescribed dose for the cleared drugs in older patient should be reduced. Adjustment in dosing is randomly practiced, where the dose of drugs is somewhat reduced in geriatric patients having impairment in hepatic metabolism.

Elimination (PH1.12, IM10.25)

Most drugs are eliminated from the body via the kidney. Reduced elimination leads to accumulation of drug substance in the body, which leads to toxicity. Aging and common geriatric disorders can impair kidney function, which leads to enhanced half-life of medication. As ageing progresses, there will be declined renal function; the altered function may be of significant degree, which affects the other physiological process. The effect of ageing on the kidney will result in reduced renal blood flow, reduced number of functioning nephrons, and reduced renal tubular secretion, which result in lower glomerular filtration rate.

The altered pharmacokinetic profile of geriatric patient shows a significant effect on the pharmacokinetic properties of drug substances, wherein it is observed that among pharmacokinetic parameters, except for the absorption rate of drug, which is probably not affected by aging, accumulation of drug substances is highly probable, leading to drug toxicity. Depending on the changes in the pharmacokinetic parameters, it is difficult to calculate the dose by considering the extent of hepatic clearance, so the appropriate measure may be prescribing low dose or closely monitoring the patient. The renally excreted drugs dose can be calculated accordingly; also, close monitoring and dose adjustment are important.

Pediatric Pharmacology

It is a branch of medicine dealing with the care of children younger than 18 years and adolescents. The term is derived from the Greek words *Pedo pais* (meaning a child) and *iatros* (meaning healer).

According to the Center for Drug Evaluation and Research, the pediatric groups are classified into four categories mentioned in **Table 14.1**.

Administering drugs to children is very important, and the pharmacology of pediatrics is necessary to understand. Characteristics that we have to look into very seriously are pharmacodynamics and pharmacokinetics. They are essential processes in the body that decide the fate of the drugs. These parameters differ between the adult and child population. Partial knowledge, improper assessment, and failure in understanding these differences and not considering these may lead to morbidity, and in some populations, mortality also can be seen due to the failure in understanding the organizational differences between neonatal and premature group of neonates.

Table 14.1 Classification of pediatric groups

Classification	Age
Neonates	Birth to 1 mo
Infants	1st mo to 2 y
Children	2 to 12 y
Adolescent	12 to 16 y

The first year is very important in an infant's life as the physiological processes influence the pharmacokinetic parameters in early life. Children in this age group need special attention and care, with emphasis on pharmacokinetics.

Pharmacokinetics

Absorption

In children, most of the drugs are usually administered orally. Oral dosage forms are manufactured at low cost and are more easy to administer and acceptable to children than using other routes of drug administration.

Changes observed during the growth of pediatric population will cause alteration in absorption due to the effect on gastric acidity, surface area of absorbing site, GI permeability, biliary function, and other important physiological functions. Similarly, different routes of administration can also affect the absorption mechanism of drugs, as there are changes taking place in muscular tissue, fat, water content, and extent of vascularization.

Distribution

Distribution process is affected by changes observed in total water concentration in the body as well as tissue fat, which may or may not be equal with the changes in body weight. Since there is a change in body composition, there may be change in plasma protein binding, growth, and development, which affect distribution. The major differences between adult and pediatric patients is in the blood flow to the organs and blood–brain barrier.

Body Composition

The total body composition and water content vary significantly between children and adults. As per the World Health Organization (WHO) formulary 2010 for children, the total body water concentration in terms of percentage is up to 80% during birth, 65% at 2 months, and 60% in a young adult male. Similarly, fat content in terms of percentage is 3% in a premature infant, 12% in neonates, 30% in 1-year-old child, and 18% in an average adult male individual, which changes as age increases. Hence, it is clear that the therapy of drug allotted for infants and neonates should consist of drugs with higher solubility in water, in order to attain high plasma drug concentration. The most important thing that has to be considered is hepatic and renal elimination before arriving at a final dose.

Plasma Protein Binding Drug

Since most of the drugs have higher affinity toward the plasma protein, especially albumin, it is observed that plasma protein binding is very low in neonates due to lower binding capacity of drug in fetal albumin. This increased quantity of unbound drugs competes with the endogenous substances such as free fatty acid and bilirubin for the albumin-binding site.

Drugs used in neonates are carefully studied for high protein binding, and the drugs with high protein binding are only considered. Since protein binding is most important, precaution should be taken while giving drugs such as diazepam, phenytoin, sulphanilamide, and salicylates in conditions like hyperbilirubinemia. There are certain disease conditions affecting the protein binding of drug, which include hepatic, renal, nephrotic, and cardiac-related disorders.

Blood–Brain Barrier

Newborn babies have larger brain; hence, it receives more amount of blood (i.e., cardiac output), which is one of the major reasons that some of the inducing agents produce their effect more rapidly in neonates. The BBB in neonates is not completely developed and functionally incomplete. Since the BBB is immature, some of the drugs that are relatively lipid insoluble can enter BBB very easily, for example, drugs such as fentanyl and morphine, and some drugs may easily penetrate into brain. Therefore, the important factor that decides the rate of transport of the drugs is lipid solubility.

Metabolism

Metabolism also is a very important process of pharmacokinetics. Metabolism of most of the drugs mainly depends on liver. Liver in neonates is not fully developed, due to which blood flow in the liver is also low. Immature liver and decreased blood flow result in decrease in the rate of metabolism. It is observed that during the early phase of birth, metabolism rate is low, but as the age increases (1–10 years), the microsomal activity increases. Therefore, phenytoin, theophylline, and phenobarbitone have shorter half-life in younger children.

Excretion

In the early stage of development in neonates, the renal function is inefficient, which may be due to immature nephrons, but as the age increases, the elimination rate increases, which is due to improved perfusion pressure and adequate osmotic load of excretory system.

Multiple Choice Questions

1. According to the regulatory authority, what is the age of geriatrics?

A. 65 years.

B. 62 years.

C. 60 years.

D. 58 years.

Answer: A

2. Which additional risk can lead to adverse drug reaction in geriatric patient?

A. Polypharmacy practice.

B. Alopecia.

C. Dementia.

D. Psoriasis.

Answer: A

The important thing in the older patients is that those with additional risk factors such as advanced age, polypharmacy practice, multimorbidities, renal failure, and cognitive impairment are at high risk of adverse drug reactions.

3. Prescribing for older patients is challenging because:

A. Of aging.
B. Complexity.
C. Systematic way of prescription.
D. Severity.

Answer: B

Prescribing for older patients is challenging because of its complexity not only for doctors but also for other paramedical staff.

4. In an older population, we can expect that drug will be:

A. Absorbed more quickly.
B. Metabolized more quickly.
C. Excreted more rapidly.
D. Excreted less readily.

Answer: D

Since the metabolism is slow in older population, there will be an obvious delay in excretion.

5. In which scenario, reconciliation of therapy should be performed:

A. On admission.
B. After transition of care.
C. Before prescribing new medication.
D. All of the above.

Answer: D

Reconciliation is the process of updating a recent medication list. This should be conducted: on admission; during routine and acute visits by provider; after transition of care; during significant changes in condition; when the goals of care change; before prescribing new medication; when the drug is discontinued if there is any need for that or as per routine orders; when considering the risks, benefits, and burden of any prescription.

6. Small changes in protein binding takes place with aging due to:

A. Increased serum albumin and decreased α1-acid glycoprotein.
B. Decreased serum albumin and decreased α1-acid glycoprotein.
C. Increased serum albumin and increased α1-acid glycoprotein.
D. Decreased serum albumin and increased α1-acid glycoprotein.

Answer: D

The extent of protein binding is the function of drug and protein concentration. Age-related variation will generally be there. Generally decreased serum albumin is evident and unaltered or increased α1-acid glycoprotein is seen in older population.

7. Due to what reason metabolism is affected in older people:

A. Increased in hepatic blood flow and reduction in liver mass.
B. Reduction in hepatic blood flow and increased in liver mass.
C. Reduction in hepatic blood flow and reduction in liver mass.
D. Increased in hepatic blood flow and increased in liver mass.

Answer: C

Recent studies reported that aging is associated with a 40% reduction in hepatic blood flow and 30% reduction in liver mass. Since the blood flow and the liver health play a major role in metabolism in the older patients, the metabolism is affected as their age prolongs.

8. What is the age of neonates?

A. Birth up to 5 days.
B. Birth up to 15 days.
C. Birth up to 1 month.
D. Birth up to 3 months.

Answer: C

9. Developmental changes in the pediatric population that can affect absorption include:

A. Secretion of acid.
B. Surface area of absorption site.
C. Biliary function.
D. All of the above.

Answer: D

Changes during development of pediatrics affect absorption, surface area of absorption, biliary function, and other important physiologic functions.

10. According to the WHO, what is the percentage of water at the time of birth?

A. 80%.
B. 70%.
C. 60%.
D. 72%.

Answer: A

As per the World Health Organization (WHO) formulary 2010 for children, total body water as a percentage of body weight is approximately 80% at birth.

11. Compared to adults, what is the percentage of cardiac output in neonates?

A. 30% higher.
B. 25% higher.
C. 50% lower.
D. 20% lower.

Answer: B

Newborn babies have larger brain; hence, it receives more amount of blood.

Chapter 15 National Health Programme

M. Vijay Kumar

PH1.55: Describe and discuss the following National Health Programmes including immunization, tuberculosis, leprosy, malaria, HIV, filaria, kala azar, diarrhoeal diseases, anemia and nutritional disorders, blindness, noncommunicable diseases, cancer, and iodine deficiency.

Learning Objectives

- Pulse Polio Immunization Programme.
- Hepatitis B vaccine.
- Japanese encephalitis vaccine.
- Measles vaccine.
- Mission *Indradhanush*.
- Revised National TB Control Programme (RNTCP).
- National Leprosy Eradication Programme (NLEP).
- National Malaria Control and Eradication Programme.
- National Filaria Control Programme.
- Kala-azar Control Programme.
- National AIDS Control Programme.
- National Programme for Control of Blindness (NPCB).
- National Iodine Deficiency Disorders Control Programme.
- National Health Programs for Nutritional Disorders.
- National Programme for Prevention and Control of Cancer, Diabetes, Cardiovascular Diseases and Stroke (NPCDCS).

Introduction

After independence, the Indian government had taken numerous steps to boost people's health in the country. Among all the measures, the most important and one of the flagship programs as far as health is concerned is the National Health Programme under the National Rural Health Mission (NRHM), intended to manage, regulate, and eradicate diseases of communicable nature, and focused mainly on improvement of sanitization and environmental condition in the society, which would consequently improve rural health.

Such health programs exist globally, and there are some agencies such as the World Health Organization (WHO), United Nations Educational, Scientific and Cultural Organization (UNESCO), and United Foundation Population Fund (UNFPA) that provide the technical data required and material assistance for the implementation of such programs.

There are large numbers of diseases that are very harmful to mankind; however, many of them can be managed and some of them can be eradicated. The government has taken up this particular initiative of focusing on communicable diseases, which are contagious and can easily spread. Here, we proceed with a list of diseases for which the government has taken necessary steps to control and eradicate.

Immunization (PH1.54)

Immunity is the most important thing in humans as far as disease control is concerned, because it is the main aspect that decides whether a disease can be controlled, and if it can be controlled, how and when and what is the time taken by the body. Obviously, if one's immune system is strong, one can easily avoid many diseases.

In 1978, the government introduced the immunization program in India—the Expanded Programme of Immunization (EPI)—by the Ministry of Human Resource and Development, which was able to cater only to the urban population. In 1985, this was revised as the Universal Immunization Programme (UIP) for implementation in a series of phases, so as to encompass various districts and cities in the country by 1989–1990.

One of the greatest impacts on the health of mankind has been due to the use of vaccines. In fact, proper vaccination plays a major role in the battle against infectious diseases.

Vaccines are basically combined drug formulations that activate the immune system to defend the individual from infectious diseases.

Under the immunization program (UIP) proposed by the Ministry of Health and Family Welfare, numerous vaccines have been provided to infants, children, and pregnant women (**Table 15.1**).

Evolution of the Program

Diseases that are protected by vaccinations under the immunization program are as follows (**Fig. 15.1**):

- Diphtheria.
- Hepatitis B.
- Japanese encephalitis.
- Measles.
- Meningitis and pneumonia.
- Pertussis.
- Polio.
- Tetanus.
- Tuberculosis (TB).

The government came up with a lot of programs for effective implementation of immunization.

Table 15.1 List of vaccines under UIP

Vaccines	Coverage by the end of 2012
BCG	29% (by 1985–1986) 87%
DPT	41% (by 1985–1986) 72%
OPV	70%
Measles	72%
TT	87%
JE vaccination (in selected high disease burden districts)	
HiB containing pentavalent vaccine (DPT + hepatitis B + HiB) (in selected states)	70%
Hepatitis B	70%

Abbreviations: BCG, bacillus Calmette–Guérin; DPT, diphtheria, pertussis, and tetanus; HiB, haemophilus influenzae type B; JE, Japanese encephalitis; OPV, oral polio vaccine; TT, tetanus toxoid; UIP, Universal Immunization Programme.
Source: Immunization division at MoHFW.

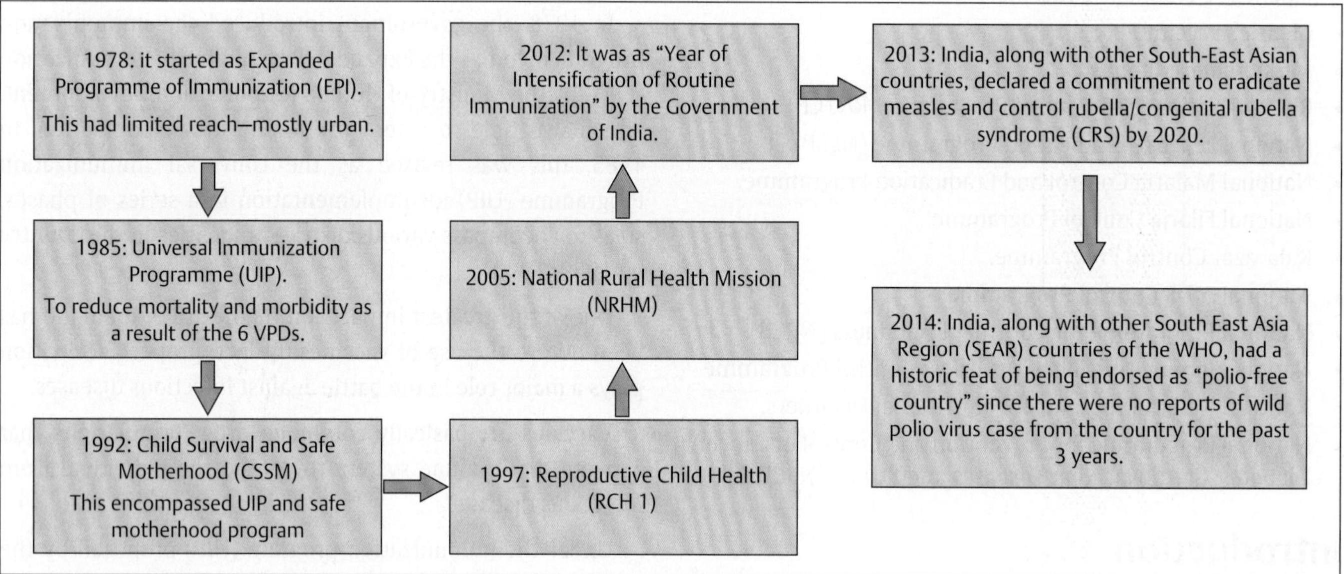

Fig. 15.1 Flowchart of evolution of the programs.

Surveillance of Vaccine-Preventable Diseases

This particular program is essential to generate an evidence base for efficient interventions. Various surveillance models are present in India, such as the Integrated Disease Surveillance Project (IDSP), that are useful for detection of early warning signals of outbreaks. Various other surveillance strategies are in place that fall under vertical national health programs targeted to control forbidden diseases. There are some other popular programs such as the National Polio Surveillance Project (NPSP), which has excelled in the surveillance of acute flaccid paralysis (AFP) and measles in India. Support in the field of technicality and training has been provided by WHO/NPSP for effective surveillance of AFP and measles. Apart from these programs, the National Immunization Schedule (NIS) is also released by the government for effective implementation.

Routine Immunization

The target of the program is to provide vaccinations to 27 million neonates annually with selected preliminary doses and to provide booster doses of UIP vaccines to nearly 100 million children of ages 1 to 5 years. Furthermore, 30 million pregnant women have been targeted for tetanus toxoid (TT) vaccination every year. About 10 million sessions of immunization are conducted for vaccinating these 157 million recipients, most of which are at the village level. According to the 2009 Coverage Evaluation Survey, 89.8% of vaccines in India are dispensed via the public sector (around 53% of the children received vaccination from outreach locations such as *anganwadi* center [25.6%], subcenter [18.9%], and other places [9.4%]), while only 8.7% contribution was made by the private sector. To reinforce routine immunization programs, the establishment of state Programme Implementation Plan (PIP) has been planned by the government. It comprises the following:

- Primary health centers (PHCs) to subcenters and outreach sessions will play a key role in supporting alternate vaccine delivery.
- Urban slums and underserved areas with inadequate services to have retired personnel carrying out the immunization programs.
- District immunization officer to be provided with mobility support and will be given extra duties to support and supervise the program.
- Two review meetings to be organized annually at the state level with the districts.
- Training to be provided to auxiliary nurse midwife, cold chain handlers, refrigerator technicians, middle-level managers, etc.
- Accredited social health activist (ASHA) workers to help mobilize children to sites carrying out immunization sessions.
- Immunization cards, cold chain chart monitoring sheets, and vaccine inventory charts to be printed.
- At immunization session site, bacillus Calmette–Guérin (BCG) vaccines are available in a multidose ampoule having 20 doses to ascertain that BCG vaccine is accessible at immunization session sites. It is also important to ascertain the supply of vaccines as well as vaccine vans and maintain and strengthen the cold chain system across the states.

Pulse Polio Immunization Programme

It was introduced in 1995 and includes children younger than 5 years to be given additional oral polio drops on fixed days in the months of December and January annually. In addition, in 1999–2000, house-to-house vaccination for all the missed children was also launched. Various studies and monitoring programs were undertaken. Consequently, in 2011, there was only one polio case in the month of January. During the polio endemic, India was declared free from it. The nation was eliminated from the list of polio endemic countries on February 25, 2012. Our country was certified as polio-free country on March 27, 2014.

Hepatitis B Vaccine

In 2010–2011, hepatitis B vaccination was launched in all states and union territories (UTs) by the Government of India. The injection of hepatitis B should be administered as intramuscular (IM) injection on specific weeks (6th, 10th, and 14th) along with preliminary rounds of DPT (diphtheria, pertussis, and tetanus) and polio vaccination. Moreover, in cases of institutional deliveries, one dose of hepatitis B is administered in less than 24 hours postbirth.

Japanese Encephalitis Vaccine

The year 2006 witnessed the launch of Japanese encephalitis (JE) vaccine, with the aim to gradually reach endemic districts. It is now getting integrated into program of routine immunization, where the campaign is to immunize children of ages 9 to 12 months and 16 to 24 months. This covers 104 endemic districts, using SA 14-14-2 vaccine.

Measles Vaccine

To control the morbidity and mortality related to measles, a second cycle of measles vaccination is under execution. The National Technical Advisory Group on Immunization (NTAGI) has recommended implementing a second dose of measles vaccine for 9- to 10-year-old children.

Pentavalent Vaccine (DPT + Hep B + HiB)

In December 2011, the government, under routine immunization program, launched the pentavalent vaccine, which consists of DPT, Hep B, and HiB, in an effort to cover vaccination of DPT, HiB, and hepatitis B in the Kerala and Tamil Nadu regions. It requires six injections to deliver primary doses. A novel antigen, namely, HiB, has been incorporated, which provides protection against haemophilus influenzae type B, which is an analogue of meningitis and pneumonia. From 2012 to 2013, this vaccine has been scaled up to six more states—Jammu and Kashmir, Haryana, Gujarat, Karnataka, Goa, and Puducherry.

Mission *Indradhanush*

The Government of India has been proactive in implementing the immunization program, but there are still a few cases of children who have been left out without vaccination or partially vaccinated. To cover such cases, Mission *Indradhanush* was launched by the government on December 25, 2014. The goal of this program was to vaccinate all children younger than 5 years by 2020, against polio, TB, diphtheria, whooping cough, tetanus, measles, and hepatitis B. Rotary International, WHO, and United Nations International Children's Emergency Fund (UNICEF) along with other donor partners technically supported this program.

Revised National TB Control Programme (PE34.4)

The TB Control Programme was implemented in 1962 in the form of district TB center models, which have been running in the country for more than 50 years. They were engaged with TB treatment and BCG vaccination.

Later, in 1992, the Indian government along with the WHO and the Swedish International Development Agency (SIDA) conducted a joint review of the National TB Programme (NTP). A detailed review revealed a few drawbacks such as insufficient revenue to achieve the goals, below-standard treatment regimens, managerial shortcomings, increased dependence on X-rays, and insufficient systematic information regarding outcomes of treatment.

In 1993, TB was proclaimed as a global emergency by the WHO, which then concocted the directly observed treatment, short-course (DOTS) and advocated that all countries should follow it. In the same year, NTP was reinvigorated by the Indian government as Revised National TB Control Programme (RNTCP). In 1997, the RNTCP strategy officially launched DOTS, and by the latter half of 2006, the program covered the entire country.

Some objectives were set during the second phase of the program (2006–2011), such as detection of cases at a global level, targets to cure, and quality and outreach services, which were attained by 2007–2008. In spite of the achievements, there were numerous cases being undiagnosed or/and mistreated, which revived the TB endemic. TB was regarded as the prime cause of illness as well as death among people with HIV/AIDS, and a multitude of multidrug-resistant TB (MDR-TB) cases were reported annually. To attain the larger long-term goal of a "TB-free India," the 2012–2017 National Strategic Plan (NSP) for TB control aimed to achieve "universal access to quality TB diagnosis and treatment for all TB patients in the community."

India's 12th 5-year plan encompassed this program. The concept of the NSP 2012–2017 was "universal access for quality diagnosis and treatment for all TB patients in the community," which targeted "reaching the unreached."

However, the aim is to eliminate TB in India by 2025, 5 years more than the global target. To that end, a framework has been made and circulated among the health care workers, doctors, and civil servants involved in health care, following the guidelines pertaining to eradication of TB in India, as devised by RNTCP under NSP for TB Elimination 2017–2025.

Organizational Structure in States

To execute the RNTCP program proposed by the government, the organizational structure constitutes of the following:

- State TB center for training and demonstration controlled by director.
- TB officer for state.
- District officer with TB center.
- Medical officer.
- Senior treatment officer for TB.
- Senior laboratory technician.
- DOTS provider.

RNTCP-Endorsed TB Diagnostic Methods

- Microscopic examination: acid-fast bacilli smear method:
    - Ziehl–Neelsen staining.
    - Fluorescence stain method under microscopy sans LED.
- Culture methods:
    - Solid media (Löwenstein–Jensen).
    - Liquid media (Middlebrook), for example, BACTEC, mycobacteria growth indicator tube (MGIT).
        - Manual semiautomatic.
        - Automatic machines.
- Rapid diagnostic molecular tests:
    - Line probe assay for *Mycobacterium tuberculosis* (MTB) complex based on polymerase chain reaction (PCR).
    - Nucleic acid amplification test based on reverse transcription (RT)-PCR.
    - Nuclear acid amplification test (NAAT) for MTB complex, for example, GeneXpert.

Targets proposed during the 12th 5-year plan:

- Identification and treatment of about 8.7 million patients with TB.
- Detecting and treating at least 200,000 patients with MDR-TB.
- Improved methods for all types of TB that can have fast diagnostic method and treatment of all types of TB cases.
- Quick accessible resources for disadvantaged communities, which are hard to reach, and groups of needy people.

Achievements of RNTCP

October 1, 2006, witnessed the launch of the second phase of the RNTCP. There has been a significant rise in the success rate of the treatment, which tripled from 25 to 88% during 1998–2013. Death rates plummeted to 4% from an initial 29%. In this program, 662 district TB centers, 2,698 TB units, and 13,209 designated microscopy centers operated within the country. More than 2,708 NGOs and 13,311 patients are also part of this program.

National Leprosy Eradication Programme (DR9.5)

The year 1955 witnessed the launch of the National Leprosy Control Programme (NLCP), supported by the central government, to attain the goal of managing leprosy by detecting cases early. The treatment with dapsone monotherapy was employed on an itinerant basis. The program was presumably initiated for the need of well-defined policies for about two decades. It gained momentum during the 4th 5-year plan; thereafter, it was executed as a centrally sponsored program.

Later, in 1983, it was named the National Leprosy Eradication Programme (NLEP) and achieved success in mitigating the burden of leprosy in the country. Leprosy was viewed as a public health problem. A targeted prevalence rate of less than 1 case/10,000 population at the national level by December 2005 was set by the National Health Policy 2002. Although the program was successful in minimizing cases of leprosy at both the state and national level, new cases kept emerging. The General Health Services (GHS) system undertook the responsibility of providing quality services to leprosy patients.

Objectives

- Prompt detection by active surveillance from the trained health workers.
- Timely treatment of cases through multidrug therapy (MDT) in centers or a nearby village of moderate-to-low endemic areas/district.
- Augmented health education and public awareness campaigns to eliminate social stigma regarding diseases.
- Suitable medical rehabilitation and leprosy ulcer care services.

Components of the Program

- Early case detection and management.
- Medical rehabilitation and prevention of disability.

- Information, education, and communication (IEC), which consists of behavior change communication capacity building in view of effective implementation of the program and increase in human resource.
- Program management.

NLEP Activities

- *Diagnosis and treatment of leprosy*: Diagnostic and treatment services (MDT) are provided at no cost by all health facilities across the country. Difficult-to-treat and complex cases and cases involving reconstructive surgery (RCS) are referred for further treatment to the district hospital. ASHA workers play a major role in creating awareness and collecting data from the villages and providing them the necessary facilities to avail the treatment for which these ASHA activists are paid with some incentives.
- *Training*: Training of general health staff (doctors, nurses, laboratory technicians, and ASHA activists) and also the district-level staff is provided to help develop requisite skills in diagnosis and management of leprosy cases.
- *Urban leprosy control*: Such practices are reported in 524 urban areas with more than 1 lakh population. It includes MDT and posttreatment follow-ups, compassionate prescription assistance, and supervision of surgical dressing.
- *IEC*: IEC activities are carried out for creating awareness and, at the same time, ensuring safety to prevent discrimination against leprosy patients. Such awareness activities are carried via mass media, advocacy meetings, rural media, and outdoor media. Interpersonal communication was the focused domain. Antileprosy fortnight is observed every year from January 30 to February 13, wherein, along with services pertaining to leprosy at the village level, IEC is also assisted.
- *NGO services under NLEP*: At present, grants have been provided from the government to NGOs (43) as a part of the survey, education, and treatment scheme. NGOs work in villages, distant areas, slums, and labor camps, and accountable activities are undertaken, namely, IEC, prevention of impairments and deformities, case detection methods, and MDT delivery.
- *Disability prevention and medical rehabilitation*: Disability correction in people afflicted by leprosy was a problem, which was addressed by RCS. The government of India has recognized 111 institutions to reinforce RCS services. Among these, 60 are government organizations and the remaining 51 are NGOs.
- Dressing cloth, protective medications, and microcellular rubber (MCR) footwear are given to prevent impairment in people with insensitive hands and feet. During 2013–2014, 69,331 persons affected by leprosy were provided with footwear. The patients are also empowered to take care of themselves by means of self-care procedure. As many as 44,412 leprosy patients were given self-care kits in that period.
- *Supervision and monitoring*: This particular program is under observation at varied levels. Monthly analysis was performed and reported via field visits by the central and state officers, and reviews meetings were held periodically at the central as well as state level. For enhanced epidemiological analysis of the disease conditions, priority has been given to detection of new case and its treatment; also, completion of grade II disability is considered for proportion and rate. From 2012 to 2013, visits have been instituted by the Joint Monitoring Team (JMT). The members of JMT included personnel from the International Federation of Anti-Leprosy Associations (ILEP), the Government of India, and the WHO annually.

Initiatives

- *Special activity in high-endemic district:* In states and UTs more than 10% population reported annual new case detection rate (ANCDR) in 209 districts. Specialized activities are undertaken for prompt detection and assessment of the whole treatment. Capacity building and extensive training and development programs through IEC, easy and ample accessibility of MDT, reinforcing district nucleus for making regular surveillance easy, supervision and review, steady follow-up for neuritis and its reaction, self-care practices, supply of MCR footwear in adequate quantity, and enhancement of RCS performance through camp approach have been carried out during 2012–2013 to decrease burdens related to the disease.
- *Disability prevention and medical rehabilitation:* All leprosy patients are provided with an amount of ₹8,000 as incentive as means of compensation to account for cost and lack of income during their stay in government-/NGO-identified hospitals for big reconstructive operation. Funding is also offered to government agencies for the purchase of supply and equipment and other ancillary expenditures incurred for the procedure (₹5,000 per RCS carried out). An additional ₹5,000 is paid for RCS done in camps.
- *Role of ASHA:* A dedicated scheme to incorporate ASHAs was launched to unfold cases of leprosy in villages for diagnosis at PHC and follow-up cases for completing the treatment. They are being given the following incentives to promote their participation:
  - Upon confirmation of diagnosis of a case: ₹100.
  - Upon completing the course of treatment of the case within stipulated time—paucibacillary leprosy case: ₹200; multibacillary leprosy case: ₹400.
- *Discriminatory laws relating to leprosy:* Within laws/acts, there are some clauses that are unfair in nature against persons afflicted by leprosy. The Ministry of Health and Family Welfare has taken up the matter with the ministries/departments/state governments concerned for the modification of various discriminatory acts/laws of this kind.

National Malaria Control and Eradication Programme (PH1.47, IM4.23)

Malaria is one of India's grave health problems. Before the launch of the National Malaria Control Programme (NMCP) in 1953, malaria contributed 75 million cases, with 0.8 million deaths annually at the time of independence. A systematic countrywide malaria prevention scheme was approved by the Bhore Committee in 1946 and was supported by the Planning Commission in 1951. Since then, the national malaria program has had a long history. The Government of India, in April 1953, launched the NMCP during the 1st 5-year plan. Following exceptional success in malaria control, this program was renamed into an eradication program in 1958, with the primary objective of completely eradicating malaria from the country.

The main activities of the program are as follows:

- Framing guidelines and policies.
- Logistics support and technical assistance.
- Execute the plan of action.
- Regular monitoring and evaluation.
- Coordinating activities with the help of the states/UTs as well as in consultation with National Centre for Disease Control (NCDC) and National Institute of Malaria Research (NIMR).
- Collaborate with the World Bank, WHO, Global Fund to Fight AIDS, Tuberculosis and Malaria (GFATM), and other agencies.
- Training to handle the situation.
- Facilitating and encouraging research in NCDC, NIMR, regional medical research centers, etc.

Objective

To reduce the transmission of malaria to a level before it reaches a stage of advanced public health problem.

Strategic Plan

- Periodic screening of all fever cases suspected for malaria by microscopy methods and other available diagnostic kits.
- Treating all *Plasmodium falciparum* cases with full course of effective artemisinin-based combination therapy and primaquine, and all *Plasmodium vivax* cases with 3 days of chloroquine and 14 days of primaquine.
- Development of infrastructure in all health institutions (PHC level and above), with more emphasis on high-risk areas. This should be supported by the availability of laboratory microscopy facility and rapid diagnostic test for emergency use and injectable artemisinin in derivatives.
- Strengthening all hospitals at district and next level in malaria endemic areas as per Indian Public Health Standards (IPHS), with facilities for treatment and management of severe malaria cases.

Antimalaria Month Campaign

Every year, the month of June is observed as antimalarial campaign month throughout the country, prior to the onset of monsoon and transmission season, to improve and enhance the extent of awareness and to encourage community participation in the campaign through mass media and interpersonal communication and intersectoral collaborative efforts with other government departments, NGOs, corporates, and voluntary agencies at the national level.

Externally Supported Projects

Additional financial support for combating malaria is provided in high malaria risk areas. The projects that are currently being implemented for malaria control are:

- Global fund–supported Intensified Malaria Control Project (IMCP II).
- World Bank–supported project on malaria control and kala-azar elimination.
- Enhanced Malaria Control Project (EMCP)
- Six crore tribal population in eight states have been supported by the World Bank. This has been implemented in 1,045 PHCs in 100 districts of the eight states.

Diagnostic Methods

- Peripheral blood smear methods are employed. Two types of smears:
    - Thick smear for sensitivity: gives the data of presence of malaria.
    - Thin smear for specificity: causative organism species identification.

National Filaria Control Programme

- *Wuchereria bancrofti* is the causative organism of filariasis. It is transmitted through mosquito bite, such as from *Culex*, *Anopheles*, *Mansonia*, and *Aedes*.
- Lymphatic filaria is prevalent in 18 states and UTs.
- In 1955, the government launched the National Filaria Control Programme. The program was primarily confined to urban areas. Nevertheless, since 1994, the program has been modified to include rural areas as well.

Training under the Program

The filaria education and research centers are under the National Institute for Communicable Diseases, Delhi, and are located at Rajahmundry (Andhra Pradesh), Calicut (Kerala), and Varanasi (Uttar Pradesh). In fact, 12 headquarters work at the state level.

The eradication of this disease was attempted through the following:

- Annual mass drug administration in a single dose for 5 years.
- Home-based treatment of lymphedema cases and upscaling of hydrocele operations.

Kala-azar Control Programme

Leishmania species (intracellular protozoan) are the causative organisms of kala-azar or visceral leishmaniasis. Kala-azar is a persistent protozoal disorder transmitted by female *Phlebotomus* sand fly bite.

It is currently a big issue in Bihar, Jharkhand, West Bengal, and some parts of Uttar Pradesh.

In light of the increasing problem, well-planned control measures were implemented to control kala-azar.

Active Case Search Plan

The incidence and frequency of cases have been on the rise from search for single case in a year to search for multiple cases every 2 months. The "kala-azar fortnight" was a good move which was effective during which there was door-to-door searching by peripheral health workers and volunteers, referring the cases complying with the case definition of kala-azar, and subjecting them to definitive diagnosis and treatment centers.

ASHA workers are being given an amount of ₹300 to recognize each case of kala-azar as well as ₹100 to ensure a proper and regular insecticide spray in the areas with high risk. Most notably, ₹500 is given to patients being treated at the hospital as compensation during the care. This amended strategy of complete elimination of kala-azar was implemented on September 2, 2014.

The incorporation of the rapid diagnostic kit into the system developed by the Indian Council of Medical Research (ICMR)—a single-dose treatment with liposomal amphotericin B, intravenously (IV) administered in 10-mg dosage—was the critical step in the new strategy. In an attempt to curtail the reservoir of infection in humans, the WHO supplies the drug at no cost.

National AIDS Control Programme

The National AIDS Committee was established in the Ministry of Health and Family Welfare in 1986 after the discovery of the country's first AIDS case. The national strategy for the prevention of AIDS was launched in 1987 by the Indian government.

As of now, the National AIDS Control Organization (NACO) is a division of the Ministry of Health and Family Welfare, offering leadership to 35 HIV/AIDS prevention and control societies for the HIV/AIDS prevention system in India. As the epidemic grew, a regional program and an organization needed to direct the program. Consequently, the first National AIDS Control Programme (NACP) (1992–1999) was introduced in India in 1992, and NACO was established to implement the program.

Timeline of the NACP

- 1992—NACP I was launched with an aim to decelerate the spread of HIV infections and minimize the impact of AIDS as well as the rates of morbidity and mortality in the country.
- 1999—NACP II was introduced for decreasing the spread of HIV infection in India, and to augment India's capacity to deal with HIV/AIDS on a long-term basis.
- 2007—NACP III was launched with the purpose of halting and reversing the epidemic over the 5-year period.
- 2012—NACP IV was implemented to speed up the reversal process and further improve India's disease response through a deliberate and well-defined integration phase over the next 5 years.

Key Strategies

- Intensifying and strengthening preventive programs, with emphasis on high-risk groups (HRGs) and vulnerable people.
- Promotion of comprehensive health care as well as increasing the access for diagnosis, treatment, support, and care.
- Expansion of the IEC services for awareness and spreading the knowledge to (a) general public and (b) HRGs, with emphasis on changes in behavior and generation of demand.
- Capacity building to face the conditions at state and national level.
- Reinforcing and equipping the strategic information management system to draw effective and useful data.

Preventive Approaches

- Increased awareness of the risk factors due to HIV infection.
- Interventions targeting sex workers, migrants, truckers, and transgenders.
- Promotion of condoms.
- Preventing the transmission of AIDS from parent to child.
- Exploring HIV counselling and testing services.
- Safety measures of blood transfusion and timeline of transfusion.
- Needle/syringe exchange programs.
- Mainstreaming of HIV/AIDS activities with all prime ministries/departments of center/state to be regarded as a high priority.

Supportive Approaches

- Free treatment via first- and second-line antiretroviral therapy (ART).
- Diagnosis in early infant stage for infants and children younger than 18 months who have been exposed to HIV.
- Aid in terms of nutrition and psychosocial support with the assistance of care and support centers for HIV/TB coordination.
- Treatment of opportunistic infections.
- CD4 laboratory research facilities and other examinations.

New Initiatives under NACP IV

- Data triangulation techniques for districts with due regard to vulnerabilities.
- Scaling up of programs addressing key vulnerabilities.
- Scaling up opioid substitution therapy for treating injecting drug users.
- Scaling up and improving migrant interventions at source, transit, and destinations along with the rollout of migrant tracking system for successful response.
- Establishing and expanding programs for transgenders by involving community-oriented and engaging approaches to resolve their vulnerabilities.
- Employer-led model to resolve migrant labor challenges, for example, female condoms programs.
- Scaling up the multidrug regimen for prevention of parent-to-child transmission, in compliance with international guidelines.
- Social security of vulnerable communities via the mainstreaming and distribution of HIV budgets among the concerned departments.
- Establishing metro blood banks and plasma fractionation centers.
- Launching the third-line ART and scaling up the first- and second-line ART.
- Demand marketing approaches directly utilizing mid-media, for example, national folk media initiative.
- Red ribbon express and buses (converging with the National Health Mission).

National Programme for Control of Blindness

In view of the progressive increase in blindness in the country, the government in the year 1976 launched the National Programme for Control of Blindness (NPCB). It is a health scheme fully sponsored by the central government, with the definite aim of decreasing the prevalence and incidence of blindness to 0.3% by 2020.

Major causes of blindness are cataract (62.6%), refractive error, glaucoma, posterior segment disorder, surgical complication, corneal blindness, and posterior capsular opacification.

Main Objectives of the Program

- To decrease the cases of blindness that can be avoided, by employing effective identification techniques with suitable diagnostic methods and treatment of curable blind in a phase-wise manner. Overall assessment of visual impairment is the most important criterion of this program.
- To design, strengthen, and execute the strategy for "eye health for all" and comprehensive universal eyecare services.
- To strengthen the Regional Institutes of Ophthalmology (RIOs) as institutions of excellence with upgraded facilities in different specialties of ophthalmology. This strategy encourages the various medical colleges and hospitals in the district and subdistrict levels. Many NGOs' private practitioners are into this program as partners.
- To promote additional human resource development and strengthen the existing infrastructure facilities with latest equipment for imparting comprehensive, high-quality eyecare across all districts of the country.
- To conduct awareness programs among the society on eyecare and promote the prevention approach, with emphasis on the consequences.
- To strengthen the research and development for prevention of blindness and visual impairment disorders.

Important steps adopted to achieve the objectives:

- Focused approach and attention given to publicizing and implementing various programs such as free surgeries.
- Eyecare programs with emphasis on including disorders other than cataracts, such as glaucoma, diabetic retinopathy, corneal transplantation, vitreoretinal surgery, and childhood blindness therapy. Such emerging diseases require urgent attention to eradicate the country's preventable blindness.
- Population screening for those 50 years or older to achieve a reduction in the backlog of blind people; successful organization of eye screening camps and transfer to fixed eyecare facilities of operating cases.
- Refractive errors represent a significant part of the blindness that can be avoided. Screening of children to recognize and manage refractive errors, and to offer free glasses to those affected and belonging to disadvantaged socioeconomic strata.
- Public–private partnerships are focused on the under-served areas. Creating ability of health care practitioners to improve their expertise and skills in providing high-quality eyecare services.
- Activities related to IEC are important and are given importance to building community understanding of eyecare.
- RIOs and medical colleges of the states to be reinforced in a phased manner.

Other than these, there are a lot of programs that came into existence and are implemented, such as eye screening camps in schools and colleges, rural camps, and eye donation campaigns. Steps are taken to collect and deliver to needy.

Initiatives

The government has undertaken numerous initiatives to control blindness in India. Some of the important initiatives are as follows:

- **Vision 2020: The Right to Sight**–A global initiative for the reduction of avoidable blindness by the year 2020.
- **Universal eye health: a global action plan 2014–2019**–According to estimates by the WHO, 285 million people were visually impaired in the year 2010, among which 39 million were blind.

Most notably, two main causes of visual loss were considered priorities, and prevention mechanisms were continuously enforced by delivering refractive care and offering cataract surgery to the vulnerable, allowing two-thirds of visually disabled people to regain good eyesight.

National Iodine Deficiency Disorders Control Programme

Human body growth is influenced by and depends on minerals and micronutrients. Among important micronutrients, iodine is the one that has gained a lot of importance. Iodine is especially required by the human body because it is essential in the synthesis of thyroid hormones. The daily requirement is 100 to 150 μg for normal growth. Iodine deficiency results in a few disorders, which are known as iodine deficiency disorders (IDDs). IDDs are one of the major health problems globally. According to the available information, more than 1.5 billion people globally are at risk of IDDs. In 1962, a goiter control system was initiated by the Government of India, focused on the value of iodized salt. The prevalence of the disease remained high at the end of three decades. Consequently, a new national initiative, the "IDD Control 1 Program," was launched nationally, which encourages the use of iodized salt. The National Goiter Control Programme (NGCP) was renamed the National Iodine Deficiency Condition Control Plan (NIDDCP) in 1992. As a national initiative, it was agreed to gradually strengthen all edible iodized salt by the end of the 8th 5-year plan.

Objectives of National Programme

- To carry out periodic surveys to estimate and analyze the extent of the IDDs.
- Common salt is replaced by iodized salt and made mandatory for the manufacturers.
- The surveys are repeated every 5 years to ensure the effect of usage of iodized salt
- Monitoring the urinary excretion of iodine and use of iodized salt.

National Health Programs for Nutritional Disorders (IM9.15)

Nutrition is the science of diet and its correlation to various stages of health. Food plays a critical role in both health and illness. Either over- or undernutrition is detrimental to health and therefore nutrition is itself a double-edged sword, because undernutrition is especially harmful in early age groups, i.e., childhood, and overnutrition is harmful in adulthood. However, both types are likely to impact all age groups in the immediate future. Some predominant diseases of malnutrition include obesity associated with excess energy consumption, anemia due to inadequate iron intake, thyroid insufficiency disorders due to iodine intake deficiency, etc.

According to the National Family Health Survey (NFHS), 96% of children up to the age of 5 years and have ever been breastfed, but only one-quarter of last-born children have ever been breastfed within 1 hour. Nearly 48% of children younger than 5 years are chronically undernourished. In India, one out of five children younger than 5 years is wasted. For their age, 43% of children younger than 5 years are underweight. As many as half (54%) of all deaths in India prior to age 5 years are associated with malnutrition. Mild-to-moderate malnutrition is causing more deaths (43%) than extreme malnutrition (11%).

Iron deficiency anemia is a significant disease in India, wherein 7 out of 10 children in the age group of 6 to 59 months are anemic. Among this, 3% are severely anemic, 40% are moderately anemic, and 26% are mildly anemic. Less than 50% of these children stay in households that use properly iodized salt. Great prevalence of nutritional deficiency in adults is depicted by the fact that 36% of women have a body mass index (BMI) less than 18.5. About 45% of all the women who are thin are moderately to severely thin, and 10% of women are overweight and 3% are obese. The “excess” and “deficiency” of nutrition are both equally detrimental and have long-term effects on health of people, families, and societies. It is therefore of extreme significance to tackle this issue in order to make the world aware of balanced eating principles.

Nutrient Types

The following categories make up the different types of nutrients:

- **Proteins:** Proteins are composed of series of chains of amino acids:
  - A few of the inherent amino acids of protein that are known as essential amino acids cannot be synthesized within the body and therefore should be explicitly obtained from food.
  - Proteins of animal origin such as milk, meat, cheese, fish, and poultry contain sufficient quantities of all essential amino acids.
  - Proteins of vegetable origin contain some of the essential amino acids in a small quantity. One gram of protein gives an energy of 4 cal.
- **Fats:** Fats and oils are important energy sources and are vital for several biological processes for which fatty acids are required.
- **Carbohydrates:** They are consumed in the form of vegetable starches and sugars; cereals are also an essential source. Energy is obtained mainly from sources of carbohydrates, especially cereals, throughout many developing countries such as India. Carbohydrate provides 4 kcal of energy per 1 gram.
- **Vitamins:** Vitamins are vital to the proper functioning of the body. Two main classes are:
  - **Water-soluble vitamins:** This group includes B-complex vitamins, especially thiamine (B1), riboflavin (B2), and niacin, and vitamin C. Whole cereals, pulses, and other vegetables are adequate sources of B-complex vitamins, while vitamin C is contained in raw fruits and vegetables. Water-soluble vitamins get lost during cooking fairly quickly.
  - **Fat-soluble vitamins:** This category includes vitamins A, D, E, and K which are present in most animal products. In emergencies, the most relevant are A and D.
    - Vitamin A: Vitamin A is involved in maintaining epithelial cell and membrane stability as well as night vision. It is present primarily in animal-sourced foods. However, one of its precursors, B-carotene derived from plants, can be transformed into vitamin A in the body.
    - Vitamin D is derived from skin upon exposure to sunlight and is found in the liver of fish and animals.

Balanced Diet Gives Health and Well-Being

Balanced diet is the only option to maintain good health, and it is viewed as one containing a variety of foods in the required quantities and proportions, which adequately meets the energy sources, amino acids, vitamins, minerals, fats, carbohydrates, and other nutrients to maintain health.

Healthy Nutrition

A balanced diet assists in defending against malnutrition in all its manifestations as well as potential noncommunicable diseases (NCDs). The concept of a healthy and balanced diet constitutes the following:

- Intake of energy (calories) must balance expenditure on energy. To stop excessive weight gain, total fat must not surpass 30% of total energy intake.
- Unsaturated fats (e.g., fish, salmon, almonds, sunflower, canola, and olive oils) are favored to saturated fats (e.g., fatty meat, butter, palm and coconut oil, milk, cheese, ghee, and lard).
- Restricting free sugar consumption (sugar-sweetened drinks, snacks, and sweets) below 10% of total energy.
- Holding salt consumption to below 5 g a day (preferably iodized salt) helps avoid hypertension and decreases the risk of heart attack, stroke, and nutritional deficiency.
- Vitamins and minerals can be obtained from fruits, vegetables, legumes, nuts, and whole grains (e.g., unprocessed corn, millet, oats, wheat, brown rice).
- The diet must include at least 400 g of fruit and vegetables daily. They could ideally be consumed both raw and fresh.

- It is best to avoid trans fats (contained in processed food, fast food, snack food, fried food, frozen food, pizza, cakes, cookies, margarines, and spreads).

Nutritional Disorders

Protein–Energy Malnutrition

Protein-energy malnutrition (PEM) more often affects children aged 6 months to 5 years. PEM has several physical and mental consequences in the short and long term, namely, stunted growth, increased susceptibility to disease, and higher mortality rates in young children. Marasmus and kwashiorkor are two main types.

Marasmus

It is a consequence is a consequence of chronic starvation. The child (or adult) affected is extremely thin (skin and bones), having used much of the fat and muscle mass to provide strength. In conditions of extreme food shortage, marasmus is the most common type of PEM. Symptoms of the condition are:

- A thin "old face."
- "Baggy pants" (the loose skin of the buttocks hanging).
- Affected children might seem alert despite their condition.
- The lower extremities do not have edema.
- Ribs are prominent.

Kwashiorkor

This tends to affect children 1 to 4 years of age. The principal symptom is edema, usually beginning with the legs and feet and extending to the hands and face in more advanced cases. Owing to edema, children with kwashiorkor can look "fat," so that their parents find them as well-fed. Other symptoms of kwashiorkor are:

- Hair changes: pigmentation loss; straightening of curly hair, easy pluckability.
- Skin lesions and depigmentation: in a few places, lightening of dark skin is visible, predominantly in the skin folds; outer layers of skin may peel off (especially on legs), and ulceration may occur; the lesions may look similar to burns.
- Children with kwashiorkor are typically apathetic, miserable, and irritable. They show no signs of hunger, and it is difficult to convince them to eat.

Iron Deficiency Anemia (PE13.5, PE13.6)

Iron is present in both animal- and vegetable-derived foods, but it is better absorbed from animal-derived ones. Foods that are relatively iron-rich include red meat (particularly liver), dark green leafy vegetables, pulses, and tubers. Iron absorption can be significantly improved by eating foods of animal origin and also by increasing the amount of dietary vitamin C. Other compounds found in cereals and tea and coffee severely impede iron absorption. Tea and coffee contain substantial amounts of absorption-inhibitors and therefore should be drunk 2 hours before or after meals rather than with them. Iron supplementation is required to reduce iron deficiency anemia prevalence.

Vitamin A Deficiency

Vitamin A deficiency is the leading cause of preventable blindness in young children worldwide and leads substantially to high mortality rates in malnourished populations of infants and young children. Most dietary vitamin A is obtained from green and yellow vegetables and fruits, particularly dark green leafy vegetables, carrots, mangoes, pumpkins, and papayas; red palm oil is an especially rich source. Vitamin A is stored in the liver.

The principal preventive measures are as follows:

- High-dose vitamin A.
- Immunizing measles.
- Promotion of breast-feeding, which must be persisted during diseases such as diarrhea.
- Development of local growth, marketing, and usage of green leafy vegetables and yellow fruits, and intake of vitamin A–rich animal products.
- Vitamin A–fortified foods, particularly those intended for vulnerable groups.
- Environmental sanitation and hygiene steps, particularly those aimed at preventing diarrheal disease.

Current Scenario

Recently, we can see the dramatic shifts in lifestyle and eating habits, as well as a worldwide decline in physical activity. There is an increase in the production and consumption of processed food. People consume more energy-intensive foods, saturated fats, trans fats, free sugars, or salt/sodium, and many do not eat enough fruits, vegetables, and dietary fibers such as whole grains.

Initiatives Taken by the Government of India

- The government has taken up several programs to tackle the burden of malnutrition in India. Midday meal scheme was initiated to boost the nutritional status of students in classes I to VIII in schools, funded by the government and industries. Cooked food is provided as a part of the scheme for the students.
- Integrated Child Development Services (ICDS) scheme was introduced in 1975 with the goal of improving the nutritional and health status of children in the age group of 0 to 6 years. Children younger than 6 years as well as pregnant and nursing mothers are given supplementary dietary nutrients. Take-home ration is being provided to adolescent girls, under the Rajiv Gandhi Scheme for Empowerment of Adolescent Girls (RGSEAG).
- The government has also launched various programs to lessen the risks of micronutrient deficiencies, such as the vitamin A prophylaxis program, wherein prophylactic vitamin A is administered to children up to 6 years of age, with early detection and treatment of deficiencies, if any.
- The Weekly Iron and Folic Acid Supplementation (WIFS) scheme is a community-based program that treats adolescents (boys and girls) with nutritional (iron deficiency) anemia. The scheme includes adolescents in classes VI to

XII of government-assisted and municipal schools as well as girls from *anganwadis* who are "out of school."

Future Approach

To promote the idea of healthy nutrition across the country, a holistic approach is required. Cross-sectoral initiatives should be taken to incorporate all age groups, in order to make people aware of the importance of healthy nutrition, keeping in mind traditional diversity in food habits and earning capacity. The initiative should be taken in schools, childcare centers, and the family right from childhood, so that basic framework of healthy eating habits is set down in the perfect age and can be inculcated in future generations well. Availability of healthy foods at low cost should be assured by policy-making and mobilizing society and health education.

National Programme for Prevention and Control of Cancer, Diabetes, Cardiovascular Diseases and Stroke

India is undergoing a major health change with a rise in the burden of NCDs, which account for over 42% of all deaths—the leading cause of death in India. Cardiovascular diseases (CVDs) will be India's leading cause of death and disability by 2020, according to a 2002 WHO report.

National Programme for Prevention and Control of Cancer, Diabetes, Cardiovascular Diseases and Stroke (NPCDCS) was established in 2010, with a priority toward improving services, and enhancing human resources, health promotion, early detection, management, and referral.

Different cells are identified and established at regional, state, and district levels to function as teams under this system, and NCD clinics are established in districts to provide early detection, care, and follow-up services for specific NCDs. There are facilities equipped with ICU, CCU, and various units to provide quality treatment for these NCDs.

The modified strategies to control and monitor these diseases are:

- Promotion of health through change in behavior and involvement of community NGOs, civil society, media, etc.
- Outreach camps are designed for opportunistic screening at all stages of the provision of health care and early identification of diabetes, obesity, and certain cancers.
- Chronic NCD care, with more emphasis on cancer, diabetes, CVDs, and stroke through early diagnosis, treatment, and follow-up through the creation of these centers.
- Capacity building for prevention, early diagnosis, treatment, operational research, and rehabilitation at different levels of health care.
- Diagnostic support and appropriate treatment offered at reasonable cost at primary, secondary, and tertiary medical care units.
- Extending support for NCD database development via an effective monitoring system, and tracking morbidity, mortality, and risk factors of NCD.

The cumulative cost of the program for the 2012–2017 period was ₹8,096 crore (the Government of India's share was ₹6,535 crore and the state government's share was ₹1,561 crore). The funds are distributed to states under NCD Flexi-Pool via state PIPs of the respective states/UTs, with a center-to-state share of 60:40 (except northeastern [NE] and hilly states, where the share is 90:10). There is the tertiary care cancer centers (TCCCs) scheme for the cancer component, which aims to establish/strengthen 20 state cancer institutes (SCIs) and 50 TCCCs to provide comprehensive cancer care in the country. The scheme provides for a one-time grant of ₹120 crore per SCI and ₹45 crore per TCCC to be used for the construction and purchase of equipment, with a center-to-state share of 60:40 (except for NE and hilly states, where the share is 90:10).

Recent Initiatives

- Integration of recommendations for the prevention and management of chronic obstructive pulmonary disease and chronic kidney disease under NPCDCS for the prevention and management of chronic respiratory and kidney disease, respectively, which are both primary causes of NCD death.
- For the early identification of diabetes, obesity, and common cancers in the community, recommendations for the implementation of "population-based screening of common NCDs" are provided to states using frontline workers' and health workers' facilities within the current primary health care program.
- Pilot project on "AYUSH integration with NPCDCS" has been launched in six districts across the country. AYUSH services and methodologies are incorporated with NPCDCS facilities for the prevention and management of common NCDs, in which yoga practice is an essential part of the intervention.
- Pilot action was undertaken under the NPCDCS and RBSK (*Rashtriya Bal Swasthya Karyakram*) platforms for the prevention and management of rheumatic fever and rheumatic heart disease in three selected districts (Gaya in Bihar, Firozabad in Uttar Pradesh, and Hoshangabad in Madhya Pradesh). This action would be slowly expanded to other districts.
- Another strategy is the amalgamation of RNTCP with NPCDCS, wherein the "national framework for joint tuberculosis-diabetes collaborative activities" has been developed to devise a national strategy for "bidirectional screening," early and quick detection, and better management of tuberculosis and diabetes comorbidities in India.

Multiple Choice Questions

1. On which weeks is the hepatitis B vaccine given?

A. 6th, 10th, and 14th week.
B. 1st, 5th, and 10th week.
C. 1st, 3rd, and 6th week.
D. 5th, 10th, and 15th week.

Answer: A

In 2010–2011, hepatitis B vaccination was generalized to all states and union territories (UTs) by the Government of India. It is to be administered as intramuscular (IM) injection at 6th, 10th, and 14th weeks to the infant along with preliminary rounds of

DPT and polio vaccinations. Moreover, in the case of institutional deliveries, one dose of hepatitis B is administered in less than 24 hours postbirth.

2. Pentavalent vaccine comprises:

A. Diphtheria, pertussis, and tetanus toxoid.
B. DPT, Hep B, HiB.
C. BCG, OPV, and TT.
D. Meningitis and pneumonia.

Answer: B

Since December 2011, the government, under routine immunization program, launched the pentavalent vaccine (DPT + Hep B + HiB) as an effort to cover DPT, hepatitis B, and HiB vaccines in Kerala and Tamil Nadu.

3. Hemophilus influenza type B (HiB) is associated with:

A. Measles and small pox.
B. Bronchiolitis and meningitis.
C. Pneumonia and meningitis.
D. Lymphoma and mumps.

Answer: C

The spectrum of Hib disease ranges from meningitis & pneumonia.

4. DOTS was launched by .... :

A. NACP.
B. NGCP.
C. RNTCP.
D. ASHA.

Answer: C

RNTCP strategy officially launched DOTS, and by the latter half of 2006, the program covered the entire country.

5. January 30 to February 13 is observed as ....:

A. Kala-azar fortnight.
B. Antiepileptic fortnight.
C. Antileprosy fortnight.
D. Anti-TB fortnight.

Answer: C

IEC activities are carried out for creating awareness and at the same time ensuring safety to prevent discrimination against leprosy patients. Such awareness activities are carried via mass media, advocacy meetings, rural media, and outdoor media. Interpersonal communication was the focused domain. January 30 to February 13 is observed as antileprosy fortnight every year, wherein, along with services pertaining to leprosy at the village level, IEC is also assisted.

6. Kala-azar is a type of ....:

A. Giardiasis.
B. Leishmaniasis.
C. Helminthiasis.
D. Schistosomiasis.

Answer: B

7. One gram of protein gives energy of .... :

A. 4.00 cal.
B. 0.40 cal.
C. 4.04 cal.
D. 0.44 cal.

Answer: A

8. Children with kwashiorkor are:

A. Apathetic.
B. Miserable.
C. Irritable.
D. All of the above.

Answer: D

Children with kwashiorkor are typically apathetic, miserable, and irritable. They show no signs of hunger, and it is difficult to convince them to eat.

9. Vitamin A is stored in .... :

A. Lungs.
B. Liver.
C. Adipose tissue.
D. Muscular tissue.

Answer: B

10. Normally, BCG vaccine is used for:

A. Rabies.
B. Tuberculosis.
C. Cancer.
D. Polio.

Answer: B

11. Which one among the following statements is not correct?

A. Vaccines stimulate active immunity.
B. Vaccines are used for long-term prophylaxis.
C. Patient receives antibodies in active immunization.
D. Patient produces antibodies in active immunization.

Answer: C

Patient receives antibodies in active immunization.

12. Smallpox vaccine was introduced by:

A. Paul Ehrlich.
B. Robert Koch.
C. Louis Pasteur.
D. Edward Jenner.

Answer: D

Edward Jenner discovered the smallpox vaccine in 1796. The smallpox vaccine was the "first vaccine" to be discovered. Smallpox is the "first and only" disease to be eradicated. The term *vaccination* was coined by Edward Jenner

Part II

Drugs Affecting Autonomic Nervous System

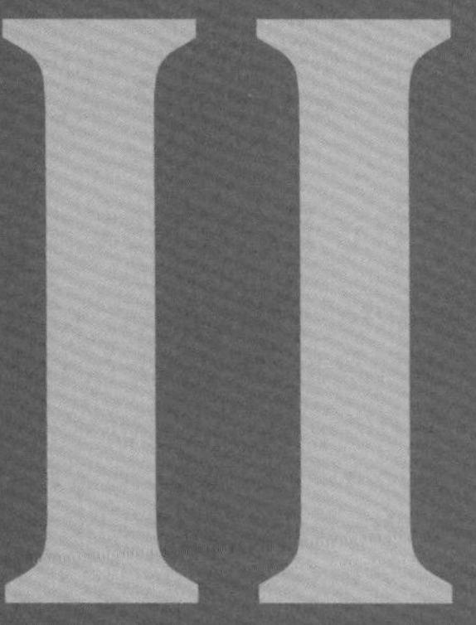

Chapter 16 Introduction to the Nervous System

D. H. Nandal, Sandeep Prakash Narwane, and Rashmi Bhaskarrao Kharde

PH1.13: Describe mechanism of action, types, doses, side effects, indications, and contraindications of adrenergic and antiadrenergic drugs.

PH1.14: Describe the mechanism of action, types, doses, side effects, indications, and contraindications of cholinergic and anticholinergic drugs.

Learning Objectives

- Process of neurotransmission.

Introduction

The nervous system, along with the endocrine system, serves a function of controlling the functions of other organ systems. It enables the organism to appreciate the external and internal stimuli and respond to them in a suitable manner. Anatomically, the nervous system is divided into the central nervous system (CNS) and peripheral nervous system (PNS). The brain and spinal cord comprise the CNS, while the remaining part of nervous system is collectively known as PNS.

The sensory organs and somatic and visceral afferent nerves form part of the afferent system, which convey the stimuli to the CNS. The CNS processes the stimuli and designs appropriate reaction. These designs of reactions are executed by the PNS. The reaction may be psychic, somatic, or autonomic. Changes in mood, attitude, thoughts, and memory form the psychic response of the CNS. The locomotion and observable behavior constitute the somatic response. The autonomic changes are seen as change in respiratory, cardiovascular, gastrointestinal, and other system functions.

A neuron is the basic functioning unit of the nervous system. It can be divided into dendrite, cell body, and axon. The dendrite of a successive neuron usually receives a signal from the preceding neuron through the release of a chemical substance, called neurotransmitter, from the axon of the preceding neuron (the process is known as neurotransmission). This neurotransmitter may have a stimulatory or inhibitory effect on the successive neuron. This stimulatory/inhibitory effect is carried along the axon of successive neuron (the process is known as conduction). A series of such neurons are at play for modulation of original stimuli. In order to carry out functions of the nervous system, the neurons have been grouped into nuclei/areas/centers. For example, the motor area, oculomotor nucleus, respiratory centre, and so on.

A neuron is basically identified on the basis of the neurotransmitter it releases. Neurons have a characteristic feature of communicating with other neurons and organ tissues via these neurotransmitters. The effector system of the neurotransmitter comprises receptors, mainly ligand-gated ion channels and G protein-coupled receptors.

The autonomic nervous system (ANS) plays a vital role in maintaining the autonomic (involuntary) physiological functions. It modulates the activities of the heart, lung, exocrine glands, and smooth muscles of viscera.

The visceral afferent nerves, sinus nerve, aortic depressor nerve, and the vagal afferents are some of the important afferent components of the ANS that take part in visceral reflexes. The cortex, hypothalamus, medulla, and spinal cord form the central part of the ANS. The efferent components of the ANS arise in the form of cranial, sacral, and thoracolumbar outflows.

The cranial (namely, the oculomotor, facial, glossopharyngeal, and vagus nerves) and the sacral outflows (the second, third, and fourth sacral segment) together form the parasympathetic system (cholinergic). The chief neurotransmitter that is released by parasympathetic neurons is acetylcholine.

The thoracolumbar outflow (the first thoracic through second or third lumbar segment) forms the sympathetic system (adrenergic). The chief neurotransmitter that is released by the sympathetic neurons is noradrenaline.

The effector autonomic fiber (both sympathetic and parasympathetic) is formed by two neurons. The cell body of the preceding neuron (preganglionic) lies in the CNS, from which the axon runs to form preganglionic fiber. This axon is connected to the cell body of the successive neuron (postganglionic) and, in turn, gives rise to its axon to form postganglionic fiber. The junction between the two neurons (pre- and postganglionic) is known as ganglion. The postganglionic fiber ends into the organ supplied by it at the neuroeffector junction. The muscle or gland on which the effect is seen is referred to as the effector cell (**Fig. 16.1**).

The Process of Neurotransmission

Neurotransmission of an impulse occurs along the gap between the axon of the preceding neuron and the cell body of the successive neuron or effector cell. This gap is known as synapse, which comprises the presynaptic membrane of the axon of the preceding neuron and postsynaptic membrane of the successive neuron or effector cell (**Fig. 16.2**). The process of neurotransmission occurs in the following stages:

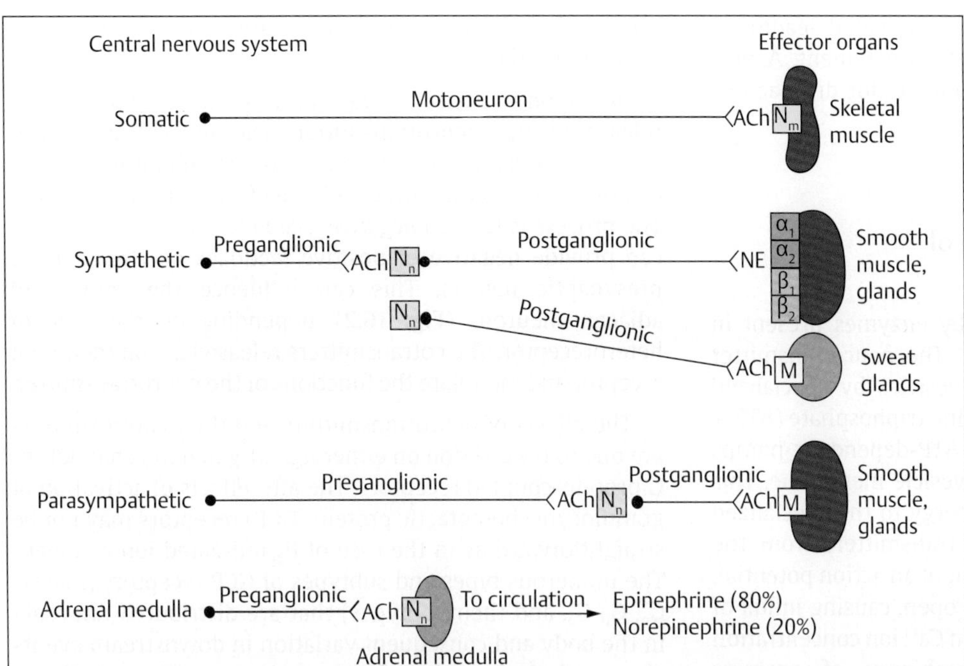

Fig. 16.1 Autonomic innervation in the body.

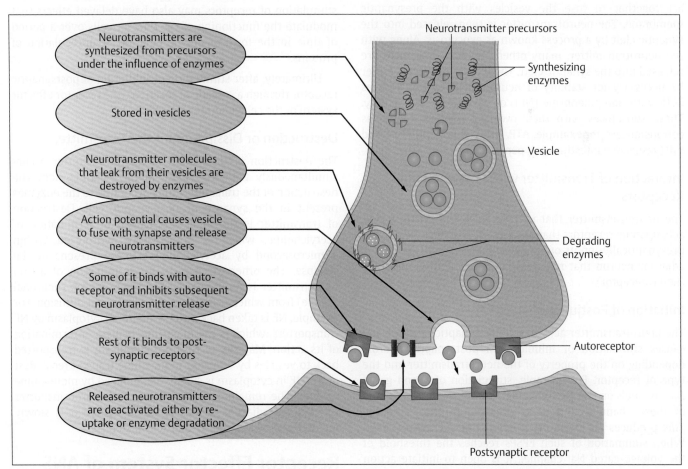

Fig. 16.2 The process of neurotransmission.

Axonal Conduction

The impulse is carried along the nerve axon by successive depolarization. The voltage-gated Na^+ channels are activated at a sufficient stimulus (threshold potential) to generate action potential. The activated Na^+ channels are opened for a fraction of milliseconds and remain refractory (resistant to activation) for a transient time. This action potential generated is transferred all along the axon by production of local circuit currents such that adjacent resting Na^+

channels (susceptible to activation) are activated, leading to propagation of an impulse without any decrement. Axonal conduction is one of the important targets for drug action, for example, local anesthetics.

Junctional Transmission

Synthesis, Storage, and Release of Neurotransmitter

Neurotransmitters are synthesized by enzymes present in the cytoplasm of the neuronal cell. The neurotransmitter thus synthesized is transported in vesicles by specialized transporters, with the help of adenosine triphosphate (ATP)–dependent transporter pumps. The ATP-dependent pumps produce proton gradient across the vesicle membrane. This electrochemical gradient provides energy to the specialized transporters to transport the neurotransmitters from the cytoplasm to the vesicles. On the event of an action potential, the voltage-dependent Ca^{++} channels open, causing influx of Ca^{++} ions into the cytoplasm. The rise in Ca^{++} ion concentration is sensed by the specialized machinery of proteins (synaptosomal-associated protein receptor—SNARE), which act together to fuse the vesicles with the presynaptic membrane. The neurotransmitter is then released into the synaptic cleft by a process known as exocytosis. Along with the neurotransmitter, many other chemical substances are released into the synaptic cleft. These substances may either be necessary for stability of neurotransmitters in vesicles (ATP with norepinephrine [NE]) or have their own activity. These substances with their own activity are known as cotransmitters, for example, ATP, NPY (neuropeptide Y), and VIP (vasoactive intestinal polypeptide).

Interaction of Transmitter with Postjunctional Receptors

The neurotransmitter that is released in the synaptic cleft acts upon its receptors that are present postsynaptically and presynaptically—on its own neuron (autoreceptor) or on the adjacent neuron that releases a different neurotransmitter (heteroreceptor).

Initiation of Postjunctional Activity

The neurotransmitter acts on the postsynaptic receptor and causes stimulation or inhibition of postsynaptic neuron, depending on the property of the neurotransmitter and the type of receptor. For example, stimulation of ligand-gated Na^+ channels on the postsynaptic membrane causes opening of these channels and entry of Na^+ ions intracellularly. This produces an excitatory postsynaptic potential (EPSP). When summation of such EPSPs reaches the threshold of the voltage-gated Na^+ channel, it is open to initiate action potential. On the contrary, stimulation of ligand-gated Cl^- channels causes opening of these channels and entry of Cl^- ions intracellularly. This produces an inhibitory postsynaptic potential (IPSP). IPSPs make the postsynaptic membrane refractory (resistant) to depolarization and initiation of action potential.

Action on an excitatory autoreceptor increases the further release of the neurotransmitter. The process is termed *positive feedback*. Similarly, action on an inhibitory autoreceptor decreases the further release of the neurotransmitter. The process is termed *negative feedback*. The heteroreceptor can provide negative or positive feedback on the adjacent presynaptic neuron. This can influence the activity of adjacent neurons (**Fig. 16.2**), depending on the type of heteroreceptor. The cotransmitters released act on their own receptor and modulate the functions of the neurotransmitter.

The effects of neurotransmitters and their cotransmitters are due to their action on either ligand-gated ion channels or G protein-coupled receptors. The aftereffects of activation of granulocyte chemotactic protein (GCP) receptors may not be straightforward as in the case of ligand-gated ion channels. The numerous types and subtypes of GCP receptors (like G_s, G_q, G_i, G_o, and their subtypes) that are distributed unevenly in the body and consequent variation in downstream events along with the interplay of cotransmitters make it a challenge to understand the pharmacology of neurotransmission. The stimulation of receptors may also have delayed effects that modulate the functioning of the effector cells over a period of time in the form of downregulation or upregulation of proteins.

Ultimately, after stimulation or inhibition of postsynaptic receptor through a cascade of reactions, the receptor effector system of the cell generates the effect.

Destruction or Dissipation of the Transmitter

The destruction or dissipation of neurotransmitter occurs simultaneously with its release in the synaptic cleft. The destruction of the transmitter may occur due to the enzymes present in the synapse or postsynaptic cell. Destruction of transmitter is the main mechanism of termination of acetylcholine, which is immediately hydrolyzed within a microsecond by acetylcholine esterase present in the synapse. The other mechanism for termination of action of transmitter is its uptake by the same neuron (neuronal uptake) from which it is released, or by lateral diffusion. For example, NE is taken back into the neuronal cytoplasm by NE transporters, which is the major mechanism of termination of its action. Majority of NE from cytoplasm is transported back to vesicles by vesicular monoamine transporter 2. Rest of the NE in cytoplasm is slowly metabolized by monoamine oxidase. The remaining small quantity of neurotransmitter is taken by adjacent tissues or blood, where it is slowly metabolized by catechol-*O*-methyltransferase.

Receptor Effector System of ANS

All the sympathetic receptors are G protein-coupled receptors. The types of receptors, their distribution, and overall effect on the organs are shown in **Table 16.1**.

Table 16.1 Types of receptors, their distribution, and overall effect on the organs

Organ	Receptor dominance	Effect
Heart		
SA node	$\beta_1 > \beta_2$	↑ in automaticity → ↑ in heart rate
	$M_2 \gg M_3$	↓ in automaticity → ↓ in heart rate (major determinant)
AV node	β_1	↑ in automaticity and conduction velocity
	M_2	↓ in automaticity and conduction velocity (dominant)
Bundle of His and Purkinje fibers	β_1	↓ in automaticity and conduction velocity
	$M_2 \gg M_3$	Little effect
Atria	$\beta_1 > \beta_2$	↑ in conductivity and force of contraction
	$M_2 \gg M_3$	↓ in contractility and ↓ AP duration
Ventricle	$\beta_1 > \beta_2$	↑ in contractility, conductivity, automaticity, and rate of idioventricular pacemakers (risk of ventricular arrhythmias)
	$M_2 \gg M_3$	Minimal ↓ in contractility
Blood vessels		
Skeletal muscles and liver	$\beta_2 \gg \alpha_1$	Dilatation (dominant); constriction
Skin and mucosa	α_1, α_2	Constriction
Coronary	$\beta_2 \gg \alpha_1, \alpha_2$	Dilatation (dominant); constriction
Cerebral	α_1	Slight constriction
Salivary	$\alpha_1, \alpha_2 \gg M_3$	Constriction (dominant); dilatation
Veins	$\beta_2; \alpha_1, \alpha_2$	Dilatation; constriction
Endothelium	M_3	Vasodilatation (↑ NO synthesis)
Eye		
Radial muscles of iris	α_1	Mydriasis
Circular muscles of iris	M_3, M_2	Miosis
Ciliary muscles	$M_3, M_2 \gg \beta_2$	Contraction for near vision (prominent); relaxation for far vision
Lacrimal gland	$M_3, M_2 \gg \alpha$	Secretion (dominant); secretion
Lung		
Trachea, bronchi	$\beta_2; M_3 = M_2$	Relaxation; contraction
Bronchial glands	$\alpha_1; M_3, M_2$	↑ ↓ secretion; ↑ secretion
Stomach and intestine		
Motility and tone	$M_3, M_2 \gg \alpha_1, \alpha_2, \beta_1, \beta_2$	↑ Motility and tone (prominent); ↓ motility and tone
Sphincters	$\alpha_1; M_3, M_2$	Contraction; relaxation
Secretion	$M_3, M_2 \gg \alpha_1$	↑ Secretion (dominant); ↓ secretion
Gall bladder and ducts	β_2; M	Relaxation; contraction
Kidney—JG cells	$\beta_1 \gg \alpha_1$	↑ Renin secretion (prominent); ↓ renin secretion
Urinary bladder		
Detrusor	$(M_3 > M_2) \gg \beta_2$	Contraction (prominent); relaxation
Trigone and sphincter	$(M_3 > M_2); \alpha_1$	Relaxation; contraction
Ureter	α_1, M	Increased motility and tone
Pancreas		
Acini	$M_3, M_2; \alpha$	↑ Secretion (prominent); ↓ secretion
β cells of islets	$\alpha_2; \beta_2$	↓ Secretion (prominent); ↑ secretion
Adipocytes	$\alpha_1, \beta_{1,2,3}; \alpha_2$	↑ Lipolysis (prominent); ↓ lipolysis

(Continued)

Table 16.1 *(Continued)* Types of receptors, their distribution, and overall effect on the organs

Organ	Receptor dominance	Effect
Miscellaneous		
Salivary gland	M_3, $M_2 \gg \alpha_1$	↑ K^+ and water secretion
Nasopharyngeal gland	M_3, M_2	↑ Secretion
Uterus	α_1; β_2	Contraction; relaxation
Male genitalia	M_3; α_1	Erection; ejaculation
Arrector pili	α_1	Contraction
Sweat gland	M_3, M_2; α_1	Generalized sweating; localized sweating
Splenic capsule	α_1; β_2	Contraction (prominent); relaxation
Adrenal medulla	N_N, M	Secretion of EPI and NE
Skeletal muscles	β_2	Increased contractility, glycogenolysis
Liver	α_1	Glycogenolysis, gluconeogenesis

Abbreviations: AP, action potential; AV, atrioventricular; SA, sinoatrial; EPI, epinephrine; JG, juxtaglomerular; NE, norepinephrine.

Multiple Choice Questions

1. Following are the attributes of sympathetic nervous system.

A. Ganglionic neurotransmitter: acetylcholine.
B. The postganglionic fibers are longer than the preganglionic fibers.
C. Thoracolumbar origin for preganglionic cell bodies.
D. All of the above.

Answer: D

The chief neurotransmitter, irrespective of the type of autonomic (sympathetic/parasympathetic) nervous system, released in the ganglia is acetylcholine. The ganglia of parasympathetic neurons reside near the organ of supply, while the ganglia of the sympathetic nervous system lie near the vertebral column. Therefore, in contrast to the parasympathetic system, the sympathetic postganglionic fibers are longer than the preganglionic fibers. The thoracolumbar outflow (the first thoracic through second or third lumbar segment) forms the sympathetic system.

2. Which of the following is an adrenergic receptor type(s) mediating pupillary dilation?

A. Beta-2.
B. Alpha-1.
C. Muscarinic.
D. Serotonergic.

Answer: B

The α1 receptors are present on the radial muscle of the iris. Stimulation of these receptors causes contraction of the radial muscles, causing pupillary dilation.

3. The sympathetic and parasympathetic systems exert functionally opposite influences on the following parameters except:

A. Heart rate.
B. Atrial refractory period.
C. Pupil diameter.
D. Intestinal motility.

Answer: B

Stimulation of sympathetic system exerts increase in heart rate by stimulation of β1 adrenergic receptors of SA node, whereas stimulation of parasympathetic system decreases the heart rate by stimulation of M2 receptors on the SA node. Similarly, the simulation of adrenergic α1 receptors on the radial muscles of the iris causes mydriasis as against miosis caused by stimulation of cholinergic M3 receptors on the circular muscles of the iris. Intestinal motility is enhanced by parasympathetic stimulation (M2, M3 mediated), while it is decreased by sympathetic stimulation (α, β). However, the atrial effective refractory period is shortened by both sympathetic and parasympathetic stimulation.

4. Cholinergic muscarinic receptor stimulation produces the following effects except:

A. Sweating.
B. Rise in blood pressure.
C. Bradycardia.
D. Urination.

Answer: B

Cholinergic muscarinic receptor stimulation in sweat glands (M3), SA node (M2), and urinary bladder (M3-mediated detrusor contraction and sphincter relaxation) causes sweating, bradycardia, and voiding of urine, respectively. However, direct stimulation of M3 in the blood vessels cause NO release, causing reduction in blood pressure.

5. The following reflexes are all autonomic except:

A. Salivary secretion.
B. Micturition.
C. Flexion of the arm following a painful stimulus.
D. Acceleration of the heart.

Answer: C

Flexion of the arm following a painful stimulus is a spinal reflex, which does not involve the autonomic system. Salivary

secretion involves both sympathetic and parasympathetic system. Micturition and acceleration of heart are predominantly parasympathetic and sympathetic reflexes, respectively.

6. The system that controls smooth muscle, cardiac muscle, and gland activity is the:

A. Somatic nervous system.
B. Autonomic nervous system.
C. Skeletal division.
D. Sensory nervous system.

Answer: B

The smooth muscle, cardiac muscle, and glands are involuntary organs and are supplied by the autonomic nervous system.

7. The parasympathetic nerves:

A. Are important in emergency conditions, for example, fight and flight reactions.
B. Play important functions in skin and skeletal muscles.
C. Tend to have longer postganglionic fibers than preganglionic fibers.
D. Are catabolic in their actions.
E. Mostly exert effects opposite to those done by the sympathetic nerves.

Answer: E

Most of the effects of stimulation of the parasympathetic system are opposite to that of stimulation of the sympathetic system. The sympathetic system plays a vital role in fight-or-flight reactions, have longer postganglionic fibers than preganglionic fibers, and are catabolic in general.

8. Stimulation of the sympathetic nervous system causes:

A. Contraction of the ciliary muscle for near vision.
B. Mostly generalized actions affecting many systems.
C. Bronchoconstriction.
D. Decreased glycogenolysis and lipolysis.
E. Increased gastric HCl and pepsin secretion.

Answer: B

Sympathetic stimulation causes a generalized effect on the body systems via the thoracolumbar outflow and adrenaline release from the adrenal glands. Sympathetic stimulation causes increase in glycogenolysis and lipolysis. Contraction of the ciliary muscle for near vision, bronchoconstriction, and increased gastric HCl and pepsin secretion are mediated by parasympathetic stimulation.

9. Which of the following may be produced by parasympathetic stimulation?

A. Acceleration of the heart.
B. Contraction of the urinary bladder wall.
C. Vascular dilatation of skeletal muscle blood vessels.
D. Dilatation of the pupil.
E. Relaxation of the gastrointestinal tract (GIT) wall.

Answer: B

Parasympathetic stimulation causes voiding of urine by contraction of the detrusor muscle (M3) in the urinary bladder. Acceleration of the heart (β1), vascular dilatation of skeletal muscle blood vessels (β2), dilatation of the pupil (α1), and relaxation of the GIT wall (α, β) are mediated by sympathetic stimulation.

10. Which of the following structures is an example where double innervation does not apply?

A. The heart.
B. The bladder.
C. The stomach.
D. The intestines.
E. The splenic capsule.

Answer: E

The splenic capsule is solely supplied by the sympathetic fibers. Adrenergic α1 receptor stimulation (which is predominant) causes contraction, while β2 stimulation causes relaxation of the splenic capsule.

Chapter 17 Cholinergic System

Prasan R. Bhandari

Learning Objectives

- Cholinesterases.
- Choline esters.
- Cholinomimetic alkaloids.
- Glaucoma.
- Anticholinesterases.
- Irreversible anticholinesterases.

Introduction

Acetylcholine (ACh) is the major neurotransmitter of parasympathetic nervous system (PSNS). Cholinergic nerves synthesize, store, and release ACh. Some of the important ACh release sites include the following (**Fig. 17.1**):

1. Ganglia: all preganglionic autonomic nervous system (sympathetic and parasympathetic nervous systems) fibers.
2. Postganglionic parasympathetic nerve terminals.
3. Adrenal medulla.
4. Brain and spinal cord.
5. Neuromuscular junction (NMJ).
6. Sympathetic postganglionic nerve terminals of sweat glands (this is an unconventional site).

Synthesis/Transmission/Metabolism of ACh

Choline goes inside the cholinergic neuron by carrier-mediated transport. Here, choline reacts with acetyl coenzyme A with the assistance of choline acetyltransferase to become ACh. The ACh is subsequently accumulated in storage vesicles. It is liberated into the synaptic cleft, after an action potential spreads to the nerve terminals. The liberated ACh interacts with cholinergic receptors on effector cell and stimulates them. In the synaptic cleft, the ACh is instantaneously metabolized by the acetylcholinesterase (AChE) enzyme.

This is depicted in **Fig. 17.2** and **Fig. 17.3**

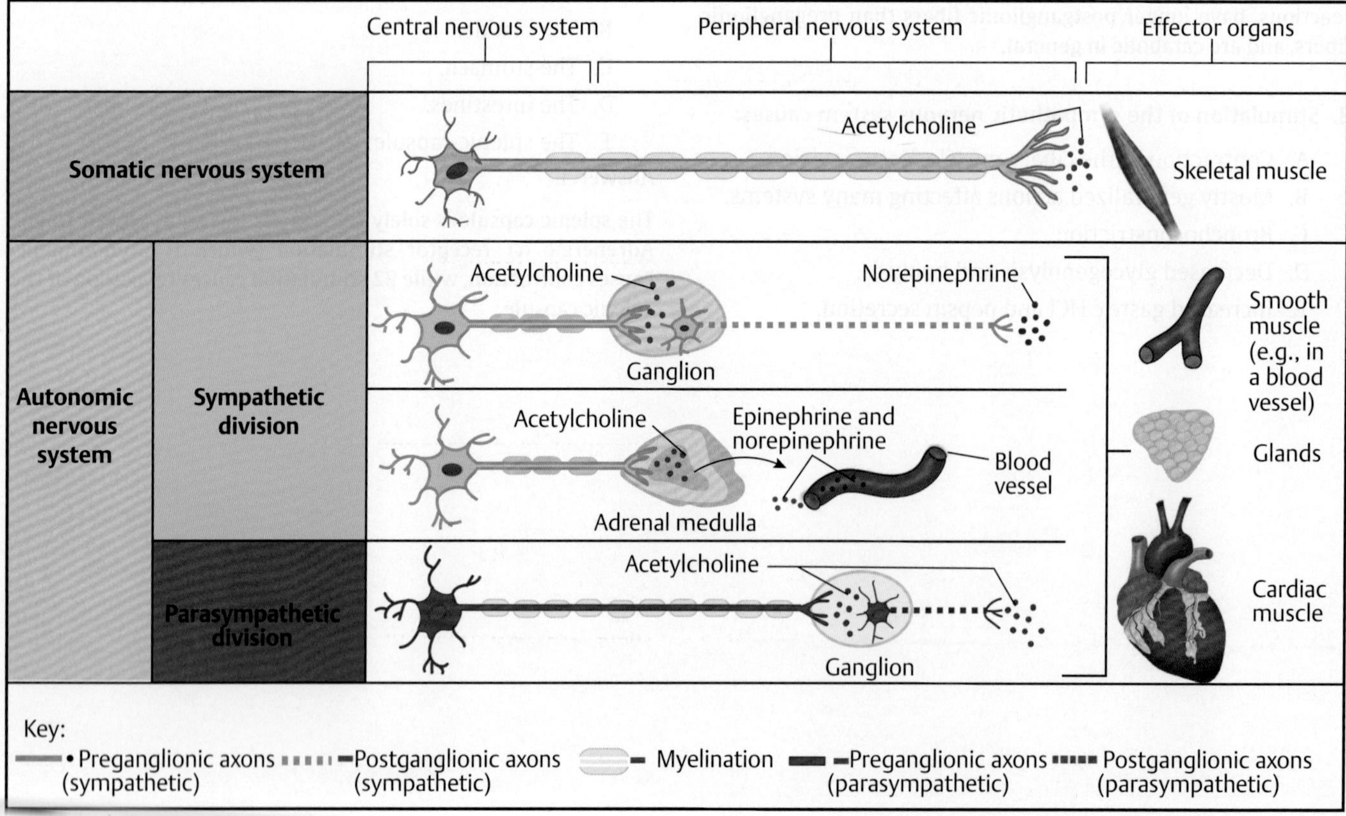

Fig. 17.1 Important ACh release sites.

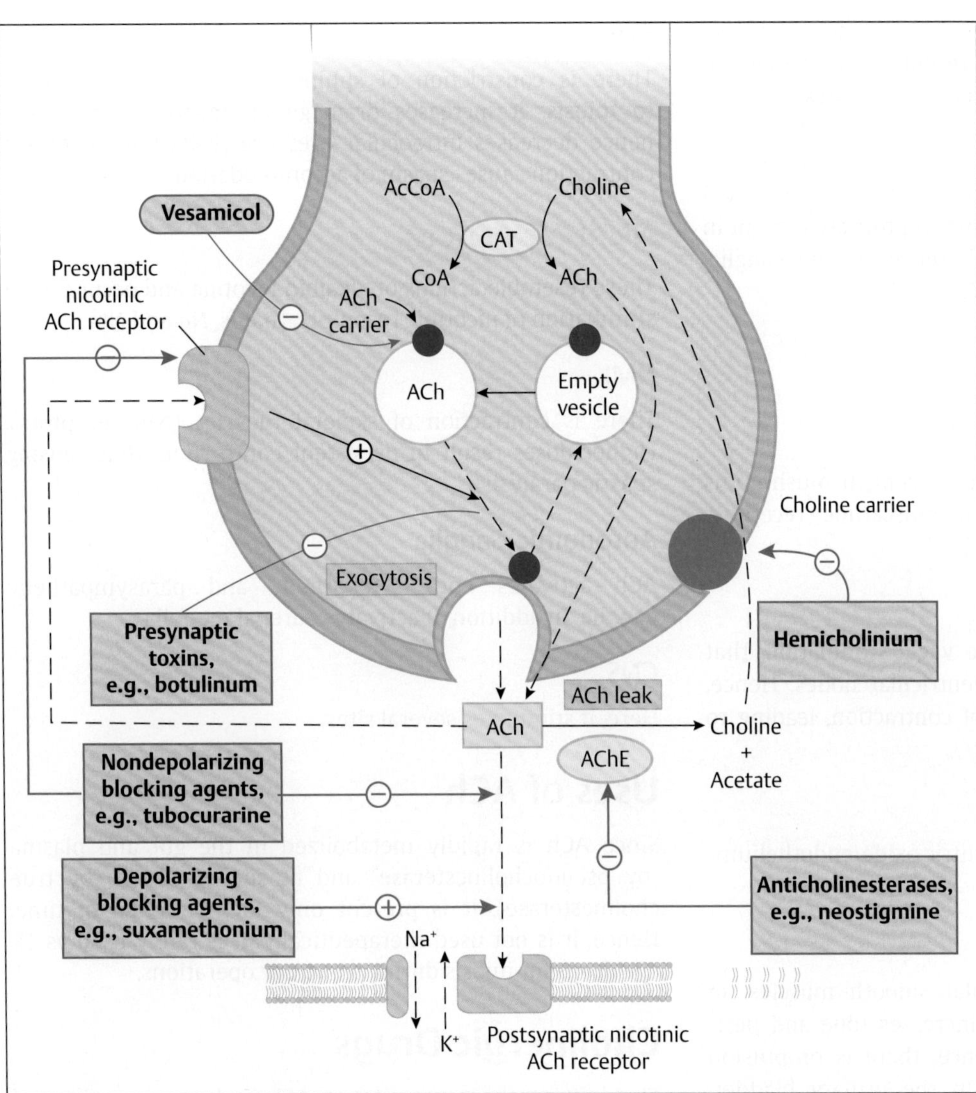

Fig. 17.2 Synthesis/transmission/metabolism of ACh.

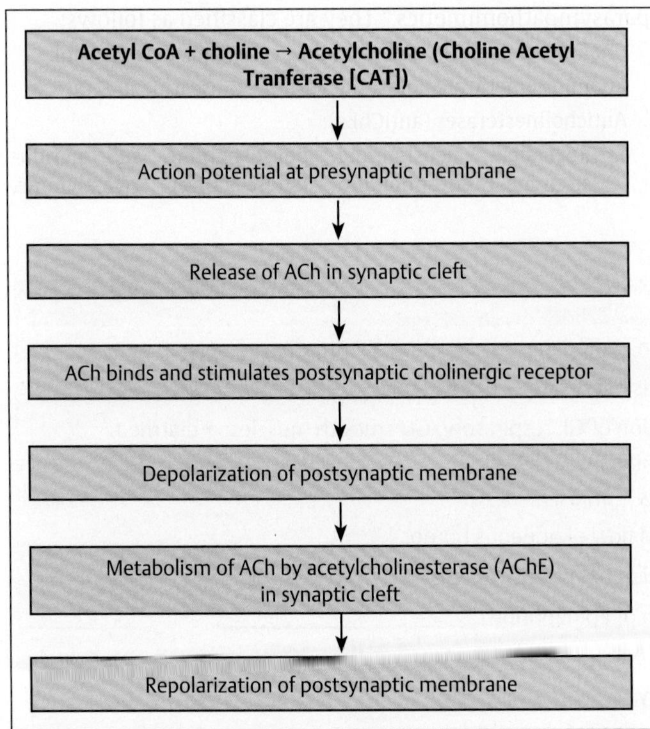

Fig. 17.3 Synthesis/transmission/metabolism of ACh.

Cholinesterases

AChE is a cholinergic enzyme primarily present at postsynaptic NMJs, mostly in muscles and nerves. It rapidly metabolizes or hydrolyzes ACh, a naturally occurring neurotransmitter, into acetic acid and choline. The primary function of AChE is to end neuronal transmission and signaling within synapses to end ACh diffusion and activation of neighboring receptors. AChE is inhibited by organophosphates and is a crucial constituent of pesticides and nerve agents.

$$\text{Ach} \xrightarrow[\text{Acetylcholinesterase (AChE)}]{} \text{Choline + Acetic acid}$$

There are two types of AChE: (1) true (AChE), present at neurons, ganglia, and NMJ, and (2) pseudo (butyrylcholinesterase), present in plasma and the liver.

Cholinergic Receptors

They are of two types: muscarinic and nicotinic. Muscarinic receptors are subdivided into five subtypes: M1, M2, M3, M4, and M5. Nicotinic receptors are of two subtypes: Nn and Nm. Muscarinic receptors are G protein–coupled receptors, whereas nicotinic receptors are ion (Na) channels and have five subunits: 2α, 1β, 1γ, 1δ. M1 receptors are present in the autonomic ganglia, gastric glands, and central nervous system (CNS). M2 receptors are present in the heart, smooth muscles, and nerves. M3 receptors are present in the exocrine glands, smooth muscles, and eye. M4 and M5 receptors are present in the CNS. Nm receptors are present in the NMJ. Nn receptors are present in the autonomic ganglia, adrenal medulla, and CNS (**Table 17.1**).

Actions of ACh

Muscarinic Actions

These resemble alkaloid muscarine present in mushrooms and occur due to stimulation of muscarinic receptors (M1–M3).

Heart

The actions on the heart resemble vagal stimulation, that is, it inhibits sinoatrial and atrioventricular nodes. Hence, it decreases heart rate and force of contraction, leading to bradycardia.

Blood Vessels

There is dilatation due to release of nitric oxide/endothelium-derived relaxing factor.

Smooth Muscles

It increases tone of all nonvascular smooth muscles. In the gastrointestinal tract (GIT), it increases tone and peristalsis, and relaxes sphincters; hence, there is propulsion and evacuation of GI contents. On the urinary bladder, the detrusor contracts and the trigone relaxes; hence, it promotes evacuation of urine.

Secretory Glands

It increases secretion of all glands, namely, lacrimal, salivary, tracheobronchial, nasopharyngeal, gastric, intestinal, and sweat.

Eye

There is constriction of sphincter pupillae, which leads to miosis. It increases drainage of aqueous humor and hence decreases intraocular pressure (IOP). Ciliary muscle contraction causes spasm of accommodation.

Nicotinic Actions

These resemble actions of alkaloid nicotine and occur due to stimulation of nicotinic receptors, that is, Nn and Nm.

NMJ

There is contraction of skeletal muscles (Nm receptors). Higher doses result in persistent contraction, thus causing spastic paralysis.

Autonomic Ganglia

ACh activates both sympathetic and parasympathetic ganglia. In addition, it activates adrenal medulla.

CNS

Here, it stimulates several sites.

Uses of ACh

Since ACh is rapidly metabolized in the gut and plasma (by pseudocholinesterase) and at site of action (by true cholinesterase), it is present only for a fraction of time. Hence, it is not used therapeutically. It is rarely used as 1% eye drops for miosis during some eye operations.

Cholinergic Drugs

They act at the same site as ACh and mimic actions of ACh; therefore, they are also called "cholinomimetics" or "parasympathomimetics." They are classified as follows:

1. Choline esters: ACh, methacholine, carbachol, bethanechol.
2. Cholinomimetic alkaloids: pilocarpine, muscarine.
3. Anticholinesterases (antiChEs):
   a. Reversible: neostigmine, physostigmine and pyridostigmine, edrophonium (short-acting), rivastigmine,

Table 17.1 Cholinergic receptors

M1	Secretory glands	Salivation, stomach acid, sweating, lacrimation
M2	Heart	Decreases heart rate → bradycardia
M3	Smooth muscle (GI/GU/respiratory)	Contraction of GI, respiratory, GU smooth muscles → diarrhea, bronchospasm, urination
	Pupil and ciliary muscle	Contracts → miosis Increased flow of aqueous humor
Nm	Skeletal muscle and plate	Contraction of skeletal muscle
Nn	Autonomic ganglia, adrenal medulla	Secretion of epinephrine Controls ANS

Abbreviations: ANS, autonomic nervous system; GI, gastrointestinal; GU, genitourinary.

galantamine, donepezil (CNS action, i.e., to treat Alzheimer's disease).

b. Irreversible: organophosphates—echothiophate, malathion, toxic nerve gases (sarin, tabun).

Choline Esters

Bethanechol

Its selectivity of muscarinic actions is seen on the GIT and urinary bladder. It is ideal in postoperative urinary retention and paralytic ileus since it has a wide safety margin and lacks nicotinic actions. Its muscarinic adverse effects are totally antagonized by atropine. In patients with urinary retention, it leads to passing of urine by contracting the detrusor muscle and relaxing the trigone sphincter. In patients with paralytic ileus, it activates peristaltic movement and enhances the tone by acting on the M3 receptors of the GIT.

Carbachol

It is utilized to manage/treat acute angle-closure glaucoma and open-angle glaucoma, in addition to treating increased IOP. It constricts the ciliary body muscle and opens the trabecular meshwork. Opening this trabecular meshwork enhances aqueous humor outflow from the eye to decrease IOP.

Uses of Other Cholinomimetics

1. Carbachol/bethanechol are resistant to metabolism by cholinesterases and hence have long duration of action.
2. Carbachol is used in glaucoma.
3. Bethanechol is used in:
   a. Urinary bladder hypotonia.
   b. Urinary retention.
   c. Postoperative paralytic ileus.
   d. Xerostomia (alternative to pilocarpine).

Adverse Reactions of Cholinomimetics

- **S**alivation.
- **L**acrimation
- **U**rination
- **D**iarrhea
- **G**I/genitourinary cramps
- **E**mesis/**e**ye (miosis)

(Mnemonic "SLUDGE.")

Cardiovascular symptoms include hypotension and bradycardia. GI symptoms are manifested as abdominal pain, diarrhea, and nausea. Genitourinary symptoms comprise uncontrolled urination. In the exocrine glands, ACh leads to gastric secretion, increased sweating, and increased salivation. Ocular symptoms include lacrimation and miosis. CNS-related symptoms include lethargy, tremor, ataxia, restlessness, and anxiety and can culminate in hypoventilation and coma. Musculoskeletal symptoms are manifested as spasms and fasciculations, weakness, paralysis, or peripheral neuromuscular respiratory failure.

Cholinomimetic Alkaloids

Pilocarpine

This drug is obtained from *Pilocarpus microphyllus* and has prominent muscarinic actions. The actions on the eye are important, which include miosis, spasm of accommodation, and decreased IOP on topical administration. It also increases sweating (diaphoresis) and salivary secretion (sialogogue). Side effects include brow ache and headache (due to spasm of accommodation and miosis). Corneal edema and retinal detachment can occur on long-term use. It is used in glaucoma as an Ocusert, a novel delivery system that releases pilocarpine for 7 days. It can also be utilized in alternation along with mydriatics (pupillary dilators) to avoid/break adhesions between the iris and lens. Other uses include xerostomia (Sjögren's syndrome) and dryness of mouth following radiation of head and neck.

Muscarine

The poisonous mushroom *Amanita muscaria* has muscarine as an active ingredient. It lacks any therapeutic application.

Arecoline

It is an alkaloid obtained from areca nut. It possesses muscarinic and nicotinic actions like choline esters.

Glaucoma

See also Chapter 91.

Aqueous humor is produced by the ciliary body and it drains via the canal of Schlemm. Any increase in IOP beyond 21 mm Hg is generally labeled as glaucoma. Increase in IOP leads to optic nerve degeneration and therefore causes blindness. Glaucoma is a condition characterized by advancing optic neuropathy, finally leading to impairment of optic nerve accompanied by loss of visual function. This is usually accompanied with increased IOP. Normal IOP ranges between 10 and 20 mm Hg. Treatment of glaucoma is generally focused at lowering the prevailing IOP either by enhancing drainage or by reducing the production of aqueous humor.

There are two types of glaucoma. In acute congestive/angle-closure/narrow angle, the iris blocks the canal of Schlemm and it should be treated urgently. Chronic simple/open-angle/wide angle has a slow onset. In patients with this type of glaucoma, long-term treatment is required and surgical treatment is usually preferred.

Drugs for glaucoma are classified as follows (**Fig. 17.4**):

1. Drugs decreasing formation of aqueous humor (all topical):
   a. β-blockers: timolol, betaxolol, levobunolol (first-line drugs).
   b. Adrenergic agonists: adrenaline, dipivefrine (used with β-blockers).
   c. α_2 adrenergic agonists: apraclonidine, brimonidine.
   d. Carbonic anhydrase inhibitors (CAIs): dorzolamide, acetazolamide (oral).

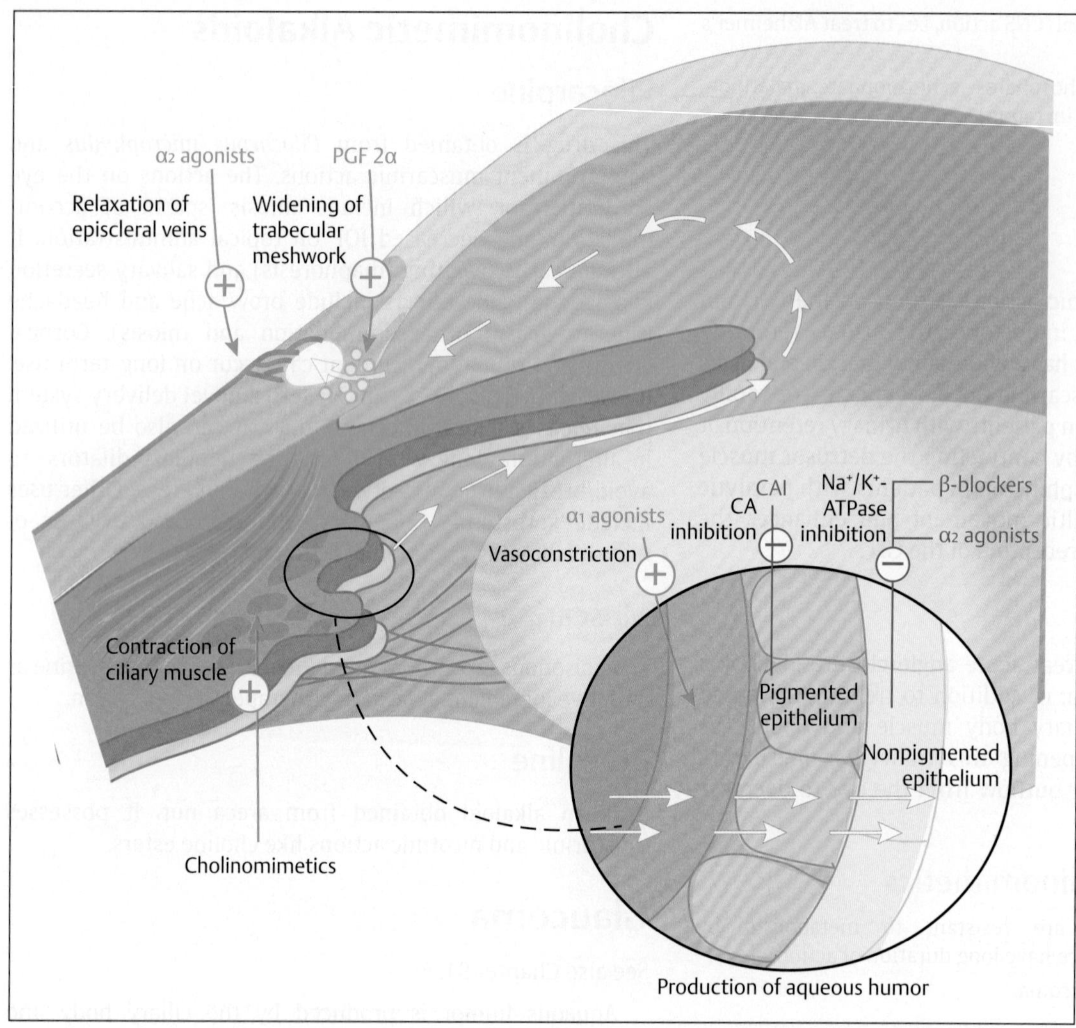

Fig. 17.4 Sites of action of antiglaucoma drugs.

2. Drugs increasing drainage of aqueous humor:
   a. Cholinergics: pilocarpine, carbachol, physostigmine, echothiophate.
   b. Prostaglandin analogs: latanoprost, bimatoprost (adjuvants).

β-Blockers in Glaucoma

They are first-line drugs, which decrease aqueous production. These agents block β-receptors in the ciliary body. There is no miosis and hence there is no headache or brow ache (unlike pilocarpine); therefore, they are preferred. These drugs cause a smooth and sustained decrease in IOP. Systemic absorption via the nasolacrimal duct can precipitate asthma, congestive cardiac failure, and heart block. Hence, these drugs are to be used carefully. Examples include timolol, betaxolol, levobunolol, and carteolol.

Timolol is commonly utilized in glaucoma due to the following reasons: (1) it does not possess local anesthetic property; (2) it lacks any action on the pupil size or accommodation; (3) it possesses a longer duration of action; (4) it is well accepted and tolerated; (5) it is cost-effective; and (6) topical timolol has a wide margin of safety and is highly efficacious. Betaxolol is a selective β_1-blocker employed for the treatment of glaucoma; however, it has less efficacy as compared to nonselective agents. β-blockers must be used carefully and are contraindicated in bronchial asthma and heart failure.

Adrenergic Agonists in Glaucoma (PH1.13)

Common adrenergic agonists are dipivefrine (a prodrug of adrenaline) and apraclonidine (analog of clonidine). Topical apraclonidine is administered as an add-on therapy in glaucoma. It has no hypotensive effect like clonidine, since it does not cross the blood–brain barrier (BBB). Apraclonidine, an α_2-agonist, decreases the production of aqueous humor and thus reduces the IOP. Dipivefrin is a prodrug of adrenaline. It infiltrates the cornea and is activated to adrenaline by corneal esterases.

Miotics

Commonly used miotics include pilocarpine and physostigmine. They constrict the pupil and thus open up the canal of Schlemm, thereby increasing drainage.

Prostaglandin Analogs

Latanoprost and bimatoprost (PGF2α, analogs) are topical prostaglandins, which are favored medications used for primary treatment in open-angle glaucoma due to their longer duration of action, better efficacy, and lesser frequency of systemic toxicity. These agents could also be employed for acute congestive glaucoma. They decrease IOP possibly by enhancing uveoscleral outflow. They generally lack any systemic side effects; however, they could lead to mild ocular irritation and iris pigmentation.

Carbonic Anhydrase Inhibitors

Normally, aqueous humor formation requires HCO_3^- ions. HCO_3^- ions are produced by carbonic anhydrase by the following reaction:

$$\begin{array}{c}\text{Carbonic anhydrase}\\ \downarrow \\ H_2CO_3 \rightarrow H^+ + HCO_3\end{array}$$

CAIs include dorzolamide (topical) and brinzolamide (topical) or acetazolamide (oral, intravenous [IV]). They noncompetitively suppress carbonic anhydrase enzyme and reduce IOP by lessening the production of aqueous humor. Since topical CAIs lack systemic side effects, they are favored over systemic CAIs in patients with chronic simple glaucoma. In patients with acute congestive glaucoma, acetazolamide is given intravenously and orally. CAIs, by suppressing the enzyme carbonic anhydrase, decreases HCO_3^- and hence decreases IOP. Oral acetazolamide causes drowsiness, hypokalemia, and anorexia. Therefore, topical dorzolamide is selected.

Osmotic Agents

In patients with acute congestive glaucoma, either mannitol (20%) IV infusion (1.5 g/kg body weight) or 50% glycerol oral (1.5 g/kg) is employed. They extract fluid from the eye into the circulation due to their osmotic effect and consequently decrease IOP.

Anticholinesterases

AntiChEs are structural analogs of ACh. The hydrolysis of ACh due to cholinesterases is inhibited. Consequently, ACh is not hydrolyzed and thus gets collected at muscarinic and nicotinic sites, causing cholinergic effects. Hence, their pharmacologic actions are like that of ACh. Thus, antiChEs are termed indirectly acting cholinergic drugs.

$$\begin{array}{c}\text{Acetylcholine} \rightarrow \text{Acetic acid + Choline}\\ \uparrow \\ \text{AntiChE inhibits} \rightarrow \text{AChE}\end{array}$$

Classification of AntiChEs

1. Reversible:
   a. Carbamates: physostigmine, neostigmine, pyridostigmine, edrophonium, donepezil, rivastigmine, tacrine, galantamine.
   b. Insecticides: propoxur (Baygon), carbaryl, aldicarb.
2. Irreversible:
   a. Organophosphates: echothiophate, malathion, toxic nerve gases (sarin, tabun).

ACh is promptly metabolized by both true and pseudocholinesterases. Since reversible antiChEs inhibit both true and pseudocholinesterases reversibly, ACh is collected and this leads to cholinergic effects.

The structure of AChE contains an anionic site and an esteratic site (**Fig. 17.5**). Reversible antiChEs, except edrophonium, bind to both anionic and esteratic sites. Edrophonium binds only to anionic site and the binding is quickly reversible; hence, it is very short-acting. Organophosphates (OP) bind only to the esteratic site but the enzyme is phosphorylated (by covalent bonds) and the binding is stable. With some OPs, the binding takes many days to be reversed, while with others it is not fully reversible at all.

Physostigmine

Physostigmine is an alkaloid obtained from the plant *Physostigma venenosum* (**Table 17.2**). It is a tertiary ammonium compound—hence, it has better penetration into tissues and also crosses the BBB. It is available as IV injection, as 0.1 to 1% eye drops, and in combination with pilocarpine nitrate 2%. It is used in glaucoma and in atropine poisoning. Its use as eye drops can cause brow ache and, on long-term use, retinal detachment and cataract.

Neostigmine

Neostigmine is a synthetic AntiChE drug. Its pharmacologic actions are marked on GIT, NMJ, and urinary bladder as compared to that of cardiovascular system or ocular tissues. It has both direct and indirect actions on skeletal muscle. Neostigmine raises ACh levels at NMJ by its indirect actions by inhibiting cholinesterases. It additionally directly activates the NM receptors at NMJ due to its structural similarity with ACh (i.e., quaternary ammonium compound). Hence, it increases muscle power in myasthenia gravis. Neostigmine is not able to penetrate the BBB and thus does not possess central side effects. It is administered either orally, or subcutaneously, or intramuscularly.

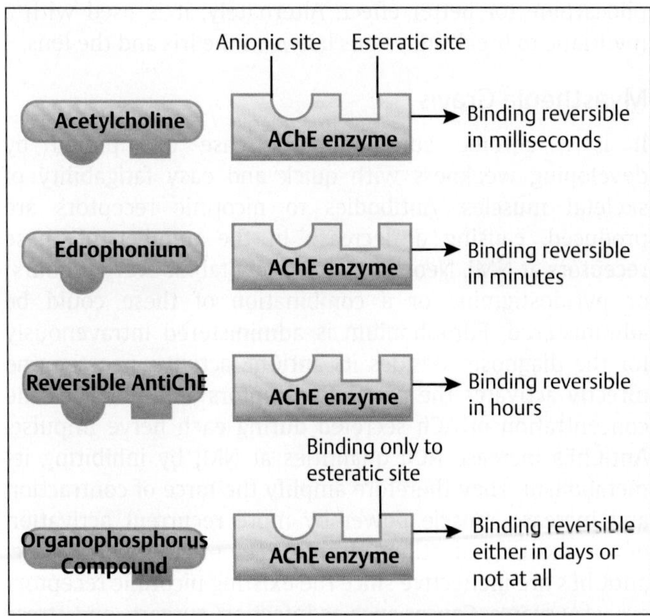

Fig. 17.5 Structure of acetylcholinesterase enzyme and actions of anticholinesterases.

Table 17.2 Differences between physostigmine and neostigmine

Physostigmine	Neostigmine
Natural (*Physostigma venenosum*)	Synthetic
Tertiary amine	Quaternary amine
Good oral absorption	Poor oral absorption
Good tissue penetration	Poor tissue penetration
Crosses BBB: CNS effects	Does not cross BBB: no CNS effects
Main indication: glaucoma	Myasthenia gravis
Used in atropine poisoning	Used in curare poisoning

Abbreviations: BBB, blood–brain barrier; CNS, central nervous system.

Edrophonium

It is a quaternary ammonium compound. It has a fast onset but short duration of action (5–15 minutes) as seen on IV administration. It is used in diagnosis of myasthenia gravis; it differentiates myasthenic crisis from cholinergic crisis. Since it has a rapid onset of action, it is preferred in curare poisoning.

Rivastigmine, Donepezil, Galantamine, and Tacrine

They are specifically used for Alzheimer's disease.

Important Contraindications

Choline esters and AntiChEs are contraindicated in bronchial asthma, peptic ulcer, ischemic heart disease, and hyperthyroidism.

Uses of Reversible AntiChE

Physostigmine causes miosis, spasm of accommodation, and a decrease IOP. It is used in glaucoma and can be used with pilocarpine for better effect. Alternately, it is used with a mydriatic to break adhesions between the iris and the lens.

Myasthenia Gravis

It is a chronic autoimmune disease exemplified by developing weakness with quick and easy fatigability of skeletal muscles. Antibodies to nicotinic receptors are produced, causing a decrease in the number of these receptors at NMJ. Neostigmine (15-mg tablet every 6 hours) or pyridostigmine or a combination of these could be administered. Edrophonium is administered intravenously for the diagnosis. Besides its antiChE activity, neostigmine directly activates the nicotinic receptors and enhances the concentration of ACh secreted during each nerve impulse. AntiChEs increase ACh quantities at NMJ by inhibiting its metabolism. They therefore amplify the force of contraction and increase muscle power by more recurrent activation of the existing nicotinic receptors. In progressive disease, antiChEs are ineffective since the existing nicotinic receptors are very scarce. Causes such as infection, surgery, and stress can lead to severe muscle weakness, termed myasthenic crisis. However, severe weakness could also be due to an excess dose of an antiChEs drug (flaccid paralysis due to more of ACh), known as cholinergic crisis. These two crises can be distinguished by giving edrophonium 2 mg intravenously. The patient instantly recovers if it is myasthenic crisis; however, the weakness aggravates if it is cholinergic crisis. Treatment of cholinergic crisis is with atropine, whereas myasthenic crisis needs a higher dose of a different anti-cholinergic drug. Other drugs used in myasthenia gravis are:

1. Glucocorticoids: prevent the synthesis of antibodies to the nicotinic receptors. These are used when antiChEs alone are not sufficient.
2. Immunosuppressants: azathioprine and cyclosporine can be utilized as substitutes to prednisolone in progressive myasthenia gravis. They suppress the synthesis of antinicotinic receptor antibodies.

Anticholinergic Poisoning

Physostigmine is used in atropine poisoning and in toxicity due to other drugs with anticholinergic activity such as phenothiazines, tricyclic antidepressants, and antihistamines. Because physostigmine crosses the BBB, it reverses all the symptoms of atropine poisoning including CNS effects.

Curare Poisoning

Skeletal muscle paralysis caused by curare can be antagonized by antiChEs. Although edrophonium has fast action, it is less effective than neostigmine.

Postoperative Paralytic Ileus and Urinary Retention

Neostigmine may be useful.

Cobra Bite

Cobra venom, a neurotoxin, causes skeletal muscle paralysis. Specific treatment is antivenom. IV edrophonium prevents respiratory paralysis.

Alzheimer's Disease

To overcome the deficient cholinergic neurotransmission, rivastigmine and donepezil are tried in Alzheimer's disease. Tacrine is another reversible antiChE tried in this disease, but it is not preferred because it causes hepatotoxicity.

Irreversible AntiChE

Echothiophate eye drops for glaucoma.

Irreversible AntiChE: Organophosphorus Compounds (PE14.3)

They are powerful, irreversible inhibitors of antiChE. Their binding is covalent to only esteratic site, and enzyme is phosphorylated; hence, binding is stable and irreversible. Reversible antiChE (except edrophonium) binds to both anionic and esteratic site. Edrophonium binds only to anionic site; hence, action is quickly reversible and short-acting. All OP compounds (except echothiophate) are highly lipid soluble and hence can be absorbed from all routes, including intact skin. Thus, OP poisoning can also occur by spraying of agricultural pesticides/insecticides.

Organophosphorus Insecticides

All organophosphorus (OP) compounds excluding echothiophate lack therapeutic applications. Echothiophate is rarely used in resistant cases of glaucoma. Organophosphorus (OP) compounds possess only toxicological significance. Organophosphorus poisoning is one of the most frequent poisoning globally. Regular OP compounds are parathion, malathion, dyflos, etc. They irreversibly inhibit cholinesterases and lead to increase of ACh levels at muscarinic and nicotinic sites.

Organophosphorus Poisoning (FM9.5)

OP compounds are used as agricultural insecticides/pesticides; hence, poisoning is frequent. Poisoning could be accidental/suicidal/homicidal. The signs/symptoms are similar to cholinergic (muscarinic, nicotinic, CNS) hyperactivity, that is, SLUDGE (**s**alivation, **l**acrimation, **u**rination, **d**iarrhea, **G**I/genitourinary cramps, **e**mesis/**e**ye [miosis]).

Signs and Symptoms

1. Central effects: restlessness, confusion, headache, convulsions, coma, and death occur generally because of respiratory failure.
2. Nicotinic effects: twitchings, fasciculations, muscle weakness, and paralysis due to sustained depolarization.
3. Muscarinic effects: bradycardia, hypotension, vomiting, salivation, intense sweating, lacrimation, enhanced tracheobronchial secretions, bronchospasm, abdominal cramps, miosis, involuntary urination, and defecation.

Diagnosis

Organophosphorus poisoning can be diagnosed by:

1. History of exposure.
2. Characteristic signs and symptoms.
3. Estimating the cholinesterase activity in the blood, which is decreased.

For the treatment of poisoning via skin, remove clothing and wash skin with soap and water. For poisoning via oral route, perform a gastric lavage and maintain blood pressure and airway patency. Atropine IV 2 mg every 10 minutes till pupil dilates/dryness of mouth is the drug of choice. Cholinesterase reactivators (e.g., pralidoxime) too can be administered. Pralidoxime combines with cholinesterase–OP complex and releases binding and frees AChE enzyme. These have to administered within minutes of poisoning (maximum 12–24 hours), since delay leads to "ageing" of enzyme, which cannot be freed. "Ageing" is due to loss of one chemical group from the complex, making the complex stable. These agents are not useful in carbamate compound poisoning, since they do not have a free site (anionic site) for binding of oximes.

Multiple Choice Questions

1. A 40-year-old woman has been managed for myasthenia gravis for many years. She presently complains of difficulty swallowing, weakness of her hands, and diplopia. She could be having a variation in response to her myasthenia therapy, that is, a cholinergic or a myasthenic crisis. The best drug for differentiating myasthenic crisis (insufficient therapy) and cholinergic crisis (excessive therapy) could be:

A. Physostigmine.
B. Pralidoxime.
C. Pyridostigmine.
D. Atropine.
E. Edrophonium.

Answer: E

Any of the cholinesterase inhibitors (choices B, C, or E) could efficiently manage myasthenic crisis. However, because cholinergic crisis is worsened by a cholinomimetic, it is proper to select the shortest-acting cholinesterase inhibitor, that is, edrophonium.

2. A 3-year-old child has accidentally swallowed a drug from her parents' medicine cupboard. The signs indicate that the drug could be an indirect-acting cholinomimetic with minimal, if at all, CNS effect and a duration of action of around 2 to 4 hours. The most probable causative agent could be:

A. Acetylcholine.
B. Neostigmine.
C. Physostigmine.
D. Pilocarpine.
E. Bethanechol.

Answer: B

Neostigmine is the ideal indirect-acting cholinomimetic. Being a quaternary (charged) substance, it has poor lipid solubility and it acts for around 2 to 4 hours.

3. During a visit for vacation, a 40-year-old man with a 9-year history of myasthenia gravis forgets to take medications. Thus, he is admitted to the casualty with signs and symptoms of difficulty swallowing, diplopia, and dysarthria. The drug that could reverse his myasthenic crisis is:

A. Neostigmine.
B. Vecuronium.

C. Pralidoxime.
D. Succinylcholine.
E. Calcium.

Answer: A

Neostigmine is the only cholinesterase inhibitor that is a suitable therapy for myasthenic crisis, which is an indirect-acting cholinomimetic. It can also be used for chronic therapy of this condition.

4. A 40-year-old farmer is admitted to the casualty department of a hospital with complaints of anxiety, sudden difficulty in breathing, and increased sweating. In his farm, he was spraying insecticide when this occurred for the past 30 minutes. The patient is administered atropine with another agent, which reactivates acetylcholinesterase along with performing an intubation. What is the other agent?

A. Propranolol.
B. Phenylephrine.
C. Pralidoxime.
D. Pancuronium.
E. Physostigmine.

Answer: C

Pralidoxime combines with cholinesterase-OP complex and releases binding, frees AChE enzyme. These have to be administered within minutes of poisoning (maximum 12–24 hours), since delay leads to "aging" of enzyme, which cannot be freed. "Aging" is due to loss of one chemical group from the complex, making the complex stable. These agents are not useful in carbamate compound poisoning, since they do not have a free site (anionic site) for binding of oximes.

5. Bethanechol is a:

A. Nicotinic blocker.
B. Muscarinic agonist.
C. α-agonist.
D. β_2-blocker.
E. β_1-blocker.

Answer: B

Bethanechol is a type of muscarinic receptor agonist that is employed clinically to treat urinary retention.

6. Which of the following is a short-acting acetylcholinesterase inhibitor?

A. Pyridostigmine.
B. Bethanechol.
C. Edrophonium.
D. Scopolamine.
E. Methantheline.

Answer: C

The structure of AChE contains an anionic site and an esteratic site (Fig. 17.4). Reversible antiChEs, except edrophonium, bind to both anionic and esteratic sites. Edrophonium binds only to anionic site and the binding is quickly reversible, hence, it is very short-acting. Organophosphates (OP) AQ8 bind only to the esteratic site but the enzyme is phosphorylated (by covalent bonds) and the binding is stable. With some OPs, the binding takes many days to be reversed, while with others it is not fully reversible at all. It is a quaternary ammonium compound. It has a fast onset but short duration of action (5–15 minutes) as seen on IV administration. It is used in diagnosis of myasthenia gravis; it differentiates myasthenic crisis from cholinergic crisis. Since it has a rapid onset of action, it is preferred in curare poisoning.

7. Organophosphate poisoning is treated with:

A. Nicotine.
B. Parathion.
C. Amyl nitrate.
D. Pralidoxime.
E. Bethanechol.

Answer: D

Pralidoxime reactivates acetylcholinesterase to reverse the effects of exposure to organophosphates, of which parathion is actually an example.

8. A 60-year-old man complains of increasing visual loss along with a sensation of pressure behind his eyes. He is diagnosed as glaucoma. To stop additional advancement of the disease and to lessen the present symptoms, the physician initiates the patient on oral acetazolamide treatment. What is its mechanism of action?

A. Enhances excretion of hydrogen.
B. Increases rate of production of bicarbonate in the aqueous humor.
C. Augments uptake of sodium in the proximal tubule.
D. Reduces reabsorption of bicarbonate.
E. Potentiates carbonic anhydrase in all parts of the body.

Answer: D

Acetazolamide is a carbonic anhydrase inhibitor. It decreases bicarbonate reabsorption in the proximal tubule. It suppresses enzyme carbonic anhydrase throughout the body, as well as the aqueous humor, which makes this medication beneficial as a therapy for glaucoma. Acetazolamide inhibits excretion of hydrogen and associated sodium uptake.

9. A 55-year-old patient develops paresthesias and intermittent nausea related with one of her drugs. She is diagnosed with hyperchloremic metabolic acidosis. The medication she is possibly consuming could be:

A. Furosemide for severe hypertension and heart failure.
B. Acetazolamide for glaucoma.
C. Hydrochlorothiazide for hypertension.
D. Mannitol for cerebral edema.
E. Amiloride for edema associated with aldosteronism.

Answer: B

The frequent side effects of acetazolamide are paresthesias and gastrointestinal distress, particularly during its long-term administration such as in glaucoma. The diagnosis of metabolic acidosis also indicates the use of acetazolamide.

Anticholinergics, Atropine, and Its Substitutes

Mayank Kulshreshtha, Rajaneesh Kumar Chaudhary, and Swetza Singh

PH1.14: Describe mechanism of action, types, doses, side effects, indications, and contraindications of cholinergic and anticholinergic drugs.

Learning Objectives

- Pharmacological actions of anticholinergics.
- Semisynthetic derivatives.
- Synthetic compounds.

Introduction

Anticholinergics are also called antimuscarinics, parasympatholytics, or cholinergic-blocking drugs. They block the effects of acetylcholine (ACh) on muscarinic receptors. Drugs that block nicotinic receptors are ganglionic blockers or neuromuscular blockers. The sites and actions of various cholinergic receptors and their respective agonists and antagonists are mentioned in **Fig. 18.1.**

Anticholinergic drugs or agents produce their effect on different systems such as circulation, respiration, alertness, and eye. These drugs are useful for the treatment of various disorders such as respiratory diseases (asthma, chronic obstructive pulmonary disorder [COPD]), Parkinson's disease, cardiovascular disease, urge incontinence, psychiatric disorders, depression, mydriasis, and allergies. There are more than 600 medications that produce some level of anticholinergic activity, and except in the case of a few drugs, experts consider the anticholinergic properties to be the cause of adverse rather than therapeutic effects.

Atropine is the main member of anticholinergic family. Apart from atropine, lots of anticholinergics are available.

Classification

A classification of anticholinergic drugs is given in **Fig. 18.2.**

Cholinergic receptors

Muscarinic

M_1 (Location: Autonomic ganglia, gastric glands, and CNS; Type: G protein coupled receptor; Agonist: Oxotremorine; Antagonist: Pirenzepine, Telenzepine)

M_2 (Location: Heart; Type: G protein coupled receptor; Agonist: Methacholine; Antagonist: Methoctramine, Tripitramine)

M_3 (Location – smooth muscles, exocrine glands and eye./ Type – G protein coupled receptor/Agonist – Bethanechol/ Antagonist-Solifenacin, Darifencin)

M_4 (Present on nerve endings in certain area of brain)

M_5 (Present on nerve endings in certain area of brain)

Nicotinic

N_M

Location: Neuromuscular junction
Type: Intrinsic ion channel
Agonist: Nicotine
Antagonist: Tubocurarine

N_N

Location: Autonomic Ganglia
Type: Intrinsic ion channel
Agonist: Nicotine
Antagonist: Hexamethonium

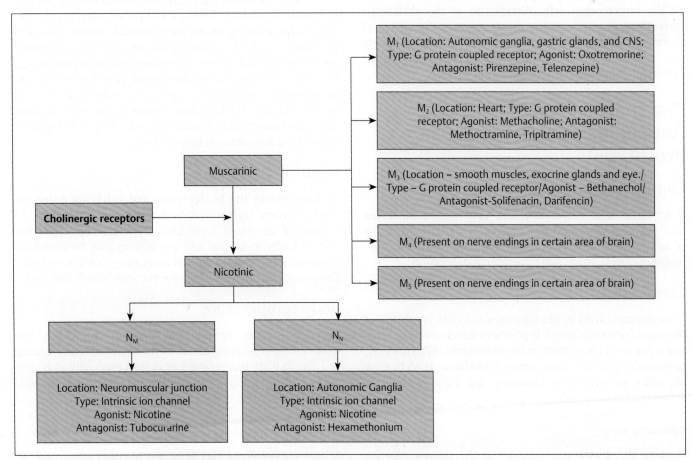

Fig. 18.1 The sites and actions of various cholinergic receptors and their agonists and antagonists.

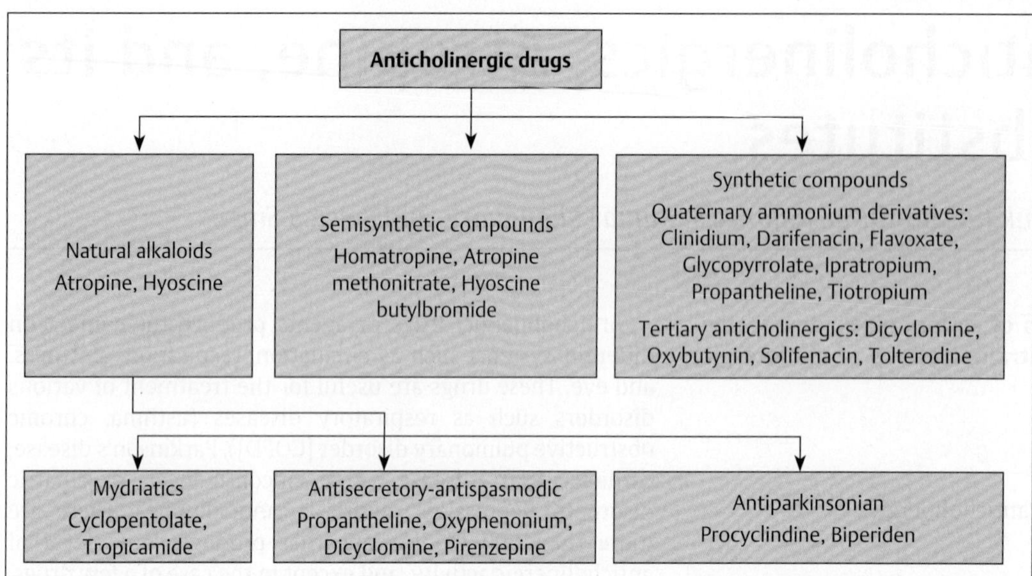

Fig. 18.2 Classification of anticholinergic drugs.

Common Mechanism of Action of Anticholinergics

The cholinergic system has two types of receptors—muscarinic and nicotinic, i.e., plasma membrane–bound G protein-coupled muscarinic receptors and ligand-gated ion channel nicotinic receptors, respectively. Nicotinic receptors are found in the postganglionic dendrites and nerve bodies of the autonomic nervous system and on the motor end plate of the neuromuscular junction. Muscarinic receptors are present on the target organ cells. Antagonism of the cholinergic system reduces or, in some cases, prevents the effects of cholinergic neurotransmission in the central nervous system and peripheral tissue. Medications with anticholinergic activity predominantly affect muscarinic receptors.

Pharmacological Actions of Anticholinergics (Atropine as Prototype)

Central Nervous System

It activates vagal, respiratory, and vasomotor centers and also suppresses tremor and rigidity of parkinsonism due to central anticholinergic effect. Additionally, it has anti-motion sickness action due to vestibular depression.

Cardiovascular System

It causes tachycardia by blocking muscarinic (M_2) receptors in the heart (sinoatrial node). It produces direct vasodilatation, and it has no marked effect on blood pressure (BP). However, tachycardia and vasomotor center stimulation tend to raise BP, while the release of histamine and direct vasodilator action tend to lower BP.

Eye

Blocking the muscarinic receptors in the circular muscles of iris atropine causes mydriasis and abolition of light reflex. As a consequence, photophobia and blurring of near vision may be precipitated. The intraocular tension tends to rise, especially in narrow-angle glaucoma; hence, it is contraindicated to administer atropine or its derivatives in such cases.

Smooth Muscles

Almost all the visceral smooth muscles are relaxed by atropine due to muscarinic receptor (M_3) blockade. Smooth muscles in the gastrointestinal tract (GIT) are relaxed and the passage of chyme is slowed; hence, constipation may occur. This action also accounts for its antispasmodic action. However, peristalsis is only incompletely suppressed, as it is primarily controlled by local reflexes and other neurotransmitters and hormones. Atropine causes bronchodilation; hence, it is safe in asthmatics. Atropine has relaxant action on ureter and urinary bladder; thus, urinary retention can occur in older males and those with prostatic hypertrophy. Relaxation of biliary tract and uterus is less marked.

Glands

Atropine blocks the M_3 receptors and markedly decreases sweat, salivary, tracheobronchial, and lacrimal secretion. As a result of decreased secretions, dryness of skin and eyes and difficulty in talking and swallowing may be observed. However, it is not efficacious in decreasing gastric secretions. Pancreatic and bile secretions are not significantly reduced.

Body Temperature

Atropine inhibits sweating as well as stimulates the temperature-regulating center in the hypothalamus, leading to a rise in body temperature as is seen especially at higher doses. Children are more susceptible to fever associated with atropine treatment.

Side Effects and Toxicity

Belladonna poisoning may occur due to either drug overdose or consumption of seeds and berries of belladonna/

datura plant. Symptoms include: dry mouth; difficulty in swallowing and talking; dry, flushed, and hot skin; fever; difficulty in micturition; constipation; and rashes. Dilated pupil, photophobia, and blurring of near vision can occur. Excitement, ataxia, delirium, and hallucinations can be observed. Palpitation, hypotension, cardiovascular collapse, and respiratory depression are also seen. Convulsions and coma occur only in severe poisoning.

Contraindications

Atropine is contraindicated in people with glaucoma and elderly males with prostatic hypertrophy since urinary retention can occur. Atropine is also contraindicated in CHF and angina pectoris (**Table 18.1**).

Pharmacokinetic

Atropine and hyoscine are better and rapidly absorbed from the GIT. When it is applied on the eye, it will freely penetrate cornea. Nearly 50% atropine is metabolized from the liver and the rest is excreted unchanged in urine. $t_{1/2}$ is 3 to 4 hours.

Semisynthetic Derivatives

Ipratropium Bromide

This drug is a selective bronchial smooth muscle relaxant administered by inhalational route. Its action lasts for 4 to 6 hours. It acts by blocking the bronchoconstrictor effect of muscarinic receptors. Mucociliary function is not depressed. Side effects include dryness of mouth, cough, scratching in trachea, and bad taste.

Tiotropium Bromide

This is a longer-acting congener of ipratropium bromide, with similar pharmacological profile.

Synthetic Compounds

Mydriatics

Cyclopentolate and tropicamide induce mydriasis within 30 to 60 minutes, which lasts about a day. They are preferred as cycloplegic for refraction testing in adults. Cyclopentolate is also used in iritis and uveitis.

Antiparkinsonian Drugs

These are drugs that have higher central:peripheral anticholinergic action ratio than that of atropine but the pharmacological profile is similar to that of atropine. They act by reducing the overactive cholinergic activity in the striatum of parkinsonian patients. They are inexpensive and quite safe. Anticholinergics are the only drugs effective in drug-induced parkinsonism. Side effects are similar to those of atropine.

Uses

- As antisecretory in preanesthetic medication when irritant general anesthetics (ether) are used.
- To treat Parkinson's disease.
- To relieve from intestinal, renal, and biliary colic.
- In the treatment of bronchial asthma, COPD, and bronchitis.
- As mydriatic and cycloplegic for refraction testing.
- As anti-motion sickness drug to control vomiting.
- As an antidote for anticholinesterases poisoning.

Role of Anticholinergics in Eye

Mechanism of Mydriasis and Miosis

The iris of the eye consists of the circular muscles (sphincter pupillae) and radial muscles (dilator pupillae). The sphincter pupillae are supplied by the parasympathetic system, and the dilator pupillae are supplied by the sympathetic system. Contraction of the dilator pupillae leads to mydriasis and that of the sphincter pupillae causes miosis. Relaxation of the dilator pupillae leads to miosis and that of the sphincter pupillae causes mydriasis. Cycloplegia results from paralysis of the sphincter pupillae, in which the near vision becomes blurred due to loss of pupillary reflex (**Fig. 18.3**).

Mydriatics

These are drugs that, upon topical instillation into the eye or systemic administration, induce mydriasis, that is, dilatation of pupils. Mydriasis is induced by either contraction of the dilator pupillae or relaxation of the sphincter pupillae. Thus, sympathomimetics and parasympatholytics produce mydriasis. These are basically used for refraction testing of the eyes. They are also used alternately with miotics to prevent the formation of adhesion between iris and lens or

Table 18.1 The differences between atropine and hyoscine

Parameters	Atropine	Hyoscine
Source	*Atropa belladonna*	*Hyoscyamus niger*
Ester of tropic acid	Tropine	Scopine
CNS effect	Excitation	Depressant
Anticholinergic action	More in heart, bronchial muscles, and intestines	More in eye and glands
Duration	Longer	Shorter
Antimotion sickness	Normal	High

Abbreviation: CNS, central nervous system.

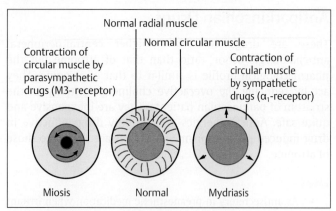

Fig. 18.3 Mechanism of mydriasis and miosis.

iris and cornea and may even break them if already formed. Examples of drugs used as mydriatics are as follows:

- **Sympathomimetics:** adrenaline, phenylephrine, ephedrine.
- **Parasympatholytics:** atropine, homatropine, cyclopentolate, tropicamide.

Miotics

These are drugs that, upon topical instillation into the eye or systemic administration, induce miosis, that is, constriction of pupils. Miosis is induced by either relaxation of the dilator pupillae or contraction of the sphincter pupillae. Thus, parasympathomimetics and sympatholytics produce miosis. These are basically used for the treatment of glaucoma.

Glaucoma

It is a group of diseases characterized by a progressive form of optic nerve damage. This may lead to visual loss. In this condition, the intraocular tension may rise. The main therapeutic approach is to reduce the intraocular tension, which may slow down the progressive damage to the optic nerve. Examples of drugs used as miotics in the treatment of glaucoma are as follows:

- **Parasympathomimetics:** physostigmine, pilocarpine, carbachol.
- **Sympatholytics:** timolol, betaxolol.
- **Carbonic anhydrase inhibitors:** acetazolamide, dorzolamide.

Multiple Choice Questions

1. Which anticholinergic drug is preferred in sedation?

A. Atropine.
B. Glycopyrrolate.
C. Scopolamine.
D. Ipratropium.
E. Neostigmine.

Answer: C

Because it has very potent central nervous system (CNS) effects with sedation property. In some patients, however, this may lead to restlessness, delirium, and difficulty in waking after short procedures.

2. Atropine is the antagonist of:

A. Acetylcholine (ACh).
B. Diazepam.
C. Lorazepam.
D. All of the above.
E. None of the above.

Answer: A

ACh because atropine is a cholinergic receptor antagonist, and ACh produces its effects through cholinergic receptor.

3. Which is not an anticholinergic drug?

A. Atropine.
B. Glycopyrrolate.
C. Scopolamine.
D. Ipratropium.
E. Neostigmine.

Answer: E

Neostigmine is an indirect-acting cholinergic drug, which inhibits the effect of enzyme cholinesterase.

4. Mechanism of atropine includes:

A. Blocking of action of acetylcholine.
B. Blocking of muscarinic receptor.
C. Blocking of nicotinic receptor.
D. Blocking of cholinergic receptor.
E. All of the above.

Answer: E

Atropine blocks the action of acetylcholine by blocking the cholinergic receptors (muscarinic and nicotinic).

5. Atropine is obtained from the plant:

A. *Atropa belladonna.*
B. *Hyoscyamus niger.*
C. Both of the above.
D. None of the above.
E. *Hibiscus rosa sinensis.*

Answer: A

Chapter 19

Skeletal Muscle Relaxants

Farhana Rahman

PH 1.15 Describe mechanism of action, types, doses, side effects, indications, and contraindications of skeletal muscle relaxants.

Learning Objectives

- Peripherally acting neuromuscular blockers.
- Centrally acting muscle relaxants.

Introduction

At the neuromuscular junction (NMJ), normally neuromuscular transmission results due to release of acetylcholine (ACh) from the postsynaptic nerve terminals. ACh receptors are present postsynaptically at the NMJ and autonomic ganglia. In the central nervous system (CNS), ACh receptors are present presynaptically. Cholinergic transmission mediates release of ACh and subsequent activation of nicotinic ACh receptors resulting in muscle contraction.

Skeletal muscle relaxants are drugs that block the neuromuscular junction or muscle fibers peripherally. They are known as neuromuscular blockers. Some drugs also block the cerebrospinal axis centrally to cause paralysis or reduce muscle tone. These drugs are known as centrally acting muscle relaxants. Curare is the plant extract obtained from *Strychnos toxifera*, *Chondrodendron tomentosum*, and related plants that possess neuromuscular blocking properties. It was used as arrow poison for game hunting by the South American tribes. The first clinically used neuromuscular blocker was tubocurarine. Classification of muscle relaxants is given below:

Classification of Muscle Relaxants

Peripherally Acting Muscle Relaxants

Neuromuscular Blocking Agents or Skeletal Muscle Relaxants

1. Nondepolarizing blockers (competitive)
   a. Long-acting (60–90 minutes)
      i. d-Tubocurarine.
      ii. Pancuronium.
      iii. Doxacurium.
      iv. Pipecuronium.
   b. Intermediate-acting (duration of action: 20–40 minutes).
      i. Vecuronium.
      ii. Atracurium.
      iii. Cisatracurium.
      iv. Rocuronium.
      v. Rapacuronium.
   c. Short-acting (duration of action: 10 minutes)
      i. Mivacurium.
2. Depolarizing blockers
   a. Succinylcholine (SCh).
   b. Decamethonium.

Directly Acting

a. Dantrolene sodium.
b. Quinine.

Centrally Acting Muscle Relaxants

1. **Mephenesin congeners**—carisoprodol, chlorzoxazone, chlormezanone, and methocarbamol.
2. **Benzodiazepines (BZD)**—diazepam.
3. **GABA mimetic**—baclofen and thiocolchicoside.
4. **Central 2 agonist**—tizanidine.

Mechanism of Action of Nondepolarizing Blockers

Nondepolarizing blockers or competitive blockers are produced from curare and related drugs. After the discovery of muscle relaxants, the practice of anesthesia has revolutionized. Initially, tubocurarine and gallamine were used, but since better drugs with lesser side effects became available, these drugs were no longer used. Nondepolarizing blockers compete with the ACh binding site on nicotinic alpha subunits in the NMJ.

The nicotinic receptor protein (N_M) has five subunits (α2, β, ε or γ, and δ), which are arranged like a chevron surrounding the Na^+ channel. Entry of an action potential in the distal motor nerve ending releases ACh from the presynaptic terminal and diffuses across the synaptic membrane. The neurotransmitter then binds to the nicotinic receptor (N_M receptor) in the postsynaptic membrane and activates Na+ channel domain. An activated receptor allows influx of Na+ ion and depolarizes the motor end plate. The membrane potential of the motor end plate changes from −100 mV (resting potential) to +40 mV (depolarized potential). The depolarizing signal which reaches the sarcoplasmic membrane signals release of Ca^{+2} (calcium) ions that facilitate muscle contraction.

Neuromuscular competitive blockers are usually thick bulky molecules that have two or more quaternary N^+ atoms that provide necessary attraction to the ACh binding site. Hence, ACh molecules released from the motor endings were not able to fuse with the N_M receptor, resulting in dropping of the magnitude of the end plate potential (EPP). When the magnitude of EPP drops below a critical level, ACh is unable to trigger propagated muscle action potential (MAP), and muscle contraction fails in response to nerve impulse.

Mechanism of Action of Depolarizing Blockers (PY3.5)

Depolarizing blockers acts as ACh receptor agonist by binding to the ACh receptor at the motor end plate and depolarize the muscle end plates by opening Na^+ channels. It produces twitching and fasciculations of muscles in two phases.

Phase I

After the drug binds the motor end plate receptor, there is a persistent depolarization of muscle end plate. During the depolarization phase, transient muscle fasciculation occurs. This depolarization phase is rapid onset and gradually declines to a repolarization state despite continuous presence of the drug at the receptor. Phase I block is replaced by phase II but the neuromuscular transmission is not reestablished.

Phase II

This phase is slow in onset, and in this phase, muscles are no longer receptive to ACh released by the motor neurons. This phase is slow in onset and also known as the desensitizing phase where the depolarizing agent finally achieves full paralysis.

Pharmacological Actions of Neuromuscular Blockers (PY3.5)

Skeletal Muscles

Intravenous (IV) injection of nondepolarizing blockers produces rapid muscle weakness followed by flaccid paralysis. Initially, small rapidly moving muscles such as those of eyes, jaws, and larynx are affected; then, paralysis spreads to limbs and trunk. Ultimately, the intercoastal muscle and, finally, diaphragm are paralyzed and respiration ceases. Usually, reverse order follows while there is recovery of muscles; hence, diaphragm is the first muscle to regain function.

Depolarizing blockers after IV injection typically produce brief muscle fasciculations, particularly over the chest and abdomen. Relaxation of the muscle occurs, reaching maximum and gradually disappearing within a brief period. Transient apnea occurs at the time of maximum muscle relaxation.

Autonomic Ganglia

Neuromuscular blockers block the nicotinic receptors present in the autonomic ganglia and cause some amount of ganglionic blockade.

Histamine Release

Tubocurarine releases histamine from the mast cells, leading to hypotension, flushing, bronchospasm, and increased respiratory secretions. Among the neuromuscular blockers, tubocurarine has the highest histamine-releasing potential. Others include doxacurium, atracurium, and SCh.

Cardiovascular System (CVS)

Due to N_M receptor blockade, there is histamine release from the mast cells and reduced venous return, leading to significant fall in blood pressure by d-tubocurarine. Heart rate might increase due to vagal ganglionic blockade. Pancuronium tends to cause tachycardia and rise in blood pressure. All newer nondepolarizing drugs, namely, vecuronium, rocuronium, and cisatracurium, have negligible effects on blood pressure and heart rate.

Gastrointestinal Tract (GIT)

Nondepolarizing blockers, due to their ganglion blocking activity, may enhance postoperative paralytic ileus after abdominal operations.

Central Nervous System (CNS)

As all neuromuscular blockers are quaternary compounds, these drugs in clinical doses do not penetrate the blood–brain barrier (BBB).

Peripherally Acting Neuromuscular Blockers

They do not cross the BBB as these are quaternary compounds. The route of administration is usually IV, although it can be given intramuscular (IM); however, orally, it is not absorbed. The duration of action and $t_{1/2}$ of vecuronium, atracurium, cisatracurium, rocuronium, and mivacurium is relatively shorter and is 20 to 40 minutes. These drugs are metabolized primarily in the plasma or liver. Pancuronium, tubocurarine, doxacurium, and pipecuronium have longer $t_{1/2}$ and duration of action is > 60 minutes. They are metabolized in the kidney.

D-Tubocurarine

d-tubocurarine is obsolete nowadays because of prominent histamine release and long duration of paralysis.

Pancuronium

Pancuronium is an aminosteroid compound which is more potent with lesser side effects. It has good cardio-vascular stability because of less ganglionic blockade. Flushing, bronchospasm, or cardiac arrhythmias also occur rarely because of low histamine releasing potential. But rapid IV injections of pancuronium might cause increase in blood pressure and tachycardia.

Adverse Effects

Patient with renal condition might experience a decrease in 30 to 50% plasma clearance, leading to prolong neuro-muscular blockade.

Dose

In critically ill patients for intubation—0.1 mg/kg with a 3- to 5-minute onset for maximal muscle relaxation. Maintenance dose of neuromuscular blockade is 0.02 mg/kg, titrated to the level of blockade.

Doxacurium

It is the most potent neuromuscular blocker, which has a longer duration of action. In patients with renal and hepatic insufficiency, duration of action is prolonged.

Dose

With a dose of 0.05 mg/kg, its duration of action is 80 to 90 minutes.

Pipecuronium

Pipecuronium is structurally related to pancuronium and vecuronium. It is devoid of cardiovascular events.

Dose

Recommended dose for endotracheal intubation is 0.07 mg/kg.

Vecuronium

Vecuronium is an aminosteroid compound like pancuronium. This drug is often used as an adjuvant with general anesthesia to facilitate endotracheal intubation and surgical relaxation. Due to its rapid distribution and considerable hepatic metabolism, vecuronium experiences a shorter duration of action. Hence, it has higher lipid solubility and is excreted mainly in bile. Because of minimal histamine release, cardiovascular stability is also better.

Adverse Effects

Few cases were reported for bronchospasm, hypotension, edema, sinus tachycardia, erythema, urticaria, flushing, pruritus, and skin rash.

Dose

For endotracheal intubation prior to surgery, 0.08 mg/kg to 0.1 mg/kg IV over 60 seconds.

Atracurium

Atracurium is indicated as an adjuvant with general anesthetics to facilitate endotracheal intubation and provide skeletal muscle relaxation during surgery or mechanical ventilation. It is a less potent and short-acting drug. Atracurium has a unique mode of elimination by spontaneous degradation from plasma known as Hofmann elimination in addition to that by cholinesterase.

Adverse Effects

Atracurium causes dose-dependent histamine release. Most common are flushing and erythema. Less commonly, more severe adverse effects can occur and include bradycardia, bronchospasm, dyspnea, hypotension, laryngospasm, tachycardia, urticaria, and wheezing.

Dose

For intubation, 0.23 mg/kg and 0.5 mg/kg for adults and children older than 2 years of age, and 0.3 to 0.4 mg/kg for children less than 2 years of age.

Cisatracurium

R-Cis enantiomer of atracurium is nearly six to eight times as potent as atracurium. It is devoid of clinically significant histamine release; hence, fewer adverse effects. Even though cisatracurium undergoes Hofmann elimination, it is not hydrolyzed by plasma cholinesterase. Hepatic metabolism is limited, so less toxic metabolite is formed. Especially for liver and kidney disease and elderly patients, currently cisatracurium is one of the preferred muscle relaxants.

Adverse Effects

Less than 1% of cases show bronchospasm, bradycardia, flushing, pruritus, myositis ossificans, hypotension, and rashes.

Dose

For neuromuscular blockade, initial intubating doses starts with 0.15 to 0.2 mg/kg IV. Maintenance dose is 0.03 mg/kg IV.

Rocuronium

Neuromuscular blocking agent is used to produce muscle relaxation in emergency situation and facilitate surgery and ventilation of the lungs. Because of its rapid action, clinically, rocuronium has major advantage than other nondepolarizing neuromuscular blockers.

Adverse Effects

Allergic reactions, residual neuromuscular weakness, myopathy, and polyneuropathy occur due to prolonged infusion of the drug.

Dose

For intubation, it is 0.6 to 1.2 mg/kg; relaxation occurs within 1 to 2 minutes, with effects lasting until 20 to 35 minutes.

Mivacurium

It is the shortest-acting neuromuscular blocker which does not need reversal. Prolonged paralysis with mivacurium can occur in pseudocholinesterase-deficient individuals. Reversal of muscle paralysis can be done by neostigmine.

Adverse Effects

Adverse effects are mainly dose-dependent. The most common adverse effects reported are cutaneous flushing about the face, neck, or chest and hypotension.

Dose

For tracheal intubation, 0.15 mg/kg is administered over 5 to 15 seconds, 0.2 mg/kg is administered over 30 seconds, or 0.25 mg/kg is administered in divided doses (0.15 mg/kg followed by 0.1 mg/kg in 30 seconds).

Succinylcholine (SCh)

The US Food and Drugs Administration (FDA) had approved succinylcholine (SCh), despite its tendency to produce muscle fasciculation, changes in blood pressure and heart rate, arrhythmias, histamine release, and K^+ efflux. These effects lead to hyperkalemia and its complications. It is the drug of choice in quick intervention and airway control where endotracheal intubation is not possible. Approximately within 5 minutes, SCh induces rapid and complete paralysis with spontaneous recovery.

Adverse Effects

Most common adverse effect is hyperkalemia. In a small percentage of population, after SCh administration, patients may manifest masseter muscle spasms (trismus). Bradycardia can be seen, especially in pediatric population due to nicotinic activation. There is also increase in intraocular pressure and malignant hyperthermia.

Dose

The US FDA approved 1.5 mg/kg IV for rapid sequence intubation.

Choice of Neuromuscular Blockers

For therapeutic use, drugs should be selected based on achieving their pharmacokinetic profile, which is consistent with the duration of any interventional procedure, minimizing cardiovascular or other side effects, with specific attention to patients with renal or hepatic failure. The characteristics which distinguish side effects and pharmacokinetic behavior are as follows:

- Chemical nature of the drug—Depending upon the degree of blockade of ganglia, block of vagal responses and histamine release, side effects of the skeletal muscle relaxant or neuromuscular blockers are exhibited.
- Duration of drug action—Depending on the necessity of the situation, long-acting, short-acting, or ultrashort-acting agents can be administered.

Drug Interactions with Neuromuscular Blockers

1. Thiopentone sodium + SCh—Should not be mixed in the same syringe, as it may lead to chemical reactions.
2. General anesthetics + SCh—Fluorinated anesthetics like halothane and isoflurane when administered with SCh may cause malignant hyperthermia in genetically predisposed individuals.
3. Anticholinesterase + competitive neuromuscular blockers—Reverse the action of competitive neuromuscular blockers.
4. Antibiotics + competitive neuromuscular blockers—Aminoglycoside antibiotics potentiate the action of competitive neuromuscular blockers. The dose of competitive blocker should be reduced in patients receiving high doses of these antibiotics.
5. Calcium channel blockers + neuromuscular blockers—Verapamil and others potentiate the action of neuromuscular blockers.
6. Diuretics + competitive blockers—May enhance hypokalemia, which would potentiate the action of competitive blockers.
7. Diazepam, propranolol and quinidine + competitive blocker—Intensifies the action of competitive blockers.

Toxicity of Neuromuscular Blockers

1. Respiratory paralysis and prolong apnea.
2. Flushing due to histamine release.
3. Fall in blood pressure and cardiovascular collapse.
4. Cardiac arrythmias and arrest.
5. Precipitation of asthma.
6. Postoperative muscle soreness and myalgia.
7. Malignant hyperthermia.

Uses of Neuromuscular Blockers

1. Neuromuscular blockers are used as an adjuvant along with general anesthesia. SCh is employed for brief procedures such as endotracheal intubation, laryngoscopy, bronchoscopy, esophagoscopy, and reduction of fractures.
2. Assisted ventilation mainly used for critically ill patients in intensive care units.
3. To avoid convulsion and trauma for electroconvulsive therapy, muscle relaxants such as SCh are used.
4. In severe cases of tetanus and status epilepticus, neuromuscular blockers are helpful in maintaining intermittent positive pressure respiration.

Directly Acting Muscle Relaxants

Dantrolene

Dantrolene sodium is a postsynaptic muscle relaxant. FDA has approved usage of this drug for the treatment of malignant hyperthermia in adult and children. Other uses of dantrolene are muscle spasticity disorders which includes stroke, spinal cord injury, cerebral palsy, and multiple sclerosis.

Mechanism of Action

Dantrolene acts intracellularly in the skeletal muscles by inhibiting Ca^{+2} release from the sarcoplasmic reticulum and limiting the capacity of Ca^{+2} and calmodulin to activate the ryanodine receptor (RYR1). Calcium concentration within each sarcomere decreases and no binding of calcium to the troponin on actin filaments occurs. This prevents exposure of the myosin-binding site on the actin, hindering actin, and myosin cross-bridging. Hence, it minimizes the excitation-contraction coupling interaction between actin and myosin within the individual sarcomere and decreases the contractibility and energy expenditure of the muscle cells.

Adverse Effects

Muscle weakness is the main adverse effect. Sedation, malaise, and light headedness can occur sometimes.

Dose

Adult and Pediatric Patients

1. *For treatment of malignant hyperthermia*—2.5 mg/kg dantrolene IV immediately.

   If the signs and symptoms of malignant hyperthermia persist, additional IV boluses of 1 to 2.5 mg/kg are indicated to a maximum cumulative dose of 10 mg/kg.

   Following the successful treatment of the initial reaction, 1 mg/kg of IV dantrolene should be provided every 6 hours for 24 hours since the last observed symptom of malignant hyperthermia to prevent a recurrence.

2. *Prophylaxis of malignant hyperthermia*—2.5 mg/kg IV over 1 minute approximately 75 minutes before surgery.
3. *Chronic muscle spasticity*—Initial dose of oral dantrolene is started at 25 mg daily for 7 days and should be titrated to the maximum individual effect. Doses are typically increased by 25 mg at a time and require monitoring for 7 days before further advancement. The maximum dose is 400 mg/day.
4. *Malignant hyperthermia*—Malignant hyperthermia is an autosomal dominant pharmacogenetic disorder of skeletal muscle calcium regulation. It is associated with excess release of calcium from the sarcoplasmic reticulum due to triggering substances (e.g., fluorinated general anesthetics such as halothane, isoflurane, sevoflurane, desflurane, enflurane alone or in combination with SCh). This may enhance entry of more extracellular calcium into the myoplasm. Increasing Ca^{+2} concentration in the myoplasm results in skeletal muscles' contractability, glycogenolysis, and increased cellular metabolism, followed by more production of heat and lactate. Affected individuals manifest hyperthermia, tachycardia, hyperkalemia with risk of cardiac arrhythmia or cardiac arrest, hypercapnia, muscle rigidity, increase in serum creatinine kinase concentration with rhabdomyolysis, and myoglobinuria with risk of renal failure.

It has been established from various research works that genetic polymorphisms of *CACNA1S*, *RYR1*, or *STAC3* genes in an individual may lead to malignant hyperthermia while administering fluorinated general anesthetics and SCh.

Quinine

Quinine minimizes the nerve stimulation by increasing the refractory period and decreasing the excitability of the motor end plates.

Uses

It decreases muscle tone in myotonia congenita.

Dose

A total of 200 to 300 mg at bedtime abolishes nocturnal leg cramps in some patients.

Centrally Acting Muscle Relaxants

These drugs are used as adjuvant with other therapy to reduce discomfort from acute painful musculoskeletal conditions. It reduces skeletal muscle tone and lessens muscle spasm by a selective action in the cerebrospinal axis, without altering consciousness. These drugs selectively depress the spinal and supraspinal polysynaptic reflexes involved in the regulation of muscle tone without significantly affecting the stretch reflex (monosynaptic pathway). To a lesser extent, polysynaptic pathways, which involve maintenance of wakefulness, are also depressed.

Centrally acting muscle relaxants have sedative property to some extent, but they do not have any effect on neuromuscular transmission and on muscle fibers. These drugs reduce decerebrate rigidity, upper motor neuron spasticity, and hyperreflexia.

Mephenesin

This was the first drug to prove centrally acting muscle relaxants in animals. It is not used clinically nowadays because of its adverse effects.

Mechanism of Action

Mephenesin reducing neuronal excitability leads to decrease in action potentials to muscle fibers, which ultimately produces a reduction in spasticity.

Adverse Effects

Orally, gastric irritation is more common. Thrombophlebitis, hemolysis, and fall in blood pressure might occur through IV route.

Dose

Used as counterirritant ointments and available as 0.5 or 10 or 1% or 30 g cream or ointment.

Carisoprodol

Carisoprodol is approved by FDA for the relief of discomfort associated with acute, painful musculoskeletal conditions. It has sedative properties along with weak analgesic, antipyretic, and anticholinergic properties.

Mechanism of Action

Muscle relaxing effect of carisoprodol is not clear. In animal studies, altered interneuronal activity in the spinal cord and the descending reticular formation of the brain were observed. Meprobamate, the primary metabolite of carisoprodol, is believed to be acting on GABA receptors and responsible for therapeutic effect and abuse potential.

Pharmacokinetics

Carisoprodol is primarily metabolized in the liver by isoenzyme CYP2C19 and excreted through kidney. Elimination half-life is 1.7 to 2 hours, and half-life of carisoprodol metabolite, meprobamate, is approximately 10 hours.

Adverse Effects

Most common adverse effects are drowsiness, dizziness, and headache. Prolonged use of the drug might cause dependence, withdrawal, and abuse potential in patients who have a history of addiction.

Dose

Orally 250 mg or 350 mg up to three times a day or at bedtime.

Chlorzoxazone

Even though chlorzoxazone is pharmacologically similar to mephenesin it has a longer duration of action and better tolerance by patients.

Adverse Effects

Commonly observed adverse effects are dizziness, drowsiness, headache, fatigue, and tremor. Hepatotoxicity and allergic reactions are rarely seen.

Dose

Combination of:

- Ibuprofen (400 mg) + paracetamol (325 mg) + chlorzoxazone (250 mg).
- Diclofenac (50 mg) + paracetamol (325 mg) + chlorzoxazone (250 mg).
- Diclofenac (50 mg) + paracetamol (500 mg) + chlorzoxazone (500 mg).
- Paracetamol (300 mg) + chlorzoxazone (250 mg).

Chlormezanone

Chlormezanone is a nonbenzodiazepine muscle relaxant. It has antianxiety and hypnotic actions. It was discontinued due to serious and rare cutaneous reactions.

Methocarbamol

Methocarbamol is used for the treatment of muscle spasms resulting from injury, musculoskeletal disorders, tetanus, and other disorders, with limited therapeutic use. The drug is better than placebo but not a superior muscle relaxant.

Dose

Available as oral and parenteral forms (IV, IM). Oral dose is 500 mg and 750 mg. Parenteral is IV or IM injection in 10-mL single-dose vials containing 10 mg/mL.

Diazepam

Diazepam acts through specific BZD receptors present in the brain, enhancing GABAergic transmission. It is mainly used for reducing muscle tone in spinal injuries and tetanus.

Dose

Orally, 5 mg TDS; for IV, 10 to 40 mg in tetanus.

Baclofen

The US FDA has approved baclofen for the management of muscle spasticity originating from multiple sclerosis, and spinal injuries.

Mechanism of Action

Baclofen is a selective $GABA_B$ receptor agonist. It primarily acts on mono- and polysynaptic neurons at the spinal cord and brain, resulting in decrease in excitatory transmitter release.

Pharmacokinetics

Baclofen is well-tolerated orally. It is secreted unchanged in urine. Plasma half-life ($t_{1/2}$) is of 3 to 4 hours.

Adverse Effects

Most common adverse effects include transient sedation, confusion, muscle weakness, vertigo, and nausea. Rare adverse effects reported were neuropsychiatric impairment, seizure, insomnia, etc.

Sudden withdrawal of the drug after chronic use may lead to hallucinations, tachycardia, and seizures.

Dose

10 mg twice daily to 25 mg thrice daily.

Thiocolchicoside

Thiocolchicoside is chemically related to colchicine. It is mainly used for painful muscle spasms like torticolis, sprains, and backache.

Mechanism of Action

Mechanism of thiocolchicoside is thought to be a GABA-mimetic and glycinergic action.

Adverse Effects

Gastric upset and photosensitivity reactions.

Dose

Orally, 4 mg thrice daily or four times a day.

Tizanidine

Tizanidine one of the most potent centrally acting muscle relaxants. Even though it has structural and biochemical similarity with clonidine, cardiovascular effects of tizanidine are mild. The FDA has approved tizanidine for the management of muscle spasticity due to multiple sclerosis and spinal cord injury.

Mechanism of Action

It acts as an agonist for the central α_2 receptor which inhibits excitatory amino acids' (like glutamate and aspartate) release in the spinal interneurons. Tizanidine also increases presynaptic inhibition of motor neurons, with the greatest effect on spinal polysynaptic pathways. The above effects are believed to be helpful in reducing the facilitation of spinal motor neurons.

Pharmacokinetics

Tizanidine is extensively metabolized in liver by CYP450: 1A2 and excreted in urine and feces. It undergoes significant first pass metabolism. Oral bioavailability is 20 to 34%. Elimination half-life is 2.5 hours.

Adverse Effects

Tizanidine is well-tolerated orally. Common adverse effects include xerostomia, drowsiness, asthenia, dizziness, hypotension, bradycardia, constipation, urinary frequency, blurred vision, dyskinesia, nervousness, hallucination, and rhinitis.

Serious adverse effects may be hepatotoxicity, severe bradycardia, QT interval prolongation, severe hypotension, syncope, Stevens–Johnson syndrome, anaphylaxis, and exfoliative dermatitis. Abrupt withdrawal of drug may cause tachycardia, rebound hypertension, and increased spasticity.

Dose

Orally available as 2 mg, 4 mg, and 6 mg capsules.

Drug Interactions

Tizanidine + ciprofloxacin or tizanidine + fluvoxamine causes hypotension and increased psychomotor impairment.

Uses of Centrally Acting Muscle Relaxants

1. Acute muscle spasm—Spasm due to overstretching of a muscle, sprain, tearing of ligaments and tendons, dislocation, fibrositis, bursitis, etc.
2. Torticollis, lumbago, backache, neuralgias.
3. Anxiety and tension—Increased muscle tone due to anxiety. Diazepam acts as an antianxiety agent and a muscle relaxant.
4. Spastic neurological diseases; for example, hemiplegia, paraplegia, spinal injuries, multiple sclerosis, and cerebral palsy.
5. Tetanus—Diazepam is effective; methocarbamol can also be used as alternative.
6. Electroconvulsive therapy (ECT)—Diazepam is effective in decreasing the intensity of convulsions resulting from ECT, without diminishing its therapeutic effect on ECT.
7. Orthopedic manipulations.

Multiple Choice Questions

1. From the list below, choose the depolarizing neuromuscular blocker most likely to be used in "rapid sequence intubation," a procedure that is done when the stomach contents have a high risk of refluxing and causing aspiration:

A. Baclofen.
B. Succinylcholine (SCh).
C. Neostigmine.
D. Homatropine.

Answer: B

SCh is a depolarizing neuromuscular blocker that is used in rapid-sequence intubation as well as other procedures. It quickly relaxes all muscles in the body, allowing a prompt intubation to prevent the reflux of gastric contents into the trachea.

2. A 22-year-old male patient being operated for hernia was anesthetized with halothane and nitrous oxide; tubocurarine was given for skeletal muscle relaxation. The patient suddenly develops tachycardia and becomes hypertensive. Generalized skeletal muscle rigidity was associated with severe hyperthermia. Laboratory values showed hyperkalemia and acidosis. This rare complication of anesthesia is most likely due to:

A. Acetylcholine (ACh) release from somatic nerve endings at skeletal muscle.
B. Activation of brain dopamine receptors by halothane.
C. Block of autonomic ganglia by tubocurarine.
D. Release of calcium from the sarcoplasmic reticulum.

Answer: D

Malignant hyperthermia is a rare but life-threatening adverse reaction that can develop during general anesthesia with halogenated anesthetics and skeletal muscle relaxants, especially succinylcholine (SCh) and tubocurarine. Release of calcium from skeletal muscle causes muscle spasms, hyperthermia, and autonomic instability. Predisposing genetic factors comprise clinical myopathy associated with mutations in the gene loci for the skeletal muscle ryanodine receptor or L-type calcium receptors.

3. The patient from the previous question should be managed immediately with:

A. Atropine.
B. Baclofen.
C. Dantrolene.
D. Edrophonium.

Answer: C

The drug of choice in malignant hyperthermia is dantrolene, which prevents liberation of calcium from the sarcoplasmic reticulum of skeletal muscle cells. Necessary measures to lower body temperature, control hypertension, and restore acid-base and electrolyte balance must be ensured.

4. A 45-year-old lady has planned to undergo laparoscopic cholecystectomy. She is a known case of hypertension and coronary artery disease. For hypertension management, she has been on angiotensin-converting enzyme (ACE) inhibitors for a long time. The anesthesiologist advised her to do some laboratory investigations. Laboratory report suggested increase in serum potassium level (hyperkalemia). Along with anesthesia (general/spinal/epidural), neuromuscular blockers are added for better outcome of the surgery. Which neuromuscular blocker has to be avoided because of hyperkalemia?

A. Vecuronium.
B. Succinylcholine (SCh).
C. Atracurium.
D. Cisatracurium.

Answer: B

One of the common side effects of SCh is hyperkalemia.

5. A 30-year-old woman was rushed to the hospital with 30% burn injury. She needs intubation for airway management. Which rapid acting neuromuscular blocker will be suitable in this case?

A. Vecuronium.
B. Rocuronium.
C. Succinylcholine (SCh).
D. Atracurium.

Answer: D

Rocuronium is one of the fastest acting neuromuscular blockers.

6. A muscarinic receptor antagonist would probably not be needed for reversal of the skeletal muscle relaxant actions of a nondepolarizing drug if the agent used was:

A. Cisatracurium.
B. Mivacurium.
C. Pancuronium.
D. Vecuronium.

Answer: C

One of the distinctive characteristics of pancuronium is that it can block muscarinic receptors, especially those in the heart. It has sometimes caused tachycardia and hypertension and may cause dysrhythmias in predisposed individuals.

7. The drug that undergoes Hofmann elimination is:

A. Atracurium.
B. Vecuronium.
C. Succinylcholine (SCh).
D. Tubocurarine.

Answer: A

Nonenzymatic degradation (Hofmann elimination) accounts for 45% of the metabolism of atracurium. The remainder is metabolized via ester hydrolysis by nonspecific esterases in the plasma which are unrelated to pseudocholinesterase. This neuromuscular blocking agent is preferred in critically ill patients as their metabolism is not affected by renal or hepatic dysfunction. A primary metabolite of Hofmann elimination of atracurium is laudanosine, which does not have any neuromuscular blocking activity, but it is a central nervous system (CNS) stimulant.

8. Prolonged apnea may occur following the administration of succinylcholine (SCh) to a patient with a hereditary deficiency of which of the following enzymes?

A. Glucose-6-phosphate dehydrogenase.
B. Plasma cholinesterase.
C. Monoamine oxidase.
D. Acetylcholinesterase.

Answer: B

Plasma cholinesterase is responsible for the rapid inactivation of SCh.

9. The clinical use of succinylcholine (SCh), especially in patients with diabetes, is associated with:

A. Antagonism by pyridostigmine during the early phase of blockade.
B. Aspiration of gastric contents.
C. Decreased intragastric pressure.
D. Histamine release in a genetically determined population.

Answer: B

Fasciculations associated with SCh may increase intragastric pressure with possible complications of regurgitation and aspiration of gastric contents. The complication is more likely in patients with delayed gastric emptying such as those with esophageal dysfunction or diabetes. Histamine release resulting from SCh is not genetically determined.

Chapter 20

Adrenergic System and Adrenergic Drugs

Prasan R. Bhandari

PH1.13: Describe the mechanism of action, types, doses, side effects, indications, and contraindications of adrenergic and anti-adrenergic drugs.

Learning Objectives

- Adrenergic system.
- Adrenergic drugs.

Adrenergic System

Adrenergic system is also called sympathetic nervous system (SNS), which is activated during stress and prepares the body for fright, flight, or fight. The actions on stimulation of SNS are multiple, such as increased blood pressure (BP), increased cardiac output, and increased heart rate. Blood is shifted from skin, gastrointestinal tract (GIT), and kidney (less important organs) to heart, brain, lungs, and skeletal muscles (more important organs). The pupils and the bronchi dilate. There is increased sweating and there is increased blood glucose because of glycogenolysis.

Distribution of SNS

It is distributed from the thoracolumbar outflow, that is, T1 to L2–L3. Their ganglia are prevertebral, paravertebral, terminal, and adrenal medulla.

Neurotransmitters

Major neurotransmitters of SNS include noradrenaline (NA) and dopamine (DA). Major neurotransmitter of adrenal medulla is adrenaline (a hormone).

Biosynthesis of Catecholamines

Three endogenous catecholamines that are present are NA, adrenaline, and DA. These are synthesized from tyrosine (**Fig. 20.1**).

Sympathetic postganglionic fibers synthesize, store, and release NA (adrenergic nerves). NA is stored in vesicles of adrenergic nerve endings. Action potential at nerve terminals releases NA by exocytosis in synaptic cleft. Binding of NA to postsynaptic receptors generates response (uptake 2). Around 80% of NA is taken back into nerve endings (uptake 1). A small fraction is metabolized by catechol-*O*-methyltransferase (COMT) in synapse. Portion of NA reuptaken by uptake 1 is metabolized by monoamine oxidase (MOA).

Norepinephrine (NE) is the primary neurotransmitter for postganglionic sympathetic adrenergic nerves. It is synthesized inside the nerve axon, stored within vesicles, and then released by the nerve when an action potential travels down the nerve. The following are the details for release and synthesis of NE.

The amino acid tyrosine is transported into the sympathetic nerve axon. Tyrosine is converted to DOPA by tyrosine hydroxylase (rate-limiting step for NE synthesis). dihydroxyphenethylamine (DOPA) is converted to DA by DOPA decarboxylase. DA is transported into vesicles and then converted to NE by DA β-hydroxylase (DBH); transport into the vesicle can by blocked by the drug reserpine. An action potential traveling down the axon depolarizes the membrane and causes calcium to enter the axon. Increased intracellular calcium causes the vesicles to migrate to the axonal membrane and fuse with the membrane, which permits the NE to diffuse out of the vesicle into the extracellular (junctional) space. DBH as well as, depending on the nerve, other secondary neurotransmitters (e.g., adenosine triphosphate) is released along with the NE. The NE binds to the postjunctional receptor and stimulates the effector organ response.

Adrenergic Receptors

They were classified by Ahlquist and are subcategorized into two types, that is, α → α1, α2; β → β1, β2, β3. The following are the actions of different adrenergic receptors (**Fig. 20.2**).

α receptor stimulation causes excitation (except GIT), whereas β receptor stimulation causes inhibition (except heart). α and β receptors are G protein-coupled receptors. α stimulation activates phospholipase C, which, in turn, generates inositol triphosphate (IP_3) and diacylglycerol. β stimulation activates adenylyl cyclase, which, in turn, increases cyclic adenosine monophosphate (cAMP) (**Table 20.1**). α2 receptors are presynaptic autoreceptors (major). Their stimulation leads to inhibition of NA release; hence, they cause a negative feedback. Postsynaptic receptors (minor) are present in brain, platelets, and pancreatic islets.

The following agents are the agonists and antagonists of adrenergic receptors:

- α_1 agonists: phenylephrine and mephentermine.
- α_1 antagonists: prazosin and terazosin.
- α_2 agonist: clonidine.
- α_2 antagonist: yohimbine.
- β_1 agonist: dobutamine.
- β_1 antagonists: atenolol and metoprolol.
- β_2 agonists: salbutamol, salmeterol, etc.
- β_2 antagonist: butoxamine.

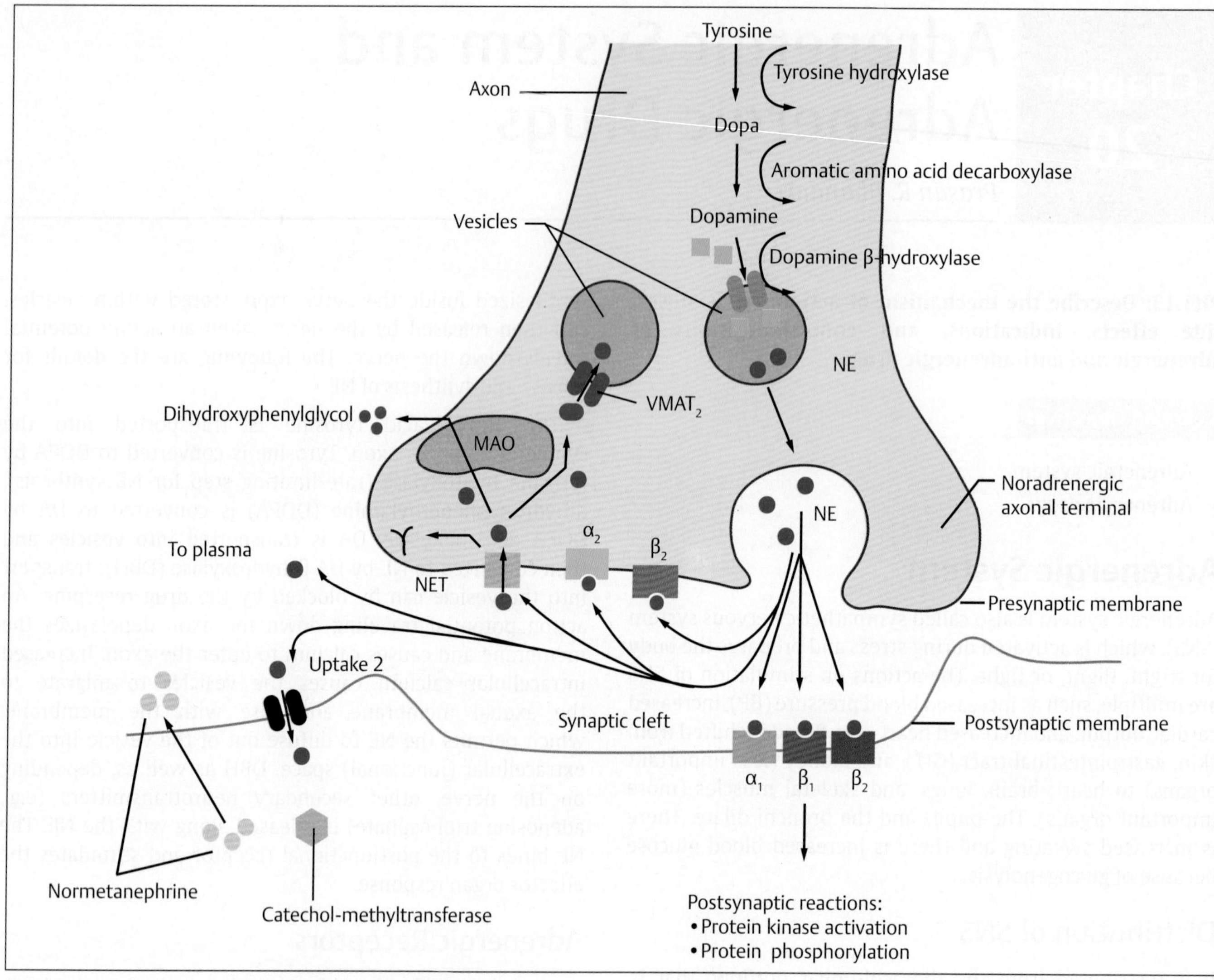

Tyrosine
Tyrosine hydroxylase
Axon
Dopa
Aromatic amino acid decarboxylase
Dopamine
Vesicles
Dopamine β-hydroxylase
NE
VMAT2
Dihydroxyphenylglycol
MAO
Noradrenergic axonal terminal
NE
α2
To plasma
β2
NET
Presynaptic membrane
Uptake 2
Synaptic cleft
Postsynaptic membrane
α1
β1
β2
Normetanephrine
Catechol-methyltransferase
Postsynaptic reactions:
• Protein kinase activation
• Protein phosphorylation

Fig. 20.1 Synthesis/storage/release/metabolism of catecholamines.

Adrenergic receptors
Alpha-1
• Vasoconstriction
• ↑ Peripheral resistance (blood flow)
• ↑ Blood pressure
• Mydriasis
• ↑ Closure bladder sphincters
Alpha-2
• Inhibits Norepinephrine release
• Inhibits acetylcholine release
• Inhibits insulin release
Beta-1
• ↑ Heart rate
• ↑ Lipolysis
• ↑ Myocardial contractility
• ↑ Renin
Beta-2
• Vasodilation
• ↓ Peripheral resistance
• Bronchodilation
• ↑ Glycogenolysis (muscle, liver)
• ↑ Glucagon release
• Relaxes uterine smooth muscle

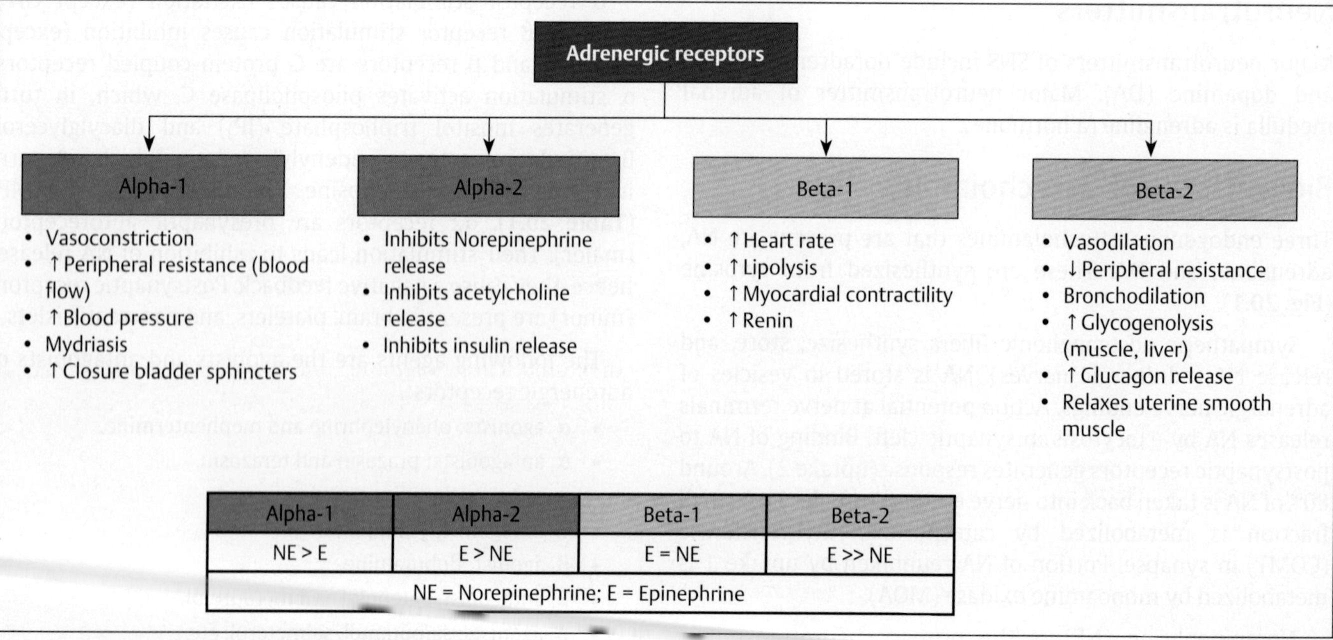

Alpha-1	Alpha-2	Beta-1	Beta-2
NE > E	E > NE	E = NE	E >> NE

NE = Norepinephrine; E = Epinephrine

Fig. 20.2 Distribution/actions of adrenergic receptors.

Table 20.1 Summary of therapeutic classification of adrenergic drugs

Agents	Drugs
Cardiac stimulants	Adrenaline, Dobutamine, Isoprenaline
Bronchodilators	Isoprenaline, Salbutamol (Albuterol), Salmeterol, Formoterol, Bambuterol, Terbutaline
Nasal decongestants	Phenylephrine, Pseudoephedrine, Phenyl propanolamine
CNS stimulants	Amphetamine, Methamphetamine, Dexamphetamine
Anorectics (is a dietary supplement or drug which reduces appetite)	Fenfluramine, Sibutramine, Dexfenfluramine
Uterine relaxant and vasodilators	Ritodrine, Isoxsuprine, Salbutamol, Terbutaline

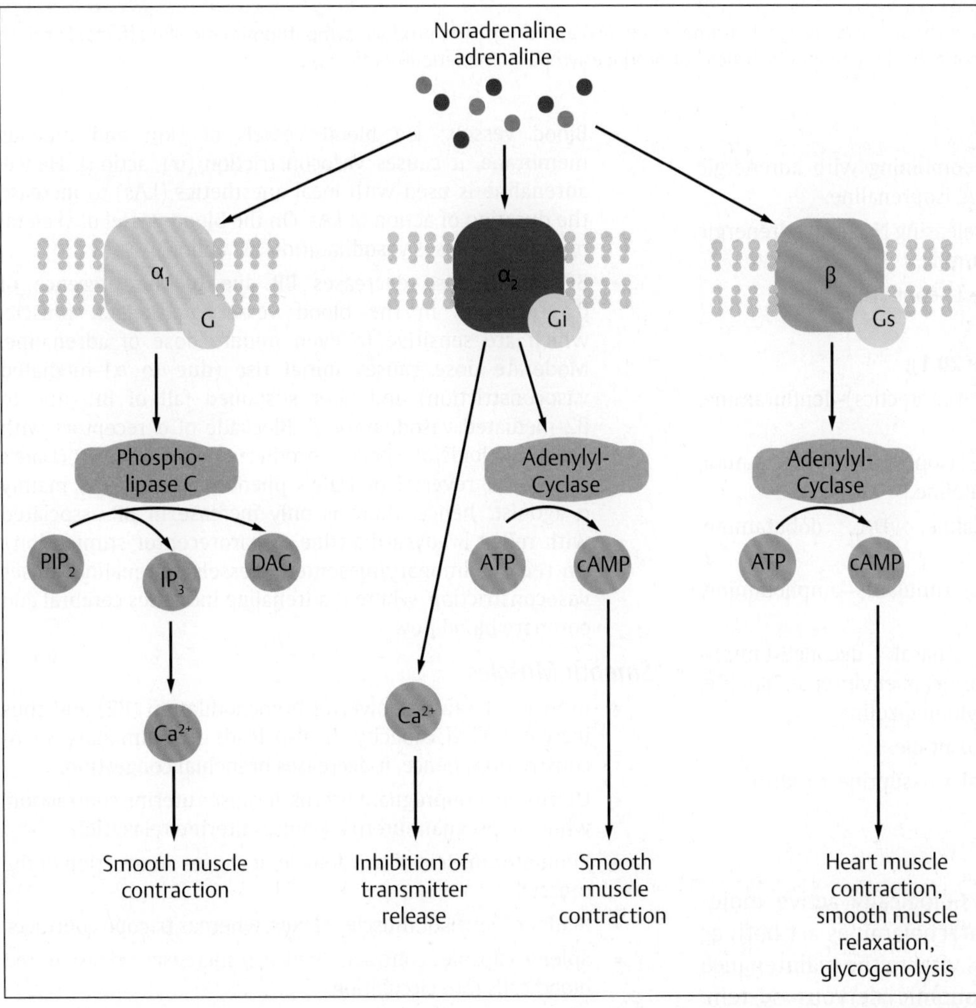

Fig. 20.3 Actions of different adrenergic receptors.

The actions on stimulation of different adrenergic receptors have been summarized in **Fig. 20.3**.

Adrenergic Drugs

Adrenergic drugs are a broad class of medications that bind to adrenergic receptors throughout the body. These receptors include α1, α2, β1, β2, and β3. Adrenergic drugs will bind directly to one or more of these receptors to induce various physiologic effects. Some drugs indirectly act at these receptors to induce certain effects. These are also known as catecholamines and sympathomimetic drugs. Adrenergic drugs must be classified based on the specific receptors they bind. Catecholamines and sympathomimetic drugs are classified as direct-acting, indirect-acting, or mixed-acting sympathomimetics (**Fig. 20.4**).

Classification

- Chemical classification—depending on presence/absence of catechol nucleus:
  - Catecholamines → natural: NA, adrenaline → synthetic: isoprenaline.
  - Noncatecholamines: ephedrine, amphetamine.

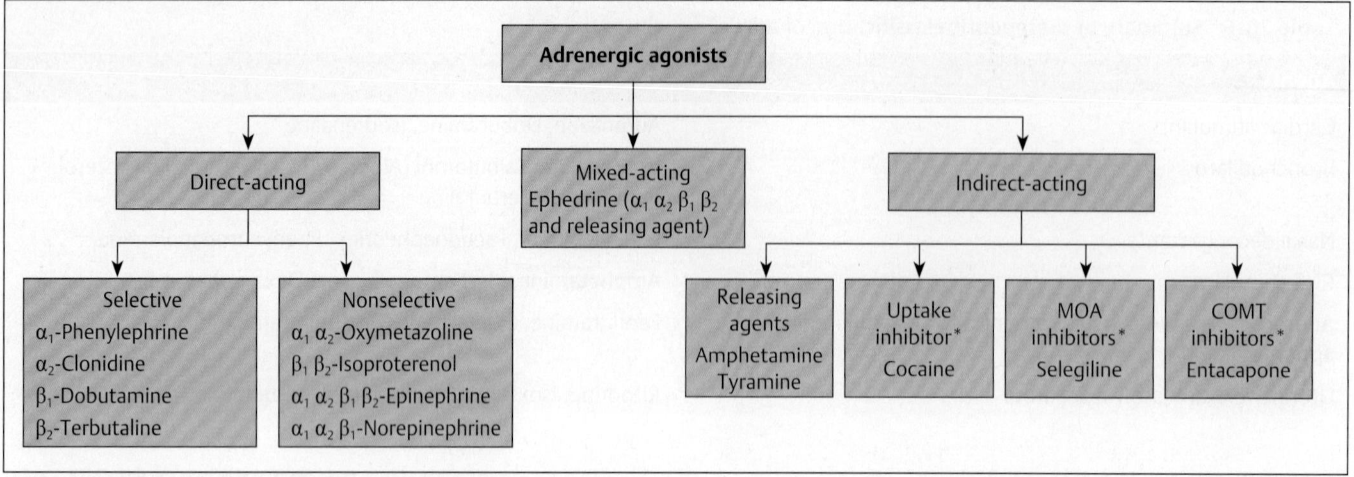

Fig. 20.4 Classification of adrenergic receptor agonists (sympathomimetic amines) and drugs that produce sympathomimetic-like effects. For each category, a prototypical drug is shown (*not actually sympathetic drugs but produce sympathomimetic-like effects).

- Based on mechanism:
  - Directly acting, that is, by combining with adrenergic receptors—NA, adrenaline, DA, isoprenaline.
  - Indirectly acting, that is, by releasing NA from adrenergic neurons—amphetamine, tyramine.
  - Mixed acting—direct + indirect—ephedrine, methoxamine.
- Therapeutic classification (**Table 20.1**):
  - Appetite suppressants (anorectics)—fenfluramine, dexfenfluramine.
  - Bronchodilators—adrenaline, isoprenaline, salbutamol, salmeterol, formoterol, terbutaline.
  - Cardiac stimulants—adrenaline, DA, dobutamine, isoprenaline, ephedrine.
  - Central nervous system (CNS) stimulants—amphetamine, ephedrine.
  - Decongestants of nose (nasal decongestants)—pseudoephedrine, phenylephrine, phenylpropanolamine, ephedrine, oxymetazoline, xylometazoline.
  - Vasopressors—NA, DA, methoxamine.
  - Uterine relaxants—salbutamol, isoxsuprine, ritodrine.

Catecholamines

DA, NE, and epinephrine are physiologically active molecules known as catecholamines. Catecholamines act both as neurotransmitters and as hormones vital to the maintenance of homeostasis through the autonomic nervous system. Physiologic principles of catecholamines have numerous applications within pharmacology. Pheochromocytoma is a catecholamine-producing neoplasm relevant to clinical medicine.

Adrenaline

Pharmacological Actions

Cardiovascular System

- Heart: It is a powerful cardiac stimulant (β1 receptor activity); hence, it increases heart rate, force of contraction (FOC), cardiac output, and conduction velocity. It increases the work of the heart as well as O_2 consumption.
- Blood vessels: On blood vessels of skin and mucous membrane, it causes vasoconstriction (α1 action). Hence, adrenaline is used with local anesthetics (LAs) to increase the duration of action of LAs. On the blood vessel of skeletal muscles, it causes vasodilatation (β2 action).
- BP: Small dose decreases BP due to the presence of β2 receptors in the blood vessel of skeletal muscle, which are sensitive to even minute dose of adrenaline. Moderate dose causes initial rise (due to α1-mediated vasoconstriction) and later sustained fall of BP (due to β2-mediated vasodilatation). Blockade of α receptors with ergot alkaloids/α blockers produces only fall of BP (Dale's vasomotor reversal or Dale's phenomenon). NA is mainly α agonist; hence, there is only increase in BP associated with reflex bradycardia (due to baroreceptor stimulation). On renal/pulmonary/mesenteric vessels, adrenaline causes vasoconstriction, whereas adrenaline increases cerebral and coronary blood flow.

Smooth Muscles

- Bronchi: it causes powerful bronchodilation (β2) and thus increases vital capacity. It also leads to pulmonary vasoconstriction; hence, it decreases bronchial congestion.
- Uterus: on nonpregnant uterus, it causes uterine contraction, while on pregnant uterus it causes uterine relaxation.
- Pilomotor muscle of hair follicle: it causes contraction of the muscle.
- Bladder: detrusor muscle relaxes, whereas trigone contracts.
- Splenic capsule: contracts; hence, it increases release of red blood cells into circulation.

Eye

It causes mydriasis due to contraction of radial muscle of iris (α1); hence, it decreases intraocular pressure (IOP).

Skeletal Muscles

Adrenaline increases neuromuscular transmission (α and β), since it increases acetylcholine release.

Metabolic Effects

It increases blood sugar, since it increases hepatic glycogenolysis. It decreases insulin release. Additionally, it increases free fatty acids due to increase in breakdown of triglycerides (β3 receptors in adipocytes).

Pharmacokinetics

Adrenaline is rapidly inactivated in GIT and liver, and hence it is not given orally. It is metabolized by MAO and COMT.

Adverse Reactions

They include anxiety, palpitations, tremors, pallor, dizziness, restlessness, throbbing headache, and increase in BP. It precipitates anginal pain in ischemic heart disease. Arrhythmias, subarachnoid hemorrhage, hemiplegia (if rapid intravenous [IV] injection), and acute pulmonary edema (since it shifts blood from systemic to pulmonary circulation) are also seen.

Contraindications

It is contraindicated in cardiovascular diseases, such as angina, hypertension, congestive cardiac failure (CCF), and arrhythmias, as well as in β-blocker therapy, since it can lead to hypertensive crisis and cerebral hemorrhage due to unopposed action of adrenaline on α1 receptors. Other contraindications include pheochromocytoma and thyrotoxicosis.

Preparations

- 1:1,000, 1:10,000, 1:100,000, solutions.
- Administration:
  - Subcutaneous (SC)/intramuscular (IM).
  - Intracardiac in emergencies.
  - Aerosol for inhalation.
  - 2% eye solution.

Uses

Anaphylactic Shock

Adrenaline is the drug of choice. It is administered in a dose of 0.3 to 0.5 mL of 1:1,000 solution IM (since SC route is not preferred in shock). It relieves laryngeal edema, bronchospasm, and reverses hypotension.

Acute Bronchial Asthma

Adrenaline is administered as SC/inhalation. Nowadays, it is not preferred, as more selective agents (such as salbutamol) are available.

Cardiac

Due to drowning or electrocution, intracardiac adrenaline is administered between the fourth and fifth intercostal space, 2 to 3 inches away from sternum. It is to be ensured that the tip of the needle is in cardiac chamber and not in the cardiac muscle, by withdrawing blood in the syringe.

To Increase Duration of Action of LA

Since adrenaline causes vasoconstriction, it decreases systemic absorption of LA and hence there is less systemic toxicity of LA; thus, it increases the duration of action of LA. For this purpose, 1:10,000 to 1:20,000 solution is utilized.

Epistaxis

It is used to control hemorrhage. In these cases, 1:10,000 to 1:20,000 solution is used. It is a topical hemostatic, since adrenaline causes vasoconstriction and is also used to reduce bleeding in tooth extraction.

Glaucoma

Topical application of adrenaline decreases IOP. Drawbacks of topical adrenaline include poor absorption, short action, and rapid metabolism. Hence, dipivefrin is preferred, which is a prodrug of adrenaline and is converted to adrenaline by corneal esterases. Dipivefrin has high-lipid solubility and hence there is good corneal penetration.

Noradrenaline

It is a natural catecholamine and is the major neurotransmitter of the adrenergic system. It acts on α1, α2, and β receptors; however, it does not act on β2 receptor. Hence, it is a direct cardiac stimulant (β1). It causes vasoconstriction of blood vessels (α1); therefore, there is an increase in systolic as well as diastolic BP. This leads to reflex bradycardia. NA is not effective orally and it cannot be given SC/IM also, as it may cause necrosis and sloughing at the site of injection. Hence, it is administered as IV infusion. It is used to increase BP in hypotensive states; however, it decreases blood flow to vital organs due to generalized vasoconstriction. Hence, it is generally not preferred.

Isoprenaline

It is a synthetic catecholamine, which is a nonselective β agonist (both β1 and β2) and has no action on α receptors. It is a powerful cardiac stimulant; hence, it has positive ionotropic, chronotropic, and dromotropic effects. Additionally, it dilates renal, skeletal, and mesenteric blood vessels, and hence there is no change in systolic BP, but diastolic BP and mean arterial pressure decrease. It relaxes bronchial and GI smooth muscles. Isoprenaline undergoes extensive first-pass metabolism, and hence it is not effective orally. Therefore, it is given parenterally or by aerosol. It is metabolized by COMT. Its uses include heart block and bronchial asthma (but selective β2 agonists like salbutamol are preferred). The adverse drug reactions (ADRs) comprise tachycardia and arrhythmias (since it is a cardiac stimulant).

Dopamine

It is a precursor of NA which stimulates dopaminergic and adrenergic receptors. Additionally, it is also a neurotransmitter in the brain. The effects of DA varies, depending on its dosage, for example, low-dose DA (1–5 μ/kg/minute IV) stimulates vascular D1 receptors in renal, mesenteric, and coronary vessels and causes vasodilation. D2 receptor stimulation in sympathetic nerve endings and cardiovascular centers cause renal vasodilation; hence, renal blood flow and glomerular filtration rate increase. Intermediate dose (5–15 μg/kg/minute IV) causes cardiac stimulation, since β1 receptors are activated. Therefore, it increases the heart rate and FOC. Higher dose of DA (20–50 μg/kg/minute IV) causes vasoconstriction and increased BP due to α1 stimulation. It has no CNS effects, since it does not cross the blood–brain barrier (BBB). It is administered IV, since it has short duration of action and is rapidly metabolized by MAO and COMT. It is used in the treatment of cardiogenic/hypovolemic/septic shock. It is especially used in patients with renal dysfunction with low cardiac output. ADRs include nausea, vomiting, palpitation, angina, headache, and sudden rise in BP.

Dobutamine

It is a derivative of DA which is a selective β1 agonist. It also activates α1 receptor in therapeutic doses. However, only FOC increases, without increase in the heart rate; hence, increase in myocardial demand is milder as compared to DA. Therefore, dobutamine is preferred over DA in cardiogenic shock. It is used in CCF, acute myocardial infarction, and following cardiac surgeries (if cardiac failure is present).

Fenoldopam

It is a selective D1 agonist which dilates coronary, renal, and mesenteric arteries. It is used in severe hypertension (as IV infusion).

Noncatecholamines

These agents are devoid of catechol nucleus, which act by direct stimulation of adrenergic receptors and indirectly by releasing NA. Compared to catecholomines, they are orally effective, resistant to MAO inactivation, and long-acting, and cross the BBB. Hence, they have CNS effects.

Ephedrine

It is an alkaloid obtained from the plant of genus *Ephedra*, which has both direct and indirect action. Repeated administration of ephedrine leads to tachyphylaxis. It increases BP by vasoconstriction and by increasing cardiac output. As it is a CNS stimulant, it leads to insomnia, anxiety, restlessness, tremors, and increased mental activity. Uses include the following:

- Bronchial asthma—but not preferred, since it causes side effects.
- Nasal decongestion—but a congener, pseudoephedrine is used.
- Mydriasis—eye drops produce mydriasis without cycloplegia.
- Hypotension—for prevention and treatment of hypotension during spinal anesthesia, administered through IM route.
- Narcolepsy (excessive daytime sedation)—as it is a CNS stimulant.
- Nocturnal enuresis (bedwetting)—since it increases bladder's holding capacity.
- Stokes–Adams syndrome—as an alternative to isoprenaline.

ADRs comprise insomnia, tremors, palpitation, and difficulty in micturition.

Amphetamine

It is a synthetic compound that has properties similar to ephedrine. Being similar to ephedrine, tachyphylaxis is seen on repeated use. Since it crosses the BBB, it produces CNS effects. It is a powerful CNS stimulant; hence, it leads to increased mental and physical activity, alertness, increased concentration, and attention span (hence, it is used in attention-deficit hyperactivity disorder [ADHD]), elation and euphoria (therefore, it can be abused), increased work capacity, increased initiative and confidence, and decreased fatigue. It increases physical performance (especially in athletes); therefore, it is a drug of dependence and abuse. High dose can lead to confusion, delirium, and hallucinations. It stimulates respiration and depresses appetite. It has weak anticonvulsant (hence, it is combined with conventional anticonvulsants to increase efficacy and decrease sedation). ADRs include insomnia, palpitations, anxiety, tremors, restlessness, confusion, and hallucinations. Psychosis is seen on repeated use. High dose can lead to angina, arrhythmias, hypertension, acute psychosis, coma, and death due to convulsion. Uses include:

- ADHD: Children with ADHD have reduced concentration and attention span, show aggressive behavior, and engage in hyperactivity. Amphetamine increases attention span and performance in school.
- Narcolepsy: Amphetamine is preferred over ephedrine. Other drugs that can be used include methylphenidate, which is an indirectly acting sympathomimetic. Modafanil stimulates central α1 receptors and also acts on GABA and 5HT receptors. It is better tolerated. Methamphetamine and pemoline, too, are alternative treatments.
- Obesity—since there is appetite suppression.
- Epilepsy—as an adjuvant to counter-sedation of antiepileptics.

Vasopressors (IM15.14)

These agents are α1 agonists, for example, NA, DA, metarminol, mephentermine phenylephrine, and methoxamine. They increase BP by increasing peripheral resistance and/or cardiac output. These agents can cause reflex bradycardia. Vasopressors are administered parenterally. Their repeated use can develop tachyphylaxis. They are used in hypotension following cardiogenic shock/neurogenic shock/spinal anesthesia.

Nasal Decongestants

Oral nasal decongestants (administered orally) include pseudoephedrine, phenylephrine, phenylpropanolamine, and ephedrine, whereas topical nasal decongestants (administered topically on nasal mucosa) are oxymetazoline, xylometazoline (Otrivin), and naphazoline. These agents are α1 agonists of blood vessels in nasal mucosa and hence they cause vasoconstriction, shrinkage, and decreased volume of nasal mucosa. Thus, it relieves nasal congestion and decreases airflow resistance. Additionally, they also decrease nasal secretions, thereby providing symptomatic relief in allergic rhinitis and upper respiratory tract infection (URTI). ADRs of orally administered agents include insomnia, tremors, and irritability. Topically (nasal drops) agents can lead to nasal irritations and nasal mucosal atrophy (due to vasoconstriction); rebound congestion (due to vasodilatation) is seen on long-term use. Tolerance can develop due to desensitization. These agents are to be used carefully in hypertensives. Phenylpropanolamine has been banned due to increased risk of hemorrhagic stroke. It is used for only symptomatic relief in allergic rhinitis, vasomotor rhinitis, sinusitis, rhinitis in URTI, and blocked eustachian tubes.

Selective β2 Stimulants

These are bronchodilators and they also cause uterine relaxation without significant cardiac stimulation. Hence, they are used for the management of bronchial asthma (as inhalation) and premature labor prevention (parenterally). ADRs generally include tremors, palpitation, and arrhythmias. Isoxuprine is specifically used for preventing/treating premature labor, threatened abortion, and dysmenorrhea. Examples of older agents are salbutamol, terbulaline, and orciprenaline. Examples of newer agents are salmeterol, formoterol, and bambuterol.

Anorectics (Appetite Suppressants) (IM14.13)

Amphetamine has anorectic effects, but it is not recommended for obesity due to its CNS side effects. Other anorectics include fenfluramine, dexfenfluramine, mazindol, and phenylpropanolamine (but has been banned). ADRs are similar to that of amphetamine. Sibutramine has been tried in obesity. It acts by decreasing uptake of NA and 5-HT. ADRs comprise insomnia, anxiety, mood changes, and hypertension. Serious ADRs could include cardiovascular deaths.

Table 20.1 provides a summary of the therapeutic uses of adrenergic drugs.

Multiple Choice Questions

1. A 25-year-old woman has frequent occurrences of angioneurotic edema accompanied by the liberation of histamine and other mediators. The physiologic antagonist of histamine on smooth muscle is:

A. Chlorpheniramine maleate.
B. Adrenaline.
C. Ondansetron.
D. Ranitidine.
E. Sumatriptan.

Answer: B

H1 receptors primarily mediate the smooth muscle effects of histamine. Adrenaline has a physiologic antagonist action that reverses histamine's effects on smooth muscle.

2. A 25-year-old man consumed a high dose of reserpine and is brought to the emergency room. His blood pressure is 45/5 mm Hg and pulse rate is 45 beats per minute. A cardiovascular stimulant that could be administered for best results is:

A. Methylamphetamine.
B. Clonidine.
C. Cocaine.
D. Norepinephrine.
E. Tyramine.

Answer: D

An overdose of reserpine leads to a severe reduction of stored catecholamine transmitter.

3. Which is true about dobutamine?

A. Dobutamine decreases peripheral resistance.
B. Acts on D1 and D2 receptors.
C. Decrease kidney circulation.
D. Has no effect on coronary circulation.

Answer: A

Dobutamine decreases peripheral resistance. Dobutamine acts by activating β1 receptors and may decrease the peripheral resistance by its minor effect on β2 receptors.

4. Which of the following concentrations of epinephrine does not correspond to the respective route of administration?

A. 1:10,000 for intravenous route.
B. 1:1,000 for inhalational route.
C. 1:1,000 for intramuscular route.
D. 1:1,000 for subcutaneous route.

Answer: B

For inhalational route, adrenaline is used in a concentration of 1:100 for treatment of bronchial asthma by nebulizer.

5. Fenoldopam is used in the management of:

A. Hypertensive emergencies.
B. Congestive heart failure.
C. Migraine prophylaxis.
D. Tachyarrhythmia.

Answer: A

Fenoldopam is a D1 agonist useful for IV treatment of hypertensive emergencies. Fenoldopam (dopamine agonist), nicardipine, clevidipine (parenteral dihydropyridine [DHPs]), enalaprilat (a parenteral ACE [angiotensin-converting enzyme] inhibitor), and trimethaphan (a ganglion blocker) are other drugs for hypertensive emergencies. They are occasionally used in other countries.

6. A child on β2 agonists for treatment of bronchial asthma may exhibit all of the following features except:

A. Tremors.
B. Hypoglycemia.
C. Hypokalemia.
D. Bronchodilation.

Answer: B

β2 agonists are the inhaled bronchodilators used for the management of bronchial asthma.

7. Which is not an endogenous catecholamine?

A. Dopamine.
B. Dobutamine.
C. Adrenaline.
D. Noradrenaline.

Answer: B

Dobutamine is an exogenous (synthetic) catecholamine.

8. Norepinephrine action at the synaptic cleft is terminated by:

A. Metabolism by catechol-*O*-methyl-transferase (COMT).
B. Metabolism by monoamine oxidase (MAO).
C. Reuptake.
D. Metabolism by acetylcholinesterase.

Answer: C

Endogenous adrenaline action is terminated mainly by reuptake.

9. Dopamine is preferred in the treatment of shock because of:

A. Renal vasodilatory effect.
B. Increased cardiac output.
C. Peripheral vasoconstriction.
D. Prolonged action.

Answer: A

Dopamine acts on D1, β1, and α1 receptors. Stimulation of D1 receptors causes renal vasodilation, which is useful clinically to improve renal perfusion in shock with oliguria.

10. Biphasic reaction on blood pressure is seen with the administration of:

A. Adrenaline.
B. Noradrenaline.
C. Dopamine.
D. Dobutamine.

Answer: A

Rapid IV injection of adrenaline in experimental animals causes a noticeable increase in both systolic and diastolic BP (at high concentration, α1 response predominates and vasoconstriction occurs even in skeletal muscles). A secondary fall in mean BP follows. Low concentrations are not able to act on α receptors but continue to act on β_2 receptors. When an α blocker has been given, only fall in BP is seen, which is called vasomotor reversal of Dale.

11. A 59-year-old man with a past history of several myocardial infarctions is admitted for breathlessness. The patient is diagnosed to have congestive cardiac failure for which a positive inotropic agent is administered. The cardiologist is worried about retaining the normal renal blood flow, hence a drug that increases renal blood flow is recommended. Which of the following agents has both of these effects?

A. Adrenaline.
B. Dopamine.
C. Isoprenaline.
D. Salbutamol.

Answer: B

Dopamine is beneficial in controlling congestive cardiac failure, since it has dual action of positive inotropic effects on the heart and maintaining blood flow to the renal tissues.

Chapter 21 Adrenergic Receptor Blockers

Shardendu Kumar Mishra

PH1.13: Describe the mechanism of action, types, doses, side effects, indications, and contraindications of adrenergic and antiadrenergic drugs.

Learning Objectives

- α-adrenergic antagonist.
- β-adrenergic antagonist (β-blockers).

Antiadrenergic Drugs

Adrenergic system is the most prominent defense program comprising various chemicals known as neuronal hormones or neurotransmitters. Being a part of the autonomic nervous system (ANS), adrenergic system acts by releasing the neurotransmitters, namely, norepinephrine (NE) or noradrenaline (NA), which act at preganglionic and postganglionic sites. The released neurohormones bind selectively with adrenoceptors, that is, alpha (α) and beta (β) receptors. NE exerts various physiological functions via the G protein-coupled receptor (GPCR) mechanistic pathway.

Adrenergic blockers or sympatholytics are the agents which are used to inhibit the action of adrenergic drugs. These agents bind competitively with adrenoceptors to prevent the action of the adrenergic agonist.

Antiadrenergic agents or sympatholytics are the agents which bind with adrenoceptor to inhibit the action of NE or adrenergic agonist (**Fig. 21.1**).

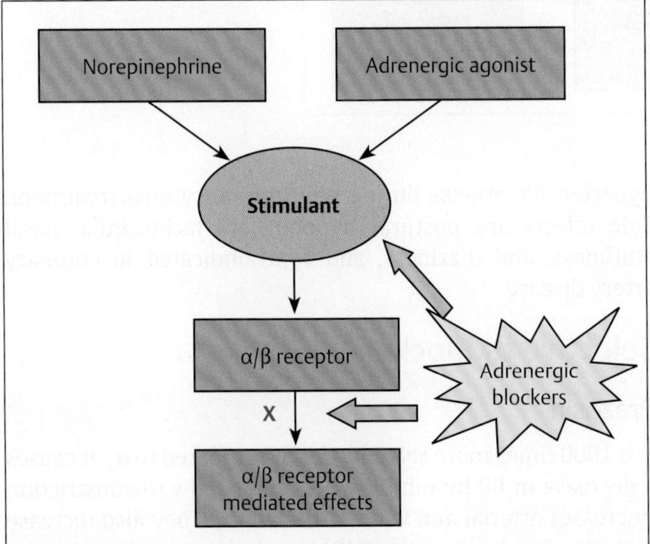

Fig. 21.1 Mechanism of adrenergic blockers.

Classification of Adrenergic Antagonist

Antiadrenergic blockers can be classified on their ability of selective or non-selective binding to adrenoceptors. Sympatholytics can be classified into two types, that is, α-blockers (**Fig. 21.2**) and β-blockers (**Fig. 21.3**).

α-Adrenergic Antagonist

These are the agents which specifically targets the blockade of α receptors. They downregulate or inhibit the actions mediated by α-agonists.

Pharmacological Actions

Selective α_1-blockers induce dilation in arteries and veins which, in turn, result in decreased peripheral resistance and venous return. Overall, α_1 blockers cause a decrease in blood pressure (BP), whereas selective α_2 blockade causes positive chronotropic effect due to the presence of baroreceptor reflexes. This elevation in heart rate may also be due to the contribution of the release of NA (**Table 21.1**).

Dale's vasomotor reversal (Sir HH Dale, 1913): *α-blockers abolish the vasopressor action of adrenaline and lead to depressor action*, that is, decrease in BP due to β_2-mediated vasodilatation.

Table 21.1 Pharmacological actions of α-blockers

Organ system	Effect
Blood vessels	BP (α_1) Reflex tachycardia (α_2)
Eye	Miosis (α_1 blockade)
Nose	Nasal congestion
GIT	Intestinal motility Diarrhea
Urinary tract	Easy micturition (used in BHP) Relaxes trigone muscles and sphincter
Vas deferens	Inhibition of ejaculation
Pancreas	Increased insulin release (α_2)
Platelets	Platelet aggregation (α_{2A})

Abbreviations: BHP, benign prostatic hyperplasia; BP, blood pressure; GIT, gastrointestinal tract.

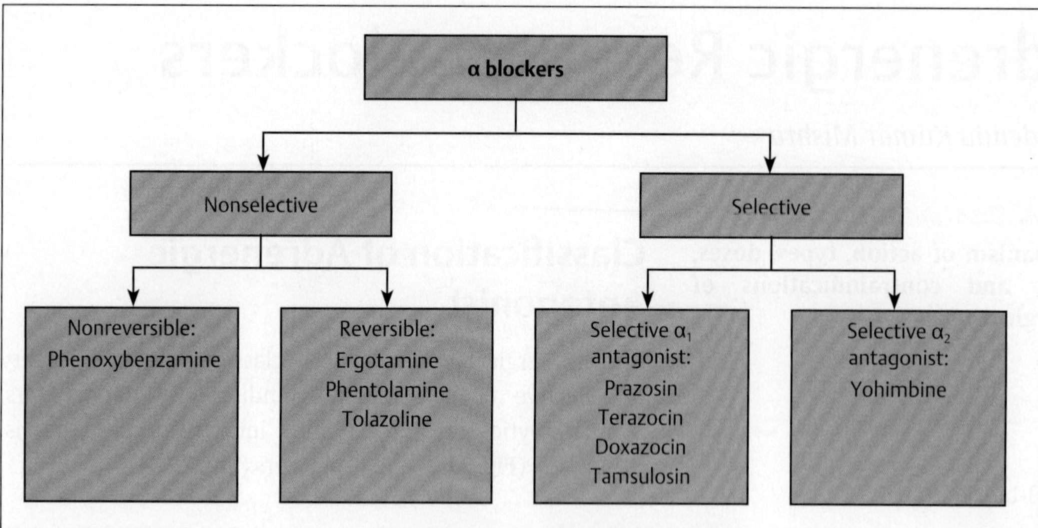

Fig. 21.2 Classification of α blockers.

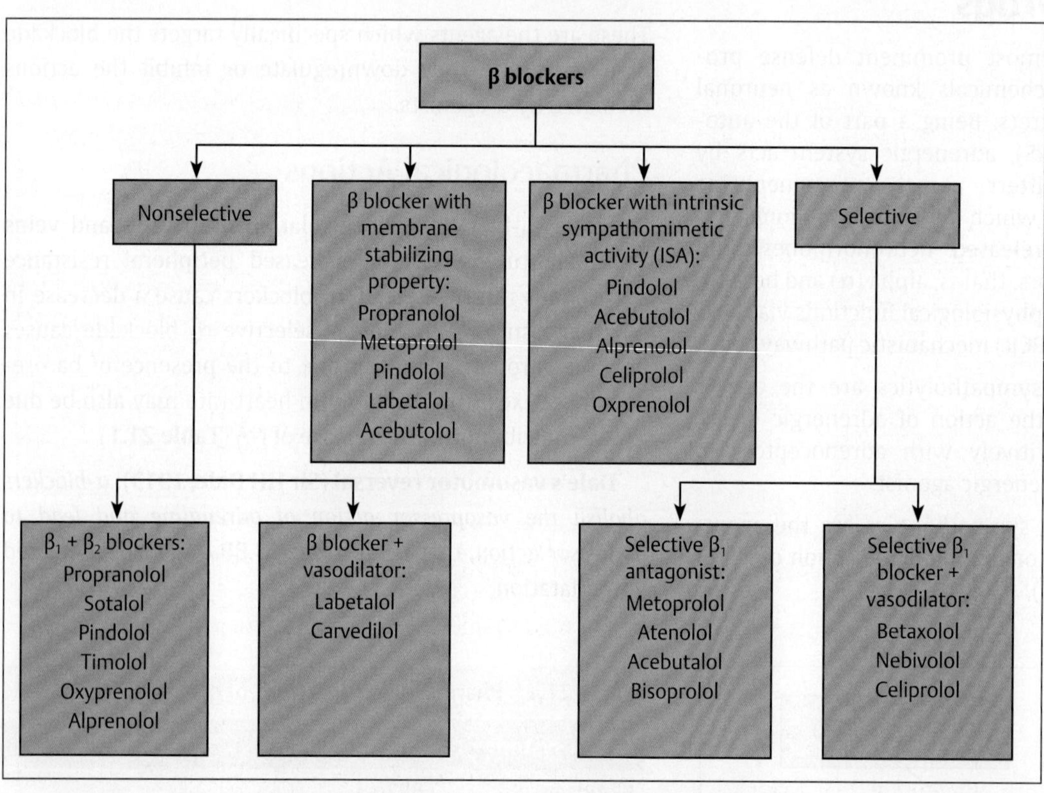

Fig. 21.3 Classification of β blockers.

Tamsulosin and silodosin are selective α_1 blockers and drug of choice for the treatment of benign prostatic hyperplasia (BHP) due to less possibility of causing postural hypotension.

Phentolamine and tolazoline are used in clonidine withdrawal and cheese reactions.

Nonselective α-Blockers

Phenoxybenzamine

It is an irreversible α-blocker. It blocks both α_1 and α_2 receptors. The long-acting agent, which causes vasodilatation and postural hypotension, is mediated through α_1 blockade. α_2 blockade causes cardiac stimulation and tachycardia due to NE release. Phenoxybenzamine is used to prevent hypertensive attacks during pheochromocytoma treatment. Side effects are postural hypotension, tachycardia, nasal stuffiness, and dizziness, and contraindicated in coronary artery disease.

Selective α_1 Blockers

Prazosin

It is 1000 times more selective for α_1 compared to α_2. It causes a decrease in BP by inhibiting α_1-mediated vasoconstriction (increases arterial and venous dilatation). They also increase high-density lipoprotein (HDL) and decrease low-density lipoprotein (LDL) and triglyceride (TG) level. α_1 blockers are the drug of choice for the treatment of BHP. Prazosin is used in the treatment of scorpion stings.

Pharmacokinetics

Absorption

Prazosin is well-absorbed through the oral route and has bioavailability of around 60%.

Distribution

Plasma concentrations of prazosin are reached in 1 to 3 hours. It is 95% bound to plasma protein (α_1 acid glycoprotein), which means only 5% of free drug is available in the circulation.

Metabolism

Metabolized in the liver.

Excretion

Excreted unchanged by the kidneys. The plasma $t_{1/2}$ is 2 to 3 hours and increases to 6 to 8 hours in congestive heart failure (CHF). The duration of action is around 8 to 10 hours in the treatment of hypertension.

Adverse Effects

- The main side effect is postural hypotension, seen with "first dose response," which is minimized with an initial low dose of 1 mg at bedtime.
- Other side effects are blurred vision, impotence, and palpitations.

Clinical Implications

- Clinically, α-blockers are used in the treatment of essential hypertension, pheochromocytoma, Raynaud's disease (peripheral vascular disease), hypertensive emergencies due to cheese reaction or clonidine withdrawal, BHP, and hypovolemic shock (phentolamine).
- Ergotamine or dihydroergotamine is preferred in migraine management, but the action is mediated due to 5-$HT_{1B/1D}$ agonistic activity.

Selective α_2 Blockers

Activation of α_2 receptor by α-agonist inhibits the release of NE. This activation, in turn, hampers sympathetic nervous system, leading to falling in BP. Yohimbine is analogue of indole alkylamine alkaloid and present in the bark of the tree *Pausinystalia yohimbe*. Yohimbine binds selectively and possesses competitive antagonism for α_2 receptors.

Yohimbine blocks α_2 receptor and stimulates sympathetic outflow, which increases BP by α_1 and β_1 mediated activity. Yohimbine also antagonizes the effects of 5-hydroxytryptamine (5-HT).

β-Adrenergic Antagonist (β-Blockers)

The β-adrenergic antagonist is the agent which competitively blocks the β-receptors and downregulates or inhibits the pharmacological action of NE or β agonist mediation through the β-receptor. Clinically, they have enormous importance due to their vast applications in the treatment of hypertension, CHF, arrhythmia, and ischemic heart diseases.

Pharmacological Actions of β-Blockers

Nonselective β-Blockers (Table 21.2)

Propranolol (Prototype β-Blockers)

Propranolol is a nonselective β-blocker with equal affinity to β_1 and β_2 receptors. It is a pure β-antagonist and never activates β-receptors like other β-blockers such as pindolol and acebutolol.

Pharmacological Actions

Heart

Propranolol decreases the heart rate, the force of contraction, which leads to reduced cardiac output (CO). Cardiac workout and oxygen consumption gradually decrease due to negative inotropic and chronotropic effects. Propranolol also has negative dromotropic effect, leading to delayed atrioventricular (AV) conduction. Exercise-mediated increase in heart rate and force of contraction are antagonized by β-blockers without affecting increased stroke volume.

At higher doses, some β-blockers have membrane stabilizing property or quinidine-like effect which means a good antiarrhythmic activity.

Blood Vessels

Propranolol inhibits vasodilatation induced by catecholamine, and fall in BP is elicited by isoprenaline. It does not have any direct action on blood vessels but decreases BP in normotensive patients. In short course treatment, propranolol increases the peripheral vascular resistance and returns to its normal value on continuous administration. It augments the release of renin from juxtaglomerular cells, which is mediated by β_1 receptors.

Respiratory System

Propranolol blocks the β_2 mediated bronchodilation, which indicates severe bronchospasm in asthmatic patients. Hence, they are contraindicated in asthma or chronic obstructive pulmonary disorder (COPD) patients.

Metabolic Effects

Propranolol attenuates glycogenolysis and may reduce carbohydrate tolerance in augmented insulin. Sometimes, it abolishes the warning sign of hypoglycemic attack (tremor, tachycardia) in diabetic patients. Hence, β-blockers should be cautiously used in diabetic patients with frequent hypoglycemic attacks. Propranolol increases LDL and TG and decreases HDL cholesterol.

Central Nervous System (CNS)

Long-term administration of propranolol induces forgetfulness and nightmares.

Local Anaesthetic

It is potent local anesthetic but clinically obsolete due to irritation at the site of injection.

Skeletal Muscles

It inhibits tremors induced by adrenaline acting on peripheral muscles (β_2 receptor-mediated).

Table 21.2 Pharmacological actions of β-blockers

Organ system	Effect
Heart	Negative chronotropic (↓ HR), inotropic (↓ FoC), and dromotropic (↓ AV conduction) effects Decreased CO O_2 demand and cardiac function reduced (↓ HR, aortic pressure)
Blood vessels	On the short course, vasoconstriction ↑ PVR, no change in BP On the long course, vasodilatation, ↓ PVR, ↓ BP
Respiratory system	Bronchoconstriction
Metabolic effect	Inhibit glycogenolysis Nonselective β blockers may ↓ HDL, ↑ LDL, TG
Eye	↓ IOP
Skeletal muscles	↓ Adrenaline mediated tremors ↓ Exercise capacity

Abbreviations: FOC, force of contraction; HR, heart rate; IOP, intraocular pressure; PVR, pulmonary vascular resistance.

Pharmacokinetics

Absorption

Propranolol is well-absorbed orally. It has low bioavailability (30%) due to high first-pass metabolism in the liver. Bioavailability of propranolol is higher when it is taken with meals because food decreases its first-pass metabolism.

Distribution

Propranolol is lipophilic and crosses the blood-brain barrier (BBB) easily. It is 90% plasma protein binding.

Metabolism

Metabolized in the liver and depends on hepatic blood flow. The hydroxylated metabolite of propranolol has β-blocking activity.

Excretion

The metabolites are excreted in the urine.

Adverse Effects

Bradycardia, CHF precipitation, prinzmetal angina, bronchial asthma, weakness, nightmares, depression, and myocardial infarction (MI) precipitation (β-blocker withdrawal).

Drug Interactions

Pharmacodynamic Interactions

1. **Propranolol and verapamil**—additive cardiac depressant effect may cause bradycardia or cardiac arrest.
2. **Propranolol and nonsteroidal anti-inflammatory drugs (NSAIDs)**—The latter decreases prostaglandin (PG) synthesis and leads to Na^+ water retention. NSAIDs decrease the antihypertensive effect of propranolol.
3. **Propranolol and sulfonylurea**—Sulfonylurea decreases blood sugar, leading to stimulation of glycogenolysis, which is augmented by propranolol and which, in turn, inhibits glycogenolysis. This may result in a hypoglycemic coma due to lack of signs such as tremors and palpitations.

Pharmacokinetic Interactions

1. The enzyme inducers (phenytoin, rifampin) can increase the metabolism of propranolol and decrease its plasma concentration.
2. The enzyme inhibitors (cimetidine, fluoxetine) can decrease the metabolism and increase the plasma concentration of propranolol.

Contraindications

It is contraindicated in case of severe depression, asthma, COPD, bradycardia, and active Raynaud's disease.

Clinical Implications

Cardiovascular Uses

1. **Essential hypertension**—β-blockers reduce CO. Atenolol is a drug of choice due to its cardioselectivity and long duration of action.
2. **Angina pectoris (classical angina)**—β-blockers reduces the workload on heart and oxygen consumption.
3. **Arrhythmias**—Sotalol, esmolol, and atenolol are very effective in paroxysmal supraventricular tachycardia (PSVT).
4. **MI**—β-blockers prevent reinfarction and ventricular fibrillation in MI. During myocardial recovering, β-blockers are administered through intravenous (IV) route, followed by oral β-blockers. It reduces the infarct size by attenuating oxygen consumption.
5. Selective β_1-blockers are preferred in patients with history of diabetes, hyperlipidemia, and bronchial asthma, as they do not precipitate the symptoms.

Central Nervous System (CNS) Uses

1. **Migraine**—Propranolol is highly useful in the prophylaxis of migraine. This activity is attributed by inhibition of 5-HT receptor in CNS by propranolol. They are not the drug of choice in the acute attack of migraine.
2. **Tremor prevention**—Propranolol prevents β_2 mediated tremors. Selective β-blockers are not useful in tremor treatment.

Endocrine Uses

1. **Pheochromocytoma**—Due to massive release of catecholamines, rise in BP causes pheochromocytoma (tumor of adrenal medulla). β-blockers should be used after α-blockade. Agents which block both α and β (labetalol) are the drug of choice for the treatment of pheochromocytoma.
2. **Thyrotoxicosis**—Propranolol inhibits peripheral conversion of T_4 to T_3 and is highly effective for thyroid storm. It also controls the palpitation, nervousness, tremor, severe myopathy, and sweating without affecting thyroid status.

Ophthalmic Uses

1. **Glaucoma**—β-blockers reduce the formation of aqueous humor, which help in the treatment of glaucoma. Timolol is preferred over other agents for the same.

β-Blockers with Intrinsic Sympathomimetic Activity (ISA)

These drugs are partial agonists at β_1 receptors apart from having β-blocking property. These are preferred in the patients who are prone to develop severe bradycardia with β-blocker therapy. Precipitation of bronchospasm does not occur with these drugs; hence it is safe to use in asthmatic agents. However, these drugs are less useful in angina (because of the stimulation of the heart by β_1 receptors). Examples of β-blockers with intrinsic sympathomimetic activity are celiprolol, oxprenolol, pindolol, penbutolol, alprenolol, and acebutolol.

β-Blockers with Membrane-Stabilizing Activity

These drugs possess Na^+ channel blocking activity. It can show antidysrhythmic action at higher doses. These drugs should be avoided in glaucoma due to the risk of corneal anesthesia. Examples are propanolol, metoprolol, labetalol, acebutolol, and pindolol.

α + β Adrenergic Blockers

Labetalol

Labetalol is a drug that acts as a competitive blocker to both α and β receptors. These agents have mixture antagonism, including the selective blockade of α_1 receptors, β_1 and β_2 receptors, and inhibition of neuronal uptake of NE. The potency of β receptor blockade is 5- to 10-fold that of α_1 receptor blockade. There are four isomers of labetalol which exert their pharmacological actions. The marketed labetalol preparation is effective as $\beta_1 + \beta_2 + \alpha_1$ blocker with weak β_2 agonistic activity. Lowering of BP (both systolic and diastolic) is due to α_1 and β_1 blockade as well as β_2 agonistic activity. Increase in CO and total peripheral resistance is seen with high doses without affecting heart rate. It also inhibits NE uptake by adrenergic nerve endings.

Labetalol is orally effective and undergoes considerable first-pass metabolism. It is an effective hypotensive and is useful in pheochromocytoma and clonidine withdrawal treatment. The major side effect is postural hypotension and failure of ejaculation.

Pharmacotherapy of Glaucoma (PH1.58)

Glaucoma is a cluster of diseases characterized by a progressive form of optic nerve damage.

It is diagnosed with raised (> 21 mm Hg) i.o.t. The pharmacotherapy of glaucoma involves lowering of i.o.t. either by reducing the secretion of aqueous humor or by enhancing its drainage. Lowering of i.o.t. augments the progression of optic nerve damage. The drainage of aqueous humor involves trabecular channels. Glaucoma is classified into two forms: open-angle glaucoma and angle-closure glaucoma.

Open-Angle Glaucoma

It is also known as wide-angle glaucoma, probably a genetically predisposed degenerative disease affecting trabecular meshwork, which is gradually lost after middle age. Hypotensive agents effective in ocular disorders are used on a long course and alleviate the majority of cases.

β-Adrenergic Blockers

Topical β-blockers are the first-line drugs, followed by $PGF_{2\alpha}$ analogs for the treatment of glaucoma. The β-blockers decrease i.o.t. by attenuating aqueous humor level without affecting pupil size or tone of the ciliary muscle. The mechanism behind the decrease in i.o.t may be attributed to down-regulation of adenylyl cyclase due to β2 receptor blockade in the ciliary epithelium. These β-blockers are lipophilic with high ocular penetration and have weak local anesthetic activity (to avoid corneal hypoesthesia and damage).

Ophthalmic β-blockers cause mild and infrequent side effects such as redness and dryness of the eye, corneal hypoesthesia, allergic conjunctivitis, and blurred vision.

Timolol is nonselective ($\beta_1 + \beta_2$) and has no intrinsic sympathomimetic activity. The ocular hypotensive action, that is, fall in i.o.t. by 20 to 35% is evident within 1 hour and persists for up to approximately 12 hours.

Advantages of Ocular β-Blockers

- No change in pupil size.
- No headache due to persistent spasm of iris and ciliary muscles.
- No fluctuations in i.o.t. as occurring with pilocarpine drops.

α-Adrenergic Agonists

Dipivefrine is a prodrug of adrenaline which crosses the cornea and is hydrolyzed by the esterases present in adrenaline. The released dipivefrine decreases i.o.t. by augmenting uveoscleral outflow and reducing aqueous formation ($\alpha_1 + \alpha_2$ receptor-mediated). Dipivefrine produces significant ocular burning and other side effects.

Apraclonidine is a clonidine analog which does not cross BBB and is used topically (0.5–1%) to lower i.o.t. This activity is mediated by less aqueous formation and α_2 and α_1 action in the ciliary body. Common side effects are itching, eyelid dermatitis, conjunctivitis, mydriasis, and dryness of the mouth.

Prostaglandin (PG) Analogs

$PGF_{2\alpha}$ at low concentration is effective to decrease i.o.t. without causing ocular inflammation. PG analogs act by increasing uveoscleral outflow and increased permeability of tissues in ciliary muscle.

Latanoprost, used topically as $PGF_{2\alpha}$ derivative, exhibits activity similar to timolol in terms of i.o.t. reduction. It reduces i.o.t. in normal pressure glaucoma. Common side effects are ocular irritation, pain, blurring of vision, and darkening of eyelashes.

The clinical approach toward treatment of open-angle glaucoma can be started as monotherapy with latanoprost or a topical β-blocker. Brimonidine/dorzolamide (carbonic anhydrase inhibitors) is used only when there are contraindications to PG analogs or β-blockers.

Angle-Closure Glaucoma

It is also known as narrow-angle glaucoma, which occurs in individuals with a narrow iridocorneal angle. The intraocular pressure remains normal until an attack is precipitated (40–60 mm Hg). The failure to decrease i.o.t results in loss of sight.

The following protocol has been known for the treatment of closed-angle glaucoma:

1. Hypertonic mannitol (20%) 1.5 to 2 g/kg or glycerol (10%): IV infused.
2. Acetazolamide: 0.5 g IV.
3. Miotic: pilocarpine 1 to 4% is instilled every 10 minutes.
4. Topical β-blocker: timolol 0.5% eye drops.
5. Apraclonidine (1%)/latanoprost (0.005%) eye drop.

Multiple Choice Questions

1. A drug that produces a pressor response is administered repeatedly by intravenous injection over a short period of time. After several injections, a tachyphylaxis occurs. What drug was most likely administered?

A. Ephedrine.
B. Epinephrine.
C. Norepinephrine.
D. Phenylephrine.

Answer: A

Ephedrine exerts most of its effect as an indirectly acting sympathomimetic, like tyramine. As it acts to release a limited store of presynaptic neurotransmitter, a form of acute tolerance to the drug develops when the releasable pool becomes gradually depleted by successive doses of ephedrine.

2. A 16-year-old patient arrives in the emergency department suffering from an anaphylactic reaction. The patient is having difficulty breathing, has severe urticaria, and is hypotensive. Which of the following is a drug of choice for treating this patient's potentially life-threatening condition?

A. Epinephrine.
B. Isoproterenol.
C. Norepinephrine.
D. Phenylephrine.

Answer: A

Parenterally administered epinephrine is a drug of choice for treating anaphylactic reactions. Its β2 effects produce bronchodilation as well as decreased release of inflammatory mediators from mast cells and basophils. Its α receptor effects produce vasoconstriction (raising the blood pressure) to counteract hypotension. Its vasoconstrictive effects on bronchial blood vessels may also reduce bronchial fluid congestion. Epinephrine is the best-studied medication for the treatment of anaphylaxis.

3. Several drugs used to treat noncardiovascular conditions have α-blocking "side effects." If epinephrine is injected into such patients, it will likely produce a change in blood pressure (BP) resembling that produced by:

A. Dobutamine.
B. Dopamine.
C. Isoproterenol.
D. Norepinephrine.

Answer: C

Epinephrine normally stimulates α1, α2, β1, and β2 receptors. If you block α-receptors, what you have left resembles isoproterenol, a nonselective β1 and β2 agonist. Under such conditions, epinephrine will produce a reduction of mean arterial blood pressure, instead of an increase. This is known classically as "epi-reversal."

4. A 27-year-old woman with a history of hypertension comes to your office to discuss her drug therapy for hypertension. Her blood pressure (BP) is currently well controlled (BP < 130/85) by a combination of enalapril (an angiotensin-converting enzyme inhibitor [ACEI]) and hydrochlorothiazide (a thiazide-type diuretic). The reason for her visit is that she is planning to become pregnant in the near future, and she is aware that ACEIs are contraindicated in pregnancy. After discussing her therapeutic options, you decide to replace her ACEI with a drug that is considered relatively safe in pregnancy, and is believed to exert its effects by multiple mechanisms including working as a false neurotransmitter. This drug is:

A. α-methyltyrosine.
B. Methyldopa.
C. Prazosin.
D. Terbutaline.

Answer: B

Methyldopa is one of several drugs commonly used for temporary replacement of ACEIs and other contraindicated antihypertensive medications during pregnancy. It is one of the older drugs available, with a fairly good track record for safety. Methyldopa is converted within the nerve terminal to α-methyl norepinephrine, which replaces norepinephrine stored in sympathetic nerve terminal vesicles. When it is released in response to sympathetic nerve stimulation, it is believed to work by several mechanisms including: (a) as a false neurotransmitter (it does not stimulate postsynaptic α1 or β1 receptors), (b) stimulates presynaptic α2 receptors to reduce sympathetic release of neurotransmitters, and (c) reduces plasma renin activity (which is normally increased by sympathetic stimulation).

5. This adrenergic receptor subtype is expressed on vascular smooth muscle at sites some distance away from sympathetic nerve terminals, and produces vasoconstrictor responses when stimulated by circulating catecholamines such as epinephrine:

A. α1.
B. α2.

C. β1.

D. Dopamine.

Answer: B

Circulating catecholamines exert a large degree of their vasoconstrictor effects by stimulating α2 receptors. "Why" α-2 receptors (vs α1 receptors) are expressed at sites distal to sympathetic nerve endings is still unclear. They both mediate the same physiological response in vascular smooth muscle. Evidence indicates that α1 receptors are located in the vicinity of sympathetic nerve terminals (strategically situated to be activated by norepinephrine coming out of nerves). Epinephrine also stimulates other adrenergic receptors (e.g., β1 and β2), but they are not involved in mediating vasoconstriction.

6. Karl is a 65-year-old man with severe hypertension who has not achieved his therapeutic goal for controlling his blood pressure (BP) after treatment with a combination of four different antihypertensive drugs for the past 6 months. Having exhausted the list of the most highly recommended drugs, his physician elects to add reserpine to his drug regimen, since it has a unique mechanism of action and remains as a therapeutic option, based upon the consensus of expert opinions for treatment of hypertension (JNC 8 guidelines, 2014). The molecular target for this antihypertensive drug is inhibition of:

A. α-adrenergic receptors.

B. Monoamine oxidase (MAO).

C. Vesicular monoamine transporter (VMAT).

D. β-adrenergic receptors.

Answer: C

Reserpine blocks VMAT. VMAT transports free intracellular catecholamines in the cytoplasm into presynaptic vesicles for subsequent release during exocytosis. Unprotected cytoplasmic neurotransmitters (that are not packed into vesicles) are available for metabolism by MAO in the mitochondria, or catechol-O-methyltransferase (COMT), which can be present in both intracellular and extracellular locations.

7. Which of the following α-blocker drug is used in the treatment of benign prostatic hyperplasia (BPH) without producing significant hypotension?

A. Doxazosin.

B. Phentolamine.

C. Tamsulosin.

D. Terazosin.

Answer: C

The α1A adrenergic receptor has been shown to mediate the contraction of human prostatic smooth muscle. Because tamsulosin has a high affinity for the α1A adrenergic receptor, it is effectively used to treat BPH. The selectivity of this compound for the prostate is reflected in the fact that there is little decrease in blood pressure (BP) after therapeutic doses of the drug.

8. Tamsulosin, a competitive α-adrenoceptor antagonist has affinity for which of the following receptors?

A. α1A.

B. α1D.

C. None of the above.

D. Both (A) and (B).

Answer: A

The α1A adrenergic receptor has been shown to mediate the contraction of human prostatic smooth muscle. Because tamsulosin has a high affinity for the α1A adrenergic receptor, it is effectively used to treat benign prostatic hyperplasia (BPH). The selectivity of this compound for the prostate is reflected in the fact that there is little decrease in blood pressure (BP) after therapeutic doses of the drug.

9. Ideal drug employed in the preoperative preparation for surgical excision of pheochromocytoma is:

A. Atenolol.

B. Phenoxybenzamine.

C. Reserpine.

D. Clonidine.

Answer: B

Phenoxybenzamine, a nonselective α-blocker, is the most common medication used to α block the patients prior to pheochromocytoma resection. However, due to increasing drug costs and increased side effects in comparison with selective α-blockers, there is a renewed interest in studying alternatives to phenoxybenzamine. Selective α-blockers such as doxazosin are also commonly used to α block the patients prior to pheochromocytoma resection. Selective α-blockers are significantly less expensive and are associated with fewer side effects than phenoxybenzamine.

10. Which of the following drugs is most effective for control of orthostatic hypotension:

A. Clonidine.

B. Fludrocortisone.

C. Esmolol.

D. Phenylephrine.

Answer: B

Fludrocortisone binds to the aldosterone receptor, which increases activity of the distal tubule of the kidney, causing enhanced sodium ion and water transport into the plasma, and increasing urinary excretion of potassium and hydrogen ions. Its effect on alleviating orthostatic hypotension is largely thought to be modulated through these actions.

11. A hypertensive patient has heart rate of 50 beats/min and is taking tablet atenolol 200 mg/day in divided doses. After anesthesia, heart rate further fell down to 40 beats/min. What will be the appropriate treatment to improve heart rate?

A. Intravenous (IV) adrenaline.

B. IV atropine.

C. IV isoprenaline.

D. Dobutamine IV infusion.

Answer: B

IV atropine increases heart rate in a dose-dependent manner in elderly patients undergoing spinal anesthesia. It reduces the incidence of hypotension and the dose of ephedrine required. Small-dose atropine may be a useful supplement in preventing spinal anesthesia induced hypotension in elderly patients.

Part III

Drugs Affecting Cardiovascular System

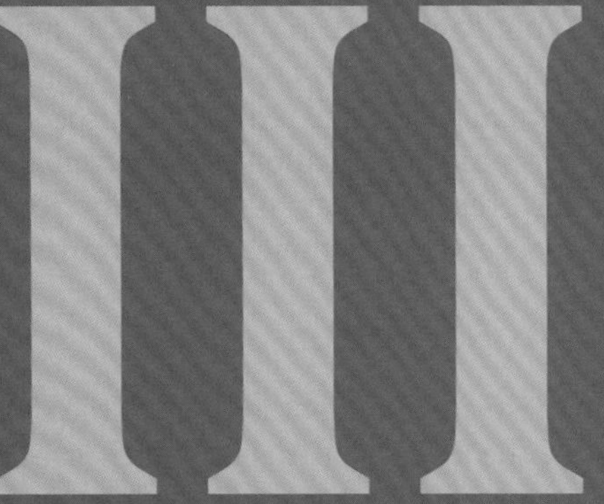

Chapter 22 Renin–Angiotensin System

Shubhadeep Sinha, Leeela Talluri, and Prasan R. Bhandari

PH1.26: Describe mechanisms of action, types, doses, side effects, indications, and contraindications of the drugs modulating the reninangiotensin and aldosterone system.

PH1.27: Describe the mechanisms of action, types, doses, side effects, indications, and contraindications of antihypertensive drugs and drugs used in shock.

Learning Objectives

- Circulating renin–angiotensin system.
- Angiotensin receptors and transduction mechanism.
- Drugs that affect renin–angiotensin system.

Introduction

At the end of the 19th century, it was demonstrated that saline extract of kidney led to pressor response. It was named renin. This discovery was beneficial in appreciating the importance of the kidney in arterial hypertension. In 1940, it was shown that renin was enzyme that acts on plasma protein α_2-globulin to produce the actual pressor substance. This pressor substance was termed hypertension by one group of workers and concurrently another different group termed it angiotonin and eventually the term recognized was angiotensin. The plasma protein substrate was labeled angiotensinogen. Later, it has been shown that renin leads to the conversion of angiotensinogen to angiotensin I (Ang I), which is inactive and converted to angiotensin II (Ang II) because of angiotensin-converting enzyme (ACE)/kininase II.

Circulating Renin–Angiotensin System

Renin is produced and stored in juxtaglomerular cells of the kidneys and liberated (exocytotic) into the circulation and converts angiotensinogen to Ang I. The level of renin present in plasma is an important limiting factor to regulate the rate of production of Ang II. Renin production is regulated by numerous physiological stimuli such as reduction in sodium concentration in the fluid of distal tubule close to macula densa and decrease in renal perfusion pressure. Renin secretion is likewise stimulated by the sympathetic system stimulation by β_1-receptors, β-receptor agonists, and prostacyclin. Ang II produced causes negative feedback inhibition of renin.

Synthesis of Angiotensin and Its Degradation

Angiotensinogen (α_2-globulin) is changed into Ang I by renin. Ang I is transformed into Ang II by ACE present in vascular endothelial cells and abundant in the lungs. Ang II is converted into Ang III, which is equipotent with respect to effect on aldosterone secretion and less potent in increasing the blood pressure (BP) and stimulating adrenal medulla (**Fig. 22.1**).

These peptides, that is, Ang III and IV, are metabolized to inactive fragments by nonspecific angiotensinases.

Local (Tissue) Renin–Angiotensin System (IM1.24)

Besides the conventional renin–angiotensin system (RAS), local RAS also exists, which may be extrinsic or intrinsic.

Extrinsic

Ang I and Ang II could also be synthesized locally on the surface of blood vessel wall within the endothelium since endothelial cells have the ability to take up the circulating renin (of renal source), angiotensinogen (hepatic source), and ACE already present in the vascular endothelial cells. Hence, local synthesis of angiotensin in cardiac tissue and blood vessels occurs, which might be of clinical importance.

Intrinsic

Several other tissues such as the brain, pituitary, kidney, adrenal gland, cardiac tissue, and blood vessels demonstrate the presence of renin, angiotensin, and ACE and hence form Ang I, Ang II, and Ang III locally. This indicates the independent presence of local RAS besides the renal/hepatic-based system, which could be of clinical importance in cardiovascular and renal system.

Angiotensin Receptors and Transduction Mechanism

Angiotensin acts on cell surface (membrane) receptors and hence has a rapid action. These are G protein–coupled receptors called AT_1 and AT_2 receptors. The majority of the effects of Ang II are facilitated via AT_1 receptor (abundant in vascular smooth muscles). The functional importance of AT_2 receptor is not well recognized, and the general effect is to reduce the vasoconstriction because of AT_1 receptor, as activation of AT_2 receptor leads to vasodilatation. AT_1 receptor has high affinity for angiotensin receptor blockers, for example, candesartan, valsartan, and losartan.

AT_1 Receptors

These are abundant in most of the tissues and mediate most of the effects of Ang II, which comprise the vascular and myocardial tissue, brain, kidney, and adrenal glomerulosa

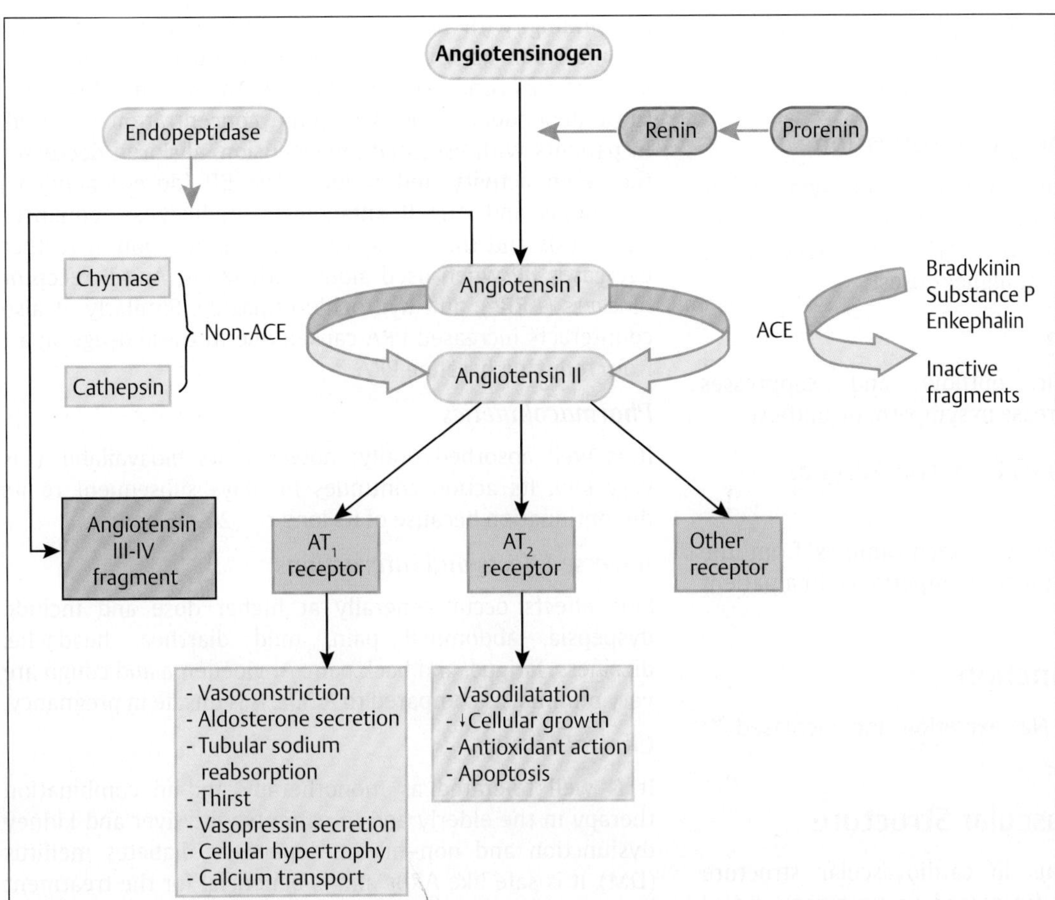

Fig. 22.1 Synthesis of angiotensin and its degradation.

cells, which liberate aldosterone. AT_1 receptor likewise mediates feedback inhibition (autoreceptor).

AT_2 Receptors

These are widely present in all the fetal tissues, but less in adults, where it is present in high concentration in vascular endothelium, adrenal medulla, reproductive tissues, and parts of the central nervous system.

Transduction Mechanism

AT_1 Receptors

They are linked with several G proteins (G_q, G_1, and $G_{12/13}$). Because of the activation of AT_1 receptor, the transducer mechanisms are varied in different tissues. However, in most of the tissues, AT_1 receptors are linked to G_q and primarily combination of Ang II and AT_1 receptor activates phospholipase C (PLC) – inositol trisphosphate (IP3)/diacylglycerol (DAG). This, in seconds, leads to intracellular Ca^{2+} release. This leads to contraction of smooth muscles, both vascular and nonvascular. Entry of calcium into cells because of activation of cell membrane Ca^{2+} channels leads to synthesis and release of aldosterone, release of catecholamines, sympathetic discharge, and positive inotropic effect on the heart.

AT_2 Receptors

These too have affinity for Ang II, but the signal transduction is different and does not involve formation of IP_3. Vasodilatation caused by stimulation of AT_2 receptor could be due to the nitric oxide–cyclic guanosine monophosphate pathways and could involve bradykinin B_2-receptor.

Functions and Pathophysiological Role

Regulation of BP

RAS is implicated in control of both short- and long-term regulation of arterial BP. Angiotensin is the primary pressor agent and it is around 40 times more potent (base on molarity) than noradrenaline in this context. For short-term control (rapid pressor response), the major mechanism is increase in total peripheral resistance because of vasoconstriction, whereas long-term regulation (slow pressor response) is due to the suppression of renal excretion of Na^+ and water and is observed in subpressor dose. It is imperative to know that there is little or no reflex bradycardia because of the pressor response of Ang II due to the reset of baroreceptor reflex control at a higher BP level.

Effect on Total Peripheral Resistance and Effect on BP

Direct Vasoconstriction

Ang II, by acting on AT_1 receptors (vascular smooth muscles), primarily constricts precapillary arterioles and likewise postcapillary venules to a certain level. Highest vasoconstriction happens in renal blood vessels and to a lesser extent in splanchnic blood vessels, causing a significant decrease in blood flow when Ang II is infused.

Facilitation of Noradrenergic Transmission

Ang II leads to noradrenergic (NA) release from sympathetic nerve terminal, suppresses the reuptake of NA into nerve terminal, helps vascular response to NA, and likewise causes a ganglionic stimulant effect at higher doses.

Central Nervous System

It enhances sympathetic outflow and suppresses baroreceptor-mediated decrease in sympathetic outflow.

Release of Catecholamines from the Adrenal Medulla

Ang II causes the liberation of catecholamines from the adrenal medulla, which might be of importance in a patient with phaeochromocytoma.

Changes in Renal Function

Ang II leads to decreased Na^+ excretion and increased K^+ excretion.

Changes in Cardiovascular Structure

The pathological alterations in cardiovascular structure could lead to hypertrophy (increased tissue mass) and/or redistribution of mass within a structure (remodeling).

Drugs That Affect Renin–Angiotensin System

Drugs that affect RAS can be categorized as follows (**Fig. 22.2**):

1. Drugs that block renin secretion, for example, clonidine, methyldopa, and β-blockers.
2. Renin inhibitors, for example, aliskiren.
3. ACE inhibitors (ACEIs), for example, captopril, enalapril, and lisinopril.
4. Ang II receptor (AT_1) blockers or antagonists, for example, losartan and candesartan.
5. Aldosterone antagonists, for example, spironolactone.

Drugs That Block Renin Secretion

Clonidine and methyldopa suppress the renin secretion due to centrally mediated decrease in neural activity to the kidneys, in addition to a direct intrarenal action. The β-blockers (e.g., propranolol) block the intrarenal and extrarenal β_1-receptors implicated in neural control of renin secretion.

Renin Inhibitors

Aliskiren

It is a low-molecular-weight, nonpeptide, competitive renin inhibitor (competing with angiotensinogen). It acts by binding with active site of renin and decreases the plasma renin activity (PRA) and subsequent changes, that is, it reduces concentration of Ang I, Ang II, and aldosterone (dose-dependent). However, renin concentration is raised. In patients with essential hypertension, aliskiren decreases the renin activity and reduces the BP (dose-dependent) like ACEIs and Ang II antagonists. It, likewise, enhances natriuresis and there is K^+ retention. In addition, it further decreases BP when used along with ACEIs, Ang II receptor blockers (ARBs), and hydrochlorothiazide. Similarly, it also counteracts increased PRA caused due to these drugs, apart from reducing baseline PRA.

Pharmacokinetics

It is well absorbed orally; however, its bioavailability is very low. Its action continues for days subsequent to its discontinuation because of its long $t_{1/2}$ (20–45 hours).

Adverse Effects and Interactions

Side effects occur generally at higher dose and include dyspepsia, abdominal pain, mild diarrhea, headache, dizziness, fatigue, and back pain. Angioedema and cough are very minimal as compared to ACEIs. It is unsafe in pregnancy.

Clinical Status

It is well tolerated as monotherapy and in combination therapy in the elderly and in patients with liver and kidney dysfunction and non–insulin-dependent diabetes mellitus (DM). It is safe like ARBs and is beneficial for the treatment of essential hypertension and other cardiovascular and renal diseases, similar to ACEIs and ARBs. It is indicated as a substitute to ACEIs/ARBs either singly or in combination in patients who do not tolerate first-line drugs. Its antihypertensive effect is similar to ACEIs (e.g., ramipril), ARBs (e.g., losartan), and hydrochlorothiazide.

Dose

The recommended dose is 150 to 300 mg once a day.

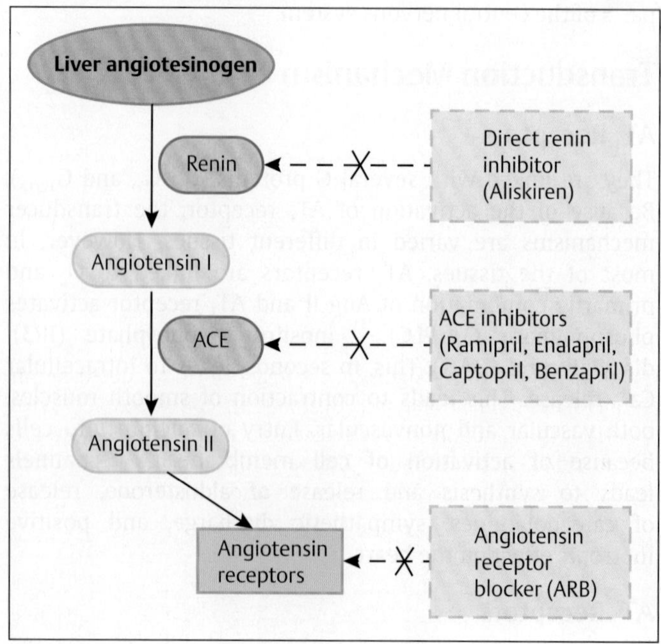

Fig. 22.2 Drugs that affect renin–angiotensin system.

Angiotensin-Converting Enzyme Inhibitors

1. Sulfhydryl (mercapto) compounds: for example, captopril.
2. Dicarboxyl compounds: for example, enalapril, lisinopril, perindopril, ramipril, trandolapril, benazepril, quinapril, and moexipril.
3. Phosphoryl compounds: for example, fosinopril.

Mechanism

1. ACE (kininase II) inhibitors competitively inhibit the conversion of Ang I to Ang II; thus, the formation of Ang II does not occur. Because Ang II is not produced, ACEIs block the vasoconstriction and secretion of aldosterone. Subsequently, there is natriuresis and diuresis.
2. Formation of Ang II is likewise inhibited in different tissues such as vascular, cardiac, and renal and this also contributes to effects of ACEIs.
3. Furthermore, there is inhibition of degradation of bradykinin. This is due to the fact that the enzyme responsible for degradation of bradykinin is ACE (kininase II). Thus, due to accumulation of bradykinin, vasodilatation occurs that contributes to antihypertensive action of ACEIs and also some of the side effects (dry cough).
4. Increased prostaglandin (PG) synthesis could likewise add to pharmacological actions, particularly antihypertensive action, since indomethacin (PG synthesis inhibitor) has been found to blunt the antihypertensive action of ACEIs.

Pharmacodynamics

Effect on BP

In Hypertensive Person/Patients

Both the systolic and diastolic BP decrease considerably in hypertensive patients, and the effect is more pronounced if there is high renin level. However, on repetitive administration or on prolonged use, patients with low renin level/activity also respond well to ACEIs. In spite of the decrease in BP, the coronary and cerebral blood flow are preserved.

In Patients with Congestive Heart Failure

ACEIs decrease both the preload and afterload.

1. Preload is decreased due to reduced circulatory volume because of natriuresis and diuresis. Since there is reduced circulated volume, there is decrease in venomotor tone and hence reduction in venous return.
2. Afterload decreases because of reduction in pulmonary vascular resistance (PVR); however, there is no reflex increase in sympathetic activity.
3. The level of aldosterone is decreased.
4. In patients with DM, ACEIs minimize nephropathy and retinopathy. Their significant effects include decrease in microalbuminuria and improvement in complications. With regard to reduction in cardiovascular complications, they are superior than other antihypertensive agents, namely, calcium channel blockers, β-blockers, and thiazide diuretics.

Pharmacokinetic Characteristics and Exceptions)

1. All ACEIs have similar uses, adverse effect profile, and contraindications. Most of the ACEIs generate active drug since they are ester-containing prodrugs and are converted to active metabolites by hepatic esterase. However, prodrugs cannot be utilized for emergency since they have delayed onset. Captopril, lisinopril (lysine derivative of enalaprilat), and enalaprilat are active drugs.
2. The duration of action of all of them is around 24 hours or more, except captopril (6–12 hours), and hence they are administered as single daily dose. Captopril is used twice a day.
3. All are tightly bound with enzymes in tissues.
4. Plasma half-life depends on elimination and slow dissociation from tissue ACE. It could be prolonged because of slow dissociation from the tissue ACE. Elimination could be biphasic (due to clearance from plasma and slow dissociation from tissues) for most of the agents.
5. It is imperative to note that the doses of all ACEIs are decreased in renal impairment/renal failure and hyponatremia, as well as with the simultaneous use of diuretics. Dose must likewise be decreased in patients with high renin level (due to any cause) like in patients with heart failure since response of ACEI is increased in patients with high renin level.

Adverse Effects

1. Cough (5–20%): It is because of the accumulation of bradykinin (due to inhibition of its degradation). It is dry cough, and occurs as early as 1 week or delayed up to few months (up to 6 months) of continuous treatment. It is more common in women and reduces within few days (4–6 days) after discontinuing the drug or using thromboxane antagonist (low dose of aspirin).
2. Skin rashes: Primarily occurs because of the sulfhydryl group and it subsides by itself. However, occasionally antihistaminics might be necessary.
3. Dysgeusia: Alteration in taste or loss of taste might occur, especially with captopril (reversible).
4. Hypotension: In hypertensive patients who have raised plasma renin concentration or sodium depleted (due to low salt intake or due to diuretics) or patients with congestive heart failure (CHF) or patients on multiple antihypertensive drugs. There is a drastic reduction in BP on initiation of therapy, that is, when the first dose is administered. First-dose hypotension is more common with captopril and fosinopril. This can be minimized by starting with very low dose and diuretics may be discontinued if patient was earlier on diuretic therapy.
5. Hyperkalemia: This does not occur when ACEIs are used singly, but more likely because of concurrent K^+ supplementation or use of K^+-sparing diuretics or nonsteroidal anti-inflammatory drugs (NSAIDs) or β-blockers or K^+-rich food (sweet lime, mango).
6. Angioneurotic edema: This occurs especially within the first few weeks of treatment and more so within the first few hours of the first dose but is not dose-related. It is manifested by swelling of nose, lips, throat, mouth, etc. Death could occur because of airways obstruction, if edema involves larynx and glottis. Discontinuation of drug and administration of adrenaline, antihistaminics, and corticosteroids are required for treatment.
7. Proteinuria might occur in patients on ACEI. However, ACEIs provide protection against proteinuria due to diabetic nephropathy. Hence, they are indicated in diabetic nephropathy and prevention of nephropathy.
8. If there is Na^+ loss or volume depletion, there is increased aldosterone and Ang II formation. This is due to compensatory mechanism. However, if ACEIs are used, they block this compensatory mechanism, leading to renal failure. Renal failure is more likely if there is bilateral renal artery stenosis, stenosis of artery of single kidney, heart failure, or dehydration due to

diarrhea or use of diuretics. However, it is reversible if adequate measures are taken in time.

9. During pregnancy (fetopathic effect): When administered during the second and third trimesters, ACEIs might lead to teratogenic effect. The fetopathic effect is partially because of fetal hypotension. It is imperative to note that ACEIs are not usually contraindicated in women of childbearing age. However, once conception is confirmed, the ACEI must be discontinued at the earliest and replaced by a safer antihypertensive agent, for example, methyldopa.

Interactions

Hyperkalemia can occur mainly when ACEIs are used with K^+-sparing diuretics or if K^+ is supplemented. Concurrent administration of antacids reduces the bioavailability of ACEIs. Antihypertensive action of ACEIs is reduced by concurrent administration of NSAIDs, including aspirin and indomethacin.

Clinical Uses

The conditions where efficacy is proved and is commonly used include the following:

Hypertension

ACEs are efficacious with better adverse effect profile and patient compliance, and have the following advantages:

1. There is no postural hypotension nor rebound hypertension.
2. These agents reverse the left ventricular hypertrophy (LVH).
3. There is no effect on the electrolytes especially hypokalemia, nor any changes in uric acid or lipids. ACEIs are safe in patients with associated disease such as bronchial asthma, DM, ischemic heart disease, CHF, and peripheral vascular disease.
4. They prevent secondary hyperaldosteronism and type II DM and provide a better quality of life.

Cardiac Failure/Left Ventricular Systolic Dysfunction

ACEIs are efficacious for the treatment of CHF and prevent subsequent changes that occur in untreated heart failure. ACEIs decrease both the preload and afterload and are beneficial in all grades of heart failure. Preload is decreased due to reduced circulatory volume, which occurs due to natriuresis and diuresis. Because of the decreased circulatory volume, there is reduced venomotor tone and thereby reduced venous return. Afterload is decreased because of reduced PVR; however, there is no reflex increase in sympathetic activity. ACEIs may reverse the ventricular remodeling by reducing preload and afterload.

Acute MI with Mild Systolic Ventricular Dysfunction

ACEIs are beneficial in patients with acute myocardial infarction (MI) when administered immediately after MI (preinfarct period) particularly in hypertensive and diabetic patients. They are beneficial in preventing the remodeling and subsequent events such as heart failure. It is recommended to administer ACEIs immediately after MI along with thrombolytic and other agents. However, they are contraindicated if there is severe hypotension or cardiogenic shock. ACEIs can be continued for long-term treatment depending on the associated disease, especially if there is CHF or if infarct is of large size.

The condition where efficacy has not yet been established include the following:

Chronic Renal Failure (Progressive)

ACEIs decrease nephropathy and protect against renal damage.

Diabetic Nephropathy

They decrease nephropathy, reduce microalbuminuria, improve endothelial function, and reduce cardiovascular complications. In DM, ACEIs provide protection against renal damage independent of antihypertensive action. With regard to reduction in cardiovascular complication, they are superior than other groups of antihypertensive agents, namely, calcium channel β-blockers and thiazide diuretics.

Patients More Prone to Ischemic Cardiovascular Events

They significantly minimize the rate of MI, stroke, and death in patients with DM and other vascular diseases (ischemic conditions).

Scleroderma Renal Crisis

It is almost a fatal and rare condition but few studies have shown marked improvement.

Diagnostic Use (Captopril Test)

This is used to test the renovascular hypertension. PRA is much higher in renovascular hypertension as compared to essential hypertension when action of Ang II is blocked by captopril.

Individual Agents

The various ACEIs available differ in potency, whether prodrug/active drug and mostly in pharmacokinetic property (extent of absorption and effect of food, plasma $t_{1/2}$, distribution in tissues, and elimination), and rest of the properties (pharmacodynamic, therapeutic, and adverse effect profile) are similar and thus they can be used interchangeably.

Captopril (Prototype)

It is a sulfhydryl-containing compound and the first orally effective ACEI introduced for clinical use, but currently, it is not preferred due to various common side effects.

Enalapril

It is a prodrug and is converted to an active metabolite, enalaprilat, which is more potent than captopril and is long acting. Food does not affect the absorption.

Enalaprilat

Enalaprilat is an active drug (metabolite of enalapril) not absorbed orally and thus it is used by IV route when oral treatment is not satisfactory.

Lisinopril

It is a lysine derivative of enalaprilat and an active drug. Its onset of action is delayed due to slow absorption and thus it is less likely to cause first-dose hypotension.

Ramipril

It is a prodrug with long $t_{1/2}$ and hence is used once a day. Its elimination is triphasic (due to distribution, elimination, and slow dissociation from tissues). Due to wide tissues distribution, its effect is more prominent on local ACE inhibition. The recommended dose is 1.25 to 10 mg once daily.

Angiotensin II (AT_1) Receptor Blockers/ Antagonists

Saralasin was the first ARB; however, it was not suitable for clinical use due to its partial agonist activity as it elicited pressor response. It has no oral bioavailability, so it had to be used by parenteral route. Subsequently, other agents have been introduced, namely, candesartan, losartan, olmesartan medoxomil, telmisartan, and valsartan.

Important Features of ARBs

ARBs have high affinity for AT_1 receptor and binds to AT_1 receptors with very high selectivity (10,000 times more as compared to AT_2 receptors). Binding of ARBs to AT_1 receptor is competitive but, even then, maximum response of angiotensin cannot be achieved in the presence of ARB.

Among the available ARBs, candesartan has the highest affinity for AT_1 receptors, while losartan has the lowest. Some ARBs also possess weak antiplatelet action due to blockade of thromboxane A_2 receptors. They inhibit most of the effects induced by Ang II and the important ones are:

1. Vascular smooth muscle contraction (vasoconstriction).
2. Release of aldosterone (kidneys) leading to altered renal function (Na^+ and water retention), antidiuretic hormone (pituitary), and catecholamines (adrenal medulla).
3. Sympathetic simulation (central and peripheral).
4. Facilitation of growth of cells of blood vessels and heart.
5. Thirst.

All the above-mentioned effects are inhibited by ARBs but they do not inhibit ACE.

Clinical Uses

Hypertension

All are beneficial, and efficacy is similar to other antihypertensive drugs, without significant adverse effects. They enhance the antihypertensive effect of other drugs.

Heart Failure

Valsartan is preferred in those who cannot tolerate ACEI (first-line drug for heart failure). Candesartan is equally effective as valsartan in reducing mortality in heart failure.

Acute MI

ARBs are equally effective as ACEIs and can be used as an alternative.

Miscellaneous

Diabetic Nephropathy

They are equally efficacious as ACEIs in preventing renal damage in type II DM and the renoprotective effect is not related to maintaining BP within normal range with these drugs. Losartan and irbesartan are commonly employed. ARBs can be considered as the drug of choice for this purpose because of better adverse effect profile as compared to ACEIs.

Stroke Prophylaxis

ARBs are better than β-blockers in reducing the stroke in hypertensive patients with LVH.

Portal Hypertension

Losartan is safer than and effective as portal antihypertensive in patients with cirrhosis of liver with portal hypertension without worsening the renal function.

Antidysrhythmic

In patients with atrial fibrillation (chronic and persistent), irbesartan was found to be effective in maintaining sinus rhythm.

Adverse Effects

There is no cough and the incidence of angioedema is less than with ACEI. Although hypotension may occur, first-dose hypotension is not seen. Hyperkalemia may occur in patients with renal disease or in those taking K^+ supplementation or K^+-sparing diuretics. They are also teratogenic (similar to ACEIs) and contraindicated in cases of bilateral renal artery stenosis as they can cause hypotension, oliguria, progressive azotemia, and, possibly, acute renal failure.

Differences between ARB and ACEIs

Both ARBs and ACEIs inhibit RAS, but by different mechanisms. Important differences in this regard between these two classes of drugs are mentioned in the following. However, the relevance of difference with regard to clinical efficacy has yet to be established.

1. ARBs do not inhibit the breakdown of substrates of ACE such as bradykinin, so there is no increase in the level of ACE substrates such as bradykinin and other substances. Thus, cough rarely occurs as side effect.
2. Activation of AT_1 receptor is more effectively blocked by ARBs because Ang II formed from non-ACE pathways is not inhibited by ACEIs. Hence, Ang II produced by other pathway may act on AT_1 receptors.
3. AT_2 receptors are activated by ARBs because, due to blockade of AT_1 (also autoreceptor) receptor, negative feedback is inhibited. Hence, there is increased renin release and increased Ang II production. On the contrary, ACEIs block the activation of both AT_1 and AT_2 receptors as Ang II is not produced.
4. Advantages of ARBs over ACEIs: first-dose hypotension, dry cough, dysgeusia, and angioedema are less likely.

Individual Agents

The various ARBs differ in potency, whether prodrug or active drug, mostly in pharmacokinetic properties such as effect of food, plasma $t_{1/2}$, generation of active metabolite, and elimination (renal, hepatic, or biliary), and rest of the properties (pharmacodynamic, therapeutic, and adverse effect profile) are similar. Thus, they can be used interchangeably.

Losartan

It generates active metabolite, which is more potent, and noncompetitively blocks the AT_1 receptor and has higher affinity for AT_1 receptor. Dose: 50 mg twice daily.

Candesartan Cilexetil

It is a prodrug and is converted to active drug. It has the highest affinity for AT_1 receptor because of slow dissociation from the receptor.

Eprosartan

It also claims to improve cognitive function.

Irbesartan

It generates active metabolite and also has antiplatelet action.

Telmisartan

Its plasma $t_{1/2}$ is very long (24 hours).

Valsartan

Its oral absorption is significantly affected by food, so it should be administered 1 hour before the meals. It is safe in renal insufficiency.

Aldosterone Antagonists

See Chapter 29.

Multiple Choice Questions

1. A prediabetic 54-year-old woman with hypertension, chronic obstructive pulmonary disease (COPD), and 2+ proteinuria is being treated with telmisartan. She complains of a rash and a mild itching since she started telmisartan. Which of the following drugs would inhibit renin–angiotensin–aldosterone system (RAAS) and be most suitable for this patient?

A. Losartan.
B. Enalapril.
C. Eplerenone.
D. Spironolactone.
E. Aliskiren.

Answer: E

Inhibition of RAAS has been shown to slow the progression of kidney damage in type 2 diabetes. Since the patient has COPD, ACEIs would be contraindicated because of the potential to worsen cough. She has demonstrated a sensitivity to an ARB; she is likely to have a sensitivity to other ARBs. Aliskiren is a small-molecule inhibitor of renin.

2. A 34-year-old woman with hypertension desires to become pregnant. Her gynecologist suggests her that she will have to switch to another antihypertensive drug. Which of the following drugs is absolutely contraindicated in pregnancy?

A. Pindolol.
B. Enalapril.
C. Methyldopa.
D. Prazosin.
E. Nebivolol.

Answer: B

ACEIs (enalapril) and ARBs have been shown to be teratogenic.

3. A 57-year-old contractor with hypertension has been treated by different physicians. He checks into the emergency department with a severe reaction. He has been taking ramipril and spironolactone. This combination is usually ill advised because of the risk of:

A. Bone loss and osteoporosis.
B. Calcium-containing kidney stones.
C. Hyperkalemia.
D. Metabolic acidosis.
E. Postural hypotension.

Answer: C

Spironolactone inhibits potassium excretion in the kidney by blocking aldosterone. Ramipril reduces Ang II levels and secondarily reduces aldosterone. The combination may increase serum potassium to dangerous levels.

4. A 67-year-old man presents with a 6-month history of dry cough. His past medical history includes a recent myocardial infarction (MI), with a past history of multidrug therapy. He does not smoke, nor has he had a history of asthma. Which of the following medication's side effect has caused the patient's symptoms?

A. Ramipril.
B. Nitroglycerin.
C. Simvastatin.
D. Digoxin.
E. Quinidine.

Answer: A

Angiotensin-converting enzyme (ACE) inhibitors cause dry nonproductive cough.

Chapter 23 Congestive Cardiac Failure

Vishal Munjajirao Ubale

PH1.29: Describe the mechanisms of action, types, doses, side effects, indications, and contraindications of the drugs used in congestive heart failure.

Learning Objectives

- Heart failure.
- Classification of drugs for heart failure.
- Drugs for acute heart failure (emergency treatment)/ parenteral drugs (hospitalized patient).
- Drugs for chronic heart failure/oral drugs.
- Miscellaneous agents in heart failure.
- Aim of treatment.

Heart Failure (IM1.24)

Heart failure is the inability of the heart to pump blood and/or decreased blood supply to different organs as per the needs. The normal heart has the ability to enhance the ability to pump the blood four to five times it pumps at rest depending on the requirement. If cardiac output (COP) is not adequate (decreased) to deliver oxygen requirement of the body, it is known as heart failure. Increased heart rate is the primary compensatory mechanism to preserve COP in heart failure (**Fig. 23.1**).

1. Systolic failure (forward failure)/pump failure (contractility): Ejection fraction is decreased. Long-term treatment is highly efficacious if the patient can be controlled by vasodilators, diuretics, angiotensin-converting enzyme inhibitors (ACEIs), angiotensin II (A-II) receptor blockers, and aldosterone antagonists.
2. Diastolic failure (backward failure): COP is decreased due to failure of sufficient relaxation of blood vessels because of stiffening of blood vessels and stiffness and hypertrophy of myocardium. Ejection fraction is normal. Response to positive inotropic agent may not be optimum. Ischemic heart disease (IHD) is the common cause and the mainstay of therapy is the treatment of the underlying cause.

Depending on COP, the cardiac failure could be:

1. Low-output failure: It is characterized by systolic dysfunction and decreased COP. In acute failures, ejection fraction is considerably reduced, for example, hypertension and IHD including acute myocardial infarction (MI). Drugs utilized for cardiac failure are effective.
2. High-output failure: In high-output failure, the body's demand is very high, so that increased COP is not adequate, for example, in patients with hyperthyroidism, beriberi, severe anemia, myocarditis, and arteriovenous (AV) shunt. Essentially, the term "heart failure" is a misnomer for such ailment since there is no heart failure; however, the body's demand is increased. Accordingly, the drugs used for cardiac failure are not efficacious in high-output failure and thus the mainstay of therapy is the treatment of the underlying cause.

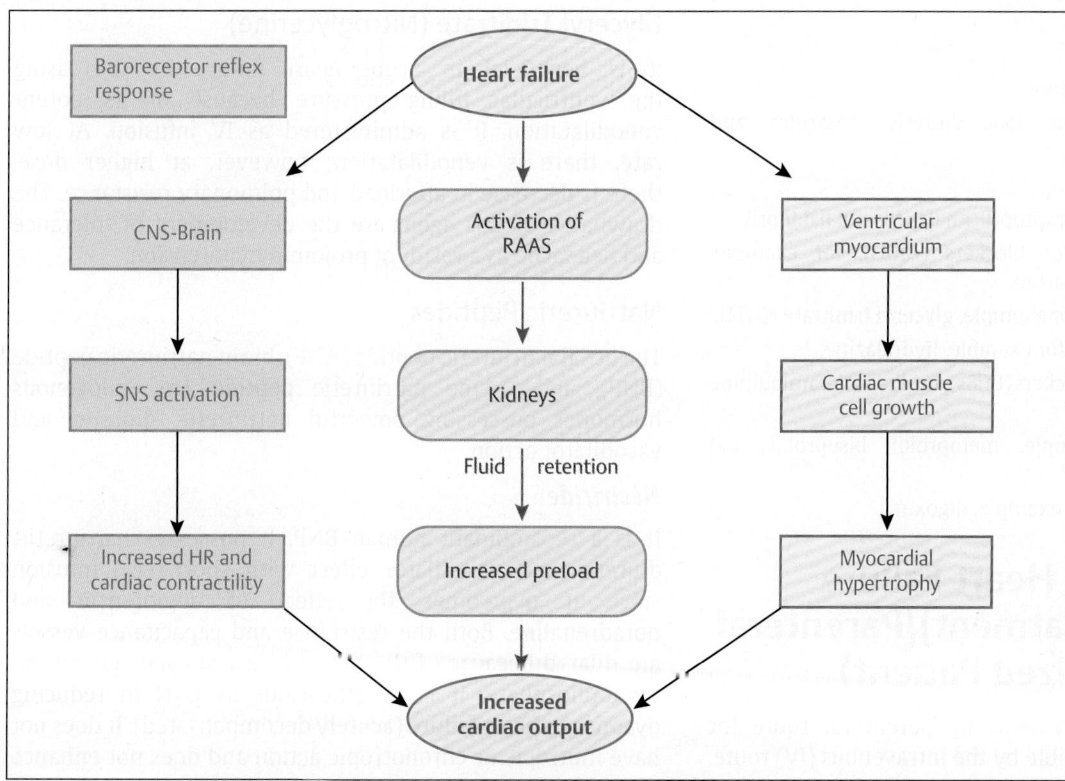

Fig. 23.1 Compensatory mechanisms during heart failure.

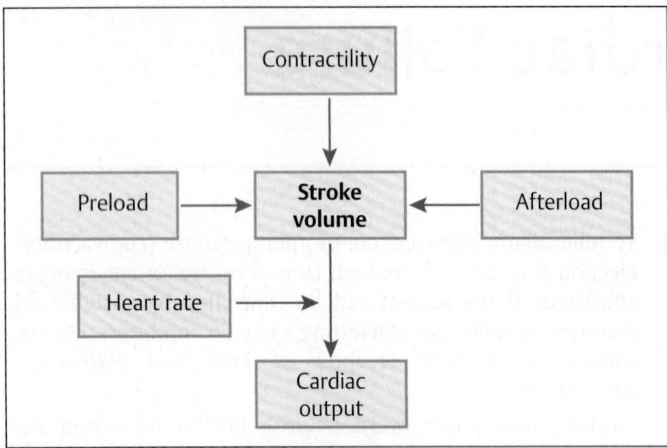

Fig. 23.2 Determinants of cardiac output.

COP can be determined by multiplying the heart rate with the stroke volume. Thus, the heart function is determined by stroke volume and heart rate and the stroke volume depends on the preload, afterload, and the myocardial contractility (**Fig. 23.2**).

Classification of Drugs for Heart Failure

1. Drugs for acute/severe heart failure (emergency treatment):
   a. Diuretics, for example, loop diuretics such as frusemide and bumetanide.
   b. Parenteral vasodilators, for example, sodium nitroprusside, nitrates, and nesiritide.
   c. Inotropic agents:
      i. β-agonists, for example, dopamine (DA), dobutamine, and dopexamine.
      ii. Phosphodiesterase (PDE) inhibitors, for example, inamrinone (amrinone), milrinone, and levosimendan.
   d. Morphine.
   e. Aminophylline.
2. Drugs for chronic heart failure:
   a. Diuretics, for example, loop diuretics, thiazides, and potassium-sparing.
   b. Vasodilators:
      i. ACEIs, for example, captopril, enalapril, and lisinopril.
      ii. Angiotensin receptor blockers (ARBs), for example, losartan and candesartan.
      iii. Nitrovasodilators, for example, glyceryl trinitrate (GTN).
      iv. Direct vasodilators, for example, hydralazine.
      v. Calcium channel blockers (CCBs), for example, amlodipine and felodipine.
   c. β-Blockers, for example, metoprolol, bisoprolol, and carvedilol.
   d. Cardiac glycosides, for example, digoxin.

Drugs for Acute Heart Failure (Emergency Treatment)/Parenteral Drugs (Hospitalized Patient)

These drugs are primarily used by parenteral route for severe heart failure, if possible by the intravenous (IV) route. Patients with chronic heart failure could develop acute failure due to some causes. The potential causes are noncompliance of drug treatment and acute MI. Additional causes could be severe exertion, high dietary salt intake, or enhanced oxygen requirement (e.g., anemia and fever). The important reason of acute failure is acute myocardial infarction and it is treated accordingly. Hence, very rapid treatment is essential, and saving life is the immediate objective of treatment.

Diuretics (PH1.24)

Loop diuretic such as frusemide is utilized in patients with severe decompensated heart failure. It is given by IV route, which offers prompt and predictable result. For this objective, frusemide should be administered as a bolus dose and repeated or as continuous IV infusion. However, response must be supervised and dose should be titrated. Frusemide 40 mg bolus is followed by IV infusion at a rate of 10 mg/hour and escalated as per the condition.

Parenteral Vasodilator

Sodium Nitroprusside

It is a powerful vasodilator and decreases both the ventricular filling pressure and systemic or arterial resistance. The onset of action is noted in 2 to 4 minutes, and it is because of the rapid formation of nitric oxide (NO). However, poor hepatic or renal function, high rate of infusion, or too rapid or prolonged use could lead to cyanide poisoning. The manifestations of toxicity include abdominal pain, mental changes, lactic acidosis, and convulsions. Hence, sodium nitroprusside must be administered only for short period. Management of toxicity is by the administration of sodium nitrite and sodium thiosulphate. The most common side effect is hypotension.

Glyceryl Trinitrate (Nitroglycerine)

It is beneficial in acute heart failure by decreasing the ventricular filling pressure because of its potent venodilatation. It is administered as IV infusion. At low rate, there is venodilatation; however, at higher dose, there is decrease in afterload and pulmonary resistance. The drawbacks of this agent are the development of tolerance and headache as a result of profound hypotension.

Natriuretic Peptides

The atrial natriuretic peptide (ANP), brain natriuretic peptide (BNP), and C-type natriuretic peptide are endogenous hormones possessing powerful natriuretic, diuretic, and vasodilator action.

Nesiritide

It is a recombinant human BNP. It possesses natriuretic, diuretic, and vasodilator effect with short-term infusion since it overcomes the effect of angiotensin and noradrenaline. Both the resistance and capacitance vessels are dilated because of the raised levels of cyclic guanosine monophosphate. It is as efficacious as GTN in reducing dyspnea in heart failure (acutely decompensated). It does not have inotropic or chronotropic action and does not enhance the chances of atrial and ventricular arrhythmias. Due to these benefits, it is chosen over inotropic agents to alleviate dyspnea in patients with refractory heart failure, mostly in patients with risk of arrhythmias. It is given as initial loading dose (2 μg/kg/min) followed by IV infusion (0.01 μg/kg/min; maximum, 0.03 μg/kg/min). Long-term therapy could cause potentially serious renal damage.

Inotropic Agents

β and/or Dopamine Agonists

Dobutamine

It is available as racemic mixture and acts on both the β_1 and β_2 receptors. Due to its action on β_1 receptors, it increases the force of contraction without comparable increase in heart rate, that is, positive inotropic effect. Because of its action on β_2 receptors, peripheral vascular resistance is reduced but not to a significant level. It is essential to mention that DA receptors are not activated by dobutamine even at very high dose. Renal blood flow is increased because of enhanced COP. It is administered in the starting dose of 2 to 3 μg/kg/min and then modified, that is, increased or decreased depending on the response, which can be evaluated by assessing COP and pulmonary capillary wedge pressure. Side effects include tachycardia, palpitation, and arrhythmia because of overdose, and dose should be decreased if side effect occurs. If a patient is being administered a β-blocker, the response of dobutamine may not be produced due to blockade of β receptors.

Dopamine

Though DA is also used for heart failure because of its inotropic effect, it has restricted usage in this situation and not preferred over dobutamine. Because of its short half-life, it is administered as IV infusion. At higher rate (10–20 μg/kg/min), it activates vascular α receptors and thus acts as "inoconstrictor" because it produces positive inotropic action and vasoconstriction.

Dopexamine

It is a synthetic agent related to DA; however, it possesses intrinsic activity at DA (D_1 and D_2) and β_2 receptors. It could be beneficial in patients with shock and severe congestive heart failure (CHF).

Phosphodiesterase III Inhibitors

Both inamrinone and milrinone are administered for short-term therapy of advanced/severe/acute heart failure. Both lead to an increase in myocardial contraction and hence there is an increase in COP. It also reduces peripheral vascular resistance because of vasodilatation. Both the PDE III inhibitors are better than other parenteral vasodilators such as sodium nitroprusside and dobutamine. This is because PDE III inhibitors produce both the actions, that is, positive inotropic effect and peripheral vasodilatation. Hence, they are also called "inodilators." Both are used by initial loading dose and subsequently by IV infusion. Both are unstable in dextrose solution.

Milrinone is more selective for PDE III and has lesser side effects and hence is preferred to inamrinone. It has a short half-life (30–60 minutes) and it is used for short-term treatment of heart failure by IV route, for example, emergency control of heart failure or before transplantation. However, milrinone has been demonstrated to increase the mortality in certain patients, especially on long-term use. Also, it is expensive.

Levosimendan is also an "inodilator," which acts by PDE III inhibition. However, it also acts by other mechanisms such as sensitizing cardiac muscle to the action of calcium (Ca^{2+}). It also acts by stimulation of ATP sensitive K^+ channel in vascular smooth muscles. It is beneficial for therapy of severe heart failure and shock.

Vasopressin Antagonists

Some patients of heart failure with acute decompensation develop hyponatremia because of enhanced vasopressin activity. Thus, vasopressin antagonists such as conivaptan could be beneficial for heart failure with hyponatremia. Tolvaptan is a selective V_2 receptor antagonist and therefore is a more appropriate agent for therapy of hyponatremia and heart failure.

Drugs for Chronic Heart Failure/ Oral Drugs

These drugs are administered primarily for mild-to-moderate heart failure and some of them, particularly digoxin, are likewise indicated for severe heart failure. The drugs are also administered by parenteral route, if necessary. The drugs utilized are DDD, that is, diuretics, dilators (vasodilators), and digoxin. Moreover, β-blockers are beneficial in a certain small number of patients.

Diuretics (PH1.24)

These agents cause improvement in congestive symptoms by decreasing the extracellular fluid volume (preload) (**Fig. 23.3**). Diuretics are not efficacious in enhancing the survival time. Nevertheless, the potassium-sparing diuretic spironolactone has been demonstrated to cause an increase in the survival time.

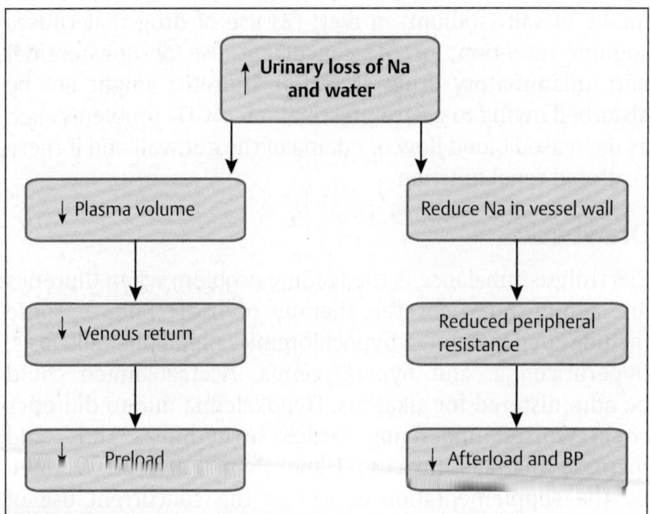

Fig. 23.3 Mechanism of action of diuretics. Na, sodium.

Loop Diuretics

These include frusemide, bumetanide, and torsemide. Frusemide is the most frequently used agent. Their effectiveness is determined by the factors responsible for their accessibility at the site of action such as the proximal renal tubular secretion and renal plasma flow. They act on ascending limb of loop of Henle by inhibiting the $Na^+–K^+–Cl^-$ symporter, a specific protein participating in ion transport in the renal epithelial cells.

Thiazide Diuretics

These include chlorothiazide and hydrochlorothiazide. They are beneficial in patients with mild heart failure to decrease the circulatory volume. They act at renal tubular epithelial cells of distal convoluted tubules by affecting $Na^+–Cl^-$ cotransporter. However, they are not efficacious if the glomerular filtration rate is less than 30 mL/min. Nonetheless, they can be administered along with loop diuretics when refractoriness develops to loop diuretics and they produce a synergistic effect.

K+-Sparing Diuretics

Triamterene and amiloride act by blocking Na^+ conductance in the epithelial cells in the collecting duct, while spironolactone and canrenone act as aldosterone antagonists. Aldosterone antagonists spironolactone and canrenone are beneficial for heart failure. These agents are less effective when used alone. However, when used along with other diuretics, they improve their efficacy and minimize the toxicity by reducing the renal loss of potassium and magnesium, that is, prevent the development of hypokalemia and hypomagnesemia.

In patients with advanced heart failure, it has been seen that the administration of spironolactone (25–50 mg/day) along with ACEIs can enhance the survival time.

The minor problems associated with spironolactone include gynecomastia in men, which could need withdrawal of drug, and hyperkalemia in few patients.

Diuretic Resistance

It could be because of: (1) poor patient compliance, that is, the patient is not consuming the drug; (2) excess intake of salt (sodium) in diet; (3) use of drug that causes sodium retention; or (4) concurrent use of nonsteroidal anti-inflammatory drugs (NSAIDs). Diuretics might not be absorbed owing to gastrointestinal tract (GIT) problems such as decreased blood flow or edema of the gut wall and if there is altered renal function.

Drawbacks

Electrolyte imbalance is the leading problem when diuretics are administered for the therapy of heart failure. These include hypokalemia, hypochloremic metabolic alkalosis, hyperuricemia, and hyperglycemia. Acetazolamide could be administered for alkalosis. Hypokalemia due to diuretics could worsen underlying cardiac arrhythmias and could increase digitalis toxicity. Hypokalemia can be rectified by the supplementation of KCl or the concurrent use of K-sparing diuretic. It is imperative to note that the use of K-sparing diuretic with ACEIs could lead to the development of hyperkalemia.

Vasodilators

ACEIs

Captopril was the first agent introduced for clinical use. Examples include enalapril, lisinopril, ramipril, quinapril, and fosinopril. A-II causes vasoconstriction and retention of sodium and water by releasing the aldosterone. Additionally, A-II leads to the secretion of ANP and endothelin, adding to increased afterload. A-II also leads to catecholamine release, vascular hyperplasia, myocardial hypertrophy, and death of myocardial cells (myocyte). These actions of A-II are accountable for remodeling of myocardium progression of disease and heart failure.

ACEIs act by two mechanisms: short term and long term.

Short-Term Mechanism

Due to decrease in formation of A-II and aldosterone and also by diminishing the sympathetic activity.

Long-Term Mechanism

ACEIs also inhibit the degradation of bradykinin since the enzyme responsible for the degradation of bradykinin is also inhibited. Hence, the bradykinin collected leads to the secretion of NO and prostaglandins, both of which are vasodilators. Bradykinin possess hemodynamic and antiremodeling action.

These dual mechanisms ACEIs cause both arterial and venous dilatations and reduction in both the systemic and pulmonary artery resistances. Hence, there is decrease of both the preload and the afterload.

ACEIs are beneficial for the treatment of heart failure of all grades (New York Heart Association [NYHA] grade I–IV). They are also administered in patients with asymptomatic left ventricular dysfunction. The initial dose should be smaller and then slowly the dose must be escalated to the desired response and the tolerated dose over days or weeks. Mild hyperkalemia could occur with ACEIs, which can be tackled by regulating the dose or by administering low-potassium diet. Dry cough could be an additional problem, and if it is so, this can be controlled by stopping the ACEI and using ARB. ACEIs possess a diuretic-sparing effect, that is, the dose of diuretics is decreased when ACEIs are used. It has been found that ACEIs increase the survival time regardless of the cause or severity of the heart failure.

A-II Receptor Blockers/Antagonist

The hemodynamic effects generated by ARB are similar to that of ACEI. The long-term benefits of ARB on renal function, hospitalization, and mortality are inadequately understood since only little studies are available.

Presently, it is appropriate to use ACEI if drugs that affect renin–angiotensin system have to be used in cardiac failure and ARB should be used as an alternative in cases where ACEI cannot be administered because of any reason. Most of the actions of A-II responsible for the heart failure are because of its action on AT_1 receptors. As ARB blocks AT_1 receptors, they inhibit all the actions of A-II and effect is sustained even if the concentration of A-II comes back to initial value because of the synthesis of A-II by other pathways. Additionally, AT_1 receptor blockade is accompanied by a compensatory increase in AT_2 receptor stimulation (vasodilatation) and this enhances the beneficial effect of AT_1 antagonist. The drawback of ARBs as compared to ACEIs is that ARBs are unable to inhibit the metabolism of bradykinin and hence the favorable effects/changes that ensue owing to accumulation of bradykinin are lacking when treated with ARBs. Therefore, it seems that the combination of ACEI and ARB would be more beneficial than either agent used alone due to their different modes of action.

Organic Nitrates

They mimic the action of NO, which is produced by the enzyme NO synthase present in endothelium of vascular epithelial cells and some other smooth muscle cells. It is responsible for the synthesis of NO by conversion of arginine to citrulline. Isosorbide dinitrate (IDN) and glyceryl trinitrate (GTN) or nitroglycerine are beneficial and safe in the therapy of heart failure. The foremost effect of nitrates is decrease in preload by producing the venous pooling of blood as a result of venodilatation. Thus, they decrease ventricular filling pressure in both the acute and chronic heart failure. Coronary flow is also improved by their selective vasodilatation in epicardial coronary vessels and this increases equally the systolic and diastolic ventricular function.

Their limitations are their reduced effect on arterial resistance, that is, afterload, and development of tolerance on repeated use, if used alone. However, if used in combination with other vasodilators such as hydralazine, their efficacy is preserved. Hydralazine diminishes the tolerance by increasing the availability of NO. Acetylcysteine, likewise, decreases the tolerance of nitrates. If nitrates are used singly, tolerance can be reduced by allowing a nitrate free blood level for around 6 to 8 hours daily. This can be achieved by missing of the dose and this must be dependent on the symptoms of the patient. IDN and GTN are valuable as adjuvant in patients with heart failure who are maintained on digoxin and diuretics. It is imperative to mention that the GTN is a drug that can be administered in several ways, including IV route, sublingual tablet, ointment, transdermal patch, and lingual spray, as per the necessity and suitability.

Direct Vasodilators

Hydralazine

It is a direct smooth muscle relaxant with unknown intracellular mechanism. Hydralazine is beneficial in heart failure by decreasing both the pulmonary and systemic vascular resistance. It causes arteriolar vasodilatation; hence, it decreases the afterload. However, it has a negligible effect on veins, that is, capacitance vessels.

Arterial dilatation leads to increase in heart rate, contractility, and increased renin activity because of sympathetic stimulation. This causes fluid and water retention and eventually loss of therapeutic benefit.

It likewise leads to vasodilatation of coronary blood vessels. Hydralazine could be chosen in patients with heart failure with renal dysfunction since it enhances renal blood flow more than the other vasodilators by decreasing the renal vascular resistance. It is beneficial in combinations with or without some venodilator such as IDN in patients with heart failure who are already taking diuretics, ACEI, and digoxin.

Headache and dizziness could be troublesome side effects, which are more if nitrates are also used simultaneously. However, these recede on regular use. Occasionally, dose modification or drug withdrawal could be essential. IV use of hydralazine does not provide any benefit over oral formulation except in emergency situation, for example, during pregnancy where other vasodilators are contraindicated.

Calcium Channel Blockers

CCBs decrease the afterload and thus they are beneficial for heart failure. However, the trials conducted to explore the beneficial effect of CCBs in cases of heart failure did not find satisfactory results. The probable reason could be due to tachycardia caused by short-acting dihydropyridine (DHP) CCBs. Additionally, drugs such as verapamil and diltiazem might cause negative inotropic action and decreased AV conduction. However, long-acting DHP CCBs such as amlodipine and felodipine can be effective since they decrease afterload, but reflex tachycardia is minimal. Hence, the long CCBs could be of benefit as adjuvant together with other agents in selected patients. However, the trials conducted have not revealed encouraging results.

β-Adrenoceptor Antagonists

These agents can aggravate heart failure since patients of heart failure are dependent on some degree of sympathetic drive to maintain adequate cardiac function. β-blockers are generally avoided in cases of cardiac failure due to fear of precipitation of heart failure. However, in selected cases in which there is obstructive outflow, for example, hypertrophic obstructive cardiomyopathy and dilated cardiomyopathy, catecholamines can produce mild-to-moderate congestive cardiac failure (CCF) and β-blockers are effective. The agents that are found not to be effective in certain patients bring benefit by improving the cardiac function and prolonging the life (reduced mortality). For this purpose, certain β-blockers can be administered in low doses vigilantly in mild-to-moderate cases of CCF and dose escalation must be small and steady contingent to the response of individual patient. The favored agents are those that cause vasodilatation (decrease in afterload) such as carvedilol, due to additional α-blocking action. The other β-blockers used for CCF are β_1-selective agents metoprolol and bisoprolol.

Possible Mechanism of Action of β-Blockers in Cardiac Failure

It is not well defined and all the β-blockers are not effective. Studies have revealed that increased sympathetic activity occurs in majority of the patients of CCF. Activation of β_1 receptors by the excess catecholamines produces toxic effect on the heart. Additionally, cardiac remodeling and myocardial cell death could also occur due to β receptor stimulation. Consequently, by inhibiting the β receptors, the above-mentioned damaging effects on heart are inhibited.

However, the agents preferred to be used are β_1-selective blockers such as metoprolol and bisoprolol and nonselective β-blockers with additional α-blocking action such as carvedilol.

It is essential to note that all the β-blockers are not suitable in cases of CCF and useful β-blockers are effective in selected cases of CCF of class II and III of NYHA.

Cardiac Glycosides

These include agents such as digoxin and digitoxin. *Digitalis* (foxglove) was used for several years and was known to Egyptians as medicinal plants. The term *digitalis* is used for all the cardiac glycosides. In 1785, William Withering, a British physician, published a book associated with details of cardiac glycosides. However, digitalis was utilized extensively without following guiding principle and precautions recommended by Withering, and this has led to several fatalities associated with the use of digoxin and has caused its disuse till the 20th century. However, in the previous decade, its first-line status is taken over by diuretics and vasodilators, mostly ACEIs. Digoxin is the prototype drug among the cardiac glycoside. All the cardiac glycosides have three components: a steroid nucleus with a lactone ring and sugars. Both the steroid nucleus and lactone ring comprise a glycone and are vital for their pharmacodynamic effects, whereas a sugar attached to carbon is significant for pharmacokinetic property.

All the cardiac glycosides have similar efficacy and safety. Certain glycosides with their sources are cited in **Table 23.1**. Only digoxin and digitoxin are used clinically, and digoxin is preferred.

Mechanism of Action

Sodium potassium pump maintains sodium outside and potassium inside of the cardiac muscle cells by continuous active transport of sodium from inside to outside and potassium from outside to inside. Hence, there is accumulation of sodium inside and increase in cytosolic Na^+ concentration. Because of increased cytosolic Na^+, the Na^+–Ca^{2+} exchange, which happens during repolarization, is decreased, causing a secondary rise in Ca^{2+}. The increase in calcium triggers the liberation of large concentrations of calcium through ryanodine receptors from intracellular stores, the sarcoplasmic reticulum (**Fig. 23.4**). Consequently, the calcium concentration increases intracellularly. This increase in intracellular calcium is adequate to combine with troponin C, which causes an interaction between actin and myosin, resulting in the contraction of myocardial muscle. The inotropic action of digoxin develops slowly even if the drug is administered by IV route.

Pharmacological Actions

The primary effects are on the cardiac tissue; however, cardiac glycosides also produce extracardiac actions. Their action is primarily because of the inhibition of sodium pump, the direct (extravagal) and also due to indirect action (vagal stimulation)

Cardiac Action

Because of both the direct and indirect action, the effect of digoxin on the heart could be considered unique as it produces positive inotropic action but negative chronotropic action, a noteworthy variance from other inotropic agents. Additionally, it has negative dromotropic action, that is, it decreases the AV conduction. The cardiac actions are more pronounced in decompensated heart as compared to normal heart.

Mechanical Effects

Force of Contraction

Increase in force of contraction (positive inotropic action) occurs. The forceful contraction leads to augmented COP, more complete ventricular emptying, decreased diastolic pressure, and diminished size of the heart (ventricles).

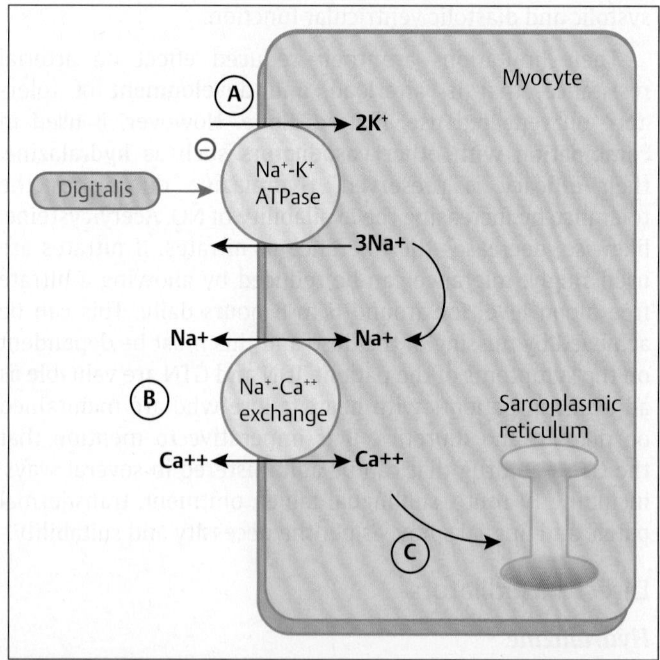

Fig. 23.4 Mechanism of action of digitalis.

Table 23.1 Some of the cardiac glycosides and their sources

Source	Part	Glycosides
Digitalis purpurea (purple foxglove)	Leaves	Digitoxin, gitoxin, gitalin
Digitalis lanata (white foxglove)	Leaves	Digoxin, digitoxin, gitoxin
Strophanthus gratus	Seed	Strophanthin-G (ouabain)
Strophanthus kombe	Seed	Strophanthin-K

These effects are more prominent in failed heart. The increased force of contraction in ventricle is due to direct action.

Rate and Rhythm

The heart rate is reduced due to both inhibition of sodium pump (increased intracellular calcium) and vagal action. AV conduction is reduced due to increased vagal activity (vagomimetic action). Besides, digoxin increases refractory period of AV node and contributes to delay in AV conduction. At higher dose, automaticity of AV node, His-Purkinje system, and ventricles is increased because of the direct action. These effects are useful in certain types of arrhythmias.

Cardiac glycosides as well as digoxin have narrow safety margin, and at somewhat higher doses, the interruption in AV conduction might be transformed into AV block, ectopic beats. Excessive increase in calcium concentration leads to afterdepolarizations and this consequently leads to ventricular ectopics and pulsus bigeminus, that is, one normal beat followed by one ectopic beat. This might be transformed into ventricular tachycardia and even ventricular fibrillation.

Electrophysiological Effects

These effects are due to direct action as well as autonomic action. The effect is on the cardiac pacemaker, atrial and ventricular muscles, and conduction fibers (**Table 23.2**).

Due to Direct Action

At therapeutic levels, there is early prolongation of action potential. Subsequently, there is shortening mainly of the plateau phase. Additional increase in dose causes abnormal generation of impulses such as delayed afterdepolarizations (DADs). When DAD crosses the threshold, it leads to ectopic beats/extrasystole. Crossing the threshold potential in His-Purkinje system leads to pulsus bigeminus.

Due to Effect on Autonomic Nervous System

Both the parasympathetic and sympathetic effects are seen based on the dose. In lower dose, parasympathetic effect is significant. These effects are more pronounced in atria and AV nodal tissue. Due to increase in vagal tone, heart rate is decreased. AV conduction velocity is slowed due to increased effective refractory period of AV node. Certain parasympathetic effects are utilized for the treatment of some arrhythmias. Sympathetic tone is decreased and this is also secondary to improvement in COP in failed heart due to digoxin. At toxic levels, sympathetic system is activated due to digoxin, leading to sensitization of myocardium and thus toxic effects of digoxin could be heightened. Due to increased effective refractory period of AV node, the excessive impulses that occur in atrial fibrillation (AF) and atrial flutter are not allowed to pass from AV node to ventricles. On this basis, cardiac glycosides reduce the ventricular rate in both the AF and flutter.

Electrocardiographic Changes

Notable ones include prolongation of PR interval, shortening of QT interval, and ST segment depression. At toxic dose, AV block may occur.

Coronary Blood Flow

This is increased secondary to increased COP.

Other Actions

Cardiac glycosides have an excitatory effect on other excitable tissues, including the smooth muscles. The effect is due to suppression of enzyme Na^+/K^+-ATPase. However, the effect is not as significant in cardiac tissue, probably due to the reason that diverse forms of enzymes are existing in different tissues and they may not be so sensitive to digitalis.

Effect on Autonomic Nervous System (Discussed Earlier)

Digoxin in low doses leads to vagal stimulation and at higher dose there is decrease of sympathetic tone and reduced vascular tone.

Renal System

There is no direct effect in normal person or in patients with CHF; however, there is diuresis in patients with CHF secondary to effect on the heart, that is, improvement of circulation and removal of excess salt and water. All these effects lead to increased urine output and reduced edema in patients with cardiac failure. It is, however, imperative to mention that edema due to any other reason does not respond to digitalis.

Effect on Blood Vessels

In normal individuals, slight rise in peripheral vascular resistance is detected due to slight direct vasoconstriction. But, in cases of CHF, there is reduced peripheral resistance due to increased COP. The increased venous pressure is also brought to normal level.

Central Nervous System Effect

Digoxin might cause disturbances in vision, manifested as blurring of vision, photophobia, and yellow, green, or blue color discrimination. Furthermore, there may be confusion

Table 23.2 Electrophysiological effects of digoxin on cardiac tissues

Tissue or variable	Effects at therapeutic dosage	Effects at toxic dosage
Sinus noted	↓ Rate	↓ Rate
Atrial muscle	↓ Refractory period	↓ Refractory period, arrhythmias
Atrioventricular node	↓ Conduction velocity, ↑ refractory period	↓ Refractory period, arrhythmias
Purkinje system, ventricular muscle	Slight ↓ refractory period	Extrasystoles, tachycardia, fibrillation
Electrocardiogram	↑ PR interval, ↓ QT interval	Tachycardia, fibrillation, arrest at extremely high dosage

and mental disturbances and chemoreceptor trigger zone (CTZ) stimulation.

GIT

Nausea, vomiting (partly central nervous system effect), anorexia, and diarrhea. Stimulation of CTZ at higher dose contributes to vomiting.

Gynecomastia

It is rare, but could occur in men who are on digitalis therapy, and breast enlargement may occur in women.

Pharmacokinetics

The cardiac glycosides differ in pharmacokinetics. The three main agents are digoxin, digitoxin, and ouabain; but the most frequently used cardiac glycoside is digoxin. The bioavailability of different brands of digoxin from different manufacturers (including generic drug) fluctuates and all the cardiac glycosides as well as digoxin have low therapeutic index (narrow safety margin). Bioavailability from capsule form might be more than tablets (**Table 23.3**). Consequently, if a patient is sustained on digoxin therapy, the digoxin must be used only from a particular manufacturer, that is, same brand, and in the same dosage form (capsule or tablet), or else toxicity or loss of therapeutic effect might ensue contingent on high- or low-bioavailability preparations, respectively. They produce pain on subcutaneous (SC) and intramuscular (IM) administration due to their irritant nature. Hence, they are not used by SC or IM route. Digoxin may be used via either oral or IV route.

Digoxin is preferred over digitoxin because it has rapid quicker onset of action, dose adjustment takes less time, and cases of toxicity can be tackled without difficulty by discontinuation of drug. However, because of a very long half-life of digitoxin and high binding with plasma protein, more time is required for dose adjustment and to attain steady-state plasma concentration. Furthermore, there is more likelihood of toxicity due to cumulative effect; thus, it is occasionally used for maintenance therapy.

Clinical Status

Digoxin is the most commonly used cardiac glycoside.

Cardiac Failure

Digoxin is beneficial for patients not responding to first-line agents, for example, diuretics and vasodilators such as ACEIs and ARBs. It is indicated in patients who are symptomatic in spite of treatment with first-line drugs. It is administered in patients with left ventricular failure and CCF. It acts due to direct action on myocardium to increase the force of contraction and at the same time reduce the heart rate (bradycardia), that is, increasing the efficiency of heart. Its onset of action is about 5 to 30 minutes as compared to other inotropic agents such as dobutamine (1 min) and milrinone (3 min). Hence, digoxin is not suitable for the treatment of acute heart failure. It is preferred and should be reserved for patients with heart failure with associated AF.

It can be administered by either oral route or IV route. IV is used if urgent action is required such as during emergency or in unconscious patients or if a patient cannot take the drug orally due to any reason such as vomiting. Digoxin has narrow therapeutic index, and toxicity can occur, which can be minimized by giving a maintenance dose (0.125–0.25 mg) when treatment is commenced. This is the current clinical practice whenever digoxin is indicated, unlike digitalization, which was practiced earlier. The full clinical benefit is usually observed within 1 week.

The beneficial effects of digoxin are clinically evident from the following features: dyspnea and cyanosis (if present) are relieved due to reduced pulmonary congestion; increased urine output and reduced body weight due to reduction in peripheral edema; tachycardia and palpitation are relieved due to reduced heart rate (however, heart rate less than 60/minute can be considered as sign of overdose); and pain due

Table 23.3 Pharmacokinetic effects of digoxin and digitoxin

Parameters	Digoxin	Digitoxin
Onset of action	Shortest and fastest	Delayed and longer acting
Oral absorption	75%	> 90%
PPB	25%	> 90%
Half-life	1–2 d	4–6 d
Metabolism	Excreted unchanged by the kidney	By the liver, so safe in renal insufficiency
Caution	Renal insufficiency	Hepatic diseases
Administration	Oral, IV	Oral
Daily maintenance dose	0.125–0.5 mg	0.05–0.02 mg
Daily elimination	35%	10–15%
Plasma concentration:		
• Therapeutic	0.5–1.4 ng/mL	15–30 ng/mL
• Toxic	> 2 ng/mL	> 35 ng/mL
Generally used for	Routine treatment and emergency	Maintained

Abbreviations: IV, intravenous; PPB, plasma protein binding.

to enlargement of liver (tender hepatomegaly) is relieved due to reduced systemic venous pressure.

It is indicated to reduce the ventricular rate in patients with AF, for which it is considered the drug of choice. In AF, the ventricular rate is very high (300–500/min) and irregular. Digoxin indirectly increases the vagal activity. The beneficial effects are due to vagal effect on AV node, decreasing the conduction through it by prolonging the effective refractory period on AV node. Thus, it reduces the number of ectopic impulses from atria to ventricle and this effect ultimately decreases the ventricular rate. Additionally, β-blockers (atenolol) and CCBs (verapamil) can be used as alternatives or combined with digoxin if digoxin alone does not produce the desired response.

Atrial Flutter

In atrial flutter, the ventricular rate is high (200–300/min) but not as high as in AF. However, it is regular and may be associated with AV block. Digoxin transforms atrial flutter to AF by shortening the effective refractory period of atria. When atrial flutter is converted to fibrillation, the treatment is same as mentioned earlier for fibrillation. It is safer to use anticoagulant prior to the use of digoxin.

Paroxysmal Supraventricular Tachycardia and AV Nodal Tachycardia

Supraventricular tachycardia and AV nodal tachycardia are also terminated by digoxin. It is not preferred presently due to its delayed onset and toxicity and the availability of very rapidly acting and better agents such as adenosine, β-blockers (atenolol), and CCBs (verapamil).

The onset of antiarrhythmic action takes several hours even if digoxin is administered by IV route. This is due to slow distribution to the site(s) of action, slow binding of digoxin with Na^+/K^+-ATPase, and also gradual rise in cytosolic calcium concentration. The signs of antiarrhythmic effects are prolongation of PR interval and slowing of the ventricular rate in AF.

Adverse Effects

All the cardiac glycosides possess a narrow safety margin and toxicity is not infrequent. Nevertheless, the incidence of digoxin toxicity has decreased currently due to reduced use of digoxin, as presently it is not the first-line agent for heart failure. If toxicity occurs, plasma concentration monitoring and consequently dose decrease are essential.

Cardiac

Cardiac arrhythmias might occur owing to digoxin, such as atrial and ventricular ectopics. Sinoatrial node and AV node conduction defects could also occur. It is imperative to mention that if there is arrhythmia in a patient on digoxin therapy, the first possibility of arrhythmia could be because of digoxin toxicity and this should be ruled out before thinking about other possibility. Accordingly, potassium level must be assessed instantly whenever there is arrhythmia because toxicity of digoxin is higher if there is hypokalemia, which could be due to any cause including diuretics. The commonest arrhythmia due to digoxin is atrial tachycardia with 1:2 or 1:3 AV block.

Sinus Bradycardia or AV Block

This might occur but is temporary. Atropine 0.6 to 1.2 mg via IM or IV route may be administered.

Ventricular Tachyarrhythmia

This occurs because of increased AV junctional automaticity and is generally due to potassium reduction. It is treated with potassium administration by oral route or IV depending on the patient's condition. Potassium must be administered only after assessing the serum level.

Ventricular Arrhythmias

Lignocaine is preferred and phenytoin (slow IV) is an alternative since both these agents produce membrane-stabilizing action by blocking the sodium channels and have insignificant effect on AV nodal conduction.

For Supraventricular (Atrial) Arrhythmia

β-blockers (propranolol, atenolol) could be beneficial for supraventricular tachycardia either orally or IV depending on the patient's condition.

Others

Central Nervous System

Dizziness, mental confusion, malaise, fatigue, delirium, or altered cognitive function may occur.

Ocular Disturbances

Halos, photophobia, and blurred vision may occur. Disturbance of color vision may occur and this includes yellow, green, or blue color discrimination (chromatopsia).

GIT

Anorexia, nausea, vomiting, and abdominal pain partly due to gastric irritation on oral use may occur.

Gynecomastia

Gynecomastia may occur in males. Also, breast enlargement in women may occur with long-term use due to estrogenlike action because of structural resemblance of digitalis with estrogen.

Precautions

Since the effective plasma concentration and toxic concentration of digoxin are well established, the therapeutic drug monitoring is essential in suspected cases that are not responding or in cases showing toxicity of digoxin. Plasma concentration can be measured by digoxin antibodies by radioimmunoassay method. These antibodies can also be used for acute toxicity.

Acute Digoxin Toxicity

Acute toxicity could occur because of overdose (toxic) or as a result of drug interactions or other factors such as hypoxia, hypokalemia, hypomagnesemia, or hypercalcemia. The manifestations of toxicity include nausea, vomiting, and hyperkalemia. The toxic concentration of digitalis may cause any type of arrhythmias but specific one is atrial tachycardia with AV block.

Treatment of Overdose/Toxicity

It depends on the symptoms, type of arrhythmias, and potassium administration if hypokalemia. Digoxin should be discontinued. The drug for various types of arrhythmias mentioned earlier can be used depending on arrhythmias. For severe digoxin toxicity, the infusion of digoxin-specific binding fragment of the antibody to digoxin is used. It is effective and acts by inactivating the digoxin in plasma.

Digoxin Antibodies (Digoxin Immune Fab)

Digoxin antibodies can be used as specific antidote (digoxin immunotherapy) in cases of severe digoxin intoxication, which may prove fatal if not treated promptly. Purified fab fragment (Digibind) binds with digoxin, digitoxin, and other cardiac glycosides obtained from plants and significantly reverses toxicity and increases their renal excretion. About 40 mg (content of one vial) of antibody neutralizes 0.6 mg of digoxin accumulated in the body during toxicity. It does not show immunogenicity.

Interactions and Precautions

1. If there is reduced plasma potassium concentration (i.e., hypokalemia), the effect of digoxin and other cardiac glycosides are enhanced and may attain toxic concentration, which is clinically significant and causes cardiac arrhythmias. Thus, hypokalemia should be avoided while using digoxin, and in cases of digoxin toxicity, if serum potassium level is low, K^+ should be supplemented. Drugs that can cause hypokalemia should better be avoided with digoxin, such as diuretics (loop diuretics) other than K^+-sparing diuretics, amphotericin B, and corticosteroids. Conversely, hyperkalemia reduces the effect of digoxin by inhibiting the binding of digoxin to Na^+/K^+-ATPase. This is because both digoxin and potassium inhibit binding of each other to Na^+/K^+-ATPase.
2. Calcium increases the toxic effects of digoxin by causing overload of intracellular calcium and thus facilitates digoxin-induced arrhythmias.
3. Reduced magnesium level may cause arrhythmias and thus hypomagnesemia should be avoided.
4. Broad-spectrum antibiotics such as tetracyclines increase the plasma concentration of digoxin by inhibiting the metabolism of digoxin by bacterial flora in the gut.
5. Antiulcer drugs reduce the absorption of digoxin, for example, antacids, proton pump blocker (omeprazole), and sucralfate (absorbs digoxin).
6. Plasma concentration of digoxin is increased in renal impairment, in the elderly, and in patients with hypothyroidism due to reduced clearance.
7. AV block caused by digoxin is increased by β-blockers, verapamil, and disopyramide.
8. Digoxin may lead to complete heart block when used in patients with already existing partial AV block.
9. Sympathomimetic drugs such as adrenaline and isoprenaline may cause arrhythmia by increasing the pacemaker activity. Succinylcholine and anticholinesterase may also cause cardiac arrhythmias.

Miscellaneous Agents in Heart Failure

Vasopeptidase Inhibitor

Omapatrilat increases the level of natriuretic peptide and reduces the formation of A-II. Omapatrilat is orally active antihypertensive. It is useful in heart failure and improves the cardiac function in heart failure patients. Its adverse effects are angioedema, cough, and dizziness.

Endothelin Receptor Blockers

They have been shown to have short-term benefits but the long-term usefulness is not yet known. Bosentan is a nonselective endothelin antagonist used orally and proved useful in animal models of heart failure; however, clinical trials have shown discouraging results. Currently, it is indicated for pulmonary hypertension.

Aim of Treatment

The aim is to reduce morbidity and mortality.

General Measures

An important measure is salt restriction to the extent of 3 g/day; however, severe restriction may cause hypokalemia, hyponatremia, metabolic alkalosis as a result of depletion of chloride, and suppressed appetite leading to reduced muscle mass.

Definitive Treatment

This is to find out the underlying cause of heart failure such as IHD, chronic uncontrolled hypertension, and valvular heart disease, and should be corrected as far as possible, including the surgical intervention. It depends on the pathophysiological factors as depicted in **Fig. 23.5.**

Symptomatic Treatment

1. To provide relief from symptoms:
   a. To relieve the congestion by using diuretics and venodilators.
   b. Precipitating factors such as infection and fever should be identified and treated.
   c. Avoidance of drugs that increase sodium overload, for example, NSAIDs and sodium salt of antibiotics such as carbenicillin.
2. To prevent and/or reverse disease progression and reduce mortality.
3. To prevent and reverse the myocardial dysfunction/ventricular dysfunction by reducing the afterload and increasing the contractility. ACEIs (e.g., enalapril), ARBs (e.g., losartan), β-blockers (e.g., carvedilol, bisoprolol, metoprolol), and aldosterone antagonist (spironolactone) can be used for such purpose based on the evidence provided by various studies.

Guidelines for the management of heart failure are depicted in **Fig. 23.6.**

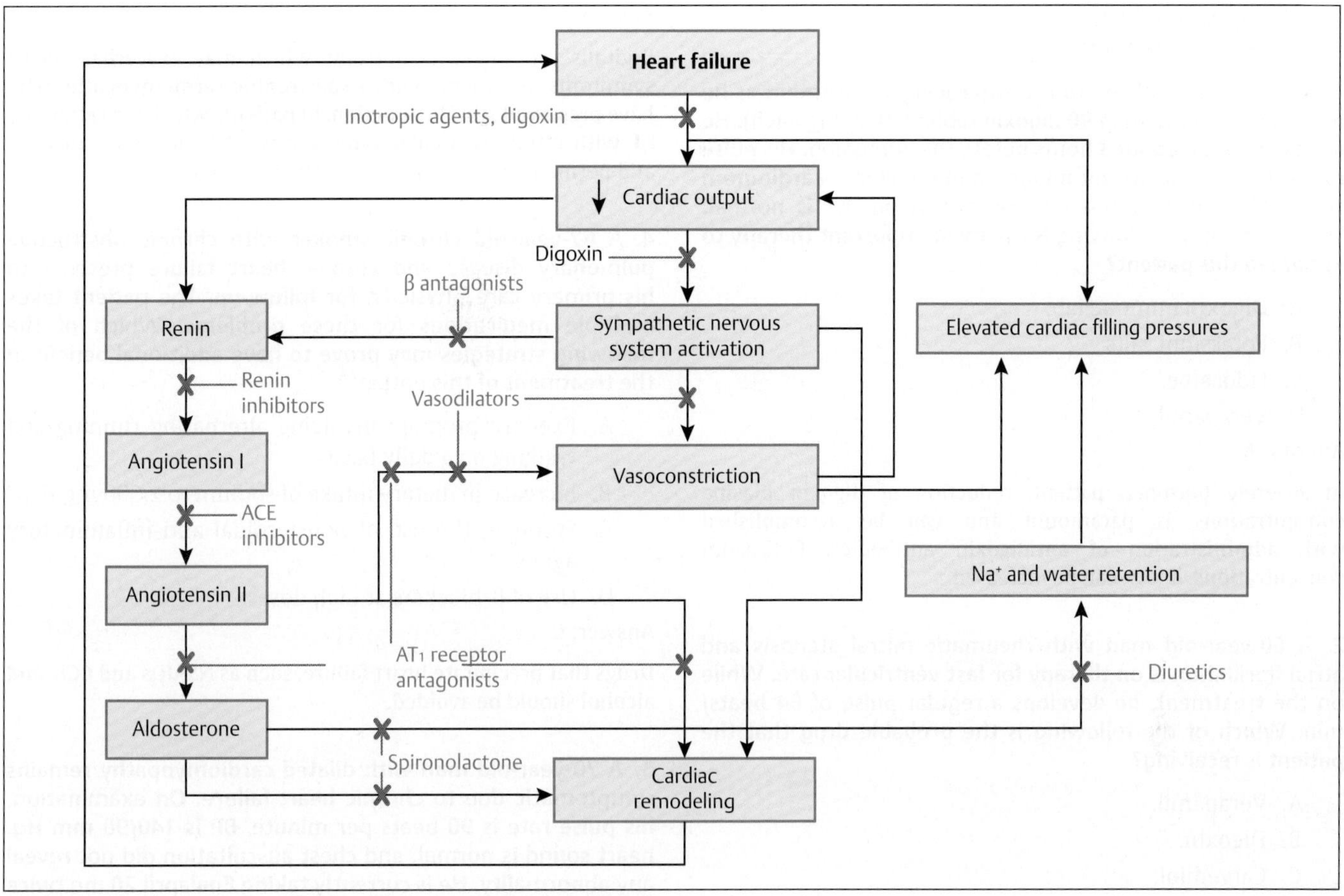

Heart failure
Inotropic agents, digoxin
Cardiac output
Digoxin
β antagonists
Renin
Sympathetic nervous system activation
Elevated cardiac filling pressures
Renin inhibitors
Vasodilators
Angiotensin I
Vasoconstriction
ACE inhibitors
Angiotensin II
Na⁺ and water retention
AT1 receptor antagonists
Diuretics
Aldosterone
Spironolactone
Cardiac remodeling

Fig. 23.5 Treatment of cardiac failure based on pathophysiology.

Stage D Refractory symptoms requiring special intervention
Stage C Structural disease, previous or current symptoms
Stage B Structural heart disease, no symptoms
Stage A High risk with no symptoms
Hospice
VAD, transplantation
Inotropes
Aldosterone antagonists, nesiritide
Consider multidisciplinary team
Revascularization, mitral-valve surgery
Cardiac resynchronization if bundle-branch block present
Dietary sodium restriction, diuretics, and digoxin
ACE inhibitors and β-blockers in all patients
ACE inhibitors or ARBs in all patients; β-blockers in selected patients
Treat hypertension, diabetes, dyslipidemia; ACE inhibitors or ARBs in some patients
Risk-factor reduction, patient and family education

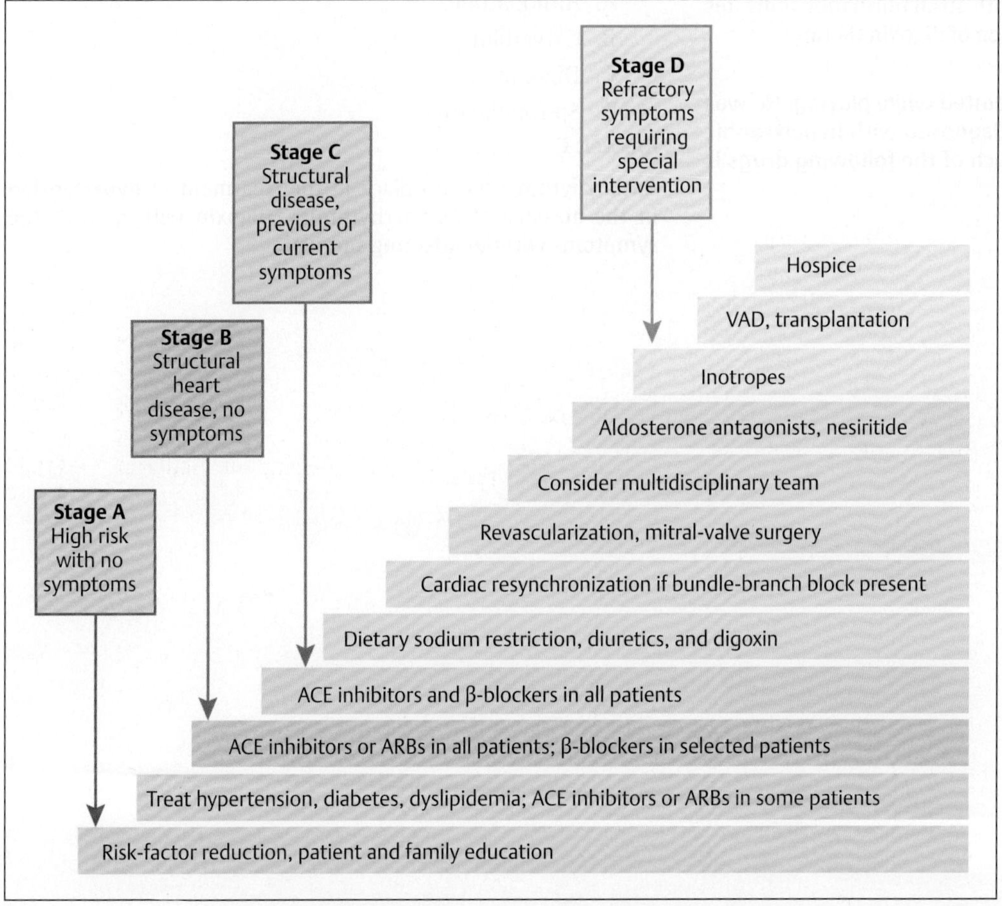

Fig. 23.6 Stages of heart failure along with its management.

Multiple Choice Questions

1. A person is admitted to the emergency department as he has ingested more than 90 digoxin tablets (0.25 mg each). He has taken them about 3 hours before the admission. His pulse rate is 50 to 60 beats per minute, and the electrocardiogram shows third degree heart block. His serum K+ is normal. Which one of the following is the most important therapy to initiate in this patient?

A. Digoxin immune fab.
B. Potassium salts.
C. Lidocaine.
D. Verapamil.

Answer: A

In severely poisoned patient, reduction of digoxin plasma concentrations is paramount and can be accomplished with administration of antidigoxin antibodies. Potassium concentrations, if low, can be increased.

2. A 60-year-old man with rheumatic mitral stenosis and atrial fibrillation is on therapy for fast ventricular rate. While on the treatment, he develops a regular pulse of 64 beats/min. Which of the following is the probable drug that the patient is receiving?

A. Verapamil.
B. Digoxin.
C. Carvedilol.
D. Propranolol.

Answer: B

Slow ventricular rate in a patient with atrial fibrillation indicates complete heart block—a complication of digoxin therapy.

3. A 30-year-old football player fainted while playing. He was admitted to a hospital and was diagnosed with hypertrophic obstructive cardiomyopathy. Which of the following drugs is contraindicated in this patient?

A. Propranolol.
B. Captopril.
C. Losartan.
D. Digitalis.

Answer: D

Digitalis can increase inotropy, which may exacerbate heart symptoms in patients with hypertrophic cardiomyopathy who have preserved systolic function. In patients who have refractory AF with rapid ventricular rates, atrioventricular node ablation and permanent pacing are alternative options.

4. A 67-year-old chronic smoker with chronic obstructive pulmonary disease and chronic heart failure presents to his primary care physician for follow-up. The patient takes multiple medications for these problems. Which of the following strategies may prove to have additional benefit in the treatment of this patient?

A. Exercise program involving alternating running and walking on a daily basis.
B. Increase in dietary intake of sodium to 2,000 mg/d.
C. Stopping the use of nonsteroidal anti-inflammatory agents.
D. Use of β-blockers at high doses.

Answer: C

Drugs that precipitate heart failure, such as NSAIDs and CCB, and alcohol should be avoided.

5. A 70-year-old man with dilated cardiomyopathy remains symptomatic due to chronic heart failure. On examination, his pulse rate is 90 beats per minute, BP is 140/90 mm Hg, heart sound is normal, and chest auscultation did not reveal any abnormality. He is currently taking Enalapril 20 mg twice daily. Which of the following drugs could be considered to optimize his therapy?

A. Amiodarone.
B. Carvedilol.
C. Digoxin.
D. Spironolactone.

Answer: C

Antiarrhythmic has no place in the treatment of hypertension in the absence of any arrhythmias. Digoxin will improve the symptoms without affecting survival.

Chapter 24 Antianginals and Drug Treatment of Myocardial Infarction—1

Nishigandha Suresh Jadhav

PH1.28: Describe the mechanisms of action, types, doses, side effects, indications, and contraindications of the drugs used in ischemic heart disease (stable, unstable angina, and myocardial infarction), peripheral vascular disease.

Learning Objectives

- Antianginal drugs.
- Nitrates.

Ischemic Heart Disease (IM2.15, IM2.20, IM2.23)

Ischemic heart disease (IHD) is defined as the condition developed due to slowly progressive insufficiency of coronary circulation. Angina pectoris is the primary symptom of IHD.

Angina Pectoris

It is defined as the clinical manifestation of transient episodes of reversible myocardial ischemia, and usually it is experienced as suffocating substernal pain in the chest, often radiating to the left shoulder, flexor aspect of left arm, neck, jaw, or epigastrium. Symptoms often last for 1 to 5 minutes.

This pain is elicited by accumulation of metabolites due to imbalance in myocardial oxygen supply and demand. In silent myocardial ischemia, ischemic episodes occur without any pain.

Clinical Forms of Angina Pectoris

Table 24.1 presents the various forms of angina.

Factors Influencing the Myocardial Oxygen Demand and Supply (Fig. 24.1)

Heart rate, contractility, and ventricular wall tension are the three factors that determine the myocardial oxygen demand. Coronary blood flow and regional myocardial blood flow determine the myocardial oxygen supply.

Local myocardial metabolism also regulates coronary blood flow. Coronary blood flow is determined by the luminal radius of the coronary artery, as blood flow is inversely proportional to the fourth power of artery's luminal radius. The progressive decrease in vessel radius due to atheromatous plaque can impair the coronary blood flow, which reduces myocardial oxygen supply and precipitates the symptoms of angina when myocardial oxygen demand increases, as seen with exertion (increase in heart rate). Autonomic nervous system also plays a role in coronary blood flow by affecting

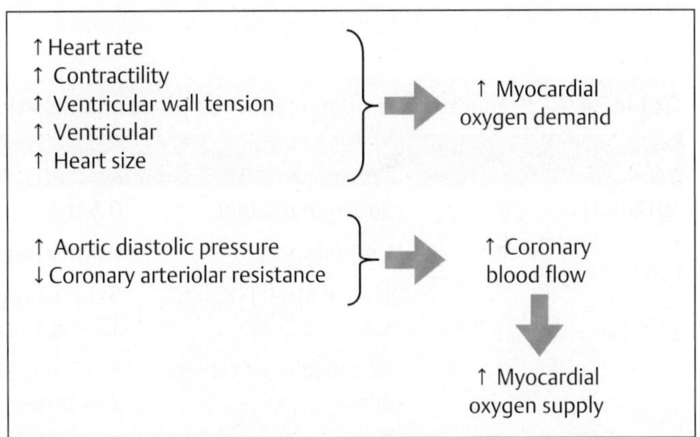

Fig. 24.1 Factors influencing the myocardial oxygen demand and supply.

Table 24.1 Forms of angina

Stable/classical/exertional/atherosclerotic angina	Unstable/crescendo/preinfarction/acute coronary syndrome	Prinzmetal/variant/vasospastic angina
▪ Most common (90%) type ▪ Ischemic attack on exertion, emotions, meals ▪ No symptoms at rest ▪ Symptoms due to reduced myocardial oxygen supply or increased oxygen demand ▪ Fixed atheromatous stenosis of larger coronary arteries leads to acidic metabolites' accumulation, causing stimulation of myocardial pain mediating nerve endings	▪ Recurrent attacks of angina at minimal exertion or even at rest ▪ Progressive atheromatous narrowing of coronary artery ▪ In acute coronary syndrome, there is dislodging of coronary plaque that triggers local platelet aggregation and thrombosis, which causes coronary occlusion causing non-STEMI	▪ Episodes of recurrent localized acute coronary vasospasm ▪ Pain during rest or sleep and is usually not related to exercise ▪ Vasospastic angina may deteriorate into unstable angina

Abbreviation: STEMI, ST-segment elevation myocardial infarction.

its vascular tone. Oxygen-carrying capacity of red blood cells may also affect myocardial oxygen supply.

Risk Factors for Ischemic Heart Disease

Patients with hypertension, diabetes mellitus, anemia, thyrotoxicosis, obesity, heart failure, cardiac arrhythmias, acute anxiety, and heavy cigarette smoking are prone to precipitation of angina symptoms.

Antianginal Drugs

Classification

1. **Nitrates:**
   a. Short acting (rapid onset)—glyceryl trinitrate (GTN; prototype), isosorbide dinitrate (IDN; sublingual), amyl nitrite.
   b. Long acting (slow onset)—IDN (oral), isosorbide mononitrate (IMN), erythrityl tetranitrate, pentaerythritol tetranitrate.
2. **β-blockers**—propranolol, metoprolol, atenolol, bisoprolol, celiprolol.
3. **Calcium channel blockers**—verapamil, diltiazem, amlodipine.
4. **Potassium channel openers**—nicorandil.
5. **Miscellaneous drugs:**
   a. **Cytoprotective drugs**—trimetazidine, ranolazine.
   b. **Bradycardic drugs**—ivabradine.
   c. **Antiplatelet drugs**—aspirin, clopidogrel, dipyridamole.
   d. **HMG CoA reductase inhibitors**—statins.

Nitrates

Organic nitrates are polyalcohol esters of nitric acid, whereas organic nitrites are esters of nitrous acid. Nitrates mimic the actions of endogenous nitric oxide by releasing or forming nitric oxide within the tissues.

Preparations of nitrates used in ischemic heart disease are nitroglycerin (NTG), IDN, IMN, erythrityl tetranitrate, pentaerythritol tetranitrate, etc. (**Table 24.2**).

Nitroglycerin

Plasma $t_{1/2}$ of NTG is 2 minutes and peak blood levels are attained in 3 to 6 minutes when it is administered by sublingual route. When given orally, hepatic biotransformation reduces the bioavailability, which can be overwhelmed by administering large dose orally (5–15 mg). Sustained-release capsules of large dose can be used for chronic prophylaxis of angina. Bioavailability is increased to 70 to 90% by transdermal patch.

Isosorbide Dinitrate

It can be used both in acute attack of angina by sublingual route and in chronic prophylaxis of angina by oral route. Plasma $t_{1/2}$ is 40 minutes but may be increased to 6 hours when sustained-release capsules are used.

Table 24.2 Preparation of organic nitrates—dose and duration of action

Drug	Preparations	Dose and route	Duration of action	Onset of action
NTG/GTN	Sublingual tablet	0.5 mg	15–30 min	1–2 min
	Lingual spray	0.4 mg per spray	10–30 min	Peak 3–6 min
	Transdermal patches	5- or 10-mg patch for 12–16 h per day	Maximum 24 h	30–40 min
	SR capsules or tablets oral	5–15-mg SR capsules 2–4 times daily	4–8 h	15–30 min
	Ointment (2%)	Topically to skin 4–8 hourly	3–8 h	30–120 min
	IV	5–20 μg/min, maximum of 400 μg/min	Transient	Immediate
IDN	Sublingual tablet	2.5–10 mg	1–2 h	5–15 min
	Chewable tablet	5–10 mg	–	1/2–1 h
	Oral tablet or capsule	10–20 mg	2–4 h	15–45 min
	SR capsules or tablets	10–40 mg	6–10 h	60–90 min
IMN	Sublingual tablet	10–40 mg	6–10 h	15–30 min
	Oral	10–40 mg		
Erythrityl tetranitrate	Sublingual tablet	5–10 mg	2–4 h	5–15 min
	Oral	10–30 mg	4–6 h	15–30 min
Pentaerythritol-tetranitrate	Oral	10–20 mg	3–5 h	30 min
	SR capsules or tablets	80 mg	8–12 h	20 min

Abbreviations: GTN, glyceryl trinitrate; IDN, isosorbide dinitrate; IMN, isosorbide mononitrate; IV, intravenous; NTG, nitroglycerin; SR, sustained release.

Isosorbide Mononitrate

It is an active metabolite of IDN. It has a higher oral bioavailability as it undergoes little first-pass metabolism. It is longer acting and its $t_{1/2}$ is 3 to 6 hours.

Erythrityl Tetranitrate and Pentaerythritol Tetranitrate

These are the longest-acting nitrates used only for chronic prophylaxis of angina.

Routes of Administration of Nitrates in Angina

Sublingual Administration

Because of its rapid onset of action, sublingual NTG and other nitrates can be used to terminate acute attack of angina. An initial dose of 0.3-mg NTG often relieves the pain within 3 minutes and is the mainstay of therapy for relieving acute coronary vasospasm.

Transdermal Application (Ointment/Patches)

NTG ointment (2%) applied to skin (2–2.5 cm) also acts within 15 minutes and may produce its effects, which last for 3 to 8 hours. Ointment is useful particularly for nocturnal angina, which develops within 3 hours after patient goes to sleep.

Transdermal NTG patch starts working in 30 to 40 minutes, with improved bioavailability of 70 to 90%. A free period of about 8 hours should be kept between two transdermal applications of NTG ointment or patch to avoid development of tolerance.

Buccal/Transmucosal Administration

Preparations are kept under upper lip above the incisors, which are absorbed through gingival mucosa and can be used for short-term prophylaxis of angina. Relief comes within 2 to 5 minutes.

Intravenous Infusion

If anginal pain persists, intravenous (IV) infusion (10 µg/min) of NTG can be given, with maximum of 200 µg/min until anginal pain is relieved.

Oral Administration

Oral administration is preferably used for prophylaxis of angina. The major disadvantage of this route is extensive first-pass metabolism. Sufficient large doses should be used to increase plasma concentration.

Mechanism of Action

The nitrate receptors at vascular smooth muscles possess sulfhydryl (-SH) group, which causes enzymatic denitration of organic nitrates to nitrite and nitric oxide (NO). NO activates cytosolic guanylyl cyclase (GC). Cytosolic GC converts GTP to cyclic guanosine monophosphate (cGMP), which, through protein kinase G, causes dephosphorylation of myosin light chain (MLC). Reduced availability of phosphorylated MLC interferes with activation of myosin and reduces the binding of myosin with actin to produce contraction, which indirectly causes relaxation of smooth muscle cells (**Fig. 24.2**).

Pharmacokinetics

Organic nitrates are lipid-soluble. There is low bioavailability of most nitrates by oral route due to first-pass metabolism, so sublingual route is preferred for acute attacks. Therapeutic blood levels are reached within minutes after sublingual route. Nitrates are inactivated in the liver by glutathione-organic nitrate reductase. Mitochondrial aldehyde dehydrogenase plays a role in biotransformation of nitrates. Amyl nitrite is obsolete now due to its unpleasant odor and shorter duration of action. IDN is inactivated at one-sixth of the rate of NTG. Enzymatic denitration is followed by formation of glucuronide conjugate. IMN has excellent bioavailability (100%), as its dose does not undergo first-pass metabolism. It has longer $t_{1/2}$ of 3 to 6 hours.

Pharmacological Effects

Fig. 24.3 shows the pharmacological effects of nitrates.

Adverse Effects

Due to the vasodilator effect (postural hypotension), severe throbbing headache (due to dilatation of meningeal vessels), transient episodes of dizziness, sweating, weakness, flushing (due to dilatation of cutaneous vessels of face), fainting, and palpitation can occur. All these effects are accentuated by standing immobile and alcohol intake, and the severity can be decreased with the help of the laying down posture. Methemoglobinemia seen with high doses is a rare adverse effect. Monday morning disease/sickness is also observed. GTN manufacturing factory workers develop headache and dizziness on Monday and Tuesday, which gradually disappears by Friday and again reappears on next Monday while resuming work. Other adverse effects include tolerance and zero-hour effect (**Box 24.1**) and acute coronary syndrome (coronary artery spasm—this occurs on being away for 1 to 3 days after chronic exposure to nitrates).

Box 24.1 Features of nitrate dependence and zero-hour effect

Nitrate dependence: Develops due to sudden withdrawal of nitrates after prolonged administration. Spasm of coronary and peripheral blood vessels is seen in such cases. Threat of increasing episodes of angina is present due to reduced threshold after withdrawal of nitrates. Hence, gradual withdrawal of nitrates is advisable to reduce these symptoms.

Zero-hour effect: More than 12-hour gap between the removal of patch in night and the application in next morning may cause rebound angina in morning before next patch application, which is called zero-hour effect. Ischemic changes in ECG can be correlated with clinical symptoms during this period. Intermittent application of transdermal patch can avoid this rebound effect.

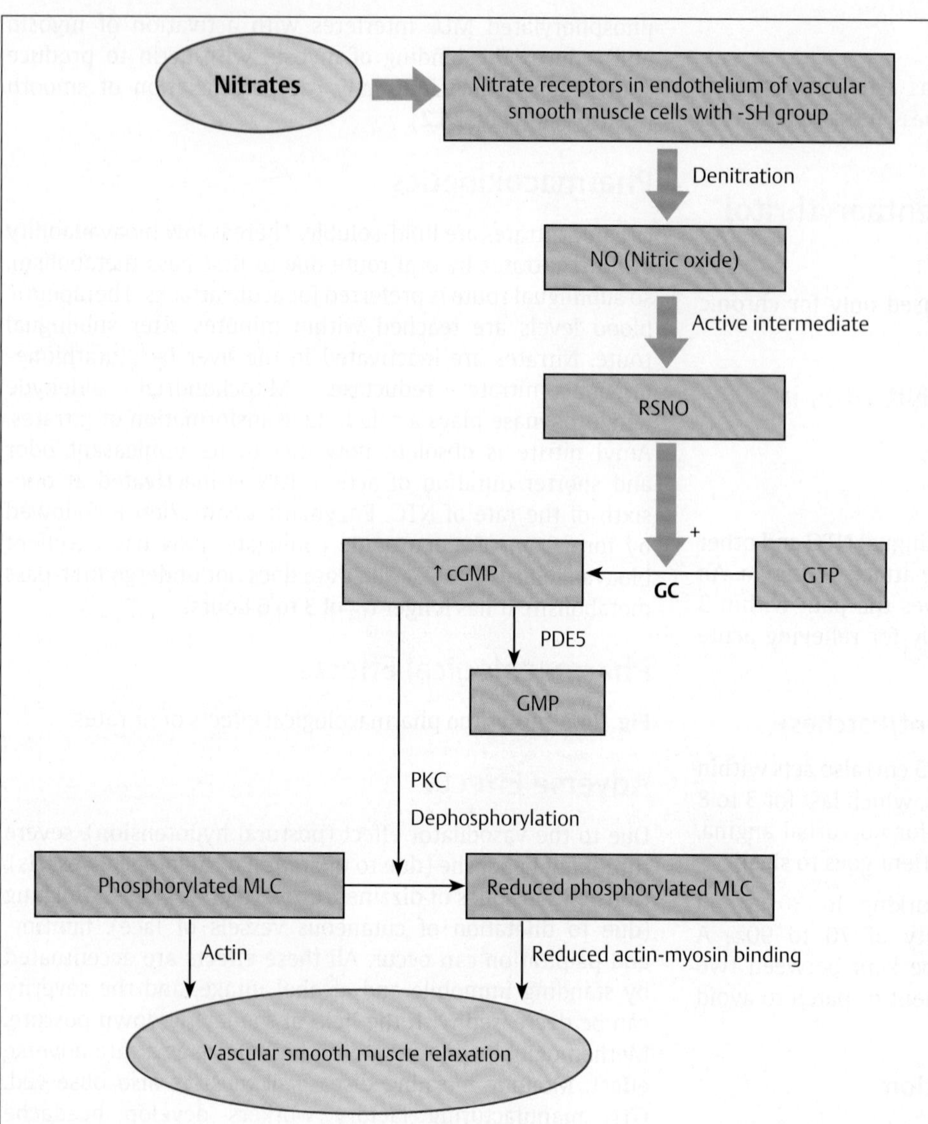

Fig. 24.2 Illustrative demonstration of mechanism of action of nitrates. MLC, myosin light chain; RSNO, S-nitrosothiols; cGMP, cyclic guanosine monophosphate; GTP, guanosine triphosphate; PKC, protein kinase C

Nitrate Tolerance

It is defined as the cessation of pharmacological effects of nitrates in a dose- and duration-of-exposure-dependent manner when they are used continuously in high dose. Degree of tolerance depends upon the dose of drug used and the duration of exposure (**Fig. 24.4**).

Ways to Avoid Nitrate Tolerance

Nitrate-Free Interval

Maintenance of gap of 8 to 12 hours between the two administrations of nitrates is an effective method to avoid development of tolerance. In the case of transdermal patches, removing patch at night and again applying in morning may prevent tolerance. Some patients may develop nocturnal angina due to this practice, which can be minimized by administration of other class of antianginal drugs at bedtime (NTG ointment).

Use of Other Drugs

Use of sulfhydryl donors (acetylcysteine or methionine) may also help prevent development of tolerance by providing –SH group, which stimulates production of cGMP. Hydralazine, due to its antioxidant property, attenuates superoxide function and increases bioavailability of nitric oxide. Use of other drugs before nitrate administration, such as angiotensin-converting enzyme (ACE) inhibitors, thiazides, and carvedilol, can also decrease the chances of nitrate tolerance.

Indications in IHD

Angina Pectoris

Role of Nitrates in Management of Acute Episodes of Angina

Nitrates cause systemic venodilation and therefore reduce myocardial wall tension and oxygen requirements. They also dilate epicardial coronary capacitance vessels, thereby increasing blood flow in collateral vessels.

Nitrates in Various Clinical Forms of Angina

In exertional angina/stable angina, nitrates cause venous dilatation, which reduces preload and end diastolic

Nitrates

Vasodilatation

Redistribution of blood flow to ischemic regions (by inhibiting platelet aggregation)

Coronary vasodilatation

Venous dilatation

Dilate collaterals

Arteriolar dilatation

(Predominant action)

Reduces afterload

Decrease in coronary arteriolar resistance

Reduces preload

Reduces aortic resistance to left ventricle

Increases coronary blood flow

Reduces ventricular end-diastolic pressure

Increase myocardial oxygen supply

Decrease in myocardial wall tension

Decrease in myocardial oxygen demand

Symptomatic relief in angina

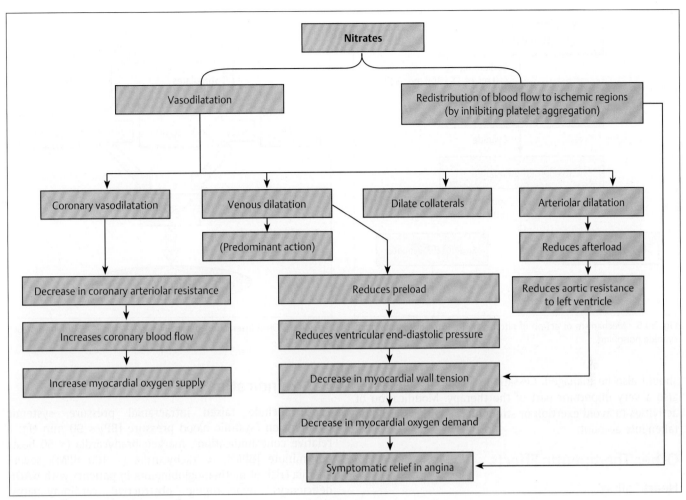

Fig. 24.3 Pharmacological actions of nitrates.

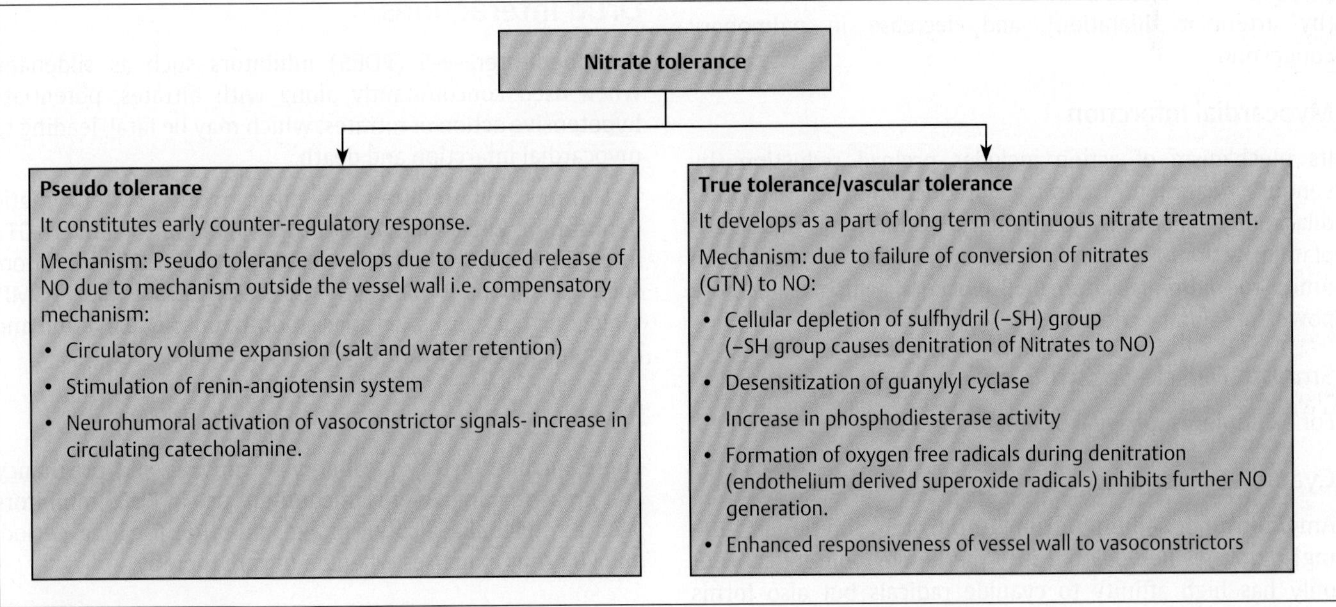

Fig. 24.4 Nitrate tolerance.

ventricular pressure and size and hence reduces myocardial oxygen demand. In variant angina, nitrates relax smooth muscles of epicardial coronary arteries and thus relieve spasm. In unstable angina/acute coronary syndrome, nitrates dilate epicardial coronary arteries and thus reduce myocardial oxygen demand and decrease platelet aggregation (antiplatelet action).

Risk factor management includes treatment or elimination of coexisting illness such as diabetes mellitus and hypertension. Dietary and drug therapy of dyslipidemias

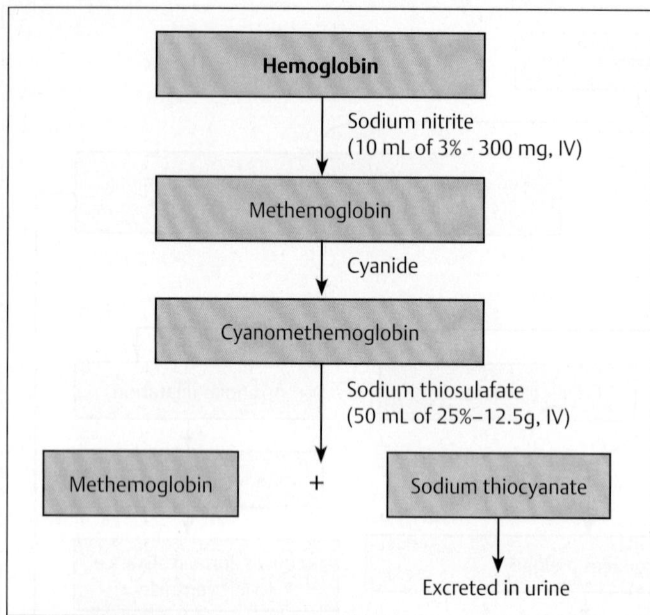

Fig. 24.5 Mechanism of action of nitrates and nitrites in treatment of cyanide poisoning.

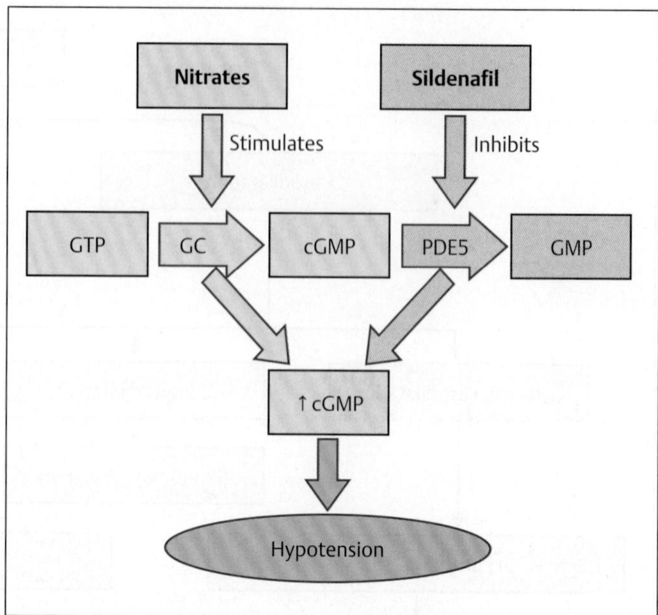

Fig. 24.6 Drug interaction between nitrates and PDE5 inhibitors such as sildenafil.

should also be managed. Cessation of cigarette smoking is also a very important part of the therapy. Modification of activities to avoid exertion or strenuous activities should be taken into account.

Other Therapeutic Effects

Heart Failure

The beneficial actions of nitrates in these cases involve preload reduction (by venous dilatation), afterload reduction (by arteriolar dilatation), and decrease in pulmonary congestion.

Myocardial Infarction

Its mechanism of action includes preload reduction (by venous dilatation), afterload reduction (by arteriolar dilatation), decreased pulmonary congestion, and anti-platelet action. Nitrates should not be used if hypotension limits the administration of β-blockers, which have more powerful salutary effects.

Smooth Muscle Spasm

For example, esophageal or biliary spasm.

Cyanide Poisoning

Amyl nitrite or sodium nitrite (10 mL of 3% solution IV [300 mg]) converts hemoglobin into methemoglobin, which not only has high affinity to cyanide radicals but also forms cyanmethemoglobin. Subsequent administration of sodium thiosulfate (50 mL of 25% solution [12.5 g]) reacts with cyanmethemoglobin to form sodium thiocyanate, which is excreted in urine (**Fig. 24.5**). Hydroxocobalamin and dicobalt edetate are alternative antidotes used in cyanide poisoning (as chelating agents).

Contraindications

These include raised intracranial pressure, systemic hypotension (systolic blood pressure [BP] < 90 mm Hg; a relative contraindication), marked bradycardia (< 50 beats per minute [BPM]) or tachycardia (> 100 BPM), severe anemia (risk of methemoglobinemia in patients with NADH deficiency), hypertrophic obstructive cardiomyopathy, recent stroke, or cardiac arrest.

Drug Interactions

Phosphodiesterase-5 (PDE5) inhibitors such as sildenafil, when used concomitantly along with nitrates, potentiate hypotensive action of nitrates, which may be fatal, leading to myocardial infarction and death.

Nitrates get reduced to nitric oxide by enzymatic denitration, which activates intracellular GC to convert GTP into cGMP. PDE5 metabolizes cGMP to GMP. PDE5 inhibitors such as sildenafil indirectly increase intracellular cGMP, which further causes vascular smooth muscle relaxation and hypotension (**Fig. 24.6**).

Precautions

These include history of allergy to nitrates and pregnancy and breastfeeding. Avoid concomitant use of PDE5 inhibitors such as sildenafil, alcohol intake, standing for long period, and vigorous exercises when on nitrate therapy.

Multiple Choice Questions

1. A 47-year-old laborer, a chain smoker, known case of diabetes mellitus and hypertension presented to the OPD with history of retrosternal chest pain radiating to left arm. The problem began a month before and occurred two to three

times a week, with pain increasing on exertion and relieving on rest and never exceeding 15 minutes. His physical findings were normal except for blood pressure (BP) 160/100 mm Hg. Blood reports were normal including liver function tests (LFTs). Most probable diagnosis is:

A. Pneumothorax.
B. Peptic ulcer.
C. Angina pectoris.
D. Esophageal rupture.

Answer: C

The clinical symptoms and signs such as episodic retrosternal chest pain radiating to left arm, increasing on exertion, and relieving by rest with normal ECG findings are typical of angina pectoris.

2. A 55-year-old woman presented to the emergency department with crushing substernal chest pain radiating to left shoulder. Diagnosis was made on clinical finding and ECG changes. Sublingual nitroglycerin was given for the treatment. The most probable mechanism that NTG would have acted would be:

A. Decrease preload.
B. Increase afterload.
C. Coronary vasoconstriction.
D. Increase myocardial wall tension.

Answer: A

The clinical scenario is typical of angina pectoris. Nitrates predominantly cause venodilation, which reduces preload and ventricular end diastolic pressure, which, in turn, decreases myocardial wall tension and myocardial oxygen demand.

3. A 45-year-old male patient is on an antianginal medication that increases cGMP levels in vascular smooth muscles. Which of the following action is responsible for the effect?

A. Increase binding of calcium to calmodulin.
B. Inactivation of aldehyde dehydrogenase.
C. Inhibition of phosphodiesterase-5.
D. Release of nitric oxide.

Answer: D

Among the antianginal drugs, nitrates act by denitration to nitric oxide, which gets converted to intermediate reactive nitrosothiol, which, in turn, activates guanylyl cyclase (GC). GC metabolizes GTP to cGMP and increases intracellular cGMP in vascular smooth muscle cells. Cyclic GMP stimulates protein kinase G and causes dephosphorylation of phosphorylated myosin light chain. This reduces actin–myosin binding and thus relaxes vascular smooth muscles, that is, vasodilatation.

4. A 50-year-old male patient was diagnosed to be suffering from acute attack of angina in an emergency department based on his clinical symptoms and ECG changes. You were advised to give nitrates by senior resident doctor. Which of the following routes of drug administration will you prefer for immediate relief of this acute attack?

A. Oral.
B. Transdermal patch.
C. Ointment.
D. Sublingual.

Answer: D

For immediate relief of acute episode of angina, sublingual route is preferred. Sublingual nitroglycerin acts within 1 to 2 minutes and peak blood levels are attained in 3 to 6 minutes. $t_{1/2}$ of sublingual nitroglycerin is 2 minutes.

5. Which of the following is the longest acting preparation of nitrates?

A. Pentaerythritol tetranitrate.
B. Isosorbide dinitrate.
C. Amyl nitrite.
D. Glyceryl trinitrate.

Answer: A

Pentaerythritol tetranitrate and erythrityl tetranitrate are longer acting preparations of nitrates. Action of pentaerythritol tetranitrate lasts for about 8 to 10 hours, whereas action of erythrityl tetranitrate lasts for 4 to 6 hours.

6. Nitroglycerin can be administered by all of the following routes except:

A. Intramuscular.
B. Intravenous.
C. Sublingual.
D. Transdermal.

Answer: A

Nitroglycerin can be administered by via sublingual, transdermal patch and ointment, oral, and intravenous routes.

7. Which of the following drugs can be used for the treatment of acute attack as well as chronic prophylaxis of angina pectoris?

A. Sublingual glyceryl trinitrate.
B. Isosorbide dinitrate.
C. Erythrityl tetranitrate.
D. Pentaerythritol tetranitrate.

Answer: B

Isosorbide dinitrate can be used for relief of symptoms of acute episode of angina by sublingual route (peak action in 5–8 min) and can also be given by oral route for prophylaxis of angina.

8. A young man presented to the emergency department with cyanotic appearance, hypotension, headache, and shortness of breath with a history of development of symptoms after intravenous injection of some drug. The drug that caused these symptoms most probably would be:

A. Sodium chloride.
B. Sodium nitrite.
C. Sodium thiosulfate.
D. Sodium thiocyanate.

Answer: B

The clinical scenario is typical of methemoglobinemia. Hemoglobin is converted to methemoglobin by sodium nitrite (10 mL of 3% solution–300 mg intravenously).

9. A 45-year-old male patient brought to casualty was diagnosed to be having cyanide toxicity. He was on nitroprusside therapy. You were advised to give intravenous sodium nitrite to combat this toxicity. The most probable mechanism by which sodium nitrite exerted beneficial effect in this case would be:

A. Facilitation of formation of cyanocobalamin.
B. Direct chelation of cyanide.
C. Conversion of hemoglobin to methemoglobin.
D. Conversion of methemoglobin to hemoglobin.

Answer: C

Refer to the explanation provided for question 8.

10. A 40-year-old male patient came to psychiatric outpatient department for some problem, and some drug was prescribed by the doctor. The patient hid history of being on nitrate therapy for angina. The patient developed severe hypotension after taking that drug. Which of the following drug would have been prescribed?

A. Fluoxetine.
B. Ranolazine.
C. Sildenafil.
D. St. John's wart.

Answer: C

Nitrates get reduced to nitric oxide, which activates intracellular guanylyl cyclase (GC). GC converts GTP to cGMP. Phosphodiesterase-5 (PDE5) metabolizes cGMP to GMP. PDE5 inhibitors such as sildenafil thus indirectly increase intracellular cGMP, which further causes vascular smooth muscle relaxation and hypotension (potentiates action of nitrates).

11. A patient of angina on nitrate treatment is advised to avoid PDE5 inhibitors concomitantly due to risk of profound hypotension. The most probable underlying cellular mechanism would be:

A. Decrease binding of calcium to calmodulin.
B. Inhibition of guanylyl cyclase.
C. Increase intracellular GMP.
D. Increase intracellular cGMP.

Answer: D

Refer to the explanation provided for question 10.

12. A patient with angina is on nitroglycerin (NTG) transdermal patch therapy for chronic prophylaxis. He keeps the patch applied for 24 hours a day, except for few minutes during baths every day. Which of the following effect is prone to occur with this practice of round-the-clock administration of this or other long-acting nitrate preparations?

A. Paradoxical vasoconstriction leading to accelerated hypertension.
B. Development of tolerance in dose- and duration–of-exposure-dependent manner.
C. Development of zero-hour effect phenomena.
D. Development of nitrate dependence.

Answer: B

In this scenario, the patient is applying transdermal patch continuously round the clock every day. Such continuous use of nitrate leads to cessation of pharmacological effects in a dose- and duration-of-exposure-dependent manner, known as nitrate tolerance.

13. A patient is on prophylactic nitrate therapy for angina since a long period. Now, the patient complains of episodic symptoms of angina even after continuing nitrate therapy. Which of the following mechanism is not attributed for the development of this effect?

A. Increased sensitization of guanylyl cyclase.
B. Cellular depletion of sulfhydryl (SH) group.
C. Formation of superoxide radicals.
D. Neurohumoral activation of vasoconstrictor signals and increased responsiveness to vasoconstriction.

Answer: A

Cessation of pharmacological effects of nitrates on continuous round-the-clock administration is known as nitrate tolerance. True tolerance develops due to failure of conversion of nitrates to nitric oxide. Probable underlying mechanisms are desensitization of guanylyl cyclase, cellular depletion of sulfhydryl (-SH) group, formation of superoxide radicals, and enhanced responsiveness to vessel wall to vasoconstriction.

14. You came across a patient in the medicine outpatient department who is on nitrate therapy for angina since a long period. Now, the patient complains of episodic symptoms of angina even after continuing nitrate therapy. You diagnosed it to be nitrate tolerance. Which of the following ways will not help you to further avoid and treat the nitrate tolerance?

A. Sudden withdrawal of nitrates.
B. Nitrate-free interval of 8 to 12 hours.
C. Use of sulfhydryl (SH) donors such as methionine.
D. Use of angiotensin-converting enzyme (ACE) inhibitors before nitrate administration.

Answer: A

Sudden withdrawal of nitrates leads to nitrate dependence and thus should be avoided.

15. A 55-year-old male patient presented to the emergency department with acute onset of suffocating chest pain radiating to left shoulder. He gave history of being on nitrate therapy for angina pectoris since several years, which he stopped abruptly recently without physician consultation. Which of the following phenomenon is responsible for his symptoms?

A. Development of tolerance in dose- and duration–of-exposure-dependent manner.
B. Development of zero-hour effect phenomenon.
C. Development of nitrate dependence.
D. Development of Monday morning syndrome.

Answer: C

In this scenario, the patient is on nitrate therapy since a long period and he abruptly stopped therapy without physician consultation. Such abrupt withdrawal of nitrates leads to nitrate dependence. Spasm of coronary and peripheral blood vessels may develop. There is risk of increasing episodes of angina due to reduced threshold after abrupt withdrawal of nitrates. Gradual withdrawal of nitrates is advisable to reduce these symptoms.

Chapter 25

Antianginals and Drug Treatment of Myocardial Infarction–2

Upinder Kaur and Sankha Shubhra Chakrabarti

PH1.28: Describe the mechanisms of action, types, doses, side effects, indications, and contraindications of the drugs used in ischemic heart disease (stable, unstable angina, and myocardial infarction), peripheral vascular disease.

Learning Objectives

- Ischemic heart disease.
- Pharmacologic treatment of stable angina.
- Pharmacologic treatment of NSTE-ACS (NSTEMI and unstable angina).
- Management of STEMI.
- Calcium channels and their blockers.

Ischemic Heart Disease (IM2.15, IM2.20, IM2.23)

Ischemic heart disease (IHD) refers to a state of imbalance between the heart's oxygen demand and supply. The most common cause of IHD is coronary artery atherosclerosis. Other less common etiologies include coronary vasospasm, coronary artery thrombus/emboli, and congenital anomalies of coronary arteries. Broadly, IHD is categorized as stable angina, acute coronary syndrome (ACS), and variant angina. ACS encompasses ST-segment elevation myocardial infarction (STEMI) and non-ST segment elevation ACS (NSTE-ACS). The latter, in turn, is categorized into unstable angina and NSTEMI (**Fig. 25.1**)

Risk Factors of IHD

1. Smoking.
2. Diabetes mellitus.
3. Hypercholesterolemia: elevated low-density lipoprotein (LDL) cholesterol levels.
4. Hypertension.
5. Obesity.
6. Family history of premature atherosclerotic disease (<55 years in male, <65 years in female).
7. Hyperhomocysteinemia.

Stable Angina

Classic attacks of stable angina manifest as chest pain, which usually occurs when oxygen demand of the heart exceeds the oxygen supply. The obstruction of coronary artery flow is fixed due to atherosclerosis, and attacks are precipitated during some exertional activity such as exercise and climbing stairs or during sexual activity. Chest pain is of squeezing or crushing type, substernal in location, and may radiate to jaw, both shoulders, and both arms. The attacks typically last for 2 to 5 minutes and are relieved by rest. Anxiety, palpitations, and sweating are some of the other associated features. Treadmill test or stress electrocardiogram (ECG)/ echocardiography (ECHO) is done in patients with stable angina to confirm the presence and severity of ischemia. In stress testing, clinical, ECG, and blood pressure (BP) findings are recorded with progressive increase in workload. Occurrence of ST-segment depression is a sign of ischemia. Additionally, stress ECHO and stress cardiac magnetic resonance imaging (MRI) are some of the imaging techniques performed in patients with stable angina, which estimate the degree of ischemia, left ventricular function, and ejection fraction.

Acute Coronary Syndrome

Chest pain of unstable angina is not relieved at rest; rather, it can start at rest. Attacks last for more than 10 minutes, may be of recent onset (< 2 weeks) with severe intensity, and display a crescendo pattern, that is, increase in frequency and severity with time. Pathologically, rupture of atherosclerotic plaque or erosion of plaque on the background of coronary vasoconstriction, followed by platelet aggregation and

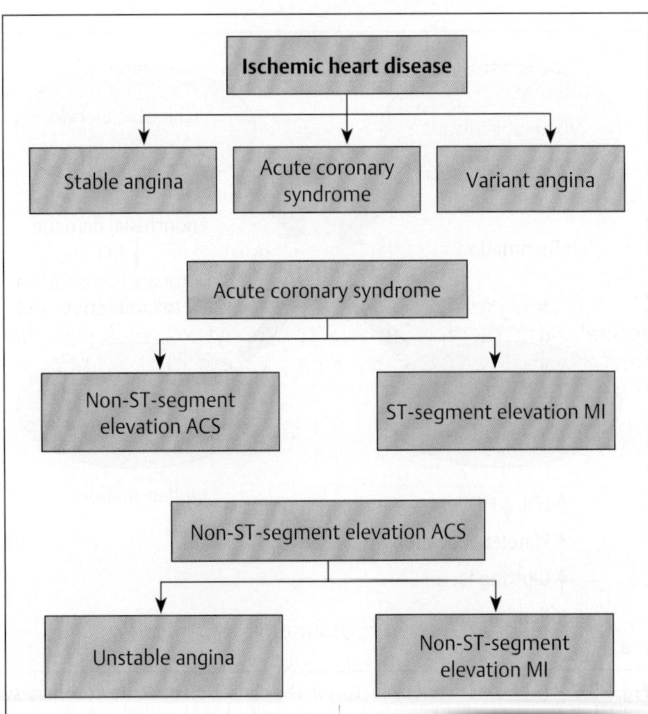

Fig. 25.1 Classification of ischemic heart disease. ACS, acute coronary syndrome; MI, myocardial infarction.

accumulation of clotting factors, leads to the formation of occlusive coronary artery thrombus. This results in abrupt cessation of coronary artery flow and precipitates the anginal attacks. When the myocardium gets damaged and there is release of biomarkers, such attacks constitute MI. While STEMI and NSTEMI can be differentiated by ECG findings, NSTEMI and unstable angina are differentiated by the levels of these cardiac markers. Thus, abrupt cessation of coronary artery flow leading to cardiomyocyte necrosis and elevated cardiac markers is MI.

Anginal Equivalents

Sudden onset of weakness, nausea, dyspnea, and epigastric distress are some of the other clinical features of IHD that can occur in the absence of chest pain. They are also known as anginal equivalents. Chest pain is often absent in patients with type 2 diabetes mellitus and elderly patients with IHD, and these patients can present with sudden-onset weakness, mental confusion, dyspnea, nausea, vomiting, and arrhythmias as the only manifestations of IHD.

Variant Angina/Prinzmetal's Angina

This is a rare form of angina seen in young adults. Anginal pain of variant angina can occur at rest as in the case of ACS. Focal vasospasm of epicardial coronary artery is the classic pathology behind variant angina. Peripheral vascular disease, smoking, and migraine are some of the risk factors linked with variant angina.

Pathophysiology of Angina

The role of various atherogenic factors is given in **Fig. 25.2a** and the disease progression of ACS is summarized in **Fig. 25.2b**.

Treatment of Ischemic Heart Disease

The treatment of IHD is broadly divided into two categories: nonpharmacological and pharmacological.

Treatment of Hypertension

The recent American College of Cardiology/American Heart Association (ACC/AHA) 2019 guidelines define normal BP as a systolic BP < 120 mm Hg and diastolic BP < 80 mm Hg. Elevated BP refers to a systolic BP of 120 to 129 mm Hg, whereas stage I hypertension is a systolic BP of 130 to 139 mm Hg or a diastolic BP of 80 to 89 mm Hg. It is believed that a systolic BP 20 mm Hg more than the normal or a diastolic BP 10 mm Hg more than the normal doubles the risk of dying because of cardiovascular diseases. Therefore, BP lowering is recommended at these cutoffs. Lifestyle modifications such as salt restriction, relaxation therapies, adequate physical activity, and fiber- and potassium-rich diet are recommended for stage I hypertension if 10-year atherosclerotic cardiovascular disease (ASCVD) risk calculated by pooled cohort equation (available online) is < 10%. When risk is ≥ 10% and in stage II hypertension, pharmacological treatment of hypertension is required.

Treatment of Dyslipidemia (PH1.31)

Increased level of LDL cholesterol is one of the major risk factors in the causation of IHD. Oxidized LDL is internalized into macrophages and responsible for foam cell formation, which results in atherosclerotic plaques. Dietary cholesterol restriction is advised in all patients with one or more risk factors of ASCVD. LDL goal of less than 70 mg/dL is desired in patients with documented ASCVD and multiple risk factors. Statins should be used for primary prevention of ASCVD if ASCVD risk is 7.5% or more. Fibrates such as fenofibrate are

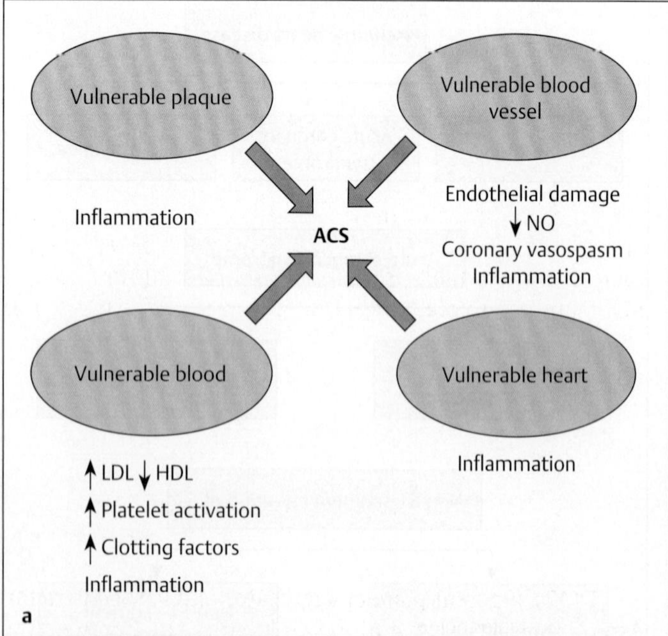

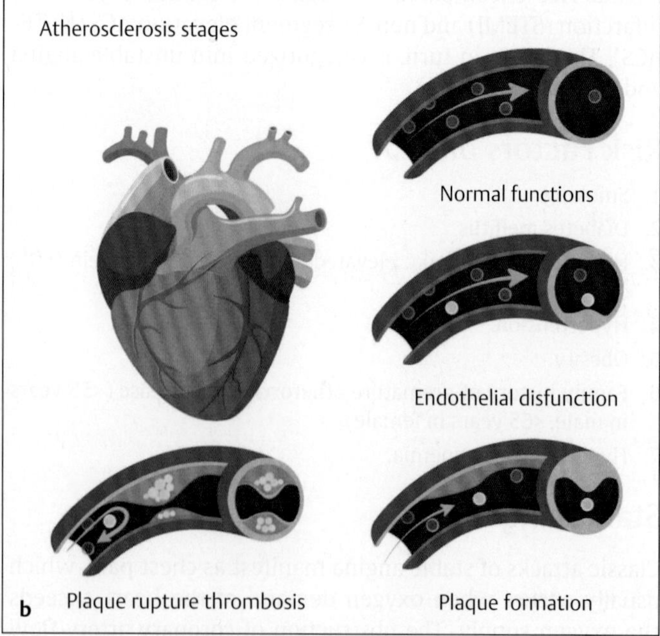

Fig. 25.2 **(a)** Role of various factors in the causation of acute coronary syndrome (ACS). Vulnerable plaque has lipid-rich core surrounded by thin fibrous cap, vulnerable blood vessel is prone to endothelial damage and vasospasm, vulnerable blood has elevated lipid levels, high platelet reactivity, and increased inflammatory markers, and vulnerable heart is prone to ischemia and inflammation. **(b)** Stages of atherosclerosis leading to coronary artery disease.

used in patients with elevated plasma triglyceride levels not responding to dietary restrictions or with significantly high triglyceride levels of 500 mg/dL or higher.

Physical Activity

Moderate level of physical activity in the form of 150 minutes of moderate walk/week or 75 minutes of brisk walk/week is useful for primary prevention of IHD. In persons with established cardiovascular diseases, such strenuous exercises should not be started suddenly. Gradual adaptation of physical activity and adoption of isotonic exercises are useful for secondary prevention of IHD. Activities that precipitate angina can be accomplished by slow adaptation and titration of exercise level.

Treatment of Diabetes Mellitus

Elevated blood sugar level directly as well as indirectly, through glycated end products and creation of oxidative stress, exacerbates the risk of coronary heart disease. Lifestyle modifications such as caloric restriction, physical activity, and use of metformin can reduce the blood sugar level as well as decrease cardiovascular risk. Among newer antidiabetics, injectable liraglutide and sodium dependent glucose co-transporter 2 (SGLT2) inhibitors have additional benefit of improving cardiovascular outcomes.

Treatment of Obesity (IM14.13)

Dietary restrictions of 500 to 1,000 calorie per day can bring about 0.45 to 1 kg weight loss/week. This should be complemented by physical activities of 200 to 250 minutes/week for the primary prevention of CVD in obese individuals. Pharmacologic treatment for weight loss should be given if the body mass index (BMI) is ≥ 30 kg/m^2 or if comorbidities are present in persons with BMI ≥ 27 kg/m^2. Orlistat, topiramate/phentermine, bupropion/naltrexone, lorcaserin, and liraglutide are examples of pharmacological agents used in the management of obesity, each carrying a unique mechanism of action.

Cessation of Smoking

Smoking is one of the major and independent risk factors in the causation of IHD. Proper counselling and motivation, use of pharmacologic agents, such as bupropion and varenicline, and substitution therapies, such as nicotine gums, nicotine transdermal patch, and nicotine lozenges, are used for nicotine deaddiction.

Other Risk Factors Correction

Other IHD precipitating risk factors are thyrotoxicosis, anemia, vitamin B_1 deficiency, and tachycardia, which should be corrected.

Pharmacologic Treatment of Stable Angina

For Symptom Relief in Acute Episode

Short-acting nitrates such as glyceryl trinitrate (GTN) and isosorbide dinitrate (IDN) are given sublingually for the relief of chest pain. Nitrates, by increasing cGMP in vascular smooth muscle, act as preferential venous dilators; they reduce preload and hence cardiac work. In addition, they favorably distribute blood to ischemic areas. Symptom relief occurs within 5 minutes.

For Prophylaxis against Symptoms

Long-acting nitrates, sustained release (SR) preparations of GTN, IDN, isosorbide mononitrate, and pentaerythritol tetranitrate are given to prevent the occurrence of anginal attacks. Dosing is given in a way that ensures a nitrate-free period of at least 8 hours. Nitrate-free period prevents the development of tolerance to nitrates.

β Blockers

Cardioselective β1 blockers such as metoprolol and bisoprolol reduce the heart rate (HR) and cardiac load and prevent exercise- or stress-induced cardiac ischemia. Blood flow to subendocardial region increases because of favorable redistribution.

Calcium Channel Blockers

Verapamil and diltiazem reduce the HR and cardiac load. They are used if patients are intolerant to β blockers or in patients in whom β blockers cannot be used such as patients with asthma, peripheral vascular disease, and insulin-dependent type 1 diabetes. Nifedipine immediate release (IR) tablets should be avoided because of the risk of reflex sympathetic tachycardia. The risk is less with SR tablets of nifedipine and long-acting dihydropyridines (DHPs) such as amlodipine and felodipine.

Angiotensin-Converting Enzyme Inhibitors and Angiotensin Receptor Blockers

Enalapril, lisinopril, and ramipril are some examples of angiotensin-converting enzyme inhibitors (ACEIs). These drugs do not relieve the anginal pain but reduce recurrent ischemia. They are used in patients with stable angina and associated chronic kidney disease (CKD), diabetes, hypertension, or left ventricular dysfunction (LVD). ACEIs reduce the ventricular remodeling and hence prevent the progression of LVD. Angiotensin receptor blockers (ARBs) such as olmesartan, losartan, and telmisartan are used if ACEIs are not tolerated because of adverse effects such as cough or angioedema.

Antiplatelets

Aspirin

Aspirin at low doses (75–300 mg) acts by irreversibly and nonselectively blocking the enzyme cyclooxygenase (COX) in platelets. This reduces the generation of thromboxane A2 (TXA2), a potent platelet aggregator and vasoconstrictor. Aspirin thus acts as an anti-ischemic agent and improves the coronary artery blood flow.

Clopidogrel

This antiplatelet drug is a prodrug and requires CYP2C19 for activation. The drug blocks adenosine diphosphate (ADP) receptors (P2Y1 and P2YAC, also known as P2Y12) located on the cell surface of platelets. Blockade of P2Y1, a GPCR (G_q type), and P2YAC, respectively, results in decrease in intracellular calcium and increase in cAMP in platelets. Both phenomena inhibit platelet aggregation.

Statins (PH1.31)

These hypolipidemic drugs act by reversibly inhibiting the HMG-CoA reductase enzyme, the rate-limiting enzyme of cholesterol synthesis. The resulting decrease in cholesterol levels causes increased expression of LDL receptor on cell surfaces, thus facilitating cholesterol uptake into hepatic and peripheral tissue cells. This reduces the serum levels of LDL cholesterol and reduces atherosclerotic plaque formation. In addition, statins have pleiotropic actions independent of reduction in cholesterol levels. These include endothelial protective action, anti-inflammatory action, antioxidant action, reduction in fibrinogen levels, and prevention of rupture of atherosclerotic plaques. Atorvastatin, rosuvastatin, and simvastatin are few examples of members of this class. Hepatitis and myalgias are the common adverse effects of statins.

Other Drugs

Ranolazine

This drug inhibits late Na channels involved in indirect calcium influx in cardiomyocytes. The resulting decrease in calcium decreases the cardiac workload. Ranolazine also inhibits rapidly activating potassium channels (IK_r channels). Nausea, constipation, and prolonged QT are the common adverse effects. The drug is given at the dose of 500 to 1,000 mg twice a day orally.

Ivabradine

This is a newer antianginal drug that mainly inhibits the funny channels (hyperpolarization activated cyclic nucleotide gated [HCN] channels) located in the sinoatrial (SA)/atrioventricular (AV) node and reduces the Na influx in conducting cells. It is given in anginal patients with persistent tachycardia not responsive to β blockers. Blurring of vision, visual disturbances, and seeing bright-colored lights, also known as phosphenes, are the common adverse effects of ivabradine. Blockade of HCN channels in retina is thought to be responsible for these adverse effects. The drug can also precipitate atrial fibrillation in susceptible individuals and therefore should be given cautiously in at-risk individuals. Ivabradine is given at the dose of 5 to 10 mg once or twice a day.

Trimetazidine

The drug has several uncertain mechanisms. Inhibition of ketoacyl thiolase, an enzyme involved in fatty acid oxidation, shifts the cardiac metabolism toward glucose, which is less energy consuming. Also, the accumulation of Na, Ca, and free radicals is reduced. Gastrointestinal disturbances, liver toxicity, agranulocytosis, and thrombocytopenia are the adverse effects of trimetazidine. Additionally, the drug has been found to cause or aggravate Parkinsonian features.

Nicorandil

This drug is an opener of adenosine triphosphate (ATP)-sensitive K^+ channels located on vascular smooth muscle cell. The resulting hyperpolarization causes vascular smooth muscle relaxation, thus reducing afterload as well as preload. Oral ulcers, headache, and hypotension are the common adverse effects of nicorandil. The drug is given at the dose of 10 to 20 mg twice daily.

Pharmacologic Treatment of NSTE-ACS (NSTEMI and Unstable Angina)

Nitrates

As described, nitrates such as GTN and IDN are given for the symptomatic treatment of chest pain. A total of three doses are given sublingually at 5-minute intervals. Intravenous (IV) GTN is started if there is no response.

Morphine

If there is no response to nitrates, IV morphine at the dose of 2 to 5 mg can be given at 5-minute intervals, with simultaneous monitoring of the HR and BP. Apart from reducing chest pain, morphine has negative chronotropic action and blunts the effects of sympathetic overactivity on heart. It also reduces anxiety and apprehension and calms the patient.

Oxygen

This is given in cases of hypoxia and low saturation levels of O_2 in the blood. Also, bicarbonate supplementation is given to correct the acidosis if present.

β Blockers

IV use of β blockers followed by shift to oral route, depending on the clinical improvement, is a crucial step in reducing reinfarction, reischemia, and arrythmias. Metoprolol, carvedilol, and propranolol are some examples of β blockers that can be used in NSTEMI. Cardioselective (β-1) blockers are preferred over nonselective β blockers, as the latter produce multiple unwanted adverse effects.

Calcium Channel Blockers

Verapamil and diltiazem should be used in patients with NSTEMI if β blockers cannot be used or are not tolerated because of adverse effects. Calcium channel blockers (CCBs) should only be used if there is no ventricular dysfunction or heart failure. Nifedipine should be avoided in patients with NSTEMI, as it has been found to increase mortality.

Antiplatelets

Dual antiplatelet (aspirin and clopidogrel) are given to patients with NSTE-ACS requiring medical or interventional therapy. The therapy is continued for at least 1 year with monitoring of the risk of bleeding. Aspirin and clopidogrel are given as loading dose (300 mg each), followed by a maintenance dose of 75 to 150 mg/day. Another irreversible ADP receptor antagonist, prasugrel, is superior to clopidogrel in patients requiring percutaneous coronary intervention (PCI) and can be given as a substitute to clopidogrel, along with aspirin 75 to 100 mg. The risk of bleeding with prasugrel is more than clopidogrel. Prasugrel is avoided in patients with a history of stroke and should be used carefully in patients with weight less than 60 kg, elderly ≥ 75 years of age, and those with renal failure. Ticagrelor, a reversible ADP receptor antagonist, is also superior to clopidogrel in reducing cardiovascular death and MI. The drug can be given in patients requiring PCI as well as those requiring medical therapy. Dyspnea, hypotension, ventricular pauses, and increase in serum uric acid are the major adverse effects of ticagrelor. Increase in adenosine levels as a result of inhibition of adenosine reuptake by ticagrelor is thought to be the mechanism behind these adverse effects. Cangrelor is another reversible ADP receptor blocker. It is given intravenously to select patients requiring PCI. The risk of bleeding with cangrelor is more than clopidogrel and should be watched over. Triple antiplatelet therapy with addition of a third antiplatelet agent such as Gp IIb–IIIa inhibitors (abciximab, eptifibatide, tirofiban) can be advised in selected patients if there are signs and symptoms of ischemia relapse or there is no remission despite dual antiplatelet therapy. PCI is usually required in such patients.

ACE Inhibitors/ARBs

These drugs should also be started as soon as possible after an NSTE-ACS because they have also been shown to produce short-term benefits apart from the disease-modifying benefits that come with their long-term use. Rates of reischemia are reduced with these drugs. These drugs are generally preferred if patient has concomitant hypertension, diabetes, CKD, congestive heart failure, or left ventricular disease.

Aldosterone Antagonists

Spironolactone and eplerenone are known aldosterone antagonists. They reduce aldosterone-induced salt and water retention, and by modifying the role of angiotensin, reduce ventricular remodeling. In addition, the effect of sympathetic activity on the heart and blood vessels is also reduced. They should ideally be used in patients with NSTEMI and heart failure or uncontrolled hypertension. Their use should be avoided if creatinine clearance is less than 50 mL/min. Serum potassium needs to be monitored frequently with the use of aldosterone antagonists.

Statins (PH1.31)

High-dose statins are given to patients with NSTE-ACS. As discussed earlier, the beneficial effects of statins come because of LDL-lowering and pleiotropic effects. Liver function and creatine phosphokinase (CPK) monitoring may be required at times. Other drugs such as the NPC1L1 inhibitor ezetimibe and PCSK9 inhibitors (such as alirocumab and evolocumab) are used if LDL cholesterol lowering is not achieved with the optimal dose of statins.

Anticoagulants

Heparin, low-molecular-weight heparin (LMWH), fondaparinux, and bivalirudin are the parenteral anticoagulants used in patients with NSTE-ACS. Heparin is given as IV bolus followed by infusion. LMWH and fondaparinux are given by the subcutaneous route. Bivalirudin is given by the IV route. Fondaparinux is generally given to patients with NSTE-ACS not requiring coronary intervention as the risk of factor XII–mediated thrombosis of the catheter increases with fondaparinux.

Other Drugs

Drugs such as diuretics (furosemide) are given if MI is accompanied by heart failure. Likewise, dopamine/dobutamine/noradrenaline infusion is given in MI patients with shock.

Supportive Therapies

These include benzodiazepines such as clonazepam and diazepam to sedate the patient, and laxatives such as lactulose or stool softeners, which can be given to prevent or treat constipation. Drugs with anticholinergic properties and H2 blockers that can cause or aggravate delirium in elderly patients should be avoided.

Coronary Reperfusion Therapy

If symptoms of NSTE-ACS do not resolve despite the optimal dose of the above-mentioned drugs or if symptoms recur, stress testing shows evidence of ischemia, or patient has diabetes and significant LVD, then PCI followed by stenting is done. Dual antiplatelets are given for at least 1 year following PCI.

Management of STEMI

The main aim of treatment of a patient diagnosed with STEMI is to restore the coronary blood flow and prevent the progression of infarction. Although perfusion is restored spontaneously in some patients, use of pharmacological or interventional approaches expedites the opening of the blocked coronary artery. Rapid recognition of symptoms and rapid start of reperfusion therapy is the backbone of the STEMI management armamentarium. MI is complicated by the development of ventricular fibrillation (VF) and congestive heart failure. Since VF is the major cause of early mortality in patients with STEMI, rapid defibrillation to maintain the heart rhythm may be crucial step to prevent death. The coronary reperfusion therapies can be medical or interventional and are described in the following.

Medical Reperfusion

Fibrinolytics are the cornerstone of medical reperfusion therapy. These include plasminogen activators and recombinant tissue plasminogen activators (tPAs). These drugs should not be used in the presence of any active pathological bleed, history of hypersensitivity reactions to these agents, and hypertensive urgency or shock. Presence or history of any intracranial bleed, any intracranial neoplasm, and cerebrovascular lesion are some of the absolute contraindications for the use of fibrinolytic therapy.

For reasons unknown, fibrinolytics are not used in patients with NSTEMI or unstable angina. Their use is rather associated with increase in mortality. This is the major difference in the management of STEMI and NSTE-ACS.

Streptokinase

Streptokinase is obtained from β-hemolytic Streptococci and *Escherichia coli*. It activates plasminogen and converts fibrin to degradation products. It can also activate kinins, which are responsible for transient lowering of BP. Other adverse effects include allergic reactions. The drug is given at the dose of 1.5 million units as IV infusion over 1 hour.

Anistreplase

It is the acylated derivative of streptokinase–plasminogen complex.

Alteplase

It is a recombinant tPA. It is better than streptokinase in restoring tissue perfusion and reducing cardiovascular mortality. It is given as a 15-mg IV bolus followed by a dose of 50-mg IV given over 30 minutes and another dose of 35 mg given over the next 1 hour.

Reteplase

It is a derivative of recombinant tPA. It is administered as two boluses, separated by an interval of 30 minutes. Dose of each bolus is 10 million units over 2 to 3 minutes.

Tenecteplase

It is derived from recombinant tPA by the change of glycosylation site and addition of tetraglycine linker in its structure. These changes make the drug longer-acting. Tenecteplase is administered as a single IV bolus at the dose of 0.53 mg/kg over 10 seconds.

Other Drugs

Morphine

As described for NSTE-ACS, morphine is used intravenously for chest pain. It also lessens the effect of sympathetic activity on the heart and produces a negative chronotropic effect.

Oxygen

This is administered if saturation levels of oxygen are low in the blood.

Nitrates

GTN or IDN is given sublingually for up to three doses to relieve anginal pain in STEMI. They reduce the preload and preferentially redistribute the blood to ischemic areas. If no relief occurs despite three doses, IV infusion of GTN is initiated.

Anticoagulants

To prevent the progression of thrombus, the following anticoagulants are used:

1. **Heparin**: This is administered at the dose of 70 U/kg IV followed by 12 to 15 U/kg/hour to maintain a target activated partial thromboplastin time (aPTT) of two to three times the control value.
2. **LMWH**: Enoxaparin and dalteparin are some of the examples of LMWH. They are given subcutaneously twice daily. Dose of enoxaparin is 1 mg/kg or 100 IU/kg twice daily and that of dalteparin is 120 IU/kg twice daily.
3. **Fondaparinux**: This parenteral factor X inhibitor can be given in those patients with STEMI not requiring PCI at a dose of 2.5 mg once a day subcutaneously.
4. **Bivalirudin**: It is a direct thrombin inhibitor given intravenously in patients with STEMI.

Antiplatelets

As described for NSTEMI management, aspirin loading dose of 300 mg followed by maintenance dose of 75 to 150 mg/day is given to patients with STEMI. By inhibiting COX enzyme, aspirin reduces TXA2 formation, thus interfering with platelet aggregation. Another antiplatelet and ADP receptor inhibitor, clopidogrel, is also given with aspirin. Dual antiplatelet therapy is continued for at least 1 year post MI. Prasugrel is a newer antiplatelet and an irreversible ADP receptor blocker with a faster onset of action compared to clopidogrel. It can be given as a substitute to clopidogrel in patients with STEMI requiring PCI. It is administered at the loading dose of 60 mg followed by 10 mg. As mentioned earlier, prasugrel, compared to clopidogrel, is better in reducing cardiovascular death but carries a high risk of bleeding and is costlier. Ticagrelor is a reversible ADP receptor blocker and may increase the levels of adenosine in circulation. Given orally, initially at the loading dose of 180 mg followed by 90 mg twice daily, it is also superior to clopidogrel in reducing cardiovascular death. Dyspnea, bleeding, hypotension, increase in serum uric acid levels, and transient ventricular pauses may be seen with ticagrelor in the initial few days of treatment. Ticagrelor can be given to STEMI patients requiring PCI or medical intervention. Cangrelor is another reversible ADP receptor blocker. It is given intravenously in patients requiring PCI.

β Blockers

Metoprolol, propranolol, and carvedilol may be given initially by IV route followed by oral route, depending on the clinical condition of the patient. They should be avoided if the HR is less than 60/min, if the systolic BP is less than 90 mm Hg, if the patient has a second degree or higher AV conduction block, a history of asthma, or in the presence of acute decompensated heart failure. β blockers reduce the

HR and hence the cardiac load, increase the distribution of blood to subendocardial region, lessen the development of ventricular arrythmias, and reduce the chances of reischemia and reinfarction.

ACEIs/ARBs

These drugs are used particularly if there is underlying hypertension, LVD, CKD, or diabetes. They have acute short-term as well as long-term benefits in patients with STEMI. Glomerular filtration rate should be monitored with these agents.

Statins (PH1.31)

Atorvastatin, rosuvastatin, and simvastatin are examples of LDL cholesterol–lowering drugs, which are given to patients with STEMI. High-dose atorvastatin at 40 to 80 mg once a day for initial period of 1 to 2 weeks followed by a standard dose of 10 mg once a day is used. Liver function monitoring and serum CPK estimation is done if the patient shows signs or symptoms of hepatitis and myalgias, respectively, with the use of these drugs. Other LDL cholesterol–lowering drugs are ezetimibe and PCSK9 inhibitors, which will be discussed in Chapter 50 Drugs Used in Dyslipidemias.

Supportive Therapies

Antianxiety/sedative drugs and stool softeners should be administered to sedate the patient and relieve constipation, respectively.

Interventional Reperfusion Therapies

PCI followed by stenting is done for one- or two-vessel disease, and coronary artery bypass grafting (CABG) is done for three-vessel disease or if the left main coronary artery is involved or in patients with diabetes. PCI is better than medical reperfusion therapy using fibrinolytics in opening blocked coronary arteries, particularly when the clot is mature, that is, after 2 to 3 hours of formation. PCI can also be done under situations when fibrinolytics cannot be used or if symptoms or signs of STEMI do not resolve despite the use of fibrinolytics. **Table 25.1** summarizes the various treatments of stable angina, NSTE-ACS, and STEMI, with key differences.

Treatment of Variant Angina

Since the main pathology responsible for variant angina is coronary artery vasospasm, therapies targeted at relieving the spasm and producing vasodilation are useful. CCBs such as nifedipine, verapamil, and diltiazem form the cornerstone of therapy of variant angina. β blockers should better be avoided as they can aggravate coronary spasm.

Statins should be used, as atherosclerotic plaque is found near the site of vasospasm in many cases.

Nitrates are useful for the treatment of anginal pain. Aspirin should be avoided as the use of aspirin shifts the arachidonic acid pathway towards leukotrienes. Patients with variant angina have abnormal reactivity of blood vessels toward leukotrienes, serotonin, and epinephrine.

Coronary revascularization can be done in selected patients with focal obstruction of coronary artery. Cessation of smoking should be done alongside.

Calcium Channels and Their Blockers

Types of Calcium Channels

1. Voltage-gated calcium channels (VGCCs).
2. Store-operated calcium channels.
3. Ligand-gated calcium channels.
4. Receptor-operated calcium channels.
5. Transient receptor potential vanilloid channels.
6. Leak-sensitive and stretch-sensitive calcium channels.

Table 25.1 Various available treatment options for stable angina and ACS patients, along with the key differences

Drugs	Stable angina	NSTEMI/unstable angina	STEMI
Morphine	×	✓	✓
Nitrates	✓	✓	✓
Anticoagulants	×	✓	✓
Antiplatelets	✓	✓	✓
Fibrinolytics	×	×	✓
ACEIs	✓	✓	✓
ARBs	✓	✓	✓
β blockers	✓	✓	✓
Verapamil, diltiazem	✓	✓	✓
Nifedipine IR	✓ (with β blockers)	×	×
Ivabradine, trimetazidine, ranolazine, nicorandil	✓	✓	✓
Statins	✓	✓	✓

Abbreviations: ACEI, angiotensin-converting enzyme inhibitor; ACS, acute coronary syndrome; ARB, angiotensin receptor blocker; IR, immediate release.

Table 25.2 shows the classification of VGCCs. These channels are composed of five subunits: α_1, α_2, β, γ, and δ. α_1 lines the ion channel pore. $\alpha_2\delta$ is a dyad. Drugs that block each type of VGCCs are also mentioned in **Table 25.2**. Another way of classifying VGCCs depending on the duration of depolarization is as follows: **Cav1**: L-type (long-lasting type); **Cav2**: N, P/Q, R; **Cav3**: T-type (transient type). L-type CCBs are, in turn, divided into three classes, as shown in **Fig. 25.3**. Specific cardiovascular properties of L-type CCBs are given in **Table 25.3**.

Classification of Calcium Channel Blockers

Fig. 25.3 shows three major classes of L-type CCBs and the individual members of each class. DHPs are further categorized into four generations.

1. **First generation:** nifedipine, nicardipine–maximum risk of reflex sympathetic activity, edema, and hypotension.
2. **Second generation:** nifedipine SR, benidipine, efonidipine, nilvadipine, felodipine, nimodipine.
3. **Third generation:** amlodipine, barnidipine, azelnidipine, nitrendipine–less risk of reflex sympathetic activity.
4. **Fourth generation:** cilnidipine, lacidipine, lercanidipine–least risk of reflex sympathetic activity, edema, and hypotension.

Pharmacodynamics

Verapamil and diltiazem preferentially block L-type Ca channels located in the heart on cardiomyocytes and conducting tissues. Decrease in intracellular calcium, in turn, decreases calcium-induced calcium release from sarcoplasmic reticulum of cardiomyocytes. The decrease in cellular calcium in cardiomyocytes and SA/AV node results in a negative inotropic and a negative chronotropic effect, respectively. The decrease in the HR produced by these two drugs reduces the cardiac load, justifying their role in stable and unstable angina. Since the drugs have negative inotropic effect also, they should be avoided in patients with established or impending heart failure and significant LVD.

The members of DHP class, on the other hand, preferentially block the calcium channels located on vascular smooth muscle, leading to vasodilation. The resulting fall in peripheral vascular resistance reduces the afterload, thereby reducing the cardiac stress. Because of the same reason, they are also preferred in anginal patients with underlying hypertension. Nifedipine, amlodipine, and nicardipine are few examples of this class of CCBs. Their use in various types of angina is described in the following section.

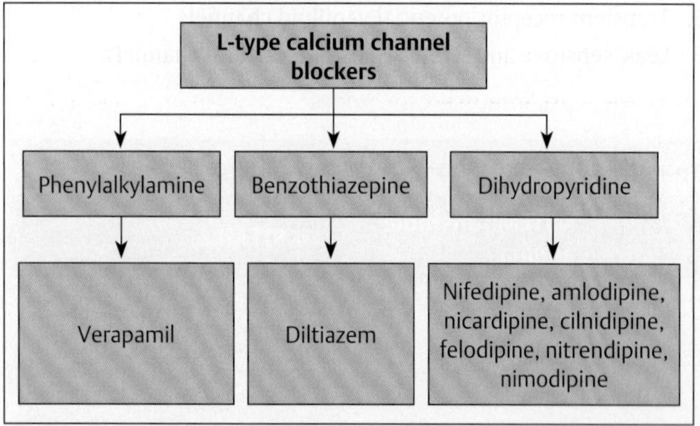

Fig. 25.3 L-type calcium channel blockers.

Pharmacokinetics

Pharmacokinetic properties of CCBs are mentioned in **Table 25.4**. Due to variable first-pass metabolism, bioavailability of CCBs varies from 15 to 90%, with nitrendipine and felodipine having the lowest and amlodipine having the highest bioavailability. Elimination $t_{1/2}$ is short for nifedipine (2–4 hours), while it is highest for amlodipine (40–50 hours). Thus, amlodipine has the longest duration of action as well as highest bioavailability (> 90%) among all the CCBs. Felodipine and nitrendipine have maximum plasma protein binding (99%). Nicardipine shows nonlinear pharmacokinetics.

Individual Drugs

Nifedipine

The drug is used in stable angina, variant angina, and hypertension. β blockers should be given with nifedipine to counter the reflex sympathetic tachycardia. Because of the risk of reflex tachycardia, the use of nifedipine should be avoided in patients with ACS. Nifedipine is available as IR tablets, SR tablets, and as fixed-dose combination (FDC) with atenolol. The risk of reflex tachycardia is less with SR forms compared to the IR forms.

Amlodipine

This drug has the advantage of a long $t_{1/2}$, which makes once-daily dosing possible. Also, the risk of reflex tachycardia and symptoms such as flushing and headache are less with this drug as compared to nifedipine. Amlodipine is commonly used for treatment of hypertension. Its main adverse effect is pedal edema, which is reversible and improves with the cessation of the drug use. Edema can be prevented to a considerable extent by asking the patients to avoid

Table 25.2 Types of VGCCs, their location, and specific blockers

VGCCs	Location	Drugs that block VGCCs
L-type	Cardiomyocyte (role in plateau phase of action potential), SA, AV node (for pacemaker activity, phase 0)	Verapamil, diltiazem, amlodipine
T-type	SA, AV node (role in prepotential), thalamic-cortical neurons	Ethosuximide, trimethadione, valproate
N-type	Neurons (role in neurotransmitter release)	Gabapentin, lamotrigine, pregabalin, conotoxin

Abbreviations: AV, atrioventricular; SA, sinoatrial; VGCCs, voltage-gated calcium channels.

Table 25.3 Cardiovascular properties of prototype drug of each class of L-type CCBs

	Verapamil	Diltiazem	Nifedipine
Effect on BP	–	–	↓
Effect on HR	↓	↓	↑
Reflex sympathetic activity	–	–	↑
Effect on blood vessels	–	–	Smooth muscle relaxation
Ca channel blockade	+	+	++
Frequency or use dependence	++	–	–
Effect on SA/AV node conduction	↓	↓	↑
Effect on cardiac contractility	↓ ↓	↓	Reflex ↑
Use in stable angina	✓	✓	✓ with β blockers
Use in unstable angina	✓	✓	Avoid
Use in variant angina	–	–	✓

Abbreviations: AV, atrioventricular; BP, blood pressure; CCB, calcium channel blocker; HR, heart rate; SA, sinoatrial.

Table 25.4 Pharmacokinetics of calcium channel blockers

Drug	Bioavailability	Half-life ($t_{1/2}$)	Dosing	Plasma protein binding	Route of metabolism	Active metabolite
Verapamil	20–30%	3–5 h	Thrice daily	90%	Hepatic	Yes
Diltiazem	40%	4–5 h	Twice or thrice daily	70–80%	Hepatic	Yes
Amlodipine	60–90%	40–50 h	Once daily	93%	Hepatic	No
Felodipine	20%	10–15 h	Once daily	99%	Hepatic	No
Nicardipine	35%, nonlinear pharmacokinetics	8–9 h	Thrice daily	96%	Hepatic	No
Nifedipine	40–50%	2–4 h	Thrice daily	95%	Hepatic	No
Nitrendipine	15–25%	8 h	Thrice daily	>99%	Hepatic	No

keeping the limbs in dependent position. Amlodipine is also renoprotective and reduces the occurrence of proteinuria in patients with diabetes and CKD. It is given at the dose of 5 to 10 mg once a day.

Nimodipine

This DHP is preferred in patients with subarachnoid hemorrhage (SAH), as it prevents the secondary vasospasm of cerebral arteries, thereby reducing the neurologic deficit seen in patients with SAH. The drug is given at the dose of 60 mg every 4 hours for a period of 21 days, to be started preferably within 96 hours of SAH.

Nitrendipine

This CCB increases the release of NO from endothelial cells, thus causing additional vascular smooth muscle relaxation.

Benidipine

This is a long-acting DHP and also a blocker of T-type Ca channels. It is approved for patients with angina and hypertension.

Cilnidipine

This DHP is mainly used for hypertension. It is a blocker of L-type, T-type, and N-type calcium channels. Like amlodipine, the drug is renoprotective. Chances of pedal edema are less compared to amlodipine. It is given at the dose of 5 to 10 mg once or twice a day.

Drug Interactions

Verapamil, diltiazem, and nifedipine are metabolized by CYP3A4. Enzyme inhibitors such as erythromycin, isoniazid, grapefruit juice, cimetidine, fluconazole, itraconazole, and voriconazole can increase their concentration. Likewise, enzyme inducers such as rifampicin, phenobarbitone, carbamazepine, and St John's-wort can decrease their concentration. Verapamil is a potent inhibitor of CYP3A4 and P-glycoprotein. It can therefore increase the concentration of concomitant drugs such as digoxin and cyclosporine, and statins such as atorvastatin.

Verapamil/diltiazem should be avoided with β blockers as the risk of AV block increases. Verapamil/diltiazem should also be avoided with simultaneous use of ivabradine. Dose of verapamil should be reduced by 30 to 50% in severe liver disease. Caution should be advised in moderate liver disease. Dose reduction should also be carried out in end-stage renal disease. The starting dose should be low in elderly patients because of age-related changes in liver function.

Uses

1. IHD: stable angina, unstable angina, and variant angina:
   a. Stable angina: Among CCBs, verapamil, diltiazem, and, if required, members of DHP class such as nifedipine are used in patients with stable angina because of their cardiac load-reducing potential. To block the reflex tachycardia seen with members of DHP class, these drugs are often combined with β blockers such as atenolol. One such FDC commonly available is that of nifedipine and atenolol.
   b. Vasospastic angina: Because of the potential to relax the coronary blood vessels, members of DHP class form the first line of therapy for patients with vasospastic angina.
   c. Unstable angina: Verapamil and diltiazem can be used in patients with unstable angina. It is better to avoid the use of short-acting members of DHP class, as the reflex tachycardia associated with them is thought to increase mortality.
2. Hypertension: Members of DHP class such as amlodipine, cilnidipine, and nifedipine are used for lowering BP in hypertensive individuals. They are also preferred in patients with both angina and hypertension.
3. Arrhythmias: Because of suppressant effect on SA and AV node, verapamil and diltiazem are used for the treatment of supraventricular and atrial arrhythmias.
4. Peripheral vascular disease (Raynaud's disease).
5. Prophylaxis of migraine: The vasodilator action of CCBs such as verapamil and diltiazem is useful in the prevention of cerebral hypoxia. The drugs are therefore used for reducing the frequency and severity of migraine attacks, generally in patients intolerant to β blockers.
6. To reduce proteinuria in CKD patients.
7. Ergot-induced vasospasm: Although rarely observed nowadays, ergot compounds such as ergotamine and ergotoxine in toxic doses are known to produce vasospasm in the lower limbs. The vasodilator action of CCBs is useful in restoring the limb perfusion in such settings.
8. Hypertrophic cardiomyopathy.
9. Select patients with pulmonary arterial hypertension.

Adverse Effects

Aggravation of urinary retention, **B**radycardia, **C**onstipation, **D**ry mouth, **E**dema, **F**lushing, **G**ERD (gastroesophageal reflux disease), aggravation of **H**yperglycemia (remember by ABCDEFGH).

Edema is common with DHP class because of its dilatory action on precapillary sphincters, smaller arterioles, and capillaries. Aggravation of hyperglycemia, tachycardia, sweating, anxiety, and tremors are seen commonly with DHP class because of their tendency to increase reflex sympathetic activity.

Contraindications and Precautions

1. Because of negative ionotropic action, verapamil and diltiazem should not be used in patients with poor left ventricular function or congestive heart failure.
2. The drugs should also be avoided if the HR is less than 60/min.
3. Nifedipine is also to be avoided in patients with heart failure as reflex sympathetic activity can be detrimental for the heart.
4. The reflex increase in norepinephrine associated with nifedipine use can disturb the glycemic control in diabetic patients.
5. All CCBs can aggravate urinary retention and gastro-esophageal reflux. The drugs therefore should be used cautiously in patients with benign prostatic hyperplasia and GERD.

Rationale for Using Antianginal Drugs Together

β Blockers + Nitrates

β blockers reduce the reflex tachycardia associated with nitrates, while nitrates reduce the unopposed α receptor-mediated increased ventricular filling caused by β blockers.

CCB + Nitrates

CCBs decrease the afterload, while nitrates reduce the preload.

Dihydropyridine (Nifedipine) + β Blocker (Atenolol)

Atenolol blocks the reflex tachycardia caused by nifedipine.

β Blockers + CCB + Nitrates

β blockers reduce the reflex tachycardia, CCBs decrease the afterload, and nitrates reduce the preload.

Multiple Choice Questions

1. A 54-year-old man presented to the medicine OPD with a chief complaint of on and off exertional chest pain for the last 1 year. There is no history of diabetes or hypertension, but the patient smokes twice a week. ECG shows some evidence of cardiac ischemia. What treatment will you prescribe for his chest pain?

A. Oral morphine.
B. Oral pantoprazole.
C. Sublingual IDN and maintenance oral nitrates.
D. Oral nicorandil.

Answer: C

This seems to be a case of coronary artery disease (stable angina). Sublingual use of nitrates is the treatment of choice for cardiac cause of chest pain. Oral sustained release tablets of nitrates are used for prophylaxis of angina.

2. A 68-year-old man with stable angina was referred to the geriatric OPD for uncontrolled tremors and difficulty in

walking for the last 1.5 months. On examination, bilateral tremors were present, and a slowness of gait was observed by the treating geriatrician. Pharmacologist opinion was sought by the geriatrician to review the drug history of the patient for the last 3 months after which one antianginal drug was removed from the treatment. The patient returned after 3 weeks with normal gait and complete disappearance of tremors and without any aggravation of chest pain. Which drug do you think the geriatrician must have removed?

A. Nicorandil.
B. GTN.
C. Ivabradine.
D. Trimetazidine.

Answer: D

This is a classic case of drug-induced Parkinsonism. Among antianginal drugs, trimetazidine has been linked with the worsening of or onset of Parkinsonian features. The geriatrician therefore stopped the use of trimetazidine. Mere discontinuation of the culprit drug can correct the symptoms of drug induced Parkinsonism as was seen in this case. The patient should, however, be watched for the risk of occurrence of Parkinsonism in future.

3. A 69-year-old hypertensive man presented to the emergency OPD with severe chest pain radiating to the jaw and left shoulder for the last 40 minutes. The patient had taken four doses of sublingual IDN before visiting the emergency but without any improvement. Investigations revealed elevated cardiac troponins (20 times the normal upper limit) and elevated brain-type natriuretic peptide (BNP) levels. ECG was normal. What is the treatment of choice for this patient?

A. Patient should be sent to general physician for immediate start of anticoagulants.
B. Patient should be sent to a cardiologist and fibrinolytic therapy should be started.
C. Patient should be managed in emergency only with the intravenous infusion of β blockers.
D. Patient should be sent to cardiologist and PCI would be the best therapy.

Answer: D

This seems to be a case of NSTEMI with a possibility of heart failure. PCI is the treatment of choice in this case.

4. A 56-year-old man visited the cardiology OPD for exertional chest pain which is uncontrolled on nitrates. The doctor prescribed him nicorandil tablet to be taken twice daily. What is the proposed mechanism of action of this drug in angina?

A. Ca channel blocker.
B. ATP-sensitive K channel opener.
C. ATP-sensitive K channel closer.
D. Na channel blocker.

Answer: B

Nicorandil is an ATP-sensitive potassium channel opener and dilates the epicardial coronary arteries, thus improving the blood flow.

5. Which of the following antianginal drug is a potent CYP and P glycoprotein inhibitor carrying the risk of drug interactions?

A. Isosorbide dinitrate.
B. Nicorandil.
C. Metoprolol.
D. Verapamil.

Answer: D

Verapamil is a potent inhibitor of CYP3A4 and the efflux protein, P-glycoprotein. Thus, the dose of concomitant drugs such as statins, digoxin, and anticoagulants need to be decreased.

6. A 55-year-old patient visits the medicine OPD with on and off headache. On examination, he was found to have BP of 170/100 mm Hg. The doctor prescribed him nifedipine tablet at the dose of 20 mg thrice daily. Which of the following hemodynamic change is expected to happen in the patient with this medication?

A. Decrease in blood pressure and increase in heart rate.
B. Decrease in blood pressure and decrease in heart rate.
C. Increase in blood pressure and increase in heart rate.
D. Increase in blood pressure and decrease in heart rate.

Answer: A

Nifedipine is a CCB acting on blood vessels. It therefore dilates the blood vessels, causing a decrease in BP and reflex increase in heart rate.

7. An obese 69-year-old patient with a history of diabetes and hypertension is admitted in the medicine ward with chief complaints of sudden onset of generalized weakness and fluctuating mental status. His BP was 126/80 mm Hg and pulse rate 86/minute and regular. Routine investigations were normal except for high random blood sugar of 260 mg/dL. ECG showed ST elevation in anterior chest leads (V1–V3). Cardiology opinion was taken, and patient was given a single bolus dose of fibrinolytic. Which fibrinolytic drug the patient must have received?

A. Streptokinase.
B. Reteplase.
C. Alteplase.
D. Tenecteplase.

Answer: D

This seems to be a case of STEMI presenting atypically (without chest pain) in elderly diabetic patient. Among the fibrinolytics mentioned, only tenecteplase is given as a single bolus injection over 10 seconds.

8. All of these drugs given in patients with MI are inhibitors of ADP receptors on platelets except:

A. Ticagrelor.
B. Clopidogrel.
C. Prasugrel.
D. Eptifibatide.

Answer: D

Eptifibatide is inhibitor of Gp IIb–IIIa receptor on platelets.

9. A 57-year-old asthmatic patient was admitted to the emergency department with severe chest pain and sweating at rest, onset of which happened a night back. ECG showed ST segment changes suggestive of ischemia, but cardiac markers were normal. Which of the following drug is to be avoided for the management of this patient?

A. Morphine intravenous/oral.
B. Metoprolol intravenous/oral.
C. Nitrate sublingual.
D. Diltiazem oral.

Answer: B

This seems to be a case of unstable angina. Since he is also asthmatic, all β blockers should be avoided in this patient, as there is a chance of precipitation of bronchospasm.

10. Compared to clopidogrel, which antiplatelet drug has been found to increase the risk of intracranial bleed in patients with stroke/transient ischemic attack (TIA)?

A. Ticagrelor.
B. Aspirin.
C. Prasugrel.
D. Dabigatran.

Answer: C

Prasugrel is a newer ADP receptor blocker. The drug, compared to clopidogrel, increases the risk of intracranial bleed in patients with a history of stroke or TIA and is therefore to be avoided in them. The drug is also used cautiously in patients with age > 75 years, renal failure, and body weight < 60 kg.

11. Which of the following antianginal drug is also used in the prophylaxis of migraine?

A. IDN tablet.
B. Ivabradine.
C. Verapamil.
D. Nicorandil.

Answer: C

Among antianginal drugs, nonselective β blockers and CCBs are used in the prophylaxis of migraine.

12. A 74-year-old male patient is admitted to the geriatric ward with altered mental status. Routine investigations were normal except for cardiac markers that showed 25 times elevated troponin T levels. Echocardiography showed signs of wall motion abnormality. ECG was normal, however. All of the following are used in the management of this patient except:

A. Aspirin.
B. Rosuvastatin.
C. Alteplase.
D. Ramipril.

Answer: C

This seems to be a case of NSTEMI. Fibrinolytics (alteplase) are avoided in patients with NSTE-ACS. Fibrinolytics are given in the acute management of STEMI, pulmonary embolism, and stroke.

13. All of these are rate-controlling drugs in angina except:

A. Metoprolol.
B. Diltiazem.
C. Ivabradine.
D. Nifedipine.

Answer: D

Nifedipine increases the heart rate by increasing reflex sympathetic activity.

14. A 59-year-old male patient is admitted in the general medicine ward with chief complaints of anorexia and dyspnea. Dyspnea is present for the last 2 days and is not relieved by rest. Routine investigations are normal except for elevated brain-type natriuretic peptide (BNP) levels and low-oxygen saturation levels (SO_2 of 90%). All of these are given in the management of this patient except:

A. Furosemide.
B. Nitrates.
C. Diltiazem.
D. Statins.

Answer: C

The patient seems to be suffering from acute congestive heart failure. Diltiazem and other L-type CCBs are avoided in the settings of congestive heart failure as they are negatively inotropic and depress the cardiac contractility.

15. Which of the following CCBs has the longest $t_{1/2}$ (half-life) and therefore is given once daily?

A. Amlodipine.
B. Verapamil.
C. Diltiazem.
D. Nifedipine.

Answer: A

Amlodipine has the longest $t_{1/2}$ of 40 to 50 hours and is given at the dose of 5 to 10 mg once daily.

16. Which CCB is used in subarachnoid hemorrhage to prevent neurologic deficit?

A. Amlodipine.
B. Diltiazem.
C. Nimodipine.
D. Cilnidipine.

Answer: C

Nimodipine is the CCB of choice in patients with SAH. It is a cerebrovascular selective CCB.

Chapter 26 Antihypertensives

Prasan R. Bhandari

PH1.27: Describe the mechanisms of action, types, doses, side effects, indications, and contraindications of antihypertensive drugs and drugs used in shock.

Learning Objectives

- Categories of hypertension.
- Diuretics.
- Angiotensin-converting enzyme inhibitors.
- Angiotensin (AT_1) receptor blockers/antagonists.
- Sympatholytic drugs.
- Calcium channel blockers.
- Vasodilators.
- Drug therapy of hypertension.

Introduction

Hypertension (HT) is the commonest cardiovascular disease in which there is continued rise of blood pressure (BP). Both the systolic and diastolic BP are significant, and increase in either has harmful effect. If systolic BP is 210 mm Hg or higher and diastolic BP is 120 mm Hg or higher, it is considered as severe HT. Systolic BP is due to circulatory volume and heart rate, whereas diastolic BP is due to peripheral vascular resistance.

Categories of Hypertension

As per the Seventh Joint National Committee (JNC) on HT, degrees of HT can be categorized as shown in **Table 26.1**.

Types of Hypertension (IM8.14, IM8.15)

Primary/Essential/Idiopathic

In most patients (>90%), the cause of HT is not detected and it is termed essential/primary/idiopathic HT. These patients are not curable; however, they are well controlled throughout the life with appropriate drug treatment and nonpharmacological measures. Treatment is lifelong virtually in all the patients with selected exceptions.

Table 26.1 Degrees of hypertension

Category	BP (mm Hg)	
	Systolic	Diastolic
Normal	<120	<80
Prehypertension	120–139	80–89
Hypertension stage I	140–159	90–99
Hypertension stage II	>160	>100

Note: If diastolic BP is more than 120 mm Hg, it is known as hypertensive crisis, which is further subdivided into hypertensive urgency (if there is no evidence of organ damage) and hypertensive emergency (if there is evidence of organ damage).

Secondary Hypertension

In lesser number of patients (<10%), there is persistent rise in BP secondary to some disease and hence it is termed secondary HT. Causes of secondary HT include cardiovascular anomalies such as coarctation of aorta, renal diseases such as glomerulonephritis, polycystic kidney, renal artery stenosis, endocrine disorders such as pheochromocytoma, steroid-secreting tumors, Cushing's disease, thyrotoxicosis, and other causes such as polycythemia vera and toxemia of pregnancy. If the cause is known, the definite treatment (often curative) is treatment of the cause besides symptomatic treatment for short duration.

Uncontrolled Hypertension

The continuous elevation in BP, whether mild to moderate or severe, has several serious harmful effects especially with severe HT, which comprise endothelial injury causing thickening of intima and occlusion of arteries (atherosclerosis). This is labeled as malignant HT and it is responsible for numerous complications such as renal failure (because of macrovascular occlusion), brain damage (hypertensive encephalopathy), and retinopathy (hypertensive hemorrhage, exudates and edema of optic disc) besides changes in the heart. Long-term uncontrolled HT could lead to complications, although it might not be severe. These complications cause damage to several organs and increase mortality. The complications occur over a prolonged period and the rate of these alterations is proportional to the severity of HT; hence, HT is termed *silent killer*. If malignant HT is not controlled, it leads to the development of microangiopathic hemolytic anemia, secondary to severe endothelial damage, besides other complications.

Classification of Antihypertensive Drugs

These are based on mechanism and/or site of action (**Fig. 26.1**):

1. Diuretics:
   a. Thiazides: hydrochlorothiazide, chlorthalidone, indapamide.
   b. Loop diuretics: furosemide, torsemide, bumetanide.
   c. K^+-sparing diuretics: spironolactone, amiloride, triamterene.
2. Angiotensin-converting enzyme inhibitors (ACEIs): captopril, enalapril, lisinopril, ramipril, perindopril, fosinopril.
3. Angiotensin II receptor blockers (ARBs)/antagonists: losartan, olmesartan, valsartan, candesartan, telmisartan.

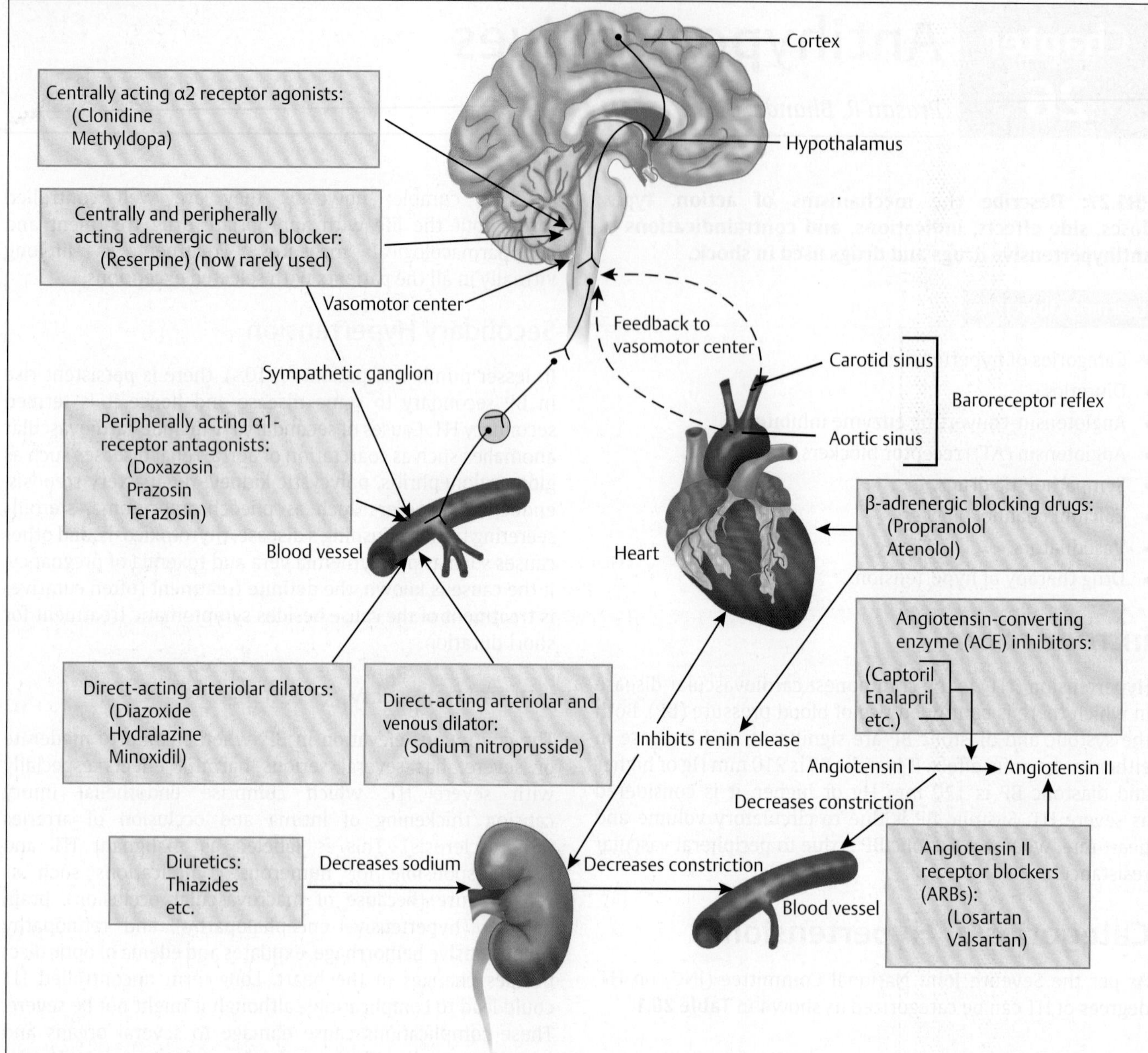

Fig. 26.1 Classification and sites of action of antihypertensives.

4. Sympatholytics:
   a. Centrally acting: clonidine, methyldopa, guanfacine.
   b. Ganglion blockers: trimethaphan.
   c. Adrenergic neuron blockers: reserpine, guanethidine.
   d. Adrenergic receptor blockers:
      i. α-blockers: phenoxybenzamine, phentolamine prazosin, terazosin, doxazosin.
      ii. β-blockers: propranolol, atenolol, metoprolol, esmolol.
      iii. α + β-blockers: labetalol, carvedilol.
5. Calcium channel blockers (CCBs): nifedipine, amlodipine, nimodipine, nicardipine, verapamil, diltiazem.
6. Vasodilators:
   a. Arteriolar dilators: hydralazine, diazoxide, minoxidil.
   b. Arteriolar + venodilators: sodium nitroprusside.

Diuretics (PH1.24)

Diuretics have antihypertensive effect even when used singly, that is, as monotherapy. When administered along with other hypertensives, their efficacy is enhanced, for example, hydrochlorothiazide, indapamide, chlorthalidone.

Thiazides

They are discussed in details in Chapter 29 and their important aspects related with antihypertensive action are mentioned here.

Mechanism

1. Short term (diuretic action): There is loss of sodium and water; however, diuretic effect is decreased on long-term use.

However, the antihypertensive effect is maintained even if the diuretics are used alone.

2. Long term (decrease in peripheral vascular resistance [PVR]): The decrease in PVR occurs on long-term use and is dependent on the functioning kidneys. The effect is due to reduced intracellular levels of calcium as a result of reduced sodium concentration in vascular smooth muscles. Additionally, there is decreased affinity of receptors in vessel wall and cells are resistant to contractile stimulus.

The antihypertensive efficacy is lost if sodium intake is raised. Efficacy of thiazide is likewise lost when glomerular filtration rate (GFR) is less than 20 mL/min, for example, in patients with renal insufficiency.

Hydrochlorothiazide is one of the commonly administered thiazides. It has been demonstrated that the initial daily dose of hydrochlorothiazide should be 12.5 mg, and this can be raised to 25 mg daily. A further increase in dose does not increase the efficacy if the drug is used alone. A dose of more than 25 mg/day exposes the patient to side effect. Hence, if the dose of 25 mg/day does not reduce the BP to desired level, then the drug of another class could be added instead of increasing the dose.

The main problem with thiazide is hypokalemia. This can be prevented by K^+ supplementation or using thiazide in combination with K^+-sparing diuretics such as spironolactone or amiloride. Combination of thiazide with ACEI or ARB also decreases the loss of potassium and thus prevents hypokalemia. However, ACEI or ARB must not be combined with K^+-sparing diuretics as this could lead to dangerous hyperkalemia in certain patients.

When sympatholytics and/or vasodilators are used, there is increase in circulatory volume; hence, thiazides are especially beneficial in combination with sympatholytics and/or vasodilators.

Generally, 2 to 4 weeks are necessary for the response to be achieved and maximum response is achieved in around 10 to 12 weeks. Hence, increment of dose should be made only after 2 to 4 weeks.

Adverse Effects

1. Hypokalemia is dose-dependent. Cardiac arrhythmias (ventricular) could occur due to hypokalemia.
2. Gout due to hyperuricemia.
3. The level of low-density lipoprotein, and hence the ratio of low-density lipoprotein to high-density lipoprotein, is increased, which is correlated with ischemic heart disease (IHD) and mortality.
4. Hyperglycemia might develop with thiazides and the level of glycosylated Hb is increased in patients with diabetes mellitus (DM). Hence, thiazides should be avoided in hypertensive patients with DM.
5. Sexual impotence and muscle cramps are the other adverse effects.

K^+-sparing diuretics such as triamterene and spironolactone could be combined with thiazides to prevent hypokalemia and to facilitate antihypertensive effect as well.

Angiotensin-Converting Enzyme Inhibitors

Drugs that affect the renin–angiotensin system can be categorized as follows:

1. Drugs that block renin secretion, for example, clonidine, methyldopa, and β-blockers.
2. Renin inhibitors, for example, remikiren and aliskiren.
3. ACEIs, for example, captopril, enalapril, and lisinopril.
4. Angiotensin receptor (AT_1) blockers or antagonists, for example, losartan and candesartan.
5. Aldosterone antagonists, for example, spironolactone (Chapter 29).

The details of these drugs are discussed in Chapter 22 and the important aspects of ACEIs and angiotensin receptor blockers in the context of their use in HT are mentioned here.

ACEIs

They are efficacious and have favorable adverse effect profile and hence they improve patient compliance. They have the following benefits:

1. No postural hypotension and no rebound HT.
2. Reverses left ventricular hypertrophy (LVH).
3. No effect on electrolytes, for example, hypokalemia and metabolites such as uric acid and lipids.
4. Safe in patients with comorbid bronchial asthma, DM, IHD, congestive heart failure (CHF), and peripheral vascular disease.
5. Prevent secondary hyperaldosteronism and type II DM.
6. Better quality of life than other antihypertensive drugs.

They are among the first-line antihypertensives as they are well tolerated. They are used to treat all grades of HT due to all causes. Diuretics increase their efficacy. K^+-sparing diuretics should not be combined as the combination can lead to hyperkalemia. Special indications include:

1. HT with LVH.
2. HT with DM, as it slows nephropathy.
3. HT with renal diseases as it slows glomerulosclerosis.
4. HT with IHD and post–myocardial infarction (post-MI) patients.

For severe HT, they are used in combination with CCBs/diuretics/β-blockers.

Adverse Effects

1. Persistent dry cough: It occurs due to increased bradykinin levels and is common in women; hence, it may require discontinuation of ACEI. ARB can be used as alternative in such situations.
2. Hypotension: It occurs at initiation of therapy, and this is called as first-dose phenomena. Therefore, start with small dose. If the patient is on diuretics, stop diuretics.
3. Hyperkalemia: It is more common in patients on K^+-sparing diuretics/K^+ supplements.
4. Reversible dysgeusia (altered taste sensation).
5. Angioneurotic edema (0.1% incidence): It is manifested as swelling of the lips, nose, larynx, and bronchospasm. This occurs due to increase in bradykinin. ACEI is immediately

stopped in such cases. Severe cases are treated with adrenaline and corticosteroids.

6. Skin rashes.
7. Teratogenicity.
8. Acute renal failure in patients with renal artery stenosis.
9. Neutropenia and proteinuria in patients with collagen diseases.

Significant aspects concerned with the use of ACEIs in HT are discussed in the following:

1. They prevent the metabolism of bradykinin and substance P; thus, several side effects occur due to accumulation of these substances, such as dry cough.
2. Angioedema is a rare but serious and potentially fatal side effect and ACEI should be discontinued once signs of angioedema are manifested.
3. GFR may be reduced in patients with comorbid renal disease or bilateral renal artery stenosis. A balance is required for potential risk of reversible drug-induced impairment of GFR versus inhibition of renal disease progression.
4. In certain patients with the initial dose, there is substantial drop in BP, that is, first-dose hypotension due to exaggerated response in increased pretreatment plasma renin activity. Hence, treatment should be started with a low dose especially in patients with a highly active renin–angiotensin system, for example, a patient with diuretic-induced volume contraction or congestive cardiac failure (CCF).
5. Doses of all ACEIs are decreased in renal dysfunction/renal failure and hyponatremia and with the simultaneous use of diuretics.
6. When ACEIs are used, there is very minute elevation of K^+ level because of attenuation of aldosterone production. This is not clinically significant in usual therapeutic doses when used alone. However, there are chances of significant hyperkalemia in patients with renal insufficiency, with K^+-sparing diuretic, when potassium is supplemented from outside, with nonsteroidal anti-inflammatory drugs (NSAIDs), when used in β-blockers, and in patients with diabetic nephropathy.
7. ACEIs are fetopathic and hence must be avoided in pregnancy, especially in the second and third trimesters.

Angiotensin (AT1) Receptor Blockers/Antagonists

In contrast to ACEIs, these agents do not prevent degradation of bradykinin and substance P. Hence, there is no accumulation of these substances. There are two types of angiotensin receptors:

1. AT_1: Present in the vascular and myocardial tissue, brain, kidney, and adrenal glomerulosa cells, which secrete aldosterone.
2. AT_2: Present in the adrenal medulla, kidney, and central nervous system (CNS). These could be important in vascular development.

AT_1 receptor also mediates feedback inhibition (autoreceptor).

Adverse Effects

Adverse effects are similar to those of ACEIs, which occur because of the inhibition of formation of angiotensin II. However, since the angiotensin receptor antagonists do not prevent degradation of bradykinin and substance P, there is no accumulation of these substances. Hence, side effect because of the accumulation of these substances does not occur or are less frequent with these drugs (e.g., dry cough). Angioedema, too, is very rare. Additionally, there is no first-dose hypotension.

Uses

Angiotensin receptor antagonists are as effective as ACEIs when administered in appropriate doses for the treatment of HT. However, like ACEIs, they are less effective in low-renin patients. They increase the antihypertensive effect of other drugs. If BP is not adequately controlled with AT_1 antagonist alone, then a small amount of hydrochlorothiazide or other diuretic significantly increases the efficacy. Likewise, if adequate response is not achieved with hydrochlorothiazide, addition of AT_1 antagonist produces significant reduction in BP. When used as antihypertensive, they do not alter the heart rate, there is no effect on cardiovascular reflexes, and there are no metabolic alterations (blood sugar level or lipid level). They do not alter insulin sensitivity when used in diabetic patients on insulin therapy.

Sympatholytic Drugs

Central Sympatholytic: α-Methyldopa

Mechanism

It is a prodrug and is converted to α-methyl noradrenaline (NA) at both peripheral nervous system and CNS. It is stored in storage vesicles in place of NA. Hence, α-methyl NA is released instead of NA and it is equally potent vasoconstrictor as NA peripherally. However, in the CNS α-methyl NA formed acts as α_2-receptor (presynaptic) agonist and mediates a negative feedback inhibition of sympathetic outflow. α-methyl NA acts at rostral ventrolateral medulla and inhibits the release of NA (**Fig. 26.2**).

Pharmacological Actions

The peripheral vascular resistance is decreased by α-methyldopa because of central action. The decrease in concentration of NA corresponds with the fall in BP. On long-term administration, there is sodium and water retention and this is responsible for the loss of antihypertensive effect. However, this can be overcome by simultaneous use of diuretics.

Pharmacokinetics

It is well and rapidly absorbed on oral administration by active amino acid transport. Therapeutic effect is delayed (6–8 hours) because of the time required for active transport of drug to the CNS and conversion into active metabolite in CNS as it is a prodrug. The plasma levels do not correlate with the therapeutic effect as therapeutic effect is due to the formation of active metabolite in the CNS. Although its $t_{1/2}$ is about 2 hours, the therapeutic effect is prolonged (24 hours) because of the accumulation of active metabolite in the adrenergic neurons in the CNS.

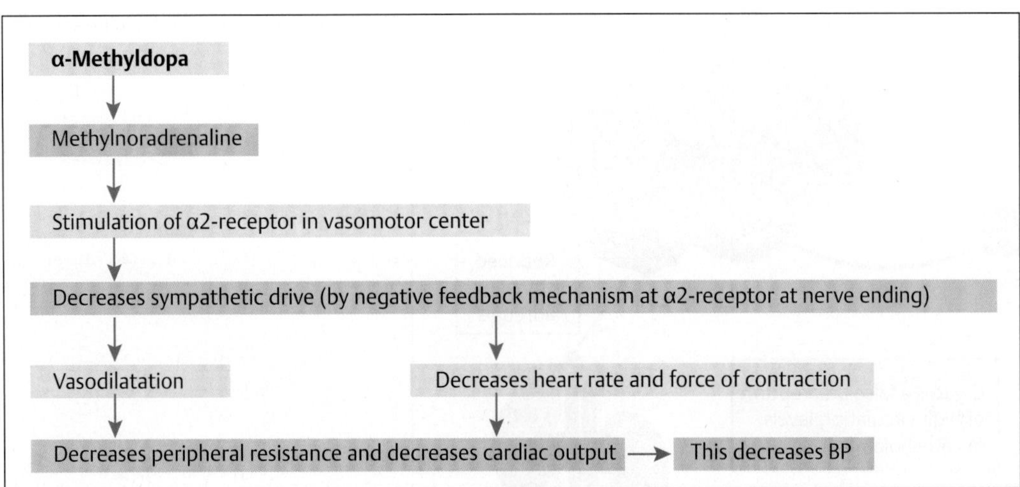

Fig. 26.2 Mechanism of action of α-methyldopa.

Adverse Effects

Sedation

Transient sedation is caused due to the stimulation of α_2-receptor in the area of brain stem responsible for wakefulness and alertness. Psychomotor slowing and depression might also occur. This can be prevented by administering it as a single dose at bed time.

Xerostomia (Dryness of Mouth)

It is because of inhibition of salivation due to stimulation of α_2-receptor in the salivation control center in the medulla (brain stem).

Others

1. Reduced libido, parkinsonism, and hyperprolactinemia causing gynecomastia and galactorrhea could occur.
2. Chronic use of α-methyldopa causes positive Coombs test in approximately 15% of patients, which might lead to difficulty in crossmatching in blood transfusion.

Present Clinical Status

Essential Hypertension

α-Methyldopa is neither a first-line agent nor preferred as monotherapy for the treatment of essential HT because of its frequent side effects. However, it is beneficial in the treatment of hypertensive patients with comorbid IHD. It decreases LVH in patients with diastolic dysfunction.

It is administered in patients with HT when other drugs are not able to control the BP in combination with diuretics.

Hypertension in Pregnancy

It is an efficacious as well as safe antihypertensive for both the fetus and the mother when administered during pregnancy and hence is preferred. Methyldopa can also be given by intravenous (IV) route.

Interaction

Tricyclic antidepressants inhibit the active uptake of methyldopa into adrenergic neurons and hence reduce its antihypertensive effect.

α_2-Receptor Agonists

Examples include clonidine, guanabenz, and guanfacine.

Clonidine was initially developed in the 1960s as a nasal decongestant because of its α_2-agonistic effect, which causes vasoconstriction in nasal mucous membrane. Subsequently, it was observed that it possesses antihypertensive action because of its central action and hence is used for the treatment of HT.

Mechanism

The precise mechanism of antihypertensive action of clonidine and other related α_2-receptor agonists is not clear. It acts probably as an α_2-receptor agonist (α_{2A}-presynaptic autoreceptor) in the brain stem and hence reduces the central sympathetic outflow and BP (**Fig. 26.3**).

Pharmacokinetics

The absorption of clonidine is extremely good by oral route and bioavailability is around 100%. Maximum antihypertensive effect is observed in 2 to 3 hours and the duration of action ranges between 8 and 24 hours.

When administered as transdermal patch, the steady-state concentration is achieved in 3 to 4 hours and the duration is around 7 days; when the patch is removed, the effect is lost in approximately 6 to 8 hours gradually. This happens over several weeks, and during this phase BP could rise.

Present Clinical Status

Essential Hypertension

Clonidine is neither a first-line agent nor preferred as monotherapy for the treatment of essential HT because of its frequent and troublesome CNS side effects such as sedation and dryness of mouth. Presently, clonidine is administered for the treatment of patients with severe HT not responding to other currently available and commonly used drugs. It is used with suitable diuretic for this purpose.

It is combined with vasodilator such as hydralazine to preserve its antihypertensive effect. However, presently

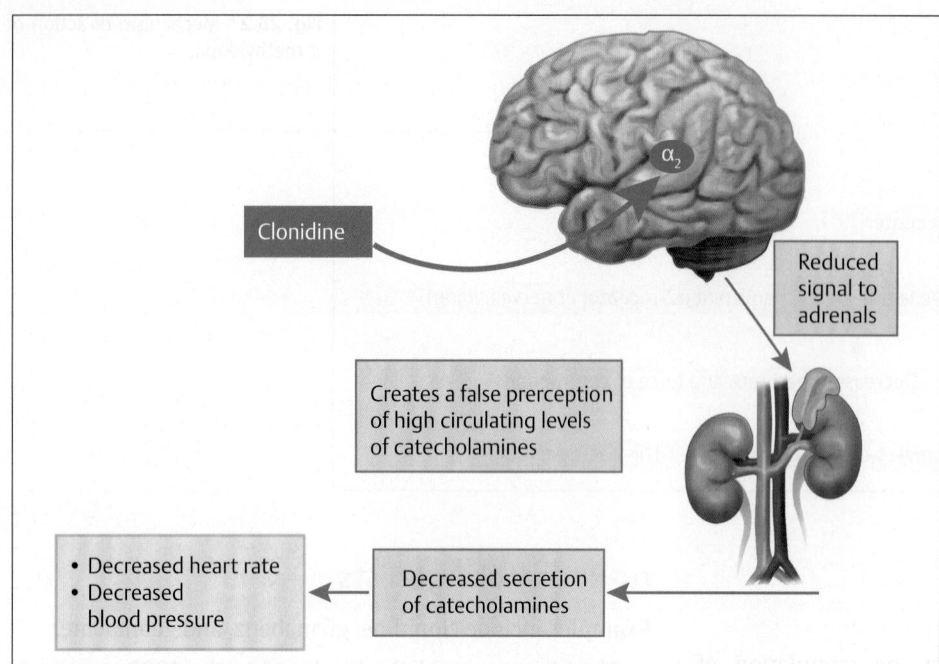

Fig. 26.3 Mechanism of clonidine action.

β-receptor blockers are preferred over clonidine for this purpose.

Other Uses

Drug Addiction

It can be administered for the treatment of acute opioid withdrawal syndrome. Chronic exposure to opioid causes decreased noradrenergic activity. On sudden discontinuation of morphine, there is abrupt increase in NA activity, which is suppressed when clonidine is administered. Clonidine is also utilized to decrease craving for opioids and alcohol and to facilitate deaddiction in cigarette smokers.

For Pain Relief

Clonidine can be administered to relieve severe cancer pain (epidural, 30 µh/h) as an alternative to morphine. It could also be used for postoperative pain; however, it is not preferred.

Diarrhea

In patients with diabetic autonomic neuropathy, it is effective probably because of the facilitation of absorption of salt due to its α_2-mediated action.

Menopause

It is beneficial in decreasing hot flushes associated with menopause.

Preanesthetic Medication

It can be administered for smooth induction of anesthesia and it decreases the need of general anesthetic. It is also beneficial in stabilizing the BP fluctuation during anesthesia.

Clonidine could similarly be administered for migraine prophylaxis and for mania. However, it is not preferred due to the availability of better agents.

Diagnostic Use

Clonidine is used for the diagnosis of pheochromocytoma. For this purpose, clonidine is given in a dose of 0.3 mg, and 3 hours after, plasma levels of NA are measured. If there is lack of suppression of plasma concentration of NA to less than 0.5 ng/mL, it indicates the presence of pheochromocytoma.

Forms and Dosages

Transdermal Patch (Extended-Release)

1. Dosage: 0.1, 0.2, and 0.3 mg/day. Change the patch after every 7 days.
2. Indications: HT, smoking cessation, cyclosporine nephrotoxicity, menopausal flushing, and opioid withdrawal.

Tablet (Immediate-Release)

1. Dosage: 0.1, 0.2, and 0.3 mg.
2. Indications: HT, acute HT, opioid withdrawal, and pheochromocytoma.

Tablet (Extended-Release)

1. Dosage: 0.1 mg.
2. Indications: alcohol withdrawal, smoking cessation, restless legs syndrome, attention deficit hyperactivity disorder, Tourette's syndrome, menopausal flushing, dysmenorrhea, postherpetic neuralgia, and psychosis.

Adverse Effects

Due to Pharmacological Actions

CNS Side Effects

Sedation is the most common. Other effects include sleep disturbance, nightmares, restlessness, and depression in higher doses.

Cardiovascular System

Bradycardia and cardia arrest in patients with preexisting cardiac disease with conduction defect.

Xerostomia (Dryness of Mouth)

Dryness of mouth could be associated with dry nasal mucosa, dry eye, and painful swelling of parotid glands.

Contact Dermatitis

This occurs when it is administered as a transdermal patch.

Due to Sudden Withdrawal of Drug

Abrupt withdrawal of clonidine and related drugs causes withdrawal syndrome manifested as a severe increase in BP. Other symptoms include headache, tremors, sweating, and tachycardia. These are because of rebound increase in sympathetic activity (increased plasma and urinary concentration of adrenaline). These generally happen within 24 hours following abrupt discontinuation of drugs. Treatment of withdrawal syndrome is by administration of same dose of clonidine on which the patient was maintained. Drugs preferred to be used are either sodium nitroprusside infusion or α-blocker or combination of α- and β-blockers or labetalol having both the α- and β-blocking action.

Interactions

3. Diuretics enhance the antihypertensive effect of clonidine and hence are combined with it.
4. Tricyclic antidepressant reduces the antihypertensive effect of clonidine probably by inhibiting active uptake of clonidine in neurons.

Guanabenz and guanfacine are similar to clonidine with regard to mechanism and actions, and produce equally effective antihypertensive effect.

Other Clonidinelike Drugs

Apraclonidine and brimonidine are also selective α_2-agonist and used topically for treatment of glaucoma. Dexmedetomidine is a selective α_2-agonist used as an anesthetic adjuvant.

Moxonidine

It is a centrally acting selective agonist at imidazoline I1 receptor and has more prominent action at this receptor apart from $\boldsymbol{\alpha}_2$-receptors. It is long-acting and causes less drowsiness (less sedation) as compared to clonidine. More importantly, rebound HT is less likely and hence it is preferred to clonidine for mild-to-moderate HT.

Reserpine

It is an alkaloid obtained from the root of the plant *Rauwolfia serpentina*, a plant indigenous to India. It was one of the common and highly effective drugs used for the first time on large scale.

Mechanism

It acts mostly peripherally and also centrally by combining with storage vesicles of the nerve endings. The function of storage vesicle is inhibited after reserpine combines by depleting the NA in the vesicle. This is achieved by releasing all the NA content into the cytoplasm and further inhibiting the reuptake of released NA into storage vesicles, that is, intragranular/intravesicular uptake. The released NA is metabolized by the MAO present in the cytoplasm of nerve endings. Hence, on nerve depolarization, NA is not released since the stores are depleted; thus, there is no impulse propagation. Dopamine is also depleted. Action of reserpine returns only when new vesicles are synthesized, which takes about few days to few weeks. Thus, it is one of the examples of hit-and-run drug. Depletion of mainly NA and also dopamine (DA) causes sympatholytic and antihypertensive effects.

Pharmacological Actions

Due to its sympatholytic action, the cardiac output and peripheral vascular resistance are gradually decreased on long-term use of reserpine. However, sodium and water retention is observed on prolonged use, causing loss of antihypertensive effect.

Pharmacokinetics

This is not yet clear because of nonavailability of methods to estimate low levels of reserpine and its metabolites. Reserpine is tightly bound with the storage vesicle and this binding is irreversible. This is responsible for its effects, and hence plasma concentration does not correlate with its concentration at the site of action and its therapeutic effect.

Clinical Uses

Hypertension

Its advantage is that it is inexpensive and efficacious and a very good antihypertensive drug. It is administered as single daily dose and hence there is good patient compliance. Because of the availability of newer agents in the last few years, the use of reserpine has declined. The reason attributed is its serious CNS side effects, which include depression and suicidal tendency. However, these are actually due to its toxic effects when toxic dose is used, which is much higher (>2.5 mg/day). This dose is rarely needed for the antihypertensive action. It is very significant to note that the antihypertensive effect of reserpine is produced in daily doses of 0.1 to 0.25 mg and even lower dose of 0.05 mg produces antihypertensive effect when it is used with diuretic.

Disadvantages

1. The maximum antihypertensive effect is observed after several weeks of regular use.
2. When used singly on long term, there is retention of sodium and water, leading to loss of antihypertensive effect. However, this can be avoided if it is administered with diuretics such as hydrochlorothiazide (thiazide group).
3. Rarely, depression could be seen on prolonged use if daily dose is higher than 1.0 mg. However, this dose is rarely used clinically.

Clinical Status

On the basis of the above-mentioned facts, it can safely be used for the treatment of mild-to-moderate HT in combination with diuretic in the daily dose of 0.05 to 0.25 mg. However, it should immediately be discontinued once signs of depression appear in patient on reserpine therapy. It is found to be a good antihypertensive in combination of diuretics or with other drugs such as β-blocker or **α**-methyldopa or vasodilator.

Adverse Effects

CNS

1. Sedation is very common, and nightmares could occur. Depression has been reported and might develop on prolonged use if higher doses (>2.5 mg) are administered.
2. Extrapyramidal side effects such as Parkinson's disease might develop because of depletion of dopamine in the corpus striatum even in usual therapeutic antihypertensive doses.

Others

Nasal congestion, abdominal cramps, diarrhea, increased acid secretion, and peptic ulceration.

Precautions

1. It is contraindicated in patients with depression or a history of depression.
2. Precaution should be taken in patients with a history of peptic ulcer.

Ganglion Blocker

Trimethaphan

Trimethaphan was earlier utilized in hypertensive patients. However, it is seldom utilized currently due to serious and many intolerable side effects and availability of better drugs.

Adrenergic Neuron Blocker

Guanethidine

Guanethidine was administered earlier for many years for the treatment of severe HT. It acts by multiple mechanism, that is, by displacing NA from storage vesicles, it inhibits nerve impulse coupled release of NA and blocks the uptake of NA in axonal membrane. It is no longer used for HT due to comprehensive sympatholytic action and availability of many better agents for all grades of HT. Some of the troublesome side effects are postural hypotension, diarrhea, and inhibition of ejaculation.

Adrenergic Receptor Blocker (For Details, Refer to Chapter 21)

α-Blockers

Prazosin and other α-blockers and their use in HT are discussed in detail in Chapter 21.

β-Blockers

β-blockers were used for the treatment of angina and their details are discussed in Chapter 21. However, their important aspects in the context of antihypertensive treatment are briefly discussed here.

β-blockers effectively control the BP as monotherapy and long-acting agents could be administered once a day, which is highly convenient and improves the patient compliance. The antihypertensive effect is observed over 1 to 2 weeks. The commonly administered nonselective β-blocker is propranolol, whereas the cardioselective (β_1-blocker) are atenolol and metoprolol.

Mechanism

The possible mechanisms that contribute to antihypertensive effect include the following:

1. Cardiovascular system: reduced contractility of myocardium:
   a. Reduced heart rate.
   b. Reduced cardiac output.
2. Renin release inhibition.
3. Alteration in sympathetic outflow at CNS level.
4. CNS altered baroreceptor sensitivity.
5. Increased PGI2 biosynthesis.

Additional Actions

Some of the β-blockers have additional α-receptor-blocking property such as labetalol (α- + β-blocker) and carvedilol. Carvedilol (α- + β-blocker) in addition has direct vasodilator property.

Labetalol is a suitable agent for emergency control of severe HT because of pheochromocytoma and also due to cheese reaction. It is also beneficial for moderate essential HT not responding to other β-blockers. It is considered safe in pregnancy.

Carvedilol is also administered in patients with associated CCF where its additional vasodilator property also contributes to beneficial effect apart from β-blocking action.

Benefits of β-Blockers

β-Blockers have the following advantages when used as monotherapy to control HT:

1. They do not lead to postural hypotension.
2. There is no sodium and water retention on long-term use.
3. Long-acting agents such as atenolol are convenient; thus, there is improved patient compliance.
4. They are suitable for young but nonobese patients.
5. They increase survival and prevent stroke in patients with HT.
6. They have additional benefit/suitability for patients with associated conditions such as:
   a. Cardiovascular disease such as classical angina, post-MI patients (reduces mortality), and select cases of CHF.
   b. Other diseases such as migraine.
   c. Pregnancy, for example, atenolol and labetalol.

Drawbacks of β-Blockers

1. Their antihypertensive action is delayed for around 1 to 2 weeks.
2. Rebound HT could develop on abrupt discontinuation.
3. They have to be avoided in patients with associated:
   a. Cardiovascular disease such as variant angina and certain cases of CHF.
   b. Other conditions such as DM, bronchial asthma, obesity, and Raynaud's phenomenon, but cardioselective (β_1-selective),

for example, atenolol and metoprolol, can be used in these conditions. However, it is better to avoid all the β-blockers unless there is no choice because cardioselectivity of β-blockers is relative and at higher dose this is lost.

Calcium Channel Blockers

The details of CCBs are mentioned in Chapter 25. The points relevant for the treatment of HT are mentioned here. They decrease the total peripheral vascular resistance. Dihydropyridine (DHP) CCBs such as nifedipine and amlodipine are preferred because of their significant arteriolar vasodilatation, whereas verapamil and diltiazem are preferred for the treatment of dysrhythmias (paroxysmal supraventricular tachycardia [PSVT]). CCBs are also beneficial for the treatment of isolated systolic HT.

Increased venous return causes increase in cardiac output because of peripheral vasodilatation. Increased venous return is beneficial in improving diastolic function in patients who are susceptible to develop left ventricular failure. In hypertensive patients with cardiomyopathy, the increased venous return is beneficial in improving diastolic function. LVH is the important actor causing the diastolic dysfunction. Ventricular diastolic function is not improved by CCBs. Long-term use of CCBs reduces left ventricular mass and, in this aspect, they are less efficacious as compared to the ACEIs and α-methyldopa; however, they are more effective than the diuretics. CCBs are equally effective antihypertensive as β-blockers and diuretics.

Adverse Effects

These include headache, flushing, dizziness, and peripheral edema. Dizziness and flushing are less with long-acting agents such as amlodipine. Some side effects are due to the relaxation of nonvascular smooth muscles such as gastroesophageal reflux (due to inhibition of contraction of lower esophageal sphincter (LES); verapamil and nifedipine cause constipation. Retention of urine is seldom seen. Inhibition of sinoatrial (SA) node by diltiazem and verapamil could cause bradycardia and SA node arrest especially in patients with SA node dysfunction and this effect is aggravated by β-blockers.

Benefits

1. CCBs are preferred in low-renin patients and the elderly as monotherapy.
2. They do not modify exercise tolerance and do not alter the plasma lipid levels and plasma concentration of uric acid or electrolytes unlike diuretics.
3. They do not affect male sexual function.
4. CCBs are safe in patients with DM, bronchial asthma, gout, hyperlipidemia, and renal dysfunction.
5. They are beneficial in isolated systolic HT in the elderly. They control BP and decrease cardiovascular complications.
6. Verapamil and diltiazem are of advantage in patients with comorbid PSVT, atrial fibrillation, and atrial flutter due to their antiarrhythmic effect.
7. DHP CCBs such as nifedipine can be administered during pregnancy; however, they delay the labor and hence must be discontinued prior to the labor.

Drawbacks

1. In hypertensive patients with comorbid IHD and post-MI patients, CCBs of all the groups, that is, DHP, verapamil, or diltiazem, do not improve survival and usually are not preferred. The agents preferred are β-blockers and ACEIs since they enhance the survival of hypertensive patients with IHD.
2. Short-acting agents such as nifedipine are not preferred for treatment of essential HT since they cause fluctuation in BP and increase in sympathetic activity with each dose interval. However, slow release or sustained release preparation can be utilized.

Interactions

1. Antihypertensive effect of CCBs is potentiated with ACEIs, methyldopa, and β-blockers; this could be combined with these drugs if CCBs alone are producing inadequate response.
2. Bradycardia produced by CCBs such as verapamil and diltiazem is potentiated by β-blockers.
3. Quinidine and CCB could lead to excessive hypotension.

Vasodilators

Vasodilators are efficacious antihypertensives. However, if they are used alone, their effect is lost in due course of time. This is due to several compensatory mechanisms. To counteract the compensatory mechanism or to maintain the efficacy of vasodilators on prolonged use, they are used along with other agents. The most appropriate agents are the diuretics, and another group consists of β-blockers.

Diazoxide

It was developed as a byproduct in search of thiazides. These agents cause relaxation of vascular smooth muscles. It acts by activating ATP-sensitive K^+ channel and thus there is hyperpolarization leading to relaxation of smooth muscles and consequently there is vasodilatation. It only causes arteriolar vasodilatation, thus leading to increased sympathetic activity. Because of the increased sympathetic activity, there is increase in heart rate and myocardial contractility, leading to increase cardiac output. Additionally, retention of salt and water occurs because of enhanced sympathetic activity and increased secretion of renin. All these factors contribute to loss of hypertensive effect of diazoxide.

It is used as an alternative to sodium nitroprusside in patients with hypertensive emergencies where sodium nitroprusside cannot be used or facility for IV infusion or monitoring is not present. Diazoxide can be administered as IV bolus. It can also be administered as IV infusion (15–30 mg/min). Since diazoxide enhances the sympathetic activity, it is avoided in hypertensive patients with comorbid IHD, coarctation of aorta, and arteriovenous shunts. Diazoxide is likewise beneficial in inoperable cases of insulinoma.

Adverse Effects

Salt and Water Retention

This is due to reflex increase in sympathetic activity and renin release. This can be countered by reducing the salt and water intake.

Hyperglycemia

This occurs because of inhibition of release of insulin. This is due to blockade of calcium channels as a result of opening of K^+ channels in β-cells of islets of Langerhans. It is problematic only in patients with Non-insulin-dependent diabetes mellitus (NIDDM) maintained on insulin-releasing oral antidiabetic drugs.

Myocardial Ischemia

Due to reflex sympathetic increase in myocardial contractility and heart rate, increased blood flow occurs to nonischemic region, that is, coronary steal.

Others

Cerebral ischemia can develop if there is severe reduction in BP. It has a uterine relaxant effect and hence may prevent labor if administered for hypertensive crisis at term.

Hydralazine

It is a vasodilator and effective antihypertensive agent. However, it is not beneficial if used as a monotherapy for the treatment of HT because of the development of rapid tolerance, that is, tachyphylaxis (loss of therapeutic effect on repeated administration). This occurs due to salt and water retention, and reflex tachycardia is a troublesome side effect. However, it is beneficial if combined with other antihypertensive to prevent the above-mentioned side effects. It is used with diuretic for prevention of development of tolerance and β-blocker to prevent reflex tachycardia.

Hydralazine is a direct smooth muscle relaxant with unknown intracellular mechanism. It leads to arteriolar vasodilatation and does not have effect on veins, that is, capacitance vessels. Because of arterial dilatation, there is increased heart rate, contractility, and increased renin activity due to sympathetic stimulation. This causes fluid and water retention and ultimately there is loss of therapeutic effect as discussed earlier. Increased contraction of myocardium could likewise occur because of the release of NA from sympathetic nerve terminal.

It causes vasodilatation of coronary, cerebral, and renal arteries. Since the effect on venous blood vessels is negligible, it does not cause postural hypotension, that is, the fall in BP observed is equal in both the supine and standing position.

The action continues for approximately 12 hours, although the $t_{1/2}$ is short (1 hour). This could possibly be due to its tight binding with the vascular tissues. It is metabolized by acetylation in the gut and liver. The genetic variation in this process has been demonstrated, that is, certain patients are fast acetylators and hence need a higher dose, while some of them are slow acetylators. Thus, the bioavailability varies from 30% in slow acetylators to 15% in fast acetylators.

Adverse Effects

1. Common side effects occur because of the extension of pharmacological actions, which include nausea, anorexia, headache, sweating, flushing, tachycardia, and palpitation. Angina and arrhythmias might be precipitated in patients with comorbid IHD because of sympathetic stimulation and increased oxygen demand.
2. Allergic reactions such as drug-induced systematic lupus erythematosus (SLE) or SLE-like syndromes manifested as fever, skin rashes, myalgia and arthralgia could be seen at highest doses or prolonged use especially in slow acetylators. They are reversible on stopping the drug; however, corticosteroids may be needed in certain patients.
3. Peripheral neuropathy may occur. This is probably due to the formation of hydrazone compound by combining hydralazine with pyridoxine. Pyridoxine is effective in such neuropathy.

Clinical Uses

Severe Hypertension

It is used along with other agents such as diuretics and β-blockers.

Hypertension during Pregnancy

Hydralazine can safely be administered for the treatment of HT in pregnancy. During hypertensive emergency in pregnancy, it can be administered by IV route.

Heart Failure

It is beneficial in heart failure by decreasing the afterload. However, it is more beneficial if it is used along with some venodilator (decrease in preload) such as organic nitrates.

Precautions and Contraindications

Precaution is required in elderly patients and patients with IHD since myocardial ischemia could occur because of enhanced sympathetic activity.

Minoxidil

It was found to be effective for the treatment of severe HT and in cases that are resistant to other drugs. Minoxidil is inactive itself and is converted into active form minoxidil N-O sulfate by enzyme sulfotransferase in the liver. Minoxidil sulfate activates and opens the ATP-sensitive potassium channels in vascular smooth muscles. This leads to the efflux of K^+, which causes hyperpolarization and ultimately relaxation of smooth muscles (vasodilatation). Because of vasodilatation, there is reduction in BP.

Minoxidil causes only arteriolar vasodilatation and increases blood flow to the skeletal muscles, skin, gut, and heart. The increased blood flow is maximum in the heart and minimum in the CNS.

Minoxidil causes renal vasodilatation but excessive vasodilatation may cause decrease in renal blood flow because of systemic hypotension. Renal dysfunction secondary to elevated BP is improved.

Adverse Effects

Retention of Salt and Water

Its long-term administration enhances the circulatory volume because of salt and water retention. Therefore, there is loss of therapeutic effect and hence it must be combined with other drugs such as diuretics.

Hypertrichosis

Long-term administration causes growth of hairs on body including the face, back, arms, and limbs, which is embarrassing to women. This is possibly because of the activation of K^+ channels.

Cardiovascular Side Effects

Minoxidil causes sympathetic stimulation; for example, hydralazine causes tachycardia, palpitation, and increased oxygen demand. Hence, it could aggravate angina and arrhythmias in patient with comorbid IHD due to sympathetic stimulation.

Clinical Uses

Hypertension

It is preferred to be used in patients with severe HT in both adults and children who are not responding or poorly responding to other antihypertensive drugs. When minoxidil is used singly, it causes fluid retention and reflex increase in heart rate. Therefore, it should not be used as monotherapy and must be combined with diuretics and/or β-adrenoceptor blocker.

Other Uses

Topically, it is administered as 2% solution for the male pattern baldness.

Fenoldopam

Fenoldopam is racemic and its pharmacological action is produced by R-isomer. It acts by stimulating DA receptors (selective D_1 agonist) and dilates peripheral arteries. However, it does not stimulate adrenergic (α and β) receptors. It dilates renal and mesenteric blood vessels and also the coronary arteries. Fenoldopam is an effective agent in reducing BP in severe HT. It is equally efficacious as sodium nitroprusside in its BP-lowering effect and its advantage is that it does not cause cyanide or thiocyanate poisoning. However, it is slow in onset. It has a very short half-life (10 minutes) and hence is administered as continuous IV infusion. It is beneficial for short-term control of severe HT in conditions where rapid antihypertensive effect is needed. Reflex tachycardia, flushing, and headache could occur as side effects. Fenoldopam must be avoided in glaucoma since it increases intraocular tension. It is important to note that fenoldopam is not used for the treatment of hypovolemic shock, although it dilates renal and mesenteric blood vessels similar to dopamine, since it causes hypotension.

Sodium Nitroprusside

Sodium nitroprusside is spontaneously converted to nitric oxide by reducing agents such as glutathione (**Fig. 26.4**). The onset of action is 2 to 4 minutes and it is because of the rapid conversion of cyanide to NO. Additionally, there is formation of cyanide that is rapidly metabolized to thiocyanate in the liver and excreted through the kidneys (**Fig. 26.5**). However, if there is poor hepatic or renal function or if rate of infusion is high and too rapid or after prolonged use, it might lead to cyanide poisoning. Hence, sodium nitroprusside must only be administered for shorter period. The action of sodium nitroprusside is terminated following its metabolism. Nitroprusside enters erythrocytes and is transformed into methemoglobin and nitroprusside radical (unstable) by electron transfer from hemoglobin. The nitroprusside radical is converted into cyanide, which remains in bound form in the erythrocyte. However, the free form enters the plasma and proves toxic by affecting the cytochrome enzyme system. Cyanide is converted to thiocyanate. Plasma thiocyanate value indicates the toxicity.

Clinical Uses

Hypertensive Emergencies

It is administered to rapidly lower the BP.

To Produce Controlled Hypotension

It is used during certain surgical procedure with the aim to prevent bleeding.

Refractory Congestive Cardiac Failure

It is used to enhance cardiac output in acute heart failure as an emergency measure and in short-term management.

Ergot Toxicity

It is used as long as vasoconstriction persists.

Other Situation

Situations where short-term reduction in preload and afterload is useful, for example:

1. Dissection of aorta.
2. Post acute MI.

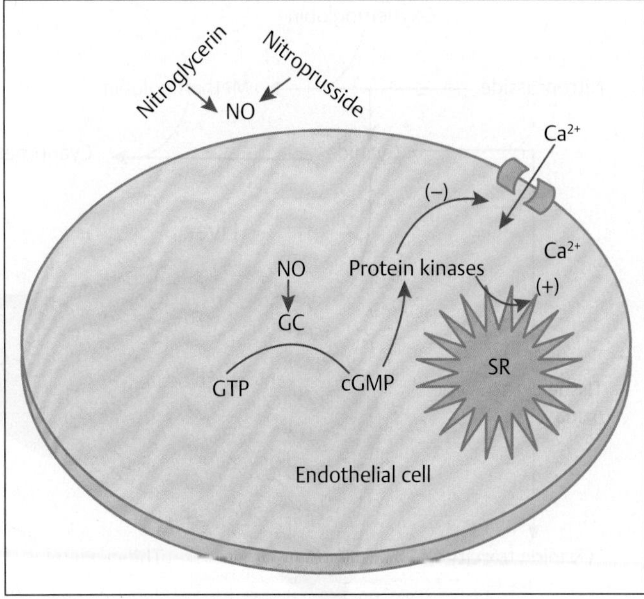

Fig. 26.4 Mechanism of sodium nitroprusside.

Adverse Effects

Hypotension

This is a common side effect.

Cyanide and Thiocyanate Poisoning

This is due to conversion of sodium nitroprusside to cyanide and thiocyanate. Usual manifestations include abdominal pain, mental changes, lactic acidosis, and convulsions.

Treatment of Cyanide Poisoning

Cyanide poisoning can be treated by either of the following:

1. If the diagnosis is definite, then dicobalt edetate is the treatment of choice. Dicobalt acetate, after combining with cyanide, forms a nontoxic stable complex (**Fig. 26.5**).
2. Sodium nitrite converts hemoglobin (Hb) to methemoglobin (MetHb), which is capable of taking cyanide due to ferric ion and forms the cyanMetHb. This is followed by sodium thiosulfate that converts the cyanide to thiocyanate, which is excreted in urine. Amyl nitrite inhalation can also be used. Oxygen should also be administered.

Both the nitrates and nitrites can convert Hb to MetHb. However, nitrates cause hypotension due to profound vasodilatation but no hypotension occurs in the dose used for cyanide poisoning with nitrite. Hence, it is preferred for this purpose. When the diagnosis is not certain, the use of thiosulfate with oxygen is a safe method of treatment. Methylene blue in usual doses can be administered for the treatment of cyanide poisoning.

The metabolism of cyanide and thiocyanate depends on sulfur-containing substances in the body such as thiosulfate. Hence, the exogenous administration of sodium thiosulfate together with sodium nitroprusside enhances the metabolism of cyanide and thiocyanate. This can prevent their accumulation, thus preventing such toxicity in patients in whom the rate of infusion was higher or the drug was administered for prolonged period. It is important to note that efficacy of sodium nitroprusside remains unaffected with the simultaneous use of sodium thiosulfate.

Drug Therapy of Hypertension

Goals of Therapy

The aim of treatment is to decrease morbidity and mortality, and in this context, there is immediate goal and long-term goal.

Immediate Goal

It is to control the BP, both the systolic and diastolic, and maintain it within the normal range. This should be achieved with minimum possible drugs and in the lowest possible dose without causing hypotension and thus maintaining the quality of life.

Long-Term Goal

To prevent complications, which could be:

1. Immediate life-threatening ones, such as MI and stroke.
2. Damage to other target organs such as the heart. This could lead to LVH, angina, arteriosclerotic peripheral vascular disease, dissecting aneurysm, retinopathy, and nephropathy, and these ultimately increase mortality.

Besides drug treatment, the risk factor must be controlled and, in this context, several nonpharmacological measures should be undertaken, as discussed in the following.

Nonpharmacological Treatment

1. Decrease in body weight if overweight.
2. Salt restriction.
3. Exercise/physical activity.
4. Reduction of daily consumption of alcohol.
5. Intake of fruits and vegetables.
6. Management of stress and anxiety.

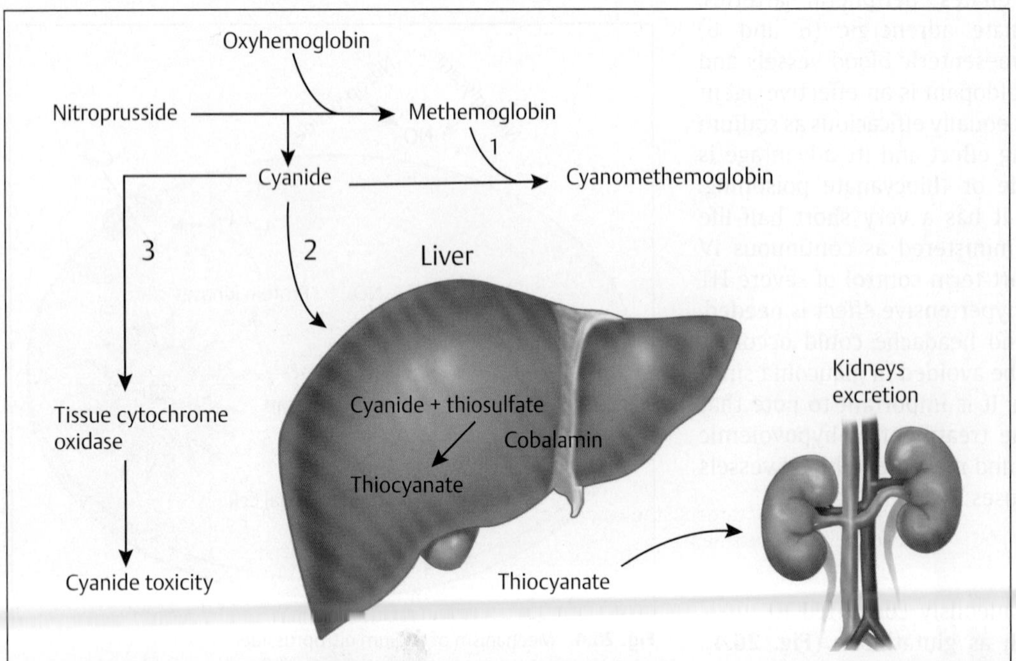

Fig. 26.5 Metabolism of sodium nitroprusside.

7. Others:
   a. Avoid tobacco.
   b. Increase dietary fibers.

Principles of Drug Therapy

Presently, there are four important groups of antihypertensive drugs that are utilized for the routine treatment of essential HT. On the basis of several studies/clinical trials, it has been demonstrated that all are equally efficacious in controlling BP and hence the choice depends on other factors, which comprise patient factors such as age, physiological condition (pregnancy), and associated disease, etc. The different classes of drugs include β-blockers, CCBs, ACEIs, and angiotensin receptor blocker (ARB). There is another group that is equally effective and their use at present has been reduced to a single group treatment and these are the thiazide group of diuretics. Considering this also, there are five classes if single-drug therapy is prescribed.

Stage I Hypertension

Single-drug treatment is recommended from any of the five groups. Thiazide is appropriate for most of the patients; however, β-blockers, ACEIs, ARBs, and CCBs may also be administered.

The treatment must be initiated with lowest possible dose (initial dose) and then increased gradually. BP must be monitored to titrate the dose and finalize the dose required for maintenance. The algorithm for the management of HT is depicted in **Fig. 26.6**.

Stage II Hypertension

Initiate treatment with two antihypertensive drugs that act by different mechanisms or from different groups, for example, thiazide and vasodilator. For inadequate response, increase the dose of individual drug one by one. If the desired response is not achieved by adjusting the dose, then change one of the drugs.

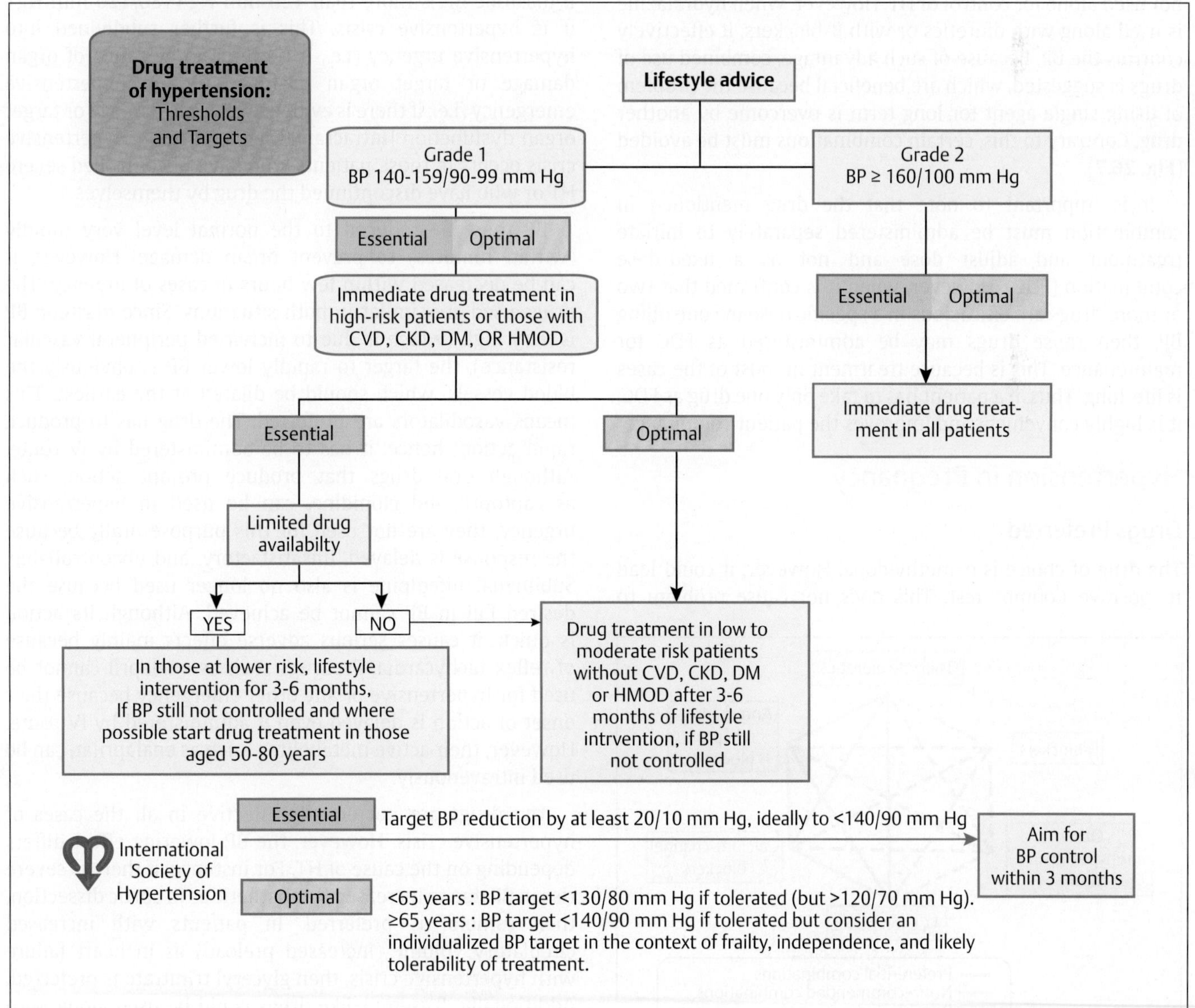

Fig. 26.6 Management algorithm for hypertension. CVD, cardiovascular disease; CKD, chronic kidney disease; DM, diabetes mellitus; HMOD, hypertension-mediated organ damage.

Studies have demonstrated that at stage I, majority of the patients (about two-thirds) are controlled with a single drug. In stage II, generally two drugs control the BP. However, in certain cases, in spite of using the maximum dose of two drugs, BP is not controlled. These patients then require a third drug to be added.

Those patients in whom BP is not controlled in spite of using three drugs (including one diuretic) in maximum doses are categorized as "resistant HT."

Combined Use of Drugs in Hypertension

When there is HT and a drug is used alone to control BP, frequently several compensatory mechanisms try to overcome the effect of the drug, leading to loss of antihypertensive effect. When direct vasodilator such as hydralazine is used singly over long term, there is compensatory increase in retention of sodium and water. This increases the circulatory volume. Additionally, there is tachycardia and there is increased renin activity. All these effects lead to loss of therapeutic effect. Hence, hydralazine is not used alone for control of HT. However, when hydralazine is used along with diuretics or with β-blockers, it effectively controls the BP. Because of such advantage, combined use of drugs is suggested, which are beneficial because the problem of using single agent for long term is overcome by another drug. Contrary to this, certain combinations must be avoided (**Fig. 26.7**).

It is important to note that the drug mentioned in combination must be administered separately to initiate treatment and adjust dose and not as a fixed-dose combination (FDC). However, when it is confirmed that two or more drugs are efficacious in a specific dose in controlling BP, then those drugs may be administered as FDC for maintenance. This is because treatment in most of the cases is life-long. Thus, if a patient has to take only one drug as FDC, it is highly convenient and improves the patient compliance.

Hypertension in Pregnancy

Drugs Preferred

The drug of choice is α-methyldopa. However, it could lead to positive Coombs test. This does not cause problem to the fetus. The drug preferred in emergency is hydralazine administered by IV route. The other useful drugs are: cardioselective β-blocker atenolol, metoprolol, acebutolol, and labetalol (α- + β-blocker). These could be used when the above-mentioned drugs cannot be used due to any valid reason. DHP and CCBs (nifedipine) could be administered; however, CCBs possess uterine relaxant action. Hence, CCBs must be discontinued before the labor. Magnesium sulfate is used for eclampsia.

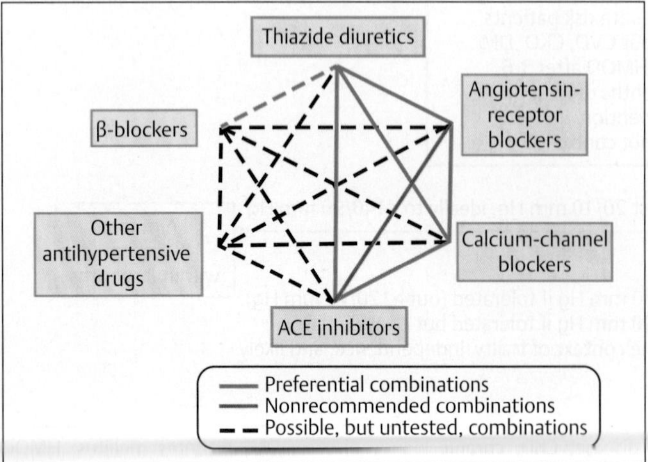

Fig. 26.7 Combinations of antihypertensives.

Drugs Contraindicated

All other drugs should be avoided, that is, ACEIs, ARBs, and diuretics are contraindicated. ACEIs could lead to oligohydramnios, growth retardation, renal and pulmonary abnormalities, and risk of fetal damage. Diuretics, by decreasing the circulatory volume, alter the uteroplacental perfusion, causing fetal damage and damage to placenta, and this may lead to abortion and stillbirth.

Hypertensive Crisis

If diastolic BP is more than 120 mm Hg (180/120 mm Hg), it is hypertensive crisis. This is further subdivided into hypertensive urgency (i.e., if there is no evidence of organ damage or target organ dysfunction) and hypertensive emergency (i.e., if there is evidence of organ damage or target organ dysfunction [intracranial hemorrhage]). Hypertensive crisis occurs in those patients who have uncontrolled severe HT or who have discontinued the drug by themselves.

BP must be reduced to the normal level very rapidly (within minutes) to prevent organ damage. However, it can be decreased within few hours in cases of urgency. The drugs used are similar in both situations. Since diastolic BP is very high (which is due to increased peripheral vascular resistance), the target to rapidly lower BP is obviously the blood vessels, which should be dilated at the earliest. This means vasodilators are preferred. The drug has to produce rapid action; hence, it has to be administered by IV route. Although oral drugs that produce prompt action, such as captopril and clonidine, can be used in hypertensive urgency, they are not used for this purpose orally because the response is delayed, unsatisfactory, and uncontrollable. Sublingual nifedipine is also no longer used because the desired fall in BP cannot be achieved. Although its action is quick, it causes serious adverse effects mainly because of reflex tachycardia. Prodrugs such as enalapril cannot be used for hypertensive or any other emergency because their onset of action is delayed even if administered by IV route. However, their active metabolites, such as enalaprilat, can be used intravenously.

The drugs are not equally effective in all the cases of hypertensive crisis. However, the BP-lowering effect differs depending on the cause of HT. For instance, if there is severe rise in BP due to increased sympathetic as in aortic dissection, then esmolol is preferred. In patients with increased circulatory volume (increased preload) as in heart failure with hypertensive crisis, then glyceryl trinitrate is preferred. Additionally, frusemidelike drugs could be used along with other vasodilators to prevent volume expansion. Sodium nitroprusside may be administered with all these drugs, if required. The BP must be decreased by approximately 25% of its initial value and diastolic BP should not be lowered beyond 110 to 100 mm Hg. Subsequent reduction of BP could be achieved over a period of several weeks by appropriate oral medication. The drugs used commonly for hypertensive crisis are discussed in details in Chapters 21 to 26 and in the section Vasodilators earlier in this chapter. However, the relevant aspect regarding their use in hypertensive crisis is discussed briefly in the following.

Direct Vasodilators (See Above)

Refer to Interactions section under Calcium Channel Blockers.

IV Infusion

Sodium Nitroprusside

It rapidly (immediate onset) reduces the BP. It is the drug of choice to treat hypertensive crisis since it is both venodilator and arteriolar dilator, it acts within few minutes, desired effect is achieved by adjusting the rate of infusion, response is predictable, and effect is over whenever infusion is discontinued.

Glyceryl Trinitrate

It has a significant venodilator action and hence is preferred when preload reduction is desired, for example, in patients with acute LVF, MI, and post cardiac surgery. A drawback is the development of tolerance within 24 hours of regular use.

Fenoldopam

It is administered as continuous IV infusion for short-term control of severe HT. However, it must be avoided in patients with glaucoma since it raises intraocular tension.

IV Bolus

Diazoxide

It is a direct vasodilator and is preferred in situations where there is no facility for IV infusion. With the use of bolus dose, the BP is reduced in half a minute and the peak effect is observed in 4 to 5 minutes. It may also be administered as IV infusion.

Enalaprilat

It is an active ACEI and can be administered in hypertensive emergency associated with acute LVF since it decreases both the preload and afterload.

Sympatholytic Drugs

β-Blockers (Esmolol)

It is an ultrashort-acting ($t_{1/2}$ of 8 minutes) β-blocker. Its onset of action is in 5 to 10 minutes and the effect lasts for about 20 minutes. It is preferred when there is increased sympathetic activity in situations such as aortic dissection and perioperative and postoperative HT. Its disadvantage is bradycardia.

α-Blockers (Phentolamine)

It is administered to rapidly reduce BP. However, it is preferred in hypertensive emergency caused due to pheochromocytoma or cheese reaction or because of abrupt clonidine withdrawal. Phentolamine is short acting (10 minutes) and is repeated as per requirement.

α- + β-Blockers (Labetalol)

It is preferred in patients with severe (malignant) HT, for example, pheochromocytoma.

Central Sympatholytic

Clonidine is particularly beneficial if hypertensive crisis occurs because of abrupt discontinuation of clonidine itself.

Others

Frusemide

It can facilitate the action of other above-mentioned drugs to decrease the BP. It reduces the circulatory volume, which could have increased in certain patients with heart failure including pulmonary edema. However, precaution is required to prevent hypovolemia.

Pulmonary Hypertension

Contrary to systemic HT, pulmonary HT associated with other diseases is more common than idiopathic cases except in premature newborn.

Causes

1. Raynaud's disease.
2. Endothelial dysfunction; this may also lead to pulmonary artery emboli
3. Hypoxemia due to any reason.
4. Familial (familial primary pulmonary HT).
5. Drug induced, for example, dexfenfluramine.
6. Occluded pulmonary arteries due to emboli or in sickle cell disease.

Treatment

As most of the cases are secondary to certain diseases, the treatment is primarily the treatment of cause except in idiopathic cases. Symptomatic improvement occurs from administration of anticoagulant, oxygen, digoxin, and diuretics. Vasodilators are effective. However, vasodilators with additional action such as those that antagonize the endothelins to facilitate actions of nitric oxide or with antiproliferative action are more beneficial and are thus preferred, for example, epoprostenol, as compared with drugs with only vasodilator action such as nifedipine.

Following drugs are also beneficial:

1. Prostaglandin (PG) analogues: Epoprostenol is a PG analogue that leads to vasodilatation and also possesses antiproliferative action. Iloprost by inhalation is another alternative.
2. Bosentan: It is nonselective endothelin antagonist used orally. It is hepatotoxic; hence, liver function test is important while the patient is being treated.
3. Nitric oxide: It is administered for primary pulmonary HT in newborn by inhalation.
4. Sildenafil: It acts by potentiating the action of nitric oxide due to inhibition of phosphodiesterase.
5. Pulmonary surfactant: Beractant and poractant are derivatives of physiological pulmonary surfactant, which prevent

the collapse of alveoli. They can directly be administered to tracheobronchial tree through endotracheal intubation for the treatment of pulmonary HT in newborn.

Failure of Antihypertensive Treatment

It has been observed that despite the best treatment, there is failure of antihypertensive therapy or BP is not optimally controlled as desired. In such situations, the cause of failure must be evaluated and managed accordingly. However, some of the causes of failure of antihypertensive treatment are as follows:

1. Improper diagnosis.
2. Improper selection of drug, dose, and duration for onset of antihypertensive effect, for example, antihypertensive effect of β-blocker is delayed.
3. Inadequate patient compliance.
4. Risk factors not changed, for example, salt restriction, alcohol, diet, weight reduction, exercise, etc.
5. Combination of drugs in which one drug could decrease/block the antihypertensive effect of the other drug, for example, effect of clonidine is blocked by prazosin. Drug combination where synergistic effect is not obtained; if two drugs with the same mechanism are administered, then synergistic effect will not occur.
6. Drugs that enhance circulatory volume, for example, use of vasodilator alone for long term.
7. Concurrent administration of other group of drugs that increase the BP.
8. Concurrent administration of corticosteroids, NSAIDs, and other drugs that raise the circulatory volume.
9. Drug interaction antagonizing the action of several antihypertensive agents.

Multiple Choice Questions

1. The antihypertensive action of which of the following drugs is due, in part, to diminished degradation of bradykinin?

A. Enalapril.
B. Losartan.
C. Aliskiren.
D. Fludrocortisone.
E. Furosemide.

Answer: A

Inhibition of ACE reduces not only the formation of the active metabolite angiotensin II, but also the proteolytic breakdown of the potent vasodilator. This contributes significantly to the antihypertensive action of ACEIs. The remaining drugs do not alter bradykinin metabolism.

2. A 54-year-old woman is diagnosed with congestive heart failure (CHF). You prescribe captopril, a medication proven to reduce her mortality. This agent delivers several benefits to patients with CHF. Which of the following effects is caused by this drug?

A. It has a high affinity for angiotensin II receptors.
B. It promotes increased peripheral vascular resistance.
C. It decreases cardiac output and increases afterload.
D. It causes venodilation and induces natriuresis.
E. It increases preload.

Answer: D

ACEIs cause venodilation and induce natriuresis, thereby reducing preload. A high affinity for angiotensin II receptors represents the mechanism of action of angiotensin receptor blockers. ACEIs counteract increased peripheral resistance, increase cardiac output, and decrease afterload.

3. A prediabetic 52-year-old woman with chronic obstructive pulmonary disease (COPD), hypertension, and 2+ protein urea is being treated with losartan. She complains that she has had a rash and a mild itching since she started losartan. Which of the following drugs would inhibit renin–angiotensin–aldosterone system (RAAS) and be most suitable for this patient?

A. Captopril.
B. Enalapril.
C. Aliskiren.
D. Eplerenone.
E. Spironolactone.

Answer: C

Inhibition of RAAS has been shown to slow the progression of kidney damage in type 2 diabetes. Since the patient has COPD, ACEIs would be contraindicated because of the potential to worsen cough. She has demonstrated a sensitivity to an ARB; she is likely to have a sensitivity to other ARBs. Aliskiren is a small-molecule inhibitor of renin.

4. A 40-year-old woman was being treated for chronic moderate hypertension. When she went on a vacation and forgot her pills, her blood pressure rose markedly and she was admitted to the emergency service with blurred vision, severe headache, and retinal hemorrhages. A drug that is most likely to be followed by rebound hypertension if stopped suddenly is:

A. Atenolol.
B. Clonidine.
C. Labetalol.
D. Losartan.
E. Prazosin.

Answer: B

Of the drugs listed, only clonidine, an α_2-agonist, is associated with severe rebound hypertension if stopped suddenly. It is speculated that this effect is due to downregulation of α_2-receptors.

5. A 32-year-old woman with hypertension wishes to become pregnant. Her physician informs her that she will have to switch to another antihypertensive drug. Which of the following drugs is recommended?

A. Atenolol.
B. Captopril.
C. Methyldopa.
D. Prazosin.
E. Propranolol.

Answer: C

Methyldopa is often recommended in pregnant patients because it has a good safety record.

6. A 16-year-old boy is brought to the hospital by ambulance with serious head injuries following a car accident. His blood pressure is 220/170 mm Hg. Fundoscopy reveals retinal damage, and you administer nitroprusside via infusion. Control of the hypertension requires 72 hours and you notice the patient becoming increasingly fatigued and nauseous. The mostly likely cause of these symptoms is:

A. Production of thiocyanate from nitroprusside.
B. Negative inotropic activity of nitroprusside.
C. Renal precipitation of nitroprusside.
D. Accumulation of nitroprusside because of its long half-life.
E. Production of hydroxocobalamin.

Answer: A

The toxicity of nitroprusside is caused by the release of cyanide and the accumulation of thiocyanate.

7. A 75-year-old woman, who is admitted for the management of her recent stroke, develops increased blood pressure, up to 195/105, with a heart rate of 95. Her physician is worried about the possibility of cerebral hemorrhage into the preexisting infarct and decides to administer a fast-acting vasodilating agent, which is also commonly used for severe decompensated congestive heart failure (CHF). Which medication did the doctor use?

A. Nitroprusside.
B. Furosemide.
C. Dobutamine.
D. Losartan.
E. Digoxin.

Answer: A

Nitroprusside is a vasodilating agent that can be used in hypertensive emergencies.

8. Which of the following drugs is genetically associated with slower metabolism in European Americans and African Americans than in most Asians?

A. Cimetidine.
B. Hydralazine.
C. Propranolol.
D. Rifampin.
E. Succinylcholine.

Answer: B

Hydralazine, such as procainamide and isoniazid, is metabolized by *N*-acetylation, an enzymatic process that is slow in about 20% of Asians and in about 50% of European Americans and African Americans.

9. The antihypertensive drug that causes decreased libido and impotence is:

A. Atenolol.
B. Enalapril.
C. Prazosin.
D. Diltiazem.

Answer: A

Diuretics have maximum risk of causing sexual dysfunction followed by β-blockers. Atenolol, metoprolol, and carvedilol have high risk, whereas nebivolol has minimum risk of erectile dysfunction. ACEIs decrease the risk.

10. Which of the following statements about diazoxide is false?

A. It acts by causing prolonged opening of ATP-dependent K channels in β-cells.
B. It can cause severe hypoglycemia.
C. It can be used to treat patients with insulinoma.
D. It is used as an antihypertensive agent.

Answer: B

It can cause severe hypoglycemia. Diazoxide cause hyperglycemia and not hypoglycemia. Diazoxide is an effective and relatively long-acting parenterally administered arteriolar dilator that is occasionally used to treat hypertensive emergencies. It acts by opening ATP-sensitive potassium channels. The most significant toxicity from diazoxide has been excessive hypotension. Diazoxide inhibits insulin release from the pancreas (probably by opening potassium channels in the cell membrane) and is used to treat hypoglycemia secondary to insulinoma. Occasionally, hyperglycemia complicates diazoxide use, particularly in persons with renal insufficiency.

11. α-Methyldopa is primarily used for:

A. Pregnancy-induced hypertension.
B. Renovascular hypertension.
C. First-line agent in hypertension.
D. Refractory hypertension.

Answer: A

α-Methyldopa was widely used in the past but is now used primarily for hypertension in pregnancy.

Chapter 27 Pharmacotherapy of Shock

D. Thamizh Vani and Dipti Sonawane

PH1.27: Describe the mechanisms of action, types, doses, side effects, indications, and contraindications of antihypertensive drugs and drugs used in shock.

Learning Objectives

- General principles in management of shock.
- Management of hypovolemic shock.
- Management of cardiogenic shock.
- Management of septic shock.
- Management of anaphylactic shock.
- Management of neurogenic shock.

Shock

Shock (circulatory failure) is a clinical syndrome characterized by inadequate or poor perfusion of tissues, with a relatively or absolutely not sufficient cardiac output. There is an impairment of supply of oxygen and nutrients to the critical body organs such as brain, heart, liver, kidneys, and also the gastrointestinal tract (GIT), which is immediately life-threatening. It is usually associated with acute decrease in effective circulating blood volume (hypotension). The oxygen perfusion in shock fails to meet the metabolic demands of tissues. The result is regional hypoxia, which leads to lactic acidosis in peripheral tissues due to anaerobic metabolism. Ultimately, it leads to multiorgan failure. In case of uncompensated shock, the end result of these mechanisms may involve impaired cellular metabolism, production and release of damage-associated molecular patterns (DAMPS), and death. A recent study on shock has shown an increased permeability of GI mucosa to enzymes of pancreas, which play a role in microvascular inflammation and failure of organs.

The term shock is also used in a condition where there is a usually benign and transient vasovagal attack, which is a result of sudden decrease of venous return to the heart caused by neurogenic vasodilatation and subsequent peripheral pooling of blood. This occurrence is seen immediately following severe pain, trauma, or an emotional overreaction due to fear, sorrow, or surprise. It lasts for few minutes or seconds, and the patient experiences brief unconsciousness, sinking sensation, weakness, clammy and pale hands and feet, rapid and weak pulse, and low blood pressure.

Classification of Shock

Circulatory shock may be classified as:

Hypovolemic Shock

This occurs due to loss of blood or dehydration. It is also known as cold shock. The causes are internal or external hemorrhage, loss of fluids and electrolytes due to excessive vomiting or diarrhea, loss of plasma due to burns, fluid loss in diabetes mellitus, diabetes insipidus, or excessive use of diuretics.

Cardiogenic Shock

The pumping ability of the heart is decreased because of some abnormality in heart such as myocardial infarction, cardiac arrhythmias, congestive heart failure, or mechanical defects such as severe valvular dysfunctions.

Septic Shock

It is a type of distributive shock in which abnormal distribution of blood flow in the smallest blood vessel results in inadequate supply of blood to organs and tissues. It results secondary to bacteremia where bacteria multiply, circulate in blood, and release toxic products. It is associated with marked vasodilation due to peripheral arteriolar paralysis and is also called warm shock. Gram-negative bacteria release endotoxins which produce shock due to marked vasodilation, reducing peripheral resistance, depressing myocardial contractility, and increasing capillary permeability.

Anaphylactic Shock

This occurs due to severe allergic hypersensitivity reaction. Large quantities of histamine and histamine-like substances are released which manifests as marked vasodilation, increased capillary permeability, exudation of fluid, angioneurotic edema, and bronchoconstriction. It occurs in conditions such as bee or wasp sting, and exposure or ingestion of allergens such as pollen, chemicals, or drugs.

Neurogenic Shock

This occurs due to marked reduction in sympathetic vasomotor tone and pronounced increase in vagal tone, producing vasodilation, hypotension, bradycardia, and syncope. The causes are traumatic spinal cord injury or adverse event during epidural or spinal anesthesia.

Obstructive Shock

There is impairment of ventricular filling during diastole phase due to some external pressure on heart. The causes are cardiac tamponade, tension pneumothorax, constrictive pericarditis, and pulmonary embolism.

Septic shock, anaphylactic shock, and neurogenic shock are also called low-resistance or vasogenic or distributive shock due to vasodilation and decrease in cardiac output. Blood volume may be normal.

Compensatory mechanisms are immediately set into motion, and they try to maintain blood flow. These are as follows:

1. Baroreceptor reflex—Hypotension results in decrease in discharge from arterial baroreceptors and leads to vasoconstriction.
2. Chemoreceptor reflex—Hypoxia and acidosis stimulate chemoreceptors, which excite vasomotor center and produce vasoconstriction.
3. Ischemic response by central nervous system (CNS) causes powerful sympathetic stimulation.

Regardless of cause, marked activation of sympathetic system occurs due to fall in blood pressure. This causes increase in rate and force of cardiac contraction and peripheral vasoconstriction. These may maintain cerebral blood flow and blood pressure in the initial stages. Blood flow to other organs may be decreased. This subsequently leads to impaired urine production and metabolic acidosis.

Symptoms and sign in shock due to compensatory mechanisms are as follows:

- Pale, cold, moist skin, increased sweating.
- Cyanotic tinge of skin.
- Tachycardia, and fall in blood pressure produces thin, thread pulse.
- Increased rate and force of respiration.
- Oliguria.
- Restlessness and apprehension.

The central venous pressure is reduced in hypovolemic and anaphylactic shock and elevated in cardiogenic shock. It is unpredictable in neurogenic or septic shock. This important distinction is quite helpful when physical signs are confusing.

When shock is in progressive stage and not treated adequately, a vicious cycle of positive feedback mechanisms set in and passes into refractory shock where all therapeutic interventions are ineffective.

General Principles in Management of Shock

Treatment of shock consists of efforts to correct hemodynamic abnormalities and reverse underlying pathogenesis. Initial therapy of shock involves basic life support measures. The initial management in shock involves volume replacement. Maintaining blood volume is essential and monitoring of hemodynamic parameters should be done. If shock is caused by hemorrhage, best possible treatment is whole blood transfusion. If a person is in shock due to loss of plasma, administration of plasma is the best therapy. When cause of shock is dehydration, administration of appropriate electrolyte solution can correct it. Normal hematocrit cannot be restored by plasma, but human body can stand a decrease in hematocrit to about half of normal before consequences are serious. Therefore, it is reasonable to use plasma in emergency conditions. Plasma substitutes such as dextran can be used if plasma is unavailable. Hypovolemia should be corrected by administration of intravenous (IV) fluids. If adequate response is not obtained by these measures, vasoactive drugs should be used to improve blood pressure and flow.

Sympathomimetic drugs have proven to be especially beneficial in neurogenic shock, where sympathetic nervous system is severely depressed, and in anaphylactic shock, where excess prominent role is played by excess histamine. The vasodilating effect of histamine is opposed by sympathomimetic drugs and is considered lifesaving. β-receptor agonists increase heart rate and force of contraction, and α-receptor agonists increase peripheral vascular resistance.

Head-down position is the first essential step in the treatment of many types of shock, especially in hemorrhagic and neurogenic shock. Patient should be placed with their head at least 12 inches lower than their feet. This helps in promoting venous return and increasing cardiac output.

Treatment with Glucocorticoids

Glucocorticoids are given to patients in severe shock for many reasons. Experiments have shown that glucocorticoids frequently increase the strength of the heart in the late stages. They stabilize lysosomes in tissue cells and prevent release of lysosomal enzymes into the cytoplasm. This prevents deterioration usually caused by them. The metabolism of glucose by severely damaged cells is aided by glucocorticoids.

Management of Hypovolemic Shock

Immediate whole blood transfusion or blood substitutes such as group O negative or group specific packed red blood cells (RBC) should be given. Rapid infusion of isotonic saline or Ringer lactate through large bore IV lines is required for severe dehydration. In traumatic brain injury patients, use of hypertonic saline and dextran increases the survival rate.

Dopamine may be needed as inotropic support after fluid replacement for adequate ventricular performance. Dopamine infusion (2–3 μg/kg/min) acts on renal (D1) and cardiac b1 receptors, and increases cardiac contractility, rate and glomerular filtration. It promotes dilation of splanchnic and renal vascular beds. Phenylephrine can be used alternatively to dopamine in patients who are at risk of tachyarrhythmias. Use of phenoxybenzamine, an α blocker, intravenously can help to counteract vasoconstriction, and shift blood from pulmonary to systemic circulation and from extravascular to vascular compartment. This helps to improve cardiac output.

Use of vasopressors such as norepinephrine is not recommended, as circulating catecholamines are already accompanied by strong reflex vasoconstriction.

Supplemental oxygen should be provided to support respiratory functions.

Crystalloids

Crystalloid solutions are isotonic to plasma and contain electrolytes. These solutions do not alter chemical balance and increase circulatory volume. Sodium chloride 0.9% is the most commonly used. Other solutions are Ringer lactate and Hartmann's and glucose solutions. Crystalloids need to be administered in larger volumes than colloid. Only one-third infused stays in intravascular space and two-thirds move into tissues. This causes side effects such as peripheral and pulmonary edema. Excess infusion of sodium chloride 0.9% can lead to renal dysfunction and reduced glomerular filtration rate (GFR) due to hypochloremic acidosis by its high chloride content. Normal saline with 5% glucose is used as maintenance fluid. Its main function involves replacing lost water and not restoring intravascular volume.

Plasma Expanders (PH1.25)

They exert colloidal osmotic or oncotic pressure, characterized by high molecular weight, and retain fluid in the vascular compartment when infused intravenously.

A plasma expander should:

1. Exert oncotic pressure similar to plasma.
2. Remain in circulation without leaking or should not be disposed rapidly.
3. Should not cause allergy or fever.
4. Should be pharmacodynamically inert.
5. Should be stable.
6. Easily sterilizable and cheap.
7. Should not interfere with blood grouping or cross-matching.

Plasma expanders are primarily used as substitutes of plasma in conditions such as acute phase burns, hypovolemic and endotoxic shock, extensive tissue damage, and severe trauma. They can be used temporarily till whole blood is arranged. In burns, only albumin can be used for maintenance of fluid volume. Other plasma expanders cannot be used, as proteins also leak out with fluids for several days.

Colloids

Colloids are gelatinous solution that maintain high-osmotic pressure and are too large to pass capillary membranes. So, colloids stay longer in intravascular spaces compared to crystalloids. They are used to correct low blood volume due to loss of blood or plasma. Human plasma or reconstituted albumin is used. Albumin is expensive while plasma carries risk of transmitting AIDS and hepatitis. Therefore, synthetic colloids are often used.

Human Albumin

They are obtained from pooled human plasma and do not interfere with blood group or coagulation. Albumin preparation is heat treated; therefore, it does not transmit hepatitis or AIDS. A total of 100 mL of 20% albumin is equivalent in osmolarity to 400 mL fresh frozen plasma and 800 mL whole blood. Crystalloid solution must be infused for added benefit. Albumin is used in burns, hypovolemia, shock, hypoproteinemia, acute liver failure, dialysis, and also before cardiopulmonary bypass for diluting blood along with crystalloids.

Dextran

It is the most commonly used plasma expanders. It is a polysaccharide obtained from sugar beet. It is present in two forms–Dextran 70 (MW 70,000) and Dextran 40 (MW 40,000). Dextran 70 is more commonly used as 6% in dextrose or normal saline. Duration of action lasts more than 24 hours, and it is oxidized or excreted by glomerular filtration. Disadvantages are it may interfere with blood grouping or cross-matching, may trigger anaphylactic reaction, and may also interfere with coagulation prolonging bleeding time.

Dextran 40

It acts more rapidly than Dextran 70. It is used as 10% solution in dextrose/normal saline. It prevents RBC sludging by reducing blood viscosity, seen in shock, coating RBCs, and maintaining their electronegative charge. Duration of action is very short, as it is rapidly filtered by glomerulus and gets concentrated in tubule–obstruction may occur. Dose should not exceed 20 mL/kg in 24 hours. It is relatively cheap and can be stored for many years.

Polygeline (Degraded Gelatin Polymer)

It is a polypeptide with MW 30,000 and is similar to albumin. Duration of action is 12 hours, and it does not have disadvantages. It is more expansive than dextran. It is used for priming of dialysis and heart lung machines. Rigor, flushing, and urticaria may occur.

Hetastarch

It is a complex mixture of ethoxylated amylopectin of various sizes of average MW 4.5 lac. As much as 6% hetastarch exerts oncotic pressure similar to albumin. Duration of action lasts for more than 24 hours. No other drugs should be added to infusion, as it is incompatible with all drugs. It also accelerates erythrocyte sedimentation. This property has been used to improve harvesting of granulocytes. Adverse effects are fever, vomiting, itching, swelling of salivary glands, and mild chills. Anaphylactoid reactions may occur. Use in patients with preexisting renal dysfunction is avoided.

The contraindications to plasma expanders are severe anemia, cardiac failure, liver disease, pulmonary edema, and renal insufficiency. Plasma expanders do not have the capacity of carrying oxygen.

Management of Cardiogenic Shock

Therapy is aimed at improvement of peripheral blood flow. Definitive therapy, such as emergency cardiac catheterization, followed by surgical revascularization or angioplasty may be done. Mechanical left ventricular assist devices may also help to maintain coronary perfusion and cardiac output in patients with severely ill status. Smaller amount of fluid replacement is required in cardiogenic shock. In patients whose cardiac output is severely impaired, blood pressure begins to fall which, in turn, leads to vasoconstriction and activation of sympathetic outflow. This leads to increased peripheral vascular resistance and further fall in cardiac output. Medical intervention is required to optimize preload, myocardial contractility, and afterload. Drugs such as nitrates and diuretics reduce preload. Sympathomimetic drugs increase force of contraction of heart. Some drugs have disadvantages like isoproterenol, which increases myocardial oxygen demand and is a chronotropic agent. Norepinephrine increases peripheral resistance and epinephrine increases heart rate and predisposes to arrhythmias. Dopamine is an effective inotropic which causes mild increase in heart rate. It also promotes renal arterial dilation, which preserves renal function. After adequate fluid replacement, dopamine or dobutamine can be instituted. Dobutamine 2.5 µg/kg/min IV provides inotropic support. It increases contractility and decreases afterload, due to reflex reduction in sympathetic tone. Dopamine infusion (2–3 µg/kg/min) can also be used. Norepinephrine 2 to 4 µg/min is used in refractory cases without increase in systemic resistance. If systolic blood pressure cannot be maintained by up to 15 µg/min, increasing the dose much further is not beneficial.

Management of Septic Shock

Urgent measures are required to treat infection and provide hemodynamic and respiratory support. Due to associated capillary leak to extravascular space, large volumes are required for resuscitation. Empirical antibiotic treatment can be started with meropenem IV, or ticarcillin with clavulanic acid, until blood culture reports come in.

Continuous invasion of recombinant-activated protein C, drotrecogin alpha (activated) 24 µg/kg/h for 96 hours, improves mortality in severe septic shock with organ failure. Vasopressin is gaining widespread acceptance in treatment of septic shock. It causes peripheral vasoconstriction by acting on V1 receptors and reduces NO synthesis. It stimulates cortisol production and potentiates effects of catecholamines. Hydrocortisone 50 mg four times a day along with fludrocortisone 50 µg OD for 7 days decrease the formation of prostaglandins and NO and also reduce the dose of vasopressors. They also prevent adrenal insufficiency. Inotropes like adrenaline, dopamine, and dobutamine can also be used in certain patients.

Furosemide may be used to maintain proper urine output. Maintenance of blood glucose levels in normal range is also important.

Management of Anaphylactic Shock

Patient should be put in reclining position and oxygen at high-flow rate should be administered. Cardiopulmonary resuscitation should be done if required. Adrenaline along with supportive measures is the treatment of choice. Adrenaline is given 0.5 mg (0.5 mL of 1 in 1000 solution for adult, 0.3 mL for 6–12 years old child, 0.15 mL for up to 6 years) intramuscularly (IM). Repeat every 5 to 10 minutes till improvement is seen. Adrenaline causes bronchodilation and counteracts effects of histamine and other mediators released from basophils and mast cells. Adjuvants such as antihistamines and glucocorticoids are also used. H1 antihistaminic chlorpheniramine 10 to 20 mg IM/slow IV is given. Hydrocortisone sodium succinate 200 mg is added in severe or recurrent cases, followed by oral prednisolone for 3 days.

Management of Neurogenic Shock

Treatment is same as hypovolemic shock. Norepinephrine or phenylephrine can be given after fluid replacement to maintain arterial pressure and vascular resistance. If hypotension is very severe, vasoconstricting drugs are required to maintain adequate cerebral perfusion. α agonists such as norepinephrine, phenylephrine, midodrine, mephentermine, ephedrine, metaraminol, epinephrine, and methoxamine have been used for this purpose. This approach is helpful in patients after spinal anesthesia or trauma. Steroid treatment is given for spinal cord injury causing spinal shock and aimed at reducing the extent of paralysis. Methylprednisolone improves neurological outcomes, if administered within 8 hours, in a regimen of bolus 30 mg/kg over 15 minutes with maintenance of 5.4 mg/kg/h for 23 hours. There was significant improvement in motor outcomes.

Management of Shock in Pregnant Woman

Treatment differs in two important respects: first, normal physiologic changes occur in most organ systems during pregnancy; second, mother and fetus both are vulnerable. Therefore, obstetric critical care involves simultaneous assessment and management of mother and fetus who have different physiological profiles. For sedation, meperidine and fentanyl are commonly used. Critically ill patients require vasoactive drugs. Ephedrine is the drug of choice to treat hypotension in pregnant patients as it is known to increase blood pressure and uterine blood flow. Dobutamine, epinephrine, and norepinephrine adversely affect uterine blood flow and should be avoided.

Management of Shock in Pediatrics

Children in shock are at risk for both hypoglycemia and hypocalcemia. These conditions should be rapidly identified and corrected. For hypoglycemia, replacement with dextrose IV is done. The dose is 0.5 to 1 g/kg. Hypocalcemia is corrected by 10 to 20 mg/kg calcium chloride at a rate which does not exceed 100 mg/min.

Multiple Choice Questions

1. In pharmacological management of shock, the primary objective is:

A. Maintenance of adequate renal perfusion.
B. Maintenance of adequate central nervous system (CNS) perfusion.
C. Maintenance of adequate hepatic perfusion.

Answer: B

We must ensure adequate blood supply to vital organs such as brain and heart. Brain cannot tolerate hypoxia for more than 8 minutes; therefore, shock should be corrected, so that perfusion to brain occurs.

2. Which sympathomimetic drug given to a patient in cardiogenic shock promotes renal arterial dilatation?

A. Dopamine.
B. Epinephrine.
C. Isoproterenol.

Answer: A

Dopamine is an effective inotropic which causes less increase in heart rate. It also promotes renal arterial dilation, which preserves renal function. After adequate fluid replacement, dopamine or dobutamine can be instituted.

3. A patient presents to the emergency room with a history of ingestion of drug followed by swelling of eyelids, angioedema, and difficulty in breathing. What is the drug of choice to be administered?

A. Dobutamine.
B. Ephedrine.
C. Adrenaline.
D. Phentolamine.

Answer: C

Adrenaline along with supportive measures is the treatment of choice. Adrenaline causes bronchodilation and counteracts effects of histamine and other mediators released from basophils and mast cells.

4. A patient presented with hemorrhagic hypovolemic shock? What caution is required if dextran is used?

A. Electrolyte abnormalities.
B. Pancreatitis.
C. Inhibition of coagulation cascade.
D. Risk of infection.

Answer: C

Disadvantages are it may interfere with blood grouping or cross-matching, may trigger anaphylactic reaction, and also interfere with coagulation, prolonging bleeding time.

5. The rationale behind the use of dopamine as a treatment of shock in a 38-year-old driver who was thrown from the vehicle in an accident is:

A. Impermeability to blood–brain barrier (BBB).
B. Long duration of action.
C. Oral administration.
D. Potentiates hypotension.

Answer: A

Impermeability to BBB. No adverse effects to brain will occur, and it increases cardiac output, thereby improving blood flow.

6. A patient is diagnosed with septic shock. Which of these should be administered first in septic shock?

A. Corticosteroids to reduce inflammation.
B. Antibiotics to treat underlying infection.
C. Vasopressors to increase blood pressure.
D. Intravenous (IV) fluids to increase intravascular volume.

Answer: D

IV fluids to increase intravascular volume. Due to associated capillary leak to extravascular space, large volumes are required for resuscitation.

7. Which of the following statements concerning intravenous administration of 5% albumin is true?

A. For a short time, it remains intravascular, then it crosses into interstitial space.
B. For a short time, it remains intravascular, then it crosses into intracellular space.
C. All of it remains in intravascular space until it is eliminated from body.
D. All of it remains in interstitial space until it is eliminated from body.

Answer: A

The hemodilution lasts for a shorter time when albumin is administered to individuals with normal blood volume. Albumin is distributed throughout the extracellular compartments, more than 60% of the body albumin pool is located in the extravascular fluid compartment.

8. A patient presents to the ER with tachycardia and pale, clammy skin. He was diagnosed to be in a state of compensatory shock. Which of the following is least likely to aggravate an existing vasoconstrictive state?

A. Dopamine 15 µg/kg per minute.
B. Dobutamine 10 µg/kg per minute.
C. Norepinephrine 8 µg per minute.
D. Epinephrine 8 µg per minute.

Answer: B

Dobutamine acts on dopamine receptors as well as β_1 receptors and causes vasodilatation.

9. After onset of hypovolemic shock, what is the important goal of therapy at 24 hours in a patient which may improve mortality?

A. Normalization of heart rate and blood pressure.
B. Normalization of base deficit and urine output.
C. Normalization of body and skin temperature.
D. Ensuring 30% hematocrit.

Answer: B

This improvement proves that all organs are well-perfused and reversibility of shock has occurred.

10. A 54-year-old patient enters ER. ST elevation is noted with inferior myocardial infarction (MI). Systolic blood pressure is 70. Lungs are clear. What is the best therapy for shock?

A. Intravenous (IV) fluids.

B. Nitroglycerine.

C. Digoxin.

D. Diltiazem.

Answer: A

Patient needs a little fluid to fill the right side of his heart, since the lungs are clear. If lungs show crackles and signs of pulmonary edema, then fluid is contraindicated.

Chapter 28 Antiarrhythmic Drugs

Vivek Jain

PH1.30: Describe the mechanisms of action, types, doses, side effects, indications, and contraindications of the antiarrhythmics.

Learning Objectives

- Cardiac arrhythmias.
- Cardiac action potential.
- Classification of arrhythmia:
  - Class I drugs.
  - Class ID (miscellaneous).
  - Class II agents.
  - Class III agents.
  - Class IV agents.

Cardiac Arrhythmia

A healthy human heart always beats with its own rhythm, which originates from the autorhythmic fibers of the right atrium called sinoatrial (SA) node. For the patient and physician, the heart rhythm serves as an indicator of well-being and disease. When the heart rhythm is disrupted due to ischemia, sympathetic stimulation, myocardial scarring, inherited variation in ion channel or other genes, and ingestion of drugs that affect heart conduction, it may result in cardiac arrhythmia. The clinical signs of cardiac arrhythmia are strong or fast heartbeat (palpitations), fluttering, dizziness, drowsiness, shortness of breath, tiredness, lack of energy, major discomfort when exercising, near-fainting, fainting, and chest pain.

Cardiac Action Potential

The resting membrane potential of the myocardium is approximately −90 mV, which results from an unequal distribution of ions (high Na^+ outside, high K^+ inside). There are five phases of the cardiac action potential (AP) (**Fig. 28.1a, b**).

Phase 0 (Rapid Depolarization)

In this phase, rapid inward movement of Na^+ occurs due to the opening of voltage-gated sodium channels (Nav). This leads to variation in resting membrane potential from −90 to +15 mV.

Phase 1 (Initial Rapid Repolarization)

This phase leads to inactivation of sodium channels and influx of Cl^-.

Phase 2 (Plateau Phase)

In this phase, there is slow but prolonged opening of voltage-gated calcium channels; it brings about contraction.

Phase 3 (Repolarization)

In this phase, closure of calcium channels is initiated and K^+ efflux starts through potassium channels. In addition, inactivated sodium channels return to resting phase.

Phase 4 (Diastole)

This phase leads to restoration of ionic concentrations by Na^+/K^+-activated ATPase (adenosine triphosphatase) and, finally, restoration of resting potential.

Important Electrocardiographic Parameters

- P wave represents atrial depolarization.
- PR interval equals the delay of conduction through the atrioventricular (AV) node.
- QRS complex represents ventricular depolarization.
- T wave represents ventricular repolarization.
- QT interval equals duration of AP in the ventricles (**Fig. 28.1c**).

Classification of Arrhythmia

Automaticity is the property of cardiac cells to generate spontaneous APs. The SA node normally displays the highest intrinsic rate. All other pacemakers are referred to as subsidiary or latent pacemakers because they take over the function of initiating excitation of the heart only when the SA node is unable to generate impulses or when these impulses fail to propagate.

Abnormal automaticity includes both reduced automaticity, which causes bradycardia, and increased automaticity, which causes tachycardia. Arrhythmias caused by abnormal automaticity can result from diverse mechanisms.

Researchers have shown many schemes to classify the mechanisms of cardiac arrhythmias (**Fig. 28.2**). Conventionally, these have been divided into nonreentrant and reentrant activity. However, mechanism of arrhythmias can also be classified on the basis of its origin and occurrence at the cellular and tissue levels. Another classification, based on dynamics and focused on the trigger-tissue substrate interactions, divided arrhythmogenic mechanisms into reduced and excess along with unstable calcium cycling.

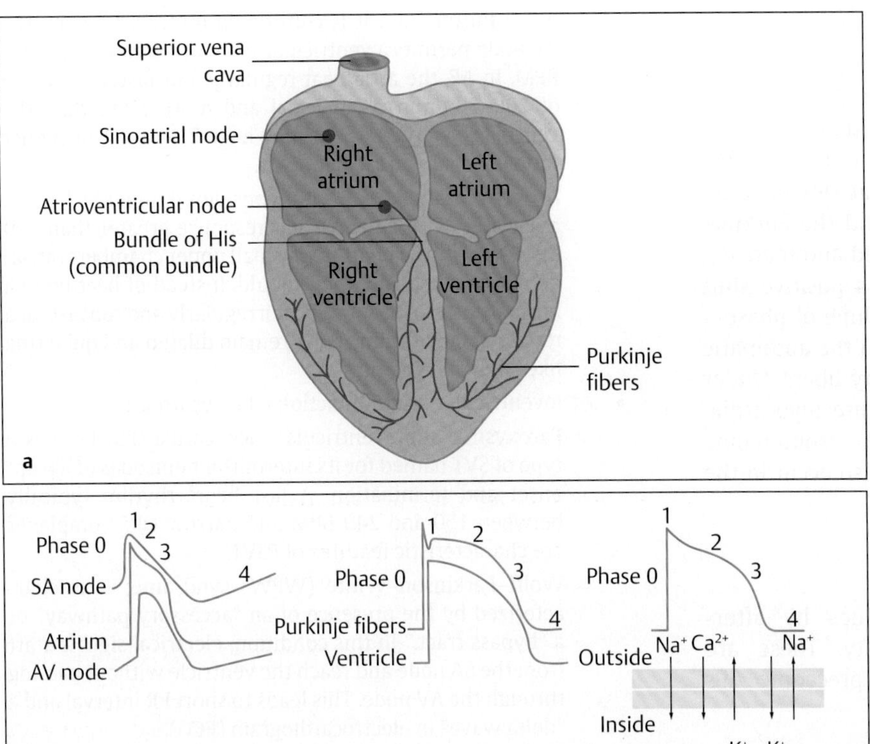

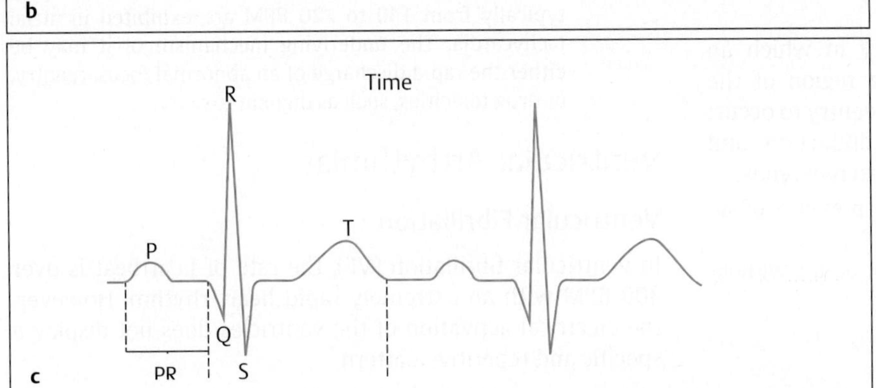

Fig. 28.1 **(a)** Normal cardiac conduction. **(b)** The cardiac activity in the sinoatrial (SA) node and the Purkinje fibers. **(c)** The normal ECG.

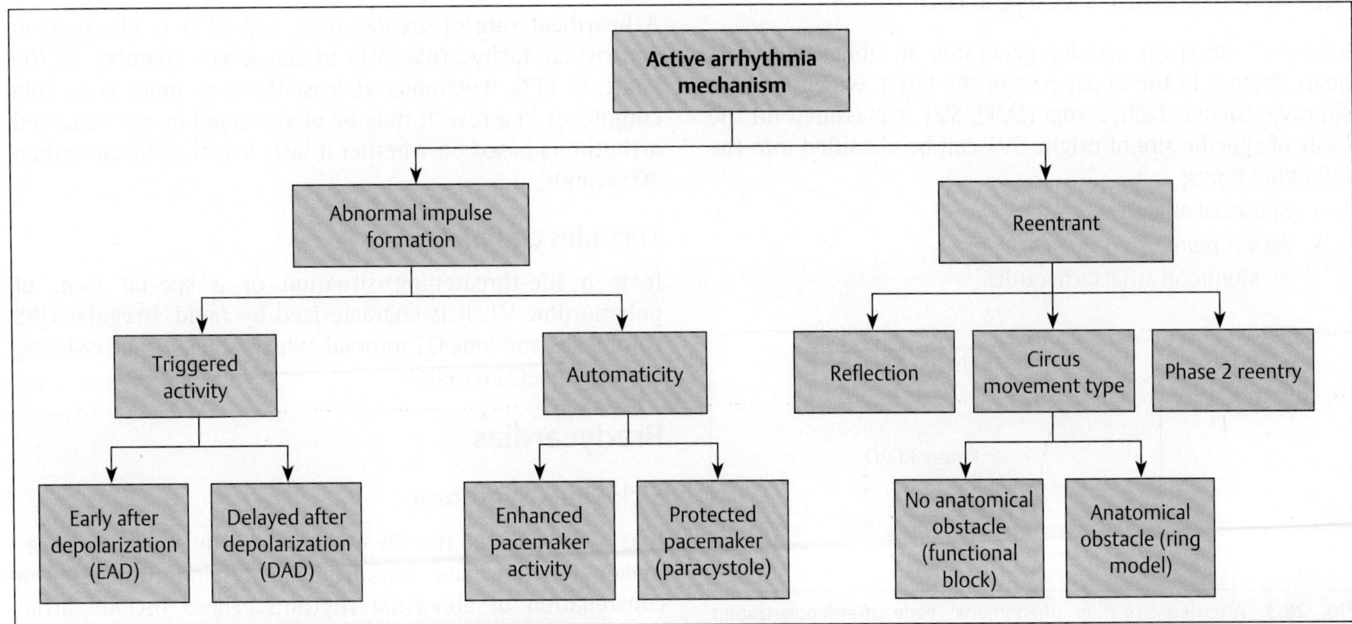

Fig. 28.2 Classification of mechanisms of cardiac arrhythmias.

Automaticity

Enhanced Automaticity

In the human heart, the normal rate of discharge of the SA node is between 60 and 100 beats per minute (BPM). However, subsidiary pacemakers discharge at slower rates. The AV node discharges at 40 to 60 BPM and the Purkinje fibers discharge at 20 to 40 BPM. In enhanced automaticity, a negative shift in the threshold potential, a positive shift in the maximum diastolic potential or the slope of phase 4 depolarization may increase pathologically in the automatic fibers or such activity may appear in ordinary fibers. Under the conditions of recent cardiac surgery, acute myocardial infarction (MI), digitalis toxicity, and isoprenaline administration, enhanced automaticity can also occur in the AV node.

Triggered Activity

The premature activation of cardiac tissues by after-depolarizations results in triggered activity. These are depolarizations triggered by one or more preceding APs (**Fig. 28.3**).

Reentry

Reentry is continuous circulating electricity in which an impulse reenters and repetitively excites a region of the heart. Three requirements are necessary for reentry to occur: (1) an abnormal electrical circuit; (2) slow conduction; and (3) unidirectional block. Reentry is divided into two types:

- Circus type: reentry that occurs in the presence of an obstacle, around which an AP can travel.
- Reflection or phase 2 reentry: reentry that occurs without an obstacle.

Types of Arrhythmia

Supraventricular Tachycardia

Improper electrical activity generates an abnormally fast heart rhythm in the upper part of the heart, which leads to supraventricular tachycardia (SVT). SVT is classified on the basis of specific site of origin. SVT can be classified into the following types:

- Sinoatrial origin.
- Atrial origin:
  - Multifocal atrial tachycardia.

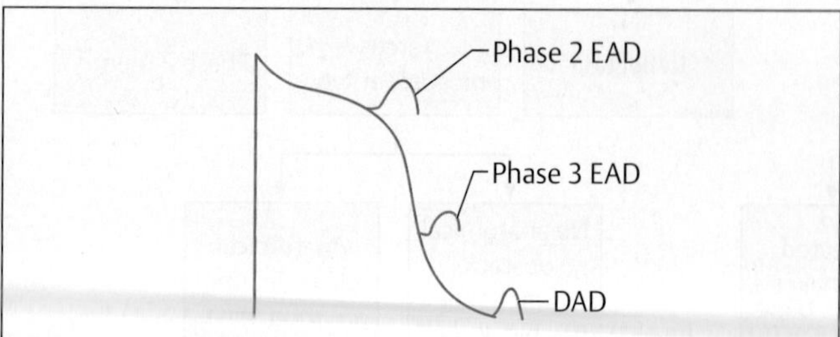

Fig. 28.3 Afterdepolarization phenomena: early afterdepolarization (EAD) occurs early (phase 2) or late (phase 3), and delayed after-depolarization (DAD) occurs during phase 4 of the action potential.

  - Atrial flutter (AF): It is considered under SVT when the AV node permits a ventricular response greater than 100 BPM. In AF, the atria beat regularly, but faster (at a rate of 200–300/min) than usual and more often than the ventricles, so the patient may have 2:1 to 4:1 or higher ratio of atrial:ventricular beats.
  - Atrial fibrillation (AFib): It is considered under SVT when associated with a ventricular response greater than 100 BPM. In AFib, the heart's two small upper chambers (atria) do not beat the way they should. Instead of beating in a normal pattern, the atria beat irregularly and too fast (at a rate of 350–550/min). Atria remain dilated and quivering like a bowl of gelatin.
- Atrioventricular origin (junctional tachycardia):
  - Paroxysmal supraventricular tachycardia (PSVT): It is a type of SVT named for its intermittent episodes of abrupt onset and termination. A fast heart rhythm typically between 150 and 240 BPM and narrow QRS complexes are characteristic features of PSVT.
  - Wolff–Parkinson–White (WPW) syndrome: It is characterized by the presence of an "accessory pathway" or a "bypass tract." In this condition, electrical signals start from the SA node and reach the ventricle without passing through the AV node. This leads to short PR interval and a "delta wave" in electrocardiogram (ECG).
  - Atrial tachycardia: Very regular heart rates ranging typically from 140 to 220 BPM are exhibited in atrial tachycardia. The underlying mechanism of it may be either the rapid discharge of an abnormal focus, reentry, or drug toxicities, such as digoxin toxicity.

Ventricular Arrhythmias

Ventricular Fibrillation

In ventricular fibrillation (VF), the rate of heartbeat is over 300 BPM with an extremely rapid heart rhythm. However, the electrical activation of the ventricles does not display a specific and repetitive pattern.

Ventricular Tachycardia

A heartbeat rate of greater than 120 BPM is observed in ventricular tachycardia (VT) in the lower chamber of the heart. In ECG, it exhibits at least three or more wide QRS complexes in a row. It may be of sustained or nonsustained arrhythmia based on whether it lasts less than or more than 30 seconds.

Torsades de Pointes

It is a life-threatening situation of a special form of polymorphic VT. It is characterized by rapid, irregular QRS complexes and long QT interval, which appear to be twisting around the ECG baseline.

Bradycardias

Sick Sinus Syndrome

It is a disorder of the SA node caused by impaired pacemaker function and impulse transmission, producing a constellation of abnormal rhythms. These include atrial bradyarrhythmias, atrial tachyarrhythmias, and, sometimes, bradycardia alternating with tachycardia, often referred to as "tachy-brady syndrome." These arrhythmias may result in palpitations and tissue underperfusion, leading to fatigue, lightheadedness, presyncope, and syncope.

Atrioventricular Block

Vagal influence or ischemia may lead to depression in conduction through AV node and bundle of His.

First-Degree AV Block

In first-degree AV block, the P waves always precede the QRS complexes, but there is a prolongation of the PR interval. That is, the PR interval will be greater than 200 ms in duration without any dropped beats.

Second-Degree AV Block

It occurs when there is intermittent atrial to ventricle conduction. That is, the P waves are sometimes related to the QRS complexes.

Third-Degree (Complete) AV Block

In third-degree, or complete, heart block, there is an absence of AV nodal conduction, and the P waves are never related to the QRS complexes. In other words, the supraventricular impulses generated do not conduct to the ventricles.

Classification of Antiarrhythmic Drugs

In 1969, Singh and Vaughan William classified antiarrhythmic drugs on the basis of four major possible modes of actions, which modify Na^+, K^+, and Ca^{2+} channel function and intracellular mechanisms regulated by adrenergic activity. This landmark classification explained actions of four proposed classes on cardiac AP components, their relationship to clinical effects, and therapeutic utility in various arrhythmias (**Table 28.1**).

Class I Drugs

Class I antiarrhythmics exhibit membrane-stabilizing activity by blocking Nav (**Fig. 28.4**). Nav is responsible for mediating myocyte depolarization.

Class IA

In cardiac AP, class IA drugs slow the rate of rise of phase 0 (V_{max}) and prolong the ventricular effective refractory period (ERP). Drugs of this class impair the membrane sodium channel function, thereby decreasing the number of channels available for membrane depolarization. However, resting membrane potential is not altered by class IA drugs. These drugs slow down the conduction velocity because they decrease V_{max}.

Slope of phase 4 depolarization decreases due to class I agent, in pacemaker cells, especially those that arise outside of the SA node.

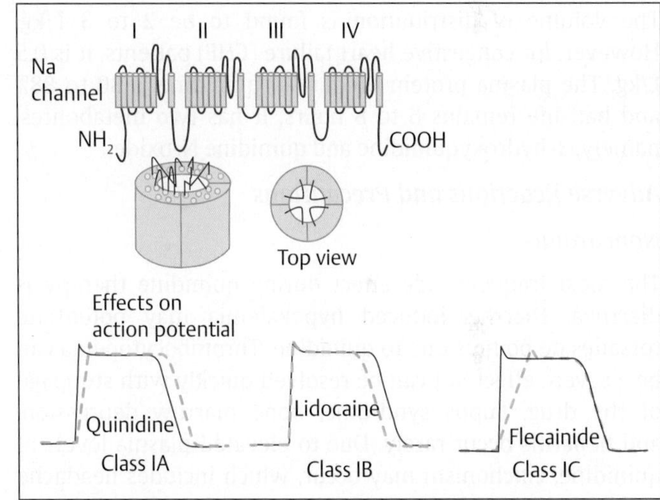

Fig. 28.4 Sodium channels and class I antiarrhythmics.

Table 28.1 Classification of antiarrhythmic drugs

Class	Action	Drugs	Clinical effects
I (Na^+ channel blockers)			
IA	Moderate decrease of V_{max} of phase 0	Quinidine, procainamide, disopyramide, moricizine	QRS widens; conduction slowed down; ERP increased; APD increased
IB	Minimum decrease of V_{max} of phase 0	Lidocaine, mexiletine, tocainide, moricizine	ERP increased; APD shortened
IC	Marked decrease of V_{max} of phase 0	Propafenone, flecainide	QRS widens; conduction slowed down
II (β-blockers)	Antiadrenergic agent	Nonselective: propranolol (class I action as well), nadolol β_1 selective: atenolol, bisoprolol, esmolol, metoprolol, sotalol	Prolong ERP
III (K^+ channel blocker)	Agents widen AP, prolong repolarization and ERP	Amiodarone, dronedarone, dofetilide, ibutilide, sotalol	Prolong ventricular AP
IV (calcium channel blocker)		Verapamil, diltiazem	On AV node: conduction slow; increase in ERP

Abbreviations: AP, action potential; AV, atrioventricular; ERP, effective refractory period.

Quinidine

Quinidine, extracted from the bark of the cinchona tree and similar plant species, is an optical isomer of quinine. Across cellular membranes, quinidine dampens the excitability of skeletal muscles and cardiac region by blocking sodium and potassium currents. It prolongs cellular AP and decreases automaticity. Quinidine also blocks neurotransmission mediated by α-adrenergic and muscarinic receptors. It augments PR and QT interval and broadens the QRS complex. It also changes the shape of T wave, suggesting its effect on repolarization.

Mechanism of Action

Quinidine acts on sodium channels on the neuronal cell membrane, limiting the spread of seizure activity and reducing seizure propagation. The antiarrhythmic actions are mediated through effects on sodium channels in the Purkinje fibers.

Pharmacokinetics

The volume of distribution is found to be 2 to 3 L/kg. However, for congestive heart failure (CHF) patients, it is 0.5 L/kg. The plasma protein binding of quinidine is 80 to 88% and half-life remains 6 to 8 hours. It has two metabolites, namely, 3-hydroxyquinidine and quinidine N-oxide.

Adverse Reactions and Precautions

Noncardiac

The most frequent side effect during quinidine therapy is diarrhea. Diarrhea-induced hypokalemia may potentiate torsades de pointes due to quinidine. Thrombocytopenia can be a severe effect but can be resolved quickly with stoppage of the drug. Lupus syndrome, bone marrow depression, and hepatitis occur rarely. Due to elevated plasma levels of quinidine, cinchonism may occur, which includes headache and tinnitus.

Cardiac

Marked QT interval prolongation and torsades de pointes occur at therapeutic or even subtherapeutic plasma concentrations.

Drug Interaction

It should be taken on an empty stomach. It is a strong inhibitor of CYP2D6.

- Quinidine prolongs $t_{1/2}$ of propafenone. It also inhibits conversion of codeine to morphine.
- Concurrent use of quinidine and warfarin increases the serum concentration of (R)- and (S)-warfarin.
- Acebutolol may increase the arrhythmogenic activities of quinidine.
- Aceclofenac may decrease the excretion rate of quinidine, which could result in a higher serum level.
- Quinidine may increase the hepatotoxic activities of acetaminophen.
- When quinidine and digoxin are given simultaneously, the serum concentration of digoxin can be raised due to displacement from tissue binding and inhibition of P-glycoprotein-mediated renal and biliary clearance of digoxin.
- Marked fall in blood pressure (BP) in patients receiving vasodilators.
- Hypokalemia caused by diuretics may increase the risk of torsades de pointes.
- With verapamil, β-blockers, and K^+ salts, it can induce synergistic cardiac depression.

Uses

It is used for the treatment of cardiac dysrhythmias, ventricular pre-excitation, AF and AFib, and arrhythmia of ventricular origin. It is also indicated for pseudobulbar effect and malaria caused by *Plasmodium falciparum*. However, it is seldom used now due to risk of adverse event such as torsades de pointes and sudden cardiac arrest.

Dose

The recommended dose is 200 to 300 mg orally every 6 to 8 hours.

Procainamide (PH1.17)

It is an orally active derivative of local anesthetic procaine with less central nervous system (CNS) action. It stabilizes the neuronal membrane by inhibiting the ionic fluxes required for the initiation and conduction of impulses, thereby effecting local anesthetic action. The mechanism of action of it is similar to that of procaine and quinidine. It decreases phase 0 depolarization and impulse conduction. However, it prolongs the APD, ERP, QRS complex, and QT interval. Nonetheless, when compared to quinidine, it causes less suppression in ectopic automaticity, depression of contractility, and AV conduction. It does not possess antivagal action and α receptor blocking activity, which suggests less fall in BP. Nevertheless, due to ganglionic blockade on higher dose, it causes fall in BP.

Pharmacokinetics

It has absorption of almost 75 to 95%, and oral bioavailability reaches close to 75%. The plasma protein binding is found to be 15 to 20%. It is metabolized in liver, and converts into *N*-acetyl-3-hydroxyprocainamide (NAPA) by acetylation. NAPA does not have any Na^+ channel–blocking activity but blocks K^+ channel and prolongs APD. Plasma $t_{1/2}$ is relatively short (2.5–4.5 hours).

Adverse Reactions and Precautions

Hypotension, AV block, ventricular tachyarrhythmias, intraventricular block, and complete heart block are reported as acute cardiovascular system reactions. If severe prolongation of the QRS complex and QT interval occurs, then the drug dosage must be reduced or even stopped.

Nausea and vomiting do occur, but gastrointestinal tract tolerance of procainamide is better than quinidine. At higher doses, weakness, mental confusion, and hallucination are reported.

Hypersensitivity reactions are rashes, fever, angioedema, and clinical lupus erythematosus–like syndrome in slow acetylators on long-term use.

Drug Interactions

- Abacavir and acarbose could diminish the excretion rate of procainamide, which might result in an elevated serum level.
- Acebutolol and zonisamide may increase the arrhythmogenic activities of procainamide.
- Hepatic clearance of procainamide may augment by concurrent use of alcohol.
- Procainamide, when used with aminoglycosides, may enhance the neuromuscular blocking activity and respiratory depression potential of the aminoglycosides.

Contraindications

In patients with bronchial asthma, procainamide should be used cautiously. It should not be used in patients who have shown hypersensitive reaction to procaine or procainamide.

Prolonged administration should be accompanied by hematological studies, since agranulocytosis may occur.

Uses

Procainamide administered intravenously is indicated for supraventricular arrhythmias, VT, life-threatening ventricular arrhythmias, and pre-excited AFib. However, it is not suitable for prolonged oral therapy because of poor efficacy and high risk of systemic lupus erythematosus.

Dose

Intravenous (IV) loading dose: 100 to 200 mg/dose or 15 to 18 mg/kg infused slowly over 25 to 30 mg/min.

Maintenance dose: 1 to 4 mg/min by continuous IV infusion.

Disopyramide

Disopyramide is a type 1A antiarrhythmic drug (i.e., similar to procainamide and quinidine). Disopyramide at therapeutic plasma levels shortens the sinus node recovery time, lengthens the ERP of the atrium, and has a minimal effect on the ERP of the AV node. Little effect has been shown on AV nodal and His-Purkinje conduction times or QRS duration. However, prolongation of conduction in accessory pathways occurs. It has no effect on α- or β-adrenergic receptors but possesses anticholinergic property and antivagal action.

Pharmacokinetics

Bioavailability of oral disopyramide is about 80%. It has about 50 to 65% plasma protein binding. In healthy men, about 50% of a given dose of disopyramide is excreted in the urine as unchanged drug, about 20% as mono-N-dealkylated metabolite, and 10% as the other metabolites. Plasma $t_{1/2}$ is 4 to 10 hours. In patient with MI and renal insufficiency, $t_{1/2}$ is increased.

Adverse Reactions and Precautions

Hypotension, CHF, and conduction disturbances are major adverse effects. Anticholinergic side effects such as dry mouth, blurred vision, urinary retention, and constipation are also seen. However, disopyramide causes less gastrointestinal effects. CNS stimulation and hallucinations are rare.

Contraindications

It is contraindicated in sick sinus, cardiac failure, and prostate hypertrophy.

Drug Interactions

- The metabolism of (R)-warfarin can be decreased when combined with disopyramide.
- Adenosine could augment the arrhythmogenic potential of disopyramide.
- Amphetamine might amplify the CNS depressant action of disopyramide.
- Unlike quinidine, disopyramide does not raise the plasma concentration of digoxin in patients receiving a maintenance dose of the cardiac glycoside.
- The therapeutic efficacy of disopyramide can be increased when used in combination with rosuvastatin.
- The serum concentration of metformin can be increased when it is combined with disopyramide.

Uses

It is used for the treatment of documented ventricular arrhythmias such as sustained VT, ventricular pre-excitation, and cardiac dysrhythmias. It is also used for maintenance therapy of AF and AFib.

Dosage

The recommended dose is 100 to 150 mg orally.

Class IB (PH1.17)

Drugs of class IB block Na^+ channel more in inactivated stage than open state but do not delay channel recovery (channel recovery time < 1 s). The characteristic feature of this class IB compounds is that they diminish the duration of AP and ERP of the Purkinje fibers. However, rate of depolarization and conduction velocity in ventricular myocardium are affected the least.

Lidocaine (Lignocaine)

Since its discovery, lidocaine has become an exceptionally frequently used medicine for local anesthesia. Additionally, it also established as popular antiarrhythmic drug in intensive care units. The cations of lidocaine reversibly bind to the sodium channels from the inside and block them, which will ultimately not depolarize and will thus fail to transmit an AP.

On sinus rate, lidocaine produces no effect. In atrium, AP amplitude, atrial muscle excitability, and membrane responsiveness are all reduced by lidocaine. ERP remains the same or is increased; however, APD of atrial muscle fibers is not altered by lidocaine. Furthermore, lidocaine minimally affects both the conduction velocity and the ERP of the AV node. In the Purkinje fibers, lidocaine produces significant shortening of the APD and ERP and slows phase 4 depolarization (low-dose effect). Nonetheless, by abolishing one-way or two-way block, it can suppress reentrant ventricular arrhythmia.

Succinctness of atrial AP and lack of lidocaine effect on channel recovery suggest its inefficacy in atrial arrhythmia.

Lidocaine does not usually alter the PR, QRS, or QT interval, although the QT may be reduced in a few patients.

Pharmacokinetics

As a result of a high degree of first-pass metabolism, the oral bioavailability is about 30 to 40%. The onset of action is 5 to 15 minutes when given intramuscularly (IM). The $t_{1/2}$ of late elimination phase is around 1 to 2 hours. It may prolong in CHF because of decrease in volume of distribution and hepatic blood flow. Additionally, lidocaine crosses the blood–brain and placental barriers, presumably by passive diffusion.

Adverse Drug Reaction and Precaution

It has dose-related neurological toxicity such as nausea, paresthesias, drowsiness, disorientation, blurred vision, twitching, fits, and nystagmus. Practically, lidocaine possesses the least cardiotoxic potential; however, high dose may cause cardiac depression and hypotension.

Drug Interactions

- The metabolism of lidocaine can be reduced when combined with hydroxychloroquine and omeprazole.
- The serum concentration of lidocaine can be augmented when it is combined with sotalol.
- No food interactions found with lidocaine.

Contraindications

Lidocaine is contraindicated in the presence of second- or third-degree heart block, since it may increase the degree of block.

Uses

Apart from its local anesthetic use, it is clinically utilized for the treatment of arrhythmia of ventricular origin. It is used only for selected cases of MI. It suppresses VT due to digitalis toxicity.

Dose

Lidocaine is given only by IV route, 50 to 100 mg bolus, followed by 20 to 14 mg every 10 to 20 minutes or 1 to 3 mg/min infusion.

Tocainide

This newer drug is a primary amine analog of lidocaine with antiarrhythmic potential useful in the management of ventricular arrhythmias. Tocainide binds preferentially to the inactive state of the sodium channels in the Purkinje fibers. It has similar electrophysiologic properties as produced by lidocaine, but dissimilar from procainamide, quinidine, and disopyramide. It produces a slight depression in His-Purkinje conduction as well as a slightly delayed enhancement of AV node conduction during atrial pacing.

Pharmacokinetics

The oral bioavailability is 100%. Onset of action is 0.5 to 2 hours; plasma $t_{1/2}$ is 10 to 12 hours. It is primarily metabolized in hepatic region (85%) via CYP2D6 and CYP1A2.

Adverse Drug Reactions and Precaution

Light-headedness, dizziness, paresthesias, and tremor are mild in intensity. Overall, approximately 20% of patients discontinue prescribed tocainide therapy because of such adverse effects. Pulmonary fibrosis is also a serious immune-based side effect reported with it. Agranulocytosis and thrombocytopenia are examples of blood dyscrasias associated with this drug.

Drug Interactions

- Simultaneous use of tocainide with other class IB antiarrhythmic drugs may shoot up its toxicity without significant gain in antiarrhythmic efficacy.
- Tocainide may augment the arrhythmogenic properties of acebutolol.
- The metabolism of tocainide can be reduced when combined with ciprofloxacin.

Contraindications

Patients who are hypersensitive to tocainide or to amide-type local anesthetics should not be exposed to tocainide. The presence of second- or third-degree heart block in the absence of an artificial pacemaker also contraindicates the use of tocainide.

Uses

Tocainide is indicated for the treatment of symptomatic ventricular arrhythmias refractory to more conventional therapy. Serious noncardiac side effects limit its use in life-threatening arrhythmias patients.

Dose

Initial: 400 mg orally every 8 hours.

Maintenance: 1,200 to 1,800 mg/day in three divided doses.

Mexiletine

It is an orally active but narrow therapeutic index antiarrhythmic agent with similar pharmacological properties to those of tocainide and lidocaine. Mexiletine has fast onset and offset kinetics, which suggests that it has more effects at faster heart rates and little or no effect at slower heart rates. It shortens the AP duration, decreases refractoriness, and reduces V_{max} in partially depolarized cells with fast response APs. In the Purkinje fibers, automaticity is reduced by diminishing phase-4 slope and by increasing threshold voltage. The decrease in ERP is of lesser magnitude than the decrease in APD, which results in an increase in the ERP/APD ratio. However, in ischemic Purkinje fibers, by reducing the rate of phase 0 depolarization, it may convert one-way block to two-way block.

Pharmacokinetics

The oral bioavailability is 90%. Plasma $t_{1/2}$ is 15 hours. In patients with severe renal function impairment, it may be prolonged by up to 35 hours.

Adverse Drug Reactions and Precaution

Fine tremor of the hands followed by dizziness and blurred vision are manifested as the first signs of toxicity. IV mexiletine can produce sinus bradycardia, widening of the QRS complex, and hypotension. Some other side effects are ataxia, confusion, nausea, and vomiting. These effects can be decreased by lowering the dose or administering the drug with food.

Contraindications

Mexiletine is contraindicated in the presence of cardiogenic shock. Also, it should not be used in patients with preexisting second- or third-degree heart block in the absence of a cardiac pacemaker.

Drug Interactions

Mexiletine may augment the arrhythmogenic properties of sotalol.

Uses

Parenteral mexiletine is utilized in postinfarction sinister ventricular arrhythmia as an alternative to lidocaine.

Dose

Mexiletine is given 100 to 250 mg IV over 10 minutes, or 150 to 200 mg thrice a day with meals.

Class IC

The drugs in class IC have the most potent Na^+ channel blocker action in open state, with longest recovery time (>10 s). Therefore, they exhibit rate-dependent block. They produce marked depression in the rate of rise of the membrane AP, prolong PR interval, and widen QRS complex. However, they have minimal effects on the duration of membrane AP and ERP of ventricular myocardial cells. Chronic administrations of these drugs may have high proarrhythmic potential.

Propafenone

Propafenone is a class IC antiarrhythmic drug with local anesthetic effects and a direct stabilizing action on myocardial membranes. It blocks Na^+ channel and slows down the conduction. It also has L-type calcium channel blocker and a weak β-receptor blocker. Propafenone causes SA node blocking activity with delay in recovery time while producing minimum effect on SA node cycle length. Both APD and ERP are prolonged by propafenone in atrium.

Propafenone can slow down the atrial rate in patients with AF, AFib, or tachycardia, resulting in a change from 4:1 or 2:1 AV block to 1:1 AV transmission, with a subsequent increase in the ventricular rate. At AV node, conduction is slowed down by IV infusion of propafenone. In His-Purkinje fibers, it depresses impulse transmission and also blocks retrograde as well as anterograde conduction in bypass tract of WPW syndrome.

Pharmacokinetics

The oral absorption is about 90%. Plasma protein binding is nearly 90%. The $t_{1/2}$ is 2 to 10 hours. It is metabolized primarily in the liver, where it is converted into two active metabolites, 5-hydroxypropafenone and N-depropylpropafenone. It is metabolized mainly by CYP2D6, a poor drug metabolizer, and increased exposure to it may lead to cardiac arrhythmias and exaggerated β-adrenergic blocking activity.

Adverse Drug Reactions and Precaution

Blurred vision, nausea, vomiting, bitter taste, and constipation are some common side effects. It can worsen asthma and CHF due to β-receptor blocker activity.

Drug Interactions

- Grapefruit products may change its metabolism; that is why, patients should avoid such products.
- The metabolism of (R)-warfarin can be decreased when combined with propafenone.
- The metabolism of propafenone can be diminished when combined with fluvoxamine, which ultimately augments the plasma concentration of propafenone.

Contraindications

Propafenone is contraindicated in the presence of severe or uncontrolled CHF; cardiogenic shock; SA, AV, and intraventricular disorders of conduction; sick sinus syndrome; chronic obstructive pulmonary disorder; asthma; and hepatic and renal failure cases.

Uses

It is approved for the treatment of AFib, paroxysmal AFib, and PSVT. It is also used for prophylaxis and treatment of ventricular arrhythmia, reentrant tachycardia AV node, and accessory pathway.

Dose

The recommended dose is 150 mg twice a day.

Flecainide

Flecainide was initially developed for its local anesthetic action and afterward found to have antiarrhythmic effects. Flecainide blocks fast inward sodium channels, which shortens the APD through the Purkinje fibers. It also prevents delayed rectifier potassium channels from opening, prolonging the action potential through atrial and ventricular muscle fibers. Besides this, it reduces calcium release from sarcoplasmic reticulum by blocking ryanodine receptor opening, which ultimately reduces depolarization of cells. However, flecainide does not possess β-blocker property.

Pharmacokinetics

The absorption is unaffected by food. The bioavailability is about 80 to 90%. Plasma protein binding is nearly 90%. The $t_{1/2}$ is 12 to 30 hours. Flecainide crosses the placenta, with fetal levels reaching approximately 70% of maternal levels.

Adverse Drug Reactions and Precaution

Light-headedness, dizziness, unsteadiness, faintness, visual disturbances, blurred vision, nausea, headache, and dyspnea are some side effects of flecainide. Flecainide can prolong PR and QRS interval, and worsening of heart failure as well as an increased risk of proarrhythmia has also been reported.

Drug Interactions

- Flecainide may increase digoxin concentrations on concurrent administration.
- Lidocaine may increase the arrhythmogenic activities of flecainide.

Contraindications

In patients with preexisting second- or third-degree heart block, flecainide is contraindicated.

Uses

It suppresses ventricular extrasystole, VT and WPW tachycardia, and prevents recurrences of AF and PSVT. It is preserved for life-threatening sustained VT in patients not having associated CHF.

Dose

It is used orally 50 to 150 mg.

Class ID (Miscellaneous)

Ranolazine

Ranolazine is a piperazine derivative and originally developed for angina pectoris. Ranolazine inhibits sodium (late current) and potassium ion channel currents. Due to its activity of L-type calcium channels, it possesses weak vasodilator property and also results in least direct effect on AV nodal conduction. Ranolazine also exerts antagonistic activity toward the a_1 and b_1 adrenergic receptors and inhibition of fatty acid oxidation. It diminishes AP recovery time and early afterdepolarization (EAD)-induced triggered activity. It can prolong QT interval.

Pharmacokinetics

Its absorption is unaffected by food. The bioavailability is about 76%. Plasma protein binding is nearly 62%. The $t_{1/2}$ is 7 hours. The mean apparent volume of distribution of ranolazine is reported to be 53.2 L. From the administered dose, about one-fourth of the dose is excreted in the feces, while three-fourths of the dose are excreted through kidney. It is metabolized via CYP3A4.

Adverse Drug Reactions and Precaution

Weakness, dizziness, postural hypotension, headache, constipation, and dyspepsia are the side effects caused by ranolazine.

Drug Interactions

- The serum levels of ranolazine can be augmented when it is combined with lidocaine or verapamil.
- The serum levels of sotalol and procainamide can be raised when it is combined with ranolazine.

Contraindications

It should be not given to patient taking CYP3A4 inhibitors.

Uses

It is used for VT.

Class II Agents

The primary action of this class of agents, that is, β-blockers, is to suppress adrenergic-mediated ectopic activity. These drugs diminish phase-4 depolarization and, thus, depress automaticity, prolong AV conduction and ERP, and decrease heart rate and contractility. The multiple effects of these drugs, electrophysiological changes, and clinical uses are given in **Table 28.2**. However, their pharmacokinetics, adverse events, drug interaction, and contraindication have already been discussed in Chapter 21 Adrenergic Receptor Blockers.

Class III Agents

Class III agents diminish the outward potassium current during repolarization of cardiac cells by blocking the potassium channels. Without altering phase 0 depolarization or the resting membrane potential, these agents prolong the APD. Also, they prolong the ERP, thereby increasing refractoriness (**Fig. 28.5**).

Amiodarone

Amiodarone is highly lipophilic, long-acting drug. It contains iodine and is structurally related to thyroxine. It shows class I, II, III, and IV actions, as well as α-blocking activity. Its dominant effect is prolongation of the AP duration and the refractory period for cardiac cells (myocytes) by blocking K^+ channels. Therefore, cardiac muscle cell excitability is reduced, preventing and treating abnormal heart rhythms. In addition, amiodarone may produce steatogenic changes in the liver or other organs due to augmenting the activity of peroxisome proliferator–activated receptors. Due to the presence of iodine in amiodarone, it has been found to bind to the thyroid receptor. This results in inhibition of peripheral conversion of T_4 to T_3, potentially leading to amiodarone-induced hypothyroidism or thyrotoxicosis.

Contraindications

It is contraindicated in patients who are already suffering from thyroid disorders.

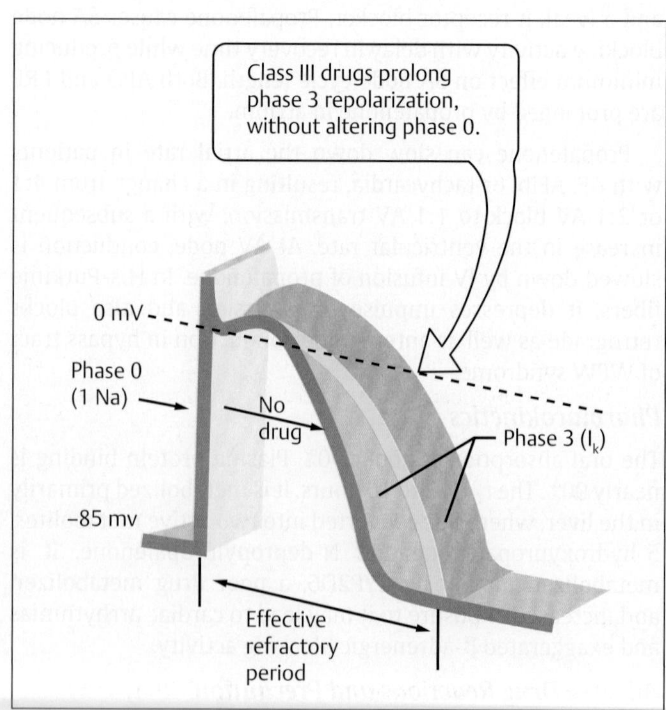

Fig. 28.5 Representing class III electrophysiological changes.

Table 28.2 Electrophysiological changes and clinical uses of β-blockers

Drug	Effect	Electrophysiological changes	Clinical uses
Acebutolol	Weak inherent sympathomimetic action and β-adrenergic antagonist	It decreases conduction velocity of SA node, AV node, and atria.	Ventricular arrhythmias, ventricular ectopy
Betaxolol	I_{CaL} in addition to class IIB antagonism	Decrease in automaticity in SA node. Sinus rate decreased	Supraventricular (AFib, AF, atrial tachycardia), arrhythmias
Carteolol	Increased nitric oxide production in addition to class IIA antagonism	Decrease in automaticity in SA node. Sinus rate decreased	Supraventricular (AFib, AF, atrial tachycardia), arrhythmias
Carvedilol	Possible antioxidant activity; I_{CaL}, RyR_2-Ca^{2+} channel, and a_1-adrenergic in addition to class IIA antagonism	Decrease in automaticity in SA node. Sinus rate decreased	Supraventricular (AFib, AF, atrial tachycardia), arrhythmias
Celiprolol	Increased nitric oxide production, partial b_2-adrenergic agonist, and weak a_2-adrenergic antagonist effects in addition to class IIB antagonism	Decrease in automaticity in SA node. Sinus rate decreased	Supraventricular (AFib, AF, atrial tachycardia), arrhythmias
Esmolol	b_1-adrenergic receptor inhibitors	It decreases conduction velocity of SA node, AV node and atria. It increases PR interval	AFib, AF, automatic tachycardias, arrhythmia associated with anesthesia
Metoprolol	b_1-adrenergic receptor inhibitors	Decrease in automaticity in SA node. Sinus rate decreased	Supraventricular (AFib, AF, atrial tachycardia), arrhythmias
Nebivolol	Increased nitric oxide production in addition to class IIB antagonism	Decrease in automaticity in SA node. Sinus rate decreased	Supraventricular (AFib, AF, atrial tachycardia), arrhythmias
Nadolol	Nonselective β-blocker	Decrease in automaticity in SA node. Sinus rate decreased	Used in treatment of long QT syndrome, used in catecholaminergic polymorphic ventricular tachycardia
Propranolol	Membrane-stabilizing effect in addition to class II action	It decreases conduction velocity of SA node, AV node, and atria. It increases PR interval.	Premature ventricular contractions, supraventricular arrhythmias, postoperative ventricular arrhythmias, WPW syndrome, used in treatment of long QT syndrome
Sotalol	Also blocks inward rectifier K^+ channel	It decreases conduction velocity of SA node, and AV node. APD and ERP also increased. PR and QT interval also prolong.	Ventricular arrhythmias, ventricular fibrillation, polymorphic VT

Abbreviations: AFib, atrial fibrillation; AF, atrial flutter; SA, sinoatrial; VT, ventricular tachycardia; WPW, Wolff–Parkinson–White.

Drug Interactions

- Amiodarone can raise digoxin and warfarin levels by diminishing their renal clearance.
- Inducers and inhibitors of CYP 3A4, CYP 2C9, and CYP 1A2, respectively, decrease and increase amiodarone levels.
- Additive AV block can occur in patients receiving β-blocker or calcium channel blocker.

Uses

It is used for recurrent hemodynamically unstable VT and recurrent VF. As per the direction of Food and Drug Administration (FDA), this drug should only be given in those conditions when other drugs are not tolerated by the patient or when they are clinically documented and have not responded to normal therapeutic doses of other antiarrhythmic agents. WPW tachyarrhythmia is terminated by suppression of both normal and aberrant pathway.

Amiodarone is suitable for chronic prophylactic therapy due to long duration of action. Aside from propranolol, it is the only antiarrhythmic drug that is able to reduce sudden cardiac death in the long term.

Dose

Amiodarone is mainly used orally 400 to 600 mg/day for few weeks, followed by 100 to 200 mg once a day for maintenance therapy.

Dronedarone

It is noniodinated and a less lipophilic congener of amiodarone. It is also a multichannel blocker. It inhibits delayed rectifier and other types of K^+ channel, L-type Ca^{++} channel, and inward Na^+ channel. It also possesses more marked noncompetitive β-blocking activity in comparison to amiodarone. In contrast to amiodarone, it is very less interfering with the thyroid function.

Dronedarone increases myocardial APD and ERP and slows AV conduction. QT interval is also prolonged by it moderately (10 ms on average).

Compared to amiodarone, dronedarone, with shorter elimination half-life and low-tissue accumulation, has shown a faster onset and offset of actions. In contrast to amiodarone, it does not cause hypothyroidism, pulmonary fibrosis, and peripheral neuropathy.

Drug Interactions

Inducers and inhibitors of CYP 3A4 and CYP 2D6, respectively, decrease and increase dronedarone levels.

Contraindications

It is contraindicated in second-/third-degree AV block, moderate-to-severe CHF, and permanent AF.

Uses

Dronedarone is indicated for the management of AFib in patients with sinus rhythm with a history of paroxysmal or persistent AF to reduce the risk of hospitalization.

Dose

The recommended dose is 400 mg twice a day.

Dofetilide

It is considered as a pure class III agent because it only blocks potassium channel. It prolongs APD and ERP by selectively blocking rapid component of delayed rectifier potassium channel. It can be used as a first-line antiarrhythmic agent in patients with persistent AFib and heart failure or in those with coronary artery disease.

Drug Interactions

Dofetilide may increase the arrhythmogenic activities of lidocaine and sotalol.

Contraindications

The drug should not be used in patients with advanced renal failure or with inhibitors of renal cation transport.

Ibutilide

It is newer agent used by IV for the rapid conversion of AFib or AF of recent onset to sinus rhythm. It slows down cardiac repolarization by binding to and altering the activity of hERG potassium channels, delayed inward rectifier potassium (I_{Kr}) channels, and L-type (dihydropyridine sensitive) calcium channels. It prolongs the APD and increases both atrial and ventricular refractoriness. Ibutilide slows down conduction through the AV node; however, there is no change in the PR interval on ECG. Ibutilide increases the ERP of ventricular myocytes and the Purkinje fibers but has no clinically significant effect on QRS duration. However, there is a risk of QT prolongation.

Drug Interactions

- Ibutilide may increase the arrhythmogenic activities of sotalol.
- Lidocaine may increase the arrhythmogenic activities of ibutilide.

Contraindications

Ibutilide should not be used in those with a history of torsades de pointes as well as in those using other QT-prolonging drugs. Further, hypersensitivity to ibutilide, uncorrected hypokalemia, hypomagnesemia, and pregnancy or breastfeeding are contraindications to the use of this drug.

Uses

Ibutilide is approved for the chemical cardioversion of recent-onset AFib and AF.

Vernakalant

Vernakalant is a novel aminocyclohexyl ether drug developed by Cardiome Pharma as an antiarrhythmic drug. It exerts a frequency- and voltage-dependent I_{Na} block, including inhibition of the late sodium current, which is probably the most important of its electrophysiological effects with regard to termination of AF. It also inhibits the early-activating K^+ channels (I_{Kur}; I_{to}) and I_{KACh}. I_{Kur} and I_{KACh} are currents that are specific to the atrium and cause prolongation of atrial rather than ventricular refractoriness and may contribute to the efficacy of the drug. However, vernakalant also blocks the rapidly activating potassium current I_{Kr}, which accounts for mild QT prolongation. QRS widening due to I_{Na} blockade also contributes to QT prolongation.

Drug Interactions

- Vernakalant may increase the arrhythmogenic activities of sotalol.
- Lidocaine may increase the arrhythmogenic activities of vernakalant.

Contraindications

Vernakalant is contraindicated in those with a history of torsades de pointes as well as in those using other QT-prolonging drugs.

Uses

The drug is designed for rapid termination of acute-onset AF in a patient with no or minimal heart disease and some forms of structural heart disease, including stable coronary heart disease, left ventricular hypertrophy, or mild heart failure. In 2010, vernakalant was approved by the European Union for cardioversion of AF that was less than 7 days in duration or for postoperative AF less than 3 days in duration.

Class IV Agents

The primary action of this class of drugs is to block Ca^{++} mediated slow channel inward current. Two antianginal drugs, namely, verapamil and diltiazem, also exhibit antiarrhythmic potential. However, dihydropyridines (e.g., nifedipine) do not share antiarrhythmic efficacy and may precipitate arrhythmias. However, other details such as pharmacokinetics, drug interactions, contraindication, and side effects are discussed in the antianginal chapter (Chapter 25).

Verapamil

Verapamil blocks both activated and inactivated L-type calcium channels. Thus, its effect is more marked in tissues that fire frequently, those that are less completely polarized at rest, and those in which activation depends exclusively on the calcium current, such as the SA and AV nodes. At therapeutic dose, it prolongs AV nodal conduction time and ERP consistently. Verapamil usually slows down the phase-4 depolarization in SA node, which results in bradycardia, although its hypotensive action may seldom result in a small reflex increase of SA rate. Verapamil can suppress both EAD and delayed afterdepolarization (DAD) and may abolish slow responses arising in severely depolarized tissue.

Uses

PSVT is the major arrhythmia indication for verapamil. Adenosine or verapamil is preferred over older treatments (propranolol, digoxin, edrophonium, vasoconstrictor agents, and cardioversion) for termination. However, IV verapamil bears a risk of marked bradycardia, AV block, hypotension, and cardiac arrest. Thus, it should be not used in PSVT patient with preexisting CHF or hypotension.

Verapamil dose dependently reduces the ventricular rate in AFib and AF ("rate control"). It only rarely converts AFib and AF to sinus rhythm.

Prophylaxis uses of verapamil in post-MI patients have not shown reduction in mortality. Moreover, its IV injection to patient of VT can precipitate VF; consequently, it is contraindicated.

Diltiazem

It produces similar direct cardiac action as exhibited by verapamil. Nevertheless, less marked actions are shown on bradycardia and depression on cardiac contractility.

It is preferred over verapamil for the rapid control of ventricular rate in AF or AFib, because it can cause less hypotension or myocardial depression and is easily titrated to the target heart rate. Another advantage associated with it is that it can be used in the presence of mild-to-moderate CHF. It is also an alternative to verapamil for treatment of PSVT (**Fig. 28.6**).

Ivabradine

As per the latest classification, ivabradine is considered under class 0 antiarrhythmic drug. It is an hyperpolarization-activated cyclic nucleotide-gated (HCN) channel blocker. In SA node, it selectively inhibits the "funny" channel pacemaker current (I_f) in a dose-dependent manner, resulting in a lower heart rate and thus more blood flow to the myocardium. At a dose of 30 to 40 mg, ivabradine exhibits a linear dose-dependent heart rate–lowering activity (bradycardic effect). At higher doses, the concentration of ivabradine tends to plateau, reducing risk of serious sinus bradycardia. It has been shown that the metabolite of ivabradine lowers heart rate as well, contributing to ivabradine's overall effect.

Pharmacokinetics

To reduce variability in systemic exposure, it is suggested to take ivabradine with meal. Administration with food slows down absorption by 1 hour but increases systemic absorption by 20 to 30%. Bioavailability of ivabradine is about 40%. Plasma protein binding of ivabradine is 70%. It is extensively metabolized by oxidation in the gut and by cytochrome P450 3A4 enzyme in the liver. Plasma half-life of ivabradine is 2 hours.

Adverse Drug Reactions

Nausea, vomiting, visual disturbances, bradycardia, extrasystole, and prolonged PR interval are side effects caused by ivabradine.

Contraindications

It should not be concurrently used with drugs that increase QT interval and that inhibit CYP3A4. It is also not used in sick sinus and AFib if the heart rate is less than 60/min.

Uses

It can be used in inappropriate sinus tachycardia.

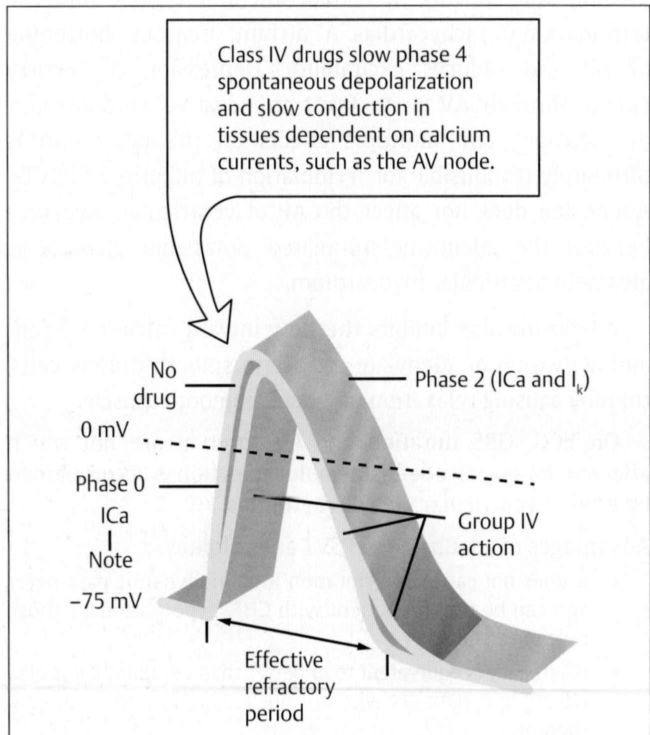

Fig. 28.6 Representing class IV electrophysiological changes.

Magnesium Sulfate

Magnesium sulfate may be effective in terminating refractory ventricular tachyarrhythmias, particularly polymorphic VT. Digitalis-induced arrhythmias are more likely in the presence of magnesium deficiency. When a rapid response is intended, magnesium sulfate can be administered intravenously.

Drugs for PSVT

In hemodynamically stable patients with regular rhythm but undetectable P waves, Valsalva's maneuver, carotid sinus massage, splashing ice cold water on face, hyperflexion, or IV adenosine might be used to slow down the ventricular rate or convert the rhythm into sinus rhythm and thus aid in the diagnosis. If IV adenosine does not work, then IV or oral calcium channel blockers (verapamil/diltiazem) or β-blockers (esmolol) should be used.

To prevent recurrence, oral therapy with verapamil, diltiazem, or propranolol alone or combined with digoxin may be prescribed.

Adenosine

It is a nucleoside that is composed of adenine and d-ribose. Adenosine is a component of DNA and RNA and also a neurotransmitter.

In myocytes of atria, SA node, and AV node, adenosine receptor (a type of G-protein-coupled receptor) is found. After activation, this receptor opens acetylcholine-sensitive outward potassium current. This leads to hyperpolarization of the resting membrane potential on SA node, prolongation of ERP, and slowing of conduction at AV node and the termination of tachycardias. At atrium, it causes shortening of AP and reduces excitability. Depression of reentry circuit through AV node leads to negative chronotropic, dromotropic, and inotropic effects on the heart and is ultimately responsible for termination of majority of PSVTs. Adenosine does not affect the AP of ventricular myocytes because the adenosine-stimulated potassium channel is absent in ventricular myocardium.

Adenosine also inhibits the slow inward calcium current and activation of adenylate cyclase in smooth muscle cells, thereby causing relaxation of vascular smooth muscle.

On ECG, QRS duration and QT interval are not much affected. Rarely, an adenosine bolus injection is accompanied by AFib or ventricular tachyarrhythmias.

Advantages of adenosine in PSVT are as follows:

- It does not cause deterioration in hemodynamic parameter and can be used in patient with CHF, hypotension, or those receiving β-blockers.
- Its efficacy is equivalent to or better than verapamil. It is also effective in patients who are not responding to verapamil therapy.
- It is safe in wide QRS tachycardia; however, verapamil is unsafe.
- Its action lasts for 1 minute.

Adverse Drug Reactions

It produces chest pain, fall in BP, transient dyspnea, flushing, and bronchospasm.

Contraindications

It is contraindicated in asthmatic patients.

Drug Interactions

Methylxanthines such as caffeine and theophylline are competitively antagonized by adenosine. It is potentiated by dipyridamole (blockers of nucleoside transport). However, atropine is not able to block adenosine.

Uses

It can be utilized to produce controlled hypotension during surgery. In certain diagnostic and interventional procedures, it can be used to induce brief coronary vasodilation.

Drugs for AV Block

As an interim measure for acute or transient AV block, drugs are used. However, the definitive treatment of chronic heart block is pacing with an implanted cardiac pacemaker.

Atropine

Atropine is used when AV block is due to vagal overactivity such as digitalis toxicity. The dose of atropine in this case remains 0.6 to 1.2 mg IM.

Sympathomimetics

Adrenaline and isoprenaline can be utilized in partial heart block by shortening of ERP of conducting tissue and facilitating AV conduction.

In third-degree AV block, these agents can be used to maintain a sufficient idioventricular rate till external pacemaker can be implanted.

Selection of an Antiarrhythmic Drug

Only detection of arrhythmia does not indicate requirement of treatment. The main aim of the therapy is to improve patient cardiovascular function either by controlling ventricular rate or by restoring sinus rhythm. Clinical objectives and management of various arrhythmias are discussed in **Table 28.3**.

- Diagnosis by ECG.
- Find out the possible etiology of arrhythmia and its mechanism.
- Select appropriate antiarrhythmic drug that suits to underlying mechanism of arrhythmia.
- Varied range of antiarrhythmic activity of drugs.
- Pharmacokinetic parameter of the drugs.
- Hemodynamic effects of the drugs.
- Choose the one that may cause least adverse events and shows less proarrhythmic potential.

Table 28.3 Choice of antiarrhythmic drugs for various cardiac arrhythmia

Type of arrhythmia	ECG changes	Clinical objective	Treatment
PSVT	Paroxysmal supraventricular tachycardia (PSVT)	Termination of PSVT Prevention of recurrence	IV adenosine/verapamil/diltiazem/esmolol Oral verapamil/diltiazem/propranolol/sotalol
AF	Atrial flutter with variable AV conduction	Reversal to SR Ventricular rate control	Cardioversion, radiofrequency ablation, propafenone (after rate control with verapamil/propranolol), propranolol/verapamil/diltiazem + digoxin or amiodarone
AFib	Atrial fibrillation	Reversal to SR (for paroxysmal/persistent AF) Maintenance of SR Ventricular rate control (for permanent AF/during recurrence of AF) Urgent ventricular rate control	Cardioversion IV amiodarone Sotalol/propafenone/amiodarone/Dronedarone/disopyramide Oral verapamil/diltiazem/propranolol + digoxin IV esmolol/verapamil/amiodarone
WPWS	Delta wave I H PR interval < 12 ms	Termination Maintenance Narrow QRS Wide QRS	Radiofrequency ablation, cardioversion Propafenone/procainamide Propafenone + verapamil/propranolol or Amiodarone/sotalol
VF		Termination Recurrence prevention	Defibrillation + amiodarone (IV) Amiodarone (oral)/propranolol
VT		Suppression Abolition Maintenance therapy	Propranolol/amiodarone (oral) IV Amiodarone + propranolol or cardioversion or propafenone/lidocaine (IV) Amiodarone/sotalol Implantable defibrillator
Torsades de pointes		Maintenance therapy	IV magnesium sulfate; isoproterenol infusion, cardiac pacing, and intravenous atropine
Sick sinus syndrome		Termination Maintenance therapy	Permanent pacemaker implantation Class I and class III agents

Abbreviations: AFib, atrial fibrillation; AF, atrial flutter; IV, intravenous; SA, sinoatrial; PSVT, paroxysmal supraventricular tachycardia; VT, ventricular tachycardia; WPWS, Wolff–Parkinson–White syndrome.

Table 28.4 Drugs prolonging QT interval

Antimicrobials Erythromycin Clarithromycin Moxifloxacin Fluconazole Ketoconazole	**Antipsychotics** (all have some risk) Risperidone Fluphenazine Haloperidol Pimozide Chlorpromazine Quetiapine Clozapine
Antiarrhythmics Dronedarone Sotalol Quinidine Amiodarone Flecainide	**Antidepressants** Citalopram/escitalopram Amitriptyline Clomipramine Dosulepin Doxepin Imipramine Lofepramine
Others Methadone Protein kinase inhibitors, e.g., sunitinib Some antimalarials Some antiretrovirals Telaprevir Boceprevir	**Antiemetics** Domperidone Droperidol Ondansetron/Granisetron

- Vigorous therapy is required for the following cases:
  - Life-threatening arrhythmia such as torsades de pointes, sustained VT, and VF.
  - Arrhythmia that is causing hypotension, activity limitation, breathlessness, or cardiac failure.
  - If palpitation is marked, such as in the case of torsades de pointes, AF, PSVT, and sustained VT.
  - When simple arrhythmia may convert into more severe ones; for example, after MI (warning arrhythmias).

Proarrhythmic Potential of Drugs

Most antiarrhythmic drugs may themselves cause serious arrhythmia when used for long term. Antiarrhythmic drugs such as flecainide and moricizine have high proarrhythmic potential. However, some other classes of drugs also possess arrhythmogenic potential. A list of drugs that may increase the QT interval is given in **Table 28.4**.

Multiple Choice Questions

1. A 65-year-old Indian woman, on physical examination, was found to have a regular heart rate of 123 BPM. She has a blood pressure of 126/73 mm Hg, respiratory rate of 19/minute, and temperature of 97.4 F. After careful examination of her electrocardiogram, it is determined that her rhythm is consistent with sinoatrial nodal reentrant tachycardia (SANRT). She has a past medical history of hypothyroidism and hyperlipidemia. Which of the following is NOT considered a feature of SANRT on an electrocardiogram?

A. Heart rate usually between 100 and 150 BPM.
B. Abrupt onset and termination.
C. A frequent premature atrial complex at the initiation or termination of the tachycardia.
D. An irregularly irregular rhythm.

Answer: D

SANRT has a regular rhythm on an electrocardiogram. An irregularly irregular rhythm is commonly used to describe atrial fibrillation on an electrocardiogram.

2. A 63-year-old woman presents to the emergency department of AIIMS, New Delhi, in acute distress from a rapid heart rate and chest pain. She is diagnosed with supraventricular tachycardia (SVT). A 6-mg dose of IV adenosine is given and then she converts back to a normal sinus rhythm. Where does adenosine act on the heart and what is the mechanism of action of adenosine?

A. AV node, increases efflux of K1.
B. AV node, increases influx of K1.
C. SA node, decreases intracellular Ca21.
D. SA node, increases efflux of K1.

Answer: A

Adenosine causes a transient (less than 15 s) heart block at the AV node. This is achieved because adenosine inhibits adenylyl cyclase, which reduces cAMP and causes the efflux of K1 from cardiac cells. This leads to hyperpolarization and decreased intracellular Ca21. Adenosine is commonly used to treat SVT.

3. A patient is admitted in AIIMS, Jodhpur, and diagnosed with ventricular tachycardia following an acute myocardial infarction (MI). The condition is life-threatening and needs to be controlled immediately. Choose the drugs from below for fast control of the patient condition:

A. Dobutamine.
B. Digitalis.
C. Quinidine.
D. Lidocaine.

Answer: D

Lidocaine is the best agent. Lidocaine does not slow down conduction and has little effect on atrial function.

4. A 55-year-old woman has had repeated episodes of atrial fibrillation. She is receiving quinidine and phenytoin to manage the atrial fibrillation. She is also on estrogen replacement therapy and a low-dose therapy of diazepam for insomnia. Due to urinary tract infection, she has been also receiving ciprofloxacin. The reason for her visit to the hospital is that she has been having ringing in the ears, blurred vision, nausea, and headache. She informs the doctor that she is also having trouble hearing sound. The most likely agent for this drug toxicity is:

A. Both ciprofloxacin and estrogen.
B. Estrogen and phenytoin.
C. Phenytoin only.
D. Quinidine only.

Answer: D

Cinchonism is the adverse event of constituents present in cinchona tree such as quinidine and quinine. All the mentioned effects in the given question are characteristics of cinchonism.

Part IV

Renal Pharmacology

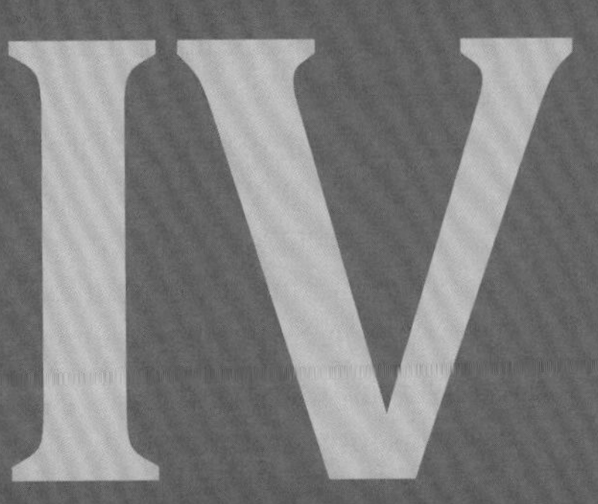

Chapter 29 Diuretics and Antidiuretics

Prasan R. Bhandari

PH1.24: Describe the mechanisms of action, types, doses, side effects, indications, and contraindications of the drugs affecting renal systems including diuretics, antidiuretics (vasopressin), and analogues.

Learning Objectives

- Physiology of urine formation.
- Diuretics.
- Antidiuretics.

Physiology of Urine Formation

The kidney has one of the major regulatory and excretory functions. The important functions of the kidney include the following:

1. Regulatory: acid–base, fluid, and electrolyte balance.
2. Excretory: waste nitrogenous products.
3. Hormonal: activation of vitamin D and formation of renin and erythropoietin.

The normal glomerular filtration is around 180 L/day, of which 99% is reabsorbed. The total urine output is approximately 1 to 1.5 L/day. The processes involved in urine formation include glomerular filtration, tubular reabsorption, and active tubular secretion. The nephron is the functional unit of the kidney. The sites of nephron along with its actions is depicted in **Fig. 29.1**.

Proximal Convoluted Tubule

It reabsorbs 100% glucose, 85% sodium bicarbonate, and 65% Na, K, Ca, and Mg. Chloride is passively transported along with sodium. It also reabsorbs amino acids and other organic solutions. Water is reabsorbed proportionately, to maintain isotonic tubular fluid. Na is transported by four ways: Na^+/H^+ exchanger/Na^+–H^+ antiporter (depends on carbonic anhydrase [CA]), direct entry, Na^+ and K^+ transport along with glucose, amino acids, and phosphates, and specific symporters. Osmotic diuretics act at the proximal convoluted tubule (PCT). Adenosine A1 receptor antagonists also act at the PCT and collecting duct (CD).

Loop of Henle

The thin descending limb is impermeable to Na. Water is reabsorbed by osmotic forces and hence fluid is hypertonic. Osmotic diuretics also act here. Thick ascending limb (TAL) actively reabsorbs 25% of filtered Na and Cl^- by Na^+/K^+/2Cl cotransporter. Water is not reabsorbed. Loop diuretics block Na^+/K^+/2Cl cotransporter, and hence they decrease NaCl reabsorption. Ca and Mg are also reabsorbed.

Distal Convoluted Tubule and Collecting Duct

In the early distal tubule, 10% NaCl is reabsorbed by Na^+-Cl^- transporter/symporter and it is impermeable to water. This transporter is blocked by thiazides. Apical calcium channel and basolateral Na/Ca exchanges reabsorb calcium. In the late distal tubule and CD, Na is actively reabsorbed and Cl and H_2O diffuse passively. K^+ is secreted in exchange for Na^+. This is controlled by aldosterone. K^+-sparing diuretics act here. Fluid absorption at CD is controlled by antidiuretic hormone (ADH). ADH controls water channels known as aquaporins. ADH secretion is controlled by plasma volume and serum osmolality. Atrial natriuretic peptide, renin–angiotensin–aldosterone system, and prostaglandins (PGs) also locally control renal function.

Diuretics

Classification based on site of action:

1. Drugs acting on the PCT:
   a. Carbonic anhydrase inhibitor (CAI): acetazolamide.
2. Drugs acting on TAL of the loop of Henle:
   a. Loop diuretics: furosemide, torsemide, ethacrynic acid.
3. Drugs acting on the early distal tubule:
   a. Thiazides: chlorothiazide, hydrochlorothiazide, polythiazide.
   b. Thiazidelike: chlorthalidone, indapamide, metolazone.
4. Drugs acting on the late distal tubule and CD:
   a. Aldosterone antagonists: spironolactone, eplerenone.
   b. Direct Na^+ channel inhibitors: amiloride, triamterene.
5. Drugs acting on the entire nephron (but mainly the loop of Henle):
   a. Osmotic diuretics: mannitol, glycerol.

Classification based on efficacy:

1. High efficacy: loop diuretics—furosemide, torsemide, ethacrynic acid.
2. Medium efficacy:
   a. Thiazides: chlorothiazides, hydrochlorothiazide.
   b. Thiazidelike: chlorthalidone, indapamide, metolazone.
3. Low efficacy:
   a. Potassium-sparing: spironolactone, eplerenone, triamterene, amiloride.
   b. CAIs: acetazolamide.
   c. Osmotic diuretics: mannitol, glycerol, urea.
   d. Methylxanthines: theophylline.
4. Newer diuretics:
   a. Vasopressin antagonist: conivaptan.
   b. Adenosine A1 receptor antagonist: rolofylline.

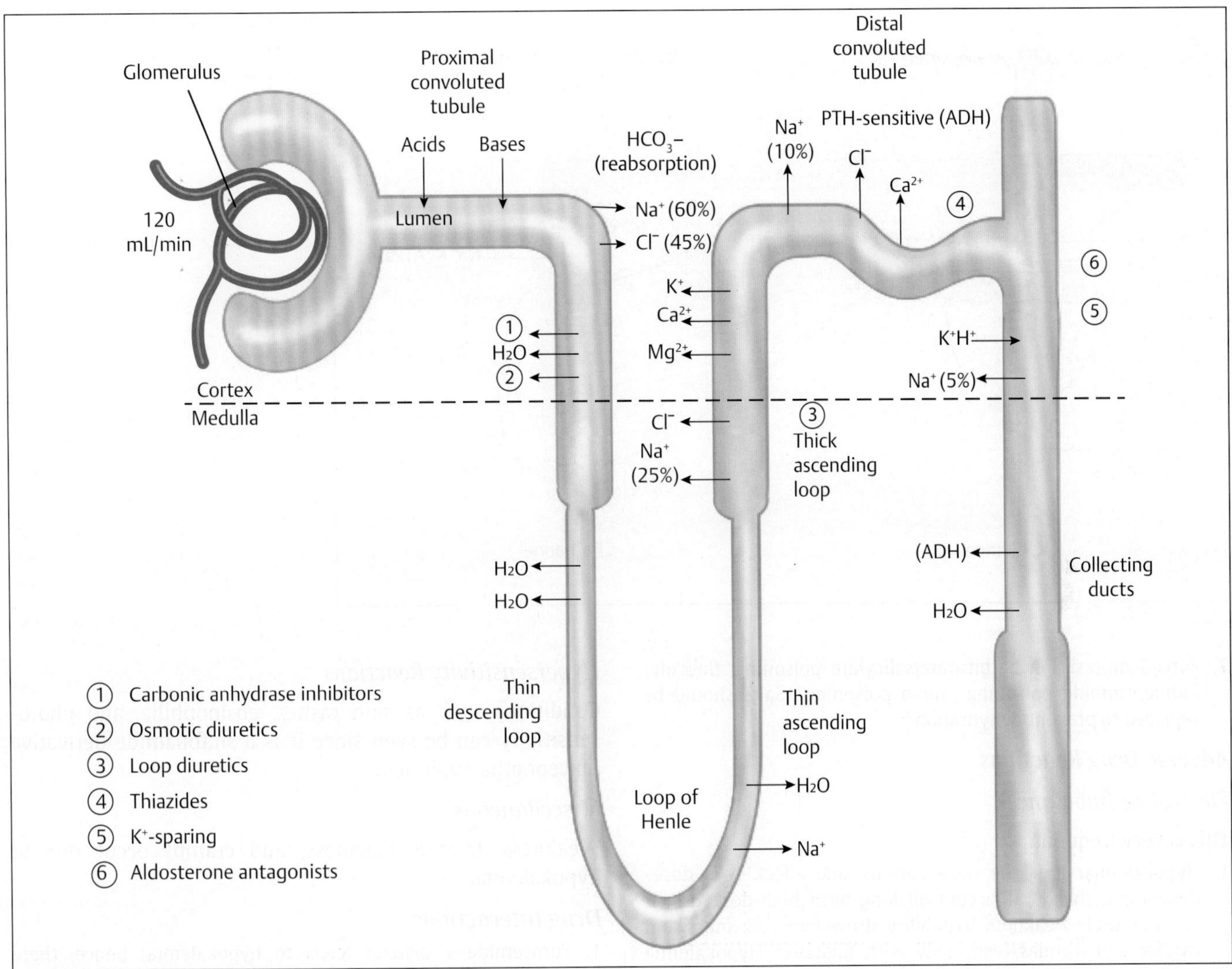

Fig. 29.1 Actions of different sites of nephrons and diuretics.

High Efficacy/High Ceiling/Loop Diuretics

These are furosemide (frusemide), torsemide, and ethacrynic acid.

Furosemide

It is a sulfonamide derivative, which blocks the function of $Na^+/K^+/2Cl$ cotransporter/symporter from the luminal side of TAL (**Fig. 29.2**). This inhibits NaCl reabsorption and hence increases Na and Cl excretion. It also increases excretion of K^+, Ca^{2+}, and Mg^{2+}, but Ca^{2+} is reabsorbed in the distal convoluted tubule (DCT); hence, there is no hypocalcemia. High Na^+ load that reaches the DCT is reabsorbed in exchange for K^+; hence, there is hypokalemia. Long-term use can lead to hypomagnesemia. It is also a weak CAI; therefore, it increases excretion of HCO_3^- and PO_3^{3-}.It also the increases renal blood flow and increases renin release. It causes venodilation and thus decreases left ventricular filling pressure, thereby relieving congestive cardiac failure (CCF) and pulmonary edema. Furosemide also stimulates PGE2 synthesis; hence, there is decreased salt reabsorption, leading to diuresis. Hence, it is a powerful and highly effective diuretic. Pharmacokinetics profile includes a rapid gastrointestinal (GI) absorption and a rapid onset of action, that is, 2 to 5 minutes after intravenous (IV) administration and 30 to 40 minutes after oral administration. The duration of action is about 2 to 4 hours.

Other Loop Diuretics

Torsemide is long-acting and hence given as once daily dose. Ethacrynic acid has more adverse effects, that is, it is ototoxic, and hence not used nowadays.

Uses

1. Edema of hepatic, renal, or cardiac origin.
2. Acute pulmonary edema.
3. Cerebral edema, but IV mannitol is preferred.
4. Acute renal failure, since it increases urine output and it is useful in impending renal failure.
5. Hypertension associated with CCF/renal failure, hypertensive emergencies. Thiazides are preferred for primary uncomplicated hypertension.
6. Acute hypercalcemia and hyperkalemia, as it increases Ca^{2+} and K^+ excretion. Simultaneous replacement of Na^+ and Cl^- is done to avoid hyponatremia and hypochloremia.

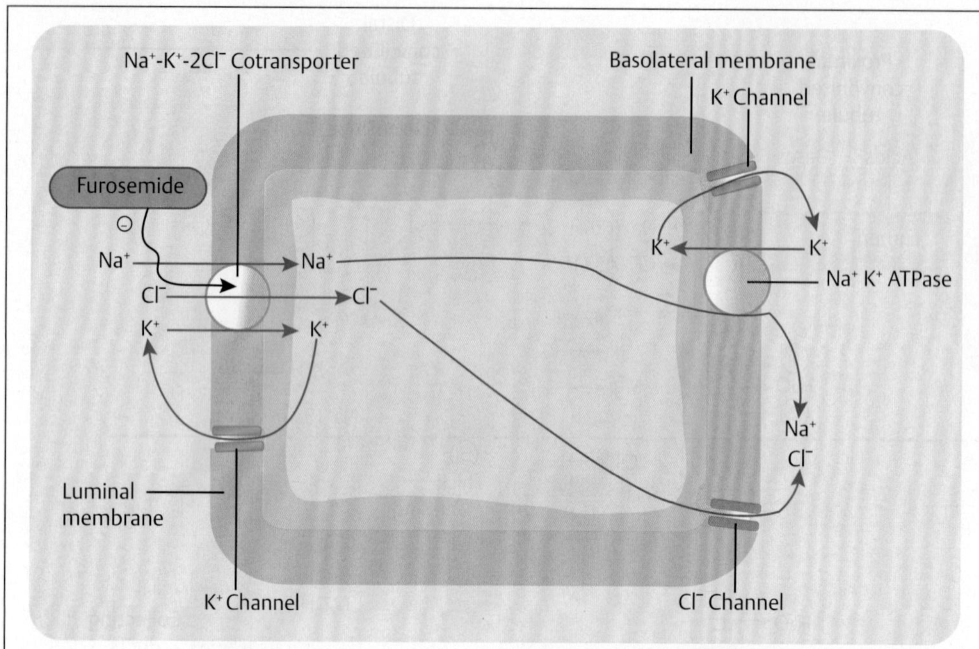

Fig. 29.2 Mechanism of action of furosemide.

7. Forced diuresis, in barbiturate/salicylate poisoning, fluoride/iodine/bromide poisoning (anion poisoning). Salts should be replaced to prevent dehydration.

Adverse Drug Reactions

Electrolyte Imbalances

This is very frequent.

1. Hypokalemia: It is the most serious side effect. It is dose-dependent, that is, it occurs on long-term high-dose use. It causes muscle weakness, irritability, drowsiness, dizziness, and cardiac arrhythmias (especially with digitalis). Hypokalemia can be prevented by using K^+-sparing diuretics (spironolactone, amiloride, triamterene), K^+ supplementation, and high K^+ diet.
2. Hypokalemia with metabolic acidosis: Since less K^+ is available for exchange with Na^+ at the DCT, more Na^+/H^+ exchange occurs and hence there is loss of H^+. This leads to metabolic alkalosis.
3. Hyponatremia occurs due to increased Na^+ loss.
4. Hypocalcemia is seen since there is increased Ca^{2+} loss; hence, long-term use will lead to osteoporosis.
5. Hypomagnesemia occurs since there is increased Mg^{2+} loss; thus, oral Mg supplements should be given.
6. Hypovolemia and hypotension occur due to loss of H_2O.

Metabolic Changes

These include the following:

1. Hyperglycemia: due to decreased insulin secretion.
2. Hyperlipidemia: increase in low-density lipoprotein and triglyceride levels.
3. Hyperuricemia: due to decreased excretion of uric acid, thereby leading to gout; patients may require allopurinol.

Ototoxicity

This is manifested as deafness, vertigo, and tinnitus. It occurs due to toxic effect on hair cells of the inner ear and it is dose-dependent. It is common with IV use and in patients with renal impairment. Hence, avoid other ototoxic drugs during treatment, such as aminoglycosides and cyclosporine.

Hypersensitivity Reactions

Conditions such as skin rashes, eosinophilia, and photosensitivity can be seen since it is a sulfonamide derivative (except ethacrynic acid).

Miscellaneous

Weakness, fatigue, dizziness, and cramps occur due to hypokalemia.

Drug Interactions

1. Furosemide + digoxin leads to hypokalemia; hence, there is increased binding of digoxin to Na^+/K^+/ATPase, leading to digoxin toxicity.
2. Furosemide + aminoglycosides causes increased ototoxicity.
3. Furosemide + nonsteroidal anti-inflammatory drugs (NSAIDs): NSAIDs inhibit renal PG synthesis and therefore cause Na^+ and H_2O retention; hence, this decreases efficacy of diuretics.
4. Furosemide + lithium leads to hyponatremia, which increases lithium absorption in the PCT and hence leads to lithium toxicity.
5. Furosemide + K^+-sparing diuretics is synergistic, as it has decreased efficacy and decreased adverse drug reaction (ADR), since furosemide decreases K^+ and K^+-sparing diuretics increase K^+, and hence there is no change in K^+ levels.
6. Probenecid decreases efficacy, since it competes for tubular secretion.

Contraindications

1. Toxemia of pregnancy since it decreases fetal circulation.
2. Hepatic cirrhosis, since increased NH_3 levels causes hypokalemia and alkalosis, which worsen hepatic coma.

Medium Efficacy (Thiazides and Thiazidelike Diuretics)

Thiazides include chlorothiazide and hydrochlorothiazide, while thiazidelike diuretics include chlorthalidone, indapamide, and metolazone. These diuretics are of medium efficacy, since 90% of filtered Na is already reabsorbed before reaching the DCT. They bind to Cl side of Na^+-Cl^- symport and block them in the early DCT, thereby increasing the excretion of Na and Cl (**Fig. 29.3**). Thus, more Na reaches the late DCT; hence, there is increased exchange with K^+. Hence, there is K^+ loss, leading to hypokalemia. It also has a weak CAI activity and thus there is loss of HCO_3^-. There is net loss of Na^+, K^+, Cl^-, and HCO_3^-. They decrease Ca^{2+} excretion (unlike loop diuretics) and hence there is hypercalcemia. It is given orally and it has a longer duration of action (6–48 hours, as compared to loop diuretics). Thiazides have a peculiar paradoxical action. It decreases glomerular filtration rate (GFR) and urine output in diabetes insipidus (DI). Patients with DI do not respond to ADH and excrete large volume of dilute urine.

Uses

Hypertension

They are first-line drugs.

Congestive Cardiac Failure

They are given in mild-to-moderate cases.

Hypercalciuria and Renal Stones

They are used since they decrease Ca^{2+} excretion.

Diabetes Insipidus

There is a paradoxical benefit, since they decrease GFR and plasma volume.

Adverse Reactions

Electrolyte Imbalance

Hypovolemia, hyponatremia, hypomagnesemia, dehydration, hypotension, hypokalemia, and hypercalcemia.

Metabolic Disturbances

Hyperglycemia is seen since they decrease insulin secretion. It is common with long-term long-acting thiazides. Hyperlipidemia and hyperuricemia can also occur.

Impotence

Because of this side effect, not preferred in young men.

Allergy

Skin rashes, photosensitivity, etc.

Chlorthalidone is a long-acting thiazide. Indapamide and metolazone are potent, long-acting thiazide diuretics and have lesser ADRs and are used in hypertension.

Potassium-Sparing Diuretics

These include aldosterone antagonists such as spironolactone and eplerenone and direct inhibitors of Na channels such as triamterene and amiloride.

Spironolactone

It is a low-efficacy diuretic, a synthetic steroid, chemically similar to aldosterone. Aldosterone increases Na reabsorption through Na channels in the late DCT and CD. It decreases K^+ secretion. They bind to specific mineralocorticoid receptor (MR) in cytoplasm. This hormone–receptor complex (mineralocorticoid receptor aldosterone [MR-AL]) enters nucleus and it directs synthesis of aldosterone-induced proteins (AIPs). AIPs retain Na and excrete potassium. Spironolactone competitively blocks MR and prevents formation of AIPs. Thus, the net effect is increased Na excretion and increased K retention (**Fig. 29.4**). They are most effective when aldosterone levels are high. Thus, it decreases K^+ excretion due to other diuretics (loop/thiazides). It increases excretion of Ca^{2+}. It is given orally as microfine powder to increase bioavailability (75%). It has high

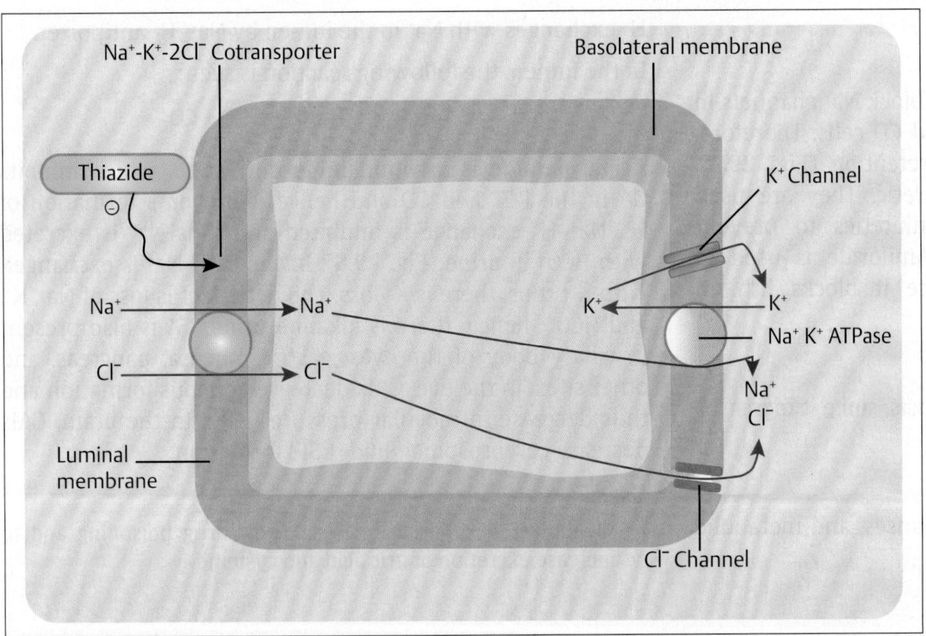

Fig. 29.3 Mechanism of action of thiazides.

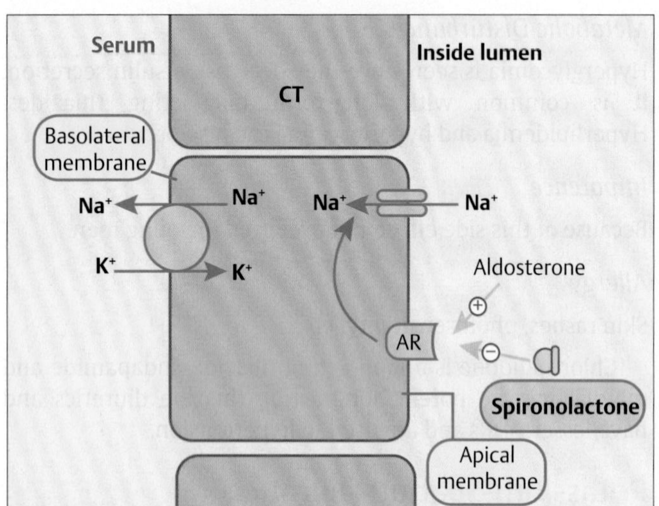

Fig. 29.4 Mechanism of action of spironolactone.

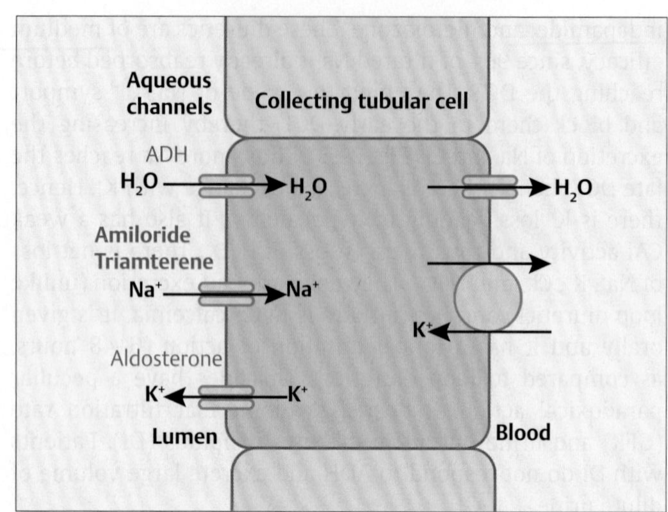

Fig. 29.5 Mechanism of action of amiloride and triamterene.

plasma-protein binding. Active metabolite of spironolactone is canrenone. Canrenone has a long $t_{1/2}$ of about 18 hours, while spironolactone has a $t_{1/2}$ of 1 to 2 hours.

Uses

It is given in edema associated with secondary hyperaldosteronism (CCF, hepatic cirrhosis, nephrotic syndrome). It is also combined with loop/thiazide diuretic to prevent hypokalemia and increase efficacy in hypertension. It can be used in Conn's syndrome, which is a resistant hypertension due to primary hyperaldosteronism.

Adverse Drug Reactions

Hyperkalemia occurs especially in patients with renal impairment, and those on concurrent angiotensin-converting enzyme inhibitors, angiotensin II receptor blockers, β-blockers, NSAIDs, etc. Endocrine disturbances comprise gynecomastia, impotence, decreased libido, and menstrual disturbances, since it binds to androgen and progesterone receptors and hence interferes with steroidogenesis. It can also cause metabolic acidosis.

Amiloride and Triamterene

They are directly acting agents, which block Na^+ channels in luminal membrane of the late DCT and CD cells. Therefore, they increase Na excretion and K^+ retention (**Fig. 29.5**). They are low-efficacy K^+-sparing diuretic. They are used in combination with loop/thiazide diuretics to prevent hypokalemia and increase efficacy. Amiloride is used in lithium-induced nephrogenic DI since it blocks lithium transport through Na^+ channels in CD.

Uses

Amiloride aerosol is used in cystic fibrosis, since it increases mucociliary clearance.

Adverse Drug Reactions

This includes hyperkalemia, GI disturbances, and metabolic acidosis.

Potassium Canrenoate

It is a prodrug, which is activated to canrenone. Canrenone is the active metabolite of spironolactone. It can be given parenterally and it has fewer hormonal disturbances.

Eplerenone

It is an analog of spironolactone and has greater selectivity for MR and fewer hormonal imbalances. It is use in hypertension as monotherapy/combination and also in CCF. It is more expensive than spironolactone.

Differences between furosemide, thiazide, and potassium-sparing diuretics are provided in **Box 29.1**.

Carbonic Anhydrase Inhibitors

Acetazolamide

In tubular cell, the following reaction occurs:

$$H_2O + CO_2 \xrightarrow{CA} H_2CO_3 \rightarrow H^+ + HCO_3^-$$

H^+ exchanges with Na^+ in the lumen by Na^+–H^+ antiporter.

In the lumen, the following reaction is seen:

$$H^+ + HCO_3^- \rightarrow H_2CO_3 \underset{CA}{\rightarrow} H_2O + CO_2$$

Acetazolamide is a sulfonamide derivative, which inhibits CA in the PCT and CD and hence it prevents formation of H^+. Na^+–H^+ exchange is inhibited and thus Na^+ is excreted with HCO_3^- in urine (**Fig. 29.6**). In the DCT, Na^+ is exchanged with K^+; thus, there is K^+ loss. The net effect is loss of Na^+, K^+, and HCO_3^-; hence, there is alkaline urine. CA is also present in ciliary body of the eyes, gastric mucosa, pancreas, and other sites. In the eye, CAIs decrease aqueous formation and thus decrease intraocular pressure (IOP). In the brain, CAIs decrease cerebrospinal fluid (CSF) formation.

Uses

1. Alkalinization of urine to treat acidic drug poisoning and to increase excretion of uric acid and cysteine.

Box 29.1 Differences between furosemide, thiazide, and potassium-sparing diuretics

Thiazide	Furosemide
Medium efficacy	High
Acts on the early DCT	TALH
Inhibits Na^+-Cl^- symport	$Na^+/K^+/2Cl$ cotransport
Onset: 1 h	20–40 min
Duration of action: long, 8–12 h	8–6 h
No response on increasing dose	Dose-dependent response
Causes hyperuricemia	No change
Increases blood sugar	No change
No ototoxicity	Ototoxic
Use: hypertension	Edema
Furosemide	**Spironolactone**
Sulfonamide	Steroid
Acts on TALH	DCT and CD
$Na^+/K^+/2Cl$ cotransport blocked	Aldosterone blocker
High efficacy	Low efficacy
Quick onset (minutes)	Slow onset (days)
Hypokalemia	Hyperkalemia
Causes ototoxicity	Causes gynecomastia, hirsutism
Use: edema	Hyperaldosteronism, as adjuvant to diuretics
Caution: allergy to sulfonamides	Caution: peptic ulcer

Abbreviations: CD, collecting duct; DCT, distal convoluted tubule; TALH, thick ascending limb of the loop of Henle.

2. In acute congestive glaucoma, acetazolamide is given orally and intravenously, and dorzolamide is applied topically.
3. It is given in acute mountain sickness prevention and treatment. Mountain climbers develop pulmonary and cerebral edema, especially unacclimatized persons. Acetazolamide decreases CSF and pH of CSF.
4. In metabolic alkalosis caused by increased use of diuretics in patients with CCF, acetazolamide increases HCO_3^- excretion.
5. Miscellaneous uses include familial periodic paralysis, adjuvant in epilepsy, and hyperphosphatemia, since acetazolamide increases PO_4^{3-} excretion.

Adverse Drug Reactions

ADRs include the following: metabolic acidosis, since it causes HCO_3^- loss, and renal stones, since it increases Ca^{2+} excretion and hypercalciuria. Other side effects are hypokalemia, allergic reactions, and drowsiness.

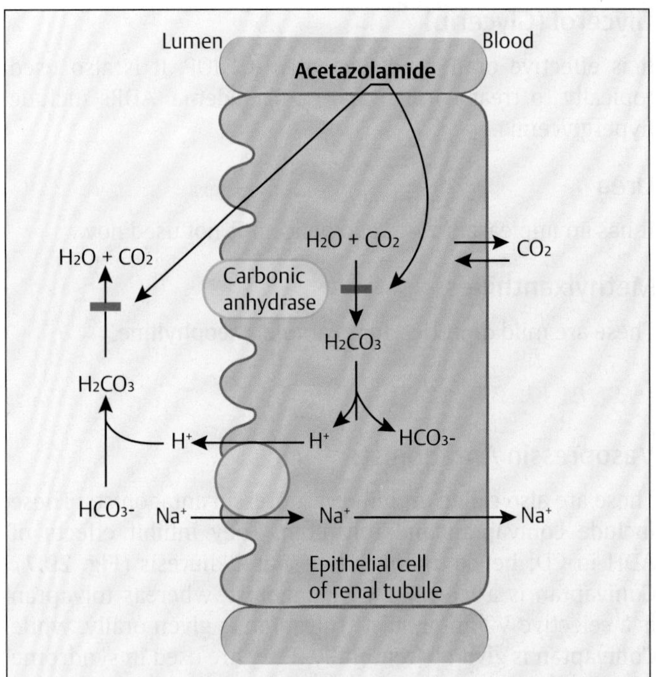

Fig. 29.6 Mechanism of action of acetazolamide.

Contraindications

It is contraindicated in hepatic disease since it precipitates hepatic coma in cirrhosis and decreases excretion of NH_3 in alkaline urine. It is also contraindicated in chronic obstructive pulmonary disease since it worsens metabolic acidosis.

Osmotic Diuretics

Examples include mannitol, glycerol, and urea.

Mannitol

It is pharmacologically inert and is given via the IV route since it is not absorbed orally. Mannitol is filtered by glomerulus and is not reabsorbed; hence, it retains water by osmotic action. Thus, there is increased excretion of water and electrolytes. Its site of action is the PCT and the loop of Henle. It is used to maintain urine volume and prevent acute renal failure in patients with massive hemolysis, shock, cardiovascular surgery, hemolytic transfusion reaction, and rhabdomyolysis. However, in patients with existing renal failure, mannitol is dangerous since pulmonary edema and heart failure can be precipitated. It decreases raised intracranial tension (ICT) following head injury and tumor, since it draws fluid from the brain to the circulation by osmotic effect. It decreases IOP in glaucoma since it draws fluid from the eye into the circulation. ADRs include dehydration. There is increase in extracellular fluid volume; hence, it leads to pulmonary edema. Therefore, it is contraindicated in pulmonary edema, CCF, chronic edema, anuric renal disease, and active intracranial bleeding.

Glycerol (Glycerin)

It is effective orally and decreases ICT/IOP. It is also used topically to treat corneal and ocular edema. ADRs include hyperglycemia.

Urea

It has an unpleasant taste and hence it is not used now.

Methylxanthines

These are mild diuretics, for example, theophylline.

Newer Diuretics

Vasopressin Antagonists

These are also called arginine vasopressin antagonists. These include conivaptan and tolvaptan. They inhibit effects of ADH in CD; hence, there is free water diuresis (**Fig. 29.7**). Conivaptan is a V1a and V2 antagonist, whereas tolvaptan is a selective V2 antagonist. Tolvaptan is given orally, while Conivaptan is given parenterally. They are used in syndrome of inappropriate ADH secretion (SIADH). Here, Vaptans increase free water clearance and correct hyponatremia.

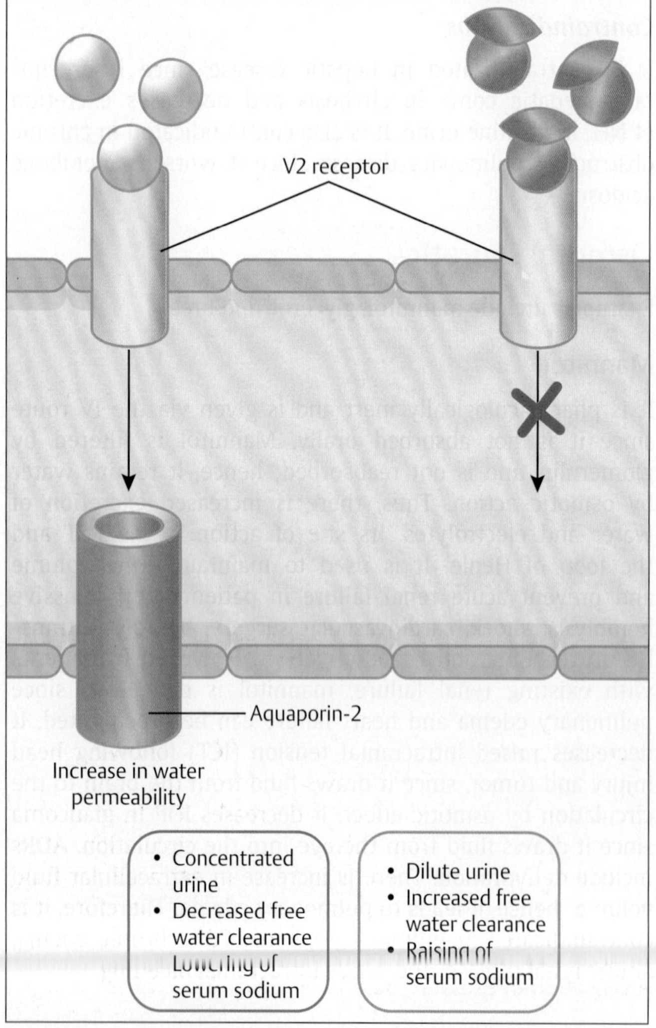

Fig. 29.7 Mechanism of action of vasopressin antagonists.

Adenosine A1 Receptors Antagonists

Rolofylline is an example. They decrease NaCl reabsorption in the PCT and CD and have been tried in CCF.

Antidiuretics

Classification

1. ADH (vasopressin).
2. Vasopressin analogs: desmopressin, terlipressin.
3. Thiazide diuretics.
4. Others: chlorpropamide, carbamazepine.

Antidiuretic Hormone (Vasopressin) (IM15.14)

It is secreted by the posterior pituitary along with oxytocin, synthesized in supraoptic and paraventricular nucleus of hypothalamus, transported along hypothalamo-hypophyseal tract to the posterior pituitary, stored in the posterior pituitary, and released in response to dehydration/increase in plasma osmolarity. There are two types of vasopressin receptors, that is, V1 and V2. V1 causes vasoconstriction, whereas V2 leads to water retention in CD. Both are G protein–coupled receptor. V1a is present in the vascular and other smooth muscles, urinary bladder, platelets, liver, and central nervous system, and V1b is present in the anterior pituitary. V2 activates adenylyl cyclase, which leads to increase in cyclic adenosine monophosphate (cAMP) and the numbers of aqueous channels in CD, thus leading to water reabsorption. V1 receptor mediates vasoconstriction, increases BP, and induces constriction of cutaneous, coronary, coeliac, and mesenteric vasculature. V1 increases GI peristalsis and uterine contraction, and V2 receptor mediates water retention. These agents can be administered via the subcutaneous, intramuscular, IV, or intranasal route. Intranasal administration leads to rhinitis and nasal mucosa atrophy, while other routes of administration cause abdominal cramps and backache. Uses mediated through V1 receptors include bleeding esophageal varices, before GI radiography since it promotes expulsion of GI gases, and asystolic cardiac arrest. Uses mediated through V2 receptor include central DI or neurogenic DI or DI of pituitary origin (lifelong treatment). In patients with nocturnal enuresis, oral/intranasal desmopressin is a short-term treatment. BP has to be monitored in these patients. They can also be used in hemophilia and von Willebrand's disease, since ADH releases factor VIII and controls bleeding. It is used for renal concentration test. If the kidneys are normal, a small dose of desmopressin increases urine concentration.

Vasopressin Analogs

Desmopressin is selective for V2 receptor. It is potent and long acting than vasopressin. It can be administered by either oral or intranasal route. Oral bioavailability is 1 to 2%, whereas intranasal availability is 10 to 20%. Other agents include terlipressin, a long-acting prodrug of vasopressin.

Thiazide Diuretics

They decrease urine output of both neurogenic and nephrogenic DI. They have paradoxical effect due to unknown mechanism.

Others

Chlorpropamide (antidiabetic) sensitizes the kidney to ADH action. Carbamazepine (antiepileptic) acts by stimulating ADH secretion.

Multiple Choice Questions

1. A 65-year-old woman has been admitted to the coronary care unit with a left ventricular myocardial infarction. She develops acute severe heart failure with marked pulmonary edema, but no evidence of peripheral edema or weight gain. Which one of the following drugs would be most useful?

A. Digoxin.
B. Furosemide.
C. Minoxidil.
D. Propranolol.
E. Spironolactone.

Answer: B

Acute severe congestive failure with pulmonary edema often requires a vasodilator that reduces intravascular pressures in the lungs. Furosemide has such vasodilating actions in the context of acute failure. Pulmonary edema also involves a shift of fluid from the intravascular compartment to the lungs. Pulmonary vasodilation and removal of edema fluid by diuresis are accomplished by furosemide.

2. A 54-year-old man develops congestive heart failure (CHF) after suffering his second myocardial infarction. His physician puts him on a regimen of several medications, including furosemide. On follow-up, the patient is found to have hypokalemia, likely secondary to furosemide use. The addition of which medication would likely resolve the problem of hypokalemia, while helping to treat the underlying condition, CHF?

A. Allopurinol.
B. Hydrochlorothiazide.
C. Spironolactone.
D. Acetazolamide.
E. Ethacrynic acid.

Answer: C

Spironolactone is commonly added to the regimen of anti-CHF medications, since it counteracts the loss of potassium caused by the loop diuretics such as furosemide. This agent is also effective in reducing the symptoms of refractory edema.

3. A 35-year-old woman presents to your office for a regular check-up. She has no complaints. On examination, her blood pressure is slightly elevated at 145/85. She is physically fit and follows a healthy diet. You decide to start her on antihypertensive therapy and prescribe hydrochlorothiazide. How does this agent work?

A. Inhibits reabsorption of sodium chloride in the early distal convoluted tubule.
B. Decreases net excretion of chloride, sodium, and potassium.
C. Increases excretion of calcium.
D. Inhibits reabsorption of sodium chloride in the thick ascending limb of the loop of Henle.
E. Interferes with potassium secretion.

Answer: A

Thiazide diuretics inhibit active reabsorption of sodium chloride in the early distal convoluted tubule of the nephron by interfering with the Na/Cl cotransporter, resulting in net excretion of sodium and water. These agents increase net excretion of chloride, sodium, and potassium.

4. A 45-year-old man with a 60-pack/year history of smoking presents to his primary care provider with loss of appetite, nausea, vomiting, and muscle weakness. His chest CT reveals enlarged hilar lymph nodes and a suspicious mass in the left hilar region. A presumptive diagnosis of lung cancer is made. Laboratory results reveal low levels of sodium, which in this setting has likely contributed to the syndrome of inappropriate ADH secretion. Which medication might be helpful for this patient's symptoms?

A. Clofibrate.
B. Conivaptan.
C. Allopurinol.
D. Acetazolamide.
E. Furosemide.

Answer: B

Conivaptan is a nonpeptide ADH antagonist and as such is useful in the treatment of SIADH, which is commonly seen in patients with lung cancer.

5. A neurosurgeon decides to start a patient on a diuretic that works by altering the diffusion of water relative to sodium (an osmotic diuretic) that is helpful in reducing cerebral edema. Which agent did the physician likely prescribe?

A. Furosemide.
B. Hydrochlorothiazide.
C. Spironolactone.
D. Acetazolamide.
E. Mannitol.

Answer: E

Mannitol is an osmotic diuretic frequently used in the management of cerebral edema caused by various insults. This agent works by altering the diffusion of water relative to sodium by "binding" the water, with a resultant reduction of sodium reabsorption.

6. A 57-year-old man develops progressive vision loss with a sensation of pressure behind his eyes. His ophthalmologist diagnoses the patient with glaucoma. To prevent further

progression of the disease and to alleviate current symptoms, the physician starts the patient on acetazolamide therapy. What is the mechanism of action of this medication?

A. Potentiates carbonic anhydrase in all parts of the body.
B. Reduces reabsorption of bicarbonate.
C. Increases excretion of hydrogen.
D. Increases rate of formation of bicarbonate in the aqueous humor.
E. Increases uptake of sodium in the proximal tubule.

Answer: B

Acetazolamide belongs to a class of medications termed carbonic anhydrase inhibitors. These agents reduce bicarbonate reabsorption in the proximal tubule. They inhibit carbonic anhydrase in all parts of the body, including the aqueous humor, which makes these agents very useful in the treatment of glaucoma. Acetazolamide inhibits excretion of hydrogen and concomitant sodium uptake.

7. A 7-year-old boy underwent successful chemotherapy and cranial radiation for treatment of acute lymphocytic leukemia. One month after the completion of therapy, the patient presented with excessive thirst and urination plus hypernatremia. Laboratory testing revealed pituitary diabetes insipidus. To correct these problems, this patient is likely to be treated with which of the following?

A. Corticotropin.
B. Desmopressin.
C. Human chorionic gonadotropin.
D. Menotropins.
E. Thyrotropin.

Answer: B

Pituitary diabetes insipidus results from deficiency in vasopressin. It is treated with desmopressin, a peptide agonist of vasopressin V2 receptors.

Part V

Drugs Affecting Central Nervous System

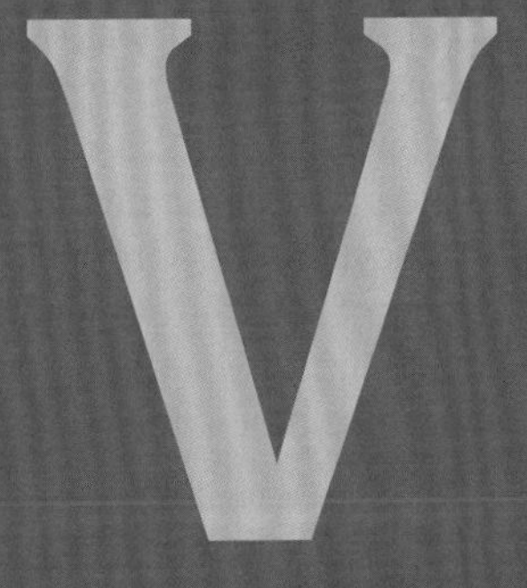

Chapter 30 Introduction to CNS

Anuja Jha

Learning Objectives

- Neurons.
- Support cells.
- Central neurotransmitters.

Introduction

This chapter introduces the basic cellular organization of the brain and actions of neurotransmitters and modulators on their respective receptors in the central nervous system (CNS). Specific pharmacotherapy of neurological and psychiatric disorders is discussed in the subsequent chapters.

The human CNS is a complex organ that regulates many daily life activities through the chemical neurotransmission process. A neuron is the primary communicating cell in this process, which is influenced and supported by a variety of cells.

Neurons

Neurons are the main signaling cells of the brain. They are classified based on the function (sensory, motor, or interneuron), location, morphology, neurotransmitter phenotype, or the class of receptors expressed. Neurons express a variety of ion channels and ion transport proteins that help in nerve impulse conduction. This conduction ultimately triggers the release of neurotransmitters in the chemical neurotransmission and transmission of information. The interneuronal communication in the CNS is known as *synapses*.

Support Cells

These include neuroglia, vascular elements, cerebrospinal fluid (CSF) forming cells, and meninges. Their function is to keep neurons in place, supply oxygen and nutrients to them, destroy pathogens, and insulate signals between the neurons.

Neuroglia cells are the most predominant support cells. They are of two types, namely, macroglia and microglia. Macroglia consists of astrocytes, ependymal cells, oligodendroglia, and radial glia. Astrocytes are the most abundant among them. Their main function is to provide energy, anchor neurons to their blood supply, and regulate the external environment of neurons by the removal of excess neurotransmitters and ions. Ependymal cells line the spinal cord and ventricular system and synthesize CSF. The oligodendroglia produces myelin, which allows nondecremental propagation of action potential through the neurons. Radial cells act as neural progenitors and scaffolds, whereas microglia acts as macrophage and protects the neurons.

Neuronal Excitability and Ion Channels

The basic principle in neurotransmission is the same as the periphery. Action potential, which is generated due to rapid change in the membrane potential, leads to the release of neurotransmitters and the transmission of information to the brain and the neurons. The flow of Na^+, K^+, and Ca^{2+} along with anion Cl^- across the ion channels (Na^+ K^+ ATPase; Na^+, Ca^{2+} exchanger, Ca^{2+}-ATPases, and Cl^- channels) helps in the generation and maintenance of the action potential. An increase in permeability to Na^+ causes depolarization and generation of the action potential. In contrast, increased permeability to K^+ leads to hyperpolarization. Changes in the concentration of Ca^{2+} lead to the release of neurotransmitters, while Cl^- helps in the maintenance of action potential.

Chemical Communication in the CNS

In neuropsychopharmacology, drugs that improve the functional status of the patients act by enhancing or blunting neurotransmission in the CNS. The main targets of these drugs are ion channels, neurotransmitter receptors, and transport proteins. Ion channels facilitate changes in excitability, which have been discussed previously. Transport proteins help in the reaccumulating of the released neurotransmitters. Central neurotransmitters and their receptors are discussed in the subsequent section.

Central Neurotransmitters

Neurotransmitters are endogenous chemicals in the brain that act to enable signaling across a chemical synapse. Small molecule neurotransmitters are synthesized in the nerve terminal, while others such as peptides are synthesized in cell bodies and transported to the nerve terminal. Synaptic vesicle stores these neurotransmitters along with other molecules such as adenosine triphosphate. Depolarization of the presynaptic nerve terminal leads to an influx of Ca^{2+} and exocytosis of neurotransmitters in the synaptic cleft. These neurotransmitters bind selectively to the receptors to initiate signal transduction events in the postsynaptic cell. There are various mechanisms to terminate the action of transmitters, including diffusion, enzymatic inactivation, and reuptake by specific transporters.

Neurotransmitters are classified based on their chemical structure and include amino acids, acetylcholine (ACh), monoamines, neuropeptides, purines, lipids, and even gases.

Amino Acids

CNS contains a high concentration of various amino acids. Among these amino acids, glutamate and aspartate produce excitation, while gamma aminobutyric acids ($GABA_A$) and glycine produce inhibition. The balance between the excitatory and inhibitory inputs determines neuronal activity.

$GABA_A$ is the main inhibitory neurotransmitter in the CNS. They act by binding to $GABA_A$ and $GABA_B$ receptors. $GABA_A$ receptors are ionotropic, ligand-gated Cl^- channels. Opening of these channels leads to hyperpolarization and reduction in membrane excitability. $GABA_A$ has several binding sites, which include the neurotransmitter GABA binding site and modulatory sites to bind benzodiazepines and barbiturates.

$GABA_B$ receptors are metabotropic G protein–coupled receptors (GPCRs). They regulate both pre- and postsynaptic activity. The presynaptic receptor acts as an autoreceptor and inhibits GABA release. Postsynaptic $GABA_B$ interacts with G_i to inhibit adenyl cyclase, activate K^+ channels, and reduce Ca^{2+} conductance and interact with G_q to increase phospholipase C activity. Baclofen, a skeletal muscle relaxant, is a $GABA_B$ agonist.

Glutamate is the main excitatory neurotransmitter in the CNS. It acts through both ionotropic and metabotropic GPCRs. Ionotropic glutamate receptors are ligand-gated ion channels and are N-methyl-D-aspartate (NMDA) or α-amino-3-hydroxy-5-methylisoxazole-4-propionate/kainate (AMPA/KA) receptors based on their synthetic ligands.

Glycine acts as an inhibitory neurotransmitter mainly in the spinal cord and brain stem. Glycine receptor is linked to Cl^- ion channel similar to $GABA_A$ and it leads to hyperpolarization. Glycine also acts as a coagonist at the NMDA receptor, which means both glycine and glutamate are required for the activation of the receptor.

Acetylcholine

ACh is mainly found in the interneurons. Both nicotinic and muscarinic receptors are present in the CNS. Nicotinic ACh receptors are ionotropic ligand-gated ion channels, while muscarinic receptors are GPCR. Activation of nicotinic ACh receptors leads to an influx of Na^+ and Ca^{2+} and depolarization. All five types of muscarinic receptors are found in the CNS. Details have been discussed in the autonomic nervous system.

Monoamines

It includes dopamine (DA), norepinephrine (NE), epinephrine (Epi), histamine, and 5-hydroxytryptamine (5HT). DA, NE, and Epi are catecholamine neurotransmitters and DA is the predominant one. There are three main DA-containing pathways in the CNS: the nigrostriatal, the mesolimbic, and the tuberoinfundibular pathways. These pathways along with DA receptors are linked with schizophrenia and Parkinson's disease. Other monoamines have been discussed in their respective chapters.

Apart from these major neurotransmitters, several peptides including angiotensin, endorphin, and vasopressin, and neuromodulatory lipids such as cannabinoids are implicated in the neurotransmission. They mainly act as a modulator rather than having direct action.

To reach the CNS, a drug has to cross the blood–brain barrier (BBB).

Blood–Brain Barrier

BBB allows selective passage of substances into the CNS from the periphery. It is made up of endothelial cells, astrocytes, and pericytes on a noncellular basement membrane.

Certain factors that regulate the passage of substances across this barrier are lipophilicity, molecular weight, charge, and plasma protein binding. A lipophilic drug and drugs unionized at physiological pH can easily permeate across this barrier, while agents with molecular weight 60,000 and above, and highly plasma protein-bound are not readily permeable. Several transporters are present in BBB, which actively transport the various substances across this. One of these transport systems that is selective for amino acids allows the movement of L-dopa across the BBB.

Certain clinical conditions such as inflammation and cerebral ischemia change the permeability of BBB and allow increased access to substances that usually do not enter into the brain in normal circumstances. Penicillin can cross the BBB in the presence of meningeal inflammation (meningitis), which is not otherwise so.

Chapter 31 General Anesthetics

Areeg Anwer Ali and Bhoomendra A. Bhongade

PH 1.18: Describe the mechanisms of action, types, doses, side effects, indications, and contraindications of general anesthetics and preanesthetic medications.

Learning Objectives

- Properties of an ideal general anesthetic agent.
- Stages and depth of anesthesia.
- Drugs used for induction and maintenance of anesthesia.
- Preanesthetic medications.

Introduction

General anesthesia is a reversible state of central nervous system (CNS) depression. It is required for a variety of medical and surgical procedures, and it is attained through the administration of one or more general anesthetic agents. General anesthetics are drugs that induce a reversible state of unconsciousness in which pain sensation is lost throughout the body. They have poor therapeutic indices in general and need a lot of attention and treatment during administration.

Routes of Administration

General anesthetics are broadly classified as inhalational and intravenous (IV) anesthetics based on their route of administration (**Table 31.1**). The selection of specific general anesthetic and the particular route of administration are based on the physicochemical, pharmacokinetic, and pharmacodynamic properties of the drug.

Properties of an Ideal General Anesthetic Agent (AS4.1)

No single anesthetic agent will provide all the desirable properties of an ideal general anesthetic agent. As a result, a variety of medications are combined to achieve the best possible general anesthesia. Adult patients are usually administered an IV injection to induce anesthesia, as it is faster and smoother, and it causes less claustrophobia, while inhalational anesthetic agent is the preferred induction anesthetic in children. The properties of an ideal inhalational anesthetic agent are shown in **Table 31.2**. Similar properties are also considered while selecting the ideal IV anesthetic agent in terms of stability, cost-effectiveness, nonirritability, low incidence of adverse effects, and presence of related pharmacodynamic properties (**Table 31.2**). In addition, the drug should be highly lipid soluble and distribute rapidly into the CNS and other tissues to allow rapid and smooth onset of action. It should be noncumulative during infusion, quickly cleared from the bloodstream and CNS, leading to fast and predictable dose-related recovery. The rapid adjustments in depth of anesthesia should also be possible.

Mechanisms of General Anesthetics

General anesthetics inhibit cortical neuronal activity that is responsible for the control of consciousness and all sensation. They possess depressant actions on all excitable tissues, including the cardiovascular system, in a wide variety of species across the animal kingdom. They cause immobility,

Table 31.1 Routes of administration of general anesthetics and anesthetic adjuncts

Routes of administration	Classes	General anesthetic agents
Inhalation	Inert gases	Nitrous oxide, xenon
	Volatile liquids (halogenated hydrocarbons)	Halothane, isoflurane, desflurane, sevoflurane, enflurane, methoxyflurane
IV	Barbiturate derivatives	Thiopental, methohexital
	Miscellaneous:	
	▪ Alkyl phenol derivative	Propofol
	▪ Carboxylated imidazole derivative	Etomidate
	▪ Phencyclidine derivatives	Ketamine
	BZDs	Midazolam, diazepam, lorazepam
	Opioids	Morphine, fentanyl
	α_2-adrenoceptor agonists	Dexmedetomidine
	Neuroactive steroids	Alfaxalone

Abbreviations: BZD, benzodiazepines; IV, intravenous.

Table 31.2 General properties of an ideal inhalational anesthetic agent

Physicochemical properties
Liquid at room temperature
High saturated vapor pressure
Low specific heat capacity
Long shelf-life with no preservatives
Light and heat resistant
Resistant to other components such as rubber, metal, plastic, and soda lime
Not flammable/explosive
Nice odor and nonirritant
Cheap
Little or no effect on the ozone layer/environment friendly
Pharmacokinetic properties
High oil:gas partition coefficient
Low MAC
Low blood:gas partition coefficient
Rapid onset and offset
Minimal/no metabolism
Nontoxic
Pharmacodynamic properties
Hypnotic, amnestic, and skeletal muscle relaxation properties
Additional properties such as anticonvulsant, antiemetic, and analgesic properties
Does not cause CNS excitation, cardiovascular or respiratory depression, and organ-specific damage
Does not cause unwanted reflexes such as laryngospasm or airway hyperactivity
Does not cause an increase in intracranial pressure
Not teratogenic
No drug interaction

Abbreviations: CNS, central nervous system; MAC, minimum alveolar concentration.

amnesia, unconsciousness, and even induce immobility in small organisms, including bacteria.

Clinical effects of general anesthetics depend on their chemical structures and their ability to localize within CNS and interact with target sites. However, the exact mechanisms of anesthetic action are still unclear. It was suggested earlier that the broad single mechanism of general anesthetics is based on physiological action, including membrane expansion, membrane perturbations, or membrane fluidization (unitary hypothesis). Later, an agent-specific hypothesis was suggested, and numerous experiments on molecular and transgenic animals investigated the number of targets for general anesthetic action. The studies led to the identification of general anesthetics' cellular and molecular mechanisms.

Effect on the Different Regions of the Central Nervous System

The inhalation anesthetics–induced immobility and inhibition of motor response to pain were found to be primarily related to the spinal cord and not to the brain, while the amnesia effect of general anesthetics was found to be linked to the hippocampus. The sedation produced by general anesthetics is associated with the neocortex and thalamus. The hypothalamus is connected with the hypnotic effect. However, as the anesthetic concentration is increased, all brain functions and parts of the CNS are gradually affected. Therefore, it is difficult to relate a single target site in the brain with the effect of general anesthetics.

Cellular Mechanisms of General Anesthesia

Many inhalation and IV anesthetics hyperpolarize motor neurons by direct action. They affect neurons at various cellular locations, but their main action is produced on the synapse, where they affect the synaptic transmission, while they have lesser effect on action potential generation and propagation.

Molecular Targets of General Anesthetics

Several studies suggested the proteins of neuronal ligand-gated ion channels as the primary molecular targets for anesthetic agents. The electrical activity of the associated ion channels is regulated by these proteins. Chloride channels (gamma-aminobutyric acid [$GABA_A$] and glycine receptors) and potassium channels (the two-pore domain [K_{2p}], voltage-gated and ATP-sensitive [K_{ATP}] potassium channels) are the general anesthetics' key inhibitory ion channel targets. Excitatory ion channel targets include those stimulated by acetylcholine (nicotinic and muscarinic acetylcholine [ACh] receptors), by glutamate (amino 3-hydroxy-5-methyl-4-isoxazol-propionic acid [AMPA], kainite, and N-methyl-D-aspartate [NMDA] receptors), and by serotonin (5-hydroxytryptamine [5-HT_2 and 5-HT_3] receptors subtypes 2 and 3). In general, the anesthetics may either enhance the activation of inhibitory postsynaptic channels or block the activation of excitatory synaptic channels.

The general anesthetics are usually grouped into three different categories, based on their relative abilities to produce unconsciousness, immobility, and analgesia and for their effect on EEG (**Fig. 31.1**). They include:

1. Etomidate, propofol, and barbiturates as IV anesthetics.
2. Ketamine as an IV anesthetic, and nitrous oxide, xenon, and cyclopropane as inhaled anesthetics.
3. Halothane, enflurane, isoflurane, sevoflurane, and desflurane as volatile halogenated anesthetics.

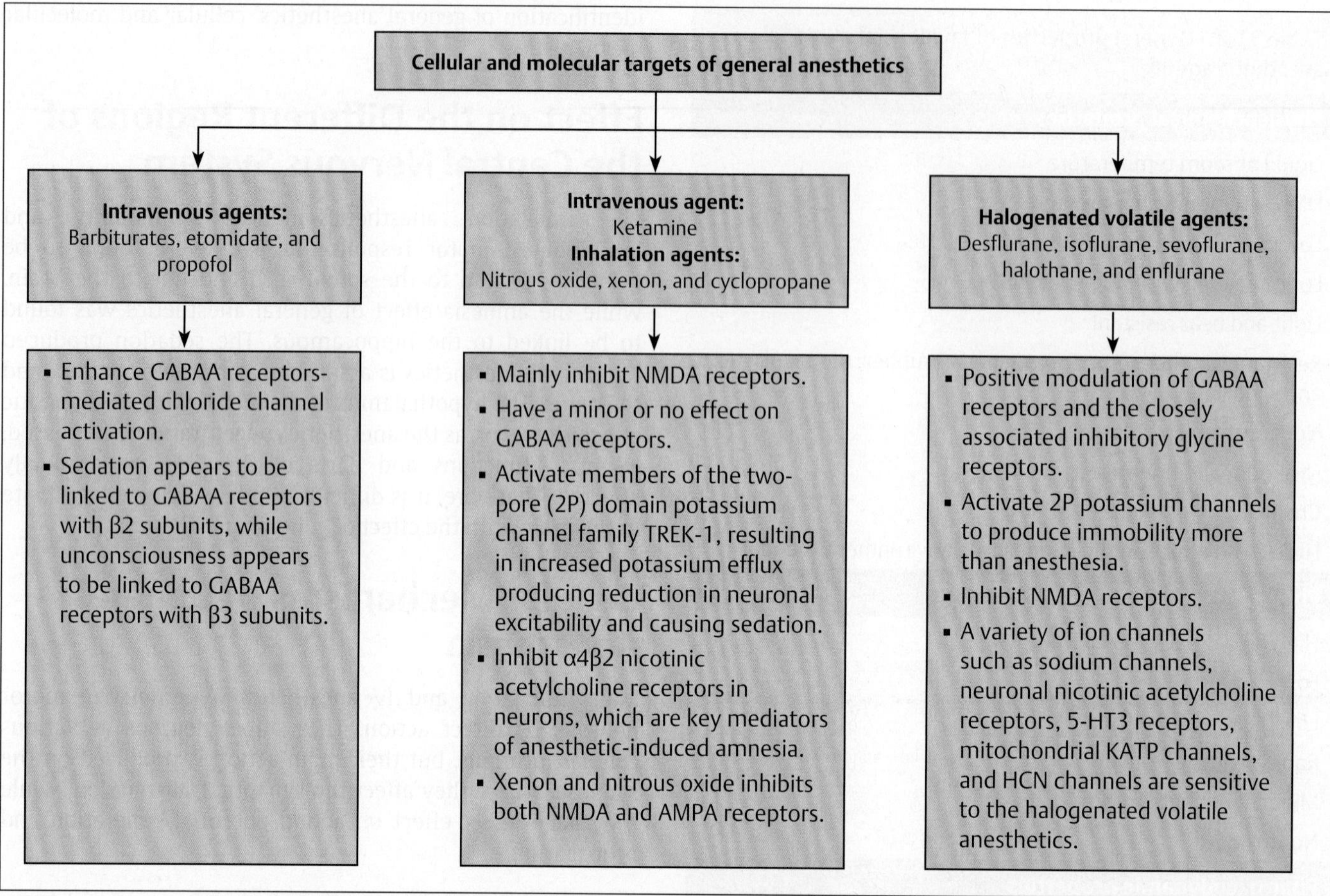

Fig. 31.1 Cellular and molecular targets of general anesthetics. 5-HT3, serotonin type 3 receptors; AMPA, α-amino-3-hydroxy-5-methyl-4-isoxazolepropionic acid; $GABA_A$, gamma-aminobutyric acid A; HCN, hyperpolarization-activated cyclic nucleotide-gated channels; K_{ATP}, ATP-sensitive potassium channels; NMDA, N-methyl-D-aspartate.

Stages and Depth of Anesthesia

General anesthesia involves three primary stages: induction, maintenance, and recovery from anesthesia. During these stages, the general anesthetics produce a neurophysiologic condition marked by five key effects: analgesia (loss of response to pain), amnesia (forgetfulness/loss of memory), suppression of autonomic reflexes, unconsciousness (hypnosis), and skeletal muscle relaxation throughout these phases. There is no single anesthetic agent that can produce the desired effects, and managing the autonomic nervous system (ANS) during surgery with only one drug is much more difficult and requires much higher concentrations. Thus, the standard practice usually involves an IV induction followed by an inhalational maintenance, which is known as balanced anesthesia. The margin between surgical anesthesia and potentially fatal respiratory and circulatory depression is quite narrow. Hence, it requires careful monitoring and adjustment of the level of anesthesia. Despite the advent of newer anesthetic agents and delivery methods, Arthur Ernest Guedel's classification for the four stages of anesthesia, which was first published in 1937, remains the most commonly used tool for assessing the depth of anesthesia or the degree of CNS depression (**Table 31.3**). Nowadays, there are different technologies for the measurement of the depth of anesthesia, which include the following: BIS monitoring, auditory evoked potentials, patient state analyzer, and approximate entropy.

Induction Phase (AS4.3)

The induction of unconsciousness in adults is usually carried out using the appropriate dose of an IV anesthetic agent such as propofol. Prior to anesthetic induction and tracheal intubation, preoxygenation is carried out for 5 minutes of normal breathing, using 100% oxygen to replace nitrogen at the alveolar level and increase the functional residual capacity (oxygen reservoir within the lungs). This delays the onset of arterial hemoglobin desaturation during apnea. Fast induction is usually initiated by using an IV bolus and slow induction by using either an IV infusion or a volatile inhalational anesthetic agent. In order to produce general anesthesia in children, nonpungent inhalational volatile agents such as sevoflurane are used. The patient progresses through different planes (a conversation can be carried on with patient at this time) till he/she reaches loss of consciousness stage/anesthetized state (**Table 31.3**). Usually, unconsciousness is produced in 30 to 40 seconds.

Maintenance Phase

It is critical to maintain stage III surgical anesthesia after induction, in which the state of analgesia, amnesia, proper

Table 31.3 Stages and depth of general anesthesia

Stages and depth of general anesthesia	Description
Stage I: Analgesia (disorientation)	▪ From the start of general anesthesia to the moment when patient loses consciousness ▪ In 1954, Joseph F. Artusio subdivided Guedel's first stage into three planes, with the patient progressing from analgesia without amnesia to analgesia with concurrent amnesia
Stage II: Excitement or delirium	▪ From loss of consciousness to the onset of automatic breathing ▪ Rapidly acting anesthetics are used to reduce the amount of time spent in this stage and get to stage III as soon as possible
Stage III: Surgical anesthesia	▪ From the beginning of automatic respiration to the paralysis of the respiratory system ▪ It is split into four planes
Plane I	From the start of automatic breathing to the end of eyeball movements
Plane II	From the cessation of eyeball movements to the initiation of paralysis of intercostal muscles
Plane III	From the beginning to the end of the paralysis of the intercostal muscles
Plane IV	From full intercostal muscle paralysis to diaphragmatic paralysis
Stage IV: Respiratory or medullary paralysis	▪ From stoppage of respiration till death ▪ The overdose of general anesthetic causes medullary paralysis with respiratory arrest and vasomotor collapse

muscle relaxation, and ANS stability must remain unchanged during the surgery under optimal surgical conditions (**Table 31.3**). Since most agents used for induction of anesthesia have a short duration of action, several inhalation and IV agents are used throughout the maintenance phase of general anesthesia. The depth of anesthesia is determined by changes in breathing pattern, eye movements, lacrimation, and muscle tone.

Emergence and Recovery Phase

Recovery or emergence from anesthesia is the gradual return of consciousness after the discontinuation of anesthetics and adjuvant agents at the completion of the surgical procedure. Majority of patients become awake and aware of their surroundings and identity within approximately 15 minutes of extubation. Usually, all patients should be responsive within 60 minutes after the last administration of any sedative, opioid, or anesthetic agent. However, the time required for return of consciousness varies, depending on different factors that include the type and duration of surgical procedure that the patient has undergone, the type of general anesthetic and analgesic agents administered (dosing, duration, and time since last administration), and patient's factors (preoperative physical and mental status, body habitus, sex, and age). Patients recovering from general anesthesia must be monitored constantly until they have regained consciousness and become aware of their surroundings and identity, their body function has been restored, and any adverse symptoms have disappeared. The elimination of anesthetic agents from the brain leads to awakening of patients. They usually respond to verbal commands when alveolar concentration of the anesthetic agent is reduced to about 30% of minimum alveolar concentration (MAC) in the absence of other hindering factors. The complete progression of patient to full postoperative recovery from anesthesia is through three phases: immediate recovery (the first 24 hours), intermediate recovery (few hours to days), and long-term recovery (few hours to weeks/months). However, many patients (especially the older population) may regain consciousness later than expected. This condition is known as delayed awakening and is characterized by persistent somnolence and unresponsiveness, during which the patient cannot be aroused. This could be due to the increased sensitivity of the patients toward general anesthetics, opioids, and benzodiazepines (BZDs).

Drugs Used for Induction and Maintenance of Anesthesia

Inhalational Anesthetics

Inhalational anesthetics are either volatile liquids or gases that diffuse rapidly across pulmonary alveoli and tissue barriers. The pharmacokinetics of inhalational anesthetics differs from that of other drugs, as they are absorbed and eliminated through the lungs.

Pharmacokinetic Principles

There are many factors that affect the occurrence and depth of anesthesia, which are discussed in the following.

Partial Pressure of the Inhalational Anesthetic in the Inspired Gas

It determines the concentration of inhalational anesthetic in the blood. Higher the inspired tension of the inhalation anesthetic, more anesthetic will be shifted to the blood. The partial pressure of the inhaled anesthetic agent in the alveoli of the lungs would be equal to the partial pressures in the patient's blood and brain at equilibrium. When the partial pressure of the inhaled gas equals the partial pressure of the end-tidal (alveolar) gas, equilibrium is reached.

Pulmonary Ventilation

It indicates the transfer of the anesthetic to the alveoli. Higher the respiratory stimulation (hyperventilation), more anesthetics will be transferred to the alveoli. Anesthetics with high-lipid solubility will dissolve easily into pulmonary blood without considerable increase in the partial pressure—thus, taking longer time in approaching the partial pressure in alveoli and leading to slow onset of action.

Alveolar Exchange

To allow inhalational anesthetics to equilibrate in the pulmonary vasculature and eventually within the CNS, effective partial pressures must be achieved within the lung's alveoli. The rapid bidirectional transfer of gases between alveoli, blood, and the CNS enables inhaled anesthetics to reach equilibrium. If the alveolar ventilation and/or perfusion are not adequate, less inhalational anesthetics exchange will occur. Except for halothane, which is metabolized in the liver (> 20%), most inhalational general anesthetics are only partially metabolized and therefore eliminated unchanged.

Solubility of Inhalational Anesthetic in Blood

The inhalational anesthetic is passively absorbed by diffusion. This depends on the blood solubility of the anesthetic agent. Anesthetics with higher lipid and blood solubility, such as halothane, have a slow induction time. The initiation of anesthetic action is determined by the solubility of the anesthetic in blood and tissue, which is dependent on the blood:gas partition coefficient. The ratio of the anesthetic agent in the blood and alveolar space at equal partial pressure is defined by the Ostwald coefficient for blood–gas. Since all inhalational anesthetics are predominantly eliminated through the lungs, lower the blood:gas partition coefficient, faster the recovery from the anesthetic effect.

Solubility of Inhalational Anesthetic in Tissue

Most of general anesthetics are equally soluble in lean tissues as in the blood, but are more soluble in fatty tissues. The inhalation anesthetic's potency is determined by its lipid solubility, which is measured by the oil:gas partition coefficient. When both phases are at equilibrium at a standard temperature and partial pressure, the oil:gas partition coefficient compares the lipid solubility of the anesthetic agent in the lipid tissues of the brain and other organs to that in alveolar air. Anesthetic agents with high MAC value have low oil:gas partition coefficient value and, thus, low potency. Since halothane has high lipid solubility, it will enter adipose tissue continuously for hours and leave it slowly. In obese patients, the recovery from anesthesia after the administration of a highly lipid soluble anesthetic might slow down, as the anesthetic will accumulate in the adipose tissue and will lead to increase in context-sensitive half-life.

Cerebral Blood Flow and Brain:Blood Partition Coefficient

The transport of the inhalational anesthetics to the CNS and their uptake into the brain depends on the cerebral blood flow (perfusion) and the lipid solubility of the inhalational agents. The brain receives 15 to 20% of total cardiac output, which makes it a highly perfused organ. Higher the brain:blood partition coefficient, greater the solubility of the inhalational anesthetic in brain. The inhalational anesthetic attain higher concentration in white matter than in gray matter.

Second Gas Effect and Diffusion Hypoxia

Nitrous oxide (N_2O) is commonly used in combination with more effective inhalational anesthetics. This is because the inhalation of nitrous oxide during induction of anesthesia may produce the second gas effect, which will enhance the speed at which the alveolar concentration of the other inhalational anesthetic is achieved, thus producing faster onset of action. The second gas effect is usually a result of the concentration effect. The rapid absorption of high concentrations of N_2O leads to its rapid diffusion, more than nitrogen and other gases, across alveolar basement membranes. It also exits rapidly from the alveoli, causing remaining alveolar gases to be concentrated, which accelerates the uptake of the volatile gases into the blood and the subsequent speedup of the onset of anesthesia.

Diffusion hypoxia, also known as Fink effect, is one of the complications that can occur during the recovery from anesthesia period when the administration of nitrous oxide ceases after prolonged use of inhalational anesthesia. Nitrous oxide, having low-blood solubility, enters the alveoli far more quickly than other anesthetics leave, causing dilution of the gaseous contents and reducing the partial pressure of oxygen in the alveoli. This results in the deficiency in the amount of oxygen reaching the tissues due to dilution of oxygen within the alveoli, causing hypoxia. The dilution of the alveolar contents aids in the elimination of other inhalational anesthetics, thus speeding wakening. It is important to monitor the patient during the first elimination phase as N_2O anesthesia is discontinued. In addition, after termination of N_2O, it is recommended to administer 100% oxygen for 10 minutes.

Minimum Alveolar Concentration

After equilibration, the alveolar concentration of the inhalational anesthetic agent equals the blood concentration and also equals to its brain concentration at a later stage. Thus, MAC is the index of potency of the inhalational agents. It is also used to compare potency among different agents. MAC represents the median effective dose (ED_{50}) value. The oil:gas coefficient is inversely related to MAC. This value represents the pulmonary alveolar concentration of the anesthetic agent at 1 atmosphere (atm) that inhibits the response (causes immobility) to a standardized painful stimulus such as surgical skin incision in 50% of patients. Any change in ambient atmospheric pressure will change MAC. The ability to respond to verbal commands can be measured as MAC-awake. MAC can also be used clinically to assess amnesia (MAC-amnesia) and autonomic response (MAC-bar). Each anesthetic has a distinct MAC value, which is affected by patient's age and declines after the age of 50. It is also affected by patient's cardiovascular status and the use of adjuvant medications. Drugs such as sedative-hypnotics, IV drugs that enhance GABA, α_2-adrenergic agonists, opioids, and local anesthetics decrease MAC. Hypoxia below 30 mm Hg, hyponatremia, acute metabolic acidosis, and acute hemorrhagic hypotension can also cause a reduction in MAC value. Factors that increase MAC will lead to decrease in the potency of inhalational anesthetic; thus, the patient will require a larger amount of the anesthetic to achieve immobility. Hypernatremia and administration of CNS stimulants such as cocaine and ephedrine increase MAC. In addition, chronic alcohol consumption and acute amphetamine use increase MAC. MAC value is expressed as the percentage at 1 atm. Nitrous oxide has the maximum MAC (105% atm), making it the least potent inhalational anesthetic agent, followed by xenon (71% atm). Halothane is highly potent as it has lower MAC value (0.75% atm). MAC varies by not more than 10 to 15% among individuals in the population and animal species.

Techniques Used for the Administration

Different techniques are used to facilitate the administration of inhalational anesthetics, depending on the condition of patient, type, and duration of surgical procedure.

Open Drop Method

This method is simple and does not require a special apparatus for its delivery, as the liquid anesthetic such as ether can be poured easily over a mask with gauze and the patient can inhale its vapor with air. This method is suitable for administering cheap anesthetics, as a lot of anesthetic vapor gets wasted in the surroundings. In addition, this method does not allow to determine the exact concentration of anesthetic that is inhaled by the patient.

Delivering the Inhalational Anesthetic via an Anesthetic Machines

The anesthesia machine is often used in conjunction with a mechanical ventilator, breathing system, suction equipment, and patient-monitoring devices, allowing for more precise control of anesthetic administration. The machine allows for the vaporization of liquid anesthetics, the composition of a mixture of oxygen, anesthetics, and ambient air, and the delivery of this mixture to the patient through a tightly fitted face mask/endotracheal tube while monitoring patient and machine parameters. The breathing system usually fulfills three main functions, which include the adequate removal of carbon dioxide (CO_2) from the patient and adequate supply of oxygen (O_2) and accurate dose of anesthetics to the patient. This can be performed either through an open, semiclosed, or closed system (closed-circuit anesthesia).

Commonly Used Inhalational Anesthetics

The most commonly used volatile anesthetics today are desflurane, isoflurane, and sevoflurane. They are frequently used in conjunction with nitrous oxide. Other volatile anesthetics are less frequently used and include halothane, enflurane, and methoxyflurane (still in use in some countries). Many researchers are exploring the use of xenon as an anesthetic, although its use is limited due to its high cost. Inhalational anesthetics have low safety margin and their toxicity depends largely on the characteristics of individual drugs and their side effects. As a result, the choice of inhalational agents is frequently based on whether the patient's pathophysiology is compatible with the drug's side effect profiles.

Nitrous Oxide

Characteristics

Nitrous oxide is known as laughing gas. It is colorless, nonflammable, and nearly odorless gas with a faint, sweet smell which is provided in steel cylinders (blue code) and must be delivered via suitable anesthetic apparatus through calibrated flow meters. It is extremely insoluble in blood and other tissues. Nitrous oxide has poor muscle relaxation property and must be accompanied with another anesthetics. It has a powerful analgesic effect with faster induction and recovery (onset of action is within half a minute and lasts for about a minute). It is expelled from the body unchanged through the lungs and does not accumulate under normal conditions.

Indications and Dosage

It is a dissociative anesthetic that is used for the maintenance of anesthesia (50–66% N_2O in 33% O_2) in combination with other anesthetic agents (as a carrier gas and adjuvant to other anesthetics: halothane, ketamine, etc.) and muscle relaxants. It is used solely in a mixture with oxygen (50% N_2O and 50% O_2) for dental and obstetric analgesia. It is also used for emergency management of injuries during postoperative physiotherapy and for the management of refractory pain in terminal illness.

Contraindications

It is more soluble than oxygen and nitrogen and, thus, diffuses freely into gas-filled spaces in the body (bowel, pneumothorax, middle ear, eye). Therefore, it is contraindicated in patients with bowel obstruction, arterial air embolism, decompression sickness, occlusion of middle ear, chronic obstructive airway disease, and emphysema.

Precautions

If administered during pregnancy, it leads to potential birth defects.

Adverse Effects

It increases pulmonary vascular resistance, nausea, and vomiting. After prolonged administration, it causes megaloblastic anemia, depressed white cell formation, peripheral neuropathy and numbness, vitamin B_{12} depletion, and psychological dependence.

Halothane

Characteristics

At room temperature, it is a volatile liquid with a sweet odor. Halothane is nonirritant, noninflammable, and light-sensitive (stored in amber-colored bottles). It provides little pain relief; thus, it is often administered with analgesics. It has high blood:gas (2.3) and high fat:blood (51) partition coefficients and takes long time for onset/offset of anesthesia, as it accumulates on prolonged administration due to solubility in fat and other body tissues. Thus, the speed of recovery may be lengthened.

Indications and Dosage

It is used for induction and maintenance of anesthesia. Halothane is a potent anesthetic and requires the precise control of administered concentration. Induction is done by using specifically calibrated vaporizer. The inspired gas concentration should be gradually increased to 2 to 4% in adult and to 1.5 to 2% in children in oxygen or nitrous oxide–oxygen mixture. Maintenance dose in adults and children is 0.5 to 2%. Halothane is the anesthetic of choice in children, and it is also the preferred anesthetic for asthmatic patients.

Contraindications

It is contraindicated in pheochromocytoma (tumor of the adrenal gland tissue), since halothane is arrhythmogenic and sensitizes the myocardium to circulating catecholamine, aggravating the patient's condition; history of unpredictable jaundice or pyrexia following a prior exposure to halothane, family history of malignant hyperthermia; increased cerebrospinal fluid pressure; and porphyria.

Precautions

At least 3 months should be allowed to elapse between each halothane re-exposure to avoid the above-mentioned complications. Care should also be taken in pregnant and breastfeeding women. In addition, the use of halothane should be avoided in dental procedures for patients under 18 years of age due to the risks of arrhythmia.

Adverse Effects

Adverse effects include arrhythmias, malignant hyperthermia in susceptible patients, bradycardia, respiratory depression, and liver toxicity in susceptible patients. It can prolong delivery and increase postpartum blood loss.

Isoflurane

Characteristics

It is a noninflammable, clear, colorless, stable volatile liquid administered by vaporizer.

It smells mildly pungent, musty, and ethereal. At 37°C, the partition coefficients for water:gas, blood:gas, and oil:gas are, respectively, 0.61, 1.43, and 90.8. MAC is 1.28%. Induction and recovery produced by isoflurane are faster than halothane. It allows a rapid change in anesthetic depth. It is mostly expelled unchanged by the lungs and only 0.2% is metabolized by CYP2E1. It is not toxic to the liver.

Indications and Dosage

It is usually used for maintenance and not for induction of anesthesia due to its irritating pungent odor. Inspired concentrations (1.5–3%) of isoflurane generate surgical anesthesia in 7 to 10 minutes when used for induction in oxygen or in conjunction with oxygen–nitrous oxide mixtures. A 1 to 2.5% concentration of isoflurane with nitrous oxide is commonly used to maintain surgical anesthesia levels. When using only oxygen to administer isoflurane, an additional 0.5 to 1% dose may be needed. Isoflurane has a relaxing effect on the muscles. Supplemental doses of muscle relaxants may be used if additional relaxation is needed. It is preferred for cardiac surgery, as it has excellent renal, hepatic, coronary, and cerebral blood flow preservation. It is also preferred for neurosurgery, as it produces little increase in the intracranial pressure as compared to other agents. It does not sensitize the myocardium to catecholamine's effects and, thus, is safe to be used in patients with pheochromocytoma.

Contraindications

It is contraindicated in sensitivity and hypersensitivity to isoflurane or to other halogenated anesthetics agents, genetic susceptibility to malignant hyperthermia, and latent and overt neuromuscular diseases (Duchenne's muscular dystrophy) in pediatric patients, as it might lead to hyperkalemia and subsequent cardiac arrhythmia and death.

Precautions

It can be used during pregnancy only if the possible risk to the fetus outweighs the benefits. When administering isoflurane to a breastfeeding woman, extreme caution is recommended. Since isoflurane relaxes skeletal muscles and improves the neuromuscular blocking effect of depolarizing and nondepolarizing muscle relaxants, caution should be exercised while using these drugs together.

Adverse Effects

It causes profound respiratory depression, arrhythmia, and dose-dependent decrease in blood pressure. In patients with coronary artery disease, it leads to coronary steal phenomenon (diversion of blood from collateral dependent myocardium to normally perfused areas) and myocardial ischemia. It may also cause malignant hyperthermia, hepatitis, postoperative shivering, nausea, and vomiting. It can produce carbon monoxide when it reacts with desiccated carbon dioxide (CO_2) absorbents, which can increase carboxyhemoglobin levels in vulnerable patients.

Desflurane

Characteristics

It is a nonflammable, colorless, highly volatile liquid at room temperature (boiling point = 23°C) that necessitates the use of a special active-temperature controlled vaporizer due to its high vapor pressure. At 37°C, the partition coefficients are blood:gas = 0.424, olive oil:gas = 18.7, and brain:gas = 0.54. Desflurane has a low lipid solubility and a very low blood and tissue solubility. As a result, anesthesia induction and emergence are both very rapidly achieved (5–10 minutes in the absence of sedative drugs). Desflurane allows the better control of depth of anesthesia (MAC is 7.3%). The anesthetic is almost five times less potent than isoflurane. MAC decreases with increasing age and with administration of opioids or BZDs. The anesthetic is mostly excreted unchanged by the lungs and just 0.02% of the anesthetic is metabolized in the liver and excreted in urine. Desflurane reacts with desiccated CO_2 absorbents in the same way as isoflurane does.

Indications and Dosage

It is usually used for maintenance and not for induction of anesthesia, as it causes irritation to air passage, provoking coughing, salivation, breath-holding, and laryngospasm. Desflurane is used for inpatients and outpatients surgical procedures. Because of its rapid onset of action and recovery, it is most often used for outpatient day care surgery procedures. In adults, the usual starting dose for induction is 3% desflurane and it is increased by 0.5 to 1% increments every two to three breaths. Desflurane in carrier gas (O_2 or N_2O/O_2) is administered at approximately 0.5 to 1 MAC after induction in adults with an IV anesthetic agent (thiopental or propofol). The anesthetics is administered for maintenance of surgical anesthesia in adults at concentrations of 2.5 to 8.5% with or without N_2O. The MAC of desflurane is reduced by 16% when BZDs (midazolam 25–50 µg/kg) are administered, and by 50% when opioids (fentanyl 3–6 µg /kg) are administered. As a result, the dosage should be changed appropriately.

Contraindications

Same as with isoflurane.

Precautions

In patients with intracranial space-occupying lesions, the anesthetic should be administered at 0.8 MAC or less (in combination with a barbiturate induction and hyperventilation, thereby maintaining cerebral perfusion pressure). In patients with coronary artery disease, it should not be used alone for anesthetic induction (it should be combined with IV opioids and hypnotics). It can only be used during pregnancy if the possible benefits outweighs the risks to the fetus. Care should be taken while administering to breastfeeding women.

Adverse effects

The anesthetic stimulates catecholamines release and produces similar cardiovascular effects to isoflurane. It causes hypertension and tachycardia on rapid administration. It can also increase the heart rate in concentrations above 1 MAC. Desflurane can cause malignant hyperthermia and sensitivity hepatitis in susceptible patients. It can also increase postoperative nausea and vomiting (PONV).

Sevoflurane

Characteristics

It is a noninflammable, clear, colorless, stable, sweet smelling, nonpungent liquid administered by vaporizer with intermediate properties between isoflurane and desflurane.

At 37° C, the partition coefficients are blood:gas = 0.63 to 0.69, water:gas = 0.36, olive oil:gas = 47 to 54, and brain:gas = 1.15. The MAC values for sevoflurane decrease with age and when nitrous oxide is administered. The MAC of sevoflurane in oxygen for a 40-year-old adult is 2.1%, making it roughly half as potent as isoflurane. The low blood and tissue solubility allows for rapid induction and changes in anesthetic depth, and its rapid emergence from anesthesia is due to rapid removal through the lungs. As a result, patients may need pain relief after surgery.

Indications and Dosage

Sevoflurane is used for induction of anesthesia (especially in children) and in patients who are prone to bronchospasm due to its nonirritating nature. It is also used to maintain general anesthesia in adult and pediatric patients during inpatient and outpatient surgery. Sevoflurane is the preferred anesthetic for neurosurgical patients with elevated intracranial pressure, as it causes minimal cerebral vasodilation in comparison to other agents. IV induction agents, such as short-acting barbiturates or other agents, are typically administered first, followed by sevoflurane inhalation. Sevoflurane induction is normally accomplished with oxygen or a mixture of oxygen and nitrous oxide, and doses of up to 5% sevoflurane in adults and 7% in children produce surgical anesthesia in less than 2 minutes. Further, the dosage of sevoflurane should be personalized and titrated based on the age and clinical status of the patient and the administration of other medications. For maintenance of anesthesia, concentrations of 0.5 to 3% sevoflurane in presence or absence of nitrous oxide will sustain the surgical levels of anesthesia. However, during the maintenance of anesthesia with sevoflurane, the dosage of nondepolarizing muscle relaxants is likely to be reduced. Due to its high cost, and the need for high-flow open or semiclosed system, sevoflurane is not used for routine procedures.

Contraindications

Same as with isoflurane and desflurane.

Precautions

When maintaining anesthesia with increasing sevoflurane concentrations, caution should be taken because it reduces blood pressure and induces respiratory depression in a dose-dependent manner. This occurs more rapidly as compared with other volatile anesthetics and can be regulated by reducing the inspired concentration of sevoflurane. Sevoflurane should be used with caution in patients with renal insufficiency, patients who are susceptible to QT prolongation, and pediatric patients with Pompe's disease, as it can cause arrhythmia. Sevoflurane should be used with caution if administered during obstetric anesthesia, as it can increase the risk of uterine bleeding due to its relaxant effect. Because of the risk of ventricular arrhythmia, sympathomimetic agents such as isoprenaline, adrenaline, and noradrenaline should be used with caution when combined with sevoflurane.

Adverse Effects

Emergence delirium after pediatric anesthesia is frequently associated with the use of sevoflurane. The anesthetic can also trigger seizures (rarely), and dystonic movements have been observed in children. When sevoflurane is exposed to desiccated CO_2 absorbents (soda lime and barium hydroxide lime), it produces carbon monoxide, which leads to heat, smoke, and/or spontaneous fire in the anesthesia machine. Additionally, many decomposition products such as methanol, formaldehyde, compound A or fluoromethyl-2,2-difluoro-1-(trifluoromethyl) vinyl ether, and compounds B, C, D, and E are formed, with compound A being the key degradation product causing renal injury. Sevoflurane might cause malignant hyperthermia in susceptible individuals (can be managed by IV dantrolene sodium).

Enflurane

It is a noninflammable, clear, colorless, odorless, volatile liquid administered by vaporizing. The anesthetic is a fluorinated ether and a structural isomer of isoflurane. Enflurane is very potent and stable, and it was one of the most commonly used inhalation anesthetic drug during the 1970s and 1980s for the maintenance of general anesthesia. However, the anesthetic induced seizure activity and severe hepatic injury (rare) and caused increased cardiodepressant effects as compared to the newer halogenated anesthetics that show a better pharmacokinetic profile. Therefore, enflurane used decreased tremendously.

Xenon

Characteristics

Xenon is a colorless, nonflammable, heavy, and odorless inert gas, which is available in fewer quantities in the atmosphere. Therefore, it is very expensive, as it needs to be extracted from the air (by fractional distillation of liquefied air) for its anesthetic use. The advancement in manufacturing technology and the use of low-flow circuit systems that allow recovering and recycling of the exhaled xenon in the operating room atmosphere might decrease its cost and increase its use. In Europe, xenon is licensed for use in adult anesthesia. It is nonirritant to the airway and does not cause ozone depletion or environmental pollution. It has a potent intraoperative analgesic activity and an adequate hypnotic effect with lack of metabolism in the liver or kidneys. Its partition coefficients at 37°C are blood:gas = 0.12 (the least soluble gas that may be used for anesthesia and results in a very rapid onset and recovery from anesthesia) and oil:gas = 1.9 (higher than the lighter noble gases). The MAC of xenon in in adults is 71% and higher in children (1-year-old, MAC = 92%).

Indications and Dosage

When combined with 30% oxygen, xenon produces surgical anesthesia. In adult, xenon can be used as a monoanesthetic agent, whereas in children it can be probably used as an additive to other anesthetics. Xenon was also reported to induce anesthesia faster than sevoflurane. Usually, propofol is additionally administered for supplementation of xenon anesthesia. Xenon is used in "day-surgery" outpatient settings and critical care medicine (for clinical examination) because of its rapid emergence from anesthesia potential.

Contraindications

Due to its high relative density and viscosity, xenon causes elevation in pulmonary resistance and increase in airway pressure. As a result, it is not recommended for patients with severe chronic obstructive pulmonary disease or in premature babies.

Precautions

At concentrations greater than 60%, xenon rises the cerebral blood flow and causes retention of significant amounts of the gas in the bowels and fatty tissues. Therefore, caution should be taken in patients with high intracranial pressure or bowel obstruction.

Adverse Effects

Xenon causes minimal respiratory depression, has minimal cardiovascular side effects, and preserves baseline blood pressure. It is a well-tolerated anesthetic in older population. No long-term side effects have been reported. Xenon might lead to increase in PONV.

Intravenous Anesthetics

IV anesthetics are a class of fast-acting compounds that cause a state of impaired awareness and loss of consciousness in one arm-brain circulation period (around 11 seconds) after IV injection. The hydrophobic nature of IV drugs helps them to preferentially diffuse into the highly perfused and lipophilic tissues of the brain and spinal cord, resulting in a rapid onset of action. They are widely used for induction of anesthesia in adult patients because of these characteristics.

Pharmacokinetics

The IV drug travels from the injection site (usually the arm) to the brain during the induction stage, where it causes the desired effect. When a drug is administered by IV bolus administration, it enters the bloodstream, and a fraction of it binds to plasma proteins, leaving the remainder unbound, which moves to the cerebral circulation, where it passes along a concentration gradient from the blood into the brain. Unbound, lipid-soluble, and unionized molecules easily cross the blood–brain barrier. Later on, the drug begins to diffuse into tissues that have less blood supply. The diffusion of the drug continues throughout the body until the partial pressure of the drug within the various tissues is equivalent to the partial pressure of the drug within the lungs. In general, the potency of IV anesthetics is determined by the drug's free plasma concentration at equilibrium, which in 50% of patients eliminates the response to surgical incision.

Commonly Used Intravenous Anesthetics

The most widely used IV anesthetics are propofol, etomidate, ketamine, and barbiturates (e.g., thiopental). In most cases, propofol is used to induce anesthesia, while etomidate is used in cases of hemodynamic instability. Ketamine, a powerful psychedelic and dissociative drug, is mainly used in emergency medicine. It also has additional sympathomimetic and analgesic effects. In patients with high intracranial pressure and/or head trauma, thiopental and other barbiturates are preferred.

Propofol

Characteristics

Propofol is usually formulated as a 1 or 2% emulsion and is known as milk of amnesia. It should be administered within 4 hours of opening the sterile containers to prevent bacterial contamination that leads to patient's infection/sepsis. Propofol is a substituted phenol, while fospropofol is a prodrug that is converted to propofol in vivo by endothelial alkaline phosphatase. On IV injection, the lipid emulsion causes significant pain (it can be minimized by administration of lidocaine) and hyperlipidemia (HL), while the aqueous emulsion containing the fospropofol is less painful and does not cause HL.

Indications and Dosage

Propofol is the most frequently administered induction agent for general anesthesia. It can be used for maintenance of anesthesia of patients older than 2 months. The drug is used not only for sedation of intubated, mechanically ventilated ICU patients but also for procedural sedation during monitored anesthesia care. Propofol is an ultrafast-acting agent and its induction dose in healthy adults is 2 to 2.5 mg/kg every 10 seconds until induction onset. In pediatric patients, propofol is administered at 2.5 to 3.5 mg/kg dose over 20 to 30 seconds. The rapid distribution after an IV bolus dose into the brain and highly perfused lipid-rich tissues leads to its fast onset of action (usually within 15 seconds with loss of consciousness in 40 seconds from the start of injection). A rapid reawakening within 10 minutes after a single dose of propofol is related to its rapid redistribution. Due to the pharmacokinetic profile of propofol, the drug can also be administered as continuous infusions for maintenance of general anesthesia. In healthy adults younger than 55 years, propofol infusion dose is 6 to 12 mg/kg/h. Propofol is used off-label for the management of refractory status epilepticus in children and adults and PONV.

Contraindications

Propofol is contraindicated in hypersensitive patients to the drug or to the components of the emulsion, especially soybean oil and egg lecithin.

Precautions

Propofol doses should be lowered to half in the elderly, debilitated, or patients with severe systemic disease (ASA-PS III) or severe systemic disease that poses a persistent threat to life (ASA-PS IV), according to the American Society of Anesthesiologists (ASA) physical status (PS) classification system. Propofol may potentiate CNS, respiratory depression–causing medications, and blood pressure–lowering medications. Caution is advised while using these drugs and other agents that cause the prolongation of the QT interval.

Adverse Effects

The most common reaction is a transient local pain at the site of injection, which can be reduced by IV administration of lidocaine before the bolus of propofol. Cardiorespiratory depression is more likely to occur at higher propofol blood concentrations, and anesthesia induction is associated with arterial hypotension, with little or no change in heart rate and cardiac output and apnea in both adults and pediatric patients. In order to reduce the undesirable cardiorespiratory effects, slow infusion/slow injection techniques are preferred when monitored anesthesia care sedation is initiated. On prolonged, higher dose infusion in young and head-injured patients, propofol triggers a rare and potentially fatal complication known as propofol infusion syndrome (PRIS), which is characterized by metabolic acidosis, HL, rhabdomyolysis, and enlarged liver. Few incidences of a green tint urine have been reported.

Barbiturates

Characteristics

The most commonly used barbiturates in general anesthesia are thiopental, thiamylal, and methohexital. All of these barbiturates are available as racemic mixtures and formulated as sodium salts. They are combined with sodium chloride or sterile water to make IV injection solutions, which should be prepared fresh before use. Thiopental is a potent anesthetic but a weak analgesic. Barbiturates should not be used solely for painful procedures, as they require supplementary analgesic (opioids or N_2O) administration during anesthesia. They have weak muscle relaxation property. Thiamylal is approximately equipotent to thiopental, while methohexital is threefold more potent. When given by IV route, they produce mild pain on injection, especially methohexital.

Indications and Dosage

The barbiturates are usually used as alternative induction drugs for patients who are allergic to propofol, since propofol has largely replaced methohexital for outpatients' procedures that require a quick return of awareness. Other uses include providing cerebral protection during incomplete brain ischemia by lowering cerebral metabolism in a dose-dependent manner, as well as facilitating electroconvulsive therapy and epileptic foci detection during surgery. Thiopental is also used to reduce high intracranial pressure. It is an ultrashort-acting thiobarbiturate, which is generally administered as a bolus induction dose of 3 to 5 mg/kg. The drug is highly lipid soluble and quickly diffuses into vessel-rich areas such as the brain, causing unconsciousness in 10 to 30 seconds and a 1-minute peak effect. The anesthetic effect lasts for 5 to 8 minutes. The induction dose is usually higher in neonates and infants (5–8 mg/kg) and lower in elderly and pregnant patients (1–3 mg/kg). Since premedications such as BZDs, opiates, or α_2-adrenergic agonists cause additive hypnotic effects, doses of drugs can be further reduced by 10 to 50%.

Contraindications

Barbiturates should be avoided in patients with respiratory obstruction or acute asthma because they can cause laryngospasm and bronchospasm. They should also be avoided in patients with hypovolemia or shock because they can cause significant reductions in cardiac output and blood pressure. They are also contraindicated in patients with hypersensitivity reactions to barbiturates and in patients with porphyria (a group of genetic disorders that result from a buildup of porphyrins in the body, negatively affecting the skin or the nervous system), as they induce the delta aminolevulinic acid synthase, which is involved in porphyrin production pathway.

Precautions

They should be administered with caution in patients with adrenocortical insufficiency, cardiovascular disease, hypovolemia, severe hemorrhage, burns, status asthmaticus, and myasthenia gravis. During anesthetic induction, lowering the alkalinity of the solution by combining the barbiturate with acidic solutions, lactated Ringer's solution, or water-soluble drugs may cause the barbiturate to precipitate as free acid, causing IV-line occlusion. Thus, it is preferable to delay the administration of drugs such as muscle relaxants and other drugs until no more barbiturate is left in the IV tubing.

Adverse Effects

Barbiturates in general can cause apnea, coughing, chest wall spasms, laryngospasm, and bronchospasm. In patients with hypovolemia or shock, they can cause severe reductions in cardiac output and blood pressure. Additionally, barbiturates decrease appetite and cause hypokalemia/hyperkalemia.

Etomidate

Characteristics

It is a substituted imidazole derivative, available as a d-isomer, poorly soluble in water, and is provided as 2 mg/mL solution in 35% propylene glycol. It is also formulated as an aqueous solution. Etomidate does not have analgesic activity; thus, suitable analgesics should be administered prior to its use in procedures involving painful stimuli.

Indications and Dosage

It is a rapidly acting sedative-hypnotic that is often used for rapid sequence intubation (RSI) and anesthesia induction in patients at risk of hypotension. Cardiovascular stability is maintained with etomidate induction doses, with a small increase in heart rate and little to no reduction in blood pressure or cardiac output. As a result, etomidate is preferred in patients with coronary artery disease, cardiomyopathy, cerebral vascular disease, or hypovolemia. In addition, induction with etomidate is associated with a temporary decrease in cerebral blood flow by 20 to 30% and reduction in cerebral oxygen utilization. Thus, it is used as a protectant against cerebral ischemia. Etomidate can be used to supplement other anesthetics (such as nitrous oxide in oxygen), and also during anesthesia maintenance for short operative procedures such as dilation and curettage or cervical conization. The drug has a rapid onset (usually within 1 minute) and short duration of action (3–5 minutes) following induction doses of 0.2 to 0.6 mg/kg injected over a period of 30 to 60 seconds in adults and in pediatric patients older than 10 years.

Contraindications

It is not recommended for patients who have had hypersensitivity reactions to the drug or any of the formulation's ingredients. Long-term infusions of etomidate are not recommended due to its prolonged suppression of adrenocortical steroid synthesis.

Precautions

Etomidate should be used with caution in patients with sepsis and other critical conditions. In patients with liver cirrhosis and esophageal varices, the volume of distribution and elimination half-life of etomidate are nearly double the original values. Therefore, caution should be taken while administering the drug in those patients and in patients who have already received neuroleptic, opioids, or sedative agents (the dose of etomidate should be reduced). The administration of etomidate in elderly patients, particularly those with hypertension, may cause decreased heart rate, cardiac index, and mean arterial blood pressure. As a result, the drug's dosage should be decreased, and renal function should be monitored.

Adverse Effects

Etomidate cause transient inhibition of adrenal steroid synthesis, lasting 6 to 12 hours following bolus administration. Methoxycarbonyl-etomidate is an ultrashort-acting analog which is rapidly metabolized and does not produce prolonged adrenocortical suppression. Etomidate may cause hyperventilation/hypoventilation, apnea of short duration (5–90 seconds), laryngospasm, hiccup, and snoring. It is painful on injection and causes myoclonic movements. Premedication of either BZDs or opiates may minimize the myoclonic movements, whereas lidocaine administration may reduce the pain. It also causes moderate lowering of intracranial pressure and intraocular pressure, nausea, and vomiting.

Ketamine

Characteristics

Ketamine is a water-soluble general anesthetic agent which is available as 10, 50, and 100 mg/mL. It is a slightly acidic (pH 3.5–5.5) sterile solution for IV or intramuscular (IM) injection. It is supplied as a racemic mixture of two optical isomers (*S* [−] and *R* [+]) which is metabolized in liver to norketamine and has less CNS activity. Ketamine is a rapid-acting agent that produces a hypnotic state known as dissociative anesthesia, which is marked by profound analgesia, unresponsiveness to commands, and amnesia. The patients have their eyes open, move their limbs involuntarily, and experience normal pharyngeal-laryngeal reflexes, normal or slightly improved skeletal muscle tone, cardiovascular and respiratory stimulation, and, occasionally, a transient and minimal respiratory depression. Other drugs such as phencyclidine, nitrous oxide, and phencyclidine can also produce dissociative anesthesia.

Indications and Dosage

Ketamine is a suitable anesthetic for diagnostic and surgical procedures of the eye, ear, nose, and mouth, and for RSI in hemodynamically compromised, shocked, and hypotensive patients in emergency setting, due to its sympathomimetic hemodynamic effects. It is also administered for patients at great risk of bronchospasm (due to its bronchodilating property and profound analgesia), and as induction agent for some pediatric procedures and in children with congenital heart disease (with right to left shunt). Ketamine is an effective agent in facilitating endotracheal intubation in emergency setting as prehospital and battlefield medicine. It is also used to facilitate sedation and analgesia during local or regional anesthetic procedures, and it is an essential adjuvant analgesic for the management of refractory cancer pain. Usually, the IV dose of 1 to 1.5 mg/kg or IM dose of 2 to 4 mg/kg will produce dissociative anesthesia. The dissociative effect of ketamine makes it ideal for its use in procedural sedation, thereby allowing the completion of short, painful procedures (abscess incision and drainage, burn debridement, graft and dressing changes, etc.). The onset of action of ketamine is rapid (less than 5 minutes), and the patient regains consciousness within 10 to 15 minutes. Redosing with smaller aliquots of ketamine (0.5 mg/kg) will maintain the patient in a trancelike state for longer procedures. The retrograde amnesia might last longer with a recovery time ranging from 45 and 120 minutes. Additionally, ketamine is used for veterinary purposes as anesthetic and analgesic agent in animals, and research is going on to determine the effective use of ketamine as a rapid-acting antidepressant for the management of resistant depression.

Contraindications

Ketamine is contraindicated in patients who are hypersensitive to the drug or to any of the ingredients in the formulation, and in those patients younger than 3 months. It is also contraindicated in patients with cardiovascular disease such as unstable angina, hypertension, or raised intraocular pressure. The drug should not be administered in patients with severe liver disease such as cirrhosis and in patients with poorly controlled psychosis such as schizophrenic patients.

Precautions

The IV dose of ketamine should be given slowly over a period of 60 seconds to avoid the enhanced pressor response of ketamine and occurrence of transient respiratory depression or apnea. After the completion of outpatient procedures, they should be released after the recovery from ketamine anesthesia with the assistance of a responsible adult. Caution should be taken while administering ketamine to chronic alcoholics and acutely alcohol-intoxicated patients, and also to patients with preanesthetic raised cerebrospinal fluid pressure, seizures, or pulmonary or upper respiratory infection (might lead to gag reflex and laryngospasm).

Adverse Effects

It causes systemic effects including elevated heart rate, hypertension, and cardiac output due to sympathetic nervous system stimulation. A major drawback of its use is that it induces emergence reactions, which are characterized by unpleasant dreams, hallucinations, and long-term psychotomimetic effects during the emergence of anesthesia. This can be managed by the administration of BZDs or propofol.

Alfaxalone

It is a synthetic neuroactive steroid that was reintroduced in a new formulation in 2001. It is used for induction and maintenance of anesthesia in animals, and it has a rapid onset of action. The formulation is clear, aqueous, colorless, and nonirritating with a shelf life of 28 days after opening. Alfaxalone produces its anesthetic action through the activation of $GABA_A$. It is administered by IV and IM routes (off-label) as part of a sedation protocol. It has a satisfactory muscle relaxation activity and no analgesic effect and might cause respiratory depression and apnea.

Anesthetic Adjuncts (AS5.4)

Anesthetic adjuncts are considered to be an integral component of general anesthetic drug regimen. The desired effect of the anesthetics and adjunct medications is obtained at a lower dose than if the drugs were administered alone, thereby reducing patient risk and increasing patient's comfort and safety.

Sedative/Hypnotic/Anxiolytic Drugs

Benzodiazepines

As adjuncts and preanesthetic medications, BZDs such as midazolam, diazepam, and lorazepam are administered preoperatively to produce sedation, hypnosis, anxiolysis, anterograde amnesia, anticonvulsion, and central muscle relaxation for smooth induction phase, but no analgesic effect is observed. BZDs are widely used to induce procedural sedation (conscious sedation) during outpatient medical or dental procedures (wisdom tooth extractions) or procedures that enable the patient to return home the same day (endoscopy or colonoscopy procedures, biopsies, and uncomplicated surgical procedures lasting less than 1 hour). They function by interacting with GABA receptors to enhance inhibitory neurotransmission. Each clinical effect is mediated by a different GABA receptor subtype. Sedation, anterograde amnesia, and anticonvulsion symptoms are modulated by α_1 receptors, while anxiolysis and muscle relaxation are modulated by α_2 receptors. Lorazepam is widely used as an adjunct to regional anesthesia because of its potent anxiolytic and sedative effects. Due to their high-lipid solubility, both diazepam (0.3–0.6 mg/kg) and midazolam (0.2–0.4 mg/kg) readily cross the blood–brain barrier after IV administration of sleep-inducing doses, and their CNS effects start within 2 to 3 minutes. Lorazepam (0.04 mg/kg), which is moderately lipid-soluble, has a slightly longer onset of action (10–20 minutes). Drowsiness, sleepiness, and dizziness are the most commonly reported side effects of BZDs. The drugs cause minimal cardiovascular depressant effects, but all have potential respiratory depressant effect, especially when IV administered. Thus, the respiratory response needs to be monitored regularly. In elderly or obese patients, as well as in patients with liver impairment, the sedative effect of BZDs may be prolonged. Furthermore, BZDs can be related to a higher risk of postoperative cognitive dysfunction in the elderly, since they are more sensitive and have slower recovery from BZDs' effect. For controlling anaphylactic/anaphylactoid reactions from BZD administration, a thorough evaluation of the patient's clinical history, as well as the detection of early signs and symptoms in the perioperative period, is crucial. In an emergency, the antagonist flumazenil may be IV administered to reverse the side effects of these drugs.

Analgesics

Opioid Analgesics

Opioids (fentanyl, sufentanil, alfentanil, meperidine, remifentanil, and morphine) have a wide range of uses in anesthesia. They exert their primary analgesic activity by interacting mainly with the μ opioid receptors, thereby reducing the anesthetic requirement and minimizing the hemodynamic changes. They are one of the most commonly used preanesthetic medications and adjuncts during surgical procedures for induction and maintenance of anesthesia, as well as for reduction of immediate postoperative pain and long-term postoperative pain management. Opioids are extremely successful at regulating the ANS's responses to surgical stimulation. They have different durations of action (remifentanil produces analgesia within 1–2 minutes and has the shortest duration of around 10 minutes), and their dose can be effectively titrated, according to the individual patient's responses (remifentanil is administered as IV infusion in 0.5 mg/kg/min, followed by 0.25–0.5 mg/kg/min). However, the excessive doses of opioids prolong the recovery of susceptible patients from anesthesia, thereby elevating the risk of postoperative ventilatory depression. In addition, the IV opioid anesthetic causes hypotension exacerbation, bradycardia, somnolence, urinary retention, constipation, nausea, vomiting, and itching. The risk of adverse effects increases in elder patients and in patients with comorbidities. This can be managed through dose reduction, opioid-sparing, or multimodal analgesia.

An alternative technique for anesthesia, which can be well-tolerated even in elderly patients who are considered at high risk of general anesthesia, is the use of neuroleptic analgesia. Neuroleptic analgesia (neurolept analgesic) is an anesthetic process that involves combining a major neuroleptic sedative/antipsychotic agent (droperidol) with a potent opioid analgesic (fentanyl) to produce a detached, pain-free, semiconscious, nonreactive state under which the patient follows instructions meaningfully and remains completely unconcerned and pain-free. Fentanyl is a potent, synthetic opioid analgesic that is highly lipophilic with short duration of action (30–50 minutes), while droperidol is a dopamine antagonist that has been used as sedative and anesthetic adjunct during induction and maintenance of general anesthesia and as an adjunct to regional anesthesia, in addition to its antiemetic use. Butyrophenones and haloperidol are the other dopamine antagonists that are used for the same purpose. During neuroleptic analgesia, droperidol maintains tissue perfusion and prevents surgical shock by blocking α-adrenergic receptors and causing vasodilation. It also potentially increases the analgesic effect of fentanyl and other opioids. Usually, the adult dose of droperidol is 2.5 to 5 mg by IM or IV routes and fentanyl is administered at doses of 0.05 to 0.4 mg by IM or IV routes for ocular surgery. The dose is decreased for children's surgeries. Neuroleptic analgesia provides many advantages in addition to the stable circulatory system conditions (stable blood pressure, pulse rate, and myocardium functions) and intraocular pressure. It also minimizes the need for postoperative analgesics and provides smooth emergence from anesthesia with no PONV.

Nonopioid Analgesics

The most frequently used nonnarcotic analgesic is acetaminophen (paracetamol), which can be given orally or injected through an IV line. This drug is commonly used to relieve postoperative pain, usually in combination with the narcotic analgesics such as hydrocodone. Other medications such as the nonsteroidal anti-inflammatory drugs (NSAIDs; e.g., ketorolac) are also used in the postoperative setting. They are administered either as an IV or IM injection. However, their use is limited in the operative setting due to the increased risk of bleeding following some surgical procedures. In addition, NSAIDs increase the risk of heart attacks, stroke, and high blood pressure, especially in patients with heart disease.

α_2-Adrenergic Agonist

Dexmedetomidine is used as an adjuvant to general anesthetic medications, as it has the unique ability to produce sedation and analgesia even at higher doses, thereby enhancing the anesthesia produced by other anesthetic agents. The drug does not cause significant respiratory depression. As a result, it is indicated for short-term sedation (< 24 hours) of critically ill adult patients as well as sedation of nonintubated patients during surgical procedures. Dexmedetomidine activates the presynaptic central α_2-adrenergic receptors on the subtype α_{2A}, which are located on the brain and the spinal cord. On activation, the noradrenaline release is inhibited, and the propagation of pain signals is terminated with induction of light sedation. Since it does not induce consistent slowing of cortical EEG frequencies or unconsciousness, dexmedetomidine is useful for awake craniotomy cases that enable patients to interact with surgeons during cortical mapping. It is usually administered at a dose of 2.5 µg/kg by IM injection for premedication use or IV at a loading dose of 1 µg/kg over 10 to 20 minutes, followed by infusion of 0.2 to 0.7 µg/kg/h as a maintenance dose. The rate of infusion can be increased at 0.1 µg/kg/h increments or higher. The drug is also indicated for use as a sedative and analgesic in dogs and cats. Dexmedetomidine produces a mild decrease in blood pressure and heart rate. It also causes nausea and dry mouth. The effects of dexmedetomidine can be reversed by α_2-adrenergic receptor antagonist atipamezole. It is contraindicated in patients with hypotension, second- or third-degree heart block, and acute cerebrovascular conditions.

Neuromuscular Blocking Agents

Neuromuscular blocking agents (NMBAs) are usually administered at the induction of anesthesia to relax the muscles of the jaw, neck, and airway in order to facilitate the endotracheal intubation and laryngoscopy. They are also used as anesthetic adjuncts and are combined with anesthetics to provide an adequate surgical field. NMBAs also improve the outcomes in mechanical ventilation. The choice of NMBA and the dose depend on the drug's duration of action, type of surgical procedure, patient-specific clinical variables, and the use of other medications. The two types of NMBAs modulate signal transmission in skeletal muscles differently. The depolarizing NMBAs (such as succinylcholine) function as agonists at nicotinic receptors, opening ion-gated channels and causing muscular fasciculation until the ion potential is depleted, paralyzing the muscles. Nondepolarizing NMBAs (pancuronium, vecuronium, rocuronium, atracurium, and cisatracurium) block ACh at the motor endplate and are competitive antagonists at nicotinic receptors. This prevents propagating the action potential and sensitivity of muscle cells to motor nerve impulses, resulting in muscle paralysis that begins with small, fast-twitch muscles in the eyes and ends progressively through other muscles to the diaphragm. The sequence of recovery from neuromuscular blockage is in the reverse order. Succinylcholine is administered at a dose of 1 to 1.5 mg/kg for tracheal intubation in adults, which produces profound block within 60 seconds. Within 3 minutes, the recovery from the neuromuscular blockage is achieved and it is complete within 12 to 15 minutes. With a faster onset and a shorter duration, succinylcholine is preferred for RSI. Rocuronium in larger doses is an alternative to succinylcholine for RSI. As compared to succinylcholine, the drug has fewer side effects and contraindications, and it is six to eight times less potent than vecuronium (0.1 mg/kg with 3 minutes onset of action and 30 minutes duration of action). Rocuronium is given at a dosage of 0.6 mg/kg, which results in intubating conditions within 60 to 90 seconds. Succinylcholine causes bradycardia, hyperkalemia, and severe myalgia. It is contraindicated in patients with a history of malignant hyperthermia and in patients at high risk of developing hyperkalemia and those with recent burns, spinal cord injuries, and myopathies. Nondepolarizing NMBAs induce histamine release, which leads to hemodynamic instability (hypotension and tachycardia), bronchospasm, and urticaria. Inhaled anesthetics can interact with the nondepolarizing NMBAs; therefore, their doses must be adjusted accordingly. The effect of NMBAs can be reversed either by increasing the concentration of ACh in the synaptic junction or by enhancing the elimination of the drug or its metabolism. Acetylcholinesterase inhibitors such as neostigmine or edrophonium are used to reverse the action of nondepolarizing NMBAs. The reversal drugs are administered along with the muscarinic receptor antagonists (glycopyrrolate or atropine) to counterbalance the muscarinic activation due to the inhibition of acetylcholinesterase.

Preanesthetic Medications (AS3.6)

Preanesthetic medications are used before the administration of the anesthetic agents in order to ease anesthesia and make it safer for the patients. One or more medications with different activities are administered for sedation, to reduce anxiety and apprehension before the surgery and to cause amnesia. They help in enhancing the analgesic action of anesthetics and in attaining a synergistic effect for smooth and rapid induction of anesthesia, so that less anesthetic is required. The following are the drugs that are used as preanesthetic medications.

Sedative/Hypnotic/Anxiolytic Drugs

BZDs such as diazepam or lorazepam at oral doses of 5 to 10 mg and 2 mg, respectively, are administered as preanesthetic medications for tranquility and smooth induction of anesthesia. The role of BZDs is described in detail in the anesthetic adjuncts section.

Other drugs such as neuroleptics, which include chlorpromazine (25 mg, IM), haloperidol (2–4 mg, IM), or triflupromazine (10 mg, IM), are also used occasionally to calm down the patients prior to surgery, facilitate smooth induction, and relieve nausea and vomiting.

Opioids

To alleviate the anxiety and apprehension of the surgery, opioids such as morphine at a dose of 10 mg IM or pethidine (50–100 mg, IM) are administered as preanesthetic medications. Other uses of opioids in general anesthesia are described in detail in the anesthetic adjuncts section.

Antiemetics

PONV is one of the most frequently encountered problems in anesthesia practice, with a peak in the immediate postoperative hours. Different drug classes are employed to minimize the risk of PONV, as discussed in the following:

5-HT_3 Receptor Antagonists

Ondansetron (4–8 mg, IV) is the antiemetic of choice as it has minimal side effects such as headache and constipation.

D_2 Receptor Antagonists

Metoclopramide (10–20 mg, IM) is used for its prokinetic gastric-emptying efficacy to reduce the chances of reflex and aspiration prior to emergency surgery. The drug might cause extrapyramidal side effects (parkinsonism, tardive dyskinesia, etc.) and motor restlessness. Domperidone (10 mg oral) is also as effective as metoclopramide with no extrapyramidal side effects.

Antihistaminic Drugs

Promethazine (50 mg, IM) is an occasionally used preanesthetic medication for its sedative, antiemetic, and anticholinergic properties. Antihistaminic drugs may cause drowsiness, xerostomia, and urinary tract issues. Promethazine is contraindicated in young children as it causes respiratory depression, leading to apnea and death.

Anticholinergics

Traditionally, the administration of anticholinergic agents prior to general anesthesia was employed to reduce the oropharyngeal and tracheobronchial secretions produced by irritating inhalational anesthetics in the past. However, the practice of administering anticholinergics has continued to some extent, even with the use of modern anesthetics that cause less irritation. Additionally, anticholinergics are used to produce sedation/amnesia and prevent reflex bradycardia. Atropine or scopolamine (hyoscine) at a dose of 0.6 mg or 10 to 20 µg/kg IM/IV are used for their antisialagogue effect. Scopolamine also produces sedation. Atropine and scopolamine can lead to central anticholinergic syndrome (reduction of central anticholinergic activity) and tachycardia, which can be managed by the administration of 1 to 2 mg physostigmine by IV route. In addition, glycopyrrolate (0.2–0.3 mg or 5–10 µg/kg IM/IV) is also used for its antisialogogue property with no central effects.

H_2 Receptor Antagonists/Proton-Pump Inhibitors

These drugs are used to prevent/minimize the aspiration of stomach's acidic contents for patients at risk of gastric regurgitation and aspiration pneumonia, such as those who are undergoing prolonged surgeries and caesarian section, morbidly obese patients, and patients with gastroesophageal reflex disease and anticipated difficult airway. Antacids are given to neutralize gastric acid. Histamine H_2 receptors antagonists such as ranitidine (150 mg) and famotidine (20 mg) or proton-pump inhibitors such as omeprazole (20 mg) and pantoprazole (40 mg) are administered to reduce the gastric acid production.

Precautions to Be Taken While Using General Anesthetics in Situations Involving Organ Dysfunctions

In spite of the continuing advancement in clinical monitoring technology used in surgery and anesthesia during the last several decades, certain patients are still more likely to develop complications and possibly even mortality than others because of many factors involved, such as age, medical conditions, organ dysfunctions, and the type of surgery they are undergoing. Although the risk of complications during anesthesia can be reduced for elective surgical procedures, it is difficult to manage the same during emergency surgeries. Anesthetics, in general, suppress cardiovascular activity to varying degrees. In addition to blunting baroreceptor regulation and a generalized decrease in central sympathetic tone, they cause a decrease in systemic arterial blood pressure due to their direct vasodilation effect and myocardial depression. Therefore, myocardial ischemia, hypertension, arrhythmias, heart failure, and hypovolemia must be controlled preoperatively. Diuretics or adrenocorticosteroid-induced potassium depletion should be corrected over several days to minimize the preoperative risk of arrhythmias. Following the induction of anesthesia, it is essential to maintain the airway and monitor the respiratory function, as all the general anesthetics diminish or abolish the ventilatory drive and the reflexes that maintain the patency of the airway, causing respiratory depression and hypercarbia, which is more prominent with isoflurane. Careful management should be considered in patients with severe emphysema who are undergoing lung volume reduction surgery (LVRS). Usually, the patients are prepared for the surgery by quitting smoking and optimization of expiratory flow, which is achieved with the use of inhaled corticosteroids and the administration of long-acting bronchodilators (tiotropium, salmeterol, and formoterol) or the short-acting β-agonists. These medications might lead to tachycardia. Since anesthetics can cause regurgitation and vomiting with risk of pulmonary aspiration, preoperative fasting for elective surgeries is highly recommended, although it cannot be planned for emergency surgeries. Thus, either endotracheal intubation with sedation and local anesthesia or intubation following rapid induction of anesthesia and neuromuscular blockage can be used for emergency surgeries. However, rapid anesthesia and intubation is a cardiovascular risk in the elderly and the critically ill patients. The release of fluoride, bromide, and other metabolites of halogenated hydrocarbons can affect the functions of the liver and kidneys, leading to toxic effects, especially if these metabolites accumulate with frequently repeated administration of anesthetics. Acute or chronic liver dysfunction affects the body's response to anesthesia and surgery, and can also cause new reactions. Patients with liver disease are normally examined by gastroenterologists and hepatologists prior to surgery in order to optimize their condition. Glycemic control is one important aspect of the perioperative management, and it is preferable to withhold the oral hypoglycemic drugs in the morning on the day of surgery, since fasting diabetic patients have low blood glucose concentration. Depending on their duration of action, few antidiabetic drugs such as chlorpropamide can be stopped 1 to 2 days before the surgery. As for the insulin-dependent diabetic patients, IV infusion of glucose and the reduction in the usual dose of insulin is required before surgery. If insulin is not provided, free fatty acids are mobilized from adipose tissues and metabolized to ketones by the insulin-deficient liver, which can lead to life-threatening ketoacidosis.

Multiple Choice Questions

1. A 52-year-old woman was admitted to the emergency operation theater for gallbladder removal under general anesthesia. Which of the following statements is correct regarding the mechanism of action of general anesthetics?

A. Amnesia is related to the effect of general anesthetics on the spinal cord.

B. All inhalational anesthetics have a single molecular target.

C. Barbiturates activate the two-pore domain potassium channel.

D. Xenon inhibits N-methyl-D-aspartate (NMDA) and α-amino-3-hydroxy-5-methyl-4-isoxazolepropionic acid (AMPA) receptors.

Answer: D

General anesthetics produce their effects through variable mechanisms of action at cellular and molecular levels. They trigger central nervous system neurodepression by enhancing inhibitory neurotransmission and decreasing excitatory neurotransmission. Xenon inhibits NMDA and AMPA receptors.

2. A patient was administered an intravenous anesthetic for induction and maintenance of anesthesia. The drug was potent at producing unconsciousness and sedation through GABAA receptors-mediated chloride channel activation. On recovery, the patient had very low incidence of postoperative nausea and vomiting. Which one of the following anesthetic agents was administered to this patient?

A. Cyclopropane

B. Propofol.

C. Xenon.

D. Isoflurane.

Answer: B

Propofol is a sedative/hypnotic anesthetic that is given intravenously for the induction and/or maintenance of anesthesia. The drug suppresses neuronal excitability by increasing GABA-mediated chloride channel activation and prolonging inhibitory postsynaptic currents. Induction takes 30 to 40 seconds after administration and is smooth. Propofol produces rapid unconsciousness with fast recovery and it is associated with a lower incidence of postoperative nausea and vomiting as compared to other anesthetic agents.

3. A 65-year-old patient has a history of dementia and abnormal hemodynamic parameters including low blood pressure. He underwent a colostomy and a surgical debridement of decubitus ulcers. The patient was administered 0.2 mg/kg of an inducing anesthetic agent X, and 0.01 mg/kg alfentanil and 1 mg/kg succinylcholine for a balanced general anesthesia. Maintenance of anesthesia was carried out using sevoflurane, cisatracurium, and alfentanil. The patient remained hemodynamically stable throughout the surgery, which lasted for 40 minutes. He had a normal uneventful recovery 10 minutes after the end of surgery. Which one of the following is the inducing anesthetic agent X?

A. Propofol.

B. Etomidate.

C. Enflurane.

D. Isoflurane.

Answer: B

Etomidate is mainly used to induce anesthesia in cardiac compromised patients who are at risk of hypotension.

4. A 65-year-old man with no previous neurologic history had uncomplicated colectomy performed under general anesthesia for the treatment of ulcerative colitis. During surgery, he developed mild tachycardia, which was painful, and was administered several doses of drug X intraoperatively. The patient was not awake enough to be extubated after 6 hours of the surgery. Upon withholding drug X for the next 3 hours, the patient regained consciousness and is safely extubated. To which one of the following drug classes does drug X belong?

A. Nonsteroidal anti-inflammatory drugs.

B. Anticholinergics.

C. Bronchodilators.

D. Opiates.

Answer: D

Failure to awaken after a surgery performed under general anesthesia is a common reason for urgent neurologic consultation in the hospital. Opioids are extremely effective at regulating the autonomic nervous system's responses to surgical stimulation. In this case, the patient was administered several doses of opioids (leading to overdose) to control the pain as mild tachycardia was believed to be the cause for pain during the surgical procedure. However, precautions have to be taken in old patients as they have increased sensitivity toward general anesthetics and opioids. In addition, opioids potentiate and prolong the anesthetic effect and loss of consciousness. Thus, upon withholding the drug, the patient regained consciousness.

5. A 7-year-old male child, weighing 20 kg, with Duchenne's muscular dystrophy, has to undergo surgery using general anesthesia. He is at increased risk of developing cardiac arrhythmias and rhabdomyolysis on administration of the following medications, except:

A. Propofol.

B. Desflurane.

C. Sevoflurane.

D. Isoflurane.

Answer: A

Duchenne's muscular dystrophy is an X-linked recessive hereditary condition that affects 1 in every 3,500 live male births. Chronic muscle fiber necrosis, degeneration, and regeneration can occur in cardiac and smooth muscle and also in skeletal muscle with abnormal or absent dystrophin. Heterozygous females, although not manifesting the disease, have an increased risk of cardiac disease later in life. When a patient with Duchenne's muscular dystrophy requires surgery under general anesthesia, various anesthetic issues might arise including complicated intubation, long-term neuromuscular blockade, the need for postoperative ventilation, and the risk of rhabdomyolysis, hyperkalemia, and cardiac arrhythmias from halogenated anesthetics (such as isoflurane, desflurane, and sevoflurane) and depolarizing muscle relaxants. When skeletal muscle tissue breaks down, myoglobin is released, which can damage the kidneys. Propofol is a safe anesthetic for children with Duchenne's muscular dystrophy, provided they are not allergic to the medication or the emulsion's ingredients, especially soybean oil and egg lecithin.

Chapter 32 Local Anesthetics

Areeg Anwer Ali and Syed Ayaz Ali

PH 1.17: Describe the mechanism/s of action, types, doses, side effects, indications, and contraindications of local anesthetics.

Learning Objectives

- Mechanism of action of local anesthetics.
- Pharmacokinetics and duration of action.
- Classification of local anesthetics.
- Local and systemic effects, including adverse effects, of local anesthetics.
- Techniques for local anesthesia.

Local Anesthetics

Local anesthetics (LAs) are drugs that cause reversible sensory-motor block and loss of pain sensation upon topical application or local injection in particular body area. They block nerve impulse generation and interrupt neural conduction at any part of the neuron by binding to a specific receptor site within the pore of the sodium (Na^+) channels in nerves, which results in muscular paralysis and loss of autonomic nervous system (ANS) regulation. LAs can also be combined with general anesthesia to decrease the concentration of general anesthetics and to improve postoperative analgesia. Their duration of action and dose-dependent adverse effects on the cardiovascular system (CVS) and central nervous system (CNS) restrict their use.

Differences between General and Local Anesthetics

Anesthesia is usually administered via different techniques to keep patients pain-free during surgical and medical procedures or tests. There are few major key differences between general and local anesthesia that depend on many factors such as the type of surgical procedure and health status and preference of patients. **Table 32.1** summarizes the major differences between general and local anesthesia.

Mechanism of Action

Nerve signals are transmitted as action potentials. Neurons produce and send these signals to the target tissues. When a stimulus causes the membrane potential to change to the value of the threshold potential (between −50 and −55 mV), an action potential is produced. The action potential consists of a rapid depolarization (the upstroke), followed by repolarization back to the resting membrane potential. After generating one action potential, neurons become refractory to stimuli for a period of time during which they are unable to produce another action potential. During the upstroke of an action potential, there is an influx of Na^+ ions to the cell through the channels or ionophores located within neuronal membranes as a result of electrochemical potential gradient. These channels are normally in a resting state, preventing Na^+ ions from entering. The channel becomes activated or open when the neuron is stimulated, allowing sodium ions to diffuse into the cell and cause depolarization.

The LAs bind to a receptor inside the voltage-sensitive Na^+ channel, specifically to the D4–S6 region of the α-subunit of neural sodium channels. They have a stronger affinity for Na^+ channel receptors in their active and inactivated states than in their resting states. Their binding to the receptor stabilizes the channel in the inactivated state. They interfere with the neural conduction by blocking Na^+ ions from entering neuronal membranes via the channels or ionophores, thereby increasing the duration of refractory period and reducing the probability of channel opening by increasing the channel's opening threshold. The Na^+ channel becomes inactivated after a sudden shift in membrane voltage, preventing further influx while active transport mechanisms return Na^+ ions to the exterior. The effect is concentration dependent and the administered volume of LA solution more easily blocks the required number of Na^+ channels and disrupts impulse transmission, causing impulses to slow down and then completely stop. Therefore, smaller and faster-firing neural fibers such as autonomic fibers are more sensitive to LA action, followed by sensory fibers, and finally somatic motor fibers. The channel then returns to its natural resting state after this repolarization. LAs can also inhibit potassium (K^+) channels. Other mechanisms by which LAs function depend on their interaction with G protein–coupled receptors, endothelial nitric oxide, and muscarinic receptors. The following is the order in which a loss of nerve function occurs in clinical practice: pain, temperature, touch, proprioception, and skeletal muscle tone.

True resistance to LAs, although rare, is hard to identify. Despite adequate technical administration, the failure of LA to achieve anesthesia is frequently thought to be due to technical and medication failure or local infection. However, atypical responses to LAs might be caused by mutations in sodium channels. If the condition is not recognized, it may result in toxicity from the administration of excessive amounts of LAs, especially in the case of epidural and spinal anesthesia, which require intrusive procedures to provide LAs.

Anesthetic Potency and Onset of Action

At physiological pH, LAs exist in ionized (water-soluble and lipid-insoluble) and unionized (lipid-soluble and

Table 32.1 Difference between general and local anesthesia

Parameters	General anesthesia	Local anesthesia
Site of administration and action	▪ Administered by intravenous route and inhalation techniques ▪ Acts on the central nervous system	▪ Administered locally by topical and parenteral routes into the tissues surrounding the incision ▪ Affects the peripheral nerves
Area of the body involved	▪ Suppresses pain in the whole body	▪ Suppresses pain in a part of the body
Effect on consciousness/senses	▪ Causes loss of consciousness and may affect other major organs and senses (hearing, sight, smell, etc.)	▪ Does not affect consciousness and may not affect other senses
Drug administration	▪ A qualified anesthesiologist must administer the anesthetic agent and must be present during the surgery/procedure	▪ Can be administered by the doctor without the help of an anesthesiologist
Monitoring of vital functions	▪ Careful monitoring during and after the surgery is essential as major organs' functions are also suppressed (e.g., lungs and diaphragm)	▪ Usually not required
Adverse effects and risks	▪ Systemic and major adverse effects can occur ▪ Greater risk of fatality	▪ Minor and local adverse effects can occur with few systemic toxicities ▪ Less risky
Uses	▪ Used in major body system surgeries such as heart transplant, brain surgery, and repair of hip fractures	▪ Used mostly in minor surgeries such as dental procedures (e.g., tooth extraction), circumcision, dermatological and facial enhancements, and earlobe repairs
Examples of anesthetics agents based on routes of administration	▪ Inhalation anesthetics: isoflurane, desflurane, nitrous oxide, and halothane ▪ Intravenous anesthetics: propofol, etomidate, and ketamine	▪ Injectable anesthetics: lidocaine, procaine, bupivacaine, mepivacaine, levobupivacaine, and tetracaine ▪ Surface anesthetics: benzocaine, dibucaine, lidocaine, and tetracaine

water-insoluble) forms. The ionization constant p*Ka* of LAs is the pH at which the ionized and unionized forms are available in equal amounts. Both the ionized and unionized forms of LAs are necessary for their action. They affect their interaction with membrane lipids, transport across the lipid plasma membrane, pharmacokinetics, and mechanism of action. The ionized form of an LA is essential because it allows reaching the receptor sites at the plasma membrane/axon. However, this form does not penetrate the neuronal membrane very well, where the receptor site for LAs is located. To enter the acting sites, the uncharged (unionized) molecules will primarily diffuse through the lipid barriers of nerve sheaths and penetrate through the lipid bilayers of cell membranes. The binding of LAs is reversible and their potency is proportional to its binding affinity or lower dissociation. In addition, K^+ channel blockade improves the drug's binding and, as a result, the anesthetic blockade.

Depending on their lipid solubility, LAs differ in their potency and, based on that, their concentration range varies. For example, bupivacaine is more lipid soluble and potent than articaine and it can be formulated in a 0.5% (5 mg/mL) concentration rather than a 4% (40 mg/mL) concentration for articaine. However, the 4% concentration of articaine provides a faster onset of action.

The most important factor that determines the time for onset of local anesthesia is the proportion of the molecules that are converted to the tertiary, lipid-soluble structure when exposed to physiologic pH (7.4), rather than a water-soluble state. However, it should be noted that, once the tertiary molecules are within the neuron, they are reionized to the quaternary form, which is responsible for blocking the sodium channel. The higher the p*Ka* of an LA, the fewer the molecules that are available in their lipid-soluble state. This will delay onset of action of LAs. Usually, amino-ester drugs have higher p*Ka* values with 15% or less unionized form; therefore, they are slow-acting anesthetics, except for chloroprocaine (rapid onset of 6–12 minutes despite high p*Ka*). The amino-amide drugs are fast acting as they have lower p*Ka* values. Moreover, inflamed tissues, such as in the case of an infected tooth, may have a pH as low as 6.8, favoring the quaternary, water-soluble state of the LAs. This could be the reason for the difficulty when attempting to anesthetize inflamed or contaminated tissues. Therefore, bicarbonate is usually administered to alkalinize the area and make the drug more lipid-soluble, allowing for faster penetration. For example, adding 1 mL of 8.4% $NaHCO_3$ to 10 mL of 2% lidocaine raises the pH from 6.5 to 7.2.

Pharmacokinetics and Duration of Action

Pharmacokinetic characteristics are not essential determinants of LAs' effectiveness since the drugs produce their effects locally near the site of administration, but they do have a major impact on the systemic effects and toxicity of LAs. The plasma concentration of LAs is determined by their rate of distribution in tissues and removal from the body after absorption from the injection site. LAs are usually quickly absorbed into the bloodstream from the injection site. Soluble surface anesthetics (lidocaine, tetracaine) get quickly absorbed by the mucous membranes and abraded areas of the skin, but intact skin absorbs them very little. The absorption pattern of amides is biphasic, consisting of an initial rapid phase, followed by a slow phase. Several variables must be considered when reviewing the local and systemic distribution of LAs, which include the tissue blood flow and the position of the patient. LAs, like most medications, bind to plasma proteins reversibly when circulating in the bloodstream. The duration of action of LAs varies due to differences in their affinity for plasma protein binding and the percentage of circulating protein-bound drug. The greater the affinity for protein binding, the longer the duration of neuronal blockade. Additionally, the anesthetic's affinity for protein within sodium channel also contributes further to the greater tendency of the anesthetic to maintain neuronal blockade for longer duration. Mepivacaine with 55% protein binding has shorter duration than bupivacaine with 95% protein binding. Since esters are rapidly hydrolyzed, they do not cross the placenta in substantial quantities, while the rate of transfer of amides is determined by their protein binding. The higher the binding (e.g., bupivacaine), the lower the rate of transfer to the placenta. In adults, the clearance of LAs is almost entirely hepatic, but neonates have a higher renal excretion due to the immaturity of some of the enzymes involved in their metabolism.

Most ester anesthetics have a short half-life due to rapid hydrolysis by plasma cholinesterase. However, patients with pseudocholinesterase deficiency/atypical pseudocholinesterase have slower metabolism. The liver mainly metabolizes amides and their metabolism decreases in presence of potent CYP450 inhibitors, such as ketoconazole. Allergies are uncommon with amide anesthetics since *para*-aminobenzoic acid (PABA)—the metabolite of ester anesthetics with an increased rate of allergic responses—is not formed. However, preservative chemicals (methylparaben) utilized in the manufacture of amide-type agents are converted to PABA. Patients who are allergic to ester LAs can be administered an amide LA that is devoid of preservatives. The amount of time an LA stays in close proximity to neural fibers affects the duration of anesthesia. Amides' terminal half-life varies from 100 minutes (lidocaine) to 200 minutes (bupivacaine). It can be further extended by the concomitant use of a vasoconstrictor such as adrenaline, which restricts the blood flow, thereby reducing the systemic absorption and systemic toxicity. Generally, the choice of LAs depends on several factors, which include the length of the procedure to be performed, the size and location of the area that needs numbing, patients' underlying health conditions, and medications for comorbidities. The injection of an anesthetic solution, whether with or without a vasoconstrictor, must be administered slowly (1 mL/min).

Effect, Indications, and Contraindications for Coadministration of Vasopressors with Local Anesthetics

WALANT (wide-awake local anesthesia with no tourniquet) method involves the use of vasopressors in conjunction with LAs to induce anesthesia, provide local hemostasis, and delay the absorption of LAs in the area of surgical procedure without the use of tourniquet. Despite the fact that it demonstrates significant cardiac stimulation due to its β_1 agonistic effect, in addition to its intended vasoconstrictive activity (α_1 agonistic action), adrenaline is the most commonly employed vasopressor as it provides a clear surgical field with less bleeding. Because adrenaline is unstable, an antioxidant is added to keep it from oxidizing. The preservative sodium bisulfite is the most widely used for LAs. Noradrenaline, such as adrenaline, can stimulate α_1 and α_2 receptors, but it does not interact with β_2 receptors. Furthermore, because noradrenaline acts on the cardiac β_1 receptors, it has a strong and paradoxical bradycardia effect, causing an increase in heart rate. It might also elicit a reflex stimulation of the aortic and carotid baroreceptors in response to an increase in diastolic and systolic pressures, resulting in severe bradycardia. As a result, noradrenaline is about four times less vasoconstrictive locally than adrenaline.

Vasopressors lower the danger of systemic toxicity while also extending the duration of anesthesia by decreasing tissue perfusion and creating local ischemia of the tissues. Additionally, the ischemia affects the vasa nervorum, which supply the axons of sensitive nerve fibers. This causes a significant reduction in the metabolism of nerve cells and, as a result, in the transmission of the nerve impulse, resulting in a deepening and lengthening of the anesthesia.

The dose of a vasoconstrictor is calculated differently from the dose of an LA because vasoconstrictors are expressed as a dilution ratio and are not weight-dependent. For example, 1:100,000 concentration contain 1 g of adrenaline dissolved in 100,000 mL of solvent. This concentration is most commonly used in LA solutions, and it means an LA with a 1:100,000 adrenaline concentration will be 0.01 mg/mL as adrenaline concentrations are usually stated in milligrams per milliliter (mg/mL). For the majority of small surgical operations in dentistry, the 1:200,000 or 1:100,000 solution provides sufficient duration of action. Reversal drugs such as the nonselective α-adrenergic receptor blocker phentolamine mesylate (0.2–0.8 mg) are used for specific cases (elderly patients, small children, or patients with special needs) for many dental procedures. The drugs cause vasodilation, reverse the influence of vasopressors on submucosal vessels, and enhance the absorption of LA, which shorten the duration of anesthesia.

Patients with cardiovascular disease, vascular disease, or other systemic conditions may face a life-threatening situation if vasoconstrictors are used inappropriately. Therefore, vasoconstrictors should be avoided in patients with conditions such as unstable angina, recent myocardial infarction (less than 6 months), and recent coronary artery bypass surgery (less than 3 months), and in patients who have suffered a cerebrovascular accident or stroke within the last 6 months. Vasoconstrictors are also contraindicated in patients with pheochromocytoma and severe arrhythmias and in the untreated or poorly controlled hyperthyroid patient and when a patient is receiving irradiation of bone. Patients with corticosteroid-dependent asthma may have an increased risk of sulfite allergy. The use of adrenaline in areas with terminal vessels and for local infiltration anesthesia in acral regions is contraindicated in many countries due to risk of necrosis.

The pharmacological interactions of vasoconstrictors with other medications that the patient is already taking should be avoided at all costs. Drugs such as nonselective β blockers (propranolol and nadolol), some antidepressants (tricyclic antidepressants such as imipramine and amitriptyline), general anesthetics such as halothane, thiopental, and barbiturates, and illicit drugs (methamphetamines) can cause serious interaction. Therefore, narcotic-addicted patients should be given additional care, as improper use of vasoconstrictors can result in life-threatening conditions and even deaths.

Classification of Local Anesthetics

Based on the Routes of Administration and Pharmacological Response

Injectable Anesthetics

Injectable anesthetics are preferred for certain procedures such as root canal, skin biopsy, and mole or deep wart removal, and for diagnostic tests such as lumbar puncture. The anesthetics are mainly administered for numbing the local body area and not for the management of pain only.

Agents of Low Potency and Short Duration of Action

Procaine and chloroprocaine.

Agents of Intermediate Potency and Duration of Action

Lidocaine (lignocaine), prilocaine, and mepivacaine.

Agents of High Potency and Long Duration of Action

Tetracaine (amethocaine), bupivacaine, ropivacaine, dibucaine (cinchocaine), and etidocaine.

Surface Anesthetics

The anesthetics are applied topically to the skin or mucous membranes inside of the mouth, nose, or throat as well as on the surface of the eyes. Topical anesthetics are formulated as liquids, creams, gels, patches, and sprays.

Surface anesthetics are classified as soluble or insoluble.

Soluble Surface Anesthetics

Cocaine, lidocaine, tetracaine, and benoxinate.

Insoluble Surface Anesthetics

Benzocaine, *n*-butyl *p*-butyl aminobenzoate (butamben), and oxethazaine.

Based on Chemical Structure

The commonly used LA are weak bases with amphiphilic property. The hydrophobic moiety (consists of an aromatic ring), the intermediate chain, and the hydrophilic moiety (consists of an amino terminus) are the three main components of LAs. The aromatic residue of LAs gives the drug molecule the lipid solubility property, while the ionizable amino group gives it water solubility. The intermediate chain, which can be an amide or an ester, separates the hydrophobic and hydrophilic ends and structurally classifies LAs into amino-amide type and amino-ester type.

Amino-Esters Anesthetics

Cocaine, procaine, chloroprocaine, tetracaine, and benzocaine. The p*K*a values range from 8.4 to 8.9 at 37°C.

Cocaine

It is the only naturally occurring LA and the first discovered anesthetic as a compound native to the Andes Mountains. The alkaloid cocaine is derived from *Erythroxylum coca* leaves, a native to the Andes Mountains, the West Indies, and Java. It is a good surface anesthetic that gets absorbed quickly through the buccal mucosal membrane. It was first used for ocular anesthesia in 1884. Later, the drug was used for dental surgeries. It is currently used topically in ear, nose, and throat (ENT) surgeries at a concentration of 4 to 10%. The LA activity of cocaine is due to the blocking of sodium channels in neurons and prevention of nerve impulse transmission. The systemic effects are the results of its ability to increase catecholamine levels while also blocking their reuptake in sympathetic presynaptic receptors, resulting in catecholamine accumulation in the synaptic cleft and increased receptor cell stimulation with a constant antagonism of both α and β receptors. Cocaine has a quick onset of action and a duration of 20 to 30 minutes. It causes conjunctival vessel constriction, corneal clouding, and sloughing (in rare cases due to drying and local toxicity). Its sympathomimetic activity manifests as local vasoconstriction, tachycardia, an increase in blood pressure, and mydriasis. It is generally contraindicated in patients with hypertension and ischemic heart disease due to its ability to sensitize adrenergic receptors and in patients who are more susceptible to the effects of cocaine. Cocaine is the only LA with inherent potent vasoconstrictor function. This aids in the reduction of intraoperative bleeding. The anesthetic should not be administered along with adrenaline. Cocaine has the potential to induce psychological dependence, leading to cocaine addiction as well as an increased risk of severe side effects. Cocaine misuse has resulted in death due to heart or respiratory failure.

Procaine

It is a derivative of benzoic acid. It was synthesized in 1905 as one of the first synthetic LA agents after amylocaine. Pseudocholinesterase metabolizes procaine quickly (half-life: 1–2 minutes). During dental procedures, procaine is most commonly used to numb the area around a tooth. It is often used to ease the discomfort of intramuscular penicillin injections. With benzyl penicillin, procaine forms a poorly soluble salt; procaine penicillin injected intramuscularly works for 20 to 24 hours due to slow absorption from the injection site. When there is a history of malignant hyperpyrexia, procaine is administered as a drug of choice. It is also used in patients who are allergic to amides. The anesthetic also has antiarrhythmic properties and sympatholytic and anti-inflammatory activities. It also enhances perfusion and has mood-enhancing effect. Therefore, it is used additionally to treat arthritis, cerebral atherosclerosis, dementia, depression, hair loss, high blood pressure, and sexual performance issues. Procaine lacks the euphoric and addictive properties of cocaine. It is contraindicated in pregnancy and during breastfeeding. Procaine should not be administered intravenously in patients suffering from myasthenia gravis, pseudocholinesterase deficiency, and systemic lupus erythematosus. The anesthetic interacts with digoxin, skeletal muscle relaxants, succinylcholine, sulfonamide antibiotics, and amino salicylic acid.

Chloroprocaine

In contrast to cocaine, this LA has vasodilation activity. The drug has been used for neuraxial anesthesia (epidural and spinal) as well as peripheral nerve blocks and obstetric anesthesia (pudendal and paracervical blocks). Chloroprocaine has been used in test dosages to examine the function of peripheral nerve and epidural catheters due to its short duration of action. Despite having a higher p*K*a (8.7) than lidocaine, ropivacaine, mepivacaine, and bupivacaine, chloroprocaine can provide faster epidural anesthesia as it is quickly degraded by pseudocholinesterase (low risk of systemic toxicity); therefore, it can be given in high dosages, resulting in a significant diffusion gradient that promotes early onset of action (6–12 minutes). In the nonobstetric population, a 50-mg dose of 1% intrathecal chloroprocaine is recommended. Additionally, chloroprocaine is used to detect unintentional intravascular epidural catheter insertion in pregnant and nonpregnant adults due to its low potential for systemic toxicity. The US Food and Drug Administration (FDA) recently approved a preservative-free formulation of chloroprocaine for spinal anesthesia in people undergoing short-term lower extremity and abdominal surgery, since sodium bisulfite and disodium ethylenediaminetetraacetate (EDTA) are the two preservatives that might be responsible for the reported localized neurodegenerative alterations in spinal nerve roots. The most common side effect is pain from the chloroprocaine procedural injection. Hypotension, bradycardia, nausea, and headache are the most prevalent side effects of spinal, epidural, and caudal anesthesia. Adrenaline should not be given with spinal chloroprocaine since it has been linked to flulike symptoms such as fever, nasal congestion, malaise, myalgias, arthralgias, and loss of appetite. The drug is contraindicated in patients with a known history of PABA allergic reaction and in patients with end-stage liver disease.

Tetracaine

It is a benzoate ester, which has been in use since the early 1930s. Currently, it is used as a topical ophthalmic anesthetic for short procedures on the eye's surface, as well as the ears and nose. It is also used for spinal anesthesia and to numb the skin prior to starting an intravenous injection or a procedure. Tetracaine is also available as a cream or a patch in a combination with lidocaine. The drug is listed as an essential medication according to the World Health Organization (WHO), and it is relatively cheaper than other LA agents. Tetracaine has a high lipid solubility, with a relative value of 80, making it one of the most potent LAs. It might cause CNS toxicity, which starts with numbness around the mouth, tinnitus, hazy vision, and dizziness. Due to the blocking of CNS inhibitory mechanisms, the patient might experience hyperexcitability before advancing to depressive symptoms, seizures, and comatose state, followed by hemodynamic collapse. At toxic doses, tetracaine has vasodilatory properties and reduces heart contractility in a dose-dependent manner. Furthermore, it may lengthen the PR and QRS intervals, leading to sinus bradycardia, ventricular arrhythmia, and eventually asystole. Intravascular administration of concentrated lipids (20% lipid emulsion) may be utilized to reverse the toxic effects of tetracaine by allowing the medication to be rapidly cleared from the systemic circulation.

Benzocaine

The drug is available in a variety of formulations, including solutions, sprays, creams, gels, aerosols, and lozenges in 5, 10, or 20% concentrations. The topical preparation is used for dental procedures, mild skin irritations, sore throats, sunburns, vaginal or rectal irritations, ingrown toenails, hemorrhoids, and in the treatment of a variety of other sources of minor pain and small traumas. The FDA issued a safety alert on May 2018, advising consumers not to use benzocaine-containing teething products in newborns and children younger than 2 years due to risk of methemoglobinemia, which is characterized by cyanosis, hypoxia, and dyspnea. Patients who have had severe allergic reactions to ester-type LAs should avoid benzocaine. Furthermore, benzocaine is not recommended for people who have heart arrhythmias, glucose-6-phosphate dehydrogenase (G6PD) deficiency, or poor lung function. Hypotension, bradycardia, cardiac arrest, sleepiness, dizziness, edema, allergic reactions, convulsive syncope, and seizures (specially in elder population) are some of the other side effects. Supplemental oxygen and intravenous administration of a 1% solution of methylene blue are indicated if the early signs of toxic methemoglobinemia are suspected after the use of benzocaine.

Table 32.2 provides details regarding the various maximum recommended doses and the duration of action of commonly used amino-esters anesthetics.

Table 32.2 Maximum recommended dose and duration of action of commonly used amino-esters anesthetics

Amino-esters anesthetics	Maximum dose with vasoconstrictor (mg/kg)	Duration of action with vasoconstrictor (min)
Procaine	10[a]	30–45
Chloroprocaine	14[a]	60–90
Tetracaine	1.5[b]	120–180

[a]Infiltration and subcutaneous routes.
[b]Topical skin and mucous membranes, infiltration and subcutaneous routes.

Amino-Amides Anesthetics

Lidocaine, prilocaine, bupivacaine, ropivacaine, levobupivacaine, mepivacaine, articaine, and dibucaine. Their p*K*a values range from 7.7 to 8.1 at 37°C.

Lidocaine

It is a tertiary amine derived from xylidine. It was first synthesized between 1943 and 1946 by Nils Löfgren and Bengt Lundquist. Lidocaine became popular and one of the most commonly used LAs due to its superior safety profile. The drug is frequently used in conjunction with adrenaline, which opposes the local vasodilatory effects of lidocaine, thereby extending its duration of action at the specific site. Lidocaine is an antiarrhythmic drug classified as class Ib by the Vaughan Williams classification system, and it is used to treat acute ventricular tachydysrhythmias. It can also be used to treat acute and chronic pain as an adjuvant analgesic. Other indication for lidocaine is its intravenous administration as an adjuvant to tracheal intubation during advanced airway management, where it reduces the hypertensive response to laryngoscopy and can also decrease the incidence of myalgia and hyperkalemia to succinylcholine administration.

When injected into the intercostal space, lidocaine enters the intravascular compartment at a rapid rate, followed by the caudal, epidural, brachial plexus, femoral, and subcutaneous spaces. Different preparations of lidocaine are administered in various concentrations, ranging from very diluted solutions (0.05–0.1%) via subcutaneous infiltration to 10% concentrated solution, which is topically administered for airway anesthesia, usually by spraying from a metered dose atomizer. In dental practice, lidocaine formulations containing 1 per 100,000 adrenaline or more, with or without preservatives are usually used. Additionally, EMLA is a premixed eutectic 5% cream containing 2.5% lidocaine and 2.5% prilocaine, which is commonly used to anesthetize tiny regions of skin prior to minor procedures. Also, it has been utilized as a substitute for lidocaine infiltration in some cases.

Lidocaine has a narrow therapeutic index, so patients with hepatic impairment who are receiving extended infusions may require plasma level monitoring to avoid excessively high plasma concentrations. When plasma concentrations reach toxic levels, majority of lidocaine adverse effects occur. Slurred speech, tinnitus, circumoral paresthesia, and feeling dizziness are among signs and symptoms of mild toxicity at plasma levels above 5 µg/mL. The patient may have convulsions or lose consciousness if the concentration is higher than 10 µg/mL. At 15 µg/mL, the heart and CNS become even more depressed, leading to cardiac arrhythmias, respiratory arrest, and cardiac arrest. Basic hemodynamic monitoring should be performed before and during the use of solutions containing vasopressors, particularly if there is any specific concern about the patient's cardiovascular status.

The drug is known to be more neurotoxic than other LAs, especially when directly applied to nervous tissue in high concentrations. Transient radicular irritation (TRI), a self-limiting painful condition affecting the calves, thighs, and buttocks, can occur as a result of the use of highly concentrated lidocaine (2.5–5%) for spinal anesthesia. Moreover, methemoglobinemia can result from the conversion of lidocaine to ortho-toluidine. Therefore, the drug is contraindicated if the patient is taking other medications that can cause methemoglobinemia, or if the patient has a hemoglobinopathy or another type of anemia. Lidocaine is also contraindicated as an antiarrhythmic drug if dysrhythmia occurred while using the drug as LA.

Prilocaine

It was first synthesized by Claes Tegner and Nils Löfgren in 1969. The drug is similar to lidocaine and both are formulated in the topical dermal anesthetic preparation EMLA. However, it does not promote vasodilation at the infiltration site and has a lower CNS toxicity due to larger volume of distribution. It is often used for intravenous regional anesthesia due to its low cardiac toxicity. It is also commonly used in dentistry in its injectable form. Ortho-toluidine, a prilocaine metabolite, can induce methemoglobinemia in some people, which can be treated with methylene blue. The drug is contraindicated in patients with sickle cell anemia, anemia, or symptomatic hypoxia.

Bupivacaine

It is a potent and long-acting amide-type LA. The drug is available in different concentrations: 0.25, 0.5, and 0.75%. Bupivacaine is administered by various routes, including local infiltration for postsurgical analgesia and peripheral nerve blocks for dental procedures, orthopaedic surgery, and other minor surgical procedures. It is also used in spinal anesthesia, where it is injected into the cerebrospinal fluid (CSF) to induce anesthesia for cesarean delivery and orthopaedic and abdominal surgeries. The anesthetic is very popular in obstetrics where it is used for labor pain by epidural route. It is also used by caudal block for pediatric surgery. The dosage of bupivacaine is determined by procedure, tissue's vascularity, area, number of segments blocked, depth or length of anesthesia required, and the patient's physical condition. During the administration of bupivacaine, standard monitoring procedure has to be followed. The anesthetic might cause nausea, vomiting, headache, shivering, back pain, dizziness, and sexual dysfunction and might also lead to serious side effects such as convulsions, myoclonic jerks, coma, and cardiovascular collapse. Rarely, cardiac toxicity due to L-carnitine deficiency might occur at dosages as low as 1.1 mg/kg of cutaneously administered bupivacaine. It can also lead to methemoglobinemia, which can be asymptomatic at low concentrations (1–3%). At higher concentrations (10–40%), the drug can cause cyanosis, gray skin discoloration, tachypnea, dyspnea, exercise intolerance, fatigue, and syncope. The drug is contraindicated if the patient is hypersensitive to bupivacaine or its components or to amide anesthetics and if there is an infection at the injection site. Bupivacaine may interact with ergotamine-based migraine medications, blood thinners, antidepressants, and monoamine oxidase inhibitors.

Ropivacaine

It was introduced in the market in 1997. The drug is an enantiomerically pure (S-enantiomer) bupivacaine congener with similar long duration and activity. However, it is preferred over bupivacaine as it has lower CNS and cardiotoxic potential, with reduced tendency of motor blockage as it blocks Aδ and C fibers, which transmit pain more fully than Aβ fibers, which control motor function. This is due to its low lipophilicity than other LAs, which makes the drug less likely to penetrate large myelinated motor fibers.

Ropivacaine in different concentrations has been used for surgical anesthesia and acute pain management. It is used to create an epidural block for surgeries such as cesarean sections where 0.2% ropivacaine was shown to be effective for the initiation and maintenance of labor analgesia. The drug is also utilized for local infiltration and major nerve blocks. Coadministration of opioids with ropivacaine minimizes the amount of LA required and extends analgesia without extending the duration of the motor block. The drug has also been demonstrated to be beneficial for severe refractory migraine.

Ropivacaine is a well-tolerated anesthetic. It might cause hypotension, nausea, vomiting, bradycardia, and headache, with higher incidence in the elderly population. Fetal bradycardia and newborn jaundice are the most common fetal or neonatal adverse effects following the administration of ropivacaine in women undergoing cesarean section. The drug is contraindicated in patients with a known hypersensitivity to ropivacaine or any amide-type LA.

Levobupivacaine

It was marketed in 1999. The drug is a pure S (−) enantiomer of bupivacaine, which in comparison to the parent compound causes less vasodilation and has a longer duration of action and a better safety profile. In adults, levobupivacaine is indicated for infiltration, nerve blocks, ocular, epidural, and intrathecal anesthesia. The drug is indicated for infiltration analgesia in children. Adverse effects are unlikely to occur and are linked to its ineffective administration. The possible side effects of levobupivacaine include hypotension, postoperative pain, fever, constipation, disorientation, drowsiness, slurred speech, and fetal distress. When levobupivacaine is administered with 1,2-benzodiazepine, the risk or severity of the undesirable effects can be enhanced.

Mepivacaine

It has similar properties to lidocaine, with a quick onset and a medium duration of action depending on the site of administration. The half-life of mepivacaine is 1.9 to 3.2 hours in adults and 8.7 to 9 hours in neonates. It is available in formulations containing 1, 1.5, 2, and 3%, which are usually used for local infiltration and regional anesthesia. Although mepivacaine is used in clinical practice in a similar way as lidocaine, it is not recommended for obstetric anesthesia since its effects last much longer in the fetus. Similar to other LAs, the drug causes effects on the circulatory and neurological systems with more toxicity than levobupivacaine and ropivacaine.

Dibucaine

It is a quinoline derivative and the most potent, toxic, and long-acting LA. It is applied topically on the skin to relieve itching and pain produced by some skin conditions such as scrapes, small burns, dermatitis, and insect bites, as well as to treat minor hemorrhoid discomfort and itching. Topical dibucaine ointment should not be applied to the nipple area because direct consumption by toddlers during breastfeeding has resulted in convulsions, arrhythmias, cardiovascular collapse, and death.

Articaine

It is an intermediately potent anesthetic with a short duration of action. It is classified as an amide anesthetic, but it has a thiophene ring instead of a benzene ring, which enhances its lipid solubility. It also has an extra ester group that is rapidly hydrolyzed by esterases, which speeds up its metabolism to articainic acid. As a result, it may be promptly removed from the systemic circulation via the kidney, reducing the risk of side effects. It has been used neuraxially, intravenously, ocularly, and in regional blocks. The drug is suitable and safe for operations that need a brief duration of action and a rapid onset of anesthesia, such as dental procedures and ambulatory spinal anesthesia. For adults, children older than 4 years, the elderly, pregnant women, breastfeeding women, and patients with hepatic diseases and renal function impairment, articaine appears to be the LA of choice in tissues with suppurative inflammation. Articaine use has been linked to persistent paresthesia. **Table 32.3** provides details regarding the various maximum recommended doses and the duration of action of commonly used amino-amides anesthetics.

Table 32.3 Maximum recommended dose and duration of action of commonly used amino-amides anesthetics

Amino-amides anesthetics	Maximum dose with vasoconstrictor (mg/kg)	Duration of action with vasoconstrictor (min)
Lidocaine	6–7[a]	120–240
Bupivacaine	2.5–3[b]	180–480
Ropivacaine	3–4[b]	180–480
Levobupivacaine	3[b]	180–360
Mepivacaine	6.6[b]	120 (approximately 2–4 h of anesthesia for peripheral nerve blocks)
Articaine	7[b]	60–230

[a]Infiltration route.
[b]Infiltration and subcutaneous routes.

Local and Systemic Effects, Including Adverse Effects, of Local Anesthetics

Toxicity from LAs can occur both locally and systemically.

Local Toxicity

Local toxicity is produced on neurons and myocytes, which is time- and dose-dependent. Autonomic fibers are generally more sensitive to LAs' toxic effect than somatic fibers. Additionally, nerve sheaths prevent LAs from diffusing into the nerve trunk, causing outer layer fibers to be inhibited before inner or core fibers.

When an LA is mistakenly injected intrafascicularly, it can cause nerve damage at clinical concentration levels, which might lead to axonal degeneration. To limit the possibility of nerve poisoning, care should be taken to prepare safe dilutions. The proper dilution will keep the concentration in the perineural and intraneural milieu within the therapeutic range, thereby preventing neural injury.

Additionally, LAs inhibit acetylcholine release from motor nerve terminals. They cause numbness of the skin and paralysis of the voluntary muscle supplied by the nerve when injected around it. The toxicity may also be due to the effect of preservative in LAs' formulations, which are included to keep medication molecules stable in solution. Chloroprocaine's neurotoxicity is considered to be caused by preservatives such as sodium bisulfite and ethylene glycol tetraacetic acid.

The application of a tourniquet to limit blood loss and produce a favorable operational field results in nerve fiber compression and tissue ischemia, which has a synergetic effect on LA neurotoxicity. Furthermore, tourniquet application compresses the vasa nervorum and reduces LA washout, hence prolonging nerve fiber exposure to LA.

Patient-related factors such as conditions of preexisting neuropathies, which include diabetic peripheral neuropathy, multiple sclerosis, and Guillain–Barré syndrome, enhance the likelihood of LA-induced neurotoxicity in the nerve fiber. Other conditions such as peripheral vascular diseases, which include vasculitis and hypertension, damage the microvasculature, making neurons more prone to ischemia and increasing the risk of neurotoxicity from LAs during the perioperative period.

One of the important local effects is the occurrence of muscle injury on administration of LAs via intramuscular injection. The effect is more prominent with potent and long-acting LAs such as bupivacaine. The effect on skeletal muscle is temporary, with full recovery occurring within 2 weeks of administration.

Systemic Toxicity

When any drug from LA category, administered either parenterally or topically, gets absorbed, it results into systemic responses depending on the blood levels reached in the plasma or tissue. Systemic toxicity of LAs is achieved from systemic concentrations due to high dose or unintentional intravascular injection of LAs.

LAs hamper the functions of those organs that are dependent on impulse conduction and transmission. Therefore, they produce effects on CNS, ANS, somatic nervous system, and CVS. These effects may be categorized as adverse effects of LAs. The toxic signs and symptoms of LA on the CNS appears at lower blood concentration than those on the CVS, which means that signs and symptoms of CNS poisoning come first, followed by those of the CVS. However, when a patient is under conscious sedation or a full general anesthesia, the CNS toxicity may be hidden, and the cardiotoxicity, manifested as cardiovascular collapse, may be the only symptom of the LA toxicity. The key risk factor for the development of systemic toxicity is extremes of age, either too young (4 months) or older than 70 years. Other risk factors include a preexisting impairment in heart conduction, ischemic heart disease, pregnancy, and renal and hepatic dysfunctions.

Central Nervous System Toxicity

LAs have the ability to produce two separate phases of CNS toxicity signs and symptoms: the excitatory phase followed by the depressive phase. The inhibitory neurons are the first to be blocked by LAs, leaving excitatory neurons free to operate. At large doses, all the neurons are suppressed, which are shown as flattened waves on the electroencephalogram (EEG). The metallic taste is frequently the first symptom, followed by numbness around the mouth, light headedness, dizziness, visual disturbances, disorientation, tinnitus, and agitation. During the excitatory phase, a range of effects is observed, which include shivering, muscular twitching, tremor, and generalized tonic-clonic convulsion. Later, during the depressive phase, LAs can lead to unconsciousness and death, generally due to depression of respiratory centers leading to respiratory failure. The CNS effects somewhat vary with various LAs used, with convulsive seizures being the principal life-threatening consequence of LA overdose, which is produced at lower serum concentrations of LAs if hypercarbia (elevated carbon dioxide) is present.

Cardiovascular System Toxicity

LAs directly affect the heart by blocking the voltage-gated sodium channels, subsequently leading to reduced depolarization rate of conducting cells and cardiomyocytes. Due to this, the duration of action potential and the refractory period decrease. Different LAs affect the conduction of action potential to varying degrees. Bupivacaine depresses conduction to a greater extent than lidocaine. It has a worse prognosis following cardiac resuscitation and generates cardiovascular toxicity at lower concentrations than lidocaine.

The duration of conduction in the atrium and ventricle is first prolonged by an increased plasma level of LAs, which is visible on an electrocardiogram (ECG) as PR interval prolonging and QRS complex enlargement. At a higher plasma level, spontaneous pacemaker activity is suppressed, resulting in bradycardia and sinus arrest. LAs can induce cardiac arrhythmias. Bupivacaine causes more ventricular arrhythmia than lidocaine, with a higher risk in pregnant patients. In addition, LAs have a negative inotropic effect.

With the exception of cocaine, which always causes vasoconstriction (due to sympathomimetic properties) regardless of concentration, low concentrations of LAs cause vasoconstriction, while greater concentrations cause vasodilation. Fall in blood pressure can occur due to the blockade of the sympathetic ganglia of the ANS, the achievement of high concentration at the injection site, and the local direct arteriolar smooth muscle relaxation. Higher concentration of LAs can result into cardiovascular failure.

Other adverse effects including methemoglobinemia and allergic reactions have also been reported, especially to amide LAs. However, these events have been mostly linked to preservatives (methylparaben) and antioxidants (bisulfites) in LA solutions. It is essential to follow the practice guidelines for safe regional anesthesia, which include thorough patient evaluation to identify factors that may influence absorption and biotransformation of LAs, estimation of the maximum dose, and adequate monitoring. Airway management by providing 100% oxygen is important to avoid hypoxia, hypercarbia, and acidosis, which might increase the CNS toxicity of LAs. Benzodiazepines are used to treat seizures. Drugs such as vasopressin, calcium channel blockers, and β blockers should not be used for the treatment of cardiac arrhythmias. Along with the early resuscitative procedures, 20% intralipid emulsion should be administered immediately.

Techniques for Local Anesthesia

Surface Anesthesia

Administration of LAs by injections can be uncomfortable. It might exacerbate needle phobia and create tissue edema, distorting the surgery site. All of these issues can be avoided by using topical anesthetics, which is becoming more common in clinical practice. Topical anesthetics are useful for reducing discomfort during ophthalmological, superficial dermatological, cosmetic, and laser procedures, minor surgeries, and venipuncture, among other procedures. They are highly effective in dentistry and in the treatment of lacerations, especially in children. Surface anesthetic is applied topically to the mucous membranes or abraded skin to generate surface anesthesia, where the exterior layer is anesthetized, yet there is no loss of motor function. The beginning of anesthesia and length of action are dependent on the site of application (rapid onset at mucosa and sites with thin stratum corneum), vascularity of tissues in the area applied, surface area, the type of LA, its concentration, and the dosage form. The lipophilic free bases can enter the stratum corneum without the use of specific delivery systems, whereas the salt forms of LAs require the use of special delivery systems. The medication of choice for application on mucosal surfaces is benzocaine ointment (20%). Tetracaine is the most powerful surface anesthetic medication that has been combined with 14% benzocaine as a cold spray. Tetracaine is also used to control gag reflexes during endoscopic operations. Eutectic mixture of lidocaine and prilocaine has a lower melting point (18°C) than either component alone, allowing for better penetration. It is also capable of anesthetizing skin that is intact. Another mixture is LET, containing 4% lignocaine, 0.1% epinephrine (adrenaline), and 0.5% tetracaine, which is used in treating nonmucosal skin lacerations, even in children over the age of 2. A few drops of LET are applied directly to the wound. The wound is then treated with a cotton-tipped applicator with 1 to 3 mL of the gel or solution, which is administered with firm pressure for 15 to 30 minutes. It is best to avoid applying it to end-arteriolar body parts such as the digits and contaminated or complex wounds. Many other topical formulations are available in the market. Permeation enhancers are included in LAs formulation to boost skin permeability through the stratum corneum temporarily and reversibly. Although the addition of adrenaline has no effect on the duration of topical anesthesia, the addition of phenylephrine can promote mucosal vasoconstriction and therefore lengthen the duration of topical anesthesia.

Infiltration Anesthesia

The technique of causing loss of sensation restricted to a superficial, localized area of the body is known as local infiltration anesthesia. The tissues in the area that requires anesthesia are infiltrated by injecting a low-dose diluted solution of the anesthetic agent under the skin in the area that needs to be rendered insensitive to minor surgical procedure, effectively blocking the sensory nerve terminals. When lidocaine (1%) and bupivacaine (0.25%) are used for infiltration technique, their action begins instantly and lasts for a shorter period of time than in nerve blocks.

Some of the applications of local infiltration anesthesia include: subcutaneous infiltration for intravenous placement, suturing and superficial/shave biopsy, submucosal infiltration for dental procedures, and laceration repairs. Additionally, the technique is used for wound infiltration for postoperative pain control at the incision site and intra-articular injections for arthritic joint pain control.

Conduction Block Anesthesia

In this type of anesthesia, LAs are injected surrounding the nerve trunk in order to anesthetize and paralyze the area distal to the injection. The selection of LAs and their amount is directly proportional to the desired period of action. For procedures requiring more time, bupivacaine is the choice and for short procedures lidocaine (1–2%) can be selected. LAs are usually applied in two ways to produce block anesthesia.

Field Block

The field block is produced by not injecting the LAs into the area to be operated on, but into the neighboring area. The LAs are injected by the subcutaneous route in such a way that all nerves leading to a certain field are blocked. By using low concentrations of LAs, a larger area can be anesthetized as compared to infiltration anesthesia. The technique is used in dental procedures, scalp stitching, herniorrhaphy, appendicectomy, forearm and leg operations, and so on. Examples of drugs used are lidocaine and bupivacaine.

Nerve Block (PM3.5)

It is produced by administering the LA close to the appropriate nerve trunk or plexus, thereby paralyzing the muscle that is supplied by that nerve/plexus such as radial, ulnar, palatine, pudendal, or a cord of the brachial plexus. The block is sometimes described by including the name of the nerve to be anesthetized, such as radial nerve block, ulnar nerve block, and so on. The supraclavicular nerve block has become a routine treatment for anesthetizing the brachial plexus during upper-limb procedures. Generally, nerve block remains for longer period of time as compared to field block or infiltration anesthesia, depending on the lipid solubility and protein binding of LAs. Lidocaine (1–1.5%), mepivacaine (1–2%), or bupivacaine (0.25–0.375%) might be used for blocks of 2 to 4 hours. The onset of action depends on the drug and the area to be covered by diffusion (lidocaine anesthetizes intercostal nerves in 3 minutes, but a brachial plexus block can take up to 15 minutes). The technique is used for tooth extraction and operations on eye, limb, or abdominal wall. It is also used for trauma to ribs and fracture setting.

Central Nerve Block Anesthesia (Central Neuraxial Blocks)

Central neuraxial blocks (CNBs) include spinal, epidural, combined spinal epidural, and caudal epidural injections techniques. They are widely used in the perioperative phase for obstetric anesthesia and analgesia, as well as for chronic pain management.

Spinal Anesthesia

It is one of the most commonly used techniques. It is efficient and cost-effective and achieves complete sensory and motor block, as well as postoperative analgesia. In this type of anesthesia, the solution of LAs is intrathecally injected into the subarachnoid space allowing the solution to get mixed in the CSF, thus reaching to the spinal nerve root and dorsal root ganglia. This anesthesia causes loss of sensation and relaxation of the muscles, leading to paralysis and aiding in the surgical procedure to be carried out. Spinal anesthesia is an alternative to general anesthesia, especially when the patient has significant breathing problems. The grade of anesthesia relies on various factors such as patient's pose, quantity of injection, and the rate of injection of LAs. For most procedures below the waist, the nerves that feed the hips, bottom, and legs can be numbed by the LA. This type of anesthesia is generally used during the obstetric procedures, cesarean section, operations of the legs, pelvis, and lower abdomen (e.g., removal of the prostate gland), orthopaedic procedures, etc. The LAs used in spinal anesthesia are procaine (short-acting), tetracaine (mostly used agent; its action lasts for 1–2 hours), lidocaine (1.5–5%), bupivacaine (0.5%), and ropivacaine (0.75%). The range of duration is from 60 to 150 minutes. The period of action of spinal anesthesia can be augmented by about one-third when epinephrine in a dose of 0.2 mL of 1:1,000 solution is added.

Spinal anesthesia has several advantages, especially in patients with potential airway issues and established respiratory disorders. It has a lower risk of deep vein thrombosis and less intraoperative blood loss and can prevent pulmonary aspiration in the event of an emergency.

Adverse Effects of Spinal Anesthesia

Because of the intrusive nature of spinal anesthesia, a variety of problems can develop with varying frequency.

During spinal anesthesia, LAs produces physiological blockade that engages the production of a sympathectomy with venous pooling and decreased venous return, causing decreased cardiac output and fall in blood pressure. Physiological complications include decreased heart rate, heart block, and cardiac arrest. The reduction in blood pressure can cause nausea and vomiting, indicating spinal cord ischemia. Following neuraxial anesthesia, a drop in body temperature usually occurs. As a result of a drop in core temperature, shivering can occur, especially during the postoperative phase, which increases oxygen consumption. Special attention should be paid particularly in the pediatric, obstetric, and elderly patients, because it can lead to inadequate perfusion of essential organs, coronary ischemia, and infection. Post-dural puncture headache is a persistent problem, which is most commonly observed in young patients including middle-aged women and obstetric patients. Following spinal anesthesia, TRI can occur, which usually decreases after 2 days, but it can be alarming. The use of lidocaine in presence of other contributing factors might increase the risk of developing these symptoms. A severe complication of spinal anesthesia is spinal hematoma, which necessitates immediate surgical intervention to avoid lifelong neurological damage. The risk is higher in females and patients of advanced age and patients using anticoagulant medications. By blocking all afferent nerve fibers, spinal anesthesia affects urination by causing urinary retention, preventing the patient from feeling bladder distension or urine urgency. There have been a few cases of bacterial meningitis that are linked to CNB, which could be due to technical complications during needle placement or multiple attempts to induce spinal anesthesia.

Spinal anesthesia is a challenge in patients with preexisting neurological diseases and degenerative vertebral anomalies and comorbidities, those using many medications, those having surgery for advanced cancer, and in patients with impaired immune systems and infections.

Epidural Anesthesia

In this type of anesthesia, a hollow needle and a small, flexible catheter are inserted (after numbing the insertion site) into the area between the spinal column and the outer membrane of the spinal cord, which is filled with fat, blood vessels, spinal nerve roots, and lymphatics and known as epidural space. The catheter remains while the needle is removed after the catheter has passed through it. LAs are injected into the catheter to anesthetize the body parts above and below the injection site. Epidural anesthesia is frequently used during childbirth. However, it can also be used to help manage pain following major abdominal or chest surgery. Usually, a 20-mL dose of 3% chloroprocaine and 2% lidocaine, with or without adrenaline, is the anesthetic of choice for outpatient surgeries, allowing the discharge of patient within 3 to 4 hours. Because of their extended duration of action, 0.5 to 0.75% of bupivacaine or levobupivacaine and 0.75 to 1% ropivacaine are the anesthetics of choice for inpatient surgery. **Table 32.4** mentions the difference between spinal and dural anesthesia. This anesthesia can be given by three different techniques according to the site of action.

Caudal

This type of anesthesia can be performed in the sacral hiatus where the caudal anesthesia can be done by injecting the LAs in the sacral canal. This anesthesia results in loss of sensation of the pelvic and perineal region. Generally, this technique is used for obstetric and genitourinary procedures. When slower onset of action and extended duration of anesthesia are desired, then adrenaline can be added to bupivacaine and other LAs.

Thoracic

In this procedure, LAs are injected in the central thoracic region of the vertebral column. Small volumes of LAs solution are required. The anesthesia produced by this procedure is mostly used for eliciting analgesic effect after the thoracic or the upper abdominal surgical procedures. By placing catheters in the epidural space, LAs can be administered by either continuous infusions or repeated bolus doses.

Table 32.4 Comparison between spinal and epidural anesthesia

Parameters	Spinal anesthesia	Epidural anesthesia
Site of administration	Involves the injection of LAs directly into the fluid sac	Involves the injection of LAs into the epidural space outside the sac
Route of administration	LAs and/or narcotics are injected via the spinal needle	Medications are injected via the epidural catheter
Types of needles	Spinal needles are much thinner and are easier to place	Epidural needles are thicker and are difficult to place
Onsite of action and doses	Spinal blocks work instantly; Spinal doses are smaller	Epidural block takes at least 15 min to begin its action; Epidural doses are larger and many doses of LAs can be administered to maintain anesthesia
Strength of anesthesia	Intense	Less intense
Incidence of patchy block[a]	Very low	More frequent
Spread of anesthesia	Highly expected	Less expected
Hemodynamic alterations	More prominent	Less prominent
Incidence of headache	Higher incidence of headache, which are often less severe	Lower incidence of headache, which are often more severe
Toxicity	Sudden and of less intensity	Gradual, intense, and systemic
Example of uses	Cesarean delivery and operations of the legs, pelvis, and lower abdomen, and orthopaedic procedures	The most common method of pain relief for women who request analgesia for labor; Procedures of legs, pelvis, and lower abdomen

Abbreviation: LAs, local anesthetics.
[a]Patchy block refers to a block that looks to be appropriate in extent but lacks sensory and motor effects.

Lumbar

This type of technique is used to produce anesthesia of the lower abdominal region, pelvic region, and hind limb. Large volumes of LA solution can be administered. This type of anesthetic technique is used during the obstetric procedures, cesarean section, and operations of the legs, pelvis, and lower abdomen for removal of the prostate gland.

Epidural anesthesia is generally safe; however, it can lead to hypotension, itchy skin, headache, temporary loss of bladder control, respiratory paralysis, septic meningitis, seizure, nerve damage, and caudal equine syndrome.

Intravenous Regional Anesthesia

The German surgeon August Bier first created intravenous regional anesthesia, which is known as the "Bier block," in 1908. A Bier block entails injecting LA solutions into the venous system of an upper or lower extremity that has been isolated from the central circulation by elevation, tightly wrapped elastic bandage, and a tourniquet. The procedure is used for rapid anesthetization of an extremity, usually for the upper limb and orthopaedic procedures. In addition, the technique is also used as a treatment adjunct of complex regional pain syndromes. Bier's original technique involved injecting the LA procaine in concentrations ranging from 0.25 to 0.5% using an intravenous cannula that was sandwiched between two Esmarch bandages, which served as tourniquets to divide the arm into proximal and distal sections. A nearly instantaneous onset of "direct" anesthesia occurs between the two tourniquets, as a result of local anesthesia coming in contact with nerve endings in the tissues, followed by "indirect" anesthesia not much far away from the distally placed tourniquet after a 5- to 7-minute delay, most likely caused by local anesthesia being carried to the nerve substance via the vasa nervorum, causing a normal conduction block. This approach is a result of two anesthetic methods: peripheral infiltration block and conduction block. Current clinical practice utilizes the pneumatic-type double-tourniquet preparation. Drugs such as lidocaine and prilocaine can be administered safely by this technique. However, drugs such as bupivacaine should be avoided due to its tendency to cause cardiac complications. The relative contraindications to this technique include the inability to detect peripheral veins, local skin infections, cellulitis, compound fractures, etc.

Multiple Choice Questions

1. A 43-year-old patient had a radial fracture after an accident. A catheter was inserted, and a low-dose local anesthetic infusion was administered. Which one of the following techniques is preferred for this patient?

A. Caudal epidural nerve block.

B. Supraclavicular nerve block.

C. Thoracic epidural nerve block.

D. Spinal anesthesia.

Answer: B

Regional anesthesia is a type of anesthesia that uses drugs to inhibit the sensory function of specific nerves in the limbs. There are several techniques available for surgical procedure of the upper extremities, each with its own set of advantages and disadvantages. The supraclavicular nerve block has become a standard procedure for anesthetizing the brachial plexus for upper-limb surgeries. The block is done at the level of the brachial plexus trunks, where nearly all sensory, motor, and sympathetic innervations of the upper extremity are carried in just three nerve structures confined to a very small surface area. Other regional anesthetic procedures that are commonly used for hand and wrist surgeries include digital blocks, wrist blocks, intravenous regional anesthetic blocks, and axillary blocks. The use of epidural and spinal anesthesia is most common in surgery of the lower abdomen, hips, legs, and pelvis. Moreover, epidural anesthesia is frequently utilized in labor.

2. A 35-year-old female patient developed symptoms of dizziness and systemic urticaria 30 minutes after receiving an injection of lidocaine containing adrenaline for a comprehensive dental treatment. She was administered an injection of diphenhydramine and her symptoms were resolved over 2 hours. Later, she informed the dentist that approximately, 3 years before, she was administered bupivacaine at the time of delivery of her last child, and she developed mild allergic symptoms. A local anesthetic has to be administered again after a few days to complete her dental procedure. Which one of the following local anesthetics can be administered as an alternative to avoid the allergic reactions to this patient?

A. Articaine.

B. Prilocaine.

C. Procaine.

D. Bupivacaine.

Answer: C

Allergies have been reported usually to ester-type local anesthetics as a result of hydrolysis by cholinesterase, leading to the release of the allergen metabolite PABA. On the other hand, local anesthetics of the amide-type are metabolized in the liver and, therefore, rarely cause allergic reactions. However, lidocaine and other local anesthetics, which are routinely used in dentistry, can have a variety of side effects, albeit uncommon. Allergic reactions mediated by the immune response (which are extremely rare), as well as others unrelated to the immune response, are examples of such adverse effects. This patient developed cross reactivity with the amide local anesthetic lidocaine as her history strongly suggests that she had earlier an acute hypersensitive reaction to another amide local anesthetic bupivacaine, which she has not informed the dentist about. For patients who have a history of local anesthetic allergy, a comprehensive and thorough history of allergies is required, and allergy testing, such as skin prick and/or intradermal tests, is required. The dentist can administer her ester procaine after conducting skin sensitivity test to eliminate any further reaction. Procaine is alternatively administered in patients that are allergic to amides such as articaine, prilocaine, bupivacaine, and lidocaine.

3. A 25-year-old male patient undergoing septoplasty for the correction of a deviated nasal septum was administered submucosal infiltration of lidocaine 2% with adrenaline

1:200,000. What is the main indication of adrenaline in this case?

A. Decreasing blood pressure.

B. Alleviating cardiac arrhythmias.

C. Causing vasodilation.

D. Reducing the systemic absorption and toxicity of LAs.

Answer: D

Nasal surgeries, such as septoplasty, is usually performed either under local anesthesia alone or in combination with general anesthesia. Vasoconstrictors such as adrenaline have been used in conjunction with local anesthetics to reduce intraoperative bleeding, lower the risk of systemic toxicity, and extend the duration of action of local anesthetics, where the combination of lidocaine and adrenaline is the most commonly utilized one in many surgeries. In susceptible patients, adrenaline use has been linked to severe hypertensive crisis, pulmonary edema, and reversible cardiomyopathy. It also increases the risk of cardiac arrhythmias and causes myocardial infarction, cerebral hemorrhage, and cardiac arrest.

4. A 25-year-old man with an injury in his index and middle fingers and with no other medical condition received a total of 15 mL of 1% lidocaine and 5 mL of 0.5% levobupivacaine as part of the terminalization and wound exploration procedure using adequate technical administration under ring block anesthesia. He showed no sign of anesthesia and felt extreme pain, even after using additional 10 mL of 1% lidocaine to block the median nerve and superficial radial nerve. The patient reported experiencing similar incidents during earlier visits to dentist. The procedure was abandoned and rescheduled under general anesthesia. Which one of the following is the main reason for the failure of the local anesthesia?

A. True resistance to LAs.

B. Wrong selection of LAs.

C. Presence of disease.

D. Hypersensitivity.

Answer: A

Amino-amides anesthetics such as lidocaine, bupivacaine, and levobupivacaine are a popular class of local anesthetics. Physicians have long noticed few cases of patients who do not respond to local anesthesia and experience pain even after injection of local anesthetics for minor surgical procedures. They attributed that to the condition of true resistance and not to other causes responsible for the failure of the anesthesia such as technical failure, infection, and issues related to medications. In our scenario, the patient had a clear history of previous local anesthetic failure. He had no infection and the LAs were administered from different vials. Therefore, it is a case of true resistance to local anesthetics. The etiology of complete failure of local anesthetics could be ascribed to a mutation in the sodium channels that are responsible for the activity of LAs.

5. An over-the-counter gel containing a local anesthetic was applied to the gum of a 1-year-old infant to relief teething pain. After half an hour of application, the infant turned pale, experienced shortness of breath, and had rapid heart rate. She was rushed to a nearby hospital for the management of her condition. Which one of the following local anesthetics caused the above symptoms?

A. Procaine.

B. Ropivacaine.

C. Benzocaine.

D. Levobupivacaine.

Answer: C

Benzocaine is a topical anesthetic that can be found in over-the-counter medications. When benzocaine gels, liquids, and other products are used to treat mouth and gum discomfort, they can cause the rare but significant side effect methemoglobinemia. It is a hazardous disorder caused by high levels of methemoglobin in the blood, decreasing the level of oxygen delivered through the blood, which can lead to cyanosis, hypoxia, dyspnea, and death. The FDA warns that over-the-counter benzocaine products should not be used to treat infants and children under the age of 2. Patients with diseases such as emphysema, heart disease, asthma, and bronchitis are at the highest risk of developing methemoglobinemia. Drugs such as procaine, ropivacaine, and levobupivacaine are injectable local anesthetics.

Chapter 33 Sedatives and Hypnotics

Panini Patankar and Nishtha Khatri

PH1.19: Describe the mechanism/s of action, types, doses, side effects, indications, and contraindications of the drugs that act on the central nervous system (including anxiolytics, sedatives and hypnotics, antipsychotic, antidepressant drugs, antimanic agents, opioid agonists and antagonists, drugs used for neurodegenerative disorders, and antiepileptics drugs).

Learning Objectives

- Physiology of normal sleep and sleep cycle.
- Benzodiazepines (BZDs).
- Barbiturates.
- Non-BZDs.
- Other hypnotics.

Introduction

For generations, knowledge regarding sleep and its anomalies was based on self-experience and observation of behaviour of sleeping people. From the middle of the 19th century, scientific investigation of sleep in the truest sense commenced, owing to development of instruments like EEG, plethysmography, and actigraphy. The interrelation of sleep to other physiological processes like changes in muscle tone and blood pressure was observed during this period. The real turning point in the study of sleep and sleep disorders came with characterization of different stages of sleep, with two predominant stages being rapid eye movement (REM) sleep and nonrapid eye movement (NREM) sleep.

One of the most common types of sleep disorder is insomnia. Although many drugs acting against insomnia have been developed in the past century, potassium bromide (KBr) was the earliest documented drug to be used by Hammond in the 1850s. At the beginning of 20th century, a new era for treatment of insomnia began with the synthesis of barbiturates which were the mainstay of therapy till they were largely replaced by BZDs by the second half of the 20th century. Newer drugs with actions like BZDs were the "Z" class of drugs which are commonly used today. The most recent class of drugs include melatonin agonists and orexin antagonists, which will be briefly discussed toward the end of this chapter.

Sedative: Any substance or drug attenuating the excitement and calming the subject without induction of sleep is known as a sedative. However, some degree of drowsiness may be produced. It may also be associated with decreased cognition and motor activity.

Hypnotic: Any substance or a drug which either induces or maintains sleep is known as a hypnotic.

However, both the terms are commonly used interchangeably. In general, hypnotics have quick onset and steeper dose-response curves compared to sedatives. Certain drugs like benzodiazepine class of drugs act as sedatives at lower dose and hypnotics at higher dose and hence there is considerable overlap between both the terms.

Physiology of Normal Sleep and Sleep Cycle

The complete mechanism of initiation and maintenance of sleep is still an area of active debate. It is now known that cortical activation is essential to maintaining wakefulness and lack of same leads to induction of sleep. Some of the important neurochemicals for maintenance of wakefulness include:

- Norepinephrine, which is a stimulatory neurotransmitter arising from the locus coeruleus (LC).
- Serotonin arising from the central raphe nucleus.
- Dopamine arising from the ventral periaqueductal gray matter.
- Acetylcholine (ACh) arising from the pedunculopontine tegmentum and laterodorsal tegmentum in the pontine region.
- Histamine arising from the tuberomammillary nucleus (TMN).
- Orexin arising from the perifornical area.

Despite being apparently redundant, normal behavioral functioning may require all the above-mentioned arousing systems. It is postulated that narcolepsy results from a selective loss of orexin-releasing neurons in the forebrain, which accounts for the enhanced sleepiness during the daytime, fragmented sleep, and cataplexy (sudden muscle fatigue without unconsciousness) which are characteristics of this disorder.

Sleep initiation and maintenance require suppression of all the above neurochemicals, which is normally achieved by inhibitory neurons of the ventrolateral preoptic area (VLPO). The molecular targets which activate VLPO are yet to be fully understood. Adenosine accumulation occurs in the basal forebrain during wakefulness and diminishes with ongoing sleep. Adenosine receptors are characteristically present in the VLPO, and adenosine activates VLPO neurons in vivo, thus making them reasonable candidates for sleep switching. Caffeine and theophylline act as adenosine receptor antagonists and hence have a characteristic alerting effect.

Sleep is not homogenous in nature, and as per the earlier discussion, it is divided into various stages, with the two broad phases being REM and NREM sleep (**Fig. 33.1**). Dreaming occurs during the REM sleep, while NREM sleep is considered as deep sleep and is further divided into four substages, depending upon the depth of the sleep. The binary system between the NREM and REM sleep is apparently controlled by the reciprocal inhibition between the monoamine secreting neurons and a characteristic subset of ACh-secreting neurons within the brainstem. When REM sleep is triggered, REM-on cholinergic neurons become fully active, while noradrenergic and serotonergic neurons become apparently silent. The binary switching between activity and inhibition of these neurons results in a specific cycling between NREM and REM during the sleep period.

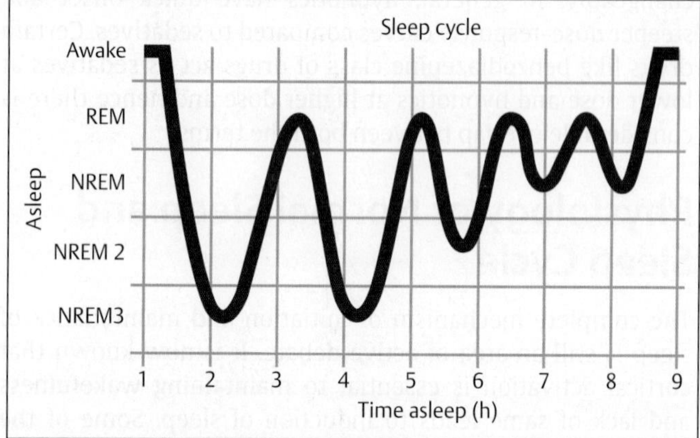

Fig. 33.1 Representation of normal sleep cycle with each cycle lasting for approximately 90 minutes and the depth and time of cycle decreasing with each successive cycle.

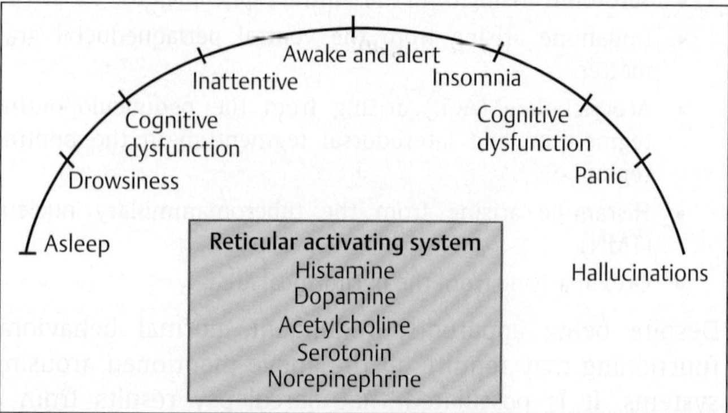

Fig. 33.2 Sleep and wakefulness spectrum.

An awake and alert person possess the appropriate balance between excessive and minimal arousal. It is essential to understand the role of the different neurotransmitters involved in the regulation of sleep. Five neurotransmitters work in synchrony to regulate arousal. These include histamine, dopamine, norepinephrine, serotonin, and ACh, all of which form a part of the ascending reticular activating system (**Fig. 33.2**). These neurotransmitters modulate the cortical arousal system in a manner like that of a rheostat on a lighting system.

The crucial role of hypothalamus in the sleep cycle regulation cannot be ignored. Hypothalamus functions like a sleep/wake switch (**Fig. 33.3**). VLPO of the hypothalamus consists of the sleep promotor region, while the TMN of the hypothalamus consists of the wake promoter region. Histamine and GABA from the TMN and VLPO, respectively, are the two most crucial neurotransmitters involved in the sleep cycle regulation. TMN, on activation, release histamine which then act on the cortex and VLPO to promote wakefulness and inhibit sleep. When VLPO becomes active, it releases GABA which acts on the TMN to cause sleep promotor activation and wake promoter inhibition. To add to this, orexin/hypocretin neurons in the later hypothalamus also play a role in the sleep/wake regulation. They stabilize wakefulness and exert an effect on the suprachiasmatic nucleus of the hypothalamus. The circadian drive leading to wakefulness is the result of input (light, melatonin, activity) to the suprachiasmatic nucleus.

Classification of Sedative-Hypnotics (PS8.4, PS8.6)

- BZDs.
- Barbiturates.
- Non-BZDs.
- Other hypnotics.

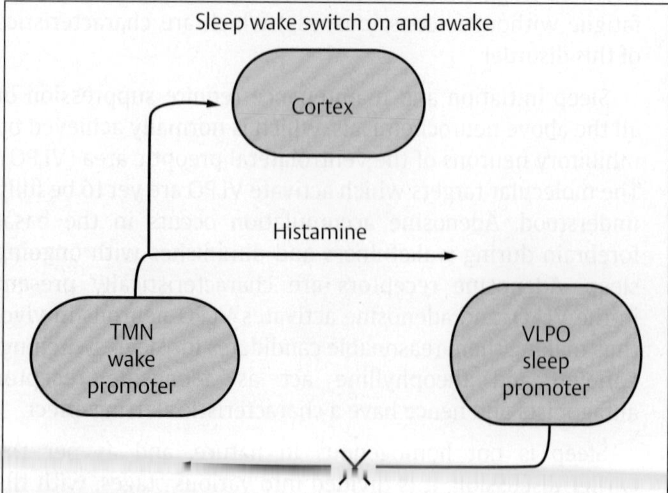

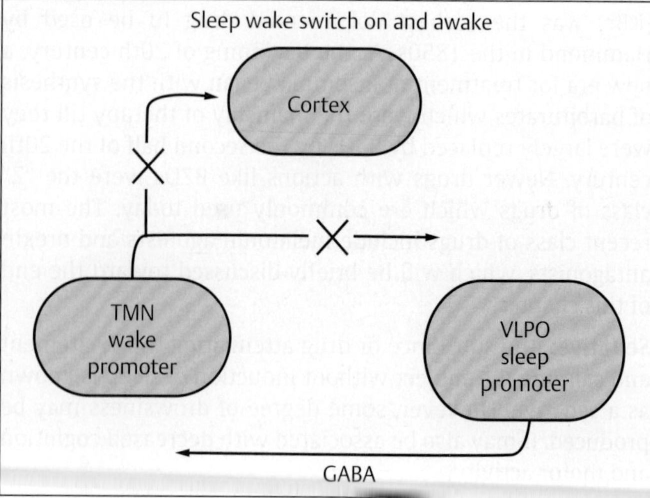

Fig. 33.3 Hypothalamic regions and their role in sleep wake regulation. TMN, tuberomammillary nucleus; VLPO, ventrolateral preoptic nucleus.

Binding Sites on GABA-A Receptor with Examples

GABA is the most abundantly present neurotransmitter in the central nervous system (CNS). It is inhibitory in nature and is found abundantly in the cortex and limbic system. There are three different types of GABA receptors, namely, type A, type B, and type C. $GABA_A$ receptors are most crucial in terms of the benzodiazepine interaction. $GABA_A$ receptors consist of five glycoprotein subunits, namely, two α subunits, two β subunits, and one γ subunit.

$GABA_A$ receptors possess multiple binding sites unique to each class of drug (**Fig. 33.4**); for example, barbiturate-binding site, benzodiazepine-binding site, and general anesthetic binding site.

Mechanism of Action of Benzodiazepines and Barbiturates (PS18.1)

Both barbiturates and BZDs act through the $GABA_A$ receptors. BZDs have affinity toward the allosteric site on the receptor (specifically $GABA_A$) which is composed of a gap created by α and γ subunits (**Fig. 33.5**). They lead to a conformational change in the receptor and cause opening of chloride channel. This brings about hyperpolarization of the cell and accounts for inhibitor effects of GABA. Barbiturates interact with a discrete allosteric-binding site on the $GABA_A$ receptor and bring about opening of the Cl^- channels. BZDs lead to increase in the frequency of opening of GABA-mediated Cl^- channels, while barbiturates increase the duration of opening of Cl^- channels. It is of due significance to know that at higher concentration barbiturates not only act on the allosteric site of $GABA_A$ receptors but can also directly activate the $GABA_A$ receptor. BZDs are safe agents compared to barbiturates and this can be attributed to the lack of direct channel activation by BZDs as well as due to their dependence on the presynaptic release of GABA at the $GABA_A$ receptor.

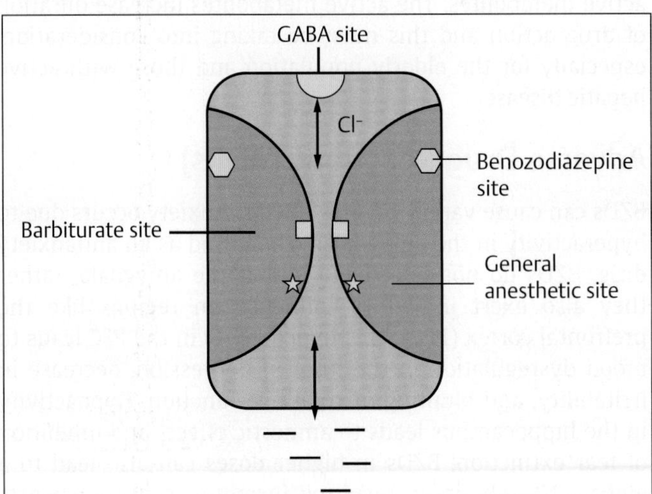

Fig. 33.4 Binding sites on $GABA_A$ receptor.

Benzodiazepines (BZDs)

BZDs are classified based on their duration of action.

Short-acting

These BZDs have an elimination half-life of < 5 hours and are primarily used for sleep induction on account of their quick onset of action; for example, midazolam, triazolam, and oxazepam.

Intermediate-acting

They have an elimination half-life of 5 to 24 hours and are primarily used as antianxiety drugs; for example, alprazolam, lorazepam, nitrazepam, and estazolam.

Long-acting

They have an elimination half-life of > 24 hours and pose a risk of accumulation especially in elderly patients and in patients with metabolic diseases; for example, diazepam, clonazepam, and flurazepam.

BZDs can also be classified based on their relative potencies.

Low-to-medium Potency BZDs

These were discovered relatively early; for example, chlordiazepoxide, oxazepam, and temazepam.

High-potency BZDs

The discovery of high-potency BZDs led to the use of BZDs in the use of various other newer psychiatric indications such as panic disorders and obsessive compulsive disorders. They may also be used as adjuncts to antipsychotics in acute mania or agitation; for example, alprazolam, lorazepam, and clonazepam.

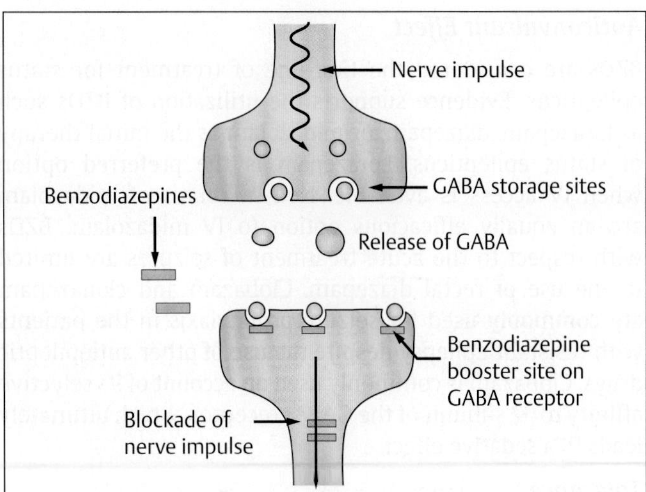

Fig. 33.5 Mechanism of action of benzodiazepines (BZDs).

Pharmacological Actions and Clinical Use

All BZDs resemble each other in their pharmacological profiles; yet, it is important to note that the individual BZDs differ from each other with respect to their selectivity. Hence, the clinical utility of the BZDs differ considerably among each other. Majority of the effects of the BZDs can be completely reversed by the use of the drug, flumazenil, which competes with both the agonists and inverse agonists at the major binding site at the $GABA_A$ receptor. BZDs produce a lesser magnitude of effect compared to barbiturates and this occurs on account of the weaker enhancing effects of BZDs.

BZDs exert effects on a variety of systems:

Central Nervous System (CNS)

Sedative-Hypnotic Effect

BZDs exert a sedative-hypnotic effect on the CNS. With increasing dose, sedative effect of BZDs progresses to hypnosis and finally to stupor. BZDs bind to α1, α2, α3, and α5 subunit of $GABA_A$ receptors. BZDs cause a variation in the sleep pattern. They lead to decrease in the latency to fall asleep and also reduce the number of awakenings. They also cause a decrease in the duration of stage 3 and stage 4 sleep (slow wave sleep) and also of the REM sleep. However, BZDs increase the total duration of sleep by enhancing the amount of time spent in stage 2 and increasing the frequency of sleep cycles.

Anesthetic Effect

These drugs are also used as anesthetics. However, BZDs do not cause true anesthesia since awareness and response to noxious stimuli still persists. They are widely used as a preanesthetic medication since they cause amnesia.

Anxiolytic Effect

It is very difficult to demarcate the boundary between the anxiolytic actions of BZDs from their sedative actions, since precise measurement of anxiety and sedation is an arduous task. BZDs also have a transient analgesic action if given by intravenous (IV) route.

Anticonvulsant Effect

BZDs are considered the first-line of treatment for status epilepticus. Evidence supports the utilization of BZDs such as lorazepam, diazepam, or midazolam as the initial therapy of status epilepticus. Lorazepam is the preferred option when IV access is available. Non-IV routes of midazolam are an equally efficacious option to IV midazolam. BZDs with respect to the acute treatment of seizures are limited to the use of rectal diazepam. Clobazam and clonazepam are commonly used for seizure prophylaxis in the patients with resistant epilepsy despite the use of other antiepileptic drugs. Clobazam is commonly used on account of its selective affinity to a2 subunit of the $GABA_A$ receptor, which ultimately leads to a sedative effect.

Tolerance

Sedative and anticonvulsant actions of BZDs are susceptible to rapid development of tolerance compared to anxiolytic and amnesic, which hardly develop any tolerance. The varied neuroadaptive mechanisms explaining tolerance include specific expression of receptor subunits and changes in the coupling along with the various intracellular changes related to the neurotropic factors.

Respiratory System

High doses of BZDs used for preanesthetic purposes cause a depression in the alveolar ventilation. This ultimately leads to hypoxia and respiratory acidosis. These effects are seen more peculiarly in individuals with an already depressed respiratory function like in the case of chronic obstructive pulmonary disorder (COPD). BZDs may cause apnea during anesthesia or when used concomitantly with opioids. Like the preanesthetic doses, hypnotic doses of BZDs can also cause hypoventilation and hypoxemia. However, in this case, the reason behind hypoxia is a decrease in the tone of the upper airway muscles and also a decrease in the ventilator response to CO_2. This effect is peculiarly seen in individuals with sleep-related breathing disorders.

Cardiovascular System

BZDs are commonly used as preanesthetic medication. They lead to lowering of blood pressure and slight tachycardia. Midazolam causes a decrease in the peripheral resistance, while diazepam leads to decrease in the workload by the left ventricle along with decrease in the cardiac output.

Pharmacokinetics (Table 33.1)

BZDs are absorbed well, orally by the alimentary tract and the IV route, and they distribute swiftly to the brain and CNS in a manner like barbiturates, owing to their high-lipid solubility. Their action is terminated by redistribution. BZDs and their metabolites have a high protein-binding capacity. Majority of the BZDs are under oxidation by the cytochrome P450 enzymes (phase I), followed by glucuronidation (phase II). Excretion occurs via urine. Few short-acting BZDs like midazolam do not produce active metabolites, but long-acting BZDs like diazepam act through the production of active metabolites. The active metabolites increase duration of drug action and this must be taking into consideration, especially for the elderly population and those with active hepatic disease.

Adverse Drug Reactions (ADRs)

BZDs can cause varied adverse effects. Anxiety occurs due to hyperactivity in the amygdala. When used as an antianxiety drug, BZDs do not selectively inhibit the amygdala, rather they also exert inhibitory influence on regions like the prefrontal cortex (PFC). This hypoactivity in the PFC leads to mood dysregulation in the form of depression, decrease in irritability, and blunting of cognitive function. Hypoactivity in the hippocampus leads to amnestic effects and inhibition of fear extinction. BZDs in higher doses can also lead to a global CNS inhibition, resulting in motor, sensory, speech, and respiratory impairments.

The ADRs due to BZDs can be classified as follows:

Table 33.1 Pharmacokinetic parameters of the different BZDs

Drug	Bioavailability PO (%)	Time to maximum plasma concentration (h)	Plasma half-life (h)	Sedative-hypnotic daily dose (mg)
Alprazolam	> 80	1–2	12–15	-
Chlordiazepoxide		0.5–4	5–30	50–100, 1 to 4 times daily
Clonazepam	90	1–4	20–40	0.25–0.5
Clobazam	95	0.5–4	35	-
Diazepam	> 90	0.5–2	20–80	5–20
Lorazepam	90	2.5	10–20	1–4
Midazolam	40	0.5–1	1–4	1–5
Oxazepam	≥ 90	1–5	6–20	15–30, 3–4 times daily
Temazepam	≥ 90	1	8–15	7.5–30

Abbreviation: BZD, benzodiazepine.

Physical

Dizziness, nausea/vomiting, speech disturbances (dysarthria, slurred speech), motor coordination abnormalities (unsteady gait, poor concentration, tremors, fatigue, excessively swift reflexes and diplopia), muscle pain, nasal congestion, sexual dysfunction, autonomic dysregulation, sensory disturbances (photophobia, hyperacusis, paresthesia, tinnitus, dysgeusia), blood dyscrasias, dependence, and seizure.

Behavioural

Weight gain, increased appetite, insomnia, impulsivity, suicidality, and aggression.

Cognitive

Sedation, fatigue, inattention, nightmares, impaired judgment, suicidal ideations, delirium, and coma.

Emotional

Depression, dysphoria, phobias, panic, euphoria, and mania.

Drug Interactions

BZDs interact with CYP3A4 inhibitors like erythromycin, ritonavir, and ketoconazole. CYP3A4 inhibitors decrease the rate of metabolism of BZDs. CYP3A4 inducers like rifampicin, carbamazepine, phenobarbital, and glucocorticoids increase the metabolism and thereby decrease the action of BZDs. Drugs with CNS depressant activity like ethanol cause further CNS depression when used with BZDs.

Therapeutic Uses of Individual BZDs

BZDs are often used for the treatment of various disorders such as insomnia, anxiety, seizure, and alcohol withdrawal. BZDs preferred for insomnia include lorazepam, temazepam, flurazepam, and triazolam. For anxiety, diazepam, clonazepam, lorazepam, oxazepam, alprazolam, and chlordiazepoxide are commonly used. BZDs employed for the treatment of seizures consist of lorazepam, diazepam, and clonazepam. Alcohol withdrawal can be treated with the aid of BZDs like chlordiazepoxide, diazepam, and oxazepam. Specific BZDs are also indicated for the treatment of other disorders such as preoperative anxiety, muscle spasm, Lennoux–Gastout syndrome, neuralgia, panic disorder, periodic limb movement disorder, and chemotherapy-related nausea/vomiting.

Therapeutic uses of individual BZDs have been depicted in **Table 33.2.**

BZD Overdose

BZD toxicity is commonly characterized by sedation and, in severe cases, there is respiratory depression along with hemodynamic stability. Supportive care supplemented with medical treatment is crucial in the management of BZD overdose. Flumazenil leads to reversal in respiratory depression in BZD toxicity patients. Flumazenil is a BZD analog which has minimal activity on its own. It acts by binding to the extracellular surface of $GABA_A$ receptors and causes competitive displacement of BZD molecules. This prevents further BZD binding. Flumazenil is contraindicated in patients with BZD tolerance and seizure disorders. It is also to be avoided in individuals with a prolonged QRS interval. Flumazenil must be administered cautiously in doses of 0.1 mg over 1 minute. The administration may be continued until a maximum dose of 1 mg is reached or until an effect is observed or toxicity develops.

Barbiturates

Classification of Barbiturates

Over 2,500 barbiturate derivatives have been synthesized so far in various universities across the globe. They have differential pharmacokinetic properties, which has made it possible to draw up a classification, based on the duration of their action. They have been classified into:

- Long-acting: phenobarbitone.
- Intermediate-acting: amobarbital.

Table 33.2 Uses of BZDs

Benzodiazepine	Insomnia	Anxiety	Seizure	Alcohol withdrawal	Other uses
Flurazepam	✓	–	–	–	–
Chlordiazepoxide	–	✓	–	✓	Preoperative anxiety
Diazepam	–	✓	✓	✓	Preoperative anxiety, muscle spasm
Clobazam	–	–	–	–	Lennoux–Gastout syndrome
Clonazepam	–	✓	✓	–	Neuralgia, panic disorder, periodic limb movement disorder
Temazepam	✓	–	–	–	–
Lorazepam	✓	✓	✓	–	Chemotherapy-related nausea/ vomiting, preoperative sedation
Oxazepam	–	✓	–	✓	–
Alprazolam	–	✓	–	–	Panic disorder
Triazolam	✓	–	–	–	–
Midazolam	–	–	–	–	Procedural sedation

Abbreviation: BZD, benzodiazepine.

- Short-acting: pentobarbitone, butobarbitone, and secobarbitone.
- Ultrashort-acting: thiopentone, methohexitone.

Based on the above classification, shorter- or intermediate-acting barbiturates were initially utilized as hypnotics, while longer-acting barbiturates found utility in terms of antianxiety and anticonvulsant drugs. Ultrashort-acting barbiturates have been useful in minor surgeries for induction of anesthesia.

Pharmacological Actions

Barbiturates, being GABAergic activators, act as general depressants for all kind of cells with maximal effect seen in CNS.

CNS

Barbiturates in general act throughout the CNS. In general, they inhibit excitation and promote inhibition. The site of inhibition may be postsynaptic, as at cortical and cerebellar pyramidal cells, substantia nigra, and thalamic relay neurons; or presynaptic, as in the spinal cord. There is an increase in inhibition primarily at the synapses where neurotransmission is mediated by GABA, especially through the $GABA_A$ receptors. Lower concentrations of barbiturates can lead to reduction in glutamate-induced depolarizations. At higher concentrations that produce anesthesia, pentobarbital leads to the suppression of high-frequency repetitive firing of neurons, because of inhibition of the function of voltage-dependent, tetrodotoxin-sensitive Na+ channels.

The effects of barbiturates on CNS are dose-dependent and they can produce wide range of effects, ranging from mild sedation at low doses to coma at high doses. Barbiturates containing a 5-phenyl substituent (e.g., phenobarbital and mephobarbital) have found to have selective anticonvulsant activity. The antianxiety effects of barbiturates are lesser compared to BZDs.

In general, the barbiturates have shown to possess a lower degree of selectivity and a narrow therapeutic index. Hence, it is not possible to achieve a desired effect without overall depression of the CNS. Perception of pain and reaction to light are relatively unimpaired until the consciousness is intact, and paradoxically, in lower doses, barbiturates lead to increase in reactions to painful stimuli. Hence, they are ineffective in producing sedation or sleep in the presence of any type of pain.

Hypnotic doses of barbiturates lead to an alteration in all the stages of sleep in a dose-dependent manner. Similar to the BZDs, these drugs lead to a decrease sleep latency along with decrease in the number of awakenings, and enhance the durations of both the REM and slow-wave sleep. On chronic use, tolerance to the effects on sleep has been observed within a few days, and the effect on total sleep time may be reduced by as much as 50% after 2 weeks of use.

Respiratory System

Barbiturates lead to depression of both the respiratory drive along with the respiratory rhythm. There is decrease in the neurogenic drive, which is like the natural sleep. However, neurogenic drive is abolished by a toxic dose, which is generally three times greater than that used to induce sleep. Toxic doses also lead to the suppression of the hypoxic drive and, to a lesser extent, the chemoreceptor drive. If barbiturates are employed as IV anesthetic agents, they may lead to coughing, sneezing, hiccoughing, and laryngospasm.

Cardiovascular System

No significant effects are seen at sedative and hypnotic doses. There may be a slight reduction in the cardiac output, heart rate, and blood pressure. There is a decrease in cardiovascular reflexes due to the partial inhibition of ganglionic transmission. This can be specifically observed in the patients suffering from right heart failure or any other condition leading to hypovolemic shock. In these patients, barbiturates can lead to excessive lowering of blood pressure. Barbiturates also impair reflex cardiovascular adjustments to inflation of the lung and hence positive pressure-respiration should be cautiously used.

Smooth Muscles

Hypnotic doses produce slight decrease in tone and motility of the bowel. Action on other smooth muscles is insignificant.

Pharmacokinetic Features

Absorption

Barbiturates are absorbed well from the alimentary tract, and its availability in CNS is directly proportional to the lipid solubility of barbiturates. Thus, thiopentone, which has high solubility in lipids, has easy access, while phenobarbitone, with lower solubility in lipids, has slower access across the blood-brain barrier in the CNS. Redistribution is another characteristic of barbiturates used as anesthetics.

Metabolism

The metabolism primarily occurs in liver through the processes involving oxidation, dealkylation, and conjugation. Their plasma $t½$ ranges from 12 to 40 hours. Barbiturates induce several hepatic microsomal enzymes and thus increases their own rate of metabolism as well as that of quite a few other drugs.

Excretion

Phenobarbitone, with lower lipid solubility, primarily shows unchanged renal excretion. The half life ($t_{½}$) of phenobarbitone ranges from 80 to 120 hours. Alkalinization of urine leads to ionization and, thus, greater excretion. This is significantly observed in case of long-acting agents.

Adverse Drug Reactions (ADRs)

Hangover was a common adverse effect post the use of barbiturates as sedatives. Chronic use leads to accumulation of barbiturates in the body, resulting in tolerance and dependence. Rarely, especially in the elderly, barbiturates paradoxically produce excitement. Idiosyncratically, barbiturates may precipitate porphyria in susceptible individuals.

Barbiturate Poisoning

Symptoms of barbiturate toxicity are variable, but most commonly include cognitive blunting, impaired consciousness, decrease in heart rate or rapid and weak pulse, ataxia, dizziness, nausea, fatigue, lowered body temperature, and dilated or contracted pupils. Fatal cases are marked by coma, hypotension (low blood pressure), and respiratory depression (decreased efforts to breathe), evidenced by cyanosis and hypotension. Pulmonary edema is another complication associated with barbiturate toxicity and contributing to respiratory depression and death. In the case of chronic abusers, severe withdrawal symptoms were observed within 8 to 15 hours of cessation. Symptoms include restlessness, tremors, hyperthermia, sweating, insomnia, anxiety, seizures, circulatory failure, and potentially death.

Supportive treatment forms the mainstay of the treatment of barbiturate toxicity, as there is no specific antidote for overdose. The first step in treatment, as with any overdose, is assessing the patient's airway, breathing, and circulation. With significant sedation and respiratory depression, intubation and mechanical ventilation may become necessary. Initial management with activated charcoal may have some utility and can be given via nasogastric tube. Patients will likely need to be admitted or observed. During recovery, the patient should receive counselling about the dangers of barbiturate misuse. Long-term barbiturate use can cause tolerance and physical dependence. Therefore, withdrawal symptoms can occur with abrupt discontinuation.

Drug Interactions

As mentioned earlier, barbiturates induce several cytochrome isoenzymes, including glucuronyl transferase, leading to the enhancement of the rate of metabolism of many drugs, resulting in the reduction in their effectiveness. Some commonly affected drugs include warfarin, steroids (including contraceptives), tolbutamide, griseofulvin, chloramphenicol, and theophylline. Barbiturates also show additive action with other CNS depressants like alcohol. Phenobarbitone leads to increase in concentration of sodium valproate.

Therapeutic Uses (Table 33.3)

Barbiturates have largely been replaced by other safer drugs like BZDs for various indications. Some of the indications where barbiturates can be used are as follows:

Insomnia

Barbiturates that were previously commonly used for this indication included amobarbital, aprobarbital, butobarbital and, rarely, phenobarbital and secobarbital. However, now they are rarely used due to serious adverse effects like respiratory depression and have been largely replaced by safer BZD and non-BZD Z drugs.

Seizures and Epilepsy

Barbiturates can be employed in emergency conditions like status epilepticus and febrile convulsions. Some barbiturates include phenobarbitone, amobarbital, pentobarbital, phenobarbitone, and primidone.

Anaesthesia

Barbiturates like Thiopentone have rapid onset of action, followed by reversal of action due to redistribution. Thus, barbiturates are mainly used for induction of anesthesia. Commonly employed barbiturates include methohexital and thiopental. Other barbiturates used for preoperative

Table 33.3 Currently employed barbiturates with therapeutic indications

Name of barbiturate	Route of administration	Therapeutic uses
Amobarbital	Oral, IM, IV	Insomnia, preoperative sedation, emergency management of seizures
Aprobarbital	Oral	Insomnia
Butobarbital	Oral	Insomnia, preoperative sedation
Mephobarbital	Oral	Epilepsy, daytime sedation
Methohexital	IV	Induction/maintenance of anesthesia
Pentobarbital	Oral, rectal, IM, IV	Insomnia, preoperative sedation, emergency management of seizures
Phenobarbital	Oral, IM, IV	Epilepsy, status epilepticus, daytime sedation
Primidone	Oral	Epilepsy
Secobarbital	Oral, rectal, IM, IV	Insomnia, preoperative sedation, emergency management of seizures
Thiopental	Rectal, IV	Induction/maintenance of anesthesia, preoperative sedation, emergency management of seizures

Table 33.4 Pharmacokinetic properties of non-BZ drugs

Drug	Onset of action (Minutes)	Elimination half-life (hours)	Duration of action	Daily dose (mg)	Active metabolites
Zaleplon	15–30	1	Short	5–10	No
Zolpidem	30	1.4–4.5	Short	2–4	No
Zopiclone	15–30	3.5–6.5	Short	3.75–7.5	Yes

sedation include amobarbital, butobarbital, pentobarbital, and secobarbital.

Non-Benzodiazepines

They are also known as "Z" drugs, and they structurally differ from BZDs but act as agonists on specific set of BZD receptors. This class of hypnotics principally includes three drugs: zaleplon, zolpidem, and zopiclone. The action of non-BZD hypnotics is selectively limited to α1 subunit containing BZD receptors. The resultant effects include hypnotic and amnesic effects, with hardly any antianxiety, muscle relaxant, and anticonvulsant effects. The abuse potential of these drugs is much lower than classical BZDs.

Pharmacokinetic Features

Brief pharmacokinetic profile of non-BZDs is given in **Table 33.4**.

Adverse Drug Reactions

Initially, Z drugs were marketed as safer alternatives to abuse liable BZDs. However, many new studies have shown concerns relating to their potential of abuse, dependence, and withdrawal over time. An enantiomer of zopiclone, that is,, eszopiclone has also been recently approved as a sedative hypnotic on account of its longer duration of action.

Tolerance and Dependence

Earlier it was believed that there is lesser incidence of tolerance and dependence as compared to BZDs. However, recent case studies and postmarketing surveillance studies have led to increase in concern due to newer discoveries pertaining to tolerance.

Some of the most common symptoms of Z-drug withdrawal are difficulty in sleeping, euphoria, anxiety, irritability, tremor, dysphasia, pain in abdomen, elevation of blood pressure, generalized seizures, and disorientation of time, place, and person.

Suicidal Behavior

This was observed with zopiclone and zolpidem.

Other Adverse Reactions

These include a characteristic metallic or bitter after taste, impaired concentration and impaired generalized alertness, psychological disturbances, and dry mouth. Besides, enhanced risk of falls in older individuals has been noted.

Therapeutic Uses

Sleep-onset insomnia is effectively relieved by zaleplon and zolpidem. They have been approved by the Food and Drugs Administration (FDA) for use for up to 7 to 10 days at a time. The $t_{1/2}$ of zolpidem is approximately 2 hours, which is enough for the common 8-hour sleep period and hence currently approved only for bedtime use. The $t_{1/2}$ of zaleplon is relatively shorter of about an hour, thus offering the possibility for safe dosing late at night, even within 4 hours of the anticipated rising time. Hence, zaleplon has wider indications with either immediate use at bedtime or when the patient has difficulty falling asleep after bedtime.

All these drugs do not disturb the sleep architecture, and along with benzodiazepines, these are currently hypnotics of choice.

Comparison and contrast between barbiturates and BZDs.

Benzodiazepines have superseded barbiturates for the following reasons:

1. Barbiturates unlike BZDs are potent enzyme inducers. Hence, drug–drug interactions are more with barbiturates as compared to BZDs.
2. Barbiturates show hyperalgesia. No hyperalgesia occurs with the intake of BZDs.
3. BZDs have a higher margin of safety as compared to barbiturates.
4. Barbiturates have an anesthetic effect and cause loss of consciousness. BZDs do cause anesthesia even at high doses.
5. Barbiturates exhibit a higher degree of tolerance as compared to BZDs.
6. BZDs possess a low-abuse liability, while barbiturates have a higher abuse liability, which cause both psychic and physical dependence.
7. Barbiturates have a greater effect on the distortion of REM sleep as compared to BZDs. Barbiturates cause a marked suppression of REM sleep; hence, on discontinuation of barbiturates, there is a rebound increase in REM sleep, thereby leading to nightmares.
8. Barbiturates cause greater respiratory depression and hypotension when compared to BZDs.
9. BZDs cause amnesia but are devoid of the automatism phenomenon. Barbiturates exhibit amnesia along with automatism. The latter may be a cause of accidental poisoning, because the patient may forget that he has taken the drug, and this could lead to drug overdose.
10. No specific antidotes are available for barbiturate poisoning, which is quite contrary to the situation with BZDs where flumazenil is available. Hence, barbiturate poisoning becomes difficult to treat as compared to BZD poisoning.

Other Hypnotics

Melatonin Agonists

Melatonin is neurohormone secreted by the pineal gland and its biosynthetic route follows a circadian rhythm. The main activities of melatonin are mediated by two receptors (named MT1 and MT2). Melatonin and especially MT2 receptor are key participants in sleep disturbances and insomnia.

Ramelteon and tasimelteon are melatonin receptor agonists currently in practice to treat insomnia, especially one due to jet lag, and it is also useful in patients who have difficulty in induction of sleep. These drugs have shown no direct effects on GABAergic neurotransmission in the brain. In polysomnography studies of patients with chronic insomnia, ramelteon resulted in reduction of the sleep latency, with no effects on sleep architecture and no rebound insomnia and without any significant withdrawal symptoms. Minimal potential for abuse is characteristic of ramelteon, and hence it is not a controlled substance. The drug shows rapid absorption postoral administration, and it undergoes high rate of first-pass metabolism, leading to the formation of an active metabolite with longer half-life (2–5 hours) than the parent drug. Although the CYP2A9 is sometimes involved in the metabolism of ramelteon, CYP1A2 isoform of cytochrome P450 is mainly responsible for its metabolism.

Insomnia

Insomnia is defined in International Classification of Sleep Disorders (ICSD)-3 as a complaint of trouble initiating or maintaining sleep, which is associated with daytime consequences and is not attributable to environmental circumstances or inadequate opportunity to sleep. Insomnia is further classified into chronic insomnia disorder, short-term insomnia disorder and other insomnia disorders. However, treatment of all the above disorders is on similar lines except for insomnia due to obstructive sleep apnea. Insomnia is often considered a disorder of hyperarousal, leading to increase in somatic, cognitive, and cortical activation.

Treatment of insomnia consists of two modalities, namely, cognitive behavioral therapy (CBT) and pharmacotherapy. CBT consists of maintenance of sleep hygiene, addressing dysfunctional beliefs, stimulus control therapy, sleep restriction, and relaxation training. Here, we are going to discuss pharmacotherapy in detail. Short- and intermediate-acting BZDs along with non-BZD "Z" drugs act as first-line of therapy. Over-the-counter antihistaminics are commonly used but are not recommended. Second- and third-line of therapies include sedating antidepressants and anticonvulsant medications. As melatonin agonists have been already briefly discussed, here the other drugs will be discussed.

Antidepressants

Tricyclic antidepressants like doxepin at antidepressant doses (150–300 mg/day) inhibits serotonin and norepinephrine reuptake and is an antagonist at histamine 1, muscarinic 1, and a1-adrenergic receptors. At low doses (1–6 mg/day), however, doxepin is quite selective for histamine 1 receptors and thus may be used as a hypnotic. Doxepin should be taken in initial doses of 6 mg (3 mg in the elderly) within 30 minutes of bedtime. It was approved by the FDA in 2010 for the treatment of sleep maintenance insomnia. Adverse effects include paradoxical worsening of depression in some cases.

Orexin Antagonists

The cells located in the hypothalamus, especially in the lateral hypothalamic area (LHA) and perifornical and posterior hypothalamus (PH), are responsible for the synthesis of the neurotransmitter orexin (also called hypocretin). Orexin A and orexin B are produced by these cells and then released at various brain areas. These areas include the monoamine neurotransmitter centers in the hypothalamic TMN(for histamine) and in the brainstem such as the (for norepinephrine), the ventral tegmental area (VTA; for dopamine), raphe nucleus (for serotonin) and the pedunculopontine tegmental and laterodorsal tegmental nuclei (PPT/LDT; for acetylcholine). Thus, it is responsible for wakefulness. Suvorexant is an orexin receptor antagonist

Table 33.5 Drugs of choice for different sleep disorders

Sleep disorder	Drug of choice
Insomnia	Short- or intermediate-acting BZDs/Z drugs/ramelteon
Obstructive sleep apnea	Modafinil: 100–400 mg (CPAP is the preferred treatment)
Idiopathic hypersomnia	Modafinil (100–400 mg)/amphetamine (5–60 mg)
Cataplexy	Selective serotonin reuptake inhibitors; e.g., fluoxetine (10–40 mg)/ tricyclic antidepressants; e.g., imipramine (25–200 mg)
Recurrent hypersomnia (Klein–Levine syndrome)	Lithium (300–900 mg)
Circadian rhythm sleep wake disorders	Melatonin/melatonin agonists
REM sleep-related parasomnia	Clonazepam (0.5–2 mg)
Sleep walking	Benzodiazepines
Sleep terror	Benzodiazepines
Nocturnal enuresis	Desmopressin 0.2 mg tablet/ 20 μg nasal sprays
Sleep-related movement disorder: restless leg syndrome	Dopamine agonists: ropinirole (0.25 mg/day); pramipexole (0.125 mg/day); rotigotine patch (1 mg/24 hr)

approved by US FDA in 2014 at a dose of 10 mg 30 minutes before going to bed. Common adverse effects include daytime somnolence and worsening of depression or suicidal ideation. Lemborexant was recently approved for insomnia in 2019.

Anticonvulsants

Gabapentin, pregabalin, and tiagabine, are rarely used to treat insomnia. Gabapentin and pregabalin act by binding to the α -2-delta subunit of N-type voltage-gated calcium channels, resulting in the decrease in the activity of wake promoting glutamate and norepinephrine systems. Tiagabine promotes sleep by inhibiting the reuptake of GABA. A relatively long t_{max} of 3 to 3.5 hours, which makes gabapentin relatively unlikely to facilitate sleep onset.

The most adverse effects associated with gabapentin include ataxia and diplopia. Pregabalin is associated with adverse effects like the dry mouth, cognitive impairment, peripheral edema along with an increase in appetite. Nausea is commonly associated with tiagabine. Gabapentin and pregabalin are specifically useful for insomnias associated with pain. Pregabalin can be considered to treat insomnia in the patients suffering from fibromyalgia, as the available evidence suggests it is effective for the same. Preliminary evidence is suggestive of utility of gabapentin for patients suffering from restless leg syndrome, leading to periodic movement during sleep.

Drug of Choice for Various Sleep Disorders

Currently, many drugs are available for treatment of various sleep disorders which we have discussed throughout the chapter. Certain disorders like various parasomnias, hypersomnias, and restless leg syndrome are beyond the scope of this chapter. However, **Table 33.5** summarizes the various drugs of choice used for treatment of various sleep disorders.

Multiple Choice Questions

1. Which of the following drugs used in treatment of insomnia facilitate the inhibitory activity of GABA, but lack anticonvulsant and muscle relaxing properties, have minimal effects on sleep architecture, and can be antagonized by flumazenil?

A. Phenobarbitone.
B. Clonazepam.
C. Ramelteon.
D. Zolpidem.

Answer: D

Nonbenzodiazepine (BZD) drugs or Z drugs facilitate GABA activity without affecting sleep architecture, and they can be antagonized by flumazenil.

2. A 21-year-old male college student complains of difficulty falling asleep at night. He asks if there is anything "mild" he can take to help him get to sleep. Which of the following hypnotics mimics an endogenous hormone?

A. Alprazolam.
B. Suvorexant.
C. Ramelteon.
D. Doxepin.

Answer: C

A hypnotic is a drug that induces sleep. Many sedatives have a hypnotic effect. Their sedation is mediated by binding to GABA receptors. Ramelteon works instead by binding melatonin receptors, mimicking the effects of melatonin. Ramelteon does not appear to lead to dependence as do many GABA modulators. Rebound insomnia does not occur with ramelteon, and it is not a controlled substance

3. A 38-year-old man with chronic anxiety and agitation is currently being treated with a long-acting benzodiazepine (BZD). He is having challenges with sleep and is referred to a sleep center for a 24-hour sleep study to further ascertain his difficulties. Which of the following is the most likely abnormality to be noted on this study?

A. Calming effect during sleep induction.
B. Hourly awakening from sleep.
C. Hypnotic effect with dreams.
D. Improved slow-wave sleep.

Answer: A

This patient is likely to experience a calming effect during sleep induction. Not all BZDs are useful as hypnotic agents, although all have sedative or calming effects. They tend to decrease the latency to sleep onset and increase stage 2 of nonrapid eye movement (non-REM) sleep. Both REM sleep and slow-wave sleep are decreased. In the treatment of insomnia, it is important to balance the sedative effect needed at bedtime with the residual sedation ("hangover") upon awakening.

4. Ramelteon, a drug prescribed for insomnia, is thought to act in the central nervous system (CNS) via:

A. Activation of benzodiazepine (BZD) receptors.
B. Activation of melatonin receptors.
C. Block of the GABA transporter.
D. Inhibition of GABA metabolism.

Answer: B

Melatonin secreted by pineal gland plays an important role in maintenance of circadian rhythm. Ramelteon is melatonin receptor agonist used in the treatment of insomnia.

5. A patient who is in comatose condition is brought to the emergency department with severe respiratory depression caused by diazepam overdosage. Reasonable intervention at this point include:

A. Administer naloxone to block the drug's effect at the receptor.
B. Provide supportive therapy until the drug effect wears off.
C. Administer flumazenil.
D. Both B and C.

Answer: D

Flumazenil is antagonist of benzodiazepine (BZD) receptor and hence after provision of supportive therapy, flumazenil administration is essential. There is no role of naloxone in treatment of BZD overdose.

6. Which of the following is classified as a long-acting barbiturate?

A. Alprazolam.
B. Phenobarbitone.
C. Pentobarbital.
D. Thiopentone.

Answer: B

Phenobarbitone has lower lipid solubility and hence a longer duration of action.

7. Which of the following drugs are used for the treatment of insomnia?

A. Doxepin.
B. Suvorexant.
C. Clonazepam.
D. All of the above.

Answer: D

Doxepin is tricyclic antidepressant with high sedation and hence used as hypnotic, clonazepam is benzodiazepine (BZD), and suvorexant is orexin antagonist which is a newer class of drug.

8. From which stage of sleep cycle can the dreams or nightmares be recollected?

A. Rapid eye movement (REM) sleep.
B. Stage II non-REM sleep.
C. Stage III non-REM sleep.
D. Stage IV non-REM sleep.

Answer: A

REM sleep is similar to wakefulness with high brain activity characterized by rapid movement of eyes, increased muscle tone, increased blood, and dreams or nightmares.

9. What is the drug of choice for circadian rhythm wake disorders?

A. Melatonin agonists.
B. Phenobarbitone.
C. Zolpidem.
D. All of the above.

Answer: A

Melatonin is responsible for normal circadian rhythm and hence melatonin agonists like ramelteon and tasimelteon are drug of choice for circadian rhythm disorders.

10. Which orexin antagonist was recently approved for the treatment of insomnia (in 2019)?

A. Suvorexant.
B. Lemborexant.
C. Eszopiclone.
D. Almorexant.

Answer: B

Lemborexant is the most recent orexin antagonist approved for insomnia by US FDA in 2019.

Chapter 34 Alcohol

Tithishri Kundu

PH1.20: Describe the effects of acute and chronic ethanol intake.

Learning Objectives

- Ethanol.
- Methanol.

Alcoholic Content in Common Alcoholic Beverages

Ethanol (C_2H_5OH) is the oldest known recreational substance in the world. The use of alcohol can be traced back to 10000 BC.

Absolute alcohol is 99% w/w ethanol, whereas the rectified spirit has 90% w/w ethanol. Methylated spirit or "denatured alcohol" can be made by mixing 95% ethanol with 5% methanol. This is available for industrial purposes and can be added to paints before use. **Table 34.1** presents the percentage of alcohol in various alcoholic beverages as well as different types of alcohol.

Table 34.1 Percentage of alcohol in various alcoholic beverages and different types of alcohol

	Percentage of alcohol present (%)
Alcoholic beverages	
Beer	6–10
Wine	15–20
Champaign (effervescent wine)	12–16
Spirit (whisky, rum, brandy)	45–50
Vodka	50–60
Types of alcohol	
Absolute alcohol	99
Rectified spirit	90
Methylated spirit/denatured alcohol	95% ethanol + 5% methanol

Ethanol (PS4.6)

Pharmacokinetics

Absorption

Absorption of ethanol occurs both from the stomach and the small intestine. Absorption of ethanol from the small intestine is rapid due to its large surface area compared to its absorption from the stomach. Therefore, the absorption of ethanol depends on various factors, for example, gastric emptying (presence of food in stomach). Delay in gastric emptying decreases ethanol absorption. In the fasting state, the peak blood alcohol level occurs after 30 to 60 minutes.

Distribution

Alcohol is distributed rapidly in the body (volume of distribution 0.5–0.7 L/kg, i.e., approximately the volume of total body water). It crosses the blood–brain barrier as well as the placenta. Concentration in the brain is very close to the concentration in the blood, as the brain receives a large proportion of total blood flow.

Metabolism

Metabolism of Alcohol to Acetaldehyde

Ethanol is metabolized to acetaldehyde mainly by the enzyme alcohol dehydrogenase (75%) present in the stomach, liver, and intestine. The oxidation reaction requires nicotinamide adenine dinucleotide (NAD^+). As limited amount of NAD^+ is present in the body, this reaction follows zero-order kinetics. Fixed amount of alcohol is metabolized (8–12 mL/hour) irrespective of the blood alcohol concentration.

When the concentration of ethanol is above 100 mg/dL in the blood, the alcohol dehydrogenase system gets saturated due to depleted NAD^+. In such conditions, the rest of the ethanol is metabolized by cytochrome P450 system (mainly CYP2E1) present in the liver. Cytochrome P450 system uses nicotinamide adenine dinucleotide phosphate hydrogen (NADPH+) instead of NAD^+. Other than CYP2E1, CYP1A2 and CYP3A4 also play an important role in ethanol metabolism.

CYP2E1 metabolism is altered by both acute and chronic consumption of alcohol. Acute and chronic consumption inhibits and induces CYP2E1, respectively. Acute alcohol intake affects the metabolism of warfarin, phenytoin, etc. Increased formation of toxic metabolite (*N*-acetyl-*p*-benzoquinone imine [NAPQI] in paracetamol) and increased susceptibility to certain toxins (CCl_4) are seen with chronic alcohol intake.

Metabolism of Acetaldehyde to Acetic Acid

Around 75 to 80% of acetaldehyde is converted to acetic acid by the enzyme aldehyde dehydrogenase present in the liver. The rest of the acetaldehyde is metabolized extrahepatically in the presence of the enzyme aldehyde oxidase. The produced acetic acid can be converted into carbon dioxide and water later. The metabolism of ethanol is presented in **Fig. 34.1**.

Excretion

Most of the ethanol (>90%) is metabolized and excreted by the liver. Only 2 to 5% is excreted through breath, urine, and

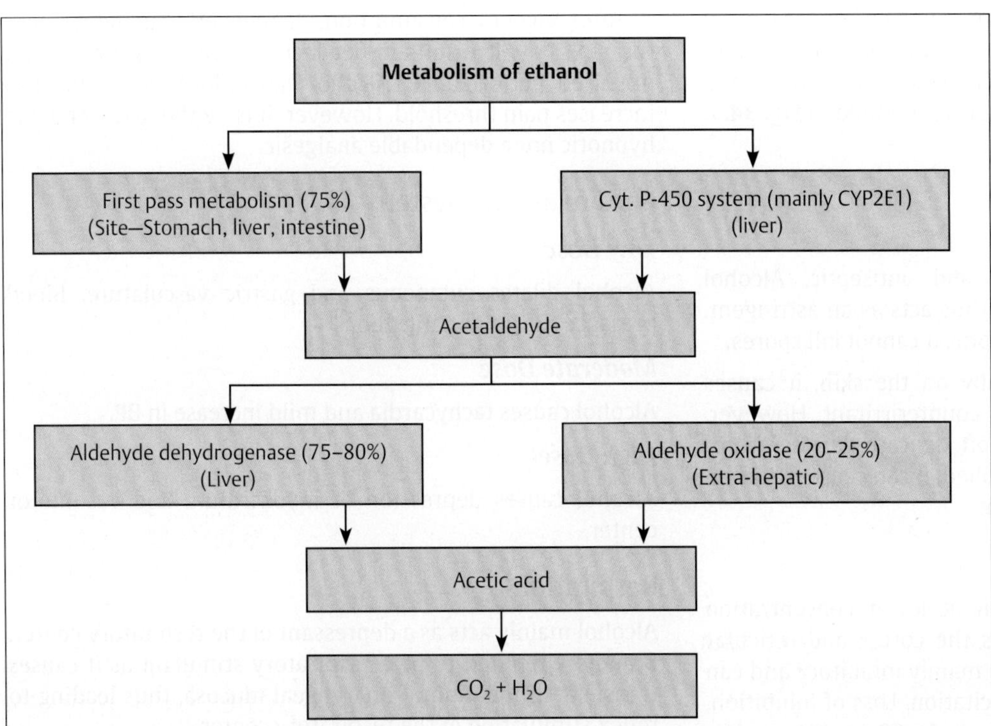

Fig. 34.1 Metabolism of ethanol.

sweat. Although it is a negligible amount, it is the basis of the breath analyzer test. It is a noninvasive screening test in which the alveolar air is exhaled into the machine. The concentration of alcohol in exhaled alcohol air corresponds to the blood alcohol level. A person with a blood alcohol level of more than 30 mg% is punishable in India.

Genetic Polymorphism

Several genetic polymorphisms protect a person against alcohol-related diseases, while other polymorphisms are responsible for the development of alcohol-use disorders (AUDs). Genetic polymorphism in the *ADH1B* gene may protect against AUDs, whereas polymorphism in the *ALDH2* gene can cause AUDs and may also increase the risk of esophageal cancer in heavy drinkers. *ADH4* gene might be responsible for alcohol dependence.

Enzyme Inhibitors in Alcohol Metabolism

Consumption of alcohol after prior intake of disulfiram can lead to inhibition of the enzyme aldehyde dehydrogenase. This can cause increased production of acetaldehyde. Accumulation of acetaldehyde can lead to flushing of the face, intense headache, nausea, vomiting, loss of consciousness, etc. Hypotension and chest pain can also be observed. Owing to the above-mentioned property, disulfiram is used in the management of alcohol dependence. However, it should only be given to extremely motivated patients.

Disulfiramlike reaction can be observed in a Chinese herbal medicine known as daidzin. It is also noted in metronidazole, tinidazole, some cephalosporins (cefotetan, cefoperazone, cefamandole), nitrofurantoin, chlorpropamide, and griseofulvin.

Fomepizole inhibits the enzyme alcohol dehydrogenase. Therefore, it is the drug of choice (DOC) in methanol and

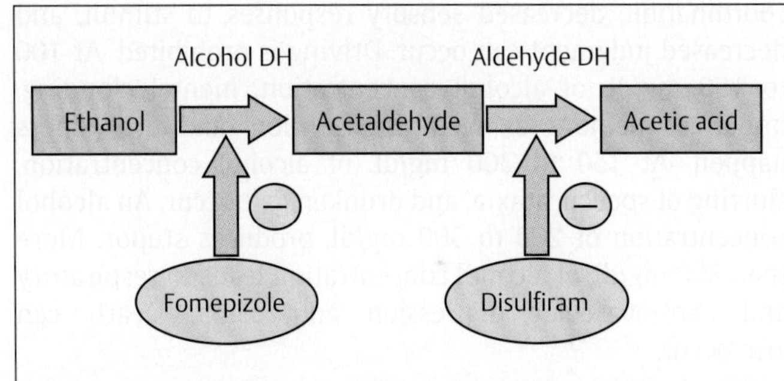

Fig. 34.2 Enzyme inhibitors in ethanol metabolism.

ethylene glycol poisoning. Enzyme inhibitors in ethanol metabolism are presented in **Fig. 34.2**.

Mechanism of Action

Alcohol acts as a central nervous system (CNS) depressant by altering the state of the membrane lipids. Recently, the action of alcohol on different receptor-operated and voltage-gated channel has come to light.

Although alcohol is a CNS depressant, its action on the $GABA_A$ receptor is different than benzodiazepine (BZD) and barbiturates. Alcohol facilitates GABA release at $GABA_A$ sites in the brain. On the contrary, barbiturate and BZD facilitate $GABA_A$ receptor-mediated Cl^- channel opening. Alcohol also inhibits *N*-methyl-D-aspartate (NMDA) receptors, causing memory loss. Alcohol augments the action of serotonin on $5\text{-}HT_3$ inhibitory autoreceptors. It acts on the nicotinic receptor present in the CNS. It also activates some K^+ channels in the brain. Ethanol inhibits voltage-sensitive Ca^{2+} channels and inhibits neurotransmitter release. Ethanol also increases the release of dopamine by augmenting β-endorphin release and also by an opioid receptor–dependent mechanism.

The abovementioned mechanism justifies the basis of alcohol dependence. Ethanol also acts on some membrane-bound enzymes, that is, Na^+/K^+-ATPase and adenylyl cyclase. The mechanism of action of ethanol is presented in **Fig. 34.3**.

Pharmacological Effects

Local Action

Ethanol acts as an astringent and antiseptic. Alcohol precipitates surface proteins and thus acts as an astringent. Although alcohol acts as an antiseptic, it cannot kill spores.

When ethanol is applied locally on the skin, it causes slight redness and also acts as a counterirritant. However, ethanol should not be applied to soft, delicate skin (scrotum) and mucous membrane. If it is applied, it can cause irritation and a burning sensation to the skin.

Central Nervous System

Ethanol is a CNS depressant. But at lower concentration (30–60 mg/dL), it mainly inhibits the cortex and reticular activating system. These areas are mainly inhibitory and can lead to apparent euphoria and excitation. Loss of inhibition, hesitation, and caution occurs first. At 50 to 100 mg/dL, symptoms such as loss of reflex, euphoria, sedation, impaired coordination, decreased sensory responses to stimuli, and decreased judgment can occur. Driving is prohibited. At 100 to 150 mg/dL of alcohol concentration, mental clouding, impaired memory as well as attention, and drowsiness happen. At 150 to 200 mg/dL of alcohol concentration, slurring of speech, ataxia, and drunken gait occur. An alcohol concentration of 200 to 300 mg/dL produces stupor. More than 300 mg/dL of alcohol concentration leads to respiratory and cardiovascular depression and coma. Death can also occur.

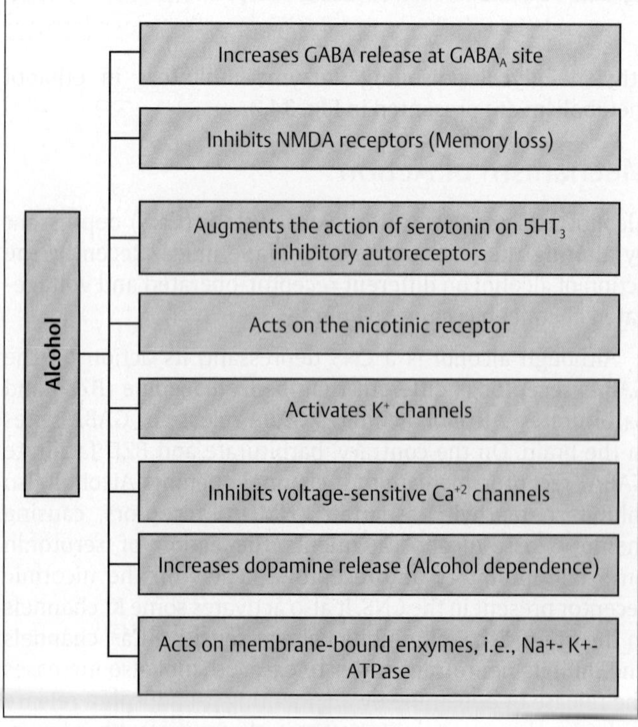

Fig. 34.3 Mechanism of action of ethanol.

After alcohol consumption, "hangover" can be present the next day. It results in headache, irritation, laziness, and impaired performance. Alcohol can induce sleep and also increases pain threshold. However, it is neither a dependable hypnotic nor a dependable analgesic.

Cardiovascular System

Low Dose

Alcohol dilates cutaneous and gastric vasculature. Blood pressure (BP) is not affected.

Moderate Dose

Alcohol causes tachycardia and mild increase in BP.

High Dose

Alcohol causes depression of myocardium and vasomotor center.

Respiration

Alcohol mainly acts as a depressant of the respiratory center. Brandy is reputed to be a respiratory stimulant as it causes transient stimulation of pharyngeal mucosa, thus leading to reflex stimulation of the respiratory center.

Liver

Alcohol redistributes peripheral fat and augments fat synthesis in the liver, causing "alcoholic fatty liver." It is a reversible condition but can progress to alcoholic hepatitis and cirrhosis. Women are more susceptible to hepatotoxicity than men.

Chronic alcoholism can lead to oxidative stress, increased lipid peroxidation, and glutathione depletion in the liver. Alcoholics are also prone to several vitamin and nutritional deficiencies. The above-mentioned mechanism is responsible for hepatotoxicity in chronic alcoholics.

Gastrointestinal Tract

In lower concentration (up to 5%), alcohol stimulates gastric acid secretion, whereas in higher concentrations (>5%), it has no effect. Chronic alcoholism is associated with gastritis. Alcohol consumption may decrease lower esophageal sphincter tone and thus lead to gastric reflux.

Chronic alcoholism is a risk factor for chronic pancreatitis. Ethanol has a direct toxic effect on pancreatic acinar cells. It also alters the permeability of pancreatic epithelial cells, causing formation of pancreatic stone and protein plugs.

Blood

Daily consumption of a small amount of alcohol decreases the oxidation of low-density lipoprotein (LDL) and increases high-density lipoprotein (HDL) cholesterol level. Thus, regular intake of alcohol can decrease the chance of coronary artery disease (CAD). Chronic alcoholism can lead to megaloblastic anemia, as it inhibits folate metabolism.

Body Temperature

After consumption of alcohol, a sense of warmth is felt, as alcohol dilates cutaneous and gastric vessels. However, intake of alcohol before a person is exposed to cold climate is not permitted, as heat loss from the body is augmented after alcohol consumption.

Skeletal Muscle

A small amount of alcohol alleviates fatigue, but chronic alcoholics are susceptible to muscle weakness and myopathy.

Sex

Consumption of mild-to-moderate amount of alcohol produces loss of inhibition and restraint and may incite sexual behavior. However, sexual performance is diminished. Chronic consumption of alcohol can cause testicular atrophy, impotence, and sterility in men and infertility in women.

Kidney

Alcohol acts as a diuretic as it inhibits antidiuretic hormone secretion, leading to less water reabsorption in nephrons.

Endocrine Effects

Alcohol consumption can cause the release of catecholamine, leading to hyperglycemia and other sympathetic effects. On the contrary, hypoglycemia is seen in acute alcoholism due to the inhibition of neoglucogenesis. Therefore, hypoglycemia associated with acute alcoholism should be treated with glucose, not glucagon.

Tolerance, Dependence, and Withdrawal Reaction (PS4.4)

Tolerance, physical dependence, and withdrawal reaction are biological phenomena associated with the chronic use of alcohol.

Tolerance

It is defined as the requirement of higher dose of a drug to produce a certain biological response. Tolerance can be divided into acute and chronic tolerance.

Acute Tolerance/Mellanby Effect

Acute tolerance in alcohol develops within a few hours. It develops due to adaptation in the CNS caused by the effects of alcohol. It is mainly pharmacokinetic tolerance.

Chronic Tolerance

Chronic tolerance develops in chronic alcoholics. Contrary to acute tolerance, it is both pharmacokinetic and pharmacodynamic types of tolerance. Chronic gastritis and mucosal inflammation can lead to a diminished rate of absorption. This is the basis of pharmacokinetic tolerance. Chronic alcoholics are susceptible to CYP2E1 induction, leading to rapid metabolism of alcohol. This is the basis of pharmacodynamic tolerance.

Cross-Tolerance

Cross-tolerance to BZD is observed in alcoholics. This tolerance is seen in abstinent alcoholics, but not in the person who is currently drinking. In those persons, alcohol has an additive effect. Overall overdose of BZD is relatively safe compared to barbiturates. However, consumption of alcohol with BZD can lead to disastrous effects.

Physical Dependence

It is the state that develops as a result of tolerance caused by resetting of the homeostatic mechanism in response to the repeated use of a drug. A physically dependent person cannot maintain the normal function without continuous administration of the drug. Psychological dependence is also observed in alcoholics characterized by craving (desire to obtain the rewarding effect of alcohol).

Mechanism of Physical Dependence

Alcohol acts via opioid-dependent system in the CNS and thus increases the level of norepinephrine and dopamine in the brain. This process is responsible for the euphoric effects of alcohol. This can also be important in the process of physical dependence. Physical dependence can be associated with upregulation and downregulation of NMDA receptor and $GABA_A$ receptor, respectively. Proliferation of the L-type Ca^{2+} channel may also play a role.

Withdrawal Reaction

It is the type of reaction that occurs in a physically dependent person after the abrupt stoppage of the drug. Increased Ca^{2+} entry through the L-type of Ca^{2+} channel and augmented neurotransmitter release might be the cause of some of the symptoms in withdrawal reaction.

Stages of Withdrawal Reaction

First Stage

The first stage of withdrawal reaction develops if a physically dependent person has gone without a drink for 8 hours. This stage is characterized by craving for alcohol, nausea, tremor, sweating, etc. Hypertension and tachycardia can also develop. Although the severe form of the first stage lasts up to 1 to 2 days, milder form can extend up to 1 to 3 months.

Second Stage

The second stage of withdrawal reaction comprises seizure and hallucination. Seizure starts 6 to 48 hours after discontinuation of alcoholic beverage. Hallucination (mainly visual) may start 12 to 48 hours after the last drink. Auditory and tactile hallucination can also be observed.

Third Stage

Delirium tremens is a rare phenomenon that is noted in the third stage of withdrawal reaction. It starts 2 to 3 days after discontinuation of alcohol. Main symptoms are confusion, agitation, fever, tachycardia, nausea, diarrhea, and dilated pupil.

Time frame of different stages of withdrawal reaction is presented in **Fig. 34.4**.

Effects of Acute Alcohol Consumption (PH1.20)

Acute alcohol intake affects several systems in the body.

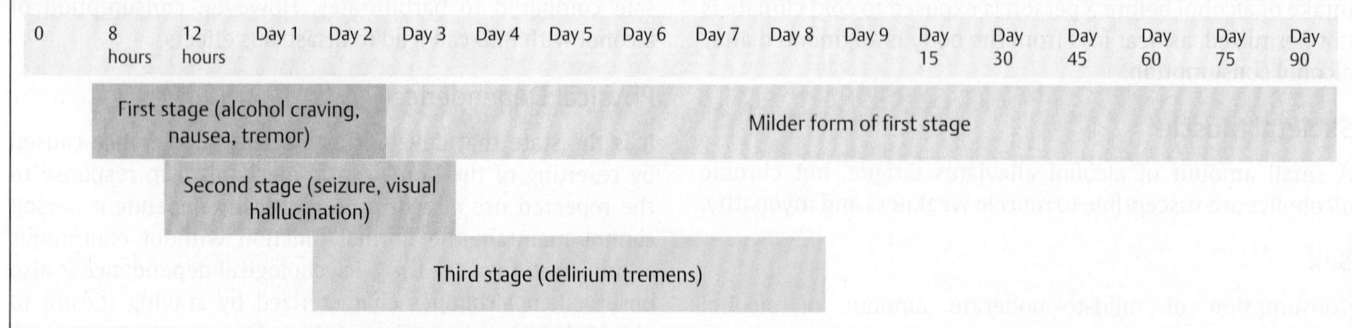

Fig. 34.4 Time frame of different stages of withdrawal reaction.

Central Nervous System

Acute alcohol intoxication can lead to decreased responsiveness, unawareness, stupor, coma, and death (explained in detail under the heading "Pharmacological Effects").

Heart

Acute intake of alcohol can cause decreased myocardial contractility, hypotension, etc. (explained in detail under the heading "Pharmacological Effects").

Kidney

Acute consumption of alcohol can be associated with diuresis. Mechanism of diuresis is explained in detail under the heading "Pharmacological Effects."

Body Temperature

Acute alcohol intake can provide a feeling of warmth to a person (explained in detail under the heading "Pharmacological Effects").

Uterus

Acute intake of alcohol can relax the uterus.

Endocrine System

Acute consumption of alcohol can cause hypoglycemia (explained in detail under the heading "Pharmacological Effects").

Sex

Acute alcohol intake can cause aggressive sexual behavior but decreased sexual performance (explained in details under the heading "Pharmacological Effects").

Calorie Intake

Alcohol is a high-calorie food without any nutritious value. One gram of alcohol produces 7 cal of energy.

Effects of Chronic Alcohol Consumption (PH1.20)

Chronic alcohol consumption affects several systems in the human body.

Central Nervous System (IM5.16)

Chronic consumption of alcohol is associated with alcoholic dementia. Chronic intake of alcohol is rarely associated with Wernicke–Korsakoff syndrome. It comprises reversible Wernicke's encephalopathy and irreversible Korsakoff's psychosis. Thiamine deficiency plays a role in Wernicke–Korsakoff syndrome.

Wernicke's encephalopathy is characterized by ataxia, paralysis of extraocular muscle, nystagmus, diplopia, blurred vision, and tremor. Prompt intravenous (IV) thiamine can prevent neurological damage. If not treated, Wernicke's encephalopathy can later progress to Korsakoff's psychosis. Korsakoff's psychosis is characterized by anterograde and retrograde amnesia.

Tolerance and Dependence

Explained in detail earlier.

Cardiovascular System

Hypertension

Chronic intake of alcohol is associated with increased systolic and diastolic BP.

Cardiomyopathy

Chronic consumption of alcohol can lead to dilated cardiomyopathy with left ventricular dysfunction. It may or may not be associated with right ventricular dysfunction.

Arrhythmia

Chronic alcohol intake can cause both atrial and ventricular arrhythmia. Atrial arrhythmias include atrial fibrillation, atrial flutter, and supraventricular tachycardia.

Stroke

Low intake of alcohol diminishes the risk of stroke and mortality due to stroke, whereas high consumption of alcohol is associated with an increased chance of stroke.

Blood

Regular consumption of a small amount of alcohol can lead to increased HDL and decreased LDL oxidation. It can also inhibit platelet aggregation. Thus, it can protect against CAD. Chronic alcohol intake can lead to impaired folate metabolism and megaloblastic anemia.

Liver

Chronic intake of alcohol is associated with the alcoholic fatty liver, which may progress to alcoholic hepatitis and cirrhosis (explained in detail under the heading "Pharmacological Effects").

Gastrointestinal Tract

Chronic consumption of alcohol can lead to impaired motility of esophagus and stomach, gastritis, and decreased absorption of vitamins and nutrients. Chronic ethanol intake is an important risk factor of chronic pancreatitis (explained in detail under the heading "Pharmacological Effects").

Endocrine System

Chronic alcohol intake can lead to alcoholic cirrhosis. It is associated with impaired metabolism of hydrocortisone and an increase in the hydrocortisone level. This can cause "pseudo-Cushing's syndrome." Chronic alcoholism can cause secondary aldosteronism and hypokalemia.

Sexual Function

Chronic alcohol consumption can cause testicular atrophy, impotence, and sterility in men and decreased libido and infertility in women.

Bone

Chronic alcohol abuse is associated with osteoporosis and increased risk of fracture. This may be due to decreased vitamin D metabolism, diminished absorption of Ca^{2+}, decreased testosterone level, and impaired hypothalamic–pituitary–gonadal axis.

Lungs

Chronic intake of alcohol can lead to acute respiratory distress syndrome and pneumonia.

Musculoskeletal System

Chronic alcohol consumption can cause myopathy. It can also decrease muscle mass and strength. It may cause gout by altering uric acid metabolism.

Cancer

Chronic ethanol intake is associated with cancer of oral cavity, esophageal carcinoma, colorectal carcinoma, breast cancer, and liver cancer.

Teratogenic Effects

Alcohol consumption in the first trimester can cause spontaneous abortion. Exposure to alcohol in pregnancy can lead to fetal alcohol syndrome, with an incidence of 3:1,000. Exposure to alcohol in the first trimester results in microcephaly, shortened palpebral fissure, flat face, thin upper lip, mental retardation, cardiac anomaly, growth retardation, etc. CNS dysfunction includes attention-deficit hyperactivity disorder, learning, memory, and language disorders. Alcohol consumption, even in the second trimester, is associated with impaired academic performance in children.

Alcohol can cross the placenta to reach the fetus. Also, fetal liver has a negligible amount of alcohol dehydrogenase. For this reason, an increase in ethanol level due to impaired metabolism can lead to the degeneration of neurons in the fetus.

Comorbidities

Mood disorder, schizophrenia, and posttraumatic stress disorder have been observed with chronic ethanol consumption.

Management of Acute Alcohol Intoxication (PH1.21, FM9.4)

1. Most patients of acute alcohol intoxication are in a disoriented state. Maintenance of patent airway is often the first measure. One must take caution to prevent the aspiration of vomitus.
2. Gastric lavage is given if the patient is brought to the hospital within 6 to 8 hours of alcohol ingestion.
3. Fluid and electrolyte balance should be maintained.
4. IV glucose infusion is given to combat hypoglycemia.
5. IV/intramuscular (IM) thiamine injection should also be given.
6. IV insulin + fructose can also be given to augment the metabolism of alcohol, but its clinical efficacy is not clear.

Management of Chronic Alcoholism (PH1.21, PH1.23, FM9.4)

Management of alcohol dependence is presented in **Fig. 34.5**.

Pharmacotherapy of alcohol dependence is a three-pronged approach. The goals are as follows:

1. To prevent relapse.
2. To decrease craving for alcohol.
3. Cognitive behavioral therapy (CBT).

Disulfiram

Earlier disulfiram-based aversion therapy was used in the management of chronic alcoholism. After prior intake of disulfiram, alcohol consumption can lead to unpleasant reactions (mentioned earlier in the chapter). This prevents patients from consuming alcohol. Thus, it prevents relapse in an alcoholic. Aversion therapy with disulfiram is associated with poor compliance in patients, possibly due to the unpleasant experience.

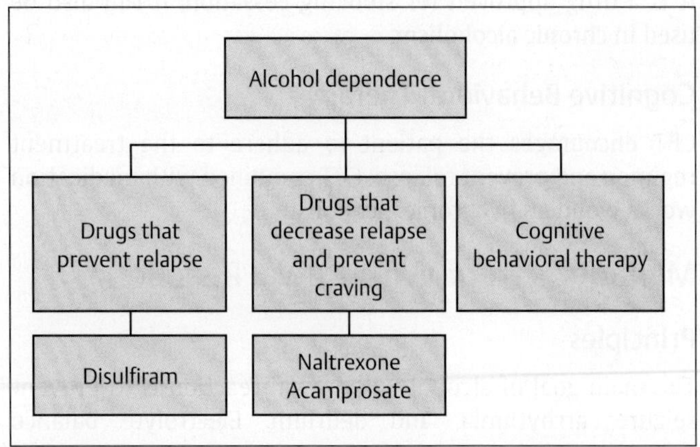

Fig. 34.5 Management of alcohol dependence.

Naltrexone

It is an opioid receptor antagonist. When a person consumes alcohol, he experiences a "kick." This euphoric feeling is responsible for the craving in chronic alcoholism. Naltrexone blocks opioid receptors in the brain, which are liable for the rewarding effects of alcohol. Thus, naltrexone can act as an anticraving drug. It also reduces relapse. Naltrexone is given at a dose of 50 mg/day. Long-acting depot preparation is also available. Adverse effects related to naltrexone are nausea (most common), dysphoria, etc. It is contraindicated in patients with depression, liver failure, etc. Naltrexone is used as an adjuvant with CBT and is the main component of treatment in most of the deaddiction centers in India.

Acamprosate

This drug acts by decreasing craving as well as preventing relapse. The mechanism of action is not clear. It is postulated that acamprosate prevents a hyperglutaminergic state. It works best in abstinent alcoholics, not in patients who are currently drinking. Mild diarrhea is a common side effect.

Newer Drugs

Topiramate

Topiramate is an anticonvulsant that decreases craving in alcoholics. The possible mechanism is due to its augmentation of the inhibitory effects of GABA.

Gabapentin

Several studies showed gabapentin, another anticonvulsant, significantly decreases craving in alcoholics.

Selective Serotonin Reuptake Inhibitor

Selective serotonin reuptake inhibitor (e.g., fluoxetine) can act as an anticraving drug by increasing serotonergic activity in the brain.

Ondansetron

Ondansetron, a 5-HT$_3$ antagonist, can also act as an anticraving drug.

Nalmefene

Nalmefene is an opioid antagonist like naltrexone. It can be used to decrease alcohol addiction in patients.

Varenicline

It is a drug approved for smoking cessation. It can also be used in chronic alcoholism.

Cognitive Behavioral Therapy

CBT encourages the patient to adhere to the treatment regimen and prevent relapse. CBT combined with medication works wonders in chronic alcoholism.

Management of Withdrawal Reaction

Principles

The main goal of alcohol withdrawal reaction is to prevent seizure, arrhythmia, and delirium. Electrolyte balance (magnesium, potassium, and phosphate) should be maintained. Vitamin B$_1$ should be given by IV/IM route.

In mild withdrawal reaction, no other drugs are necessary. In cases of severe withdrawal reaction, two basic principles are followed. Substitution of alcohol with another long-acting sedative, hypnotic drug and gradual tapering of the substitute drug after the withdrawal phase has ended.

Benzodiazepine

BZDs are the DOC in the management of withdrawal reaction. It is also helpful in preventing the progression from minor withdrawal syndrome to delirium tremens. Long-acting BZDs such as chlordiazepoxide or diazepam can be used. Short-acting BZDs, such as lorazepam and oxazepam, are commonly used in patients with liver disease, as they can be converted to inactive, water-soluble metabolites that do not accumulate in the liver. Oxazepam is prescribed at a dose of 15 to 30 mg every 6 to 8 hours. These drugs should be tapered gradually after the withdrawal phase has ended.

Carbamazepine

Carbamazepine, an antiepileptic, can also be used in the management of withdrawal syndrome. However, this drug is not as effective as BZDs.

Clonidine

Intensity of withdrawal syndrome can be diminished by clonidine, an α_2-receptor agonist. It inhibits the exaggerated transmitter release during withdrawal reaction.

Propranolol

Propranolol is a β-blocker that combats the exaggerated sympathetic effects observed during withdrawal reaction.

Drug Interactions

1. Alcohol has synergistic action with other CNS depressants (hypnotics, anxiolytics, antidepressants, opioids, antihistaminics). Chance of accidental mishap increases.
2. Acute and chronic consumption of alcohol inhibits and induces CYP2E1, respectively. Chances of hepatotoxicity increase with paracetamol due to the formation of a toxic metabolite, NAPQI, in chronic alcoholics. Metabolism of other drugs (e.g., phenytoin, tolbutamide) is also affected.
3. Disulfiramlike reaction occurs with metronidazole, tinidazole, chlorpropamide, cefoperazone, cefamandole, and cefotetan (explained in detail earlier).
4. Alcohol augments the hypoglycemic effect of insulin and sulfonylureas.
5. Alcohol also enhances gastric bleeding with aspirin and other nonsteroidal anti-inflammatory drugs.
6. Minimum alveolar concentration decreases in acute alcohol intoxication, whereas it is augmented in chronic alcoholics. Thus, less amount of inhalational anesthetic is needed in acute alcohol intoxication and more amount is needed in chronic alcoholics.
7. Hypertensive crisis is seen in patients with monoamine oxidase inhibitor after consumption of an alcoholic drink containing tyramine (beer, wine, etc.)

Uses

Local Uses

1. As antiseptic (76%) for skin.
2. Ethanol has astringent properties (precipitates proteins). Hence, it can be used in bedsores locally. It is also a component of deodorant and aftershave lotions.
3. Ethanol is also used as a counterirritant in joint ache, sprain, etc.
4. It can be injected locally around the nerves in trigeminal neuralgia and intractable neuralgia of cancer patients. It can also be injected via the epidural and subarachnoid routes. Paravertebral ethanol injection in the lumber region destroys sympathetic ganglia and thus provides relief from pain in peripheral vascular diseases involving the lower limb.

Systemic Uses

1. It is used in the treatment of methanol and ethylene glycol poisoning.
2. Ethanol can be used as an appetite stimulant. A small amount of 10% ethanol can be used as tinctures (of ginger, etc.) before any meal.

Methyl Alcohol (Methanol, Wood Spirit)

Methanol is a well-known industrial solvent found in paint remover, antifreeze, etc. It is also used as an adulterant to mix with industrial rectified spirit to make it undrinkable. Poisoning with methanol is quite common either due to the amoral mixing of methanol with alcoholic beverages or because of accidental ingestion.

Pharmacokinetics

Like ethanol, methanol is also metabolized by alcohol dehydrogenase to formaldehyde, which is further metabolized by the enzyme aldehyde dehydrogenase and produces formic acid. Metabolism of methanol also follows zero-order kinetics, but the rate of metabolism is one-seventh of ethanol.

The toxic manifestation of methanol poisoning comprises vomiting, headache, epigastric pain, disorientation, etc. Hypotension, tachypnea, and bradycardia are also observed. Retinal damage and loss of visual acuity are due to both formaldehyde and formic acid. However, formic acid is responsible for most of the toxic symptoms of methanol poisoning. Respiratory paralysis, circulatory collapse, coma, and death are also noted. Paralysis of the respiratory system is responsible for death in methanol poisoning. The fatal dose of methanol is 75 to 100 mL. Metabolism of methanol is presented in **Fig. 34.6**.

Treatment

General Measures

1. The patient should be kept in a dark room to protect the eyes from light.
2. Gastric lavage.
3. Respiratory support with ventilator.

Measures to Prevent Methanol Metabolism

Ethanol

Alcohol dehydrogenase enzyme has a higher affinity to ethanol than methanol. Therefore, ethanol is given to saturate the enzyme. Thus, metabolism of methanol is inhibited. Ethanol (10% in water) is given by nasogastric tube at a loading dose of 0.7 mL/kg, followed by 0.15 mL/kg/hour. Blood alcohol level has to be monitored regularly. Treatment has to be continued for several days until no methanol is detectable in the blood.

Fomepizole

Fomepizole is an inhibitor of the enzyme alcohol dehydrogenase. It prevents methanol metabolism. It is also the DOC for methanol poisoning. It can be administered by IV route at a loading dose of 15 mg/kg over half an hour, followed by 10 mg/kg every 12 hours until the serum methanol level is less than 20 mg/dL. Longer $t_{1/2}$, IV dosage formulation, and less chance of CNS depression are the advantages of fomepizole over ethanol. Burning pain in the infused limb, nausea, headache, and hypotension are some of the adverse effects observed with fomepizole.

Measures to Eliminate Toxic Effects of Methanol

Hemodialysis

Hemodialysis clears unchanged methanol and its toxic metabolites from the blood.

Folinic Acid

Folinic acid can be given via IV route at the rate of 30 to 50 mg every 6 hours. It increases the metabolism of formic acid and prevents retinal damage.

Sodium Bicarbonate (IV)

It can also prevent retinal damage.

Measures to Combat Acidosis and Hypokalemia

Sodium Bicarbonate

IV sodium bicarbonate can be used to combat acidosis and prevent retinal damage. It is one of the most crucial measures in the treatment of methanol poisoning.

Potassium Chloride

IV potassium chloride is administered to combat hypokalemia associated with sodium bicarbonate.

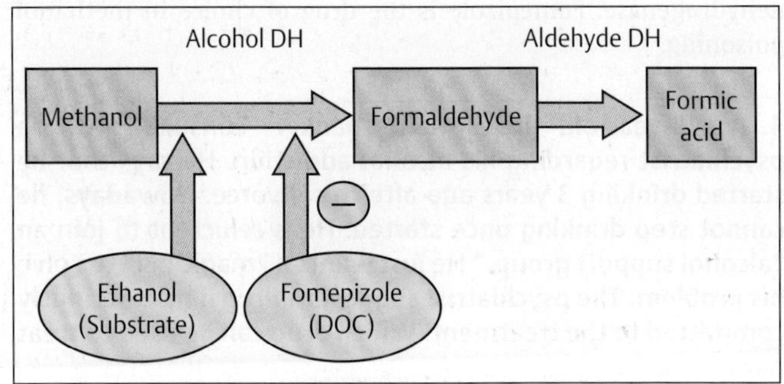

Fig. 34.6 Metabolism of methanol.

Multiple Choice Questions

1. A 30-year-old pregnant woman visits her gynecologist for a regular antenatal checkup. The doctor learns that she imbibes alcohol daily despite the pregnancy. What are the teratogenic effects that can be observed in the baby?

A. Craniofacial malformation, retarded growth, and microcephaly.
B. Congenital cardiac anomaly, growth retardation, and microcephaly.
C. Spina bifida and orofacial defect.
D. Learning defect and abruptio placenta.
E. Fetal hemorrhage and fetal bone formation defect.

Answer: B

The teratogenic effect that can be observed in the baby is "fetal alcohol syndrome." It is associated with congenital cardiac anomaly, retarded growth, and microcephaly.

2. A 40-year-old alcoholic presents to the emergency with a history of weakness and difficulty in breathing on exertion. The doctor notices pallor in the patient. His hemoglobin level is 8 g%. Peripheral blood smear shows spherocytes. Which of the following drugs can be used to treat this patient?

A. Vitamin B_6.
B. Vitamin B_{12} and folic acid.
C. Iron.
D. Erythropoietin.

Answer: A

Sideroblastic anemia is seen with the use of antitubercular drugs and alcohol. Vitamin B_6 or pyridoxine can be used to treat sideroblastic anemia.

3. A 40-year-old alcoholic is brought to the emergency after ingestion of methanol or wood spirit. He is disoriented and cannot see properly. He has high anion gap acidosis and acute renal failure. What is the suitable treatment for the patient?

A. Fomepizole.
B. Hemodialysis.
C. Ethylene glycol.
D. Flumazenil.

Answer: A

Disorientation, poor vision, high anion gap acidosis, and acute renal failure suggest methanol poisoning. The patient should be treated with fomepizole, which inhibits the enzyme alcohol dehydrogenase. Fomepizole is the drug of choice in methanol poisoning.

4. A 40-year-old investment banker consults with a psychiatrist regarding his alcohol addiction. He says that he started drinking 3 years ago after his divorce. Nowadays, he cannot stop drinking once started. He is reluctant to join an "alcohol support group." He just wants a "magic pill" to solve his problem. The psychiatrist suggests a drug if he is seriously committed to the treatment. Which drug can be used to treat him?

A. Diazepam.
B. Disulfiram.
C. Flumazenil.
D. Cognitive behavioral therapy.

Answer: B

Disulfiram can be used in strongly motivated persons who are truly committed to the deaddiction therapy. After prior intake of disulfiram, if alcohol is consumed, it can lead to unpleasant reactions, i.e., flushing of face, intense headache, nausea, vomiting, etc. Disulfiram inhibits the enzyme aldehyde dehydrogenase, leading to accumulation of acetaldehyde, which is the cause of unpleasant reactions.

5. A 42-year-old morbidly obese man is consuming whiskey for 3 days continuously after his son's recent death. He is not a habitual drinker. He is hypertensive but takes metoprolol regularly for adequate management of his hypertension. Which problem can be observed due to his binge drinking?

A. Wernicke's encephalopathy.
B. Seizure.
C. Arrhythmia.
D. Megaloblastic anemia.

Answer: C

The patient can develop arrhythmia as a result of his binge drinking.

6. A 50-year-old chronic alcoholic is brought to the emergency by the relatives. He is confused and delirious. He also has ophthalmoplegia and truncal ataxia. Which drug should be given to the patient to manage his condition?

A. Diazepam.
B. Diazepam and thiamine.
C. Chlordiazepoxide.
D. Fomepizole.

Answer: B

A history of chronic alcoholism, confusion, delirium, ophthalmoplegia, and truncal ataxia point toward Wernicke's encephalopathy. Diazepam and thiamine can be used for treatment.

7. A 27-year-old chronic alcoholic registers himself for an alcohol deaddiction program. This program is based on support-group and pharmacological therapy. He is prescribed with a drug that decreases craving for alcohol but does not cause untoward reaction if alcohol is consumed. Name the drug prescribed to the patient.

A. Disulfiram.
B. Naltrexone.
C. Fomepizole.
D. Diazepam.

Answer: B

Naltrexone is an opioid receptor antagonist that can be used for alcohol deaddiction. It decreases the craving for alcohol but does not cause unpleasant reactions like disulfiram.

8. In disulfiram-based aversion therapy, which metabolite gets accumulated?

A. Acetic acid.

B. Acetaldehyde.
C. Formaldehyde.
D. Formic acid.

Answer: B

Disulfiram inhibits the enzyme aldehyde dehydrogenase, resulting in accumulation of acetaldehyde. It brings an unpleasant reaction to the person. The person suffers from vomiting, hypotension, etc. Relapse is prevented in an alcoholic due to the unpleasantness of the reaction.

9. Disulfiram is used in the treatment of:

A. Acute alcoholism.
B. Physically dependent chronic alcoholics.
C. Psychologically dependent chronic alcoholics.
D. Both physically and psychologically dependent chronic alcoholics.

Answer: C

In physically dependent chronic alcoholics, disulfiram produces an unpleasant reaction. Thus, disulfiram is given to the strongly motivated person only who can abstain from alcohol.

10. Acamprosate is given in:

A. Acute alcoholism.
B. Chronic abstinent alcoholics.
C. A person who is currently drinking alcohol.
D. Both B and C.

Answer: B

Acamprosate is given in chronic abstinent alcoholics. It is not given to the person who is currently drinking.

11. The most common side effect of acamprosate is:

A. Diarrhea.
B. Hypotension.
C. Dysphoria.
D. Hypertension.

Answer: A

The most common side effect of acamprosate is mild diarrhea.

12. A 50-year-old chronic alcoholic has been prescribed a drug for his infection. Which drug is best suited for him?

A. Metronidazole.
B. Chlorpropamide.
C. Griseofulvin.
D. Cefixime.

Answer: D

Disulfiramlike reaction is seen in metronidazole, tinidazole, cefoperazone, cefamandole, cefotetan, nitrofurantoin, chlorpropamide, and griseofulvin.

13. Drug "T" can be used for smoking cessation. Recently drug "T" has also shown improvement in the management of chronic alcoholism. Identify the drug "T."

A. Gabapentin.
B. Nalmefene.
C. Varenicline.
D. Acamprosate.

Answer: C

Varenicline is used for smoking-cessation. Recent studies have shown that varenicline is also effective in the management of chronic alcoholism.

14. Drug "K" inhibits the enzyme alcohol dehydrogenase. It is the drug of choice in methanol poisoning. Identify the drug "K."

A. Ethanol.
B. Fomepizole.
C. Acamprosate.
D. Naltrexone.

Answer: B

Fomepizole inhibits the enzyme alcohol dehydrogenase. Thus, it prevents the metabolism of methanol in methanol poisoning. Longer $t_{1/2}$, IV dosage formulation, and less chance of CNS depression are the advantages of fomepizole over ethanol.

Chapter 35 Antiepileptic Drugs

A. Meenakumari

PH1.19: Classify antiepileptics, and write about their mechanism of action, doses, side effects, therapeutic uses, and contraindications.

Learning Objectives

- Etiology of seizures and epilepsy.
- Mechanism and clinical features of epileptic seizures.
- Antiepileptic drugs.
- Nonepileptic uses of antiepileptic drugs.
- Principles of treatment of epilepsy.
- Epilepsy and pregnancy.

Introduction

A seizure (from the Latin sacire, "to take possession of") is a transient occurrence of signs or symptoms due to abnormal excessive or synchronous neuronal activity in the brain, whereas epilepsy is a Greek word that means convulsions. It refers to a brain disorder with occurrence of spontaneous, unprovoked recurrent seizures.

Etiology of Seizures and Epilepsy

Genetic or Heredity

This is important in the etiology of juvenile myoclonic epilepsy syndrome, childhood absence epilepsy syndrome, juvenile absence epilepsy syndrome, and progressive myoclonic epilepsy syndrome.

Structural Etiology

1. Seizures due to congenital anomalies and perinatal injuries occur in the pediatric age group.
2. Mesial temporal sclerosis—Hippocampal sclerosis is the cause of focal and secondarily generalized seizures.
3. Trauma—Important cause of seizures at any age.
4. Tumors and space-occupying lesions—Any structural lesions or neoplasms involving frontal, parietal, or temporal regions cause focal seizures in middle age or later.
5. Vascular lesions—Common cause of seizures in individuals of ages 60 years and above.
6. Degenerative disorders—Alzheimer disease and other degenerative disorders cause seizures in later life.

Infectious Etiology

Infectious diseases are reversible causes of seizures at any age. They occur in acute infections like bacterial meningitis, herpes encephalitis, and chronic infections like neurosyphilis, and cerebral cysticercosis. Brain abscess may also cause seizures.

Metabolic Etiology

Hypoxia, alkalosis, hypoglycemia, hypocalcemia, hyperpyrexia, and deficiency of vitamin B_6 may cause seizures.

Immune Etiology

Autoimmune diseases like systemic lupus erythematosus (SLE) and autoimmune limbic encephalitis may cause epilepsy.

Unknown or Idiopathic (Other Causes)

1. Abrupt withdrawal of drugs of abuse such as barbiturates and alcohol.
2. Watching television, seeing disco flashes, and listening to full blast pop music.

Classification of Epileptic Seizures

Seizures can be classified based on the site of origin or on the cluster of symptoms. There are two systems of classification. The first is based on seizure types and characteristic features. The second is based on epilepsy syndromes which include etiological factors, age of onset, frequency of attacks, and clinical manifestation of epilepsy.

Focal Seizures (Previously Known as Partial Seizures)

- Focal awareness.
- Focal with impaired awareness.
- Focal-to-bilateral—tonic-clonic.

Generalized Seizures

- Generalized absence.
- Generalized myoclonic.
- Generalized tonic-clonic.

Seizures of Unknown Onset

Tonic, clonic, and atonic seizures.

Epileptic Spasms

These are seen in neonates and infants and may be due to immature central nervous system (CNS). There occurs flexion or extension of proximal muscles, including truncal muscles for a brief period. The EEG shows diffuse, giant slow waves with irregular, multifocal spikes, and sharp waves in the background.

Febrile Convulsions

They occur in infants with high temperature.

Epilepsy Syndromes

Disorders in which epilepsy is a predominant feature are referred to as epilepsy syndromes.

Three important epilepsy syndromes are given below.

Juvenile Myoclonic Epilepsy (JME)

JME is a generalized seizure disorder of unknown etiology which appears in early adolescence. It is usually characterized by single or repetitive bilateral myoclonic jerks. The myoclonic seizures are most frequent in the morning after waking up and can be provoked by sleep deprivation.

Lennox–Gastaut Syndrome

Lennox–Gastaut syndrome occurs in children and is characterized by multiple seizure types that occur concurrently with cognitive dysfunction. EEG shows slow spike waves.

Mesial Temporal Lobe Epilepsy (MTLE) Syndrome

MTLE is the most common syndrome associated with focal seizures and impairment of consciousness.

Mechanism and Clinical Features of Epileptic Seizures

John Hughlings Jackson, the father of modern concepts of epilepsy, proposed that seizures were caused by "occasional, sudden, excessive rapid and local discharges of gray matter" and that a generalized seizure resulted when normal brain tissue was invaded by the seizure activity initiated in the abnormal focus.

Focal epilepsies constitute about 60% of all epilepsies and consist of different focal seizure types. The seizure activity is restricted to a discrete area belonging to the cerebral hemisphere only.

Focal epilepsies may occur due to a cortical lesion such as a tumor, any developmental malformation, or damage as a result of trauma or stroke. It may be genetic also.

Focal seizures originate in a localized area of the brain (usually medial temporal lobe or inferior frontal lobe) with a localized focus of EEG abnormality and may or may not become generalized. The manifestations depend on the brain region or regions involved. The interictal EEG is either normal or shows epileptiform spikes, but EEG during seizure is nonlocalizing. In adults, the most common form of epilepsy is focal epilepsy, wherein the most common associated lesion is hippocampal sclerosis.

Focal Seizures without Cognitive Impairment (Focal Aware) or Simple Partial Seizures

The key feature is preservation of awareness. There may be motor, sensory, autonomic, or psychic symptoms without impairment of cognition. The patient is conscious and is aware of the event which lasts for a few seconds to a few minutes. There is sudden onset of unilateral clonic jerking of a group of muscles or a limb lasting for 30 to 90 seconds, or localized sensory disturbances like pin pricks or hallucinations, depending on the area of cortex involved.

Focal Seizures with Impaired Awareness

Complex Partial Seizures (Temporal Lobe Epilepsy or Psychomotor)

The ictal phase begins with repetitive motor activity such as lip smacking, swallowing, aimless wandering, unconscious performance of highly skilled activities such as car driving (automatisms), or motionless stare. There is amnesia for the entire period of the seizure or a postictal aphasia. The seizure focus is in the temporal lobe.

Focal Seizures Leading to Generalized Seizures

These start as focal seizures and develop into one of the generalized seizures by spreading to cerebral hemispheres. Focal seizures arising from a focus in the frontal lobe tend to become generalized. Such a seizure may be followed by postictal neurological deficit (Todd's paralysis).

Generalized Epilepsies

They make up 40% of all epilepsies and are most commonly characterized by one or more generalized seizure types.

Generalized seizures are due to (a) mutations in Ca++ channels or (b) changes in the neuronal network.

Absence Seizure (Petit Mal)

It consists of sudden impairment of consciousness without convulsive movement and loss of postural control. The patient appears to go blank for less than 30 seconds and there may be accompanying fluttering of eyelids or small chewing movements.

Myoclonic Seizure

Presents as sudden, brief, repetitive muscle contraction involving a body part or the whole body.

Tonic-Clonic Seizures (Grand Mal)

They are characterized by sudden loss of consciousness without any warning (aura), followed by generalized tonic, and finally clonic convulsive movements lasting for 1 to 2 minutes. This is followed by a period of headache, drowsiness, and sleep. The attack may be accompanied by tongue biting, frothing, and incontinence. EEG shows a generalized abnormality.

Seizures occur due to defective synaptic function. There may be a decrease in the inhibitory synaptic activity or increase in the excitatory synaptic activity to trigger a seizure. Antagonists of the GABAA receptor or agonists of different glutamate-receptor subtypes (NMDA, AMPA, or kainic acid) trigger seizures in experimental animals in vivo.

Strategies for Control of Seizure Activity

Seizures are a symptom of an underlying disorder, which may be genetic, traumatic, metabolic, inflammatory, drug-induced, or due to drug withdrawal. When a seizure occurs, it is necessary to take proper history, evaluate, and find the cause for the seizure. Antiepileptics should not be started with the occurrence of a single seizure. Treatment of the underlying cause like correction of hypoglycemia, hypoxia, or hypocalcemia is important. If the seizure is due to trauma or structural brain lesion, appropriate treatment along with antiepileptics will prevent further occurrence. Guidance to the patient on compliance to treatment, like not to stop the drug abruptly, will prevent occurrence of seizures.

Antiepileptic Drugs

They act by preventing the generation and/or spread of the seizure. Drugs for control of focal seizures act by inhibiting the voltage-activated Na^+ channels, while drugs used in petit mal seizures inhibit voltage-activated Ca^{++} channels. The agents modulating GABA transmission are effective against partial and tonic-clonic seizures. Some drugs act by multiple mechanisms.

Mechanism of Drugs in Grand Mal and Partial Seizures

Inhibition of Voltage-gated Na+ Channels

Phenytoin, carbamazepine, valproate, lacosamide, and lamotrigine preferentially block voltage-gated Na^+ channels that remain open due to repetitive neuronal firing. They prolong the duration of inactivated phase and delay its reversion to resting phase. Inhibition ultimately leads to diminished glutamate release. They thus act by:

- Blocking propagation of action potential.
- Stabilizing neuronal membranes.
- Decreasing the release of neurotransmitter glutamate, thereby reducing focal firing and seizure spread.

Enhancement of GABAergic Action

They act by increasing inhibitory neurotransmission. Drugs act by blocking $GABA_A$ receptors, inhibiting GABA transaminase and GABA uptake transporter.

Phenobarbitone and benzodiazepines activate $GABA_A$ receptors to facilitate GABA-mediated opening. Benzodiazepines increase the frequency, while phenobarbitone increases the duration of opening of Cl^- channels.

Drugs like vigabatrin inhibit the enzyme GABA transaminase and thereby increase the neuronal concentration of GABA. Drugs like tiagabine and valproate inhibit GABA uptake transporter in neurons as well as glia, increasing the availability and inhibitory action of GABA at postsynaptic $GABA_A$ receptors.

Valproic acid activates glutamic acid decarboxylase (GAD) and thus increases the synthesis of GABA.

Blockade of NMDA or AMPA Receptors

They act by decreasing excitatory neurotransmission. Felbamate involves blockade of NMDA receptors. Phenobarbital, topiramate, and lamotrigine block AMPA receptors. Valproate inhibits glutamate synthesis.

Blockade of Voltage-Gated N-Type Ca^{2+} Channels

Some drugs like lamotrigine and gabapentin act by inhibiting voltage-gated N-type Ca^{2+} channels and decreasing synaptic release of glutamate.

Selective Binding to Synaptic Vesicular Protein (SV_2A)

Levetiracetam selectively binds to SV_2A protein of synaptic vesicles in glutaminergic and GABAergic neurons.

Mechanisms of Drugs Used in Petit Mal (Absence Seizures)

Inhibition of T-Type Ca^{2+} Channels

Ethosuximide and valproate inhibit T-type Ca^{2+} channels and are useful in absence seizures.

Individual Drugs

Hydantoins—Phenytoin (Diphenylhydantoin)

Phenytoin is a hydantoin derivative and the oldest antiepileptic drug.

Mechanism of Action

Phenytoin blocks the use-dependent, voltage-gated Na^+ channels and thus inhibits the initiation and propagation of nerve impulses at therapeutic plasma levels (10–20 µg/mL). At higher doses, it reduces the influx of Ca^{2+} ions, facilitating the effect of GABA and inhibiting the effect of glutamate.

Pharmacokinetics

The pharmacokinetic properties of phenytoin are peculiar. Phenytoin is available in different oral formulations that differ in their pharmacokinetics. Bioavailability of different market preparations may differ due to differences in dissolution and other formulation-dependent factors. Therefore, when changing from one formulation to another the plasma phenytoin level may vary. Oral absorption is almost complete. Phenytoin is not given intramuscularly (IM) or intravenously (IV). When given IM, it gets precipitated causing muscle damage and necrosis. As phenytoin is poorly soluble in water, its solution is prepared in polyethylene glycol for use by the IV route. The factors which influence pharmacokinetics of phenytoin are its binding to serum proteins, the nonlinearity of its elimination kinetics, and its metabolism by hepatic cytochrome P450s (CYPs). Phenytoin is extensively bound (~90%) to serum proteins, mainly albumin. Some agents when added to the regimen can increase free phenytoin as they compete with phenytoin for binding sites on plasma proteins. Its elimination is dose-dependent and follows saturation (mixed order) kinetics. The rate of elimination of phenytoin varies as a function of its concentration. At low levels of 10 to 20 µg/mL, its elimination follows first-order kinetics with constant half-life and no fluctuations in the plasma levels. As plasma levels rise, the maximal limit of the liver to metabolize phenytoin is reached. Therefore, beyond 20 µg/mL elimination follows zero-order kinetics. Hence, a slight increase in the dose of phenytoin leads to a disproportionate increase in its plasma concentration and toxicity. Periodic assessment of plasma concentration and subsequent dose adjustments are needed. Dose increments must therefore be smaller with increasing dosage. The plasma half-life of phenytoin ranges between 6 and 24 hours at plasma concentrations below 10 mg/mL but increased to 24 to 60 hours when plasma concentration increases above 10 mg/mL. Phenytoin is metabolized mainly by CYP2C9 and to a lesser extent by CYP2C19. The principal metabolite, a parahydroxyphenyl derivative, is inactive. As its metabolism is saturable, other drugs that are metabolized by these CYP enzymes can inhibit the metabolism of phenytoin and increase its plasma concentration. Phenytoin is a potent hepatic microsomal enzyme inducer. It induces its own metabolism and metabolism of endogenous substances and drugs like warfarin and oral contraceptive pills which are metabolized by CYP. Treatment with phenytoin can increase the metabolism of oral contraceptives and lead to unplanned pregnancy due to failure of contraception. Phenytoin inhibits the metabolism of warfarin; therefore, addition of phenytoin to a patient receiving warfarin can lead to bleeding disorders. About 94% of the drug is excreted in urine.

Adverse Reactions

Adverse drug effects of phenytoin may be related to dose, route of administration, and duration of therapy.

At Therapeutic Concentration

Below are the side effects which occur at therapeutic concentration (10–20 µg/mL).

Hyperplasia/Hypertrophy of Gums

Most common (20% incidence), possibly due to alteration in collagen metabolism and poor oral hygiene. It is common in children and adolescent on chronic use. It can be minimized by maintaining good oral hygiene.

Hypersensitivity Reactions

Skin rashes (morbilliform) including Steven–Johnson syndrome may occur. SLE and fatal hepatic necrosis are rare.

Hirsutism

It is troublesome in females and young girls, as there is masculinization with coarsening of facial features and may be due to increased androgen secretion.

Hyperglycemia

This is due to inhibition of insulin release.

Hydantoin Syndrome

Fetal hydantoin syndrome consists of multiple congenital anomalies as seen in newborns of mothers who received phenytoin during pregnancy.

Hematological Reactions

Neutropenia, leukopenia, and lymphadenopathy.

Hypoprothrombinemia and Bleeding

This occurs in newborn babies of mothers treated with phenytoin due to vitamin K deficiency. Vitamin K is used for prophylaxis and treatment.

Peripheral Neuropathy

It occurs on prolonged use, particularly in old people, and is manifested as diminished deep tendon reflex of lower limbs.

Side Effects Due to Enzyme Induction

- **Osteomalacia**—mainly due to inhibition of intestinal absorption of calcium and increased metabolism of vitamin D. As osteomalacia is associated with hypocalcemia, it does not respond with administration of vitamin D alone.
- **Megaloblastic anemia**—mainly due to increased metabolism of folic acid and may come about as a result of decreased absorption and increased excretion of folic acid. This can be overcome by supplementation of folic acid.

At Toxic Concentration Toxic Effects Occur

Toxic effects occur at concentration above 20 µg/mL as the half-life of phenytoin increases. Toxicity occurs even with small increase in the dose. They manifest as CNS effects, gastrointestinal tract (GIT) effects, and intolerance.

CNS Effects

Mild toxicity consists of drowsiness, fatigue, headache, and confusion. Larger doses can cause a vestibulocerebellar syndrome characterized by vertigo, ataxia, nystagmus, and dysarthria. Nystagmus is the first sign of toxicity/overdose and can be used for dose adjustment. Ocular pain with blurring of vision, delusions, hallucinations, and other psychotic episodes are sometimes encountered. Rarely, cognitive impairment and behavioral changes may occur.

GIT Effects

Nausea, vomiting, and abdominal discomfort may occur.

Adverse Effects on IV Administration

When phenytoin is administered by IV route, adverse effects such as local edema, intimal damage, discoloration of skin, cardiac arrhythmias, and hypotension can occur. Cardiac arrhythmias and hypotension may be due to diluent. Phenytoin is precipitated in glucose and so diluted in normal saline. Rapid IV injection may cause cerebellar and vestibular toxicity. Therefore, rate of infusion should not increase 50 mg/min.

Adverse Effects When Administered during Pregnancy

Phenytoin is teratogenic and may cause congenital malformations in the newborns of mothers who received phenytoin during pregnancy. Due to folic acid deficiency, it can cause neural tube defects (spina bifida). Cleft lip, cleft palate, and microcephaly occur due to toxic epoxide metabolite. Newborns of mothers treated with phenytoin during pregnancy may develop coagulopathy due to hypoprothrombinemia and hemorrhage due to inhibition of vitamin K. Therefore, vitamin K is given prophylactically. Sometimes, when multiple congenital anomalies occur due to hydantoins (phenytoin), it is referred to as fetal hydantoin syndrome.

Therapeutics Uses

Antiepileptic Use

- Focal and generalized tonic-clonic, focal-to-bilateral tonic-clonic, tonic-clonic of unknown onset, but not generalized absence seizures (drug of second choice).
- For psychomotor seizures, it is the drug of first choice. Phenytoin is contraindicated in petit mal (absence) and myoclonic seizures.

Nonepileptic Uses

- Cardiac arrhythmias—to treat ventricular arrhythmias due to digitalis toxicity.
- To treat trigeminal neuralgia (carbamazepine is drug of choice) in diabetic neuropathy and chorea.

Fosphenytoin

Fosphenytoin sodium is a prodrug of phenytoin. It is water-soluble and can be given by IV more rapidly, unlike phenytoin which is lipid-soluble. It can also be given IM.

It causes fewer reactions. On IV injection, only minor vascular complications are produced, as it causes less damage to the intima. It can be injected at a faster rate (150 mg/min). Fosphenytoin can be injected with both saline and glucose, whereas phenytoin cannot be injected in a drip of glucose or normal saline, as it gets precipitated.

Barbiturates

Phenobarbital was the first effective organic antiseizure agent. It has relatively low toxicity, is inexpensive, and is still one of the more effective and widely used antiseizure drugs.

Mechanism of Action

Its antiepileptic activity is similar to that of diphenyl-hydantoin; in addition, it raises the seizure threshold.

1. Phenobarbitone binds to GABA receptor and acts by potentiation of synaptic inhibition by facilitating GABA-mediated opening and increasing the duration of opening of Cl^- channels.
2. It blocks AMPA receptor and inhibits glutamate-mediated excitatory effects.

Pharmacokinetics

Phenobarbitone is well-absorbed on oral administration and bound to plasma proteins (40–60%). Phenobarbitone undergoes metabolism in liver by CYPs and glucuronyl transferase enzymes. Plasma half-life is about 100 hours. Phenobarbitone induces the metabolism of drugs metabolized by these enzymes when they are coad-ministered, especially oral contraceptives which are metabolized by CYP3A4. Up to 25% of a dose is eliminated by renal excretion of the unchanged drug.

Adverse Reactions

The most frequent undesired effect is sedation, but tolerance develops during chronic medication. Excessive dosage may produce nystagmus and ataxia. Phenobarbital can produce irritability and hyperactivity in children and agitation and confusion in the elderly. Manifestations of drug allergy like scarlatiniform or morbilliform rash may occur. In the newborns of mothers who have received phenobarbital during pregnancy, hypoprothrombinemia with hemorrhage has been observed. For treatment or prophylaxis, vitamin K is effective. During chronic phenobarbital therapy of epilepsy, megaloblastic anemia, which responds to folate, and osteomalacia, which responds to high doses of vitamin D, occur.

Therapeutic Uses

1. Treatment of generalized tonic-clonic, focal-to-bilateral tonic-clonic, and tonic-clonic of unknown onset (generalized tonic-clonic) seizures.
2. Focal seizures (it is not effective for absence seizures).
3. Treatment of status epilepticus.
4. Treatment of resistant grand mal, focal cortical seizures, and hypsarrhythmia combined with phenytoin.

The daily dose varies from 60 to 180 mg given in divided doses or as a single dose at night.

The main advantages of phenobarbitone are as follows:

- It is well-tolerated by most patients.
- Its half-life is long, permitting single-dose-a-day therapy, with better compliance.
- Therapeutic drug monitoring is usually not necessary.
- It is cost-effective.

Primidone

It is a prodrug of phenobarbitone.

Pharmacokinetics

Primidone is completely absorbed on oral administration and 30% protein-bound in plasma. It is rapidly metabolized to both phenobarbital and phenylethylmalonamide (PEMA) which exerts antiepileptic activity. Primidone's $t_{1/2}$ is about 6 to 8 hours, and one-third is excreted unchanged by kidney.

Adverse Effects

Adverse effects of primidone are dose-dependent and similar to those of phenobarbital, except that pronounced drowsiness is observed early. Common adverse effects include ataxia and vertigo, both of which diminish and may disappear with continued therapy. Primidone is contraindicated in patients with either porphyria or hypersensitivity to phenobarbital.

Therapeutic Uses

In addition to its early use in patients with focal-onset or generalized epilepsy, primidone is still considered to be a first-line therapy for essential tremor along with the β-blocker propranolol.

Iminostilbenes—Carbamazepine

Carbamazepine is an iminostilbene with structural resemblance to the antidepressant, imipramine.

Mechanism of Action

Carbamazepine acts by inhibition of voltage-gated sodium channels.

Pharmacokinetics

The pharmacokinetics of carbamazepine are complex. It has limited aqueous solubility. Many antiseizure drugs, including carbamazepine itself, increase their conversion to active metabolites by hepatic enzymes.

Carbamazepine is absorbed slowly and erratically after oral administration. Approximately 75% of carbamazepine is bound to plasma proteins. It is metabolized in the liver by oxidation to an active metabolite 10-11 epoxy carbamazepine and by hydroxylation to inactive metabolites. The plasma half-life, initially 24 to 36 hours, falls to around 12 hours on chronic dosing because of autoinduction. It is a potent hepatic microsomal enzyme inducer and accelerates its own metabolism as well as that of many other lipid-soluble drugs, particularly oral contraceptives, which are also metabolized by CYP3A4. Valproate inhibits its metabolism.

Adverse Reactions

Carbamazepine produces dose-related toxicity. Stupor or coma, hyperirritability, convulsions, and respiratory depression result from acute intoxication. The more frequent untoward effects during long-term therapy include drowsiness, vertigo, ataxia, diplopia, and blurred vision. With higher doses vomiting, diarrhea and worsening of seizures may occur.

Hypersensitivity reactions like rashes, photosensitivity, hepatitis, lupus-like syndrome, and, rarely, agranulocytosis and aplastic anemia occur. More common is a transient, mild leukopenia. Water retention and hyponatremia can occur in the elderly as carbamazepine enhances antidiuretic hormone (ADH) secretion.

Carbamazepine is teratogenic and minor fetal malformations such as fingernail hypoplasia, craniofacial defects, and delayed development of fetus have been reported.

Therapeutic Uses

Antiepileptic Use

It is the drug of first choice for partial and generalized tonic-clonic seizures. Contraindicated in absence seizures.

Nonantiepileptic Use

First choice in trigeminal neuralgia, glossopharyngeal neuralgia, and postherpetic neuralgia.

It is also used in bipolar disorders.

Oxcarbazepine

Oxcarbazepine is a ketoanalogue of carbamazepine. It is a prodrug that is rapidly converted to its metabolite, eslicarbazepine. It is approved for the treatment of focal seizures in adults and children as monotherapy or as an adjunct.

Mechanism of Action

This is similar to that of carbamazepine. It is a less potent enzyme inducer than carbamazepine. Oxcarbazepine does not induce the hepatic enzymes involved in its own degradation. It reduces plasma levels of steroid oral contraceptives by inducing the enzyme CYP3A.

Adverse Effects

Hypersensitivity reactions and hyponatremia are more common with oxcarbazepine than with carbamazepine.

Succinimides—Ethosuximide

Ethosuximide is a primary agent for the treatment of generalized absence seizures.

Mechanism of Action

It inhibits low threshold T-type Ca^{2+} channels and inhibits calcium currents in the thalamic neurons, which are responsible for the generation of absence seizures.

Pharmacokinetics

Oral absorption is complete. It is metabolized in the liver and excreted by kidney. The drug obeys first-order elimination kinetics.

Adverse Effects

Common adverse effects are GI symptoms such as anorexia, nausea, and vomiting; CNS effects such as drowsiness, lethargy, euphoria, dizziness, headache, and hiccough, and skin rashes. The rare adverse effect is Parkinson-like symptoms and photophobia.

Therapeutic Uses

It is the drug of choice for petit mal epilepsy.

Dose in children of 3 to 6 years old is 250 mg and 500 mg in older children, whereas in adults, the dose is increased by 250 mg.

Valproic Acid

Valproate (*n*-dipropylacetic acid) is a simple branched-chain carboxylic acid with broad spectrum of antiepileptic activity.

Mechanisms of Action

Valproic acid has multiple mechanisms such as (i) inhibition of voltage-gated Na^+ channels or (ii) activation of glutamic acid decarboxylase (GAD), and (iii) inhibition of GABA transaminase increasing GABA activity. It also works by decreasing the release of excitatory neurotransmitter glutamate. It also blocks T-type Ca^{2+} channels.

Pharmacokinetics

Valproate is well-absorbed on oral administration. Food delays absorption. As much as 90 to 95% of valproate is bound to plasma proteins. It is metabolized in the liver. Valproate is a potent enzyme inhibitor and inhibits its own metabolism and metabolism of drugs like phenobarbitone, phenytoin, lamotrigine, and lorazepam.

Adverse Effects

Transient GI symptoms including anorexia, nausea, and vomiting are the most frequent side effects. CNS effects such as sedation, ataxia, and tremor occur infrequently and usually respond to a decrease in dosage. Rash, alopecia, and stimulation of appetite have been observed occasionally. Weight gain has been seen in some patients on chronic valproate treatment. Elevation of hepatic transaminases in plasma is seen in some patients. Thrombocytopenia and pancreatitis occur rarely. Valproic acid is teratogenic, and spina bifida in the newborn is associated with its use in pregnancy.

Therapeutic Uses

It is used in grand mal epilepsy, petit mal epilepsy, combined grand mal and petit mal epilepsy, myoclonic seizures, focal epilepsy, and also in manic depressive psychosis.

Benzodiazepines

Although benzodiazepines have antiseizure property, their drawbacks are sedation and development of tolerance.

Mechanism of Action

Benzodiazepines increase the frequency of opening of Cl^- channels, thereby increasing GABA activity.

Diazepam

It is used in status epilepticus in the dose of 20 to 30 mg given IV. It is also given IV to treat convulsions induced by local anesthetics. It is given rectally in children with risk of developing febrile convulsions prophylactically at the time of fever.

Midazolam and lorazepam are used as anticonvulsants in emergency such as status epilepticus.

Clonazepam

It is more potent and long-acting than diazepam. It is well-absorbed orally and 85% is bound to plasma proteins. Clonazepam is metabolized in liver and excreted in urine. Half-life is about 24 hours. Clonazepam is useful in the treatment of petit mal, myoclonic seizures, and infantile spasms. Sedation and dullness are the important side effects of clonazepam.

Clobazam

It is long-acting and used in partial and generalized seizures as adjunctive therapy.

Newer Antiepileptic Drugs

Lamotrigine

It is a phenyltriazine derivative with broad spectrum of antiepileptic action.

Mechanism of Action

The mechanism of action for lamotrigine is not entirely understood. It is a triazine, and research has shown that lamotrigine selectively binds sodium channels, stabilizing presynaptic neuronal membranes and inhibiting glutamate release. Researchers have not demonstrated that lamotrigine to have significant effects on other neurotransmitters such as serotonin, norepinephrine, or dopamine. There is a theory that lamotrigine may interact with voltage-activated, calcium-gated channels, contributing to its broad range of activity.

Lamotrigine is well-absorbed on oral administration and metabolized completely in the liver. Its half-life is 24 hours but reduced to 16 hours in patients receiving enzyme inducers like phenytoin, carbamazepine, or phenobarbitone. Valproate inhibits the metabolism of lamotrigine by glucuronidation and doubles its level, so dose of lamotrigine should be reduced to half in patients taking valproate.

Adverse Drug Reactions

Dizziness, ataxia, blurred or double vision, nausea, vomiting, and rash occur commonly when lamotrigine is added to other antiseizure drugs. Stevens–Johnson syndrome and disseminated intravascular coagulation are sometimes reported. Serious rash is more common in children.

Therapeutic Uses

For the treatment of focal and generalized tonic-clonic seizures in adults, a dose of 100 to 300 mg/day in divided doses as monotherapy and add-on therapy is given. It is also used for myoclonic seizures in children.

Topiramate

Topiramate is a broad-spectrum antiepileptic drug approved as initial monotherapy.

Mechanisms of Action

Topiramate has multiple mechanisms such as blockade of voltage-gated Na+ channels, GABA A receptor activation, and inhibition of AMPA receptors for glutamate. Topiramate is a weak inhibitor of carbonic anhydrase.

Adverse Drug Reactions

Although topiramate is well-tolerated, most common adverse effects are somnolence, fatigue, weight loss, and nervousness. Due to inhibition of carbonic anhydrase enzyme, renal calculi may be precipitated.

Therapeutic Uses

This is used in the treatment of newly diagnosed focal and primary generalized epilepsy. It is also used for treatment of refractory focal epilepsy and generalized tonic-clonic seizures in patients with Lennox–Gastaut syndrome as monotherapy.

Gabapentin and Pregabalin

Gabapentin and pregabalin are GABA analogs which readily cross blood–brain barrier (BBB).

Mechanisms of Action

It increases synthesis and release of GABA. They inhibit N-type Ca^{2+} channels and decrease the synaptic release of glutamate.

Pharmacokinetics

Gabapentin and pregabalin are absorbed orally and not metabolized in humans. They are not bound to plasma proteins and are excreted unchanged, mainly in the urine. Their half-lives, when used as monotherapy, are approximately 6 hours. They have no known interactions with other antiepileptics.

Adverse Drug Reactions

Side effects are somnolence, dizziness, ataxia, and fatigue.

Therapeutic Uses

It is used in treating partial seizures, generalized tonic-clonic seizures, and as adjunctive treatment of partial epilepsy. It is usually effective in doses of 900 to 1800 mg daily in three divided doses.

It is considered first-line drug for the treatment of neuralgic pain due to diabetic neuropathy, postherpetic neuralgia, and chronic pain.

Tiagabine

Tiagabine is a GABA reuptake inhibitor used as an adjunct therapy for focal seizures.

Mechanism of Action

Tiagabine reduces GABA uptake into neurons and glia and prolongs the duration of GABA presence in the synaptic space by inhibiting the GABA transporter GAT-1.

Pharmacokinetics

Tiagabine has rapid oral absorption and extensive protein binding. Its metabolism is in the liver, predominantly by CYP3A. Its $t1/2$ is about 8 hours which is shortened by 2 to 3 hours when given along with enzyme inducers like phenobarbital, phenytoin, or carbamazepine.

Adverse Effects

Side effects are dizziness, somnolence, and tremor.

Therapeutic Use

Tiagabine is useful as add-on therapy for refractory focal seizures with or without secondary generalization.

Vigabatrin

Vigabatrin is a structural analog of GABA. It is an irreversible GABA transaminase inhibitor.

Mechanism of Action

It irreversibly inhibits GABA transaminase, the major degradative enzyme for GABA, thereby leading to increased concentrations of GABA in the brain.

Pharmacokinetics

An oral dose is well-absorbed. Vigabatrin is excreted unmetabolized by the kidney. Although vigabatrin has a $t_{1/2}$ of only 6 to 8 hours, the pharmacodynamic effects are prolonged and do not correlate well with plasma $t1/2$ or the plasma concentration (Cp). Vigabatrin induces CYP2C9.

Adverse Effects

The most common side effects include weight gain, concentric visual field constriction (hence, visual field testing is mandatory), fatigue, somnolence, dizziness, hyperactivity, and seizures.

Therapeutic Use

Used as an adjunct drug for the treatment of simple and complex partial seizures, generalized seizures, and in treating drug refractory epilepsy and infantile spasm.

Levetiracetam

Levetiracetam is a piracetam derivative.

Mechanism of Action

The mechanism of action of levetiracetam is not fully understood. It binds to a synaptic vesicular protein SV2A and alters release of glutamate and GABA across the synapse.

Pharmacokinetics

Levetiracetam is absorbed completely on oral administration, partly hydrolyzed but mainly excreted in urine. $t_{1/2}$ is 6 to 8 hours.

Adverse Effects

Somnolence, asthenia, ataxia, and dizziness are the most frequent adverse effects. Behavioural and mood changes are serious but less common.

Therapeutic Use

For the treatment of refractory myoclonic, focal-onset, and generalized-onset tonic-clonic seizures in adults and children as adjunctive therapy

Zonisamide

It is a sulfonamide derivative with broad spectrum of antiepileptic activity.

Mechanism of Action

It blocks voltage-gated Na^+ channel. It also inhibits T-type Ca^{2+} channels.

Pharmacokinetics

Zonisamide is almost completely absorbed on oral administration. It is about 40% bound to plasma protein and excreted by kidney. It has a long $t_{1/2}$ (~60 hours).

Adverse Effects

Side effects are somnolence, dizziness, headache, irritability, and anorexia.

Therapeutic Use

Zonisamide is used as adjunctive therapy of focal seizures and generalized tonic-clonic seizures.

Lacosamide

It is related to amino acid serine.

Mechanism of Action

Lacosamide acts by inhibition of voltage-gated Na+ channels and collapsin response mediator protein-2 (CRMP-2).

Pharmacokinetics

Given orally, bioavailability is 100%, metabolized in the liver, and 30% is excreted unchanged.

Adverse Reactions

Headache, fatigue, dizziness, nausea, and vomiting.

Therapeutic Use

Treatment of partial seizures.

Nonepileptic Uses of Antiepileptic Drugs

Antiepileptic drugs have been used in many nonepileptic disorders with variable results. The examples are as follows:

1. Carbamazepine in trigeminal neuralgia and bipolar disorder.
2. Gabapentin in neuropathic pain syndromes, migraine/tension headache, spasticity, and social phobia.
3. Lamotrigine in neuropathic pain syndromes.
4. Primidone in essential tremor.
5. Topiramate in migraine/tension headache, essential tremor, and binge disorder.
6. Vigabatrin in spasticity.
7. Valproate in migraine/tension headache and bipolar disorder.
8. Phenytoin in digoxin-induced ventricular tachycardia.
9. Phenobarbitone in neonatal hyper bilirubinemia.

Principles of Treatment of Epilepsy

Current drugs available for treatment of epilepsies only inhibit seizures (**Box 35.1**). They do not produce total cure and are not effective for prophylaxis. Treatment is therefore symptomatic. The primary objective of anticonvulsant therapy is to suppress seizures and minimize deleterious effects from seizure attacks by providing neuroprotection.

Early diagnosis and determination of the cause of the epilepsy will help to choose the appropriate drug in the treatment of epilepsies to achieve prolonged seizure-free periods with the lowest risk of toxicity. The cost/benefit ratio of the efficacy and the adverse effects of a given drug should be considered in determining which drug is optimal for a given patient.

Treatment is started after confirmation of diagnosis by EEG, MRI, and clinical history. Treatment is started early with low doses of a single effective drug and increased gradually till there is total control of seizures or till side effects appear.

When changing from one drug to another, dose of first drug is gradually decreased and dose of second drug is gradually increased. If monotherapy fails, combination of drugs is used.

When two or more types of seizures occur in the same patient, multiple-drug therapy may be required. When using

Box 35.1 Summary of drugs used in the treatment of epilepsies

Focal and secondarily generalized tonic-clonic seizures
- Most effective agents—carbamazepine and phenytoin
- Alternative or add-on drugs—levetiracetam, gabapentin, lamotrigine, and topiramate
- Reserve drugs in the treatment of focal seizures—zonisamide, tiagabine, and phenobarbitone

Generalized tonic-clonic seizures
- First-line drugs—valproate, lamotrigine, and carbamazepine
- Add-on or alternative drugs—oxcarbazepine and phenytoin
- Reserve drugs for the treatment of generalized tonic-clonic seizures—levetiracetam, topiramate, and phenobarbitone

Absence seizures
- First-line drugs—ethosuximide and valproate
- Add-on or alternative drugs—lamotrigine, clobazam, and clonazepam
- Reserve drugs—levetiracetam, topiramate, and zonisamide

Myoclonic seizures
- Drug of choice—valproate
- Add-on or alternative drugs—levetiracetam and topiramate
- Reserve drugs—clobazam and clonazepam

Atonic seizures
- Drug of choice—valproate
- Add-on or alternative drug—lamotrigine
- Reserve drugs—topiramate and clonazepam

combination of two or more drugs, drugs with different mechanism of action such as one which blocks Na^+ channels is combined with a drug that facilitates GABA. Abrupt stoppage of therapy without introducing another drug can precipitate status epilepticus. Prolonged therapy is needed for effective seizure control. Adherence to the drug regime is most crucial for successful management. Noncompliance is the most frequent cause of failure of anticonvulsant therapy.

Measurement of plasma drug concentration at appropriate intervals facilitates the initial adjustment of dosage to minimize dose-related adverse effects without sacrificing seizure control.

Duration of Therapy

Treatment with antiepileptic drugs has to be continued for at least 2 years. Tapering and discontinuing therapy should be considered if the patient is seizure-free after 2 years; tapering should be done slowly over several months.

Febrile Convulsions

A convulsion associated with a febrile illness is experienced by some children, especially those under 5 years of age. Convulsions may occur every time with fever and few children may become chronic epileptics.

Rectal diazepam, 0.5 mg/kg given at the onset of convulsions, is the best treatment of febrile convulsions. It may be repeated 12 hourly for four doses.

In children with risk of developing epilepsy, or in recurrent cases, oral or rectal diazepam started at the onset of fever is recommended for intermittent prophylaxis.

Status Epilepticus

Status epilepticus is a neurological emergency with seizure activity occurring for > 30 minutes or two or more seizures occurring without recovery of consciousness. Characteristically, there are recurrent tonic-clonic convulsions without recovery of consciousness in between. Treatment is aimed at rapid termination of behavioral and electrical seizure activity. It is important to control seizures as quickly as possible to prevent permanent brain damage and death.

Management

1. The patient has to be hospitalized.
2. First priority is to maintain proper airway.
3. Blood pressure has to be maintained.
4. Blood glucose is estimated and hypoglycemia if present is corrected by IV injection of 20 to 50 mL of 50% dextrose.
5. Anticonvulsant Lorazepam 4 mg injected IV repeated once after 10 minutes is the drug of first choice.
6. The standard therapy till recently is diazepam 10 mg injected IV repeated once after 10 minutes but nowadays it is given only if lorazepam is not available.
7. Fosphenytoin 100 to 150 mg/min IV infusion is to be given subsequently irrespective of response to lorazepam. Continuous ECG monitoring is needed.
8. Phenytoin sodium is used when fosphenytoin is not available.
9. Phenobarbitone-sodium 50 to 100 mg IV is used as an alternative to fosphenytoin or when fosphenytoin is ineffective.
10. Refractory cases not responding to treatment with lorazepam or fosphenytoin within 40 minutes of onset of seizure activity are treated with midazolam/propofol/thiopentone anesthesia with or without curarization and full intensive care.

Importance of Plasma-Level Monitoring of Antiepileptic Drugs

Some antiepileptic drugs show good correlation between their plasma concentrations and seizure control as well as development of adverse effects. For other antiepileptic drugs, there is no correlation between their concentrations in plasma and clinical effects.

There is a good correlation between the plasma concentration of phenytoin and its clinical effect. Control of seizures is obtained with total concentrations above 10 mg/mL, while toxic effects such as nystagmus develop at total concentrations around 20 mg/mL. Even though there is no precise relationship between therapeutic results and plasma concentration of phenobarbitone, plasma concentrations of 10 to 35 mg/mL are usually recommended for control of seizures. The relationship between plasma concentration of phenobarbital and adverse effects varies with the development of tolerance.

Plasma concentrations of benzodiazepines are of limited value because tolerance affects the relationship between drug concentration and drug antiseizure effect. The plasma concentration of ethosuximide required for satisfactory control of absence seizures is 40 to 100 mg/mL. Although there is a poor correlation between the plasma concentration and efficacy of valproate, therapeutic effects are seen with concentrations of about 30 to 100 mg/mL.

Antiepileptic drug concentrations in plasma are measured to:

1. Facilitate optimizing antiseizure medication, especially when therapy is initiated.
2. After dosage adjustments.
3. In the event of therapeutic failure.
4. When toxic effects appear.
5. When multiple-drug therapy is instituted.

Epilepsy and Pregnancy

Antiepileptics use in women may affect their health in many ways. There may be contraceptive failure due to interactions of antiepileptic drugs with oral contraceptives. Antiepileptics should not be stopped abruptly even during pregnancy, as it may lead to status epilepticus and abortion consequently. Evidence suggests that antiepileptics have teratogenic effects. These may be major malformations like congenital heart defects, neural tube defects, spina bifida, cleft lip, cleft palate, or minor malformations like nail hypoplasia, low set ears and prominent lips. Use of two or more antiepileptics increases the frequency of occurrence of fetal malformations. All the newborns of mothers who received an antiepileptic drug during pregnancy should be examined for congenital abnormalities.

Phenytoin, carbamazepine, valproate, lamotrigine, and phenobarbital have been associated with teratogenic effects. Newer antiepileptics have shown teratogenic effects in animals, but whether such effects occur in humans is yet uncertain.

Antiepileptics may produce effects on vitamin K metabolism in pregnant women. Most antiepileptics that induce CYPs have been associated with vitamin K deficiency in the newborn, resulting in a coagulopathy and intracerebral hemorrhage due to deficiency of vitamin K-dependent clotting factor. Treatment with vitamin K1, 10 mg/day during the last month of gestation, has been recommended for prophylaxis.

All women on antiepileptics should receive folate supplementation 5 mg/d, starting before conception and continued throughout pregnancy to reduce the likelihood of neural tube defects in the newborn.

Precautions

1. Folic acid supplementation to the women before conception and throughout pregnancy.
2. Vitamin K given to the mother in the last month of pregnancy, and newborn after birth.

Drugs Inducing Seizures

Some drugs used for other indications can induce seizures as adverse drug reactions. They are as follows:

1. Sympathomimetics and central stimulants–ephedrine, amphetamine, terbutaline, aminophylline and cocaine.
2. Some tricyclic antidepressants.
3. Phenothiazines (antipsychotics and antihistaminics) and haloperidol.
4. Bupropion, lithium, flumazenil.
5. Withdrawal of alcohol, short-acting benzodiazepines/barbiturates.
6. Anesthetic agents such as ether, halothane, ketamine, lignocaine.
7. Analgesics–tramadol, pethidine.
8. Antimicrobial and antiviral drugs–penicillin, cephalosporins, imipenem, quinolones, INH, acyclovir, ganciclovir.
9. Immunomodulators–methotrexate, cyclosporine, tacrolimus.

Multiple Choice Questions

1. A 34-year-old woman suffers a seizure while in a shopping mall. Witnesses tell the paramedics that she lost consciousness and then had rapid contraction and relaxation of her extremities. She then awoke and was confused. The most likely diagnosis is:

A. Absence seizures.
B. Febrile seizures.
C. Myoclonic seizures.
D. Status epilepticus.
E. Tonic-clonic seizures.

Answer: E

Tonic-clonic seizures are characterized by sudden loss of consciousness without any warning (aura), followed by generalized tonic, and finally clonic convulsive movements lasting for 1 to 2 minutes.

2. A 29-year-old man with recurrent epileptic seizures presents to his primary care physician for follow-up. There is no past medical, surgical, or family history relevant to his seizures. CT scan of the head reveals normal cerebral and cerebellar structures. There is no evidence of hydrocephalus. What is the most likely explanation of this patient's seizures?

A. Alcohol-induced.
B. Iatrogenic.
C. Idiopathic.
D. Neoplastic.
E. Traumatic.

Answer: C

3. A 53-year-old woman with seizure disorder, bipolar disorder, and trigeminal neuralgia presents to her primary care physician for follow-up and treatment. She has no new complaints. Which of the following medications may serve to treat all of her earlier mentioned problems?

A. Carbamazepine.
B. Ethosuximide.
C. Felbamate.
D. Gabapentin.

Answer: A

Carbamazepine is effective for treatment of partial seizures and, secondarily, generalized tonic-clonic seizures. It is also used to treat trigeminal neuralgia and bipolar disorder.

4. A 57-year-old man with chronic liver disorder and seizures takes antiepileptic medications. Which of the following agents would be preferred?

A. Carbamazepine.
B. Valproic acid.
C. Levetiracetam.
D. Phenytoin.

Answer: C

Levetiracetam is not metabolized in the liver and hence preferred.

5. A 47-year-old man with seizure disorder presents to his primary care physician for follow-up. Because of a recent exacerbation in his seizures, he is prescribed lacosamide. Which of the following is the most likely mechanism of action of this medication?

A. Binds to collapsing response mediator protein-2.
B. Binds to GABA receptors.
C. Blockade of calcium channels.
D. Blockade of sodium channels.
E. Blockade of both sodium and calcium channels.

Answer: A

Lacosamide binds to collapsin response mediator protein-2 (CRMP-2). Lacosamide is approved for adjunctive treatment of partial seizures.

6. A 19-year-old man with a significant seizure history has various seizures including partial onset seizures, myoclonic seizures, and, occasionally, primary generalized tonic-clonic seizures. His physician prescribed levetiracetam. What is its site of action?

A. Calcium channel modulation.
B. Collapsin response mediator protein-2 (CRMP-2).
C. GABA receptors.
D. Sodium channels.
E. Synaptic vesicle protein.

Answer: E

Levetiracetam is approved for adjunct therapy of partial onset seizures, myoclonic seizures, and primary generalized tonic-clonic seizures in adults and children. It demonstrates high affinity for synaptic vesicle protein (SV2A).

7. A 68-year-old man with history of seizure disorder controlled with phenytoin presents to his dentist for routine follow-up. Which of the following findings must the dentist be concerned about and evaluate for?

A. Dental caries.
B. Exposed nerve roots.
C. Gingival overgrowth.
D. Teeth erosion.

Answer: C

Gingival hyperplasia (overgrowth), an adverse effect of phenytoin, may cause the gums to grow over the teeth.

8. A 54-year-old man with seizure disorder and chronic neuropathic pain presents to his primary care physician for follow-up. Review of his laboratory studies indicates elevated liver function tests to four times the normal levels. Which of the following agents would be preferred to manage this patient?

A. Carbamazepine.
B. Phenobarbital.
C. Phenytoin.
D. Pregabalin.

Answer: D

Pregabalin is an antiepileptic that works through voltage-gated calcium channels in the central nervous system (CNS), inhibiting excitatory neurotransmitter release. The drug has proven effects on partial onset seizures, neuropathic pain associated with diabetic peripheral neuropathy, postherpetic neuralgia, and fibromyalgia.

9. A 14-year-old boy is brought to the urgent care clinic after suffering an episode of lip smacking followed by stiffness and convulsions. His mother explains that this is the third such attack in the past 2 years and that each attack has lasted about a minute. The pediatrician prescribes carbamazepine to control his seizures. What is the mechanism of action of this agent?

A. Inhibition of calcium channels.
B. Inhibition of potassium channels.
C. Inhibition of sodium channels.
D. Potentiation of GABA receptors.

Answer: C

This patient presents with tonic-clonic seizures, which generally have an unknown cause. Carbamazepine inhibits sodium entry into cells, making them less likely to depolarize and thereby controlling the seizure.

10. An epileptic woman is being treated with an antiepileptic drug for the last 5 years. For the last six menstrual cycles, she was taking oral contraceptive pills. This time she did not start menses even after 2 weeks of stopping the pills. On examination, the gynecologist confirmed pregnancy. Which of the following drugs is responsible for the failure of contraception?

A. Phenytoin.
B. Valproic acid.
C. Ethosuximide.
D. Vigabatrin.

Answer: A

Phenytoin is a microsomal enzyme inducer, reducing the levels of estrogen in oral contraceptive pills, which is responsible for failure of contraception.

11. A young female patient employed as computer programmer is suffering from myoclonic jerks. There is no history of generalized tonic-clonic seizures. Select a suitable drug for the patient:

A. Phenobarbitone.
B. Valproic acid.
C. Carbamazepine.
D. Clonazepam.

Answer: B

Patient is suffering from myoclonic jerks which often occur after awakening or before retiring, often in combination with other seizure types. Age of onset is 5 to 20 years. Valproic acid is the drug of choice and also has no drowsiness.

12. A patient who was on antiepileptic therapy has been brought to the hospital in status epilepticus. Relatives gave history of stopping the drug since 2 days. On examination, gums were found to be hypertrophied with bleeding. On investigation, plasma drug concentration was 6 µg/100 mL. Peripheral smear showed megaloblastic anemia. What is the cause of this severe attack of epilepsy? What is the responsible drug?

A. Phenytoin.
B. Valproic acid.
C. Phenobarbitone.
D. Carbamazepine.

Answer: A

Sudden stoppage of antiepileptic drug, probably phenytoin, is the cause of status as the adverse effects like gum hypertrophy and megaloblastic anemia are associated with use of phenytoin.

13. Chronic use of which of the following drugs produces adverse effects like coarsening of facial features, hirsutism, and gingival hyperplasia?

A. Zonisamide.
B. Ethosuximide.
C. Phenytoin.
D. Tiagabine.

Answer: C

Common adverse effects of phenytoin include nystagmus, diplopia, and ataxia. With chronic use, coarsening of facial features, gingival overgrowth and hirsutism may occur.

14. Which antiepileptic drug is most likely to elevate the plasma concentration of other drugs when administered concomitantly?

A. Carbamazepine.
B. Clonazepam.
C. Phenobarbital.
D. Phenytoin.
E. Valproic acid.

Answer: E

Valproic acid, an inhibitor of drug metabolism, can increase the plasma levels of many drugs, including those used in seizure disorders such as carbamazepine and lamotrigine.

15. A young male patient suffers from a seizure disorder characterized by tonic rigidity of the extremities followed by massive jerking of the body for 1 or 2 minutes, leaving the patient in a stuporous state. Which of the following drugs is most suitable for long-term management of this patient?

A. Clonazepam.
B. Ethosuximide.
C. Lacosamide.
D. Valproic acid.
E. Pregabalin.

Answer: D

This patient is suffering from generalized tonic-clonic seizures. The drugs of choice for this seizure disorder are carbamazepine, phenytoin, or valproic acid.

Chapter 36

Antiparkinsonian Drugs and Drugs for Treatment of Alzheimer's Disease

Veena R.M., Manisha Prajapat, Jitupam Baishya, Harpinder Kaur, Phulen Sarma, and Bikash Medhi

PH1.19: Describe the mechanism/s of action, types, doses, side effects, indications, and contraindications of the drugs which act on central nervous system (CNS) (including anxiolytics, sedatives and hypnotics, antipsychotics, antidepressant drugs, antimaniacs, opioid agonists and antagonists, drugs used for neurodegenerative disorders, and antiepileptic drugs).

Learning Objectives

- Classification of parkinsonism.
- Dopamine synthesis, metabolism, and receptors.
- Classification of antiparkinsonian drugs.
- Management of Parkinson's disease.
- Drugs for the treatment of Alzheimer's disease.

Parkinson's Disease (IM19.8)

The clinical syndrome of parkinsonism was first designated by the London physician James Parkinson in 1817 as paralysis agitans or the "shaking palsy." Parkinson's disease (PD) is a progressive neurodegenerative disorder of movement that occurs mainly in the elderly.

The fundamental features are a combination of

1. Muscular rigidity.
2. Bradykinesia.
3. Tremor, mainly at rest.
4. Stooped posture and instability.

Other symptoms include anxiety, depression, hyposmia, impaired color vision, bladder hyperreflexia, and abnormalities of nociception and sleep. As the disease advances, the cognitive dysfunction and hallucinations occurs in many patients. Both the genders are equally affected. The mean age of onset and the mean duration of disease is around 65 years (range 31–85 years) and 12 years, respectively.

Classification of Parkinsonism

Parkinson disease (paralysis agitans) is primary or idiopathic Parkinsonism. The causes remain unknown or may be multifactorial, for example, genetic disposition or aging of brain due to free radical damage to dopaminergic neurons in basal ganglia.

The secondary Parkinsonism occurs from known causes and is curable. It may be due to

1. Drugs that diminish the dopamine in the brain (e.g., neuroleptic drugs—phenothiazines, butyrophenones, metoclopramide, reserpine, lithium, monoamine oxidase [MAO] inhibitors).
2. Drugs that block dopamine receptors (e.g., antipsychotic drugs such as chlorpromazine).
3. Familial early-onset PD and several gene mutations with three molecules (i) α synuclein, (ii) Parkin, and (iii) ubiquitin critical.

The basal ganglia disorders also mimic many of the clinical features mentioned in PD and is often referred to as parkinsonian syndromes, for example, striatonigral degeneration, corticobasal degeneration, and Wilson's disease.

In PD, there is degeneration of about 60 to 70% of dopaminergic neurons projecting from substantia nigra pars compacta (SNpc) to neostriatum even before the symptoms occur. The lack of dopamine due to loss of dopaminergic neurons indirectly leads to hyperactivity of cholinergic system, which is not primarily affected. There is critical imbalance between dopaminergic and cholinergic systems in the neostriatum. Other monoamines, such as noradrenaline and 5-hydroxytryptamine, are much less affected than dopamine. **Table 36.1** depicts the changes in the brain levels of neurotransmitters affected in PD.

Dopamine Synthesis, Metabolism, and Receptors

Dopamine is a catecholamine that is used as a neurotransmitter both in the CNS and the peripheral nervous system (PNS). Dopamine is synthesized in the dopaminergic nerve

Table 36.1 Neurotransmitter levels in neostriatum in the Parkinson's disease

Striatal neurotransmitter	Parkinson's disease
Dopamine	Decreased
GABA	Decreased
Glutamate	Increased
Adenosine	Decreased
Acetylcholine	Increased

Abbreviation: GABA, gamma-aminobutyric acid.

terminal from tyrosine, which is transported across the blood-brain barrier (BBB) (**Figs. 36.1** and **36.2**).

Synthesis

Phenylalanine and tyrosine are precursors of dopamine. The dietary phenylalanine is converted to tyrosine by phenylalanine hydroxylase. Tyrosine is converted into L-3,4-dihydroxyphenylalanine (L-DOPA) by tyrosine hydroxylase (TH), and L-DOPA is converted into cytosolic dopamine by aromatic amino acid decarboxylase (AADC).

Metabolism

Tyrosine crosses readily into the brain through uptake and enters dopaminergic neuronal terminal where it is converted to L-DOPA by the enzyme TH. TH catalyzes the first rate-limiting step of dopamine biosynthesis and is strongly regulated. Once generated, in the periphery, L-DOPA is rapidly converted to dopamine by AADC. In the CNS and PNS, AADC activity is very high. Unlike dopamine, L-DOPA not metabolized by AADC readily crosses the BBB and is converted to dopamine in the brain.

Metabolic Pathways

The enzymatic breakdown of dopamine to its inactive metabolites is carried out by catechol-O-methyl transferase (COMT) and MAO. MAO breaks down dopamine to 3,4-dihydroxyphenylacetaldehyde (DOPAL) which, in turn, is degraded to form 3,4-dihydroxyphenylacetic acid (DOPAC) in the CNS. Another pathway for the metabolism of DA involves the enzyme COMT, which converts it to 3-methoxytyramine (3-MT). Then, 3-MT is reduced by MAO to homovanillic acid (HVA) and eliminated in the urine (**Fig. 36.2**).

Dopamine Receptors

The actions of dopamine in the brain are mediated by a family of dopamine-receptor proteins. They have been classified into two subfamilies, termed D1 and D2.

D1 Receptor Subfamily

It includes D1 and D5 and is expressed in multiple brain regions, including the cortex, hippocampus, amygdala, and most intensively, the striatum, olfactory bulb, and SN. The D1 subfamily is excitatory. They are coupled to Gαs and Gαolf and stimulate the synthesis of the intracellular second messenger cyclic adenosine monophosphate (cAMP) and activate protein kinase A (PKA).

D2 Receptor Subfamily

This includes D2, D3, and D4, which are inhibitory. They are coupled to Gαi and Gαo and downregulate the production of cAMP by inhibiting adenylyl cyclase (AC), resulting in decrease in PKA activity. Dopamine is substrate of PKA. D2 receptor subfamily also regulates Gβγ subunits signaling, which activates PLC and produces IP3, resulting in an increase in the cytoplasmic calcium concentration, which activates receptor-operated K^+ currents.

Pathophysiology

Loss or degeneration of the dopaminergic neurons in SNpc. The accumulation of Lewy bodies, which are abnormal intracellular aggregates containing proteins like alpha-synuclein (α-syn) and ubiquitin.

Symptoms

The symptom most clearly related to dopamine deficiency is hypokinesia and rigidity, which occur immediately. Enhanced cholinergic activity due to dopamine depletion is responsible mainly for tremors. Disturbances in autonomic function and dementia are due to disturbances of other transmitters (noradrenaline, 5-hydroxytryptamine and gamma-amino butyric acid [GABA]). About 60 to 70% of neurons in SNpc are lost before symptoms occur. There is currently no cure for PD but medication can usually provide good symptom control for a long time. Therapeutic approaches to manage

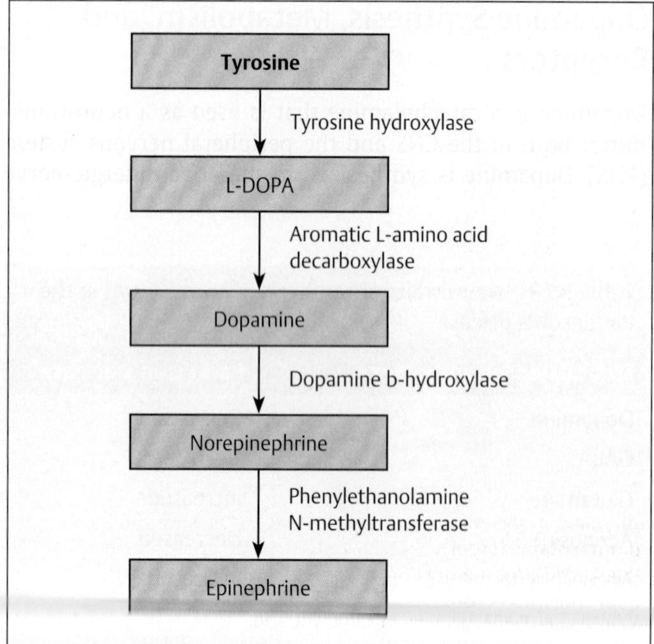

Fig. 36.1 Dopamine synthesis.

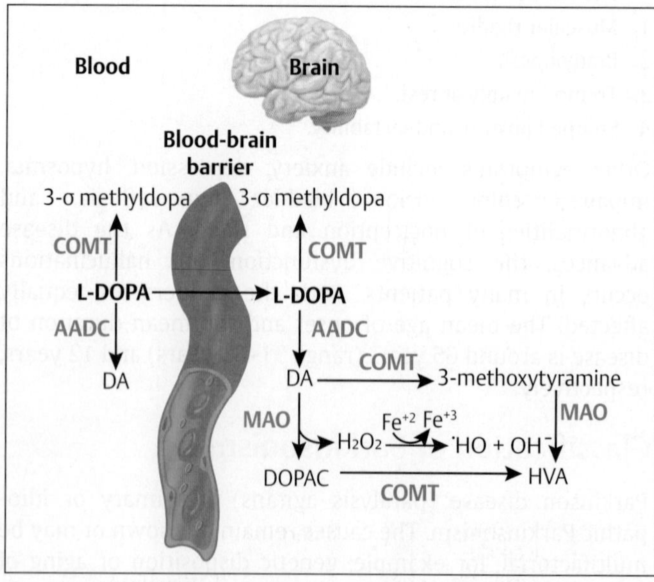

Fig. 36.2 Metabolic pathways of L-DOPA in the periphery and the brain. AAD, aromatic amino acid decarboxylase; AADC, amino acid decarboxylase; COMT, catechol-O-methyltransferase; DA, dopamine; DOPAC, dihydroxyphenylacetic acid; HVA, homovanillic acid.

PD include symptomatic therapies with the goal of slowing or stopping disease progression (**Fig. 36.3**).

Classification of Antiparkinsonian Drugs

Drugs Acting on Dopaminergic System

- Dopamine precursors: Levodopa (L-DOPA).
- Peripheral decarboxylase inhibitors: Carbidopa and benserazide.
- Dopaminergic agonists: Bromocriptyne, ropinirole, and pramipexole.
- Selective MAO-B inhibitors: Selegiline and rasagiline.
- COMT inhibitors: Entacapone and tolcapone.
- Dopamine facilitator: Amantadine.

Drugs Acting on Cholinergic System

- Central anticholinergics: Teihexyphenidyl (benzhexol), procyclidine, and biperiden.
- Antihistaminics: Orphenadrine and promethazine.
- Dopaminergic agonists: bromocriptine, ropinirole, pramipexole.
- MAO-B inhibitor: selegiline, rasagiline, safinamide.
- COMT inhibitors: entacapone, tolcapone.
- Glutamate (NMDA receptor) antagonist (dopamine facilitator)- Amantadine (Cucumber SALAD- COMT inhibitor, Selegiline, Amantadine, L-DOPA, Decarboxylase Inhibitors))

Drugs Decreasing the Cholinergic Function in Brain

- Central anticholinergics—trihexyphenidyl (benzhexol), procyclidine, biperiden.
- Antihistaminics with anticholinergic properties—orphenadrine, promethazine (**Fig. 36.4**).

Levodopa

The single most efficient drug in the treatment of PD is L-DOPA.

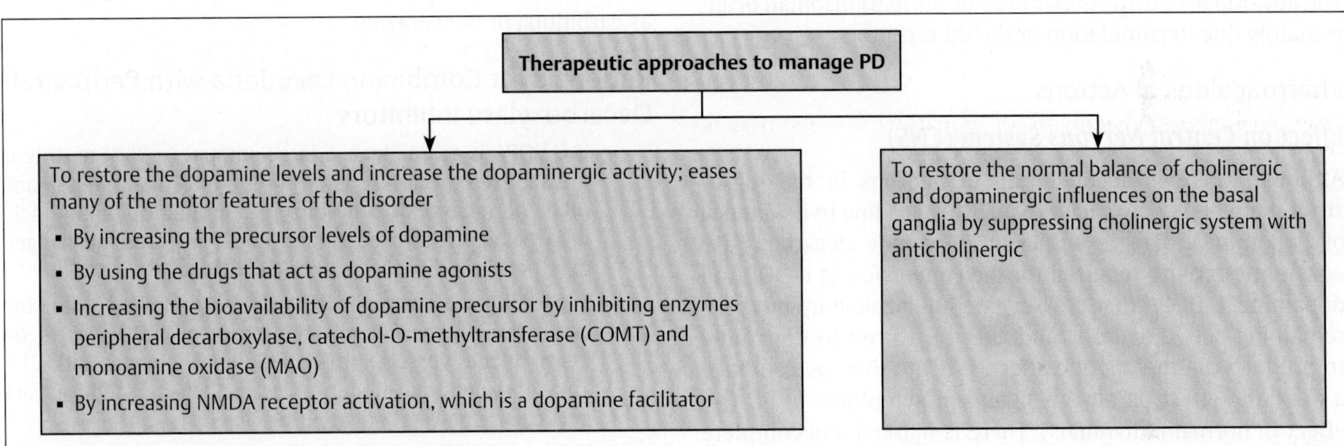

Fig. 36.3 Therapeutic approaches to manage PD.

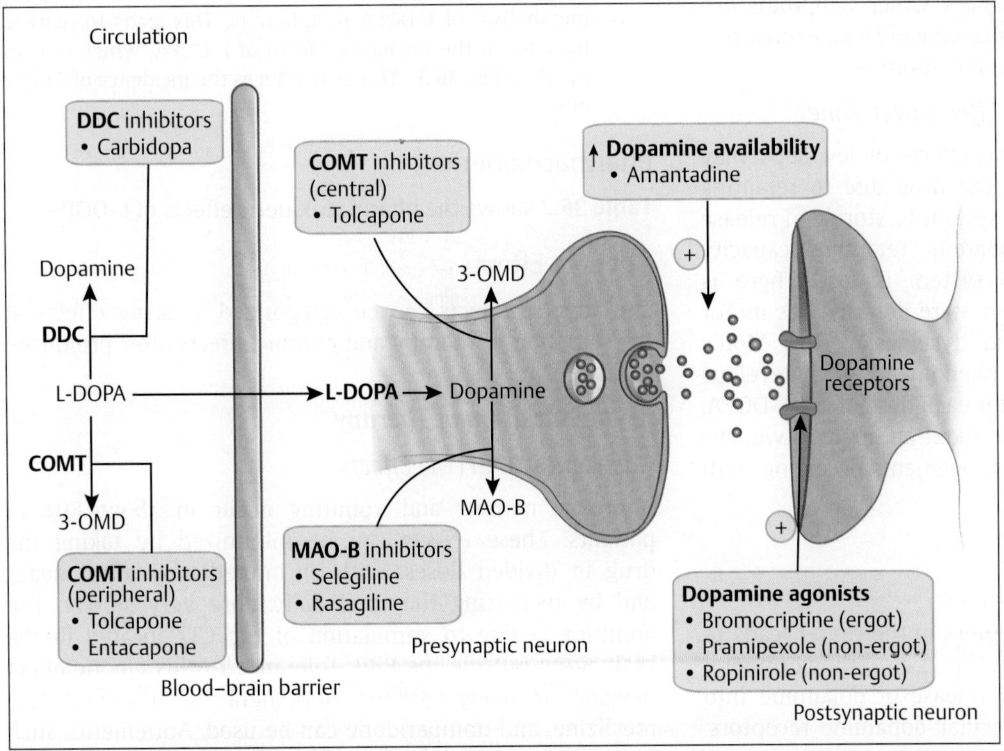

Fig. 36.4 Antiparkinsonian drugs based on their sites of action.

Mechanism of Action

Dopamine in the peripheral circulation has no therapeutic effect in parkinsonism and does not cross the BBB by itself. L-DOPA is a prodrug and is the immediate metabolic precursor of dopamine. L-DOPA is converted into dopamine in the CNS and the peripheral tissues (liver, gastrointestinal tract [GIT]) too. Approximately 95% of the L-DOPA is converted into dopamine in the peripheral tissues. About 1 to 2% of administered L-DOPA crosses to the brain and is taken up by the surviving dopaminergic neurons, converted to DA, which is stored, and released as a transmitter. This in turn activates dopamine receptors in different areas and produces therapeutic effect.

Dopamine receptor activation occurs in:

1. Corpus striatum leading to antiparkinsonian effect and resolving other secondary symptoms.
2. Pituitary leading to decreased prolactin level.
3. Limbic system leading to psychosis.

The advantage of using dopaminergic antiparkinsonian drugs is mainly due to stimulation of the D2 receptors.

Pharmacological Actions

Effect on Central Nervous System (CNS)

Although there is degeneration of neurons in the nigro-striatal tract (NST), particularly in SNpc, leading to deficiency of dopamine, there is sufficient dopamine decarboxylase enzymatic activity required for the conversion of L-DOPA to dopamine. L-DOPA that crosses the BBB is taken up by these remaining active neurons and gets converted to dopamine to produce the therapeutic effect. L-DOPA therapy can have a dramatic effect on all the signs and symptoms of PD (no effect in normal individuals). There is marked and complete improvement in hypokinesia and rigidity initially, followed by improvement in tremor early in the course of the disease but declines as the disease advances. Other symptoms like walking, writing, speaking, and masking of facial expression, self-care, and personal interest in life improve.

Levodopa (L-DOPA) Beneficial Effects over Time

In early PD, the duration of the effects of levodopa may exceed the plasma lifetime of the drug due to retaining capacity of the nigrostriatal DA system to store and release DA. On long-term use, this apparent "retaining" capacity of the nigrostriatal dopamine system is lost. There is fluctuation in the patient's motor state described as motor fluctuations and L-DOPA-related dyskinesia (LID). Motor fluctuation is the "wearing off" phenomenon that develops very commonly. Immediately after each dose of the L-DOPA, mobility improves effectively for about an hour or two. LID refers to abnormal, involuntary movements occurring with the use of levodopa.

Cardiovascular System

Postural Hypotension

Activation of the dopamine receptors in the center leads to decreased central sympathetic outflow; also, the peripheral decarboxylation of L-DOPA and release of dopamine into the circulation may activate vascular dopamine receptors. Both central and peripheral action produces orthostatic hypotension.

Tachycardia

The dopamine formed peripherally acts on β-adrenergic receptors and causes tachycardia. Tolerance develops gradually to this action.

Chemoreceptor Trigger Zone (CTZ)

Peripherally formed dopamine enters the CTZ and acts on the dopamine receptor in this area. Since dopamine is an excitatory transmitter, it induces nausea and vomiting. Gradually, tolerance develops to this action.

Other Actions

Dopamine acts on pituitary mammotropes, inhibits prolactin release, and on somatotropes, it increases growth hormone (GH) release.

In clinical practice, L-DOPA is almost always prescribed in combination with a peripheral decarboxylase inhibitors such as carbidopa or benserazide.

Rationale for Combining Levodopa with Peripheral Decarboxylase Inhibitors

- If L-DOPA is given alone, a large amount (> 95%) of drug is metabolized (decarboxylated) in the intestinal mucosa and other peripheral sites by enzyme (aromatic L-amino acid decarboxylase) into dopamine and very little unchanged drug (<1%) reaches the cerebral circulation
- In addition, dopamine formed and released into the circulation by peripheral conversion of L-DOPA acts on heart, blood vessels, other peripheral organs, and CTZ. The most common undesirable side effects produced are particularly nausea and vomiting.
- Unlike L-DOPA, peripheral decarboxylase inhibitors, such as carbidopa or benserazide, do not penetrate the CNS. They inhibit peripheral decarboxylase enzyme and thus the metabolism of L-DOPA peripherally. This leads to marked increase in the unchanged form of L-DOPA, which crosses the BBB (**Fig. 36.5**). This also reduces the incidence of GI side effects.

Pharmacokinetics

Table 36.2 shows the pharmacokinetic effects of L-DOPA.

Adverse Effects

The adverse effects can be categorized as acute effects at the initiation of therapy and chronic effects after prolonged therapy.

At the Initiation of Therapy

Gastrointestinal (GI) Effects

Anorexia, nausea, and vomiting occur in about 80% of patients. These effects can be minimized by taking the drug in divided doses, with or immediately after meals, and by increasing the total daily dose very slowly. The vomiting is due to stimulation of the CTZ located in the brain stem outside the BBB. Tolerance to this emetic effect develops in many patients. Antiemetics such as cyclizine, meclizine, and domperidone can be used. Antiemetics such

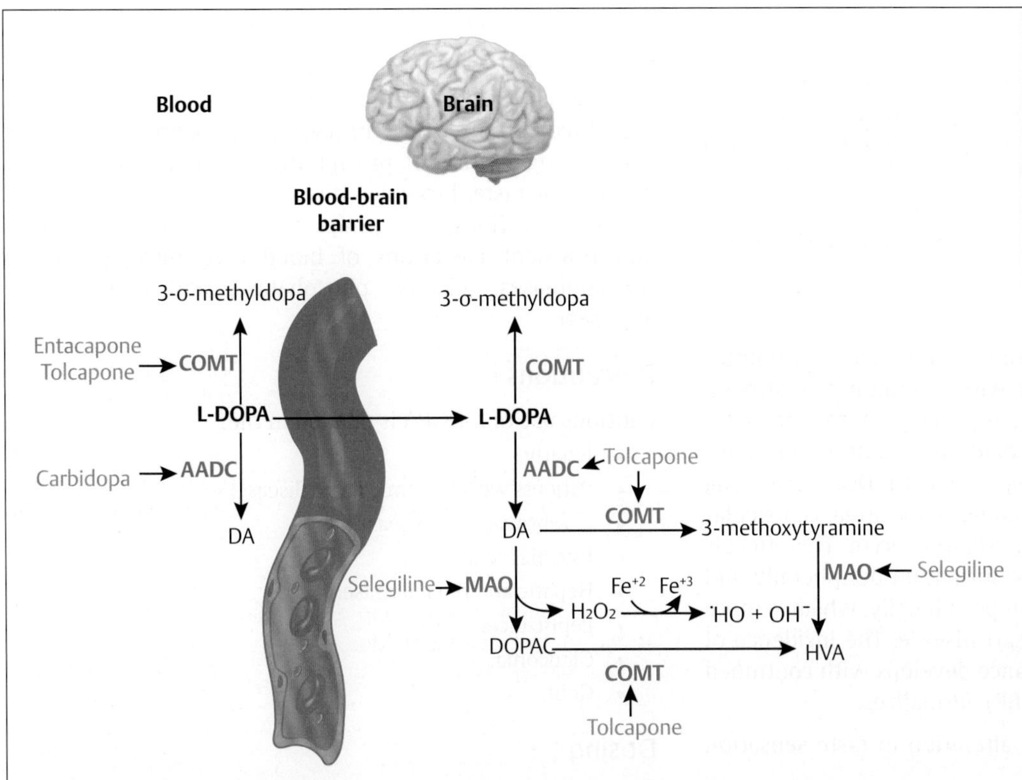

Fig. 36.5 Drugs from various classes acting on the metabolic pathway of L-DOPA to prevent its degradation in the periphery and brain. AAD, aromatic amino acid decarboxylase; AADC, amino acid decarboxylase; COMT, catechol-O-methyltransferase; DA, dopamine; DOPAC, dihydroxyphenylacetic acid; HVA, homovanillic acid.

Table 36.2 Pharmacokinetic effects of L-DOPA

PK	Effect	Implications
Absorption	L-DOPA is an amino acid derivative and thus is absorbed rapidly from the small intestine by the active transport process that is meant for absorption of aromatic amino acids. The rate and extent of absorption (bioavailability) depends on the: • Gastric juice pH • Rate of gastric emptying • Duration of time the drug is exposed to the degradative enzymes of the gastric and intestinal mucosa	Amino acids present in food compete for the same carrier for absorption. Protein-rich food delays absorption of the drug and reduces peak plasma concentrations. L-DOPA should not be taken with food specifically with protein-rich food
Distribution	Entry of levodopa into the CNS across the BBB also is mediated by a membrane transporter meant for aromatic amino acids.	Competition between dietary protein and levodopa may occur at this level too. It is best to avoid concomitant intake of levodopa and protein-rich food
Metabolism	The drug undergoes high first-pass metabolism in the CNS, GI mucosa and liver. In the brain, within the presynaptic terminals of dopaminergic neurons in the stratium, L-DOPA is converted to dopamine by decarboxylation primarily after release. Dopamine is metabolized by the actions of MAO and COMT or transported back into dopaminergic terminals by the presynaptic uptake mechanism.	Pyridoxine (vitamin B6) a cofactor for dopamine decarboxylase facilitates the conversion of levodopa to dopamine (more conversion occurs at the periphery) resulting in the lesser amount entering the brain and loss of therapeutic effect.
Elimination	Metabolites are excreted in urine mostly after conjugation.	
Peak plasma concentration *t*1/2	Concentrations of the drug in plasma usually peak between 0.5 and 2 hours after an oral dose. Short (1–3 hours).	-

Abbreviations: BBB, blood-brain barrier; CNS, central nervous system; COMT, catechol-O-methyltransferase; GI, gastrointestinal; MAO, monoamine oxidase.

as phenothiazines and metoclopramide should be avoided, as they produce acute dystonic reactions in approximately 1% of patients. These dyskinesias begin acutely after drug administration, occur most frequently in young patients, and consist of torticollis, trismus, facial spasms, opisthotonos, and oculogyric crises. When levodopa is given in combination with carbidopa, adverse GI effects are much less frequent and troublesome, so that patients can tolerate proportionately higher doses.

Cardiovascular Effects

Postural hypotension is common, but often asymptomatic, and tends to diminish with continuing treatment. Hypertension may also occur, especially in the presence of nonselective monoamine oxidase inhibitors or sympathomimetics or when massive doses of L-DOPA are being taken. Cardiac arrhythmias including tachycardia, ventricular extrasystoles and, rarely, atrial fibrillation occur. This effect is due to increased catecholamine formation peripherally and its action on β-adrenergic action peripherally, which is more in patients with preexisting heart disease. The incidence of such arrhythmias is low. Tolerance develops with continued treatment and blood pressure (BP) normalizes.

Exacerbation of angina and alteration in taste sensation can also occur.

After Prolonged Therapy

Abnormal Movements (Dyskinesias)

As much as 80% of the patients experience dyskinesias which are dose-related. The most common presentation is choreoathetosis of the face and distal. No tolerance develops to this adverse effect, but dose reduction decreases severity.

Behavioral Effects

Behavioural effects include depression, anxiety, agitation, insomnia, somnolence, confusion, delusions, hallucinations, nightmares, euphoria, increase in sexual activity, and other changes in mood or personality. Such adverse effects are more common in patients taking L-DOPA in combination with a decarboxylase inhibitor rather than L-DOPA alone because of the excessive dopamine action in the limbic system. L-DOPA is contraindicated in patients with psychotic illness. Patients should be counselled not to discontinue L-DOPA abruptly, as this can result in the parkinsonism-hyperpyrexia syndrome, which is clinically similar to neuroleptic malignant syndrome.

Fluctuations in Motor Response

In some, these fluctuations relate to the timing of L-DOPA intake, and they are referred to as wearing-off reactions or end-of-dose akinesia, and in others, fluctuations are unrelated to the timing of doses (on-off phenomenon). In the on-off phenomenon, the marked akinesia is observed during off-periods, which alternate with on-periods over few hours, during which improvement in the mobility is observed. This phenomenon most likely occurs in patients who responded well to treatment initially. This is probably a reflection of progression of the disorder.

Other Side Effects

Mydriasis and precipitation of an attack of acute glaucoma in some patients is encountered. Various blood dyscrasias, a positive Coombs' test with evidence of hemolysis and hot flushes, aggravation or precipitation of gout, abnormalities of smell or taste, brownish discoloration of saliva, urine or vaginal secretions, and priapism are also observed. Mild and transient elevations of blood urea nitrogen, serum transaminases, alkaline phosphatase, and bilirubin are also seen.

Precautions

Cautious use of L-DOPA is needed in the:

- Elderly.
- Patients with ischemic heart disease.
- Cerebrovascular disease.
- Psychiatric disease.
- Hepatic and renal disease.
- Peptic ulcer.
- Glaucoma.
- Gout.

Dosing

Treatment should begin with small doses of an immediate release (IR) L-DOPA formulation, such as carbidopa-levodopa 25/100 mg, daily with meals. If there are no side effects, the total daily dose of carbidopa-L-DOPA can be gradually increased over several weeks to a full tablet of 25/100 mg three times daily. Tolerance for the appropriate starting dose must be assessed individually.

Controlled release (CR) tablet L-DOPA preparations are not recommended as initial therapy, as they reach the brain more slowly over time. They are less completely absorbed and require a dose up to 30% higher to achieve an equivalent clinical effect. L-DOPA should not be stopped suddenly in patients with PD, because sudden withdrawal has been associated (rarely) with a syndrome resembling neuroleptic malignant syndrome or akinetic crisis.

Drug Interactions

- Phenothiazines, butyrophenones, metoclopramide: These drugs block dopamine receptors and decrease the therapeutic effect of L-DOPA.
- Pyridoxine: It enhances the peripheral decarboxylation of L-DOPA peripherally and abolishes the therapeutic effect of L-DOPA.
- Antihypertensive drugs: These drugs accentuate the postural hypotension caused by L-DOPA.
- Nonselective MAO inhibitors prevent degradation of DA. When L-DOPA is administered, dopamine degradation is prevented by MAO inhibitors. Noradrenaline is synthesized in large quantities at peripheral sites. This may cause hypertensive crisis.
- Additive therapeutic action is observed when atropine is concurrently administered with antiparkinsonian anticholinergic drugs. They also decrease the dose of L-DOPA, but retard its absorption.

Drug Holiday

The chronic treatment of PD with L-DOPA is associated with problems that include dyskinesia, on-off phenomena, hallucinosis, and possible loss of therapeutic efficacy. As a method of preventing these complications, transient withdrawal of L-DOPA is advocated. This is known as "drug holiday." A drug holiday (discontinuance of the drug for 3–21 days) may temporarily improve responsiveness to L-DOPA and alleviate some of its adverse effects but is usually of little help in the management of the on-off phenomenon. Furthermore, a drug holiday carries the risks of aspiration pneumonia, venous thrombosis, pulmonary embolism, and depression resulting from the immobility accompanying severe parkinsonism. For these reasons and because of the temporary benefits of drug, drug holidays are not recommended.

LID: comprises of a variety of involuntary movements or postures, including chorea, dystonia, ballism, and myoclonus, which correlates with the L-DOPA dosing.

- *Rx of LID*
  - *Dopaminergic drugs.*
  - *Dopamine antagonists–atypical neuroleptic drugs with selective action.*
  - *Glutamatergic antagonists–amantadine and memantine.*
  - *Drugs acting on the serotoninergic system: buspirone.*
  - *Drugs acting on the serotoninergic system: buspirone.*

MAO-B Inhibitor

Selective irreversible MAO-B inhibitors.

1. Selegiline.
2. Rasagiline.
3. Safinamide (new drug).

Role of MAO–B in PD

MAOs catalyze the breakdown of monoamine neurotransmitters including dopamine, serotonin, and epinephrine in the CNS. There are two forms of isoenzymes of MAO–(1) and (2). MAO-B. Both are also present in peripheral adrenergic structures and intestinal mucosa. They have different affinities for substrates and inhibitors. MAO-A is the major form of MAO in intestine and stomach. MAO-A is found in norepinephrine and serotonin neurons in intestine and stomach and controls the metabolic degradation of serotonin and catecholamines. MAO-B is predominantly located in brain and platelets. The isoform MAO-A controls the selective metabolic degradation of noradrenaline, adrenaline, and serotonin (5-HT), whereas MAO-B regulates the selective metabolic degradation of dopamine.

Mechanism of Action

At normal doses, selegiline selectively and irreversibly inhibits MAO-B. It also retards the breakdown of dopamine by oxidative metabolism in the striatum. Selegiline also antagonizes the dopamine reuptake from the synaptic cleft, thus increasing the dopamine concentrations in the brain. Selegiline inhibits the MAO-B-induced breakdown of dopamine by oxidative metabolism in the striatum, thus reducing the generation of potentially toxic-free radicals (**Fig. 36.6**).

Consequence of the Inhibition of MAO-B by Selegiline

This enhances the dopamine concentration in the striatum and produces clinical effect. The reduced formation of potentially toxic free radicals form can further prevent the neurodegenerative changes in PD. If given along with L-DOPA, it prolongs the antiparkinsonian effect of L-DOPA and may reduce mild on-off or wearing-off phenomena. It also reduces the declining or fluctuating response to levodopa.

At normal doses, selegiline selectively and irreversibly inhibits MAO-B. It also retards the breakdown of dopamine by oxidative metabolism in the striatum. Selegiline also antagonizes the dopamine reuptake from the synaptic cleft, thus increasing the dopamine concentrations in the brain. Selegiline inhibits the MAO-B-induced breakdown of dopamine by oxidative metabolism in the striatum, thus reducing the generation of potentially toxic free radicals.

Consequence of the Inhibition of MAO-B by Selegiline

This enhances the dopamine concentration in the striatum and produces clinical effect. The reduced formation of potentially toxic free radicals can further prevent the neurodegenerative changes in PD. If given along with L-DOPA, it prolongs the antiParkinsonian effect of L-DOPA and may reduce mild on-off or wearing-off phenomena. It also reduces the declining or fluctuating response to L-DOPA.

Pharmacokinetics

The pharmacokinetics of selegiline following an oral dose of 10 mg are highly variable as depicted in **Table 36.3**.

Dose

Selegiline

The standard dose of selegiline is 5 mg with breakfast and 5 mg with lunch. Insomnia is common when taken later during the day. A total of 20 mg is used in endogenous depression.

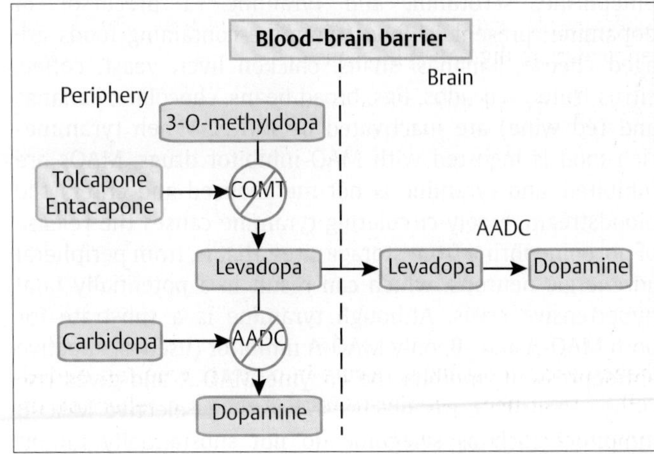

Fig. 36.6 Mechanism of action of catechol-O-methyl transferase (COMT) inhibitors.

Table 36.3 Pharmacokinetics of selegiline

Absorption	Rapidly absorbed. The absolute bioavailability of selegiline is approximately 10%.
Distribution	Apparent volume of distribution is 1854 L.
Metabolism	Partly metabolized by liver into methamphetamine and dexamphetamine, which causes insomnia and agitation.
Elimination	The oral clearance of selegiline (59 L/min) is many fold higher than the liver blood flow (1.5 L/min), indicating that extrahepatic processes are involved in the elimination of selegiline.
Plasma concentration	The mean peak plasma concentration (Cmax) is approximately 2 µg/L and the time to reach the peak is under an hour.
Half life	The elimination half-life is about 1.5 hours.

Rasagiline

Rasagiline is started at 0.5 mg once daily and then increased to 1 mg once daily, as long as it is well-tolerated.

Nausea, headache, anxiety, and insomnia are the most common side effects (due to formation of the amphetamine metabolites). Other possible adverse effects of MAO-B inhibitors are postural hypotension, confusion, accentuation of LID, and psychosis. Serious adverse reactions have rarely occurred following the concomitant use of selegiline with tricyclic antidepressants (TCADs) or selective serotonin reuptake inhibitors (SSRIs).

Drug Interactions

Selegiline interacts with

- Pethidine, which gives rise to excitement, rigidity, hyperthermia, respiratory depression.
- TCADs or SSRIs, which lead to serotonin syndrome type.
- Contraindicated in patients with convulsive disorders.

Food Interactions

"Hypertensive Crisis" or "Cheese Reaction"

Neurotransmitters such as dopamine, epinephrine, norepinephrine, serotonin, and tyramine (a precursor of dopamine) present in food (tyramine-containing foods are aged cheese, bananas, snails, chicken liver, yeast, coffee, citrus fruits, avocados, figs, broad beans, chocolate, bananas and red wine) are inactivated by MAOs. When tyramine-rich food is ingested with MAO-inhibitor drugs, MAOs are inhibited, and tyramine is not metabolized and enters the bloodstream. Freely circulating tyramine causes the release of norepinephrine from storage sites, that is, from peripheral adrenergic neurons, which can result in a potentially fatal hypertensive crisis. Although tyramine is a substrate for both MAO-A and -B, only MAO-A inhibitor (used as effective antidepressant) inhibits the enzyme MAO-A and gives rise to hypertensive crisis or cheese reaction. Selective MAO-B inhibitors such as selegiline do not substantially inhibit MAO-A, and thus there occurs the peripheral metabolism of catecholamines, which can be taken safely with L-DOPA in PD patients.

Indications and Effect of MAO-B Inhibitors on the Course of the Disease

- MAO-B inhibitor is used as initial therapy in patients at any age with very early PD and minimal signs and symptoms, looking for a small amount of benefit.
- MAO-B inhibitors are used as adjunctive therapy for patients with a fading or fluctuating response to L-DOPA. They are effective in 50 to 70% patients and allows 20 to 30% reduction in L-DOPA dose. They do not substantially inhibit the peripheral metabolism of catecholamines, thus do not exhibit the "cheese effect," and can be taken safely with L-DOPA.
- It is preferred in younger patients with early or mild PD, as they have mild antiparkinsonian and is generally well-tolerated. Not preferred in more advanced PD cases or underlying cognitive impairment, as they may increase the adverse motor and cognitive effects of L-DOPA therapy.

Rasagiline

Rasagiline is a newer selective MAO-B inhibitor with selegiline-like therapeutic effect in parkinsonism.

Advantages of Rasagiline

- In preventing MPTP-induced Parkinsonism, rasagiline is five times more potent than selegiline.
- Longer acting MAO-B inhibitor.
- Rasagiline does not give rise to undesirable amphetamine metabolites, unlike selegiline.
- Does not produce excitatory side effects if administered once a day in the morning.
- Effective in early PD. Used as adjunctive therapy in advanced PD, significantly reducing the L-DOPA-related "wearing off" symptoms.

Dopamine-Receptor Agonists

The dopamine-receptor agonists, direct agonists of striatal dopamine receptors, are an alternative to L-DOPA.

Older drugs	Newer drugs
▪ Bromocriptine	▪ Ropinirole
▪ Pergolide	▪ Pramipexole
▪ Cabergoline	▪ Apomorphine
▪ Lisuride	▪ Piribedil

Potential Advantages of Dopamine Agonists over L-DOPA

DA Agonists

- Do not require enzymatic conversion for activity.
- Even in the advanced stages, dopamine agonists stimulate the dopamine receptors in the striatum, where the neurons have lost the capacity to synthesize, store, and release dopamine from L-DOPA.
- Exert subtype selective activation of dopamine receptors involved in Parkinsonism.
- Do not depend on the functional capacities of the nigrostriatal neurons.

- Have substantially longer durations of action compared to L-DOPA.
- Are used in the management of dose-related fluctuations in motor state and is also useful in helpful in preventing motor complications.
- Modify the course of PD by reducing endogenous release of dopamine as well as the need for exogenous L-DOPA.
- Have lower incidence of the response fluctuations and dyskinesia that occur with long-term L-DOPA therapy..

Bromocriptine

It is a synthetic ergot derivative and a strong D2 agonist. Basically, bromocriptine is used in treatment of hyperprolactinemia and acromegaly.

Mechanisms of Action

It has L-DOPA-like action in CNS—D2 agonist and D1 partial agonist/antagonist. Quick improvement of PD symptoms and long-lasting therapeutic effect (1–2 hours vs. 6–10 hours).

Pharmacokinetic

The absorption from gastrointestinal tract (GIT) is variable. After an oral dose, peak plasma levels are reached within 1 to 2 hours. It is excreted in the bile and feces. The daily dose of bromocriptine for parkinsonism varies between 7.5 and 30 mg.

Adverse Effects

Vomiting, hallucinations, hypotension, and nasal stuffiness are the common adverse effects. First dose phenomenon is seen with a marked fall in BP. To minimize adverse effects, the dose is started with 1.25 mg twice daily after meals over 2 or 3 months and then increased by 2.5 mg every 2 weeks, depending on the response or the development of adverse reactions.

Bromocriptine is rarely used, as newer dopamine agonists have more pharmacodynamics and pharmacokinetics advantages. Reports of drug-induced cardiac valve fibrosis resulted in the withdrawal of pergolide from the US market in 2007.

Ropinirole and Pramipexole

Mechanism of Action

Both dopamine agonists bind selectively and strongly to D2 and D3 receptors. The drugs have negligible agonist/antagonist action at D1 receptor (seen in bromocriptine). Pramipexole, a synthetic derivative, has a seven-fold greater binding affinity to D3 dopamine receptors compared to D2 and D4 receptors. The D2 and D3 receptors are subtypes of D2 like dopamine receptor family. They belong to G protein-coupled receptors (GPCRs). These receptors are coupled to G proteins, G alpha i and G alpha o. They are inhibitory. Binding of dopamine agonists brings the confirmation changes in D2 and D3, and they act through multiple effectors:

- They inhibit AC (cAMP) activation via coupling protein Gi, resulting in a decrease in PKA activity. Additionally, they suppress the voltage sensitive Ca^{2+} currents and open the K+ channels directly via Go.

Adverse Effects

Common SE

Initial treatment causes nausea, vomiting, dizziness, postural hypotension, and ankle edema, which can be reduced rapidly by dose titration. Excessive daytime somnolence is an unfamiliar side effect, and therefore this should be avoided in drivers, factory workers and in people who require skills. Higher incidence of hallucinations and psychosis is observed in elderly patients.

Uncommon SE

These are specific to D3 agonism and can include hypersexuality, eating binges, compulsive hopping and compulsive gambling, even in patients without a prior history of these behaviors. This is due to a dysregulated dopamine-prefrontal reward system.

Dose

Prolonged release (PR) ropinirole, extended release (ER) pramipexole, and rotigotine transdermal patch. Ropinirole is started with 0.25 mg three times a day, and the maximum dose used is 24 mg per day. Pramipexole is started with 0.125 mg three times a day, and the maximum dose used is up to of 4.5 mg per day. Rotigotine is started with 2 mg/24 hr patch once a day and maximum of 8 mg/24 hr patch once a day.

Rotigotine transdermal patch is particularly convenient in PD patients with dysphagia.

Apomorphine

Apomorphine is a dopaminergic agonist, which has high affinity for D4 receptors, moderate affinity for D2, D3, and D5, and adrenergic 1D, 2B, and 2C receptors, and low affinity for D1 receptors. Apomorphine has been used as a "rescue therapy" for the acute intermittent treatment of "off" episodes in patients with a fluctuating response to dopaminergic therapy. It can be administered by subcutaneous (SC) injection.

Adverse Effects

Highly emetogenic potential and requires pre- and posttreatment antiemetic therapy. However, when apomorphine was administered with ondansetron, profound hypotension and loss of consciousness occurred; hence, the concomitant use of apomorphine with antiemetic drugs of the 5-HT3 antagonist is contraindicated.

Other potentially serious side effects of apomorphine include QT prolongation, injection-site reactions, and development of abuse characterized by increasingly frequent dosing, leading to hallucinations, dyskinesia, and abnormal behavior. Hence, apomorphine is appropriate only when other drugs such as dopamine agonists or COMT inhibitors have failed to control the "off" episodes.

Rotigotine

Rotigotine is a nonergot D3/D2/D1 dopamine receptor agonist approved for the treatment of early- and advanced-stage PD and moderate-to-severe restless legs syndrome

(RLS). Transdermal system delivery of rotigotine was approved in 2007 by the Food and Drugs Administration (FDA) for treatment of early PD, and it demonstrates dose-proportional pharmacokinetics and provides stable plasma concentrations over 24 hours. The dopamine agonist rotigotine is delivered daily through a skin patch. It provides stable plasma concentrations over 24 hours, thus more continuous dopaminergic stimulation than oral medication in early disease; its efficacy in more advanced disease is less clear. Benefits and side effects are similar to those of other dopamine agonists but reactions may also occur at the application site and are sometimes serious. The product was recalled in 2008 because of crystal formation on the patches, affecting the availability and efficacy of the agonist.

Indications and Effect of Dopamine Agonist on the Course of the Disease

- Ropinirole and pramipexole are preferred as first-line therapy in newly diagnosed patients under the age of 70 years old at present.
- Used as monotherapy for early and mild disease.
- Used as adjuvant to L-DOPA in patients with more advanced disease, as it smoothens the response to L-DOPA. These drugs are better-tolerated and have largely replaced the older agents (e.g., bromocriptine, pergolide), as the dose of these drugs requires titration more slowly.
- Used effectively in management of motor fluctuations and on/off phenomena, as they produce a more persistent period of dopamine receptor stimulation than L-DOPA due to longer duration of action of the dopamine agonists (8–24 hours) compared to L-DOPA (6-8 hours).
- They do not generate free radicals that are toxic on dopamine neurons, scavenge hydrogen peroxide, decrease excitotoxicity by suppressing subthalamic nucleus overactivity, and exert anti-apoptotic effects. They are used as neuroprotective drugs.
- Also used in RLS.

Catechol-O-Methyltransferase Inhibitors

1. Entacapone.
2. Tolcapone.
3. Opicapone (new drug).

Mechanism of Action

When L-DOPA is administered orally, nearly 99% of the drug is metabolized and does not reach the brain. In the presence of AADC, inhibition of the conversion of dopamine by carbidopa reduces and the fraction of L-DOPA in the periphery increases. In the periphery, the COMT transfers a methyl group to L-DOPA and metabolizes L-DOPA to pharmacologically inactive compounds, 3-O-methyl DOPA and 3-methoxytyramine, leading to fast elimination of L-DOPA (**Fig. 36.6**). COMT inhibitor (entacapone and tolcapone) selectively and reversibly inhibits COMT. Entacapone is active in the periphery, while tolcapone inhibits both central and peripheral COMT.

Consequences

They increase the fraction of each dose of L-DOPA that reaches the CNS, thus increasing its relative bioavailability and plasma elimination half-life, without affecting its peak plasma concentration. This leads to more stable plasma levels of L-DOPA, and the formation of 3-O-methyldopa is effectively reduced.

Pharmacokinetics

COMT inhibitors are developed to improve the pharmacokinetics of L-DOPA, and they are also used as an adjunct to combined L-DOPA and aromatic AADC inhibitor therapy.

Adverse effects include nausea, orthostatic hypotension, vivid dreams, confusion, and hallucinations. Entacapone has not been associated with hepatotoxicity and requires no special monitoring, whereas tolcapone has been associated with hepatotoxicity and requires special monitoring.

Indications and the Effect of COMT Inhibitors on the Course of the Disease

- Both drugs significantly reduce the "wearing off" symptoms; increase "on" time, decrease "off" time, allow L-DOPA dose to be reduced.
- They are not indicated in early PD cases; tolcapone is used only in nonresponders to other therapies, with appropriate monitoring for hepatic injury.
- Elevated homocysteine levels have been found in PD patients and appear to correlate with L-DOPA therapy. Addition of tolcapone resulted in a significant reduction of serum homocysteine and S-adenosylhomocysteine (SAH).

Glutamate (NMDA Receptor) Antagonist (Dopamine Facilitator)—Amantadine

Amantadine is an antiviral agent used for the prophylaxis and treatment of influenza A. Its use as antiparkinsonian drug was discovered by chance.

Mechanism of Action

Amantadine has multimodal mechanism of antiparkinsonian activity. It acts on central dopamine and noradrenaline neurons presynaptically, releases dopamine and noradrenaline from extragranular sites close to the nerve terminal, and antagonizes dopamine uptake. It blocks NMDA glutamate receptors, as NMDA glutamate receptors are excitatory, and enhances the degeneration of dopaminergic neurons in the substantia nigra (as the primary action at therapeutic concentrations). It antagonizes the effects of adenosine at adenosine A2A receptors, which are receptors that may inhibit D2 receptor function. It also possesses anticholinergic properties.

Amantadine is well-absorbed orally. It is primarily excreted unchanged in the urine by glomerular filtration and tubular secretion. It takes approximately 1 to 4 hours to achieve peak plasma concentration. The $t_{1/2}$ life is approximately 12 hours, and in patients with renal dysfunction, 18.5 hours to 33.8 days.

Amantadine is commonly introduced at a dose of 100 mg per day and slowly increased to an initial maintenance dose of 100 mg 2 or 3 times daily. Amantadine is available in an IR formulation, in 100 mg tablets or capsules, as well as ER once-daily formulations (capsules or tablets).

Adverse Effects

CNS effects include restlessness, depression, irritability, insomnia, agitation, excitement, hallucinations, and confusion. Overdose may produce acute toxic psychosis. The dermatological effects include livedo reticularis. Peripheral edema is not accompanied by signs of cardiac, hepatic, or renal disease and responds to diuretics. Other adverse reactions include headache, heart failure, postural hypotension, urinary retention, and GI disturbances (e.g., anorexia, nausea, constipation, and dry mouth).

Central Anticholinergics

- Trihexyphenidyl.
- Benztropine mesylate.
- Diphenhydramine.
- Centrally acting antihistaminics with anticholinergic properties.
  - Orphenadrine.
  - Procyclidine.

Anticholinergic drugs were the first pharmacological agents used in the treatment of PD before the discovery of L-DOPA. Compared to atropine, antimuscarinic drug, these drugs have a higher central actions compared to peripheral anticholinergic action.

Cholinergic interneurons (CINs) are the main source of acetylcholine (ACh) in the striatum. Normally, dopamine strongly inhibits ACh release from the striatum, and this critical balance between dopamine and ACh is crucial for normal motor functions. In PD, dopamine depletion produces a state of increased cholinergic activity in the basal ganglia (**Fig. 36.7**).

Mechanism of Action

There are five subtypes of muscarinic ACh receptors in the striatum that mediate the response to ACh. These muscarinic receptors arise primarily from cholinergic striatal interneurons. Like the dopamine receptors, these are GPCRs. The anticholinergic drugs are competitive antagonists of muscarinic receptors and block the receptors.

Adverse Effects

Adverse effects result from their anticholinergic properties (CNS and peripheral effects). The side effect profile is similar to atropine. Peripheral antimuscarinic side effects consist of dry mouth, blurred vision, constipation, nausea, urinary retention, impaired sweating, and tachycardia. In the elderly, sedation, memory impairment, mental confusion, blurred vision through cycloplegia, and urinary retention are more common (caution is advised in patients with known prostatic hypertrophy or closed-angle glaucoma). Dyskinesias rarely occurs. Dryness of the mouth can cause acute suppurative parotitis as a complication.

Effect of Central Anticholinergic on the Course of the Disease

Anticholinergic drugs are used as monotherapy few times for patients with PD who are ≤65 years of age with troubling tremor but do not have significant bradykinesia or gait disturbance. In mild cases, they may be used alone or used when L-DOPA is contraindicated. They can be combined with L-DOPA to lower L-DOPA dose. They are useful in patients with more advanced disease who have persistent and troubling tremor despite treatment with L-DOPA or dopamine. In drug (phenothiazine)-induced parkinsonism, anticholinergics are the drug of choice. All anticholinergics produce 10 to 25% improvement in parkinsonian symptoms lasting 4 to 8 hours after a single dose. Tremor is benefited more than rigidity; hypokinesia is affected the least. Anticholinergics are better in effectively controlling sialorrhea due to their peripheral action. Gradual withdrawal of medication is advised rather than abruptly to prevent acute exacerbation of parkinsonism and to avoid anticholinergics in older adults with PD and those with significant cognitive impairment due to increased risk of adverse effects, including cognitive impairment, constipation, and urinary retention.

Management of Parkinson's Disease

When to Start Drug Therapy

The degree of symptoms that interfere with functioning or impair the quality of life are the factors considered to initiate symptomatic medical therapy in patients with PD. No patient should be delayed or deprived of the treatment unnecessarily, as the therapeutic benefit occurs early in the disease, when the potential for sustained improvement is greatest. Patients should be reassured that the onset of motor fluctuations likely depends on the rate of progression of underlying disease, rather than choice of initial therapy.

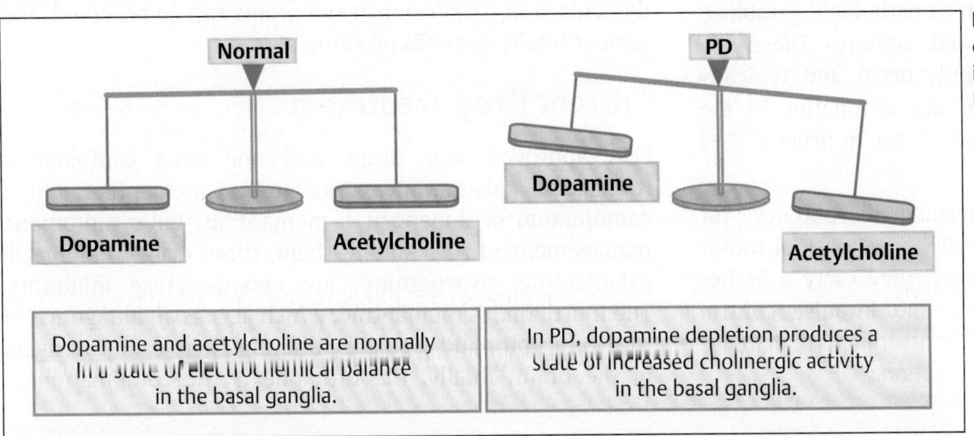
Normal
PD
Dopamine
Acetylcholine
Dopamine
Acetylcholine
Dopamine and acetylcholine are normally in a state of electrochemical balance in the basal ganglia.
In PD, dopamine depletion produces a state of increased cholinergic activity in the basal ganglia.

Fig. 36.7 Depiction of the brain levels of dopamine and acetylcholine (ACh) in normal people and patients with Parkinson's disease (PD).

How to Choose Initial Therapy

There is no single preferred therapy. The trial-and-error approach is followed which customizes treatment to the individual patient.

The four main classes of drugs that have antiparkinsonian activity are:

- L-DOPA.
- Dopamine agonists.
- MAO-B inhibitors.
- Amantadine.
- Anticholinergic drugs also have some activity, mainly for tremor.

The American Academy of Neurology recommends initiating the treatment with L-DOPA to improve motor disability or a dopamine agonist to lessen motor complications.

L-DOPA, coupled with a peripheral DOPA decarboxylase inhibitor such as carbidopa, remains the gold standard of symptomatic treatment for PD. L-DOPA/carbidopa is started with a low dose and increased slowly over 3 months and frequently evaluated. A sustained good response is observed on a daily L-DOPA dosage of 300 to 600 mg/day (usually divided 3 or 4 times daily) for 3 to 5 years or longer and then starts declining. The long-term L-DOPA is related with the development of fluctuations and dyskinesias. The fluctuations and dyskinesias are difficult to treat once they set in. The other antiparkinsonian drugs are preferred, and initiation of L-DOPA is delayed only due to these adverse effects. Dopamine agonists are commonly reserved for younger individuals (<65–70 years) who are cognitively intact. L-DOPA can be added only when the dopamine agonist (with or without an MAO-B inhibitor) no longer provides good control of motor symptoms. The patients aged 65 to 70 years who are cognitively intact are treated with a dopamine agonist before L-DOPA and add L-DOPA/carbidopa is added when necessary.

For patients with cognitive impairment and aged 70 years prone to adverse effects, such as hallucinations, from dopamine agonists. It is always wise to avoid and instead to prescribe L-DOPA/ peripheral decarboxylase inhibitor (PDI) as primary symptomatic therapy.

While adding a dopamine agonist, start at a low dose and increase slowly. Patients on dopamine agonists should be regularly asked about sleepiness, sudden onset of sleep, and impulse control disorders such as pathologic gambling, shopping, internet use, and sexual activity. These are the adverse effects which commonly occur and typically resolve with reduction in dose or discontinuation of the medication. Patients should be warned not to drive if they are experiencing undue sleepiness.

Dopamine agonists have intermediate potency for improving motor symptoms and have a lower risk of motor complications than L-DOPA; however, they carry a higher risk of somnolence, hallucinations, and impulse control disorders (ICDs), and they are not well-tolerated in older adults and those with cognitive dysfunction.

MAO-B inhibitors, amantadine, or (in younger patients) anticholinergics are preferred drugs in patients with mild symptoms.

For patients with tremor-dominant disease, anticholinergic agents are drug of choice not appropriately controlled with dopaminergic drugs. Anticholinergic medications relieves tremor in approximately 50% of patients but do not improve bradykinesia or rigidity.

Drugs for The Treatment of Alzheimer's Disease (PH1.19)

Alzheimer disease (AD) is a progressive, neurodegenerative disorder. It is a common type of dementia, which comprises 80% cases of clinical dementia cases worldwide. AD commonly affects people more than 65 years of age, however, early onset AD can be seen among patients less than 65 years of age also.

Symptoms

The symptoms of AD are categorized into three group: symptoms of cognitive dysfunction, noncognitive symptoms, and other symptoms.

Symptoms of Cognitive Dysfunction

Core clinical symptoms of AD include gradual memory decline and executive function. Short-term memory impairment and inability to retain new information are clinical hallmarks of AD, which manifest clinically as asking same question repeatedly and frequent misplacing of objects. Occasionally aphasia or visuoconstructive dysfunction may be the initial presentation. However, long-term memory, implicit, and working memory is affected only at late stage of the disease.

Noncognitive Symptoms

Noncognitive neuropsychiatric symptom occurs in mid to late stage of AD which include depression, anxiety, delusion, hallucination, apathy, disturbed social interaction, psychosis, and agitation in various degrees, depending upon disease severity.

Other Symptoms

In the late stage of AD, olfactory dysfunction, sleep disorder, dystonia, and parkinsonism symptoms can be observed, and patient totally depends on caregivers.

Current Drug Treatment

FDA approved four drugs and one drug combination (donepezil, galantamine, rivastigmine, memantine and a combination of donepezil + memantine) for symptomatic management of AD. Among them, three drugs (donepezil, galantamine, rivastigmine) are cholinesterase inhibitors. The fourth one is memantine, which acts as an antagonist of NMDA receptor and regulates different chemical messengers in the brain; finally, the fifth one is the combination of acetylcholinesterase inhibitor (AChEI donepezil) and NMDA receptor antagonist (memantine).

AChEIs are prescribed to improve the memory, judgment, language, thinking, and other cognitive-related processes. Donepezil is prescribed for all stages of AD. For mild-to-moderate stage, galantamine and rivastigmine drugs are used, but they show some side effects like vomiting, loss of appetite, nausea, etc.

Acetylcholinesterase Inhibitor (AChEI)

Donepezil

Donepezil is a reversible, noncompetitive inhibitor. Bioavailability is 100% with a Tmax of 3 to 4 hours, and steady-state concentration is achieved in 15 to 21 days of administration. Plasma protein binding (PPB) of donepezil is around 96%. It is metabolized first in liver (CYP3A4 and CYP2D6). Volume of distribution is approximately 11 L/kg for 10 mg dose. It is able to cross the BBB. In mild-to-moderate AD, the initial recommended dose is 5 mg/day, which can be increased to 10 mg/day after initial stabilization at 5 mg/day for 4 weeks. In case of moderate-to-severe disease, a higher dose of 23 mg/day (SR, to be swallowed, not crushed/chewed, OD dose, absorption not affected by timing of administration of concomitant food) is found to be safe, however, before initiation of this dose, the patient needs to be stabilized on 10 mg/day for at least 3 months.

Galantamine

The dose of galantamine is 4 to 16 mg/day twice daily. The half-life of galantamine is 6 to 8 h. It is absorbed with 100% bioavailability. The PPB is 18%, and it is also able to cross the BBB. It is metabolized by liver and excreted in urine. The ER version, initial recommended starting dose is 8 mg per day in the morning, which can be increased to 16 mg/day and 24 mg/day within 4 weeks' time in between and as per safety profile.

Rivastigmine

Rivastigmine is also known as a pseudo-irreversible AChEI. It is orally given and almost completely absorbed within 1 hour. Concomitant food lowers the absorption rate. The commonly used starting dose is 1.5 mg twice daily. After stabilization at this dose for 2 weeks, depending upon the tolerability and requirement, the dosed can be increased to 3 mg twice daily. Following this same dose increment/titration strategy, the dose can be further increased to 4.5 mg twice daily and subsequently 6 mg BD (recommended highest dose).

NMDA Antagonist: Memantine

Memantine is a noncompetitive antagonist of the NMDA. Memantine tends to function to control the excess glutamate activity; however, it has some side effects like confusion, constipation, headache, and dizziness. Memantine is given in 5 mg dose once daily and is 100% orally bioavailable.

Managing Comorbidities

As AD is a disease of the old, comorbid conditions are commonly encountered among AD patients. Presence of higher comorbidity is generally associated with worse cognitive function and poorer self-care. So, addressing these conditions are important part of routine AD care. Psychological comorbid conditions are common among AD patients, especially in advanced cases. Management of the same is important. Early recognition and treatment of comorbid medical conditions can limit neuropsychiatric and behavioral symptoms. Treatment of behavioral and psychiatric symptoms is another issue which needs to be addressed critically. Although management is a bit difficult; however, nonpharmacologic measures are the first ones to be preferred. For agitation and psychosis, atypical antipsychotics can be used; however they should be judiciously used, taking care of adverse effect profile and, more specifically, serious adverse effect profile. In case of depression or anxiety, antidepressants can be used after risk benefit assessment.

Multiple Choice Questions

1. A 56-year-old man with a strong family history of Parkinson's disease sees a neurologist for an evaluation. On examination, the neurologist observes a slight pill rolling tremor and gait abnormalities. The patient is prescribed levodopa along with the addition of carbidopa. What is the rationale for adding carbidopa?

A. Carbidopa stimulates dopamine receptors.
B. Carbidopa enhances L-DOPA absorption.
C. Carbidopa blocks peripheral COMT.
D. Carbidopa functions as a dopamine agonist.
E. Carbidopa increases L-DOPA entry into the central nervous system (CNS) by inhibiting peripheral DOPA decarboxylase.

Answer: E

L-DOPA is a prodrug and the immediate metabolic precursor of dopamine. L-DOPA is converted into dopamine mostly by decarboxylase enzymes (aromatic L-amino acid decarboxylase) in the intestinal mucosa and other peripheral sites if L-DOPA is administered alone.

In addition, dopamine released into the circulation by peripheral conversion of L-DOPA acts on heart, blood vessels, other peripheral organs and on chemoreceptor trigger zone (CTZ). Also, it produces nausea and vomiting.

Carbidopa, unlike L-DOPA, does not penetrate the CNS and inhibits peripheral decarboxylase enzyme and markedly increases the fraction of administered L-DOPA (unchanged form of dug) to cross the blood-brain barrier (BBB) and also reduces the incidence of gastrointestinal (GI) and other peripheral side effects.

2. All the statements about L-DOPA is correct except:

A. Avoid heavy protein meals when L-DOPA is administered.
B. Abrupt discontinuation of L-DOPA will not affect the patient condition.
C. Domperidone is preferred over prochlorperazine to improve nausea and postural hypotension.
D. 80% of patients receiving L-DOPA therapy for long periods will have dyskinesias.

Answer: B

Patients should be warned not to discontinue L-DOPA suddenly as this can result in the parkinsonism-hyperpyrexia syndrome and dyskinetic syndrome. Parkinsonism-hyperpyrexia is clinically similar to neuroleptic malignant syndrome.

3. The patient in the previous question returns to see his neurologist 3 years later. The patient's symptoms have progressed and he has now marked bradykinesia and an intense shuffling gait. To prevent further worsening, the neurologist prescribes a catechol-O-methyl transferase (COMT) inhibitor along with patient's L-DOPA and carbidopa. Which agent below is likely to have been added?

A. Entacapone.
B. Selegiline.
C. Ropinirole.
D. Amantadine.
E. Benztropine.

Answer: A

L-DOPA is metabolized partly by COMT; therefore, entacapone is COMT inhibitor. When entacapone is given in combination with L-DOPA and carbidopa, plasma levels of L-DOPA are higher and more constant than after administration of L-DOPA and carbidopa alone. L-DOPA/carbidopa/entacapone is useful in advanced Parkinson's disease in patients with motor fluctuations and an adjunct treatment for patients on L-DOPA. It does however increase the side effects including diarrhea, postural hypotension, nausea, and hallucinations.

4. Antiviral drug found to have antiparkinsonian properties:

A. Procyclidine.
B. Pergolide.
C. Amantadine.
D. L-DOPA.
E. Reserpine.

Answer: C

Amantadine is an antiviral agent used for the prophylaxis and treatment of influenza A. Its use as antiparkinsonian drug was discovered by chance.

5. All are true about tolcapone except:

A. Has central inhibition of catechol-O-methyl-transferase (COMT).
B. Has relatively longer duration of action compared to entacapone.
C. Has been associated with hepatotoxicity.
D. Requires special monitoring.

Answer: A

Tolcapone is a central and peripheral inhibitor of COMT. It is highly plasma albumin bound (> 99.8%), hence has a long duration of action, and its distribution is therefore restricted. Since it causes hepatotoxicity, it requires special monitoring.

6. All are true about the advantages of dopamine agonists over L-DOPA except:

A. Depends on the functional capacities of the nigro striatal neurons.
B. Does not require enzymatic conversion for activity.
C. Has substantially longer durations of action compared to L-DOPA.
D. Modifies the course of Parkinson's disease (PD) by reducing endogenous release of dopamine as well as the need for exogenous L-DOPA.

Answer: A

Dopamine agonists do not depend on the functional capacities of the nigrostriatal neurons.

7. Selegiline retards the progression of the Parkinson's disease, but it should not be used along with which of the following:

A. Meperidine.
B. Tricyclic drugs.
C. Selective serotonin reuptake inhibitors (SSRIs).
D. All of the above.

Answer: D

Selegiline interacts with pethidine and similar drugs and gives rise to excitement, rigidity, hyperthermia, and respiratory depression. Tricyclic antidepressants or SSRIs lead to serotonin-like syndrome.

8. A 71-year-old patient has had Parkinson's disease for 10 years and is currently taking pramipexole 0.5 mg three times a day, carbidopa/L-DOPA 25/100 three times a day and benztropine. His wife says that he has developed a habit of gambling and shopping. He falls asleep during the daytime. Which drug is causing these effects?

A. Pramipexole.
B. Carbidopa/L-DOPA.
C. Benztropine.
D. All the above drugs.

Answer: A

Pramipexole is a dopamine agonist that may be used in the treatment of Parkinson's disease and restless legs syndrome. It may cause spontaneous sedation and psychotic-like side effects. Excessive daytime somnolence is an unfamiliar side effect and should be avoided in drivers, factory workers, and in people who require skills. This is commonly seen in elderly patients.

9. A 67-year-old man with Parkinson's disease experiences worsening of his symptoms. He is on L-DOPA. Which medication should be added to inhibit the unopposed action of cholinergic neurons, as the disease is characterized by degeneration of dopaminergic neurons, to alleviate the patient's symptoms?

A. Benztropine.
B. Reserpine.
C. Doxazocin.
D. Timolol.
E. Tubocurarine.

Answer: A

Benztropine, an antimuscarinic agent, is used as an adjunct for the treatment of PD.

10. Memantine is:

A. Acetylcholinesterase inhibitor.
B. NMDA receptor antagonist.
C. NMDA receptor agonist.
D. None of these.

Answer: B

Memantine is a noncompetitive antagonist of the NMDA.

11. Which anti-Alzheimer's drug combination is approved by FDA?

A. Donepezil and memantine.
B. Donepezil and rivastigmine.
C. Donepezil and galantamine.
D. Rivastigmine and galantamine.

Answer: A

The FDA approved four drugs and one drug combination, that is, donepezil, galantamine, rivastigmine, memantine and a combination of donepezil + memantine for symptomatic management of Alzheimer's disease.

Chapter 37 CNS Stimulants and Drugs of Abuse

Anupam Raja, Harvinder Singh, Harish Kumar, Phulen Sarma, Ajay Prakash, and Bikash Medhi

PH1.22: Describe drugs of abuse (dependence, addiction, stimulants, depressants, psychedelics, drugs used for criminal offences).

PH1.23: Describe the process and mechanism of drug deaddiction.

Learning Objectives

- Analeptic stimulants or respiratory stimulants.
- Psychomotor stimulants.
- Xanthines.
- Opioids.

CNS Stimulant (PS4.6)

Central nervous system (CNS) stimulants are known to antagonize the range of depressive behaviors, nervousness, and anxiety. They are mostly used in the symptomatic treatment of attention-deficit disorder, narcolepsy, or excessive sleepiness. There are three categories of molecules that act as stimulant i.e., analeptic stimulants or respiratory stimulants, psychomotor stimulants, and xanthines. Examples of stimulants include methylphenidate, atomoxetine, modafinil, armodafinil, and amphetamines. Although stimulants have been effective for altering behaviors or medical conditions, some of them are abused such as cocaine and ecstasy or methylenedioxymethamphetamine (MDMA).

Generally, stimulant administration acts on glutamatergic, GABAergic, and dopaminergic neurons, resulting in global CNS hyperexcitability, and at high dose it causes convulsions. The generation of stimulation signaling in the CNS occurs mostly via the following mechanisms:

1. Potentiation of excitatory receptors (inotropic receptors, metabotropic receptors, and kainate receptors).
2. Inhibition of GABAergic receptors.
3. Alteration in neurotransmitter release.

Molecules that induce stimulation signaling in the CNS are classified into three classes considering their proposed mechanism of action and chemical structure:

1. **Analeptic stimulants**: doxapram, nikethamide, pentylenetetrazol (PTZ), strychnine, picrotoxin, bicuculline.
2. **Psychomotor stimulants**: amphetamine, methamphetamine, methylphenidate, pemoline, ephedrine, phentermine, fenfluramine, phenylpropanolamine.
3. **Methylxanthines**: caffeine, theophylline, theobromine.

Often, CNS stimulants are used primarily as respiratory stimulants to reverse the acute toxicity of CNS depressants (e.g., barbiturates). There are certain limitations of using CNS stimulants, which restrict their recommendation clinically, including: (1) they have unspecific effect on CNS depressant agents, (2) the action of CNS stimulants is so quick as compared to that of depressants, (3) they have low therapeutic window (required dose to produce the therapeutic effect against severe depression is so close to the convulsant-initiating dose that patients often end up with life-threatening complications), and (4) CNS stimulants are associated with tolerance and abuse, such as amphetamine and many of its congeners. Considering the above-mentioned limitations, it has been recommended to take supportive measures (e.g., elevation of low blood pressure and maintenance of a patent airway) with CNS depressant. Unlike antidepressants, these agents only raise the amount of CNS excitement and cannot influence depression solely, and thereby the words antidepressant and psychostimulant can be distinguished.

Analeptic Stimulants or Respiratory Stimulants

These compounds cause certain activations of the organism's mental and physical activity. They majorly excite the medulla's vasomotor and respiratory centers. Examples include doxapram, PTZ, strychnine, picrotoxin, bicuculline, and nikethamide.

Chemistry and Pharmacokinetics

Analeptic stimulants can be categorized based on their source of origin:

1. Natural molecules (e.g., picrotoxin and strychnine).
2. Synthetic molecules (e.g., doxapram and PTZ).

It is difficult to classify analeptic stimulants based on pharmacokinetics parameters due to their broad range of chemical structure. Most analeptic stimulants have quick and short response durations and show good oral absorption. Most of the drugs are metabolized in the liver rather than being eliminated unchanged by the kidneys.

Mechanism of Action

Generally, drugs of analeptic class show pharmacological activity via regulating the gamma-aminobutyric acid (GABA) receptor and altering the chloride influx to the neuronal cell. Inhibitory signaling has been principally regulated by amino acid neurotransmitters (e.g., GABA) via promoting the chloride influx.

Chloride channel facilitation can be controlled by three distinct sites: (1) GABA-binding site, (2) benzodiazepine-binding site, and (3) picrotoxin-binding site.

Clinical Uses

Analeptic stimulants were used to manage overdosage of CNS depressants, whereas some of the analeptics were also recommended to stimulate the respiratory systems after the aesthetic depression such as doxapram (Dopram). PTZ (metrazol) and strychnine have been exclusively used to activate "the electroencephalogram" experimentally and for exploring the CNS mechanisms in the spinal cord.

Adverse Effects

CNS stimulants are liable to produce adverse reactions because they have very low therapeutic window. Convulsion, coma, and death are the main adverse reactions produced by this class of stimulants. Mostly, tonic-clonic types of convulsion are the adverse effect of CNS stimulant. In certain cases, pronounced stimulation of breathing, tachycardia, and extreme pressure symptoms are followed by convulsions. Uncontrolled stimulation after unintended or deliberate strychnine absorption (in the absence of natural inhibition) leads to seizures.

Doxapram

Doxapram is a respiratory stimulant with analeptic activity. Doxapram, independent of oxygen levels, directly stimulates the peripheral carotid chemoreceptors, possibly by inhibiting the potassium channels of type I cells within the carotid body, thereby stimulating catecholamines release. This results in the prevention or reversal of both narcotic- and CNS depressant-induced respiratory depression.

Dose

The recommended dose for intravenous (IV) administration is 0.5 to 1 mg/kg for a single injection and at 5-minute intervals. The maximum total dosage by IV injection is 2 mg/kg.

Adverse Reaction

Symptoms of toxicity are manifestations of pharmacological effects of the drug. Excessive pain, skeletal muscle hyperactivity, tachycardia, and improved deep tendon reflexes can be early signs of overdose.

Strychnine

Strychnine is a terpene indole alkaloid that comes from the family of *Corynanthe* alkaloids, originating from secologanin and tryptamine. It induces excitement in all areas of the CNS. Strychnine is a competitive antagonist for inhibitory neurotransmitter glycine receptors in the spinal cord, brain stem, and higher centers. As a consequence, it improves neuronal activation and excitability, in addition to greater muscle activity.

Pharmacokinetics and Toxicokinetics

It is quickly absorbed from the gastrointestinal (GI) tract, mucous membranes, and parenteral injection sites, as well as from the oral route. Strychnine is distributed via plasma and erythrocytes, but protein binding is minor and tissue delivery happens rapidly. The absorption half-life is nearly 15 minutes and metabolism half-life is approximately 10 hours.

Dose

The lethal dose (LD_{50}) is 1.5 to 2 mg/kg orally in humans.

Adverse Reaction

Strychnine induces convulsions in decerebrate animals. Convulsions are referred to as spinal convulsions, but other areas of the CNS are also activated by doses that trigger motor manifestations in decerebrate animals. There are actually no legitimate applications of strychnine. Accidental poisoning occurs, particularly in children. The treatment of poisoning is identical to that of epileptic status.

Pentylenetetrazol (PTZ, Metrazol, Leptazol)

Pentylenetetrazole, also known as metrazol, pentetrazol (INN), pentamethylenetetrazol, Corazol, Cardiazol, Deumacard, or PTZ, is a drug previously used as a respiratory and circulatory stimulant.

It is a potent CNS stimulant, assumed to function through direct depolarization of the CNS. In addition, it interacts with GABAergic ($GABA_A$ receptor) inhibition and is anxiogenic by acting in a way similar to picrotoxin. It was also used to cause seizures during the use of single photon emission computed tomography (SPECT) scanning to identify the epileptic target as a screening technique in patients with drug-resistant epilepsy. PTZ-induced epilepsy is a proven model for studying anticonvulsant drugs in experimental animals. Several groups of drugs can regulate the different stimuli of PTZ, such as 5-HT_3, 5-HT_{1A}, glycine, *N*-methyl-D-aspartate (NMDA), and L-type calcium channel ligands.

Dose

At low doses, it acts as CNS stimulant, whereas at large doses it shows convulsion behavior similar to picrotoxin. PTZ delivered subcutaneously absorbs quickly.

Picrotoxin

Picrotoxin, also known as cocculin, is obtained from the shrub *Anamirta cocculus*. It is a noncompetitive inhibitor and acts via antagonizing the $GABA_A$ receptor/Cl^- channel due to stimulation of the CNS. Therefore, picrotoxin inhibits the permeability of the Cl^- channel and thereby promotes an inhibitory impact on a particular neuron. Picrotoxin decreases conductance across the channel by decreasing the opening period as well as the average open time. Vomiting and GI and vasomotor relaxations are caused by convulsions. Although known to be a medullary stimulant, the site of action has no selectivity. The drug of choice for picrotoxin poisoning is diazepam, which promotes GABAergic delivery. Picrotoxin is rarely absorbed orally with a short duration of action. In humans, it is highly toxic and leads to poisoning at doses as low as 20 mg. In contrast to picrotoxin, bicuculline is a competitive, light-sensitive $GABA_A$ receptor antagonist.

Psychomotor Stimulants

Psychostimulants are the most commonly used psychotropic drugs. A "psychostimulant" may be described as a psychotropic drug capable of stimulating the CNS. It induces enthusiasm, high mood, and increased alertness and excitement. The net impact of this is to accelerate brain signals. It is also possible to negatively define a psychostimulant as a substance other than a depressant or a hallucinogenic substance. Hyperkinesia, overactivity, impulsiveness, carelessness, and social change are greatly enhanced by psychostimulant. Amphetamine compound and its derivatives (e.g., dexamphetamine, methylamphetamine, and methylphenidate) are the main psychomotor stimulants. Psychomotor stimulant drugs mostly show good bioavailability via oral administration; however, some of these drugs also show beneficial effect in the injectable form. Studies revealed that a fraction of amphetamine is excreted through the urine in the unchanged form.

Amphetamine (Adderall, Benzedrine, Dexedrine)

Amphetamine, a chemical discovered more than 100 years ago, is one of the most restrictive synthetic substances. It has played a major role on brain nerve terminals to release monoamines, mostly dopamine, serotonin, and noradrenaline, by binding with presynaptic membrane transporters—responsible for the reuptake of dopamine (dopamine transporter [DAT]), serotonin (serotonin transporter [SERT]), and norepinephrine (norepinephrine transporter [NET]). In addition, it also shows inhibitory action on monoamine oxidase (MAO) at high doses; hence, to what extent it produces the therapeutics effect is questionable. A new class of G protein–based trace-amine receptors (encoded by the TAAR1 [trace amine-associated receptor 1] gene) involved in mediating direct effects has been identified in recent studies. Amphetamine is believed to be metabolized by the liver under CYP2D6. The major metabolites are potent hallucinogenic including 4-hydroxynorephedrine, 4-hydroxyamphetamine, hippuric acid, benzoic acid, benzyl methyl ketone, and p-hydroxyamphetamine. It is generally used for symptomatic management of attention-deficit disorders and narcolepsy. In addition, amphetamine is currently even used off-label for obesity, anxiety, and chronic pain. In contrast to medicinal use, it is associated with wide range of side effects such as nervousness, headaches, palpitations, insomnia, hyperpyrexia, dizziness, anorexia, hypertension, weight loss, and mouth dryness. It is a schedule II drug (high risk of misuse).

Methamphetamine

Methamphetamine, a potent psychomotor stimulant, is a sympathomimetic drug. It has higher potency than amphetamines. The main effects of this drug on the CNS are euphoria, increased energy, enhanced level of mental alertness, tachycardia, and reduced appetite; it also promotes weight loss and leads to insomnia.

Basically, methamphetamine is effective as dopaminergic and adrenergic and in higher concentration it acts as a monoamine oxidase inhibitor (MAOI). This sympathomimetic drug enters the brain and triggers a cascade by releasing norepinephrine, dopamine, and serotonin. It acts as a potent agonist for TAAR1, that is, it acts as G protein–coupled receptor that regulates the catecholamines system in the brain. The activation of TAAR1 leads to increased activity of cyclic adenosine monophosphate (cAMP), which results in the inhibition or recovering of the transport of NET, DAT, and SERT. This, in turn, triggers the transport of protein kinase A (PKA) and PKC signaling, causing phosphorylation and increasing intracellular Ca^{2+} concentration and producing an efflux of dopamine. Also, it is an agonist for α_2 adrenergic receptor and sigma receptor and inhibits MOAI affecting the CNS by promoting neurotoxicity in the brain. An IV dose of 200 mg or more is considered to be fatal and the biological half-life of this drug is approximately 4 to 5 hours. Although the route of elimination is urine, 30 to 54% remains as unchanged methamphetamine and 10 to 23% as unchanged amphetamine.

Dextromethamphetamine hydrochloride (Desoxyn), an approved drug by the FDA, is used for treating attention-deficit/hyperactive disorder (ADHD) and increased weight in adults and children. Also, methamphetamine is sometimes used for narcolepsy and idiopathic hypersomnia. Methamphetamine is quite potent for euphoriants and is also present in the form of levorotary in over-the-counter nasal decongestant products.

Physically, it affects the person in a number of ways, such as loss of appetite, dilated pupils, accelerated or slowed heartbeat, hypertension, dizziness, numbness, and dry skin. The addictive users of this drug may lose their teeth quickly in an abnormal way, causing a condition known as "meth mouth" and resulting into xerostomia (dry mouth). This drug may also lead to abrasions, genital sores, or bruxism, leading to an increased risk of sexually transmitted infections. The increased neurotoxicity, excitotoxicity, oxidative stress, protein nitration, and endoplasmic reticulum stress increases are also some of the adverse effects of methamphetamine.

Methylphenidate

It is a CNS stimulant quite similar to amphetamine and is considered to be a schedule II drug. It is usually the most prescribed medication in children. Methylphenidate is most importantly used for narcolepsy and ADHD in patients in the age range 6 to 16 years. The exact mechanism of this drug is still unclear; but generally, it is thought that it acts as a potent reuptake inhibitor of dopamine and norepinephrine and increases concentration of these neurotransmitters in extracellular space of synapse, resulting into prolonged effect. Effects of psychostimulant on stimulating receptors occur when high dose of psychostimulant causes increased norepinephrine and dopamine efflux in the brain, resulting in impairment of cognitive- and locomotory-activating effects. Lower doses are usually recommended to treat ADHD but are not correlated with locomotory-activating effects. Children with ADHD have an abnormality in DAT1 (dopamine activator transporter gene), which is overcome by the dopaminergic effect of methylphenidate.

With a peak of elevation in blood level in 1 to 3 hours, this drug is rapidly absorbed. Methylphenidate and dexmethylphenidate are available in the form of capsules for oral administration or as transdermal patch. For a long time, it is being used for the treatment of ADHD in 6- to 16-year-old children. It is also effective in treating narcolepsy.

The adverse effects usually include anorexia, insomnia, nervousness, and fever. GI effects including nausea and abdominal pain are also common. It is also contraindicated in patients with glaucoma or seizure (leads to an increased frequency of seizures).

Pemoline

It is a stimulant drug of 4-oxazolidinone class. It is a unique CNS stimulant, which exhibits the minimalistic sympathomimetic effects. Pemoline shows pharmacological aspects like amphetamines and methylphenidate. But it is the least potent to cause addictive effect on CNS. It is also used to treat ADHD and narcolepsy.

It stimulates the brain by affecting the neurotransmitters communicating the neurons. Generally, it is considered as dopaminergic and passes the blood–brain barrier, acting as a surrogate for the dopamine neurotransmitters. It is similar to amphetamine but has a slower onset of action and a long half-life of 12 to 16 hours. It usually acts by DAT inhibition similar to amphetamine. Also, it inhibits the MAO-B inhibitor by prolonging the extracellular monoamine effects.

Similar to amphetamine, it is readily absorbed in the GI tract. The half-life of pemoline is around 12 hours. The oral administration of pemoline is with an initial dose of 39.5 mg every morning and maintenance dose of 18.75 mg/day at an interval of 1 week.

Along with ADHD and narcolepsy, it is also used to enhance the motor activity and relief from drowsiness. Pemoline causes side effects on the person's body, including anorexia, stomach ache, rash on skin, irritability, nausea, dizziness, headache, insomnia, and hallucinations. Also, it causes hepatotoxicity, leading to jaundice or complete liver failure.

Ephedrine

A medication and stimulant drug was first described in 1888 in the English literature which occurs naturally in the Ephedra plant. It is an adrenergic receptor, which acts as an agonist and is basically used for its vasoconstrictive property and positive chronotropic and inotropic effects. It is commonly used in treating hypotension.

It is a direct or indirect sympathomimetic amine. It activates α- and β-adrenergic receptors as well as inhibits the reuptake of norepinephrine and increases the release of norepinephrine in nerve cells via vesicles. Due to these combined actions, large amount of norepinephrine accumulates in the synapse over a longer period of time, leading to the increased stimulation of the sympathetic nervous system. The stimulation of α_1 receptor causes increased stimulation, followed by a rise in chronotropic and inotropic effects. It causes bronchodilation by acting on the β2 receptor.

Being a sympathomimetic amine, it activates the adrenergic receptor by increasing the heart rate, blood pressure, and bronchodilation.

The IV injection of this drug is basically used for the treatment of hypotension under general anesthesia and of allergic conditions such as bronchial asthma, nasal congestions, myasthenia gravis, and narcolepsy. Ephedrine and pseudoephedrine also act as bronchodilators and promotes weight loss similar to amphetamines.

It is considered to be a dangerous natural compound by the FDA (2004/USA). It severely affects the GI tract (nausea), respiratory system (dyspnea, edema), and nervous system (insomnia, hallucination, panic, restlessness), as well as causes cardiovascular diseases (angina pectoris, tachycardia).

Phentermine

It is a sympathomimetic amine anorectic agent, which was first introduced in 1959 in combination with an antiobesity drug. It shows chemical similarity with amphetamine and hence is known as atypical amphetamine. It is classified under schedule IV drugs. This drug is basically used to treat obesity and is also available in combination with topiramate.

It is an indirectly acting sympathomimetic amine anorectic agent, which acts through release of noradrenaline from presynaptic neuron vesicle located in the lateral part of the hypothalamus. Increasing concentration of noradrenaline in synaptic cleft leads to the stimulation of β_2-type adrenergic receptors. Similar to amphetamine, it also inhibits MAOI, but its unique action of inhibitory neuropeptide Y (principal signaling pathway which induces hunger) produces a continuous flight or fright response, resulting in the reduction of hunger signals, and hence reduces obesity issues by suppressing appetite.

It shows a dose-dependent profile in terms of pharmacokinetics. The oral dose of phentermine is 15 mg and the maximum concentration of dose was reached within 6 hours.

It is generally used to reduce calories, leading to weight loss. The significant weight loss via phentermine is approved for up to 12 weeks, and more amount of weight is lost in the initial weeks.

Pulmonary hypertension and cardiac vascular diseases are some of the rarest side effects associated with this drug. Other effects include restlessness, insomnia, tremor, psychotic episodes, unpleasant taste, impotence, trouble in urination, and facial swelling.

Xanthines

An especially important class of medicines includes compounds known as xanthines, methylxanthines, and xanthins. Since they have different pharmacological properties, there is often a question of where to address them most properly in a text on pharmacology. Xanthines are considered a potent pharmacological CNS stimulant compound among all of these classes. Xanthines have permissible medicinal applications, and they are frequently present in beverages, particularly in coffee, tea, chocolate, and cola drinks. The popularity of drinks containing xanthine seems to be linked to its subtle CNS stimulant effect.

Pharmacologically, three xanthines are significant: caffeine, theophylline, and theobromine. These three alkaloids occur naturally in some plants, and they are frequently consumed as beverages prepared from these plants (infusion or decoction). Although xanthines have been shown to have good oral and rectal bioavailability, they are also administered through injection (*aminophylline* is a soluble salt of theophylline), intravenously in case of asthmatics and apnea in premature infants. In contrast to other routes of administration, intramuscular injection is generally painful. Uric acid derivatives are the main common metabolites.

Caffeine

It is a psychoactive drug of methylxanthine class, which is the most widely used CNS stimulant. It is quite similar in chemical structure to theophylline and theobromine and is a white crystalline purine. It is a bitter alkaloid extracted from coffee beans (i.e., seed of the coffee plant). The injection of caffeine citrate to premature newborn with apnea was approved by the FDA in 1999. Also, caffeine is classified as generally safe (GRAS) by the FDA.

A complex mechanism of action is regulated by body, correlating actions of respiratory, cardiovascular, and renal system along with some general cellular actions. Caffeine usually acts on cells by inhibiting nucleotide phosphodiesterase enzyme, by regulating calcium concentration, or by participating as an antagonist for adenosine receptor. In the CNS, caffeine exerts its antagonistic effect in all of the four adenosine receptor subtypes, that is, A1, A2a, A2b, and AB. Due to this, it affects the alertness and drowsiness, which is specifically due to the antagonistic effect of caffeine on the A2a receptor. Also, caffeine stimulates inotropic effect in the heart; this is due to its antagonistic action on A1 receptors of adenosine. By blocking the action of these receptors, it enhances catecholamine release, resulting in stimulation of the heart and rest of the body, or it directly exerts its effect on the blood vessels causing vasodilation. Consequently, caffeine causes rise in blood pressure.

It is readily absorbed after administrating it orally or parenterally, enhancing up to peak concentration within 30 minutes to 2 hours. Caffeine can be administered rectally, but the absorption is less efficient than in oral administration.

It is mainly used in orthostatic hypotension treatment and as a beverage in treating asthma by increasing forced expiratory volume; also, caffeine (100–130 mg) added to paracetamol and ibuprofen works as a pain reliever. It is used for both prevention and treatment of bronchopulmonary dysplasia in premature infants. In the CNS, it enhances the cognitive performance by acting as a stimulant, which reduces fatigue and drowsiness. Physically, caffeine acts as a performance-enhancing drug, also called ergogenic aids.

It badly affects GI motility and gastric acid secretion. In women after menopausal phase, high consumption of caffeine leads to degradation of bones. Increased intake of caffeine causes diuresis and natriuresis. Psychologically, it increases jitteriness, insomnia, and sleep latency and reduces coordination. Caffeinism (a condition resulting from daily intake of 1–1.5 g of caffeine) causes unpleasant symptoms such as irritation, restlessness, headache, and palpitations.

Theophylline

Theophylline, also known as 1,3-dimethylxanthine, is derived from tea. It is a smooth muscle relaxant, diuretic, and bronchodilator, and stimulates activation of the cardiac and CNS. Theophylline is a phosphodiesterase inhibitor, and blocks adenosine receptor and activates histone deacetylase. It shows structural similarity with theobromine and caffeine, and is most abundantly found in *Camellia sinensis* and *Theobroma cacao*. It is a phosphodiesterase-inhibiting drug used in treating respiratory diseases such as chronic obstructive pulmonary disease (COPD) and asthma.

Theophylline acts as a smooth muscle relaxant for the bronchial airways and pulmonary blood vessels, and reduces the responsiveness of histamine, adenosine, and allergens in airways. It competitively inhibits type III and IV phosphodiesterase (which is responsible for breaking of cAMP in smooth muscles cells). It blocks the action of adenosine-mediated bronchoconstriction by binding with A2B adenosine receptor.

It is completely absorbed after oral administration in the form of solution or solid oral dosage form and has a bioavailability of 100% when administered intravenously.

Theophylline is mainly used for relaxation of smooth muscles and eliciting positive inotropic and chronotropic effects; also, it increases renal blood flow and blood pressure and stimulates the CNS, affecting majorly the respiratory center of the medulla. As a therapeutic agent, it is used for COPD, asthma, and infant apnea.

Theophyllines have a very narrow therapeutic window. It can cause severe side effects such as nausea, diarrhea, tachycardia, and excitation in the CNS, for example, insomnia, headache, dizziness, and lightheadedness. The toxic effect of theophylline overdose includes arrhythmias, seizures, and GI effects.

Theobromine

It is a principal alkaloid present in *T. cacao* and has a weaker diuretic activity than other xanthines. It is used as a bronchodilator and vasodilator but is less potent as compared to other xanthines. It shows no stimulatory effect on the CNS; instead, it shows heart stimulation. Basically, it is used to treat angina pectoris and high blood pressure. Generally, like other xanthines, it also shows its activity by activating the vasomotor, vagal, medullary, and respiratory centers. The stimulation of a particular center is due to inhibition of phosphodiesterase (responsible for degrading the cAMP) in response to a hike in cAMP content intracellularly. In addition, theobromine activates the release of neurotransmitters by inducing the antagonistic effect on adenosine receptors, which are autacoids responsible for regulating the action of norepinephrine or angiotensin. Moreover, intake of theobromine and caffeine blocks the heart adenosine A1 receptor, resulting in increased pounding of the heart. Theobromine is present in the body even without direct consumption, as caffeine is metabolized into three primary metabolites: 12% theobromine, 4% theophylline, and 84% paraxanthine. Theobromine is used as a CNS stimulant, moderate diuretic, vasodilator, and respiratory stimulant (in neonates with apnea). Similar to caffeine, it can be effective in controlling stress and orthostatic hypotension in humans.

Theobromine poisoning, also known as chocolate poisoning, is an overdose reaction to theobromine, contained in chocolate, tea, cola, and several other foods. Median lethal (LD_{50}) doses of theobromine for cats, dogs, rodents, and mice are 0.8 to 1.5 g (50–100 g cocoa) a day.

Drug Abuse

Drug or substance abuse can be defined as the use of any chemical or medication for unintended purposes or in excessive amount or doses than prescribed; these chemicals or substances may or may not be illegal to obtain. Drug or substance abuse is widely distributed and affects the society and individual in direct or indirect ways. Causes of drug abuse are not as simple as they appear; these may differ and depend on conditions such as socioeconomic status, education stratification, peer pressure, excitement to experiment, and attempt to cope with conditions/disease by self-medication. The CNS is a major target in the human body for behavioral stabilizer or swinger substances; this induces drug-desire behavior. Drug-seeking behavior or drug desire leads to drug addiction or dependence; however, this terminology is difficult to define without considering the consequences and pattern of use of the drug or substance. Repetition of substance abuse can be said to be an addiction when individual's priority overrides the daily or normal life goals in any setup: social, family, and career settings. Addiction is promoted by the euphoria or pleasantness, which works as positive reinforcement. Euphoria property of a particular drug can be stated as abuse potential of the drug. Seeking of alternative drug in case of unavailability of addicted drug is known as psychological addiction or psychological dependence. Addiction or chronic use of a substance over significant time period leads to an increase in tolerance for the drug, which can be classified into pharmacokinetic, pharmacodynamic, or behavioral. Tolerance is directly proportional to the dose of the drug and length of time period of abuse. Withdrawal of the drug may give rise to a condition known as drug abstinence. The older term *physical (physiologic) dependence* is now generally denoted as dependence, whereas *psychological dependence* is more simply called addiction.

Epidemiological studies indicate that most drug abusers tend to abuse multiple drugs. This condition can be referred to as polydrug or coabuse, which is due to resemblance of pharmacological effects. Coabuse also leads to a condition of cross-tolerance development to a same class of drugs.

Drugs of abuse can be classified according to their chemical properties and receptor action, but pharmacological or behavioral effect may vary in chronic or acute use.

Opioids

Secondary metabolites of plants such as alkaloids have been used for medicinal or recreational purposes since ancient times. Poppy plant *Papaver somniferum* is the source of most opiates; primarily morphine. The term "opioid" is defined as morphine derivative or peptide, since it exerts morphine-like effects because of their structural similarity to morphine. Depending on the route of administration, the euphoric and pharmacological properties of the opioid vary.

Medicinal Use

Opioids are often used to manage moderate to severe pain. Chronic treatment should be monitored continuously to avoid physical dependence and tolerance development. All opioids act on opioid receptors (mu receptor, kappa receptor, delta opioid receptor) and block the nociceptive pain signals in afferent neurons of the CNS. This blockade depends on the type of opioid and its pharmacokinetic properties. For example, morphine has an onset time of 5 to 30 minutes. Bioavailability of morphine is 80 to 100% when it is administered orally; morphine is absorbed in the alkaline environment of the intestine. Oral administration is more potent than other routes of administration. In oral administration, T_{max} is 90 minutes, and in parenteral administration it is just 15 minutes. Metabolism of morphine is dominantly carried out by glucuronidation (approximately 90%) and 70 to 80% is excreted through urination within 48 hours. The half-life of morphine varies from 2 to 3 hours due to first-pass metabolism.

Intoxication or pharmacological effect is primarily euphoria. Additionally, relaxation leads to sedation, which increases the potential of drug abuse.

Acute Intoxication

Initially, users feel displeasure or regret, which results in nausea and vomiting. Warm flushing and rush in the skin and lower extremities resemble sexual orgasm behaviors. Duration of euphoria lasts for one to several minutes, which leads to sedation and relaxation. This end period is said to be on the nod. After achieving half-life, effects start dissipating, and the demand for frequent administration arises.

Tolerance and Dependence

During the first-time use of opioids, the patient feels displeasure, which is readily tolerated. This is followed by analgesic, respiratory depressant, emetic, and euphoric effects. GI and miosis effects are little and not tolerated quickly. Cross-tolerance development is a unique feature of all opioids, due to similar mechanism of action centered on opioid receptors. Tolerance development depends on frequency and dose of the abuse. For example, consumption of opioids at 4- to 6-hour intervals is quickly tolerated within a few days, whereas, in comparison, in case of twice-daily consumption, tolerance is developed in several weeks.

Physical dependence is strongly represented by abstinence syndrome after withdrawal of opioid. Abstinence syndrome includes hyperactivity, restlessness, anxiety, diarrhea, cramp, chills, fever, runny nose, lacrimation, and vomiting. Muscle and joint pain and increased heart rate and blood pressure compel the individual to craving or drug-seeking behavior. Opioid withdrawal is irritable but not life-threatening.

Treatment of Opioid Dependence

Achieving drug-free status is the primary goal, which is hardly possible without pharmacotherapy. The first step to achieve this goal is to shift the abuser from short-acting opioids to long-acting opioids—for example, from heroin to methadone. Antagonists of opioid receptor such as naltrexone can be helpful in repelling the addiction completely.

Heroin

Heroin is an illegal semisynthetic compound derived from natural opioids. Most countries categorized it under schedule I, and it has no prescription approval for medicinal purposes. It suppresses pain acutely, but also impairs cognition, sedates, and decreases respiration rate via autonomous nervous system control. It is more potent than morphine due to its high membrane permeability. The route of administration is diverse as it can be snorted, smoked, or injected. An overdose of heroin is life-threatening. Major symptoms include constricted pupils, bluish color of nails, skin coldness, confusion or loss of consciousness, low blood pressure, hard to breath, and decreased heart rate.

Oxycodone

Oxycodone-containing opioids are effectively used in moderate to severe pain management. Oxycodone is one of the most prescribed painkillers with acetaminophen and aspirin, which increases its availability and abuse potential. In a survey, these classes of opioids are common drugs involved in overdose fatalities.

Hydrocodone

Hydrocodone is a synthetic opioid indicated for cough and cold. It has more affinity to mu opioid receptor than delta opioid receptor. T_{max} is less than natural opioids; even C_{max} can be increased by the synergistic effect of food and 40% ethanol coadministration. Major intoxication effects of hydrocodone are respiratory depression, airway obstruction, bradycardia, and hypotension on overdose or abuse.

Hydromorphone

Hydromorphone is a semisynthetic, pure opioid derived from morphine by oxidation and methylation. It is more potent than its parent compound and increases the risk of overdose and abuse potential when it is taken in the form of snort, smoke, or liquid injection. Intoxication or pharmacological effects are similar to those described earlier for opioids.

Fentanyl

Fentanyl is a synthetic opioid prescribed in the management of chronic and severe pain in those patients who are tolerant of first-line opioids. It is used for short-term analgesia and in recovery of general anesthesia. It strongly binds to mu receptor and adenylate cyclase, which results in reduction in cAMP-dependent calcium influx and hyperpolarizes the nerve potential. Fentanyl is differentially absorbed via intradermal, buccal cavity, and mucosal through intranasal application. It has a high plasma protein binding affinity (80–85%). Its half-life is significantly higher than the opioids.

Codeine

Codeine was initially extracted from the poppy plant; however, currently it is synthesized from morphine. It is a less potent opioid, commonly prescribed for cough and moderate pain management. It has less adverse effect on cognition function, and only increases the threshold of pain or tolerance to pain. It decreases the intestinal motility and may lead to constipation. Similar to other opioids, the major risk of drug abuse is overdose.

Methadone

Methadone is a synthetic opioid, which acts on mu and NMDA receptor as an agonist and antagonist, respectively. This mechanism of action makes it useful for the hard-to-treat pain such as neuropathic and cancer pain; also, it is more potent than other opioids. Pharmacodynamics and pharmacokinetic activities are similar to those of other opioids. Its potency develops more tolerance, physical dependence, and addiction behavior.

Meperidine

Meperidine is a synthetic opiate derivative of phenylpiperidine class. It acts more rapidly than morphine or morphine derivatives. It is often used in acute pain management such as postoperative or labor pain. Generally, it is a second-line opioid and can be used for local and spinal anesthesia. The rapid action on smooth muscle spasm increases its abuse potential. Heavy physical dependence is hard to manage or difficult of withdrawal of meperidine reinforces the drug-seeking and addiction behavior.

Oxymorphone

Oxymorphone is a semisynthetic opiate, which is an alternative to morphine. It exerts analgesic effect on the CNS and GI and is valued for its sedative property. Respiratory depression is caused via decreasing the responsiveness of the brain stem to stimulus. The mechanism of absorption and volume of distribution of oxymorphone are not much clear in comparison to other opioids. Overdose or abuse of oxymorphone may cause deep somnolence, comma, skeletal muscle flaccidity, and respiratory depression. Dependency and addiction characteristics are similar to other opioids.

Tramadol

Tramadol is a synthetic opioid, which acts on the CNS as an analog of codeine and morphine. It causes respiratory depression, which directly affects the brain stem and reduces the responsiveness of respiratory center, resulting in increase in carbon dioxide; it also suppresses cough center. It acts via mu receptor and inhibition of serotonin and norepinephrine reuptake. Overdose or recommended dose of tramadol increases risk of convulsion or precipitates seizures. Dependence and tolerance development are similar to other opioids. Abuse may cause death due to somnolence and respiration depression.

Carfentanil

Carfentanil is an analog of fentanyl and is a more potent opioid than fentanyl and morphine by 100 and 1,000 times. It is commonly used as anesthetic in veterinary medicine. Its mechanism of action is similar to fentanyl but it is more potent in causing sedation and respiration depression. It is fatal in low doses in humans and is more addictive.

Buprenorphine

Buprenorphine is a partial agonist of mu opioid receptor often used in severe pain management where other opioids are inadequate. Opioid withdrawal pain is also managed with it. It is commonly used for its therapeutic activities such as alteration in mood, euphoria, dysphoria, sedation, and antitussive. It causes physical dependence in a manner similar to opioid, but less as compared to others when it has been withdrawn. Overdose may cause pinpoint pupils, hypotension, sedation, respiratory depression, and death.

Nicotine

Nicotine can be classified as both stimulant and depressant because of behavioral effects as influenced by mental status and expectations of the smoker. Nicotinic receptors are the target of actions, which play a major role in the CNS by stimulating dopamine release in nucleus accumbens. This is a major component of the reward system. It stimulates the release of endogenous opioids and glucocorticoids.

Tolerance and Dependence

Tolerance to nicotine is rapidly developed in the abusers with high frequency of consumption. It is strongly reinforced by reinforcement center. Short onset time of action is liable to abuse potential and creates cycle of drug abuse. Nicotine is a highly addictive drug; it increases the drug-seeking behavior and intense propensity for abuse. Almost all abusers want to quit but less than one-third attempt to do so.

Sedative Hypnotics

GABA positive allosteric modulators are medications used in the management and treatment of seizures, sedation, anxiolytic, alcohol withdrawal, and muscle spasms. These includes diazepines and barbiturate and nonbarbiturate sedatives. Secobarbital, phenobarbital, and amobarbitals are most commonly used as anxietolytic, as their attainability increases the abuse potential including diazepines. Intoxication effects of barbiturate and diazepines are similar to ethanol; they produce euphoric effect and rush in skin and extremities, and reduce insomnia and anxiety. Intoxication effects increase in dose-dependent manner. Benzodiazepines are safe CNS depressant even at higher doses but, in combination with others, enhance the effects of other drugs. Acute effects of all depressants in overdose or abuse include euphoria, reduction in anxiety, anticonvulsant activity, sedation, motor incoordination, impaired reflex response, and respiration arrest and may lead to death.

Tolerance and Dependence

Tolerance for barbiturates and benzodiazepines develops slowly in comparison to opioids. Some, but not all, of the pharmacological effects can be tolerated; this characteristic of barbiturates increases its lethality. Cross-tolerance may be seen in same classes of drugs, and lethal doses are not much higher in tolerated individual in contrast to opioids.

Dependence is developed in chronic uses of large doses, not in therapeutic doses. Dependence is very less in the case of diazepines and barbiturates in comparison to alcohol consumption. Withdrawal syndrome is mild to moderate and can be characterized by confusion, anxiety attack, seizure, sleep disruption, muscle cramps, and tremors, which may appear in 2 to 7 days after withdrawn. Benzodiazepine withdrawal is not a life-threatening condition but barbiturate and alcohols may be.

Ethanol

Ethanol is the most abused drug in the world since ancient times. Excessive consumption and procurement of alcohol, if it dominates the lifestyle, is considered alcoholism. Absorption of ethanol is totally carried out through GI tract; the rate of absorption can vary depending on the quantity consumed and the contents of gastric. Absorption of ethanol can be retarded by lipid food content. Absorption is followed by rapid distribution to the body water with blood flow. Most of the drug portion is metabolized by the liver, and it involves two enzyme system: zinc-dependent alcohol dehydrogenase and acetaldehyde dehydrogenase. Intermediate-product acetaldehyde may accumulate and cause vasodilation, facial flush, and tachycardia in some population due to insufficient activation of acetaldehyde dehydrogenase enzyme, which attain end-product acetic acid. Chronic consumption increases the activity of alcohol dehydrogenase, which metabolizes the alcohol concentration in an independent manner. The mechanism of action of alcohol, which is well studied, is mediated via $GABA_A$. NMDA ion receptors exert synergetic effect on nerve impulse suppression. It is agonist and antagonist to both receptors, respectively. As its action on the CNS can be categorized under depressant, depression of behavior may vary according to the blood concentration of ethanol. An increase in blood concentration inhibits the inhibitory interneurons. This leads to talkativeness, social inhibition, slurred speech, decreased reflexive responses, and coma. Subsequently it may lead to death due to respiratory arrest.

Sudden cessation of consumption of ethanol results in withdrawal syndrome, which can be characterized by tremors, seizures, hyperthermia, hallucinations, and autonomic hyperactivity. These effects may lead to atrial arrhythmias and ventricular tachycardia due to depressant activity of ethanol. Peripheral neuropathy and sexual organ failure can be caused due to chronic or repeated consumption of ethanol. Wernicke's encephalopathy and Korsakoff's psychosis can be observed in alcoholism behavior. Teratogenic or developmental abnormalities include fetal alcohol syndrome. Placental permeability of the ethanol plays a vital role. Disulfiram is the only pharmacological approach that is used to treat abstinence by increasing acetaldehyde concentration. It induces thirst, vomiting, hyperthermia, blurred vision, etc. Other pharmacological approaches can be mediated by serotonin uptake inhibition, dopaminergic agonists, and opioid antagonists (naltrexone).

Marijuana

Cannabis sativa plant parts (dried leaves, flowering tops) are more frequently abused in different countries by smoking. The solid dark resinous material sourced from the leaves, called hashish, which is a major constituent in marijuana, is delta-9 tetrahydrocannabinol, a psychoactive agent. Cannabinol is rapidly absorbed when the leaves are smoked than ingested orally. Absorption totally depends on lung capacity and lipid absorption. Cannabinol is highly lipophilic in nature and hence there is rapid tissue distribution. It is stored in the adipose tissue. The half-life of cannabinol is 18 hours to 4 days, and it can be located in adipose tissue even after 30 days in a person who smoked a single joint.

Cannabinoid frequently interacts with the cannabinoid receptors found in the CNS, mostly in the brain, known as CB_1 receptors. Euphoria, well-being, and happiness are initial symptoms experienced by individuals, which are followed by drowsiness, sedation, and distortion in cognition via vision, hearing, hallucination, and illusions frequently. Marijuana use also leads to increased appetite.

Dependence and tolerance develop only in heavy abusers, and there is no fatal overdose reported for marijuana. Mild to moderate withdrawal symptoms include restlessness, anorexia, irritability, short-term memory problem, and mild nausea.

Hallucinogens

Pharmacologic agents that alter the sensory perception are grouped under hallucinogens and their activity is known as hallucination. This category includes majorly lysergic acid diethylamide (LSD), mescaline, and psilocybin. Drugs that alter sensory perception at lower doses and at higher doses mimic CNS stimulatory effect. Drugs such as phencyclidine (PCP), MDMA (also known as XTC), and methylenedioxyamphetamine can be included in the subclass of hallucinogens.

Longer effects of LSD increase its abuse potential, which include euphoria, depersonalization, alertness, and minor stimulant activity. Precipitation of anxiety attacks, panic, paranoid ideation, and mood swings push the individual abuser into great emotions related to terror. Hallucination is commonly related with colors and geometric patterns. Occurrence of hangover is common in XTC/MDMA; all other properties are similar to LSD. XTC reduces the perceived intensity of psychological problems, and hallucinatory properties are shown at higher doses. MDMA effects are in dose-dependent manner: at low dose (75 mg), it shows psychotomimetic effects; at moderate dose (150 mg), it shows LSD-like effects; and at higher doses (300 mg), it shows amphetaminelike CNS stimulation effects. PCP induces hallucinatory and CNS stimulatory effects at higher doses; however, it is a dissociative aesthetic also. It produces auditory hallucination and individual believes that his/her thought, action, and efficiencies are increased. At higher doses, it produces motor incoordination, catalepsy, and depressant effect.

Tolerance to the hallucinogens develops more rapidly for LSD-like effects, even after three to four uses, and regular doses of any hallucinogen may induce tolerance. All hallucinogens exert their effect via similar action of mechanism through $5\text{-}HT_2$ receptor acting as a structural analogs of serotonin (agonism). Hence, cross-tolerance frequently develops.

Physical dependence and drug-seeking behavior are not observed in drug-free period. Hence, there is no dependence attributed to the hallucinogens. CNS stimulant may induce drug craving behavior; otherwise, there are no dependence or withdrawal symptoms observed.

Lethal and abused dose difference is quite high, and therefore there no intervention is needed. Supportive and symptomatic intervention can be made for hallucinogens. Intoxication treatment involves termination of the external stimuli (audio, and lights) and making sure the patient is in a safe environment.

Multiple Choice Questions

1. A 21-year-old boy is admitted to the emergency room at 5 am with complaints of agitation, hyperactivity, and hypersexuality. His friends report that the patient was at an all-night rave party. They say he took several pills, which they thought were "ecstasy" (methylenedioxymethamphetamine). Which of the following describes the mechanism of this "party" drug?

A. Antagonistic activity at the *N*-methyl-D-aspartate (NMDA) receptor for glutamic acid.
B. Binding to the cannabinol CB_1 receptor.

C. Increased release of dopamine and norepinephrine.
D. Mimics the action of acetylcholine.
E. Agonist at postjunctional serotonin receptors.

Answer: C

Similar to other amphetamines, ecstasy enhances the release of dopamine and norepinephrine. Its use is frequently seen in "rave" parties. Phencyclidine (PCP) is an antagonist at the *N*-methyl-D-aspartate (NMDA) receptor for glutamic acid, leading to euphoria and hallucinations.

2. A patient is admitted to the emergency because of overdose of an illicit drug. She is agitated, has disordered thought processes, suffers from paranoia, and "hears voices." Physical examination reveals tachycardia, hyperreflexia, and hyperthermia. The drug that most probably is causing the symptoms is:

A. Gamma-hydroxybutyrate (GHB).
B. Hashish.
C. Heroin.
D. Marijuana.
E. Methamphetamine.

Answer: E

The manifestations are those of high-dose abuse of dextroamphetamine or methamphetamine. There is no specific antidote, and supportive measures are directed toward protection against cardiac arrhythmias and seizures and control of body temperature.

3. Mental retardation, microcephaly, and underdevelopment of the midface region in an infant is connected with chronic heavy maternal use during pregnancy of which of the following?

A. Cocaine.
B. Diazepam.
C. Ethanol.
D. Heroin.
E. Methylenedioxymethamphetamine (MDMA).

Answer: C

Mental retardation, microcephaly, and facial dysmorphia are features of fetal alcohol syndrome produced by extreme use of ethanol during pregnancy.

4. The parents of a 10-year-old boy complains of hyperactivity at school. Additionally, he is also inattentive and impulsive at home. For his treatment, the physician gives him amphetamine-containing medication for presumed attention-deficit/hyperactivity disorder. Amphetamine acts by:

A. Inhibiting epinephrine reuptake.
B. Indirectly acting on norepinephrine receptors.
C. Blocking effects of norepinephrine.
D. Directly acting on cholinoreceptors.
E. Inhibiting serotonin reuptake.

Answer: B

Amphetamine and similar compounds are stimulants used for treatment of attention-deficit/hyperactivity disorder (ADHD). They act centrally to enhance attention span. Presently, there is no drug that inhibits reuptake of epinephrine. Blocking of the effects of norepinephrine will not lessen symptoms of ADHD.

5. Ephedra (ephedrine) increases blood pressure by:

A. Indirect action on cholinergic receptors.
B. Blockade of adrenergic receptors.
C. Stimulation of release of epinephrine.
D. Inhibition of reuptake of catecholamines.
E. Direct action on dopamine receptors.

Answer: C

Ephedrine acts indirectly to liberate norepinephrine from nerve terminals and results in effects comparable to those of catecholamines, together with elevated blood pressure. This possibly unsafe agent has been banned from the over-the-counter market due to increasing number of deaths. An example of an indirect-acting cholinergic agonist is edrophonium, which is used for diagnosis of myasthenia gravis. Adrenoceptor blockers, like atenolol, are used for the treatment of hypertension.

6. A 32-year-old lawyer is brought to the emergency room after collapsing at a party. He had developed chest pain, and an ECG revealed ventricular fibrillation, for which he was managed by cardioversion. A physical examination revealed a perforated nasal septum. His friend reveals that the patient was "doing" an illicit substance at the party. Which of the following is the most likely drug?

A. Phencyclidine (PCP).
B. γ-Hydroxybutyric acid (GHB).
C. Lysergic acid diethylamide (LSD).
D. Cocaine.
E. Marijuana.

Answer: D

Cocaine is cardiotoxic and can lead to arrhythmias, which can be life-threatening. These effects are increased when alcohol is also consumed. Cocaine leads to vasoconstriction, and snorting it results in necrosis and eventual perforation of the nasal septum.

7. Which sign or symptom is expected to happen with marijuana?

A. Bradycardia.
B. Conjunctival reddening.
C. Hypertension.
D. Increased psychomotor performance.
E. Mydriasis.

Answer: B

Two of the most typical signs of marijuana use are increased pulse rate and reddening of the conjunctiva. Reductions in blood pressure and in psychomotor performance can happen. Pupil size is *not* altered by marijuana.

8. Which statement about hallucinogens is accurate?

A. Dilated pupils and tachycardia are characteristic effects of scopolamine.

B. LSD is unique among hallucinogens where animals will self-administer it.

C. Mescaline and related hallucinogens exert their CNS actions through dopaminergic systems in the brain.

D. Teratogenic effects occur with the use of phencyclidine during pregnancy.

E. Withdrawal signs characteristic of dependence occur with abrupt discontinuance of ketamine.

Answer: A

Psilocybin, mescaline, and LSD have comparable central (via serotonergic systems) and peripheral (sympathomimetic) properties, but no actions on dopaminergic receptors in the CNS.

9. All of the following are CNS stimulants except:

A. Amphetamines.

B. Benzodiazepines.

C. Cocaine.

D. Methylphenidate.

E. Pemoline.

Answer: B

Benzodiazepines are CNS depressants, while the others are CNS stimulants.

10. Which of the following is a respiratory analeptic drug?

A. Picrotoxin.

B. Methylphenidate.

C. Caffeine.

D. Doxapram.

E. Strychnine.

Answer: D

Doxapram is a respiratory stimulant, whereas the others are just CNS stimulants. Analeptic stimulants were used to manage the overdosage of CNS depressants, whereas some of the analeptics were also recommended to stimulate the respiratory systems after the aesthetic depression such as doxapram.

11. The drug of choice for hyperkinetic children is:

A. Methylphenidate.

B. Nikethamide.

C. Caffeine.

D. Clonazepam.

E. Doxapram.

Answer: A

Methylphenidate is a CNS stimulant, quite similar to amphetamine, and is considered to be a schedule II drug. It is usually the most prescribed medication in children. Methylphenidate is most importantly used for narcolepsy and attention-deficit/hyperactivity disorder (ADHD) in patients in the age group 6 to 16 years.

Chapter 38 Antidepressants and Mood Stabilizers

Shailesh Bhosle, Biplab Sikdar, and Awanish Mishra

PH1.19: Describe the mechanism/s of action, types, doses, side effects, indications, and contraindications of the drugs that act on the central nervous system (including anxiolytics, sedatives and hypnotics, antipsychotic, antidepressant drugs, antimanic agents, opioid agonists and antagonists, drugs used for neurodegenerative disorders, and antiepileptics drugs).

Learning Objectives

- Depression.
- Antidepressants drugs.
- Clinical indications of antidepressants.
- Mood stabilizers.

Depression (PS6.4, PS6.6)

Depression is one of the most prevalent neurological conditions affecting more than 300 million people worldwide. Depression may be characterized by depressed mood, loss of interest, or pleasure in most activities for at least 2 weeks. Besides, it may be associated with altered sleep, appetite, cognitive function, and thought of wrongdoing, hopelessness, and suicide. Sometimes such a situation is also referred to as major depressive disorder. The diagnosis is primarily based on the conversation with the patient directly. In a depressed patient, the chances of other diseases such as coronary artery disease (CAD), diabetes, and stroke are more common. Association of comorbid conditions with depression worsens the quality of life in patients with depression. Anxiety is mostly associated with depression and sometimes present in patients one after another or coexist with each other.

Antidepressants are the agents that are primarily used for management of depression. Majorly, these agents work via direct or indirect elevation of synaptic biogenic amines (chiefly norepinephrine and/or serotonin) levels. The recent advancement in the research makes a more selective and safer choice of drug or psychiatric condition. Safe and effective therapy requires the proper understanding of the working principle of the agents, their pharmacokinetic properties, possible side effects or adverse effect, and drug interactions. Since the last few decades, development of antidepressants has gained wider attention. The use of antidepressants has also received attention due to their usefulness in several conditions such as generalized anxiety disorder, obsessive-compulsive disease (OCD), posttraumatic stress disorder (PTSD), panic condition, premenstrual dysphoric disorder (PMDD), neuropathic pain, and fibromyalgia.

Depression is one of the leading causes of disability, which largely contributes to the increase in the global burden of disease worldwide. Awareness regarding the prevalence of depression is not widespread due to difficulties in understanding the condition and also due to less reporting as it is a mental illness. High-income countries have higher prevalence, and this is probably due to more spending and focus on health than the poorly developed countries. It is more prevalent in women than in men. It can affect people of all ages and belonging to any country. In India, about 3.4% is affected by depression, in which urban areas contribute to the maximum number more than the rural areas, and females are more prone to develop the depressive condition. The development of depression is mainly due to the imbalance in life, relationship problems or complex social interaction, various physiological and biological factors, unemployment, loss of close ones, etc. The chronic and severe condition of depression leads to suicidal death.

Pathophysiology of Depression

Around five decades back, the first hypothesis of depression was articulated, which was based on central monoamine depletion. The primitive evidence that led to the development of the monoamine hypothesis includes: (1) the effects of reserpine on serotonin and catecholamines and (2) the pharmacological mechanisms of action of antidepressant drugs. Since the last decade, there has been a marked shift in understanding the pathology of depression (**Fig. 38.1**). In addition to monoamine hypothesis, there is evidence that glutamatergic, neurotrophic, and endocrine factors play a vital role in development of depression.

Monoamine Hypothesis

This hypothesis was proposed during the 1950s, based on the theory that depression is the impact of decreased concentration of different biogenic monoamines such as serotonin (5-HT), noradrenaline, and dopamine. It explains the reduction of monoamines and their transmission across neurons, especially in the cortical and limbic regions of the brain. This theory can be supported by an example of alkaloid from *Rauwolfia serpentina* (reserpine), which is a monoamine antagonist. Reserpine is an antagonist of monoamines used for the treatment of high blood pressure; herein, depression develops as a side effect. Reserpine mainly inhibits the uptake of monoamines at vesicles, which results in decreased brain monoamine. Also, it can be supported by the fact that the patient with depression is found with a lower concentration of 5-HT metabolites. Similarly, when serotonergic antidepressants are given in patients, they

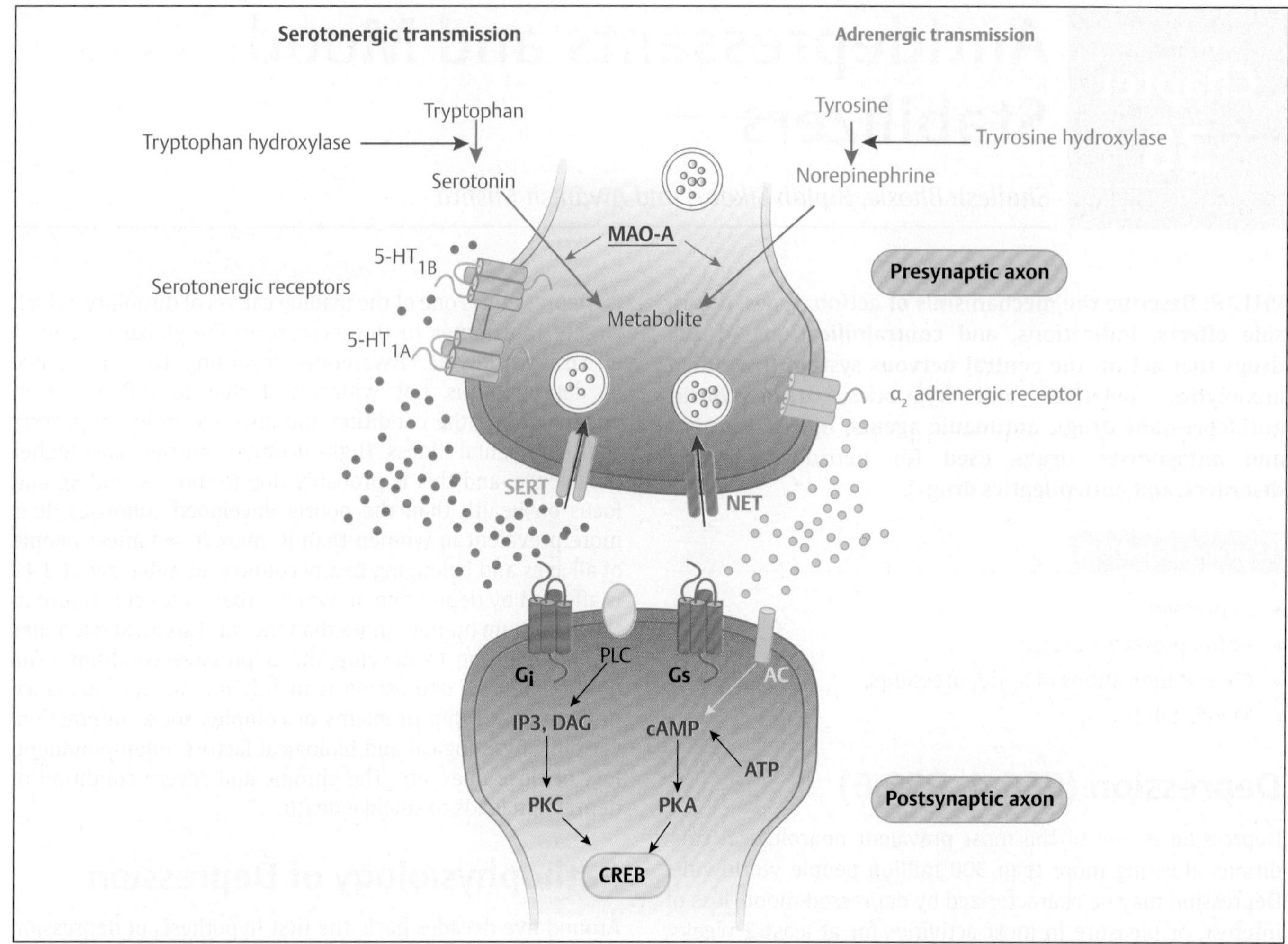

Fig. 38.1 Mechanism of action of antidepressants. 5-HT, serotonin; AC, adenylyl cyclase; CREB, cAMP response element-binding protein; DAG, diacyl glycerol; IP3, inositol trisphosphate; MAO, monoamine oxidase; NET, norepinephrine transporter; PKC, protein kinase C; PLC, phospholipase C; SERT, serotonin transporter.

rapidly recover from the depressive symptoms. Also, a diet containing tryptophan, a precursor of serotonin, reduced the symptomatic behavior of depression. Monoamine hypothesis can be supported by the shreds of evidence that all antidepressant agents increase the level of 5-HT, dopamine, or norepinephrine in the brain.

Based on this theory, the best treatment drugs for depression are the agents that increase the concentration of monoamines in the synapse. According to this, the agonist of monoamines can be used as an antidepressant agent. This theory allows the use of monoamine oxidase inhibitors (MAOIs) and tricyclic antidepressants (TCAs) in depressionlike behavior. The use of selective serotonin reuptake inhibitors (SSRIs) is found to be useful in the treatment of depression.

Neurotrophic Hypothesis

Neurotrophic factors are the agents involved in the formation of neuronal networks, and they provide neuronal plasticity. Most of the neurotrophic factors belong to the family of neurotrophins such as brain-derived neurotrophic factor (BDNF), neurotrophin-3, and neurotrophin-4. Along with these, some other factors that regulate the neuronal plasticity are insulinlike growth factors (IGF) and vascular endothelial growth factor. The involvement of the BDNF and its receptor, tyrosine kinase receptor B (TrkB), is majorly associated with the pathogenesis of depression. BDNF is the key element that is not only responsible for neuronal plasticity and resilience but also involved in neurogenesis. According to this hypothesis, the decrease in the level of BDNF leads to depressionlike symptoms, whereas the increased level of BDNF is responsible for the antidepressantlike activity.

Apart from this monoamine and neurotrophic hypothesis, the excitatory neurotransmitter glutamate is also involved in the pathogenesis of depression. Clinically, it was found that depressed patients have increased glutamate concentration in the brain.

The chemical messengers of the body (hormones) that control and regulate functioning of the body along with the nervous system also play a vital role in depression. The neuroendocrine factors or hormonal abnormalities are responsible for depressionlike behavior. Among all, the hypothalamic–pituitary–adrenal axis is found to be majorly involved in depression and its progression. An increase in the level of cortisol and adrenocorticotropin hormone is associated with depression. Fluctuations in thyroid level are also observed in patients with depressive behaviors. Approximately, 20 to 25% of depressed patients have reported thyroid dysregulation. A decrease in the level of thyroid hormone is frequently observed with depressive behavior, which gets resolved with the supplementation of the thyroid hormone. Thyroid hormones are used as conjunction therapy along with antidepressant therapy. Also, sex hormones play a role in pathogenesis of the depression. The deficit of the estrogen level has found to be one of the causes of depression in women. Similarly, in men, testosterone deficiency is linked to depressionlike behaviors.

Diagnosis of Depression

According to Diagnostic and Statistical Manual of Mental Disorders (DSM-5), the diagnosis of depression requires association of five or more symptoms within a 2-week period, and presence of either depressed mood or anhedonia has been considered as one of the major criteria. However, secondary symptoms of depression may diverge to somatic or nonsomatic clusters. The somatic issues include sleep pattern disturbances, weight gain/loss or change in appetite, poor attention, lethargy, and agitation/retardation, while nonsomatic issues include anhedonia, depressed mood, hopelessness, feeling of worthless, and suicidal thoughts. For the assessment of severity of depression, the Hamilton depression rating scale has been the most frequently used rating scale.

Antidepressants Drugs (PS10.4, PS10.6, PS11.4, PS11.6, PS12.4, PS12.6, PS13.4, PS18.1)

The major classes of antidepressant drugs include SSRIs, selective serotonin and norepinephrine reuptake inhibitors (SNRIs), MAOIs, and TCAs and related antidepressants (**Fig. 38.2**). A few number of drugs are available that do not belong to any of the above-mentioned classes and are listed as atypical antidepressants in the following.

Selective Serotonin Uptake Inhibitors

SSRIs belong to a structurally diverse group of agents that primarily cause inhibition of serotonin transporter (SERT). Fluoxetine appears to be a prototype drug of this class, which was introduced in 1988 and then went onto become one of the most prescribed antidepressants. This class of drugs was synthesized while in search of chemicals based on monoaminergic hypothesis but devoid of cholinergic, α-adrenergic, and histaminic side effects, which are common with TCAs. This class of drugs is used to treat depression, anxiety, and other mood disorders. Initially, six SSRIs (citalopram, escitalopram, fluoxetine, fluvoxamine, paroxetine, and sertraline) were approved for management of depression; recently, vilazodone and vortioxetine were also approved by the US Food and Drug Administration (FDA). The SSRIs inhibit reuptake of serotonin at the synapses both immediately and chronically. As a result, serotonin stays for longer period of time and therefore stimulates postsynaptic receptors. Activation of serotonergic receptors in different body parts may contribute to adverse effects such as gastrointestinal (GI) upset, sexual dysfunction, agitation, restlessness, and serotonin syndrome.

Mechanism of Action

The therapeutic actions of SSRIs have their basis on increasing deficient serotonin that researchers postulate as the cause of depression in the monoamine hypothesis. As the name suggests, SSRIs exert action by inhibiting the reuptake of serotonin, thereby increasing serotonin activity. Unlike other classes of antidepressants, SSRIs have little effect on other neurotransmitters such as dopamine or norepinephrine. SSRIs also have relatively fewer side effects compared to TCAs and MAOIs due to having fewer effects on adrenergic, cholinergic, and histaminergic receptors.

SSRIs inhibit SERT at the presynaptic axon terminal. By inhibiting SERT, an increased amount of serotonin (5-hydroxytryptamine or 5-HT) remains in the synaptic cleft and can stimulate postsynaptic receptors for a more extended period.

The pharmacokinetic profile of SSRIs has been summarized in **Table 38.1**.

Adverse Effects

Almost all antidepressants are associated with some potential adverse effects, which specifically depend on the subclass of antidepressants. SSRIs induce serotonergic tone not only in the brain but also throughout the body. The common adverse effects such as nausea, gastrointestinal tract (GIT) complications, and diarrhea are observed due

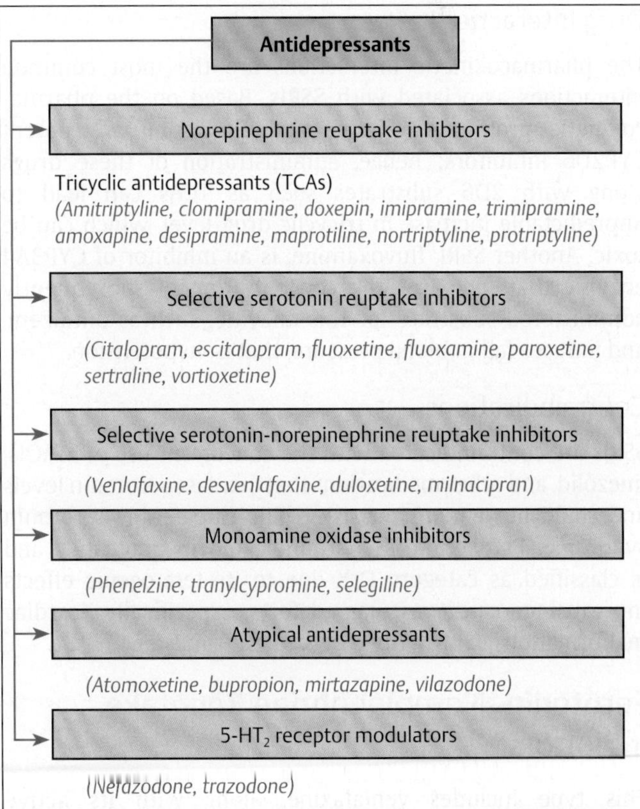

Fig. 38.2 Classification of antidepressants based on mechanism of action.

Table 38.1 The pharmacokinetic profile of SSRIs

Drug	Therapeutic dose (mg/d)	Bioavailability (%)	Active metabolite (h)	Plasma half-life (h)	Volume of distribution (L/kg)	Plasma protein binding (%)
Fluoxetine	100–300	70	180	48–72	12–97	95
Escitalopram	10–30	80	N	27–32	12–15	80
Citalopram	20–60	80	N	33–38	15	80
Fluvoxamine	100–300	90	14–16	14–18	25	80
Paroxetine	20–60	50	N	20–23	28–31	94
Sertraline	50–200	45	62–104	22–27	20	98

Abbreviations: N, no active metabolite; SSRIs, selective serotonin reuptake inhibitors.

to the induced serotonergic activity. The GI adverse effects are moderate initially, but after 1 week it tends to stabilize. Other adverse effects, such as loss of libido, is aggravated due to the increased serotonergic tone, especially in the spinal cord. These sexual activity-related adverse effects are seen as long as the patient is administered antidepressants, but it may disappear with time. In addition, the adverse effects of SSRIs include headache and insomnia or hypersomnia. Among the SSRIs, paroxetine is associated with weight gain. Upon sudden discontinuation of SSRIs such as paroxetine and sertraline, there is occurrence of discontinuation syndrome in some patients, which is characterized by dizziness and paresthesias. The FDA teratogen classification system has classified most of antidepressants as category C agents. The use of paroxetine in the first trimester is mainly associated with cardiac septal defects.

Drug Interaction

The pharmacokinetic interactions are the most common interactions associated with SSRIs. Based on the pharmacokinetic profile, paroxetine and fluoxetine are potent CYP2D6 inhibitors; hence, administration of these drugs along with 2D6 substrates such as TCAs can lead to unpredictable increase in tricyclic drug level, which can be toxic. Another SSRI, fluvoxamine, is an inhibitor of CYP3A4 enzyme that increases the concentration of subsequently administered substrate for this enzyme, such as diltiazem, and induces fall in blood pressure, that is, hypotension.

Contraindications

SSRIs are contraindicated with the concurrent use of MAOIs, linezolid, and other medications that increase serotonin levels and could put patients at risk of life-threatening serotonin syndrome. Paroxetine is contraindicated in pregnancy and is classified as category D/X due to its teratogenic effects in causing cardiovascular defects, specifically cardiac malformations, if prescribed in the first trimester.

Serotonin–Norepinephrine Reuptake Inhibitors

This type includes venlafaxine, along with its active metabolite desvenlafaxine, and duloxetine. Additionally, these SNRIs are used in pain disorders such as fibromyalgia and neuropathy, in the treatment of anxiety, and in relieving the menopausal symptoms. Venlafaxine and its active metabolite desvenlafaxine contain bicyclic ring in their structure, while duloxetine contains three cyclic rings in its structure. In the United States, milnacipran, which is an SNRI, has been approved for the treatment of fibromyalgia. Milnacipran is usually prescribed as a racemic mixture, and it contains cyclopropane ring in its structure. There is no structural similarity between the drugs belonging to this class. However, the in vivo results of venlafaxine and imipramine are similar to some extent, but among them, venlafaxine possesses more adverse effects than imipramine.

Mechanism of Action

The antidepressant mechanism by which SNRIs acts includes the inhibition of both SERT and norepinephrine transporter (NET). SNRIs initially cause the activation of 5-HT_{1A} and 5-HT_{1D} autoreceptors upon inhibition of SERT, which further results in decrease in neurotransmission of serotonin through the negative feedback mechanism till there is desensitization of serotonergic autoreceptors. Then, the increased serotonin level binds to the postsynaptic serotonergic receptors. These drugs mediate their noradrenergic action through downstream changes in gene expression, resulting in alteration of BDNF and TrkB levels and their corresponding signaling pathways. The expression of SERT is affected due to repeated administration of SSRIs, and this results in decreased neurotransmitter clearance and induced serotonergic or noradrenergic neurotransmission. SNRIs are devoid of side actions such as antihistamine, α-adrenergic blocking, and anticholinergic effects; hence, SNRIs are preferred over TCAs in cases of pain-related disorders due to their tolerability.

The pharmacokinetic profile of SNRIs has been summarized in **Table 38.2**.

Adverse Effects

All SNRIs exhibit serotonergic and noradrenergic adverse effects such as tachycardia and activation of central nervous system (CNS) including anxiety and insomnia. In addition, SNRIs are associated with some hemodynamic side effects, but these effects do not worsen in most patients. The administration of venlafaxine is associated with slight increase in blood pressure, which has been seen

Table 38.2 Pharmacokinetic profile of SNRIs

Drugs	Therapeutic dose (mg/d)	Bioavailability (%)	Active metabolite (h)	Plasma half-life (h)	Volume of distribution (L/kg)	Plasma protein binding (%)
Venlafaxine	75–375	45	9–13	8–11	4–10	27
Duloxetine	40–120	50	N	12–15	10–14	90
Milnacipran	100–200	85–90	N	6–8	5–6	13

Abbreviation: SNRI, serotonin–norepinephrine reuptake inhibitor.

Table 38.3 Pharmacokinetic profile of TCAs

Drugs	Therapeutic dose (mg/d)	Bioavailability (%)	Active metabolite (h)	Plasma half-life (h)	Volume of distribution (L/kg)	Plasma protein binding (%)
Imipramine	150–300	40	14–62	9–24	15–30	84
Clomipramine	100–250	50	54–77	19–37	7–20	97
Amitriptyline	150–300	45	20–92	31–46	5–10	90
Desipramine	150–300		33–51	11–46	–	–
Trimipramine maleate	150–300	30	16	23	–	–
Nortriptyline	50–150	–	30	16–88	–	–
Protriptyline	15–60	–	80		–	–
Doxepin	150–300	30	16	8–36	–	–

Abbreviation: TCA, tricyclic antidepressant.

in dose-dependent manner, but the same condition is not observed in the case of SNRIs. Similar to the SSRIs, these drugs are also associated with discontinuation syndrome.

Drug Interaction

As compared to SSRIs, SNRIs exhibit lesser CYP_{450} enzyme interactions. Venlafaxine and duloxetine are substrates, of which the former is an inhibitor of CYP2D6 and related isoenzymes, and the latter acts as a substrate for CYP3A4. Duloxetine inhibits CYP2D6 moderately, and so it increases the levels of TCA and other CYP2D6 substrates.

Contraindications

SNRIs should not be used in combination with MAOIs.

Tricyclic Antidepressants

Initially, TCAs were the dominant drugs of choice for depression, but after SSRIs were developed, SSRIs have become the preferred drugs. Almost all of the TCAs have tricyclic iminodibenzyl basic skeleton. In this class, imipramine is considered as a prototype drug. There are small differences between the drugs belonging to this class. There is a difference of only one methyl moiety in the propylamine side chain between imipramine and its metabolite desipramine. Due to these small differences between the structures of imipramine and its active metabolite desipramine, significant changes in their pharmacological actions have been observed, such as imipramine possesses highly anticholinergic, serotonin and norepinephrine reuptake inhibition actions, while desipramine possesses weak anticholinergic actions. Additionally, desipramine has greater tendency of inhibiting the selective norepinephrine reuptake. TCAs are preferred in patients who are not responsive to other antidepressants such as SSRIs and SNRIs. Overdoses of TCAs are lethal, which limits their use in depression. TCAs are also used in treating pain disorders, insomnia, and enuresis.

Mechanism of Action

The pharmacological actions of TCAs and SNRIs are way more similar. Basically, TCAs are thought to inhibit the reuptake of serotonin and norepinephrine. The affinities of drugs belonging to this class differ in terms of drugs. For example, clomipramine possesses greater binding affinity toward NET and lesser affinity toward SERT. Other TCAs with secondary amine, such as nortriptyline and desipramine, selectively bind to NET, but there is no evidence of them binding to SERT. Tertiary amine TCAs such as imipramine show large serotonergic effects that are counterbalanced by NET inhibitory effects of desipramine, that is, the metabolite of imipramine. Commonly, the adverse effects of TCAs are dry mouth and constipation, which are due to their potent anticholinergic effects. In addition, TCAs act as potent blockers of the H_1 histaminergic receptors. Due to these antihistaminergic effects, doxepin is extensively used in pruritus. Doxepin also acts as a hypnotic.

The pharmacokinetic profile of TCAs has been summarized in **Table 38.3**.

Adverse Effects

As discussed previously, TCAs possess anticholinergic effects, including constipation, dry mouth, bladder retention, cycloplegia, and mental confusion. The chances of the anticholinergic effects are associated prominently with the tertiary amine TCAs such as amitriptyline and imipramine over the secondary amine TCAs such as desipramine and nortriptyline. Additionally, TCAs show antiadrenergic actions such as antagonistic action on α-receptors, which finally causes orthostatic hypotension. The antihistaminergic side effects associated with TCAs include sedation and weight gain. At higher doses, TCAs cause rhythmic complications such as arrhythmia. Among all TCAs, clomipramine is associated with higher serotonergic actions that aggravate sexual side effects. Like SSRIs and SNRIs, discontinuation syndrome is commonly observed in the case of TCAs, which create flulike symptoms and cholinergic rebound that is characterized by mental confusion, anxiety, insomnia, etc.

Drug Interaction

In case of psychotic depression, synergism phenomenon has been observed with the use of TCAs and typical antipsychotics (specifically first-generation antipsychotics). The plasma concentration of TCAs is increased by the drugs, including bupropion and SSRIs, which inhibit CYP2D6 enzyme. There are various classes of drugs such as phenothiazine, class 1A antiarrhythmic agents, and other drugs associated with antihistaminic, anticholinergic, and antiadrenergic side effects that have similar adverse effects to TCAs and hence their concurrent administration may worsen the condition.

Contraindications

1. Family history of QTc interval prolongation or sudden cardiac death.
2. Hypersensitivity reactions to a TCA drug.
3. Requires caution in individuals with angle-closure glaucoma, as its anticholinergic effects may increase the risk of an acute ocular crisis.
4. Patients with CAD. However, CAD is not an absolute contraindication.

5-HT_2 Receptor Modulators

Serotonin also plays a major role in depression, so its modulation could be effective in cases of depression. Currently, there are two drugs, trazodone and nefazodone, that act through the modulation of 5-HT_2 receptors. The basic skeleton that is responsible for the antidepressant activity of trazodone is a triazolo heterocyclic ring. After administration, metabolite is generated, due to biotransformation process, as m-chlorophenylpiperazine that further acts as selective 5-HT_2 blocker. Initially, trazodone was the most preferred antidepressant, which was then dominated by the SSRIs in the 1980s. Currently, trazodone is being used as hypnotic and sedative. The major advantage of trazodone over other antidepressants is that it is devoid of dependence and tolerance. There is much structural similarity between trazodone and nefazodone. After administration, it gets transformed into its active metabolites such as hydroxynefazodone and m-chlorophenylpiperazine that further block 5-HT_2 receptors selectively. Both nefazodone and trazodone are principally used in major depressive cases, and in some instances, they are used as anxiolytics.

Mechanism of Action

Trazodone mainly targets 5-HT_{2A} and α_1-adrenergic receptors. In addition, it also inhibits SERT with lesser potency. The blockage of this serotonergic receptor produces the desired anxiolytic, antidepressant, and antipsychotic actions. Side actions of trazodone include weak presynaptic anti-α-adrenergic and moderate H_1 antihistaminic actions. The agonists of this 5-HT_{2A} receptor (e.g., lysergic acid, mescaline) can be reversely used as hallucinogenic and anxiogenic. Basically, the 5-HT_{2A} receptor is a G protein–coupled receptor present over the neocortex. Nefazodone is a potent blocker of 5-HT_{2A} receptor and a less potent inhibitor of SERT as well as NET.

Table 38.4 summarizes the pharmacokinetic profile of 5-HT_2 receptor modulators.

Adverse Effects

Adverse effects of these 5-HT_2 blockers are sedation and GI complications, out of which sedation is principally due to trazodone. Therefore, trazodone has been used for the treatment of insomnia. The GIT complications are mainly dose-dependent and their severity is less as compared to the SSRIs and SNRIs. As these drugs selectively block the 5-HT_2 receptor, there are lesser chances of sexual dysfunction. In some instances, trazodone is associated with priapism. The use of trazodone and nefazodone is associated with anti-α-adrenergic actions as well as dose-dependent reduction of blood pressure. The major adverse effect associated with nefazodone is hepatotoxicity; hence, FDA has given black box warning for nefazodone in 2001.

Drug Interaction

Due to the inhibition of CYP3A4 isoenzyme by nefazodone, the concentration of drug dependent on CYP3A4 isoenzyme is usually increased. For example, concurrent administration

Table 38.4 Pharmacokinetic profile of 5-HT2 receptor modulators

Drugs	Therapeutic dose (mg/d)	Bioavailability (%)	Active metabolite (h)	Plasma half-life (h)	Volume of distribution (L/kg)	Plasma protein binding (%)
Trazodone	150–300	95	N	3–6	1–3	96
Nefazodone	300–500	20	N	2–4	0.5–1	99

Abbreviation: N, no active metabolite.

of nefazodone causes the elevation of triazolam levels; hence, dose reduction of triazolam by 75% is employed. Similarly, on concurrent administration of nefazodone and simvastatin, there is elevation of plasma concentrations of simvastatin by 20-fold. In the case of trazodone, it is observed that it is a less potent inhibitor of CYP3A4 isoenzyme. Therefore, administration of trazodone in combination with other potent inhibitors of the same isoenzyme such as ritonavir results in the elevation of trazodone levels. As trazodone and nefazodone weakly inhibit the reuptake of serotonin, it should not be administered concurrently along with MAOIs due to drastic increase in serotonin levels, which finally result in serotonin syndrome.

Contraindications

Trazodone should be avoided in cardiovascular diseases (CVDs), arrhythmia, and serotonin syndrome, while nefazodone is contraindicated in manic episodes, patients with suicidal thought, patients with cardiovascular disorders, bleeding ulcers, seizures, and acute or chronic hepatic failure cases.

Tetracyclic and Unicyclic Antidepressants

The agents belonging to this category are random drugs that do not suit any other classes of antidepressants. These agents are widely known as atypical antidepressants, which include mirtazapine, bupropion, mirtazapine, and amoxapine. Chemically, bupropion contains cyclic aminoketone in its structure. Bupropion shares structural similarity with amphetamine; as a result, it exhibits CNS-stimulating properties. It is used to treat major depression and for smoking cessation. The off-level target of bupropion is neuropathic pain and obesity; additionally, it has proved its efficacy in relieving attention deficit hyperactivity syndrome (ADHD) symptoms. In 1994, mirtazapine was approved as an antidepressant that does not have any kind of sexual adverse effects. It contains tetracyclic ring as a basic skeleton and piperazinoazepine moiety. Other agents that have tetracyclic ring in their structure include amoxapine and maprotiline. Loxapine, an antipsychotic drug, after biotransformation releases its *N*-methylated active metabolite amoxapine. Amoxapine and maprotiline are structurally similar and hence they possess same adverse effects.

Mechanism of Action

The exact mode of action of bupropion is not clear yet. Hydroxybupropion is a metabolite of bupropion that inhibits the reuptake of norepinephrine and dopamine moderately. It induces the release of norepinephrine and dopamine presynaptically. Bupropion is not associated with any kind of serotonergic effects. Mirtazapine acts by antagonizing the presynaptic α_2 autoreceptor and induces the release of catecholamines. In addition, it blocks 5-HT_2 and 5-HT_3 receptors. Mirtazapine antagonizes H_1 receptor with greater potency and shows sedation as a side effect. Both amoxapine and maprotiline act as NET inhibitors with greater potency and as SERT inhibitors with lesser potency. Both the drugs show anticholinergic side effects. Amoxapine is a moderate blocker of D_2 receptors that are present postsynaptically; as a result, it shows various antipsychotic side effects.

Table 38.5 summarizes pharmacokinetic profile of tetracyclic and unicyclic antidepressants.

Adverse Effects

Amoxapine blocks D_2 receptors and hence symptoms similar to those of Parkinson's disease, such as muscular rigidity, akathisia, and tardive dyskinesia, occur. Maprotiline causes side effects similar to those of TCA, due to its greater affinity toward NET. In some instances, bupropion causes side effects such as insomnia, loss of appetite, and agitation.

Drug Interactions

The metabolism of bupropion is mainly carried out by CYP2B6; therefore, its metabolism is affected by drugs that are substrates for CYP2B6, such as cyclophosphamide. The metabolite of bupropion, hydroxybupropion, inhibits CYP2D6 moderately; thus, there will be elevation in levels of desipramine. It is contraindicated in patients taking MAOIs. Various CYP450 and its isoenzymes are influenced by mirtazapine as it acts as a substrate for these isoenzymes. Hence, the level of mirtazapine is elevated by drugs that inhibit these isoenzymes. The addictive behavior of mirtazapine in combination with other CNS depressants such as benzodiazepines (BZDs) has been observed due to the moderate sedative effects of mirtazapine.

Most of the interactions are common with amoxapine, maprotiline, and the agents belonging to the TCA class of antidepressants. Both amoxapine and maprotiline act as substrates for CYP2D6; therefore, they should be used cautiously with drugs that inhibit this isoenzyme. Both the drugs possess antihistaminic as well as anticholinergic effects.

Monoamine Oxidase Inhibitors

This class of antidepressants was discovered in the 1950s, but the major complications of these drugs are

Table 38.5 Pharmacokinetic profile of tetracyclic and unicyclic antidepressants

Drugs	Therapeutic dose (mg/d)	Bioavailability (%)	Active metabolite (h)	Plasma half-life (h)	Volume of distribution (L/kg)	Plasma protein binding (%)
Amoxapine	150–400	–	5–30	7–12	0.9–1.2	90
Bupropion	250–450	70	15–25	11–14	20–30	84
Mirtazapine	15–45	50	20–40	20–40	3–7	85
Maprotiline	150–225	70	–	43–45	23–27	88

their interactions and toxicity profile, which limit their use. The use of this class of drugs is mainly preferred in patients who are not giving response to other classes of antidepressants. Currently, there are two chemical classes of MAOIs, hydrazine derivatives and nonhydrazine derivatives. Agents belonging to hydrazine class are isocarboxazid and phenelzine, whereas nonhydrazine derivatives are tranylcypromine, selegiline, and moclobemide. The hydrazine derivatives and tranylcypromine are irreversible, nonselective inhibitors of MAO-A and MAO-B enzymes. The nonhydrazine derivative tranylcypromine shares structural similarity with amphetamine. Other MAOIs such as selegiline share similar metabolites with amphetamine. Due to this structural similarity, these MAOIs are associated with some CNS stimulatory actions.

Mechanism of Action

This class of antidepressants mainly increases the level of monoamine by inhibiting MAO enzyme, which is responsible for the degradation of monoamines. There are two types of MAO enzymes, MAO-A and MAO-B. The former, mainly responsible for dopamine and norepinephrine degradation, is found in the brain, placenta, gut, and liver, while the latter is responsible for serotonin and histamine and is distributed in the brain, liver, and platelets. The primary substrates of MAO-A are norepinephrine, epinephrine, and serotonin. The metabolism of tryptamine as well as dopamine is carried out by MAO-B. The nonselective and irreversible MAOIs are phenelzine and tranylcypromine. The presence of food is one of the factors responsible for the drug interactions such as displacement of moclobemide from MAO-A by tyramine. At low doses, selegiline act as an irreversible MAO-B inhibitor. It has been proved as an effective antiparkinsonian agent at low doses, whereas it acts as a nonselective MAOI at higher doses.

Table 38.6 summarizes the pharmacokinetic profile of MAOIs.

Adverse Effects

The major risk factors associated with the use of MAOIs are orthostatic hypotension and weight gain, which limit their use as an antidepressant. Among other antidepressants, the irreversible, nonselective MAOIs show frequent cases of sexual effects. Due to the resemblance in structure with amphetamine, some MAOIs cause insomnia and restlessness. The nonselective and irreversible MAOI, phenelzine, shows more sedative effects as compared with other drugs such as selegiline and tranylcypromine. Due to the inhibition of metabolic pathway of tyramine, various MAOIs show serious interactions related to food as well as to drugs belonging to the serotonergic class. All MAOIs cause discontinuation syndrome, characterized by deliriumlike condition, psychosis at some extent, excitement, and mental confusion.

Drug Interactions

All MAOIs in combination with SSRIs, SNRI, and TCAs show life-threatening interaction such as serotonin syndrome, which is mainly caused by the overactivation of serotonergic receptors located throughout the medulla and gray nuclei. The symptoms associated with serotonin syndrome are delirium, coma, hypertension, tachycardia, tremor, hyperreflexia, etc. Therefore, various drugs that can increase serotonergic activity should be avoided in combination with MAOIs. The other interaction associated with MAOIs is the increase in blood pressure. This interaction is observed when MAOIs are administered with tyramine-rich food or with sympathomimetic agents, which act as a substrate for MAO. MAOIs block the breakdown pathway of tyramine, which further causes the elevation in tyramine in serum and induces all the peripheral adrenergic actions, and finally there is dramatic increase in blood pressure. Cases of malignant hypertension and myocardial infarction have been observed in patients who took MAOIs and higher amount of tyramine-rich food additionally. Hence, patients who are on MAOIs should not ingest food containing tyramine such as cheese, soya products, and dried sausages. Similar complications have been observed with the use of sympathomimetic in patients taking MAOIs.

Miscellaneous Agents

Esketamine

It is a noncompetitive NMDA receptor antagonist. It has been approved by FDA in 2013 for treatment-resistant depression. It should be taken with an oral antidepressant. Major side effects of this medication include sedation and difficulty in attention and judgment. It has potential to be misused and abused. Therefore, restricted use of esketamine is recommended.

Brexanolone (Allopregnanolone)

It is a neuroactive steroid gamma-aminobutyric acid ($GABA_A$) receptor positive modulator and has been approved for management of postpartum depression by the US FDA in 2019. Patient taking brexanolone may experience sedation, sleepiness, sudden loss of consciousness, and dry mouth. It has very low oral bioavailability (~5%), which necessitates use of parenteral route of administration.

Table 38.6 Pharmacokinetic profile of MAO inhibitors

Drugs	Therapeutic dose (mg/d)	Bioavailability (%)	Active metabolite (h)	Plasma half-life (h)	Volume of distribution (L/kg)	Plasma protein binding (%)
Phenelzine	45–90	–	–	11	–	–
Selegiline	20–50	4	9–11	8–10	20–30	99

Abbreviation: MAO, monoamine oxidase.

Selection of Antidepressant

While selecting an antidepressant, there is little to choose in between different classes of antidepressants. The major selection should be based on the requirement of individual patient, including ongoing medications, presence of disease conditions, suicidal risk, and previous response to antidepressants. Diagnosis and management of depression in underlying medical condition appear cumbersome. Depression may appear as a comorbid condition of the medical condition or as a putative side effect of the medication used for the same. There are different medical conditions in which depression may occur as a comorbid condition, and its management has been discussed herewith.

Depression with Cardiovascular Disorders

Depression appears as a very common comorbid condition in patients with CVD. It reduces the quality of life and enhances the overall health care expenditure and mortality. Depression is present in 20 to 30% of patients with CAD, peripheral artery disease, and heart failure. Presence of depression often complicates the management of CVD by aggravating cardiovascular risk factors and diminishing adherence to healthy lifestyles. Depression also appears to worsen the risk of CVD, possibly via augmented platelet aggregation. Unfortunately, the incidence of depression in patients with CVD remains under-recognized; thus, management strategies targeting depression remain unprivileged in CVD.

TCAs are capable of inducing tachycardia, which appears as a matter of concern in patients with congestive heart failure; thus, TCAs are contraindicated in patients with bundle branch block. Besides, orthostatic hypotension has been more commonly reported with TCAs, trazodone, and MAOIs. Therefore, these antidepressants are contraindicated in depression associated with CVD. There are certain antidepressants that may have potential for QT prolongation, such as TCAs, certain SSRIs, SNRIs, and mirtazapine. The potential for QT prolongation is present in TCAs, certain SSRIs, certain SNRIs, and mirtazapine.

Owing to the low risk of drug interactions, adverse effects, and antiplatelet potential, sertraline is considered the safest choice for antidepressants for patients with ischemic heart disease. SSRIs and SNRIs are comparatively safer options for patients with heart failure. In patients with ventricular arrhythmias, bupropion appears to be a better option, as it has overall lowest risk of QT prolongation. Moreover, SSRIs may exhibit potential interaction with hepatic metabolism of anticoagulants, thereby causing increased anticoagulation.

Depression in Cancer Patients

Appropriate diagnosis and suitable management of depression in patients with cancer improves their quality of life and survival outcome. The prevalence of depression in patients with cancer is around 25%; however, in pancreatic and oropharynx cancer, this may go up to 50%. Antidepressant therapy in cancer patients has been shown to impart beneficial effect on the overall quality of life. Antidepressants may appear beneficial in mitigating depressive symptoms besides clinical depression. In acute phase of treatment with antidepressants, no differences between various antidepressants were recorded. While considering potential adverse effect, drug interactions, and heterogeneity in between studies (probably with small sample size), a generalized conclusion may not be drawn till well-defined controlled studies are performed.

Depression with Cerebrovascular Disorders

The importance of diagnosis and early management of depression in patients with neurological disorders is supported by increased prevalence and worsening effect on the quality of life and health care burden. The estimated prevalence of depression ranges from 20 to 72% after stroke, 40 to 50% in Alzheimer's disease and Parkinson's disease, up to 54% in multiple sclerosis, and around 55% in epilepsy. Generally, antidepressants remain the preferred choice for the treatment of depression in patients with Alzheimer's disease. However, there is conflicting evidence regarding cognitive outcome of antidepressants, with some observations indicating beneficial outcome, while some report worsening effect on memory. Despite the higher prevalence of depression in patients with neurological diseases, less randomized clinical trials are reported on potential of antidepressants, limiting comprehensible conclusions.

Depression with Diabetes Mellitus

Development of depression is two to three times higher in patients with diabetes mellitus, with the overall prevalence ranging from 8 to 27% depending on the degree of hyperglycemia and associated complications.Bidirectional association between depression and diabetes has also been observed, as depression may enhance the chances of development of diabetes by 60%. Higher prevalence, adverse effect on health and quality of life, and depression in diabetes remain underdiagnosed and thus undertreated. The clinical course of antidepressants in diabetes may be complicated by their potential to modulate glycemic index. TCAs may develop hyperglycemia, while SSRIs, SNRIs, and MAOIs may induce hypoglycemia.

Depression with Hypothyroidism

The association of hypothyroidism with a variety of mood problems and memory impairment has been observed. Improvement in thyroid profile (with thyroid replacement therapy) may improve underlying depressionlike symptoms; however, sometimes, use of antidepressants may be required. TCAs and SSRIs have been reported to elevate the activity of deiodinase enzyme type 2, resulting in enhanced conversion of T4 into T3 in the brain.

Depression in HIV Patients

Depression is one of the common comorbid conditions in patients with HIV infection, while effective management of the same improves morbidity and mortality in HIV patients. The diagnosis of depression in patients with HIV may be complicated by associated emotional and physiological states. The mainstay of management of depression in patients with HIV remains antidepressants. The effect of antidepressants in HIV patients is similar to non-HIV patients. Moreover, no any specific antidepressant has been reported to be superior in HIV patients. However, some psychiatric drugs have been reported to assuage depressive symptoms in HIV replication. Additionally, SSRIs and TCAs have been reported to be effective in the management of depression in patients with HIV without altering their immune status.

Clinical Indications of Antidepressants

Major Depressive Disorders

For short-term and long-term management of major depression, a wide variety of antidepressants have been approved by FDA. Acute episodes of depression may last from weeks to months, while long-term episodes of depression may last 2 years or longer. The remission of major symptoms of depression is the major goal of antidepressant medications. Use of antidepressants has been reported to achieve remission of around 30 to 40% patients in 8 to 12 weeks of treatment. If adequate response is achieved, the treatment should be continued, otherwise switching to another agent or combination of other drug may appear appropriate. Considering an example, if monotherapy fails, mirtazapine or bupropion (atypical antipsychotic) may be added to SNRIs/SSRIs for augmentation of therapeutic response. Around 70 to 80% cases of depression are able to attain improvement with alternate or add-on therapy. Once a particular therapeutic regimen achieves successful mitigation of depression symptoms, the regimen may be continued for up to 12 months to avoid risk of relapse.

Relapse cases or multiple recurrence cases may lead to development of chronic and/or pharmacoresistant depression. Therefore, for maintenance or prevention of recurrence, prolonged therapy may be necessary. In long-term treatment, SSRIs, SNRIs, and TCAs have shown beneficial effects and therefore are highly recommended in such cases. Further antidepressants may not be useful in all types of depression, for instance, patients with bipolar disorders may not be benefited with antidepressants or add-on mood stabilizers.

Cognitive behavioral therapy may appear as an alternative therapeutic strategy for management of mild-to-moderate depression. As this therapy takes longer time, it is often combined with antidepressants to improve efficacy.

Generalized Anxiety Disorders

The next major use of antidepressant appears to be in the treatment of generalized anxiety disorders. Many SSRIs and SNRIs are approved for anxiety disorders such as panic attack, OCD, PTSD, and social phobias. Moreover, BZDs provide better relief in anxiety and panic disorders than antidepressants. Nevertheless, antidepressants exhibit better efficacy (including lack of tolerance and dependence) in chronic management of anxiety as compared to BZDs. SSRIs and clomipramine, by virtue of their serotonergic mechanism, have been approved for management of OCD. In addition, SSRIs and venlafaxine are approved for management of social phobias. Besides, SSRIs are first-line drugs for the management of PTSD.

Neuropathic Pain

Chronic pain has often been reported in association with major depression. Antidepressants have been considered as first-line drug of choice for management of fibromyalgia and neuropathic pain. The agents, capable of elevating NE and 5-HT level, are often useful as analgesics. Norepinephrine appears extremely important for mitigating neuropathic pain in spinal cord. Since 1960, TCAs have been utilized for management of neuropathic pain. Highly effective antidepressants for the management of neuropathic pain are tertiary amine TCAs (imipramine, amitriptyline, doxepin), duloxetine, bupropion, and venlafaxine. Secondary amine TCAs (nortriptyline, desipramine) appear to be the next most effective drugs in managing pain. The analgesic effect of 5-HT in neuropathic pain remains unclear. SSRIs are highly recommended for depression; however, they are not recommended for neuropathic pain. Citalopram and paroxetine appear to possess modest analgesic activity; however, fluoxetine appears ineffective in such cases. The antidepressant milnacipran has been approved for the clinical management of fibromyalgia in the United States and for major depression in other countries.

Smoking Cessation

For the last two decades, bupropion is being prescribed as an adjuvant for smoking cessation. It reduces withdrawal symptoms and craving for nicotine. It appears as effective as other aids for smoking cessation such as nicotine patches and nicotine replacement therapy; however, it is less efficacious than varenicline. At lesser dose, bupropion may enhance the rewarding pathway of nicotine and self-administration; however, at higher dose, it reduces the same.

Miscellaneous Uses

Fluoxetine and sertraline are approved for the management of PMDDs, including irritable behavior, insomnia, altered mood, and other associated physical symptoms. Antidepressants have proved their efficacy in bulimia nervosa. For the last two decades, fluoxetine has been observed to reduce binge–purge cycle. Bupropion treatment has been suggested for management of obesity.

Mood Stabilizers

Mood-stabilizing agents can also be used in bipolar disorders. In addition, these drugs have been found to be effective in depression. Examples of mood stabilizers are lithium, valproic acid, and carbamazepine, of which the latter two agents are used as effective antiepileptic agents.

Lithium

The first clinical use of lithium was reported in the 19th century in a patient with gout. It was used as an alternative for sodium chloride in patients with hypertension, but it was found to be toxic, due to which it was withdrawn from the market.

Mechanism of Action

Lithium mainly suppresses inositol trisphosphate (IP_3) diacyl glycerol (DAG) signaling via decreasing the level of intracellular inositol and inhibiting glycogen synthase kinase-3, a kind of protein kinase. This kinase is helpful in almost all intracellular signaling pathways; some of them include signaling through insulin/IGF, BDNF, and WNT pathway. In various reports, it has been observed that one of the prominent mechanisms responsible for mood-stabilizing action is suppression of inositol (**Fig. 38.3**).

Pharmacokinetics

Table 38.7 summarizes pharmacokinetic profile of lithium.

Adverse Effects

The most common adverse effect associated with the use of lithium is tremor, which occurs at therapeutic doses. Apart

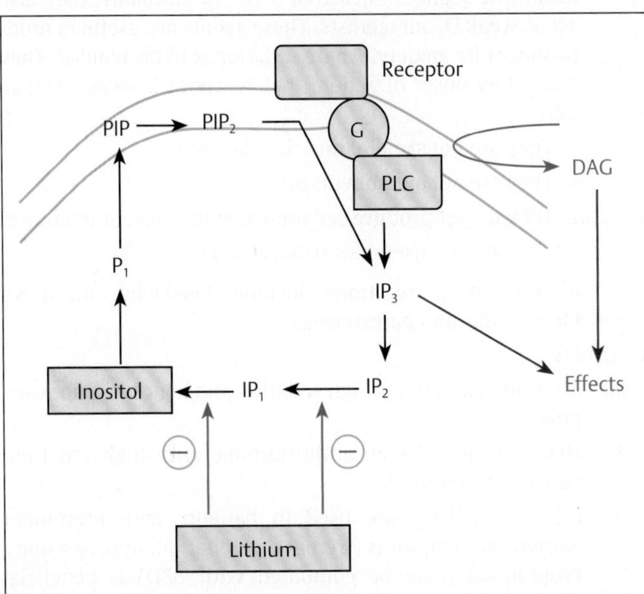

Fig. 38.3 Mechanism of action of lithium.

from this, it causes choreoathetosis, motor hyperactivity, ataxia, dysarthria, and aphasia; in some instances, psychiatric disturbances are observed, which are characterized by mental confusion. The use of lithium is associated with hypothyroidism, as it suppresses thyroid function. According to several reports, it is clear that long-term lithium administration causes renal dysfunction. Edema is the most common of all adverse effects associated with lithium use. In lactating women, upon administration of lithium, it is transported to infant via breast milk; therefore, toxicity in newborns is observed, which is manifested by lethargy and cyanosis. Lithium directly affects the process of leukopoiesis; thus, leukocytosis is related to lithium use.

Drug Interaction

There is a reduction of renal clearance of lithium by diuretics and various newer nonsteroidal anti-inflammatory drugs.

Carbamazepine

Carbamazepine is used as an alternative to lithium in cases of bipolar disorders. Structural similarities have been found between carbamazepine and phenytoin. Carbamazepine contains ureide moiety as a basic skeleton, which is common in almost all antiepileptic drugs.

Mechanism of Action

At therapeutic doses, carbamazepine antagonizes Na^+ channels; therefore, it minimizes frequent neuronal firings. In addition, it lowers synaptic transmission by acting presynapticallly.

Pharmacokinetics

Table 38.8 summarizes pharmacokinetic profile of carbamazepine.

Adverse Effects

The most common adverse effects associated with the use of carbamazepine are ataxia and diplopia. Initially, diplopia occurs, and it lasts an hour. Other adverse effects of carbamazepine are GI complaints, drowsiness, and hyponatremia. Some severe adverse effects are aplastic anemia, blood dyscrasias, and agranulocytosis. Most of these occur within 4 months of use.

Table 38.7 Pharmacokinetic profile of lithium

Drug	Volume of distribution (L/Kg)	Plasma concentration (mEq/L)
Lithium	0.5	0.6–1.4

Table 38.8 Pharmacokinetic profile of carbamazepine

Drug	Volume of distribution (L/kg)	Plasma protein binding (%)	Half life (h)	Systemic clearance (L/kg/d)
Carbamazepine	1	70	36	1

Table 38.9 Pharmacokinetic profile of valproic acid

Drug	Volume of distribution (L/kg)	Plasma protein binding (%)	Half-life (h)
Valproic acid	0.15	90	9–18

Drug Interactions

As carbamazepine is an enzyme inducer, various interactions are associated with this property of carbamazepine. Drugs such as valproic acid block the clearance of carbamazepine; hence, there is elevation of blood levels of carbamazepine. To date, no significant interactions related to protein binding have been reported.

Valproic Acid

Sodium valproate and its acid form valproic acid were used as solvents at a time when the search for more effective antiepileptic medications was on, and it was found that valproic acid itself acts as a promising antiepileptic agent. At normal body pH, valproic acid get ionized, and hence it is considered as valproate ion instead of valproic acid or sodium valproate. Basically, valproic acid is a derivative of fatty carboxylic acid, which possesses antiepileptic activity. This activity depends upon the length of carbon chain. Other derivatives of valproic acid such as amide and esters also show antiseizure activity.

Mechanism of Action

Valproic acid principally antagonizes more frequent neuronal firing at therapeutic concentrations. It mediates its protective action by blocking the excitatory NMDA receptors. In addition, it acts on GABA receptors. Valproic acid acts as a glutamic acid decarboxylase (GAD) facilitator. GAD is an enzyme that plays a vital role in synthesis of GABA. Valproate inhibits GABA transaminase enzyme at high concentrations, which ultimately means valproate stops the degradation of GABA. Another action of valproate is to inhibit histone deacetylase with which transcription of many genes are associated.

Pharmacokinetics

Table 38.9 summarizes pharmacokinetic profile of valproic acid.

Adverse Effects

The most common adverse effects of valproic acid are nausea, vomiting, and GI disturbances. At higher doses, tremor has been observed frequently. Other unwanted effects associated with the use of valproic acid are weight gain, alopecia, and increased appetite. The severe adverse effect associated with valproic acid is hepatotoxicity, which is seen in patients younger than 2 years and in those who are taking more than one medication. In several patients, reversible hepatotoxicity is observed, that is, the risk of hepatotoxicity is lower upon cessation of drug use. In addition, thrombocytopenia and teratogenic defect as spina bifida are reported in various cases.

Drug Interactions

Phenytoin bound to plasma proteins is found to be displaced by valproic acid. Additionally, the metabolism of phenobarbital, phenytoin, and carbamazepine is inhibited by valproic acid, which elevates steady-state concentrations of these drugs. Due to the inhibition of metabolism of phenobarbital, there is an intense increase in its level, which further causes coma. The clearance of lamotrigine is affected by valproic acid.

Anxiolytics (PS 8.4, PS8.6)

1. For BZDs as antianxiety agents, please refer to chapter on sedative hypnotics.
2. Non-BZDs.
   a. Buspirone, ipsapirone, gepirone: They are azapirone derivatives that act as selective 5-HT_{1A} partial agonists. 5-HT_{1A} receptors are inhibitory autoreceptors. Binding of buspirone reduces release of 5-HT. Additionally, they also act as weak D_2 antagonists. These agents are useful in mild-to-moderate anxiety, where sedation is to be avoided. They have slow onset of action, that is, about 2 weeks. Unlike BZD:
      i. They are not skeletal muscle relaxants.
      ii. They are not anticonvulsants.
      iii. They do not produce sedation, dependence, or tolerance.
      iv. They are not useful for panic attacks.

   Adverse drug reactions include headache, dizziness, tachycardia, and paresthesias.
3. Others:
   a. Meprobamate: It has high sedation and hence it is not used now.
   b. Hydroxyzine: It is an antihistaminic with high sedation; hence, it is not used.
   c. β-blockers: They are used in patients with prominent autonomic symptoms (tremors, palpitation, hypertension). Propranolol (may be combined with BZD) is beneficial before public speaking and stage performance.

Multiple Choice Questions

1. A 43-year-old woman with a history of fibromyalgia and depression presents to her primary care physician for treatment. She complains of feeling sad and worthless in addition to multiple somatic complaints. Which of the following treatments would be best for this patient?

A. Duloxetine.
B. Fluoxetine.
C. Mirtazapine.
D. Sertraline.
E. Watchful waiting.

Answer: A

Duloxetine is a serotonin/norepinephrine reuptake inhibitor that can be used for depression accompanied by neuropathic pain.

2. A 62-year-old woman with symptoms of feeling blue, sad, and without feelings presents to her primary care physician for treatment. She has a prior medical history of narrow-angle glaucoma. Which of the following treatments should be avoided in this patient?

A. Amitriptyline.
B. Bupropion.
C. Fluvoxamine.
D. Mirtazapine.
E. Sertraline.

Answer: A

Because of its potent antimuscarinic activity, amitriptyline should not be given to patients with glaucoma because of the risk of acute increases in ocular pressure.

3. A 42-year-old woman with feelings of sadness, despair, and tearfulness presents to her primary care physician for management. She has no prior medical or surgical history. Therapy with bupropion has begun. The treating physician must be aware of which of the following contraindications?

A. Anorexia.
B. Depression.
C. Seasonal affective disorder.
D. Seasonal affective disorder with mania.
E. Transient ischemic attacks.

Answer: A

Bupropion is indicated in the treatment of depression and seasonal affective disorder. This agent is not recommended for patients younger than 18 years. Contraindications include seizure disorders, anorexia, and bulimia.

4. A 68-year-old woman with a long history of sadness, gloom, and weight loss presents to her primary care physician for treatment. She is treated with a selective serotonin reuptake inhibitor (SSRI). Which of the following statements is true?

A. Maximum benefit may require 1 year.
B. Most patients require three antidepressants.
C. With adequate doses for 8 weeks, 20% of the patients respond to therapy.
D. Therapy for 2 weeks is required for mood improvement.

Answer: D

Antidepressants, including SSRIs, typically take at least 2 weeks to produce significant improvement in mood, and maximum benefit may require up to 12 weeks or more. However, none of the antidepressants are uniformly effective. Approximately 40% of patients with depression treated with adequate doses for 4 to 8 weeks do not respond to the antidepressant agent. Patients who do not respond to one antidepressant may respond to another, and approximately 80% or more will respond to at least one antidepressant drug.

5. An 18-year-old woman presents to clinic because of difficulty with school. She recently started college and is living on her own for the first time. She is constantly preoccupied with wondering if the door is locked. She checks the lock at least 20 times before she is able to leave her apartment. This often makes her late for class. She had been on selective serotonin reuptake inhibitors (SSRIs) in the past, but they are ineffective. What is the most appropriate treatment for this patient?

A. Amitriptyline.
B. Clomipramine.
C. Lithium.
D. Quetiapine.
E. Venlafaxine.

Answer: B

This patient has obsessive-compulsive disorder. Clomipramine is a tricyclic antidepressant that is also used in the treatment of obsessive-compulsive disorder. It is used as a second-line treatment when selective serotonin reuptake inhibitors fail.

6. A 27-year-old man is prescribed with an antidepressant for seasonal affective disorder. This particular antidepressant may also help him quit smoking. Which of the following antidepressants is he likely taking?

A. Bupropion.
B. Duloxetine.
C. Imipramine.
D. Sertraline.
E. Trazodone.

Answer: A

Bupropion is an antidepressant used to treat seasonal affective disorder (SAD) and is also used for smoking cessation. It is not chemically related to other known antidepressants. Although the mechanisms of action of bupropion for SAD and smoking cessation are not understood, it is known to inhibit dopamine reuptake. Interestingly, its antidepressant effect is seen even at doses too small to inhibit dopamine reuptake.

7. A 34-year-old woman with depression presents to the ambulatory care clinic with altered mental status. She is confused and unsure where she is. Her blood pressure is 240/152 mm Hg. Her creatinine is 2.93 mg/dL, which is above her baseline of 0.90 mg/dL. Her husband says she never had a problem with high blood pressure before. Everything was normal 3 hours prior to her having three glasses of wine and cheese at a party. She recently started a new medication for her depression. What is the most likely medication she started?

A. Amitriptyline.
B. Duloxetine.
C. Fluoxetine.
D. Phenelzine.
E. Trazodone.

Answer: D

Phenelzine is a monoamine oxidase inhibitor used in the treatment of depression. However, it is rarely used because of the risk of hypertensive crisis, which this patient has, after

consuming tyramine-containing foods. Wine and aged cheeses are known for containing tyramine.

8. A 53-year-old man comes to clinic for depression. He has had decreased interest and a depressed mood for the past 6 months. He also smokes half a pack of cigarettes a day. He thinks that if he could quit, it would help his mood as well. What is the most appropriate treatment for his depression and cessation of smoking?

A. Bupropion.

B. Clomipramine.

C. Imipramine.

D. Mirtazapine.

E. Sertraline.

Answer: A

Bupropion is an antidepressant that is also used for smoking cessation. The mechanism of action is an increase in norepinephrine and dopamine. It is also used for those who do not want the sexual side effects of other antidepressants.

9. A 19-year-old woman with anorexia presents to her primary care physician for follow-up. She weighs 82 lb with a body mass index (BMI) of 16.2. She says she tries to eat but is just not happy enough to eat. She has been feeling depressed for quite a while. The physician decides to start her on medication that will increase her weight and improve her mood. What is the most appropriate treatment for this patient?

A. Bupropion.

B. Maprotiline.

C. Mirtazapine.

D. Trazodone.

E. Venlafaxine.

Answer: C

Mirtazapine is an atypical antidepressant that increases the release of norepinephrine and serotonin by α_2 antagonism. It is rarely used because of the side effects of increased appetite and weight gain. However, in the case of anorexia, it is beneficial for the patient.

10. Indicate the antidepressant that blocks the reuptake pumps for serotonin and norepinephrine:

A. Amitriptyline.

B. Fluoxetine.

C. Maprotiline.

D. Phenelzine.

Answer: A

The TCAs like amitriptyline block the reuptake of both norepinephrine and serotonin (5-HT). This phenomenon being the primary mechanism of action of antidepressants brings changes in the physiological behavior of neuroreceptors. TCAs have also been reported to block muscarinic, α1 adrenergic, and histaminic receptors. However, these molecules may lead to occurrence of different side effects.

11. Which of the following antidepressants is an non-selective monoamine oxidase (MAO) blocker and produces extremely long-lasting inhibition of the enzyme?

A. Moclobemide.

B. Tranylcypromine.

C. Selegiline.

D. Fluoxetine.

Answer: B

Currently, there are two chemical classes of MAOIs, hydrazine derivatives and nonhydrazine derivatives. Agents belonging to hydrazine class are isocarboxazid and phenelzine, whereas nonhydrazine derivatives are tranylcypromine, selegiline, and moclobemide. The hydrazine derivatives and tranylcypromine are irreversible, nonselective inhibitors of MAO-A and MAO-B enzymes. The nonhydrazine derivative tranylcypromine shares structural similarity with amphetamine.

12. The principal mechanism of monoamine oxidase inhibitor action is:

A. Blocking the amine reuptake pumps, which permits to increase the concentration of the neurotransmitter at the receptor site.

B. Blocking a major degradative pathway for the amine neurotransmitters, which permits more amines to accumulate in presynaptic stores.

C. Inhibiting the storage of amine neurotransmitters in the vesicles of presynaptic nerve endings.

D. Antagonizing α_2-norepinephrine receptors.

Answer: B

This class of antidepressants mainly increases the level of monoamine by inhibiting MAO enzyme, which is responsible for the degradation of monoamines. There are two types of MAO enzymes, MAO-A and MAO-B. The former, mainly responsible for dopamine and norepinephrine degradation, is found in the brain, placenta, gut, and liver, while the latter is responsible for serotonin and histamine and is distributed in the brain, liver, and platelets. The primary substrates of MAO-A are norepinephrine, epinephrine, and serotonin. The metabolism of tryptamine as well as dopamine is carried out by MAO-B.

13. The irreversible monoamine oxidase inhibitors (MAOIs) have a very high risk of developing:

A. Respiratory depression.

B. Cardiovascular collapse and central nervous system (CNS) depression.

C. Hypertensive reactions to tyramine ingested in food.

D. Potentially fatal agranulocytosis.

Answer: C

Due to the inhibition of metabolic pathway of tyramine, various MAOIs show serious interactions related to food as well as to drugs belonging to the serotonergic class.

14. Fluoxetine has fewer adverse effects because of:

A. Mixed norepinephrine and serotonin reuptake inhibition.

B. Depleted stores of amine neurotransmitters.
C. Minimal binding to cholinergic, histaminic, and α-adrenergic receptors.
D. All of the above.

Answer: C

Unlike other classes of antidepressants, SSRIs have little effect on other neurotransmitters such as dopamine or norepinephrine. SSRIs also have relatively fewer side effects compared to TCAs and MAOIs due to having fewer effects on adrenergic, cholinergic, and histaminergic receptors.

15. Which of the following tricyclic and heterocyclic agents has the least sedation?

A. Protriptyline.
B. Trazodone.
C. Amitriptyline.
D. Mirtazapine.

Answer: A

A common problem with TCAs is sedation (drowsiness, lack of physical and mental alertness), but protriptyline is considered the least sedating agent among this class of agents. Its side effects are especially noticeable early in therapy.

16. A 30-year-old stockbroker has developed a "nervous disposition." He is easily frightened, fears about insignificant issues, and occasionally complains of stomach cramps. He grinds his teeth in his sleep. There is no history of drug abuse. Diagnosed as suffering from generalized anxiety disorder, he is given buspirone. His physician must tell the patient to expect:

A. A need to continually increase drug dosage because of tolerance.
B. A significant effect of the drug on memory.
C. That the drug is likely to take a week or more to begin working.
D. That if he stops taking the drug abruptly, he will experience withdrawal sign.

Answer: D

Buspirone is a selective anxiolytic with pharmacologic actions different from those of sedative-hypnotics. Buspirone has insignificant effects on cognition or memory; tolerance is minimal; and it has no dependence liability. Buspirone is not effective in acute anxiety because it has a slow onset of action.

Chapter 39 Antipsychotic Drugs

Nishigandha Suresh Jadhav

PH1.19: Describe the mechanism/s of action, types, doses, side effects, indications, and contraindications of drugs that act on the central nervous system (CNS) (including anxiolytics, sedatives and hypnotics, antipsychotics, antidepressant drugs, antimaniacs, opioid agonists and antagonists, drugs used for neurodegenerative disorders, and antiepileptic drugs).

Learning Objectives

- Psychiatric disorders.
- Pharmacological actions of typical/classical antipsychotics.
- Atypical or novel antipsychotic drugs.

Psychiatric Disorders

These are group of conditions that affect the mental functioning of an individual. These are broadly categorized in **Table 39.1**. The differences between psychoses and neuroses are enlisted in **Table 39.2**.

Psychoses

These are a group of mental illnesses with distortion of thought process, loss of ability to recognize reality (false belief/delusion), and perceptual distortion (false perception/hallucination).

Cognitive Disorders

The broad group of cognitive disorders includes delirium and dementia with psychotic feature. Features of cognitive disorders are confusion, defective memory, disorientation, and disorganized thought and behavior.

Functional Disorders

Memory and orientation are usually normal, but emotion, thought, behavior, and reasoning are altered.

Schizophrenia

It is the most important psychiatric disorder with split, severe personality changes with no evidence of organic cerebral damage. It usually presents in some combination of hallucinations, delusions, and distorted thinking and behavior.

Paranoid State

It constitutes persecutory and grandiose delusions with loss of insight.

Mood Disorders/Affective Disorders

This includes mania and depression.

Table 39.1 Psychiatric disorders

1. Psychoses
Cognitive disorders Functional disorders—schizophrenia, hallucinations, paranoid state/delusion, mood disorders such as depression and mania
2. Neuroses
Anxiety Phobic states Obsessive-compulsive disorder Reactive depression Posttraumatic stress disorder Hysterical

Table 39.2 Difference between psychosis and neurosis

Feature	Psychosis	Neurosis
Definition	Mental illness with distortion of thought process, loss of ability to recognize reality, and perceptual distortion	Borderline neuropsychic conditions that manifest in specific clinical phenomenon in the absence of psychical phenomena
Personality changes	Do occur	Does not affect personality
Awareness of the condition	Lost	Preserved
Empathy	Absent	Present
Contact with reality	Lost	Preserved
Organic causative factor	Present	Not present, purely functional
Language and communication	Distorted, incoherent, and irrational	Unaffected
Treatment	Antipsychotic drugs, psychological therapy, social support	Counselling, moral support, medicines, if necessary

Mania

It is characterized by elevation of mood, arousal, and energy, reduced sleep, hyperactivity, uncontrollable thought, speech, and violent behavior.

Depression

People with depression have loss of interest and pleasure, physical and mental slowing, and self-destructive ideas.

There are two types of symptoms of psychotic disorders (**Table 39.3**)—positive and negative symptoms.

These symptoms play a significant role in deciding treatment and selecting antipsychotic drugs, which have been explained later in the text.

Neuroses

These are borderline neuropsychic conditions that manifest in specific clinical phenomenon in the absence of psychical phenomena. In these conditions, an individual's ability to comprehend reality is not lost and these individuals are aware about the problem.

Anxiety

It is an unpleasant state of restlessness, uneasiness, and stress out of proportion to the impact of event and concern for future.

Phobic States

People with phobic states have persistent and excessive fear of an object or situation.

Obsessive-Compulsive Disorder

Individuals with obsessive-compulsive disorder have recurring, unwanted intrusive thoughts, feelings, sensations, and ideas, which drive them to perform some repetitive actions. This repetitive behavior may develop anxiety and distress, and interfere with social interaction, for example, washing hands or checking on things repeatedly.

Reactive Depression

It is defined as excessive disproportionate emotional and behavioral response to some physical or psychosocial stressor.

Posttraumatic Stress Disorder

It is a condition of persistent emotional stress occurring after experiencing or witnessing some distressing, terrifying event.

Hysterical

Symptoms resembling some physical illness, which occurs only in the presence of others. The basis of these symptoms is only psychic and not physical.

Pathogenesis/Hypotheses of Psychotic Disorders (Schizophrenia) (PS5.5)

1. Genetic predisposition.
2. Dopamine (DA) hypothesis.
3. 5-HT hypothesis.
4. Glutamate hypothesis.

Genetic Predisposition

Genetic studies have provided evidence for linkage of schizophrenia to loci on chromosomes 1, 5, 6, 8, 11, and 22, although not specified to any genes. Despite genetic linkage, the results of molecular studies are not conclusive. More recently, one gene encoding neuregulin-1 has been reported to be associated with schizophrenia in some European population.

In first-degree relatives, the risk is about 10%.

Dopamine Hypothesis

It was proposed by Carlson. Excessive dopaminergic activity in the limbic system is the basis of psychotic disorder. The following evidence is available: (1) postmortem studies of brains of schizophrenics revealed increased DA receptors; (2) positron emission tomography (PET) scan showed increased DA receptor density in schizophrenics; (3) most antipsychotic drugs act by blocking DA receptors in the limbic system; (4) DA agonists or DA precursors precipitate symptoms of schizophrenia; (5) overactivity of DA receptors results in positive symptoms of psychotic disorders, as shown in recent studies; and (6) levels of metabolite of DA (homovanillic acid

Table 39.3 Positive and negative symptoms of psychotic disorders

Positive symptoms	Negative symptoms
• Delusions—paranoid • Auditory hallucinations • Distortion of thought with irrational conclusions • Garbled sentences (failure to organize speech) • Abnormal and bizarre behavior (repetitive behavior, inappropriate clothing)	• Flattening of emotional response • Introvert behavior, lack of socialization • Poverty of speech (alogia) • Inability to get pleasure from any activity (anhedonia) • Apathy—lack of motivation and energy • Poor personal hygiene • Cognitive deficits—lack of attention and loss of memory

[HVA]) in cerebrospinal fluid or plasma increase initially and later decline with antipsychotic treatment.

5-HT Hypothesis

5-HT also plays a role in psychosis. The following evidence is available: (1) blockade of 5-HT_{2A} receptor facilitates DA release in nigrostriatal and mesocortical neurons; and (2) central 5-HT agonists such as lysergic acid diethylamide (LSD) produce hallucinations and sensory disturbances.

Glutamate Hypothesis

Glutamate also plays a role in psychotic disorders: (1) glutamate *N*-methyl-D-aspartate (NMDA) receptor blockers such as ketamine and phencyclidine cause hallucinations and thought disorders similar to psychotic symptoms of schizophrenia; and (2) recent studies showed that underactivity of NMDA receptors is responsible for negative symptoms of psychotic disorders (**Fig. 39.1**).

Drug Treatment of Psychiatric Disorders (PS18.1)

Psychotropic Drugs

Drugs that affect mental function are called psychotropic agents or psychopharmacological agents.

Antipsychotic Drugs

The group of drugs useful for psychiatric disorders such as psychosis are known as antipsychotic drugs or neuroleptic drugs.

Importance of Treatment of Psychiatric Disorders

Treatment of psychiatric disorders improves the overall quality of life, increases the interest in surrounding things, and improves productivity, social interaction, and self-esteem. It also adds on to sound physical health habits such as sleeping. It also increases immunity.

Hidden Cost of Not Treating Psychiatric Disorders/Adverse Effects of Not Treating Psychiatric Disorders

Neglecting or not treating psychiatric disorders rather increases stigma associated with psychiatric disorders and negative attitude toward society and vice versa. It lowers self-esteem and self-confidence, which may increase the incidence of suicidal tendency among these individuals. It also reduces productivity. If treatment is not taken properly, then the incidence of relapse and recurrence of partially or incompletely treated psychiatric disorders may increase. It deteriorates the overall quality of life.

Classification of Antipsychotic Drugs

1. Typical or classical antipsychotics (antidopaminergic drugs):
   a. Phenothiazines:
      i. Chlorpromazine (CPZ; aliphatic side chain).
      ii. Thioridazine (piperidine side chain).
      iii. Trifluoperazine (piperazine side chain).
   b. Butyrophenones: haloperidol, trifluperidol, penfluridol.
   c. Thioxanthenes: flupenthixol, thiothixene.
   d. Miscellaneous: pimozide, loxapine.
2. Atypical or novel antipsychotics (DA and/or 5-HT antagonists):
   a. Dibenzodiazepines: clozapine.
   b. Thienobenzodiazepine: olanzapine.
   c. Dibenzothiazepine: quetiapine.
   d. Benzamide: sulpiride, amisulpride.
   e. Indole derivative: sertindole.
   f. Benzisoxazole: risperidone.
   g. Others: aripiprazole, zotepine, asenapine, ziprasidone.

Pharmacological Actions of Typical/Classical Antipsychotics

Effect on Central Nervous System

The effects of CPZ differ in nonpsychotic (normal) and psychotic individuals.

Box 39.1 mentions the effects of CPZ in normal individuals.

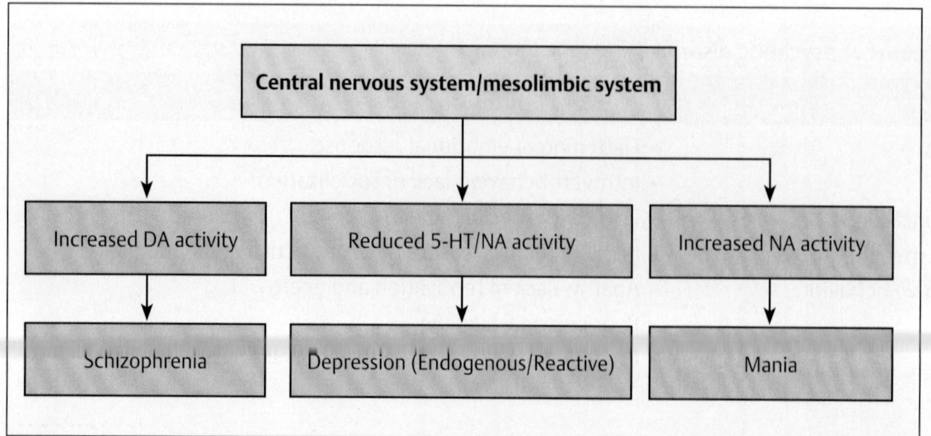

Fig. 39.1 Neurotransmitter hypothesis—correlation between neurotransmitters and psychiatric symptoms. DA, dopamine; NA, noradrenaline.

Box 39.1 Effects of CPZ in nonpsychotic (normal) individuals

- Produces unpleasant "neuroleptic syndrome"
- Indifference to external stimuli
- Psychomotor slowing, tendency to fall asleep
- Blockade of conditional response
- Paucity of thought, emotional quietening
- Minimized spontaneous movements

Effects of CPZ in Psychotic Individuals

CPZ reduces severity of psychotic symptoms such as delusions, hallucinations, anxiety, hyperactivity, abnormal aggressive behavior, and agitation. Distortion of thoughts gradually becomes normal. CPZ also normalizes disturbed sleep pattern and lowers seizure threshold. CPZ improves cognitive functions, although atypical antipsychotics are more beneficial in this regard.

Mechanism of Action of Antipsychotics

Typical or classical antipsychotics have potent postsynaptic competitive DA D_2 receptor blockade action (**Box 39.2**), although they also block presynaptic ones to a lesser extent.

The use of typical antipsychotics in the initial period increases synthesis and release of DA and its metabolites such as HVA, but prolonged use causes feedback inhibition of DA release and levels of HVA reduces to level below normal, which continues throughout the treatment.

Effect on Autonomic Nervous System

Antipsychotics affect autonomic nervous system by α- and M-receptor blocking action.

1. M-receptor blockade leads to constipation, dry mouth, urinary hesitancy, and blurred vision.
2. α-receptor blockade leads to postural hypotension.

Grading of Relative α-Blocking Activity of Antipsychotics

CPZ = triflupromazine = thioridazine > clozapine > fluphenazine > haloperidol > trifluoperazine > pimozide.

The α-blocking activity is more in less potent compounds (CPZ), whereas it is less in more potent compounds (haloperidol). CPZ produces miosis due to potent α-blocking activity.

Grading of Relative Anticholinergic Activity of Antipsychotics

Thioridazine > olanzapine > clozapine > CPZ > triflupromazine > trifluoperazine = haloperidol.

Thioridazine and olanzapine have significant anticholinergic property and thus have lesser extrapyramidal effects. These compounds produce mydriasis.

Effects of CPZ Due to Blockade of Other Receptors

H_1 receptor blockade leads to sedation.

Box 39.2 Effects of CPZ due to DA receptor blockade at various sites

- Effects of CPZ (including adverse effects) due to DA receptor blockage at various sites
- Limbic system and mesocortical area →→→→ antipsychotic effects
- Chemoreceptor trigger zone (CTZ) →→ antiemetic effects (ineffective in motion sickness)
- Hypothalamus →→→→ hypothermia
- Corpus striatum (nigrostriatal pathway) →→ extrapyramidal effects
- Anterior pituitary →→→→ hyperprolactinemia →→ adverse effects
- Cortex →→→→ sedation

Effect on Cardiovascular System

It causes postural hypotension and reflex tachycardia due to α-blocking activity. There is QT prolongation and T-wave suppression with high dose. Antiarrhythmic effects are also seen.

Local Anesthetic Effect

CPZ is a potent local anesthetic as procaine, but because of its irritant action, it is not used clinically. Other agents have some weak membrane-stabilizing action.

Effect on Hormones

Galactorrhea and gynecomastia occur due to blockade of DA receptors in the pituitary. There is reduced secretion of growth hormone, gonadotrophins, and antidiuretic hormone. Glucose intolerance also occurs.

Typical or Classical Antipsychotics Based on Their Potency

Typical antipsychotics are divided into low-potency and high-potency groups based on their effectiveness of antipsychotic effect.

High-potency agents are more selective in action due to their high affinity to D_2 receptors and hence the incidences of extrapyramidal reactions are more, and autonomic side effects are less with high-potency drugs. The reverse is observed with low-potency typical antipsychotics.

The differences are tabulated in **Table 39.4**.

Adverse Effects of Typical Antipsychotics

Central Nervous System

Confusion, lethargy, drowsiness, and sedation. Precipitation of seizures (proconvulsant effect) in epileptics, tolerance to sedative effect, and development of seizure episodes

Table 39.4 Difference between low-potency and high-potency typical antipsychotics

Parameter	Low-potency group	High-potency group
Affinity to D_2 receptor	Lesser affinity	Higher affinity
Antipsychotic effect	Less effective	More effective
Extrapyramidal reactions	Lesser incidence	Higher incidence
Sedation	More incidence	Less incidence
Postural hypotension	More incidence	Less incidence
Proconvulsant effect	More	Less
Drugs	Chlorpromazine, triflupromazine, thioridazine	Thiothixene, fluphenazine, haloperidol, perphenazine, trifluoperazine

even in nonepileptics with high dose. Low-potency typical antipsychotics (such as CPZ) are known for more adverse effects.

Autonomic Side Effects

Orthostatic postural hypotension, reflex tachycardia, and inhibition of ejaculation (common with CPZ). Dry mouth, urinary hesitancy, blurred vision, constipation, and urine retention may be seen in elderly individuals (more common with thioridazine).

Endocrine Side Effects

Hyperprolactinemia manifests differently in males and females. Gynecomastia, reduced libido, impotence, and, rarely, related infertility in males. Galactorrhea, amenorrhea, and related infertility in females infrequently occur on long-term use (probably due to reduced gonadotropin levels). Weight gain and increased appetite due to blockade of D_2 receptors in medullary-periventricular pathway (common with phenothiazines).

Hypersensitivity Reactions

These adverse reactions are not dose-related. Skin rashes, urticaria, and contact dermatitis may occur. Photosensitivity is common with CPZ. Agranulocytosis is noted to be more common with atypical agents such as clozapine. Cholestatic jaundice is common with low-potency agents. Myocarditis does occur but very rarely with atypical agents such as clozapine.

Extrapyramidal Side Effects and Their Treatment

Parkinsonism

Parkinsonism occurs due to disturbed DA–acetylcholine balance in basal ganglia due to D_2 receptor blockade. It manifests as rigidity, tremor, hypokinesia, shuffling gait, and masklike face. It generally appears on 7 to 30 days of antipsychotic treatment. Treatment is to restore the basal ganglia dopaminergic balance. DA precursor such as L-dopa is not preferred, as it may precipitate schizophrenia, albeit curing parkinsonism. The preferred treatment is to either adjust dose of antipsychotics or shift to atypical antipsychotics. Use of centrally acting antimuscarinic drugs such as trihexyphenidyl and procyclidine may also help.

Acute Muscular Dystonia

It is characterized by the bizarre muscle spasm of muscles of the tongue, face (masklike face), neck, and back. Usually, it manifests as tongue thrusting, grimacing, torticollis, and locked jaw. It is the earliest occurring extrapyramidal reaction, which occurs within hours to maximum of 1 week of therapy. It is more common after parenteral administration in female patients younger than 8 years. Although it resolves spontaneously within few hours, parenteral administration of centrally acting anticholinergic drugs such as benztropine or promethazine reverses these reactions within minutes.

Akathisia

It is one of the most commonly occurring extrapyramidal reactions with motor restlessness, that is, uncontrollable motor restlessness, feeling of discomfort, agitation, and uncontrollable desire to move out without involvement of anxiety. It generally appears between 1 and 8 weeks of therapy. Features seem like exacerbation of psychosis. Treatment involves use of benzodiazepines such as clonazepam. Other agents used are centrally acting anticholinergics and nonselective β-blockers such as propranolol. Adjusting the dose of antipsychotics or shifting to atypical agents reduces the intensity of symptoms.

Tardive Dyskinesia

It is a late-occurring (months to years after therapy) extrapyramidal reaction with characteristic involuntary, purposeless, stereotyped, repetitive, and choreoathetoid oral-buccal-lingual dyskinesias and limb movements such as chewing, pouting, lip licking, grimacing, and puffing of cheeks. It usually occurs because of neuronal degeneration and postsynaptic supersensitivity of DA receptors in striatum, which leads to decrease in cholinergic activity and gamma-aminobutyric acid (GABA). This reduction in release of inhibitory neurotransmitters leads to involuntary motor activity. This reaction is uncommon with atypical antipsychotics such as clozapine or quetiapine. Treatment involves increasing the GABA activity along with "neurolept holidays"—withdrawal of antipsychotic drugs and antiparkinsonian-anticholinergic drugs, if used. Diazepam may be added to increase the GABA activity.

Malignant Neuroleptic Syndrome

It is a life-threatening and potentially fatal extrapyramidal reaction. It occurs with high dose of the potent neuroleptics. It manifests as immobility, tremor, catatonia, rigidity, hyperpyrexia, semiconsciousness, autonomic instability with fluctuating blood pressure, myoglobinemia, and increased creatinine kinase. Treatment involves discontinuation of antipsychotic agent. Symptomatic treatment must be started immediately. Peripherally acting muscle relaxant dantrolene, given intravenously, may help.

Perioral Tremors (Rabbit Syndrome)

It is a rare variant of extrapyramidal reactions that may occur months or years after neuroleptic treatment. Characteristic presentation is rapid chewing movements (similar to rabbits and therefore the name rabbit syndrome). Treatment involves use of anticholinergic-antiparkinsonian drugs.

Drug Interactions

1. Antacids reduce absorption of antipsychotic drugs.
2. Antipsychotic drugs potentiate effect of various central nervous system depressants such as opioids, alcohol, sedative-hypnotics, antihistaminics, and anxiolytics, which may lead to overdose toxicity.
3. Antipsychotic drugs block the action of DA agonists and levodopa used in parkinsonism by DA antagonistic activity.
4. Lithium, when used along with haloperidol, enhances the neurotoxicity and precipitates neurolept-malignant syndrome.
5. Antipsychotic drugs block the nerve terminal level reuptake of antihypertensives such as clonidine and methyldopa and reduce their antihypertensive action.
6. Use of metoclopramide concurrently with antipsychotic drugs may increase the incidence of acute muscle dystonia.
7. Antipsychotics such as CPZ increase analgesic, sedative, and miotic actions of morphine, and enhance respiratory depression.
8. Enzyme inducers such as barbiturates can reduce the blood levels of antipsychotics.

Atypical or Novel Antipsychotic Drugs

Salient features of atypical or novel antipsychotic drugs are mentioned in **Box 39.3**.

Clozapine

It is the first atypical antipsychotic drug with high affinity for 5-HT_{2A} and D_4 receptors. It has partial agonistic activity at 5-HT_{1A} receptor, which leads to its anxiolytic action. Active metabolite *N*-desmethylclozapine has agonistic activity at M_1 receptor, which leads to improvement in cognitive function in schizophrenic individuals. It has weak D_2 receptor action and hence causes no or only few extrapyramidal reactions. Both positive and negative symptoms are relieved. It is most effective in refractory or resistant schizophrenia and is also an effective agent in patients with suicidal tendencies. Agranulocytosis is the most serious adverse effect. Sedation, weight gain, paradoxical hypersalivation, hyperlipidemia, seizures, hyperglycemia, and, very rarely, myocarditis are some other adverse effects noted. Negligible hyperprolactinemia is noted with clozapine.

Olanzapine

Olanzapine has spectrum similar to clozapine in blocking multiple monoaminergic, muscarinic, and histaminic receptors. Both positive and negative symptoms are reduced. It is a broad-spectrum atypical agent for schizoaffective as well as maniac disorders. Adverse effects are similar to those of clozapine, but in higher doses, it may lead to akathisia and muscular dystonia. Increased incidence of stroke in elderly individuals are observed. It has a half-life of 24 to 30 hours.

Quetiapine

It is newer short-acting atypical agent ($t_{1/2}$ of 6 hours). The spectrum of quetiapine is similar to clozapine, except it is associated with poor improvement in negative symptoms. Twice-daily dosing is required, and the major portion of dose is given at nighttime, so as to enable psychotic individuals who are insomniac to sleep. Weight gain, sedation, postural hypotension, and urinary retention or incontinence are some adverse effects. At very high dose, it may cause QT prolongation. It is also used for maintenance therapy of mania and bipolar disorders.

Risperidone

Receptor-blocking activity of risperidone is similar to that of clozapine, except risperidone is more potent D_2 receptor blocker and has weak antimuscarinic activity. Significant extrapyramidal effects and hyperprolactinemia are noted with risperidone, although less with low daily dose of less than 6 mg. Lesser incidence of weight gain and glucose intolerance is observed as compared to clozapine. Increased incidence of stroke in elderly individuals is noted. Risperidone is usually prescribed as first-line drug in schizophrenia.

Box 39.3 Salient features of atypical or novel antipsychotic drugs

- Newer or second-generation antipsychotic drugs
- Weak D_2 receptor blocking action
- Strong affinity for 5-HT_{2A} and D_4 receptors, competitively inhibiting these receptors
- Antagonistic activity at α_1, H_1, M_1 receptors
- As they have lower affinity for D_1 and D_2 receptors, the incidences of extrapyramidal side effects appear to be very low
- Significant improvement in negative symptoms occurs due to blockade of 5-HT_{2A} and D_4 receptors
- Improvement in impaired cognitive function in psychotic individuals
- Effective in levodopa-induced psychosis in patients with Parkinson's disease

Aripiprazole

It has partial agonistic activity at D_2 and 5-HT_{1A} receptors and antagonist activity at 5-HT_2 receptor. Lesser incidence of extrapyramidal effects, hypotension, weight gain, hyperglycemia, and hyperprolactinemia is seen. It is not sedating and can lead to insomnia. Constipation, light headache, dyspepsia, nausea, etc., are some noted adverse effects with aripiprazole. It is a long-acting atypical agent with $t_{1/2}$ of almost 3 days. It is useful as maintenance therapy in bipolar disorders. It relieves positive symptoms and is as effective as haloperidol. Aripiprazole is also effective as augmenting agent in resistant depression.

Ziprasidone

It is antagonist at D_2, 5-$HT_{2A, 2C, 1D}$, H_1, and α_1 receptors and has agonistic activity at 5-HT_{1A} receptor, which leads to anxiolytic action. Blockade of reuptake of 5-HT and noradrenaline (NA) leads to its antidepressant action. It is an effective agent for schizophrenia and mania associated with anxiety or depression. The half-life of ziprasidone is 8 hours. Lesser incidence of extrapyramidal effects, hyperprolactinemia, weight gain, blood glucose intolerance, etc., is seen with ziprasidone.

Zotepine

Zotepine has antagonistic activity at D_1, D_2, 5-$HT_{2A, 2C, 6, 7}$, H_1, and α_1 receptors and also blocks reuptake of NA. It relieves both positive and negative symptoms of schizophrenia. It has high first-pass metabolism with 10% bioavailability. Its half-life is 15 hours, and it is excreted in the bile. It lowers seizure threshold and increased incidence of seizures. The spectrum of use is similar to clozapine with no added specific advantages.

Advantages of Atypical Antipsychotics over Typical Antipsychotics

Box 39.4 mentions the advantages of atypical antipsychotics.

Difference between Typical and Atypical Antipsychotic Drugs

Table 39.5 mentions the difference between typical and atypical antipsychotic drugs.

Principles of Psychosis Treatment

1. Therapeutic uses of antipsychotics–psychiatric/neuropsychiatric/nonpsychiatric.
2. Selection of antipsychotic agents in various psychosis.
3. Selection of antipsychotics in special situations.
4. Selection of antipsychotics in associated diseases.
5. Typical effective doses of antipsychotic drugs.
6. Depot preparations of long-acting antipsychotics.

Therapeutic Uses

Psychiatric Indications

Although these drugs do not completely cure the psychosis, they significantly reduce the symptoms and help the individuals to manage their daily living in socially acceptable manners. These includes schizophrenia and schizoaffective disorders.

Schizophrenia

Antipsychotics have a definite role in the treatment of schizophrenia. The goal of antipsychotic therapy is symptomatic relief and functional rehabilitation of the patient. Both positive and negative symptoms are benefited with the use of antipsychotics. Efficacy of typical and atypical antipsychotics is identical against positive symptoms. When it comes to treatment of negative symptoms, the atypical antipsychotics are more effective and are the preferred agents. Antipsychotics also restore affective and motor disturbances and allow individuals to live socially acceptable lives. Memory, orientation, and judgment are only partially reduced. Recent-onset schizophrenics or those with acute exacerbations respond better to antipsychotic drugs.

Box 39.4 Advantages of atypical antipsychotics

- Newer generation antipsychotics
- Higher efficacy than typical antipsychotics
- More effective in refractory schizophrenia
- Strong affinity for 5-HT_{2A} and D_4 receptors, so good improvement in negative symptoms as compared to typical antipsychotics
- Weak D_2 action, so less incidence of extrapyramidal reactions and hyperprolactinemia as compared to typical antipsychotics
- Considered as first-line drugs for treatment of newly diagnosed schizophrenia
- These are used as drugs of choice for acute schizophrenic episode
- No serum monitoring required during the therapy with atypical antipsychotics in the case of pediatric psychosis
- Useful in treating comorbid disorders associated with psychosis
- These are useful for the treatment of bipolar disorders and depression along with psychosis and are good mood stabilizers

Table 39.5 Difference between typical and atypical antipsychotic drugs

Features	Typical antipsychotics	Atypical antipsychotics
Developmental generation	First-generation antipsychotics	Newer generation antipsychotics
Mechanism of action	Potent D_2 receptor blockade	Competitively blocks 5-HT_{2A} D_4, H_1, M_1, α_1 receptors
Action against positive symptoms	Highly effective	Highly effective
Action against negative symptoms	Weakly effective	Highly effective
Effect on refractory schizophrenia	No or weak	Highly effective
Hyperprolactinemia	Higher incidences	No or fewer incidence
Extrapyramidal reactions	Higher incidences	No or fewer incidence
Withdrawal symptoms	Fewer	Significant
Metabolic syndrome (hyperlipidemia, weight gain, hyperglycemia)	Low incidence	High incidence
Agranulocytosis, myocarditis	Not seen	More common with clozapine
Improvement in cognitive function	No or very weak	Good
Treatment of associated comorbid conditions	Less useful	Highly useful
Treatment of bipolar disorders and depression	Not or less useful	Highly useful
Treatment of pediatric psychosis	Low dose of high-potency drugs useful (haloperidol)	Atypical drugs are preferred
Treatment of generalized anxiety disorders	Not or less useful	More useful, either monotherapy or adjuvant to SSRIs

Abbreviation: SSRIs, selective serotonin reuptake inhibitors.

Choice of Antipsychotic Agents in Schizophrenia

Choice of the drug is patient-dependent, empirical, and based on type of symptoms, associated features and comorbidities, mood states, and more acceptable types of adverse effects. Mode of treatment varies from one patient to another, based on the above-mentioned features, and different patients respond differently to the same antipsychotic therapy. Atypical antipsychotics are the preferred agents nowadays with wider action spectrum and fewer adverse effects (**Box 39.5**).

High-potency typical antipsychotics such as haloperidol are preferred over low-potency ones. For long-term therapy of schizophrenia, atypical agents are preferred.

Schizoaffective Disorders

The "schizo" component of these disorders sometimes respond to antipsychotic treatment, but other drugs have to be added to the treatment according to the "affective" component. If the affective component is "depression," then antidepressants should be given along with the antipsychotic therapy. If the affective component is "mania," then lithium should be added to the neuroleptic therapy.

Neuropsychiatric Indications

Tourette's Syndrome

Tourette's syndrome manifests as tics, vocalizations, and grunts. The preferred drug for the treatment is haloperidol. Pimozide can also be used as an alternative but may increase the risk of QT prolongation.

Huntington's Disease

Haloperidol or CPZ is used to reduce progressive choreoathetosis and dementia.

Nonpsychiatric Indications

Preanesthetic Medication

Promethazine is used for preoperative sedation. A fixed-dose combination of droperidol with an opioid analgesic fentanyl is used to produce "neurolept-analgesia."

As Antiemetics

Many atypical antipsychotic drugs have antiemetic effect due to D_2 receptor blockade in CTZ and gastrointestinal tract. Prochlorperazine is used more as antiemetic than as

Table 39.6 Effective doses of antipsychotic drugs

Antipsychotic drugs	Effective therapeutic dose approx. (mg/d)[a]
Chlorpromazine	100–800
Thioridazine	100–400
Fluphenazine	1–10
Haloperidol	2–60
Clozapine	100–300
Olanzapine	2.5–20
Quetiapine	50–400
Risperidone	2–8
Ziprasidone	80–160

[a]Effective daily dose may vary from one patient to another, and the clinician should titrate the minimum effective dose for an individual.

Box 39.5 Selection of drug of choice in schizophrenia

- Predominant negative symptoms—atypical agents such as clozapine
- Violent, combative, and agitated—haloperidol, quetiapine, CPZ
- Refractory schizophrenia—clozapine (most effective), olanzapine, etc.
- Withdrawn and apathetic—trifluoperazine, fluphenazine, ziprasidone
- Elderly individuals prone to mental confusion and hypotension—haloperidol, aripiprazole, etc.
- Resistant depression—aripiprazole
- If extrapyramidal reactions must be avoided—atypical agents, clozapine
- Mood elevation and hypomania—haloperidol, quetiapine, olanzapine

antipsychotic. Domperidone and metoclopramide have very low affinity for D_2 receptors in limbic system and so have no antipsychotic action. These drugs block peripheral DA receptors and have prokinetic and gastric emptying action. Promethazine is used for motion sickness as an antiemetic due to its antihistaminic and anticholinergic (anti-motion sickness) action.

Selection of Antipsychotics in Special Situations

1. Patients with cardiovascular diseases are prone to develop hypotension; newer generation atypical agents such as risperidone and clozapine are preferred.
2. In childhood psychosis, atypical antipsychotics or low dose of high-potency typical antipsychotics are preferred.
3. Avoid olanzapine and risperidone in elderly psychotic individuals as they increase the risk of stroke. In these individuals, haloperidol or aripiprazole are preferred.
4. If compliance is the problem, then use injectable depot preparations (**Box 39.6**).

Box 39.6 Injectable depot preparations used in psychosis

- Haloperidol decanoate
- Fluphenazine decanoate
- Flupenthixol decanoate
- Zuclopenthixol decanoate or acetate
- Risperidone (in the form of carbohydrate microspheres)

Box 39.7 Selection of antipsychotic drug in schizophrenia-associated diseases

- Dementia—high-potency typical agents such as haloperidol are preferred
- Parkinson's disease—clozapine is preferred
- Depression—olanzapine along with selective serotonin reuptake inhibitors (SSRIs) such as fluoxetine. Aripiprazole may be useful in resistant depression
- Anxiety—clozapine is preferred
- Acute mania—lithium or antimanic antiepileptics (carbamazepine or sodium valproate) are preferred

Doses of Antipsychotic Drugs in Children

1. CPZ 2 mg/kg in divided doses.
2. Trifluoperazine 1 to 15 mg once a day.
3. Thioridazine 0.25 to 0.5 mg/kg once a day.
4. Fluphenazine 0.05 to 0.1 mg once a day.

Effective Doses of Antipsychotic Drugs

There are different doses for different antipsychotic drugs in different conditions (**Table 39.6**).

Selection of Antipsychotic Drug in Schizophrenia-Associated Diseases

Criteria for selection of antipsychotic drugs are mentioned in **Box 39.7**.

Multiple Choice Questions

1. A 35-year-old male patient was diagnosed with schizophrenia for which typical antipsychotics were started. Clinical antipsychotic potency of typical or classical antipsychotic drugs correlates with action at which of the following receptors?

A. Dopamine D_2 receptors.
B. α_2 adrenergic receptors.
C. Muscarinic receptors.
D. Histaminic receptors.

Answer: A

The clinical antipsychotic effect of typical or classical antipsychotic agents is because of blockade of dopamine D_2 receptors in limbic system and mesocortical area.

2. A young man was diagnosed to be suffering from schizophrenia associated with depression. The newer generation atypical antipsychotic drug was prescribed by the physician along with selective serotonin reuptake inhibitors (SSRIs). Which of the following would be the most probable mechanism of action of that antipsychotic agent?

A. Competitive dopaminergic D_2 receptor blockade.
B. 5-HT_{2A} and D_4 receptor antagonistic activity.
C. Strong agonistic activity at dopaminergic D_2 receptor.
D. Agonistic activity at α_1, H_1, M_1 receptors.

Answer: B

The patient is suffering from schizophrenia as well as depression. In such cases, atypical antipsychotic agents such as olanzapine along with SSRIs are preferred. Atypical agents such as olanzapine have high affinity for 5-HT_{2A} and D_4 receptors and act by competitive antagonism of these receptors. These agents also block α_1, H_1, and M_1 receptors. Atypical antipsychotics are weak D_2 receptor blockers.

3. A 40-year-old man was diagnosed with schizophrenia with predominant symptoms being flattening of emotional response, introvert behavior, lack of socialization, emotional blunting, alogia, anhedonia, and apathy. Appropriate antipsychotic agent was prescribed by the treating physician. Which of the following drug would have been prescribed?

A. Chlorpromazine.
B. Haloperidol.
C. Risperidone.
D. Thioridazine.

Answer: C

The patient is having predominantly negative symptoms of schizophrenia. In such cases, newer generation atypical agents are preferred. Atypical antipsychotics have higher affinity for 5-HT_{2A} and D_4 receptors, blockade of which relieves negative symptoms. Typical or classical antipsychotic drugs have strong D_2 blockade action but no appreciable blockade activity for 5-HT_{2A} and D_4 receptors and hence are not efficient enough to target negative symptoms. In the list, only risperidone is atypical antipsychotic drug and hence is the answer.

4. A 35-year-old woman was recently diagnosed with schizophrenia. A treating physician noted predominance of negative symptoms and started atypical antipsychotic drug. Antagonism at which of the following receptors may have the greatest ability to temper her negative symptoms?

A. Dopamine D_2 receptors.
B. Glutamate receptors.
C. Muscarinic M_1 receptors.
D. Serotonin 5-HT_{2A} receptors.

Answer: D

The patient is diagnosed with schizophrenia with predominantly negative symptoms. Atypical antipsychotic drugs have high affinity for serotonin (5-HT_{2A}) and D_4 receptors, antagonism of which leads to improvement in negative symptoms.

5. A young woman was recently diagnosed with schizophrenia. A high-potency drug of particular class was prescribed. Within 2 days after starting the therapy, the patient developed severe muscle cramps of neck, back, and facial muscle with torticollis and locked jaw. Which of the following drug must have been prescribed?

A. Chlorpromazine.
B. Clozapine.
C. Risperidone.
D. Haloperidol.

Answer: D

The young woman developed acute muscular dystonia shortly after the treatment with antipsychotic drug. Acute muscular dystonia is predominantly seen as an adverse effect with the typical antipsychotic agents due to their strong affinity for D_2 receptors. Among typical antipsychotics, high-potency drugs such as haloperidol have more affinity for D_2 receptors and higher incidence of developing extrapyramidal reactions than low-potency counterparts such as chlorpromazine.

6. A young male patient was diagnosed with schizophrenia and both positive and negatives symptoms were predominantly noted. A physician prescribed the appropriate drug based on symptoms of the schizophrenia. Which of the following drug would have been mostly prescribed by the physician?

A. Chlorpromazine.
B. Haloperidol.
C. Risperidone.
D. Thioridazine.

Answer: C

The patient in this case has both positive and negative predominant symptoms of schizophrenia. Typical antipsychotics, due to strong D_2 blockade, have good control on positive symptoms but they are not effective or are very less effective against negative symptoms due to lack of affinity for 5-HT_{2A} and D_4 receptors. Whereas atypical antipsychotics have strong affinity for 5-HT_{2A} and D_4 receptors and also some action against D_2 receptors too, so atypical agents have control of both positive and negative symptoms and hence are preferred drugs in newly detected schizophrenia with both positive and negative

symptoms. In the given options, only risperidone is the atypical antipsychotic agent and hence is the answer.

7. A 32-year-old man with schizophrenia is on haloperidol for the last 5 years with good response to the drug. But, recently, he developed involuntary facial movements such as pouting, chewing, grimacing, and puffing of cheeks. This adverse phenomenon would likely correspond to which of the following mechanisms?

A. Dopamine receptor sensitization.
B. Decreased synthesis of DA receptors.
C. Decreased synthesis of 5-HT receptors.
D. Sensitization of 5-HT receptors.

Answer: A

Chronic administration of dopamine receptor antagonists such as haloperidol can lead to increased density of receptors, and sensitization of receptors does occur to the drug. These involuntary movements are called tardive dyskinesia, which usually occurs years after treatment. It usually occurs because of neuronal degeneration and postsynaptic supersensitivity of dopamine receptors in striatum, which leads to decrease in cholinergic activity and GABA (gamma-aminobutyric acid). This reduction in release of inhibitory neurotransmitters leads to involuntary motor activity.

8. A 36-year-old male patient is on high-potency typical antipsychotic agent for his schizophrenia. He was responding well to the drug in terms of control of hallucinations and delusions, but he is bothered with the dry mouth he was experiencing recently. This effect corresponds to which of the following actions of that drug?

A. Antidopaminergic.
B. Antihistaminergic.
C. Antiadrenergic.
D. Anticholinergic.

Answer: D

The adverse effect of dry mouth in this case is due to the blockade of D_2 receptors at muscarinic M_1 receptors.

9. A 35-year-old man diagnosed with schizophrenia is on haloperidol and is responding well to the treatment. He reported to the physician with complaints of developing rigidity, tremor, hypokinesia, shuffling gait, and masklike face. These adverse symptoms most probably developed due to the action of haloperidol on which of the following pathways or tracts?

A. Mesolimbic pathway.
B. Nigrostriatal pathway.
C. Tuberoinfundibular pathway.
D. Medullary-periventricular pathway.

Answer: B

The adverse symptoms reported are parkinsonismlike extrapyramidal reactions of haloperidol due to blockade of D_2 receptors in nigrostriatal pathway.

10. A 32-year-old woman is diagnosed with schizophrenia. Treatment is being weighed between atypical and classical antipsychotic agents. Which of the following is an advantage of atypical antipsychotics over typical ones that helps physician to choose them over classical antipsychotics?

A. High specificity for D_2 receptor antagonism.
B. Less likely to cause new onset of diabetes.
C. Cheaper cost.
D. Lesser incidence of extrapyramidal reactions.

Answer: D

Although some extrapyramidal reactions may occur even with newer atypical agents, the incidence of these extrapyramidal reactions is very less as they have very weak D_2 receptor action.

11. A young male patient with schizophrenia is on haloperidol, a high-potency classical antipsychotic drug with a good response to the treatment. The patient showed a concern regarding the adverse effects of the drug. Which of the following adverse effect is more likely to occur with haloperidol compared to chlorpromazine, a low-potency classical antipsychotic drug?

A. Akathisia.
B. Sedation.
C. Postural hypotension.
D. Exacerbation of seizure.

Answer: A

High-potency agents are more selective in action due to their high affinity to D_2 receptors and hence the incidences of extrapyramidal reactions are more and autonomic side effects such as postural hypotension are less with high-potency drugs.

12. A 50-year-old man with schizophrenia and obesity has been shifted over to olanzapine from haloperidol as he developed tardive dyskinesia with haloperidol. He has presented to clinic for routine monitoring. Which of the following screening will you advice the patient to undergo on priority basis?

A. Tests for hemochromatosis.
B. Blood sugar levels.
C. Tests for malignancy.
D. Serum prolactin levels.

Answer: B

Atypical antipsychotic drugs such as olanzapine and others have very weak D_2 receptor affinity, so the incidence of extrapyramidal reactions and hyperprolactinemia is very less with them. But they have more metabolic adverse effects such as glucose intolerance, hyperglycemia, exacerbation of diabetes or new onset of diabetes, and weight gain. Therefore, patients should be routinely monitored for the blood glucose levels to rule out glucose intolerance or hyperglycemia. Lipid profile should also be done.

13. A 54-year-old male patient with long-standing schizophrenia has failed response with first- and second-generation antipsychotic drugs and is having persistent problems with mood disturbances, delusions, and hallucinations. Now, he is placed on clozapine. Which of the following effects the treating physician must be aware of?

A. Cholelithiasis.
B. Polycythemia.

C. Agranulocytosis.

D. Pancreatitis.

Answer: C

Approximately 20% of patients with schizophrenia have insufficient response to first- and second-generation antipsychotics. In these patients, clozapine is effective; however, its clinical use is limited to refractory schizophrenia. Clozapine can produce severe adverse effects such as bone marrow suppression with agranulocytosis, seizures, and cardiovascular adverse effects. The risk of severe agranulocytosis requires frequent monitoring of white blood cell counts.

14. A 45-year-old male patient of schizophrenia came to your clinic with the complaints that his symptoms are not relieved with your previous treatment; instead, the symptoms have flared up recently. You diagnosed it as refractory schizophrenia and prescribed atypical antipsychotic drug of choice for him. You also advised him to undergo regular screening with white blood cell counts. For which of the following adverse effect you advised white blood cell count screening tests?

A. Hyperprolactinemia.

B. Agranulocytosis.

C. Akathisia.

D. Tardive dyskinesia.

Answer: B

Atypical antipsychotic drug of choice is prescribed for refractory schizophrenia, which is clozapine. The serious adverse effect of clozapine is agranulocytosis. Regular screening of white blood cell count is required when the patient is on clozapine therapy to watch for agranulocytosis.

15. A 21-year-old woman has been diagnosed recently with Tourette's syndrome and her physician has started pimozide therapy. Now, the patient is brought to the emergency department with the complaints that she is developing tics, which appear to be different than before, along with prolonged muscle spasm of facial and neck muscles and increasing episodes of torticollis and locked jaw. Which of the following drug would be beneficial in reversing these symptoms?

A. Benztropine.

B. Bromocriptine.

C. Lithium.

D. Risperidone.

Answer: A

The patient has developed the extrapyramidal reaction due to pimozide with acute muscular dystonia–like features. Centrally acting anticholinergic drug such as benztropine would be effective in reversing these symptoms. Parenteral administration of benztropine would improve the condition within minutes.

Chapter 40 Opioid Analgesics

Ramanand Patil

PH1.19: Describe the mechanism/s of action, types, doses, side effects, indications, and contraindications of the drugs which act on central nervous system (CNS), including anxiolytics, sedatives and hypnotics, antipsychotics, antidepressant drugs, antimaniacs, opioid agonists and antagonists, drugs used for neurodegenerative disorders, and antiepileptic drugs.

Learning Objectives

- Morphine.
- Opioid antagonists.
- Mixed agonists and antagonists.

Introduction (AS8.3, AS8.4, AS8.5)

Pain or algesia is an unpleasant subjective sensation and a warning signal of structural or functional integrity impairment. It cannot be easily defined but requires prompt action. Its immediate relief boosts confidence in the physician. Each individual has variable reaction to pain and stress, and anxiety increases the perception of pain. Clinically, pain can be somatic pain, visceral pain, referred pain, etc. Somatic pain is a well-defined sharp pain, which arises from skin, muscles, bones, and joints due to inflammation. Visceral pain is an ill-defined, dull-acting pain, which arises from visceral organs due to spasm and ischemia inflammation accompanied by nausea, sweating, hypotension, etc. Referred pain is a pain centered around the cutaneous area, having spinal nerve supply as that of viscera, such as cardiac pain in the left arm. Acute pain is a usually well-defined one, occurring due to injury, burns, irritants, ischemia, etc. Chronic pain is an ill-defined pain mostly pertaining to cancer pain and neuropathic pain.

Analgesics are the drugs which relieve pain without significantly altering the consciousness. They relieve pain without tackling the cause of pain.

Analgesics are categorized into two types:

1. Morphine/opioid/ narcotic type.
2. Nonopioid/aspirin/nonnarcotic type.

Opium

In Greek, "opus" means "juice." Opium is a dark brown, gummy exudate obtained from the unripe seed capsule of the *Papaver somniferum* plant. Morphine is the most important pure opium alkaloid. "Morpheus" is the name of the Greek god of dreams. Opium contains about twenty different alkaloids comprising agonists, partial agonists, and antagonist properties.

Classification of Opioid Analgesics

Classification based on source:

1. Natural: morphine, codeine, noscapine.
2. Semisynthetic: heroin (diacetylmorphine), oxymorphone, pholcodine.
3. Synthetic: pethidine, methadone, butorphanol, tramadol, diphenoxylate, dextropropoxyphene, pentazocine, loperamide, buprenorphine.

Classification according to activity:

1. Agonists: natural (morphine, codeine) and synthetic (methadone, pethidine).
2. Antagonists: naloxone, naltrexone, nalmefene.
3. Mixed agonists-antagonists: buprenorphine, pentazocine, nalorphine, butorphanol.

Morphine

It is the most important opium alkaloid.

Mechanism of Action

Endogenous opioid peptides such as endorphins, enkephalins, dynorphins, nociceptin and endomorphins (1 and 2) are present in the brain. There are three specific G protein-coupled receptors (GPCRs) or opioid receptors such as mu (μ), kappa (κ), delta (δ), and nociceptin (N)/orphanin is a newly identified opioid receptor. Endorphins, enkephalins, and dynorphins are endogenous ligands for μ, δ and κ receptors. Periaqueductal gray area, substantia gelatinosa and spinal cord have abundant opioid receptors.

Activation of GPCRs leads to:

- Inhibition of adenylate cyclase which, in turn, leads to decreased intracellular cAMP, decrease in intracellular Ca^{2+}, and finally decreased release of neurotransmitters involved in transmission of pain such as GABA, glutamate, noradrenaline, dopamine, substance P and 5-HT.
- Facilitation of K^+ channel opening, which causes hyperpolarization and leads to decreased Ca+ entry into cells or decreased opening of Ca^+ channels and decreased neurotransmitters release.
- Inhibition of transmission of pain in dorsal horn ascending pathway.

Pharmacological Actions

Central Nervous System (CNS)

Analgesia

Morphine relieves pain without altering the consciousness. It relieves dull-acting pain better compared to sharp pain. It also increases pain threshold, alters emotional reaction to pain, and changes pain reaction as well as pain perception.

Euphoria, Sedation, and Hypnosis

Morphine causes euphoria, that is, feeling of well-being, and is a drug of abuse. It produces a highly pleasurable sensation such as a high/rush/kick. It also produces loss of rational thinking, decreases concentration, leads to colorful daydreams and feelings of detachment, and induces drowsiness, calming effect and indifference to the environment.

Respiration

Morphine depresses respiration significantly. It depresses brain stem. Sedation and indifference also make a contribution to respiratory depression. Irregular breathing occurs due to altered respiratory rhythm. There is also inhibition of neurogenic, chemical, and hypoxic drive.

Cough Center

Cough center depression by morphine reduces cough.

Nausea and Vomiting

Morphine stimulates chemoreceptor trigger zone (CTZ) in medulla and produces vomiting. But in high doses, it inhibits vomiting center; thus, there is no vomiting in case of morphine poisoning. Due to this, emetics are not recommended in poisoning.

Pupils

Toxic doses of morphine produce characteristic "pin-point" pupils. Stimulation of Edinger–Westphal nucleus of third cranial nerve (oculomotor nerve) produces centrally mediated miosis, but it does not occur with morphine eye drops.

Vagus

Stimulation of the vagus nucleus in medulla produces bradycardia.

Miscellaneous

Morphine decreases body temperature and its toxic doses induce convulsions.

Cardiovascular System

Hypotension occurs due to dilatation of peripheral blood vessels and inhibition of baroreceptor reflexes. Large doses of morphine depress vasomotor center of medulla. Hypotension can also be seen with release of histamine. Larger doses of it also produce postural hypotension and fainting.

Gastrointestinal Tract (GIT)

Morphine reduces GI motility, increases tone of atrium and first part of duodenum, increases gastric emptying time, and reduces gastric secretion. It slows down the absorption of oral drugs. Increased tone of anal sphincter, decreased intestinal secretions and motility, and inattention to defecation reflex produce severe constipation.

Other Smooth Muscles

Morphine causes spasm of sphincter of Oddi, which leads to increase in biliary pressure. This action is antagonized by atropine and opioid antagonists. In elderly and patients with prostatic enlargement, morphine produces urinary retention due to increased ureteric tone and amplitude of contractions, increased tone of sphincters, and suppression of voiding reflex. It may aggravate asthmatic attack due to bronchoconstriction as a result of histamine release.

Neuroendocrine Effects

Morphine inhibits release of gonadotropin-releasing hormone (GnRH) and corticotropin-releasing factor (CRF) which results in reduced concentration of follicle-stimulating hormone (FSH), luteinizing hormone (LH), adrenocorticotropic hormone (ACTH), and β-endorphins. Tolerance may develop on prolonged use of morphine, but it is normalized after stopping.

Pharmacokinetics

Oral absorption of morphine is slow and incomplete. It has a high first-pass metabolism and therefore bioavailability is about 20 to 40%. Morphine is metabolized by glucuronide conjugation, and its active metabolite morphine-6-glucuronide is more potent than it. Preparations are available as controlled release tablets, morphine solution, subcutaneous (SC) injections, rectal suppositories, and transdermal patches.

Adverse Effects

Adverse effects of morphine include nausea, vomiting, constipation, respiratory depression, hypotension, urinary retention, dizziness, drowsiness, mental clouding, and confusion, allergic manifestations (skin rashes, pruritus), tolerance, and drug dependence.

Tolerance

Prolonged and repeated use of morphine leads to development of tolerance to respiratory depression, analgesia, sedation, euphoria, hypotension, and emesis but not to constipation and miosis. Cross-tolerance among different other opioids also develop in individuals becoming tolerant to morphine. Tolerance occurs at receptor level of cell and hence an addict requires higher doses progressively to achieve the same effect.

Dependence

Morphine dependence occurs due to its euphoriant action, and it involves both physical and psychological dependence. Administration of antagonist or opiate withdrawal results in withdrawal syndrome. Withdrawal symptoms are seen after 6 to 12 hours of withdrawal such as intense craving of drug, lacrimation, anorexia, sweating, rhinorrhea, anxiety, restlessness, tremors, fever, abdominal colic, diarrhea, severe sneezing, yawning, mydriasis, hypertension, palpitation, severe dehydration, and bone and muscle pain. Babies born to addict mothers develop withdrawal symptoms like suckling of fists, irritability, crying, tremors, yawning, diarrhea, sneezing, fever, and vomiting.

Treatment of morphine dependence includes gradual withdrawal of morphine over a period, with substitution of oral methadone done, because it is long-acting, slowly releases from tissues, more potent, and orally effective. Start with 1 mg methadone for every 4 mg of morphine once daily, gradually taper, and withdraw completely from 6 to 10 days. Within 10 days, most of the opiate addiction is completely withdrawn. Clonidine, a central α agonist, controls autonomic symptoms of withdrawal syndrome.

Acute Morphine Poisoning

It may be due to clinical overdose and accidental, homicidal, or suicidal intension. Lethal dose of morphine is about 250 mg in nonaddicts, but addicts can tolerate higher dose of morphine. Symptoms and signs of acute morphine poisoning are respiratory depression, cyanosis, hypothermia, pinpoint pupils, shock and hypotension, and stupor and coma. Death may occur due to respiratory depression and pulmonary edema. Treatment of acute morphine poisoning includes positive pressure breathing, maintaining blood pressure (BP), gastric lavage with potassium permanganate, and specific antidote such as naloxone (0.4 to 0.8 mg) intravenously (IV) administered (IV) and repeated every 5 minutes and then every 1 to 3 hours till morphine is cleared from body.

Precautions and Contraindications

Morphine must be used with caution in respiratory dysfunctions like chronic obstructive pulmonary disorder (COPD), bronchial asthma, etc. In extremes of age, morphine is prone to cause respiratory depression. One must avoid head injuries, because it increases cerebrospinal fluid (CSF) pressure which, in turn, leads to increase in intracranial tension (ICT), marked respiratory depression, vomiting, miosis, and mental clouding. Mental clouding may interfere with diagnosis and prognosis. If given during hypovolemic shock, it may lead to hypotension, because it decreases BP. In undiagnosed acute abdomen, administer morphine only after confirmation of diagnosis, as it relieves pain without modifying underlying disease and interferes with diagnosis. Morphine also induces vomiting and spasmogenic action on GI system.

Other Opioids

Heroin

Heroin is more potent than morphine, as it has rapid onset of action and is highly lipid soluble. It produces faster euphoric effects and has high abuse liability. It is widely used as a drug of abuse.

Codeine

Codeine is a naturally occurring opium alkaloid having less potent analgesic action than morphine. Only 10% of it is converted to morphine. It is used as an antitussive, because it suppresses dry cough by depressing cough center. Respiratory depression due to codeine is less significant, but it produces constipation very frequently.

Noscapine

Noscapine is also a naturally occurring opium alkaloid. It is also used as an antitussive agent, as it suppresses the cough with no significant CNS effects, but nausea is frequent with it.

Dextromethorphan and Pholcodine

These are centrally acting antitussives that are synthetic derivatives of opioid alkaloid.

Tramadol

Tramadol is a synthetic codeine analog with weak agonistic activity. It is used as an analgesic in acute or chronic pain, postoperative pain, etc. Its analgesic action is also due to inhibition of reuptake of noradrenaline and 5-HT. Adverse drug reactions due to tramadol are nausea, drowsiness, dry mouth, dizziness, and, rarely, precipitation of seizures.

Pethidine (Meperidine)

Pethidine is a phenylpiperidine and synthetic derivative of morphine, which is similar to it but has some differences. Morphine is natural and pethidine is synthetic. Morphine is more potent than pethidine (1/10 of morphine). An analgesic dose of morphine is 10 mg compared to 100 mg of pethidine. Constipation due to morphine is high but low with pethidine. Morphine suppresses cough but not pethidine. Corneal anesthesia and anticholinergic effects are present with pethidine but absent in morphine. Toxic dose of morphine causes severe CNS depression but pethidine causes CNS stimulation due to norpethidine. Histamine release is more with morphine than pethidine.

Pethidine is preferred over morphine to relieve pain due to better oral efficacy and less spasmogenicity. It is used during labor as it causes less respiratory depression in neonate and no interference with uterine contractions. It is preferred as preanesthetic medication over morphine.

Pethidine Derivatives

Fentanyl

Fentanyl is a pethidine congener, and as an analgesic, it is 100 times more potent than morphine. It is a highly lipid soluble; hence, it has rapid onset of acting, that is, within 5 minutes. It is preferred in cardiovascular surgeries, as it causes less interference in cardiovascular functions. It does not release histamine and leads to no increase in intracranial pressure. Fentanyl in transdermal patch acts for about 48 hours.

It is used for neuroleptanalgesia in poor risk patients in combination with droperidol. Epidural fentanyl with local anesthesia is used as postoperative and obstetrical analgesia. It is also used for chronic pain. Nausea, vomiting, muscle rigidity, and respiratory depression are adverse effects that occurs due to it.

Other congeners of pethidine are sufentanil, remifentanil, and alfentanil. These are faster acting and have a rapid recovery; hence, they are preferred for short surgical procedures.

Ethoheptazine

Ethoheptazine is related to pethidine and has mild analgesic action, and less addiction liability; therefore, it is used in combination with nonsteroidal anti-inflammatory drugs (NSAIDs).

Methadone

Methadone is an orally effective synthetic opioid derivative having analgesic potency similar to morphine. It is highly bound to plasma protein (90%). It also binds to tissue protein, where there is gradual accumulation and slow release. It causes milder withdrawal reactions after discontinuation, slow development of tolerance, and less incidence of euphoria. Due to its long duration of action ($t_{½}$ 24–36 hours), it is used for management of morphine-withdrawal symptoms. It is used as an analgesic for opioid maintenance and also for substitution therapy in opioid addicts. L-alpha-acetyl-methanol (LAAM), a methadone derivative, has longer duration of action than methadone.

Dextropropoxyphene

Dextropropoxyphene is an orally effective methadone congener used for mild-to-moderate pain in combination with aspirin or paracetamol. It has a longer duration of action. Dextropropoxyphene causes mild constipation but has abuse liability and stimulates CNS in larger doses.

Uses of Morphine and Other Opioids

Analgesic (IM13.17)

Opioids are used by the following routes: oral tablet, intramuscular (IM) or SC routes, as well as transdermal, intraspinal infusion, inhalation, rectal and transmucosal routes. Morphine is one of the most potent analgesics used for symptomatic relief of various types of pain. In myocardial infarction (MI), it reduces pain and anxiety as it decreases reflex sympathetic stimulation. Opioids and atropine combination relieve spasm of sphincter of Oddi in renal and biliary colic. In smaller doses, it is used as epidural analgesia for segmental block in spinal cord, as there is neither interference with motor or autonomic functions nor systemic side effects. Pethidine is preferred over morphine for obstetric analgesia. Opioids are used during the terminal stages of cancer pain. They are used to relieve pain during fractures, pulmonary embolism, postoperative, spontaneous pneumothorax, and burns. Due to addiction liability, it should not be used for chronic pain.

Preanesthetic Medication

Pethidine is preferred over morphine as preanesthetic medication, because it provides smoother induction, reduces anaesthetic dose, allays anxiety, and affords analgesia. Opioid preanesthetic medications have disadvantages, as they cause vomiting, respiratory depression, constipation, bronchospasm, and vasomotor depression, Urinary retention interferes with pupillary response to anesthesia as it produces miosis.

Acute Left Ventricular Failure

Morphine relieves dyspnea and pulmonary edema associated with acute left ventricular failure. The mechanism of this is not clear but the hypothesis is that it reduces anxiety and reflex sympathetic stimulation, decreases work on heart, decreases peripheral resistance (shunting of blood from pulmonary to systemic circulation), and changes patient perception to reduced pulmonary function. But morphine is contraindicated in pulmonary edema, which occurs due to respiratory irritants.

Diarrhea

Pethidine congeners like diphenoxylate and loperamide are used for symptomatic relief of diarrhea.

Cough

Codeine and analogs are used as antitussives to suppress cough.

Sedative

Morphine without affecting uterine contractions decreases anxiety during threatened abortion.

Special Anaesthesia

Fentanyl is used for neuroleptanalgesia in poor risk patients in combination with droperidol. Epidural fentanyl with local anesthesia is used as postoperative and obstetrical analgesia.

Opioid Antagonists

Naloxone

Naloxone is a pure antagonist at all opioid receptors and produces no actions in normal individuals but antagonizes all actions of morphine in addicts. Action of endogenous opioids (endorphins, enkephalins, and dynorphins) are also antagonized by it. It has high first-pass metabolism after IV administration, and duration of action is about 3 to 4 hours. It is used in morphine poisoning, for diagnosis of opioid dependence (as it precipitates withdrawal symptoms), for reverse neonatal asphyxia due to opioid use during labor, and also for stress-induced hypotension or shock reversal.

Naltrexone

Naltrexone is a pure opioid antagonist having longer duration of action of around 1 to 2 days. It is effective orally and more potent than naloxone. It is used for opioid blockade therapy in postopioid addicts and also in cases of alcohol dependence.

Nalmefane

Nalmefene is an orally effective long-acting opioid antagonist which is more potent than naltrexone.

Mixed Agonists and Antagonists

Pentazocine

Pentazocine is a kappa (K) receptor agonist and weak mu (μ) receptor antagonist. When compared, 20 mg of morphine is equal to 10 mg pentazocine. Also, it causes less respiratory depression, sedation, constipation, and biliary spasm compared to morphine. It is contraindicated in MI because it increases BP and heart rate. It is used in postoperative and chronic pain due to its less abuse liability. Pentazocine is administered orally as well as parenterally. Adverse reactions due to pentazocine use includes nausea, sweating, nightmares, dizziness, dysphoria, anxiety, hallucinations, and on long-term use, tolerance and dependence.

Nalbuphine

Similar to pentazocine, it is also a kappa (K) receptor agonist and weak mu (μ) receptor antagonist but more potent than pentazocine. The ceiling dose of nalbuphine is 30 mg. It is used as an analgesic for moderate and severe pain. It produces dysphoria at higher doses and less psychotomimetic effects.

Buprenorphine

Buprenorphine is a synthetic thebaine congener having high-lipid solubility. It is a partial mu (μ) receptor agonist and weak kappa (κ) receptor antagonist. Buprenorphine is more potent than morphine (25–35 times) and has slow onset but has longer duration of action. It produces less respiratory depression, tolerance, and dependence but has mild withdrawal symptoms. It is used as maintenance drug in opioid addicts and in terminal stages of cancer pain. It is administered by SC, IM, and sublingual routes.

Nalorphine

Nalorphine is an agonist-antagonist opioid. It causes dysphoria due to its k-agonist action at low doses. It also produces respiratory depression at low doses, and therefore not used as an analgesic. At high dose, it produces antagonist action, and due to this property, it is used in acute morphine poisoning and also for diagnosis of opioid addiction.

Meptazinol

Meptazinol is a shorter-acting partial opioid agonist used for obstetric analgesia. It causes less respiratory depression and no euphoria.

Multiple Choice Questions

1. A postgraduate surgery student is posted in rotation in general surgery, colorectal surgery, cardiothoracic surgery, trauma surgery, and surgical oncology units during junior resident first year. During these rotations for control of chronic pain in patients, he used to order morphine, keeping in mind the adverse effects and contraindications of it. Among those mentioned below, which one is the absolute contraindication to opioid?

A. Acute pulmonary edema.
B. Myocardial infarction.
C. Closed head injury.
D. Renal and biliary colic.

Answer: C

Opioids are contraindicated in head injury as they increase cerebral vascular pressure, which leads to increase in intra-cranial pressure and may cause hemorrhage or herniation.

2. A 7-year-old male child having persistent cough, fever (low grade) and vomiting after prolonged coughing spells is admitted to the hospital. After admission treatment is started and throat swab is sent for culture sensitivity, throat swab culture comes negative. After treatment, fever is resolved but slight cough still remains, and he is discharged with over-the-counter opioid antitussive. Among those mentioned below, which antitussive is prescribed?

A. Loperamide.
B. Dextromethorphan.
C. Tramadol.
D. Diphenoxylate.

Answer: B

Dextromethorphan is an easily available over-the-counter drug. This is used as an antitussive without analgesic properties and has limited abuse potential at recommended doses.

3. Codeine is a naturally occurring opium alkaloid having less potent analgesic action than morphine. About only 10% of it is converted to morphine. It is used as an antitussive because it suppresses dry cough. Among those mentioned below, which statement is correct regarding this?

A. Suppress the medullary cough center.
B. Suppresses cough by triggering the vagal reflex.
C. Stimulate mucus production and expectoration.
D. Cause diarrhea.

Answer: A

Codeine acts centrally at medullary cough center to decrease the sensitivity of the cough center and suppresses dry cough.

4. An unresponsive heroin addict is brought to the casualty having respiratory depression and pinpoint pupils. Fingerstick glucose is measured immediately and found to be normal. It was diagnosed to be a heroin overdose case. Among those mentioned below, which is the most appropriate agent to administer at this point?

A. Penicillamine.
B. Insulin.
C. Atropine.
D. Naloxone.

Answer: D

Naloxone is an opioid receptor antagonist and drug of choice in (history and clinical findings show it is an opioid overdose case).

5. For a workup of suspected pulmonary tuberculosis an intravenous (IV) drug abuser in a methadone maintenance program is admitted to the hospital. After admission, he has complaints of diarrhea and cramping. Stool sample was sent but result is negative. Among those mentioned below, which drug is prescribed for diarrhea?

A. Propantheline.
B. Loperamide.
C. Codeine.
D. Kaolin.

Answer: B

Loperamide effectively controls diarrhea in such conditions and is a good choice.

6. A pure opioid antagonist has longer duration of action of around 1 to 2 days. It is effective orally and more potent than naloxone. With a single oral dose in opioid addict's treatment programs, it has been proposed as a maintenance drug which blocks the injected heroin effects for about 48 hours. Which of the following is that drug?

A. Naltrexone.
B. Amphetamine.
C. Dextropropoxyphene.
D. Buprenorphine.

Answer: A

Naltrexone is a longer-acting opioid antagonist than naloxone and its duration of action is around 1 to 2 days. In opioid addict's treatment program, a high degree of client compliance would be required for naltrexone.

Part VI
Autacoids

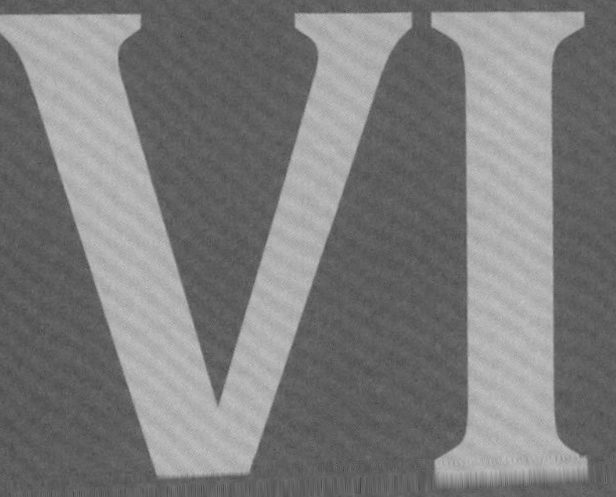

Chapter 41 Histamine and Antihistaminics

Jameel Ahmad, Bushra Hasan Khan, and Prerna Singh

PH1.16: Describe mechanism/s of action, types, doses, side effects, indications, and contraindications of the drugs that act by modulating autacoids, including: antihistaminics, 5-HT modulating drugs, nonsteroidal anti-inflammatory drugs (NSAIDs), drugs for gout, antirheumatic drugs, and drugs for migraine.

Learning Objectives

- Histamine.
- Histaminic receptors.
- Pharmacological actions of histamine.
- Classification of H1 receptor antagonists.
- Mechanism of action of H1 receptor antagonists.
- Therapeutic uses of H1 receptor antagonists.
- Adverse effects of H1 receptor antagonists.

Histamine

Histamine, meaning tissue amine (histo: tissue), is an autacoid widespread in plant and animals. The term autacoid comes from the Greek "autos" (self) and "akos" (relief or healing substance). Sir Henry Dale and his coworkers in the early 1900s had identified histamine as a mediator of biological function. Windausa and Vogta in 1907 synthesized histamine. Histamine is a naturally occurring imidazole derivative. Its widespread biologic activities are mediated through activation of specific cell-surface receptors. Histamine as such has no significant clinical applications, but agents that inhibit different histamine receptors have important therapeutic applications.

Location of Histamine

Histamine is present in practically all tissues, with significant amounts in the lungs, skin, blood vessel, gastrointestinal (GI) tract, liver, and placenta. It also occurs as a component of venom and in secretions from insect stings. The predominant sites of histamine storage are mast cells and basophils.

Biosynthesis and Storage of Histamine

Histamine is a low-molecular weight amine synthesized from the decarboxylation of the amino acid L-histidine by the enzyme L-histidine decarboxylase (HDC), a rate-limiting enzyme (**Fig. 41.1**). Histamine cannot be generated by any other known enzyme except the HDC. In stomach, histamine is synthesized by enterochromaffin-like cells (ECL), where it plays an important role in gastric acid secretion.

In the mast cells, it is held in intracellular specific granules as an inactive complex made up of histamine, the polysulphated anion heparin, along with anionic protein. If histamine is not stored, it is rapidly inactivated by the enzyme amine oxidase. The turnover of histamine is fast in nonmast cells because of its continuous release.

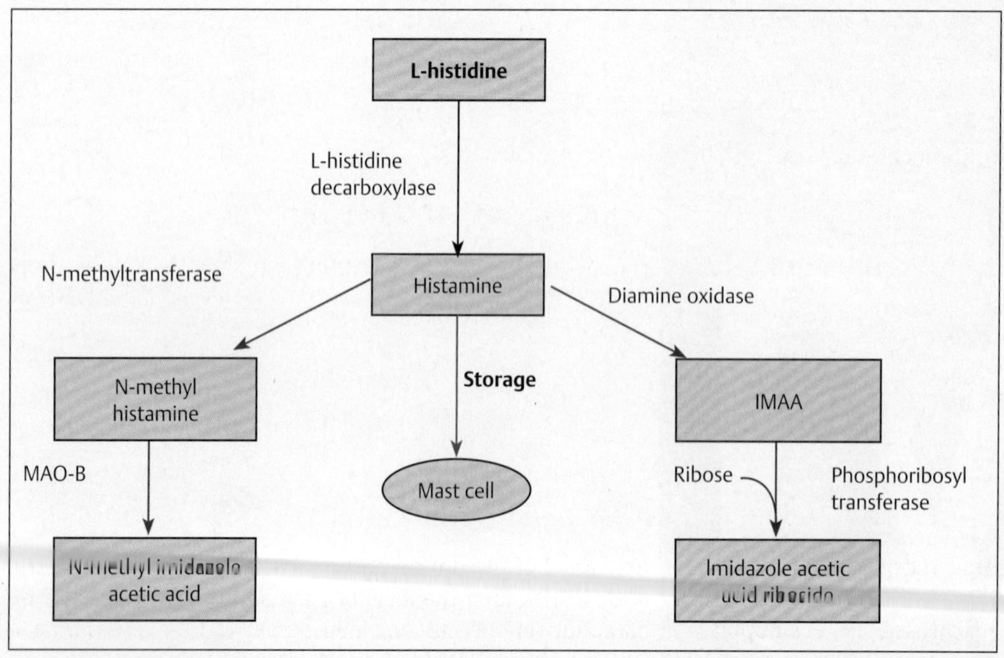

Fig. 41.1 Biosynthesis and metabolism of histamine. MAO, monoamine oxidase; IMAA, imidazole acetic acid.

Release of Histamine

The store of histamine can be released from mast cells by exocytosis during inflammatory or allergic reactions. However, the replenishment of the histamine may take days or weeks after secretion from mast cell or basophil. Histamine can be immunologic release or due to chemical or mechanical injury to mast cells.

Immunologic Release

The Fc region of immunoglobulin E (IgE) becomes bound to mast cells and basophil, and upon binding of this IgE's paratopes to an appropriate antigen, there is a release of histamine and other inflammatory mediators from these cells. Histamine release by this mechanism is a mediator in immediate (type I) allergy reactions such as acute urticaria and hay fever.

Chemical and Mechanical Release

Certain drugs like morphine, d-tubocurarine, polymyxin B, succinylcholine, radiocontrast, and vancomycin can directly release histamine from heparin-protein complex, within the mast cells, by a nonreceptor action without an immunological reaction. The red man syndrome (RMS) occurs with rapid infusion of vancomycin. Histamine release in the mast cells is inhibited by increasing cyclic AMP. Therefore, any drug or agent which can increase cyclic AMP concentration can inhibit the histamine release from mast cells, for example, adrenaline, ketotifen, and disodium cromoglycate.

Metabolism of Histamine

Histamine metabolism occurs by extracellular oxidative deamination of the primary amino group by diamine oxidase, also known as histaminase (peripheral tissues only), or by intracellular methylation of the imidazole ring by histamine-*N*-methyltransferase (HMT) in the brain and periphery. *N*-methyl histamine so produced is further metabolized by monoamine oxidase (MAO B) to *N*-methyl imidazole acetic acid. In the other pathway, diamine oxidase metabolizes the histamine into imidazole acetic acid (**Fig. 41.1**). Histamine is inactive orally because ingested histamine is degraded by the liver.

Histaminic Receptors

The biological activities of histamine are mediated through differential expressions of four known types of histamine receptors (H1, H2, H3, and H4). H1 and H2 have wide distribution in comparison to H3 and H4 receptors. Ash and Schild in 1966 were the first who differentiated the histamine receptors into H1 and H2. Burimamide was the first H2 blocker developed by Sir James Black in 1972. Lovenberg and colleagues in 1999 cloned and termed H3 receptor. Very recently, the fourth histamine receptor subtype was identified by Oda and colleagues in 2000 and named as H4 receptor. These receptors are expressed in eosinophils, mast cells, bone marrow, peripheral blood, neutrophils, and basophils. These are also present in small intestine, heart, colon, and lung. H4 receptors may play some roles in allergic inflammation. H4 receptors reveal 40% homology with H3 receptors. All these histamine receptors belong to the G protein-coupled receptor (GPCR) family. H3 receptors are predominantly presynaptic receptors.

Distribution, intracellular mechanism of action agonist, and antagonist/inverse agonists of histamine receptors have been shown in **Table 41.1**.

Pharmacological Actions of Histamine

Histamine released in response to stimuli exerts powerful effects on the nervous system, cardiovascular system, secretary tissues, smooth muscles of the GI tract, bronchiolar smooth muscles, inflammatory cells, and other cells.

Cardiovascular System

Many pharmacological actions observed on the cardiovascular system are mediated through H1 and H2 receptors. The positive ionotropic effect of histamine on the heart is observed by the activation of both H1 and H2 receptors. H1 receptors are responsible for changes in vascular permeability as a result of endothelial cell contraction, and dilatation of arterioles and postcapillary venules. Small doses of histamine produce vasodilatation by release of nitric oxide from endothelium, which is mainly mediated by H1 receptor. Separation of endothelial cells induced by the histamine can lead to transudation of fluids into perivascular space.

H2 receptor stimulation also causes dilatation of arterioles and postcapillary venules, resulting in a fall in blood pressure (BP). Positive chronotropic and ionotropic effects may be seen as reflex action due to fall in BP on histamine injection/infusion.

H1 receptors have a higher affinity than H2 receptors for histamine. Hence, with low doses of histamine, only H1 receptor mediated actions are observed. Rapid intravenous (IV) injection of histamine can cause decrease in systolic and diastolic BP, which has early, short-lasting H1 effect and slow but persistent H2 effect.

Nonvascular Smooth Muscles

The activation of H1 receptors in smooth muscle cells mediate bronchoconstriction and vascular permeability in the lungs. Their activation can also enhance the bronchiolar, salivary, and lacrimal secretions. Guinea pigs are very sensitive to histamine and death may occur due to histamine toxicity; however, human asthmatics are very sensitive to histamine.

Gastric Acid Secretion

Activation of the proton pump (H^+K^+ATPase) secretes gastric acid (HCl), and at the level of parietal cell, it is regulated by paracrine, endocrine, and neurocrine factors. The stomach mucosa contains two important types of tubular glands

Table 41.1 Characteristic features of histaminic receptors

Receptor	Distribution	Mechanism of action	Partial agonist	Partial antagonist/ inverse agonist
H1	Smooth muscle (bronchial, intestine, uterus)—contraction Blood vessels—vasodilation, increased capillary permeability CNS—neurotransmitter Sensory nerve ending—itching, pain Adrenal medulla—catecholamine release	Gq protein coupled (↑ Ca^{2+}; ↑ NO and ↑ cGMP)	Histaprodifen 2-methyl histamine	Mepyramine Cetirizine Chlorpheniramine Triprolidine
H2	Gastric glands—acid secretion Blood secretion vasodilation, increased capillary permeability Heart—positive ionotropic, positive chronotropic effect CNS—neurotransmitter	Gs protein coupled (↑ cAMP)	4-methyl histamine Dimaprit Amthamine	Cimetidine Ranitidine Nizatidine Famotidine
H3	Brain—decrease presynaptic histamine, ACh and NE release PNS—decrease histamine release Blood vessels—vasodilation	Gi protein coupled (↓ cAMP; ↑ MAP kinase)	R-α-methyl-histamine, Imetit, Immepip	Tiprolisant, Clobenpropit
H4	Basophil, eosinophils, neutrophils Bone marrow WBC chemotaxis	Gi protein coupled (↓ cAMP; ↑ Ca^{2+})	Clobenpropit Imetit Clozapine	Thioperamide

Abbreviations: ACh, acetylcholine; CNS, central nervous system; PNS, peripheral nervous system; NE; norepinephrine; WBC, white blood cell.

(oxyntic glands, the hallmark of which is parietal cells, and pyloric glands, the hallmark of which is the gastrin or G cells). Enterochromaffin-like (ECL) cells in the gastric pits of the stomach luminal epithelium secrete histamine in response to gastrin released by neighboring G cells. The secreted histamine acts on parietal cells to stimulate the release of gastric acid (**Fig. 41.2**). Histamine released from ECL cells acts as a paracrine mediator and diffuses from its site of release to nearby parietal cells, in order to cause the activation of H2 receptors. H2 receptors play a dominant role in the activation of proton pump because acetylcholine and gastrin exert their effect partly directly by stimulating the parietal cell (muscarinic, M3 and cholecystokinin receptors, CCK2) and partly indirectly by releasing histamine from histaminocytes. In the parietal cells are present two pathways, and the H2 receptors activate proton pump by generating cAMP through the activation of Gs-adenylylcyclase-cyclic AMP-PKA pathway. Acid secretion follows the circadian pattern, as the highest-level acid occurs during the night and the lowest levels during the morning hours.

H2 receptors blockers, for example, cimetidine, ranitidine, and famotidine are effective in reducing gastric acid secretion. As antiulcer medicines, these H2 receptor antagonists had achieved major market blockbuster status in the 1980s.

Histamine-induced contraction of smooth muscles of guinea pig ileum is often employed as a standard bioassay for histamine. This effect may be mediated by H1 receptors and large doses of histamine have been reported to cause diarrhea in humans.

Central Nervous System

Intracerebroventricular injections are required to produce central nervous system (CNS) effects, as histamine does not penetrate the brain. H1 receptors are abundant in hypothalamus. Postsynaptic H1 receptors in CNS are involved in the maintenance of wakefulness. H1 receptor antagonists developed initially show the known side effects of sedation, diminished alertness, and somnolence. In adrenal medulla, the H1 receptors can elicit the release of catecholamines.

In CNS and autonomic nervous system (ANS), the H3 receptors are presynaptically located as an autoreceptor controlling the synthesis and release of histamine. Their activation stimulates the negative feedback mechanism that reduces the release of histamine.

Peripheral Nervous System

Histamine is also a stimulant for peripheral sensory nerve endings and mediates pain and itching. The urticarial response to stimuli-like insect bite is also an H1-mediated effect of histamine.

Anaphylaxis

H1 receptors are involved in many pathological processes of allergy such as allergic rhinitis, atopic dermatitis, urticaria, and anaphylaxis.

Anaphylaxis is a severe, systemic allergic reaction which occurs due to systemic release of histamine and other pharmacologic mediators. The common causes of

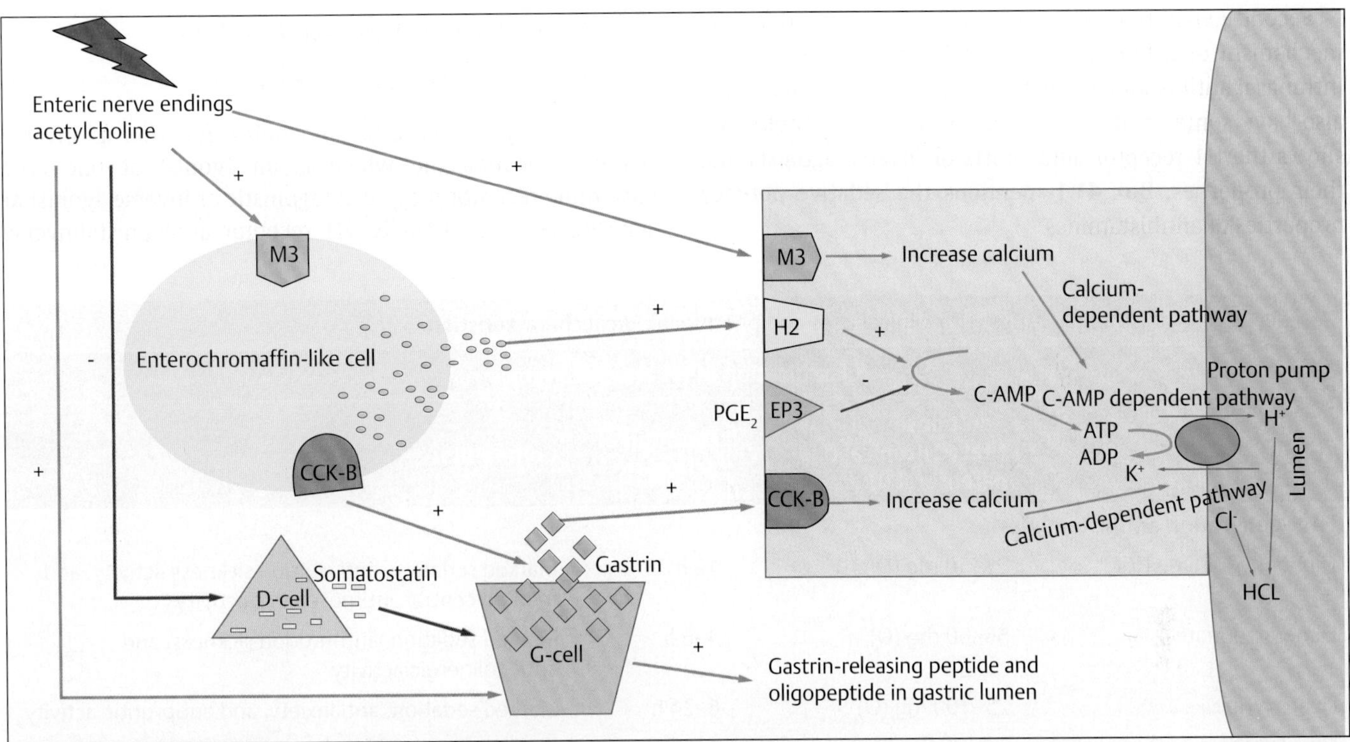

Fig. 41.2 Mechanism of histamine in gastric acid secretion.

anaphylaxis are IgE-mediated sensitivity to drugs, certain foods, and bee stings. Histamine release and other mediators cause dilatation of small blood vessels, increasing vascular permeability, and escape of plasma from the circulation. The patient can develop laryngeal edema, bronchoconstriction, and hypotension. Adrenaline is a life-saving agent which acts as a physiological antagonist of histamine. H1 receptor antagonist, H2 receptor antagonist, and corticosteroids are usually required for treating an anaphylactic reaction. Preloaded syringes of epinephrine are nowadays available for administration in patients of anaphylactic shock.

Triple Response

Histamine is known to cause the "triple response" of Lewis if injected intradermally and to act via H1 and H2 receptors to produce vasodilation and increased vascular permeability. The triple response consists of:

- Red spot: due to capillary dilatation.
- Flare: redness in the surrounding area due to arteriolar dilatation, which is mediated by axon reflex.
- Wheal: due to exudation of fluid from capillaries and venules.

H1 receptor blockers can effectively block the increased capillary permeability, edema, and wheal formation caused by histamine.

Mast Cell-Stabilizing Properties

Some second-generation H1 receptor antagonists (e.g., cetirizine, fexofenadine, olopatadine, Ketotifen, and others) have shown mast-cell-stabilizing and anti-inflammatory properties.

Antihistaminics

Antihistamines are a class of agents which antagonize the action of histamine, mediated by the H1 receptor.

Histamine has been known to mediate various physiological and pathological conditions. Many H1 receptor antagonists have clinical applications such as in rhinitis and urticaria. Most H1 receptor "antagonists" are actually inverse agonists at H1 receptors.

Classification of H1 Receptor Antagonists

H1 receptor antagonists are conventionally termed as antihistaminics. There are first-generation and second-generation H1 receptor antagonists.

Nonsedating second-generation H1 receptor antagonists were developed in the 1980s. First-generation antihistamines are lipophilic molecules that are associated with side effects largely because of their ability to cross the blood–brain barrier (BBB). Second-generation H1 receptor antagonists are more lipophobic molecules with certain advantages such as lack of sedation and cognitive impairment. These drugs also have lower affinity for nonhistamine receptors and higher selectivity for binding to H1 receptors. Therefore, second-generation H1 receptor antagonists produce no or minimal anticholinergic effects.

Another demerit of the first-generation H1 blockers is that many drugs are administered three to four times a day, but the second-generation H1 blockers have a longer duration of action.

Second-generation H1 blockers have an additional mechanism of action apart from H1 receptor antagonism. Intranasal antihistamines such as azelastine and olopatadine also have some mast-cell-stabilizing properties. **Table 41.2** shows the H1 receptor antagonists or inverse agonists and their properties. **Box 41.1** mentions the sedative potency properties of antihistamines.

Mechanism of Action of H1 Receptor Antagonists

In fact, many H1 receptor antagonists function as inverse agonists. A molecule which is an agonist at one type histamine receptor may be antagonistic or inverse agonist at another receptor. Usually, H1 receptor antagonists/inverse

Table 41.2 Antihistaminic drugs with clinical uses and pharmacological characteristics

Classification of H1 antihistaminics			
Agents	**Adult dose Oral (O)/topical (L)/ parenteral (I)**	**Duration of action**	**Comments**
First-generation antihistaminics			
Diphenhydramine HCl	25–50 mg (O/L/I)	12 h	Marked sedation, anti-motion sickness activity, and marked central antimuscarinic activity
Dimenhydrinate	50–50 mg (O)	4–6 h	Marked sedation, anti-motion sickness, and anticholinergic activity
Hydroxyzine	25–100 mg (O)	6–24 h	Marked sedation, antianxiety, and antipruritic activity
Doxylamine	1.5–25 mg (O)	4–6 h	
Promethazine HCl	12.5–50 mg (O/I)	4–6 h	Marked sedation, antiemetic, anti-motion sickness activity
Pyrilamine maleate	7.5–30 mg (O)	4–6 h	Very specific H1 antagonist
Cyproheptadine HCl	1–6.5 mg (O)	4–6 h	Sedation, antiserotonin, and anticholinergic activity
Pheniramine maleate	25–50 mg (O/I)	4–6 h	
Clemastine fumarate	1.34–2.68 mg (O)	12 h	
Meclizine HCl	25–50 mg (O)	12–24 h	Antivertigo
Chlorpheniramine maleate	4 mg, 12 mg (SR) (O)	24 h	Less prone to drowsiness
Cinnarizine	25–75 mg (O)	6–8 h	Antivertigo, weak antihistaminic activity
Triprolidine	2.5–5 mg (O)	4–6 h	
Doxepin HCl	10–150 mg (O), 5% (L)	6–24 h	Sedation, antidepressant, and topically used for atopic dermatitis
Carbinoxamine maleate	4–8 mg; 6–16 mg (O/SR)	3–6 h	Mild-to-moderate sedation
Brompheniramine maleate	2 mg (O)	3–6 h	
Cyclizine HCl	50 mg (O)	4–6 h	Sedation, anti-motion sickness activity
Cyclizine lactate	50 mg (injection)	4–6 h	Anti-motion sickness activity, antiemetic, antivertigo
Second-generation antihistaminics			
Fexofenadine HCl	60–180 mg (O)	12–24 h	
Cetirizine HCl	5–10 mg (O)	12–24 h	Mast cell-stabilizing, anti-inflammatory, and minimal anicholinergic activity
Levocetirizine HCl	2.5–5 mg (O)	12–24 h	More potent than cetirizine, mast cell-stabilizing, anti-inflammatory, and minimal anticholinergic activity
Loratadine	10 mg (O)	24 h	Longer action, mast cell-stabilizing, and anti-inflammatory minimal anticholinergic activity
Desloratidine	5 mg (O)	24 h	Mast cell-stabilizing, anti-inflammatory, and minimal anticholinergic activity
Ebastine	10 mg (O)	24 h	
Olopatadine HCl	0.1–0.2% eye drops (L)	6–12 h	Mast cell-stabilizing and anti-inflammatory properties (allergic conjunctivitis)

(Continued)

Table 41.2 (*Continued*) **Antihistaminic drugs with clinical uses and pharmacological characteristics**

Agents	Adult dose Oral (O)/topical (L)/ parenteral (I)	Duration of action	Comments
Acrivastine	8 mg (O)	6–8 h	Less sedative
Alcaftadine	0.25% 1 drop/eye (L)	16–24 h	Anti-inflammatory properties (allergic conjunctivitis)
Bepotastine besilate	10 mg (O), 1.5%, 1 drop/eye (L)	8 h	Mast cell-stabilizing and anti-inflammatory properties, and leukotrienes inhibitor effects
Ketotifen fumarate	(0.025%) 1 drop/eye (L)	8–12 h	Noncompetitive and inverse agonist of H1 receptor, mast cell-stabilizing, and weak anticholinergic effects
Mizolastine			
Azelastine HCl	0.14 mg/spray 2 sprays/nostril; 1 drop/eye (L)	12–24 h	Mast cell-stabilizing and anti-inflammatory properties
Epinastine	(0.05%), 1 drop/eye (L)	8–12 h	Mast cell-stabilizing and anti-inflammatory properties

Box 41.1 Sedative/potency properties of antihistamines

Antihistamines · Classification	
Generation I	**Examples**
Most sedative, Most potent:	Dlphenhydramine, Dlmenhydrlnate, Hydroxyzine, Promethaiine
Moderate sedative, Moderate potent:	Pheniramine, Meclizine, Buclizine, Cyproheptadine, Cetrizine
Less sedative, Less potent:	Chlorpheniramine, Mebhydrolinc, Dimethindone, Clemastine
Generation II	**Examples**
Mainly antiallergic:	Levocetrizine, Loratadine, Desloratadine, Fexofenadine
Antivertigo, Antimigraine:	Flunnarizine, Cinnarizine

agonists have reversible competitive binding to H1 receptor. Mepyramine, also known as pyrilamine, is an H1 receptor inverse agonist. First-generation H1 receptor antagonists may block muscarinic receptors producing antimuscarinic effects.

Certain second-generation H1 receptor antagonists have shown mast cell-stabilizing and anti-inflammatory properties. The postreceptor mechanism of the four known subtype histamine receptors has been briefly mentioned in **Table 41.1**.

Therapeutic Uses of H1 Receptor Antagonists

Histamine has as such no therapeutic indications except betahistine, an orally active histamine analog, which is used to control vertigo in a dose of 8 to 16 mg. It helps in the vertigo of Meniere's disease possibly by causing vasodilation and improvement of blood flow to the labyrinth and also to the brain. It may precipitate peptic ulcer and asthma.

Allergic Disorders (DR14.5)

Urticaria and angioedema represent the same pathophysiologic process occurring at different levels of the skin. In urticaria without symptoms of anaphylaxis or angioedema, the oral antihistamines are among the preferred drugs, as histamine is the primary mediator in such diseases. Angioedema may be precipitated by the release of histamine but can be result of activation of bradykinin and other vasoactive substances. First- and second-generation H1 antihistamines are effective, but second-generation, long-acting, and nonsedating H1 antihistamines are preferred because of their side effects with increased daily dosing. The H2 receptor antagonist and CysLT1 receptor antagonist are important forms of add-on therapy in such patients.

Antihistaminics do not influence antigen and antibody reaction but block the effects of histamine. Chronic urticaria may need doses up to four times higher than that approved for treating rhinitis.

Allergic Rhinitis

Allergic rhinitis may be characterized by nasopharyngeal itching, sneezing, and rhinorrhea. The second-generation, long-acting H1 antihistaminics (fexofenadine, loratadine, desloratadine, cetirizine, levocetirizine, Azelastine, and olopatadine) are among the preferred agents because older H1 antihistaminics can produce sedation, psychomotor impairment, and anticholinergic effects (visual disturbance, urinary retention, and constipation). The sedation has been reported in 50% of patients with the first-generation H1 receptor blockers. These drugs are more lipophilic than newer H1 antihistaminics. Intranasal glucocorticoids are the most potent drugs for allergic rhinitis. Azelastine is available as a nasal spray. Azelastine, antazoline, and olopatadine are also used topically as eye drops for allergic conjunctivitis.

Anaphylaxis

Anaphylaxis is a severe, systemic allergic reaction caused by the systemic release of histamine and other pharmacologic mediators. Antihistaminic-like chlorpheniramine (IV) is a useful adjunct or ancillary agent to epinephrine in acute hypersensitivity reaction (type 1) like an acute anaphylactic shock. Epinephrine, the treatment of first choice, provides both α and β adrenergic effects, resulting in vasoconstriction and bronchial smooth-muscle relaxation, and relieves angioneurotic edema of the larynx and bronchospasm.

Bronchial Asthma

In bronchial asthma, leukotrienes and other mediators play a more important role than histamine. Allergic rhinitis and asthma share some common mediators, but previous studies have reported that antihistamines may dry the secretions in the upper and lower respiratory tracts. Therefore, the therapeutic efficacy of H1 receptor blockers to alleviate comorbid asthma symptoms, particularly in patients with allergic rhinitis, needs to be established. However, the histamine release inhibitors (disodium cromoglycate and nedocromil sodium) which are different from histamine receptor blockers have been used in the treatment of bronchial asthma.

Pruritus

Pruritus or itch is a frequently described symptom of many cutaneous and systemic diseases. It can range from mild to severe and may be intermittent or chronic. Diphenhydramine and hydroxyzine may be used. Second-generation antihistamines, cetirizine, loratadine, and fexofenadine can be administered in the morning due to their nonsedating effects.

Nausea and Vomiting of Pregnancy

Nausea and vomiting in pregnancy, colloquially referred to as morning sickness, is often undertreated due to fears of possible teratogenic effects. The combination of doxylamine succinate, pyridoxine hydrochloride, and dicyclomine hydrochloride was approved by Food and Drugs Administration (FDA) in 1956 for the treatment of nausea and vomiting in pregnancy. In the 1970s, a number of lawsuits were filed alleging congenital defects. In April 2013, FDA reapproved doxylamine succinate 10 mg and pyridoxine hydrochloride 10 mg as a delayed-release combination for nausea and vomiting in pregnancy.

Cough and Common Cold

Spontaneous cough is triggered by stimulation of sensory nerve endings. The stimulus can be chemical and mechanical to initiate the cough reflex. The drugs with anticholinergic and sedative effects have been therapeutically exploited to provide symptomatic relief in patients of common cold and cough. Diphenhydramine, promethazine, and chlorpheniramine like drugs may provide symptomatic relief in some patients. These drugs do not affect the course of illness, but their anticholinergic action reduces the rhinorrhea of common cold.

Parkinson's Disease

Parkinson's disease is characterized by an imbalance between acetylcholine and dopamine in the striatum that controls extrapyramidal activity. In patients of parkinsonism, the selective degeneration of nigrostriatal tract results in a decrease in the dopaminergic activity and a relative increase in the cholinergic activity in the striatum. The drug with prominent central anticholinergic action like promethazine and diphenhydramine can be used in early Parkinsonism, but these are not preferred due to their marked sedation.

Acute Muscle Dystonia

Acute muscle dystonia or extrapyramidal side effects may occur with the use of certain drugs, for example, metoclopramide, antipsychotic drugs, and phenothiazines. Metoclopramide has central antidopaminergic (D2) action, which is responsible for its antiemetic effects. However, this D2 receptor blockade in the corpus striatum causes a relative increase in cholinergic activity. The drugs with prominent central anticholinergic property (e.g., promethazine and diphenhydramine) have been used for drug-induced acute muscle dystonia. Levodopa like antiparkinsonian drugs act by increasing dopamine activity in striatum but are not effective in drug-induced parkinsonism because dopamine receptors are already blocked.

As Sedative

Promethazine has been employed among children as a sedative. However, the FDA has issued warning against the use of promethazine HCl in children younger than 2 years due to the risk of fatal respiratory depression.

Preanesthetic Medication

Promethazine for its anticholinergic, sedative, and antiemetic effects has been used in preanesthetic medication.

Motion Sickness

Motion sickness is inducible in many people with a functioning vestibular apparatus. The vestibular apparatus sends nauseating signals to the vomiting center when the body is in motion. The drugs which possess anticholinergic, antimuscarinic, and CNS depressant activities are effective in motion sickness (e.g., promethazine, dimenhydrinate, cyclizine, and meclizine). Promethazine possesses additional antiemetic properties, which also contribute to its efficacy in motion sickness; however, sedation is the major side effect. These drugs can be used as prophylaxis for motion sickness, and administered about 1 hour before the anticipated travel because they are much less effective after nausea and vomiting have set in. Hyoscine (scopolamine) is an antimuscarinic agent often used in motion sickness.

Second-generation antihistamines, for example, cetirizine and fexofenadine, without CNS depressant effect are ineffective for treating motion sickness.

Vertigo

Meclizine, dimenhydrinate, promethazine, and cinnarizine are frequently prescribed from the antihistamine group of agents. Cinnarizine has been used to treat vertigo, tinnitus, nausea, and vomiting of Meniere's disease.

Adverse Effects of H1 Receptor Antagonists (Fig. 41.3)

Sedation, diminished alertness, motor incoordination/alteration of psychomotor functions, and tendency to fall asleep are common among first-generation antihistaminics. These are widely distributed in the body and easily cross the BBB. Therefore, these drugs should be avoided during driving a vehicle or operating machinery.

Dryness of mouth and respiratory passages, urinary hesitancy, dysuria, diplopia, blurring of vision, and constipation are related to the anticholinergic action of first-generation antihistamines.

Leucopenia, agranulocytosis, and hemolytic anemia, are very rare side effects reported with use of H1 antagonists.

Topical application of these drugs may cause allergy such as dermatitis and photosensitivity. Almost 20% of patients on intranasal azelastine and somewhat fewer on olopatadine have been found to report a bitter taste. Sometimes, systemic absorption of intranasal azelastine can cause sedation in patients.

Cyproheptadine, an H1 receptor antagonist, has been found to stimulate appetite, resulting in weight gain.

Acute poisoning/acute intoxication with H1 antihistamines results in symptoms very similar to those of anticholinergic poisoning, and also shows a remarkable similarity to that of atropine poisoning. It may cause CNS excitatory effects, hallucinations, ataxia, incoordination, tremors, flushing, and convulsions. Very high dose can cause respiratory and cardiovascular failure, which can lead to death.

Contraindications of H1 Receptor Antagonists

The H1 receptor antagonists are relatively contraindicated in any patient with QT prolongation due to the risk of potentially fatal cardiac arrhythmias.

Urinary retention in patients with an obstructed bladder neck and increased ocular pressure in primary angle closure may occur due to anticholinergic effects of antihistaminics.

H1 Receptor Antagonists in Children

First-generation H1 antihistamines on regular use may impair learning and school performance of children because of their sedative effects; however, it is still not clear about how common these effects are truly.

FDA issued a public health advisory in January 2008 which specified that fixed dose combinations (FDCs) containing antihistamines, decongestants, antitussives, and expectorants should not be used in children below 2 years of age due to life-threatening adverse events.

H1 Antihistamines in the Elderly

First-generation H1 antihistamines should be avoided in elderly patients for their sedative and anticholinergic effects, particularly in the presence of existing cognitive decline. Therefore, second-generation antihistamines are preferred for elderly patients (>65 years of age).

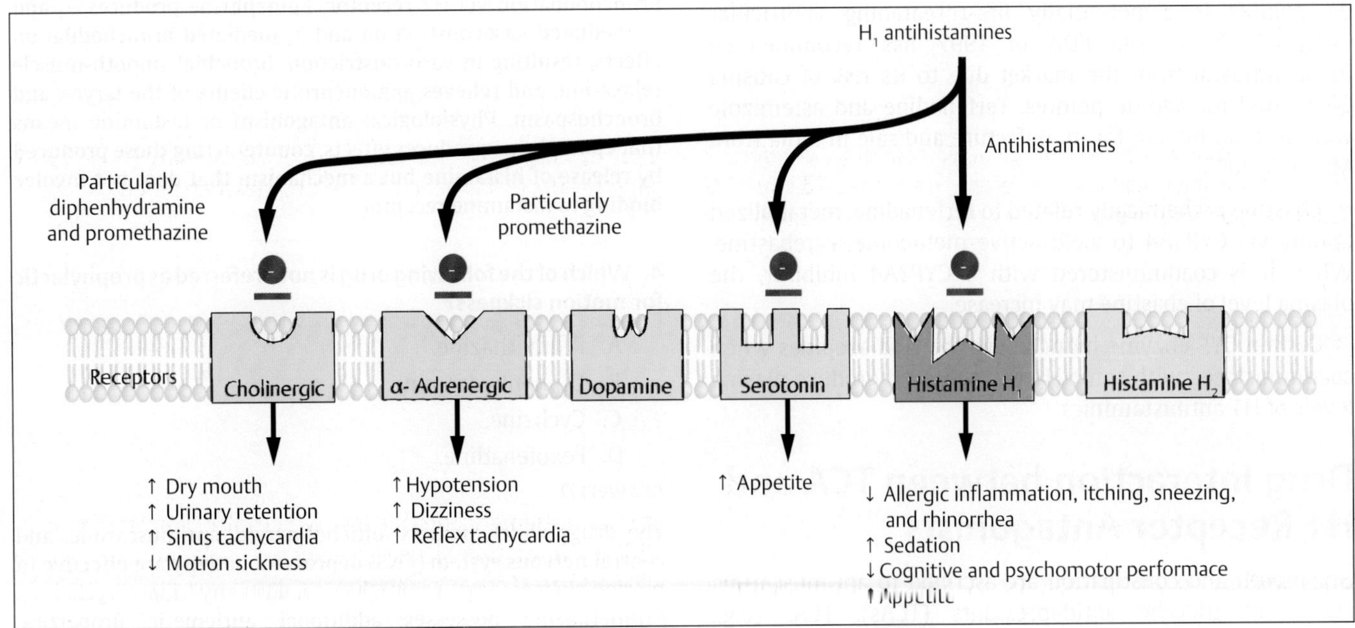

Fig. 41.3 Adverse effects and uses of antihistamines.

Antihistaminics in Pregnancy and Lactation

First-generation antihistamines are lipophilic drugs. Some animal studies with hydroxyzine, cyclizine, azelastine, hydroxyzine, fexofenadine, and promethazine have shown their teratogenic effects, but human studies have not shown teratogenicity so far with these agents.

Drugs such as chlorpheniramine, cetirizine, and loratadine were not found to have a teratogenic effect in animal studies. Recently published reviews concluded that antihistamines are unlikely to be strong risk factors for major birth defects. Loratadine and cetirizine have been found to be nonteratogenic in studies to date. Both these drugs are pregnancy category B agents. For treatment of nausea and vomiting in pregnancy, in April 2013, FDA reapproved doxylamine succinate and pyridoxine hydrochloride as a delayed-release combination.

Although a minimal amount of H1 receptor antagonists is excreted in the breast milk, yet they can cause drowsiness in the nursing infant.

CYP450 Enzyme Inhibitors and H1 Receptor Antagonists

H1 antihistamine interactions are essentially of a pharmacokinetic nature: the triggering agent induces changes in the absorption and/or metabolism of the H1 antihistaminic. Clinically significant drug interactions can occur during multiple drug therapy involving drug metabolism in which cytochrome P450 isoenzymes play a significant role.

Second-generation antihistaminics such as terfenadine and astemizole are metabolized by specific CYP3A4 subtype of P-450 enzymes. CYP3A4 microsomal enzyme inhibitors (erythromycin, ketoconazole) can elevate the plasma level of terfenadine and astemizole, which may lead to *torsade de pointes*, a form of polymorphic ventricular tachycardia. It is associated with prolongation of the QT interval due to blockade of cardiac K^+ channels (HERG; IKr). Torsade de pointes is a potentially life-threatening ventricular tachyarrhythmia. The FDA in 1997 has recommended its withdrawal from the market due to its risk of causing QT-related torsade de pointes. Terfenadine and astemizole were also prohibited for manufacture and sale in India from March 5, 2003.

Ebastine is chemically related to terfenadine, metabolized mainly via CYP3A4 to yield active metabolite, carebastine. When it is coadministered with a CYP3A4 inhibitor, the plasma level of ebastine may increase.

Certain CYP enzyme inducers like benzodiazepines when coadministered with some H1 receptors may reduce plasma levels of H1 antihistaminics.

Drug Interaction between TCA and H1 Receptor Antagonists

Dry mouth and constipation are ascribed to antimuscarinic effects of tricyclic antidepressants (TCAs). TCAs (e.g., iprindole, and mianserin) are very potent H1 receptor antagonists. This effect on the H1 receptor may contribute to the sedative effects of certain antidepressant drugs. Doxepin, a tricyclic antidepressant, produces a potent hypnotic effect, presumably via antagonism of H1 receptor.

Multiple Choice Questions

1. Histamine is synthesized by which enzyme/enzymes?

A. N-methyl transferase.
B. Diamine oxidase.
C. L-histidine decarboxylase.
D. L-histidine decarboxylase and tryptophan hydroxylase.

Answer: C

Histamine is synthesized from the decarboxylation of the amino acid L-histidine by the enzyme L-histidine decarboxylase. Histamine cannot be generated by any other known enzyme except the L-histidine decarboxylase.

2. H1 blocker with marked anticholinergic activity is?

A. Cetirizine.
B. Fexofenadine.
C. Ebastine.
D. Diphenhydramine.

Answer: D

Certain first-generation antihistaminics exhibit high cholinergic properties.

3. Which of the following is not true about epinephrine?

A. α_1 adrenergic effects.
B. Physiological antagonist to histamine.
C. β_2 adrenergic effects.
D. Bronchodilation via H2 receptor.

Answer: D

Bronchodilation via H2 receptor. Epinephrine produces α_1 and α_2 mediated vasoconstriction and β_2 mediated bronchodilation effects, resulting in vasoconstriction, bronchial smooth-muscle relaxation, and relieves angioneurotic edema of the larynx and bronchospasm. Physiological antagonism of histamine means that epinephrine produces effects, counteracting those produced by release of histamine but a mechanism that does not involve binding to histamine receptor.

4. Which of the following drug is not preferred as prophylactic for motion sickness?

A. Promethazine.
B. Diphenhydramine.
C. Cyclizine.
D. Fexofenadine.

Answer: D

The drugs which possess anticholinergic, antimuscarinic, and central nervous system (CNS) depressant activity are effective in motion sickness (e.g., promethazine, dimenhydrinate, cyclizine). Promethazine possesses additional antiemetic properties, which contribute to its efficacy in motion sickness; however,

second-generation H1 antagonists (Fexofenadine and others) do not have such effects.

5. Drug when coadministered with CYP3A4 microsomal enzyme inhibitor can cause torsade de pointes is?

A. Chlorpheniramine.

B. Astemizole.

C. Cetirizine.

D. Doxylamine.

Answer: B

Second-generation antihistaminics such as astemizole are metabolized by specific CYP3A4 subtype of P-450 enzymes. CYP3A4 microsomal enzyme inhibitors can elevate the plasma level of astemizole, leading to torsade de pointes, a form of polymorphic ventricular tachycardia due to a blockade of cardiac K^+ channels (HERG; IKr).

6. The H1 receptor antagonist that can be prescribed to patients of allergic rhinitis as nasal spray is?

A. Azelastine.

B. Levocetirizne.

C. Terfenadine.

D. Loratadine.

Answer: A

Azelastine possesses maximum topical activity, and it is administered as nasal spray for allergic rhinitis.

7. What is not correct about histamine receptors?

A. H4 receptors reveal about 40% homology with H3 receptors.

B. H3 receptors are predominantly postynaptic receptors in the CNS.

C. All histamine receptors are G protein-coupled receptor.

D. Postsynaptic H1 receptors are involved in the maintenance of wakefulness.

Answer: B

H3 receptors are predominantly postynaptic receptors in the central nervous system (CNS). In CNS and autonomic nervous system, the H3 receptors are presynaptically located as an autoreceptor and control the synthesis and the release of histamine. Their activation stimulates the negative feedback mechanism that reduces the release of histamine.

8. Drug-induced acute muscle dystonia is relieved by?

A. Ebastine.

B. Promethazine.

C. Scopolamine.

D. Fexofenadine.

Answer: B

Acute muscle dystonia or extrapyramidal side effects may occur with the use of certain drugs, for example, metoclopramide and phenothiazines. Metoclopramide acts through D2 receptor antagonism and produces central antidopaminergic (D2) action. Certain H1 receptor antihistaminics, for example, promethazine have a significant central anticholinergic effect.

9. Histaminergic receptor with a dominant role in the activation of proton pump is?

A. H4 receptor.

B. H3 receptor.

C. H2 receptor.

D. H1 receptor.

Answer: C

H2 receptors activate proton pump by generating cAMP through the activation of Gs-adenylylcyclase-cyclic AMP-PKA pathway.

10. Doxepin, a tricyclic antidepressant, produces a potent hypnotic effect presumably via?

A. Antagonism of H1 receptor.

B. Antagonism of H2 receptor.

C. Antagonism of H3 receptor.

D. Antagonism of H4 receptor.

Answer: A

Tricyclic antidepressants (TCAs), for example, iprindole and mianserin are very potent H1 receptor antagonists. This effect on the H1 receptor may contribute to the sedative effects of certain antidepressant drugs.

Chapter 42

Serotonin (5-Hydroxytryptamine) Agonists and Antagonists, Ergot Alkaloids, and Drug Treatment of Migraine

Nishita H. Darji, Suhani V. Patel, and Vishalkumar K. Vadgama

PH1.16: Describe mechanism/s of action, types, doses, side effects, indications, and contraindications of the drugs that act by modulating autacoids, including antihistamines, 5-HT modulating drugs, NSAIDs, drugs for gout, antirheumatic drugs, and drugs for migraine.

Learning Objectives

- 5-Hydroxytryptamine (serotonin) and its agonists and antagonists.
- Ergot.
- Triptans.
- Migraine headache.
- Migraine management.

5-Hydroxytryptamine (Serotonin) and Its Agonists and Antagonists

5-Hydroxytryptamine (5-HT) is derived from serum and possesses vasoconstrictor action; hence, it was named "serotonin." Another substance called "enteramine" was identified to cause vascular smooth muscle contraction within the gut mucosa. Later on, Erspamer, a scientist, studied in detail both of these and identified enteramine as 5-HT. 5-HT is an important neurotransmitter that acts within the central nervous system (CNS) as well as in periphery. It is widely distributed in plants and animal tissues such as fruits (pineapple, pear, banana), vegetables (tomato), and insect stings (scorpion, wasp). In human beings, the highest concentration of it is found in the gut mucosa, platelets, and CNS.

Synthesis, Storage, Release, and Metabolism of Serotonin

Synthesis

The synthesis of 5-HT is a two-step process. In the first step, the amino acid L-tryptophan is converted into 5-hydroxytryptophan with the help of the enzyme hydroxylase. In the second step, 5-hydroxytryptophan undergoes decarboxylation by the decarboxylase enzyme and gives 5-HT. The decarboxylase enzyme is nonspecific, as it can also act on catecholamines (CAs) and convert dihydroxyphenylalanine (DOPA) to dopamine.

Storage and Release

5-HT is stored in the storage granules with the help of vesicular monoamine transporter 2 (VMAT2) and then gets released upon arrival of action potential.

Reuptake

5-HT action is terminated mainly by reuptake via an amine pump "SERotonin Transporter" (SERT), which is a Na^+-dependent carrier present at the membrane of platelets and serotonergic nerve endings. Therefore, the free form of 5-HT is not present in the circulation. Platelets that lack nucleus cannot synthesize 5-HT, but they acquire it by passing through intestinal blood vessels. SERT pump is inhibited by selective serotonin reuptake inhibitors (SSRIs) and tricyclic antidepressants (TCAs). After reuptake, a portion of 5-HT is taken up within storage vesicles by VMAT2 such as CA. Reserpine inhibits vesicular uptake of 5-HT by blocking VMAT and thus leads to depletion.

Metabolism

The remaining 5-HT undergoes oxidative deamination by monoamine oxidase (MAO) enzyme, mainly the subtype MAO-A. In this process, 5-HT is converted into 5-hydroxyacetaldehyde. Majority of 5-hydroxyacetaldehyde is further converted into 5-hydroxyindoleacetic acid (5-HIAA) with the help of the enzyme aldehyde dehydrogenase, while some of it is converted into 5-hydroxytryptol by aldehyde reductase. 5-HIAA is excreted in the urine, which can be used in carcinoid syndrome diagnosis (**Fig. 42.1**).

Serotonergic (5-HT) Receptors

In 1957, Gaddum and Picarelli classified 5-HT receptors into main two types based on contraction of gut muscle—musculotropic (D type) and neurotropic (M type), which are blocked by phenoxybenzamine and morphine, respectively. Presently, on the basis of molecular characterization and cloning of the receptor, there are seven main types of 5-HT receptors, namely, 5-HT_1, 5-HT_2, 5-HT_3, 5-HT_4, and 5-HT_{5-7} (**Table 42.1**). The 5-HT_{5-7} receptors are cloned and found to

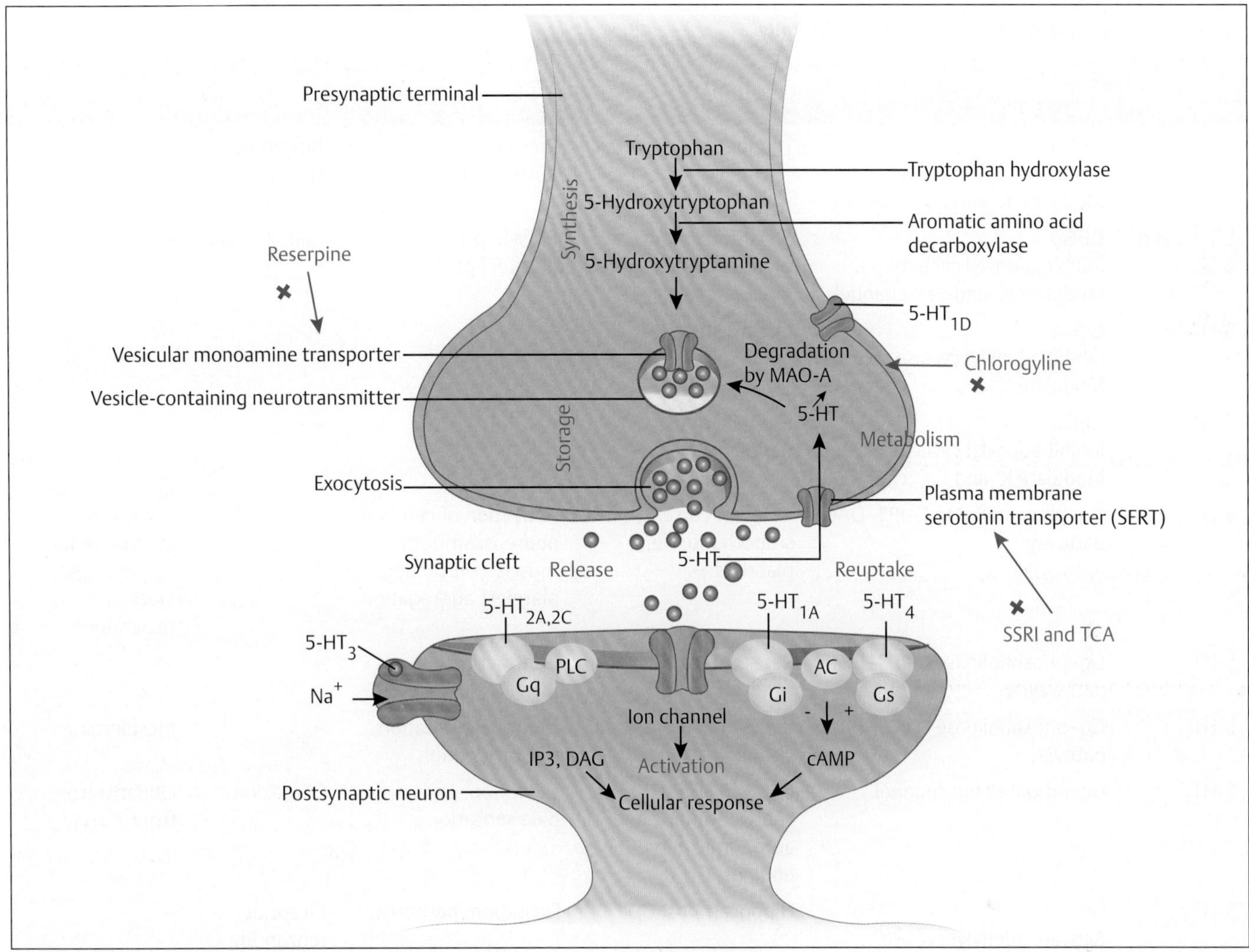

Fig. 42.1 Synthesis, storage, release, and metabolism of serotonin.

be like 5-HT_4 receptors, but their functions are yet not fully understood.

5-HT_1 Receptors

This 5-HT_1 receptor family comprises five members, namely, 5-HT_{1A}, 5-HT_{1B}, 5-HT_{1D}, 5-HT_{1E}, and 5-HT_{1F}. All of them act via Gi/Go protein and inhibit adenylyl cyclase as well as modulate K^+ and Ca^{2+} channels. This family of receptors principally function as autoreceptors and inhibit firing or release of 5-HT from presynaptic nerve terminals.

5-HT_{1B} and 5-HT_{1D} receptors are thought to be very similar and have attained a major therapeutic role. These subtypes of 5-HT_1 receptors are present in cranial blood vessels and supposedly cause vasoconstriction and peptide-mediated neuroinflammation. Drugs acting on these receptor subtypes are helpful in migraine therapy (details are given later in this chapter). The 5-HT_{1D} receptor is present in basal ganglia and substantia nigra where it regulates dopaminergic pathway. It also leads to release of noradrenaline from adrenergic nerve terminals. The functional role of other subtype of 5-HT_1 receptors is undefined till date. Notably, recently, agonists at 5-HT_{1F} receptor are tested for management of acute attack of migraine.

5-HT_2 Receptors

There are three subtypes of 5-HT_2 receptors, that is, 5-HT_{2A}, 5-HT_{2B}, and 5-HT_{2C}, all of them being postsynaptic. These receptors act through Gq protein–phospholipase C–IP3–DAG pathway and inhibition of K^+ channels, leading to depolarization of neurons. 5-HT_2 receptors, located within the limbic system, are involved in psychosis and so 5-HT_2 antagonists such as clozapine are used therapeutically for negative symptoms of schizophrenia.

5-HT_3 Receptors

They are expressed mainly in the CNS and gastrointestinal tract (GIT). This is the only serotonergic receptor that acts via ligand-gated ion channel. They mediate vomiting through chemoreceptor trigger zone (CTZ) and nucleus tractus solitarius (NTS) centers of the brain. Peripherally, they augment peristalsis and pain sensation. Antagonists at 5-HT_3 are clinically used as antiemetic drugs.

5-HT_4 Receptors

5-HT_4 receptors act via Gs protein, activate adenylyl cyclase, and ultimately increase cAMP level. They are also located

Table 42.1 Serotonin receptors and its subfamily

Receptor/ subtypes	Mechanism	Location	Function	Agonist	Antagonist
5-HT_{1A}	Gi/Go Inhibit adenylyl cyclase Modulate K^+ and Ca^{2+} channels	Hippocampus, cortex	Presynaptic autoreceptor	Buspirone, gepirone, ipsapirone	–
5-HT_{1B} and 5-HT_{1D}	Gi/Go Inhibit adenylyl cyclase Modulate K^+ and Ca^{2+} channels	Substantia nigra, globus pallidus, cranial blood vessels	Presynaptic autoreceptor	Sumatriptan	–
5-HT_{1E}	Gi/Go Inhibit adenylyl cyclase Modulate K^+ and Ca^{2+} channels	Cortex, striatum	–	–	–
5-HT_{1F}	Gi/Go Inhibit adenylyl cyclase Modulate K^+ and Ca^{2+} channels	Hippocampus, periphery	–	–	–
5-HT_{2A}	Gq–phospholipase C–IP3–DAG pathway	Cerebral cortex, smooth muscle, platelets	Activation of cerebral neurons, smooth muscle contraction, platelets aggregation	–	Ketanserin, cyproheptadine, methysergide, clozapine, risperidone
5-HT_{2B}	Gq–phospholipase C–IP3–DAG pathway	Rat stomach fundus	Contraction	–	–
5-HT_{2C}	Gq–phospholipase C–IP3–DAG pathway	Substantia nigra, choroid plexus	Neuronal excitation, CSF production	–	Mesulergine
5-HT_3	Ligand-gated ion channel	CTZ and NTS center, somatic and autonomic nerve endings, GIT	Excitation, peristalsis, pain sensation	Quipazine	Ondansetron, tropisetron
5-HT_4	Gs Activate adenylyl cyclase Increase cAMP	Hippocampus, GIT	Excitation, peristalsis	Cisapride, renzapride	–
5-HT_5	Gi/Go Inhibit adenylyl cyclase	Hippocampus, cortex	Unknown	–	–
5-HT_6	Gs Activate adenylyl cyclase Increase cAMP	Hippocampus, striatum	Excitation	–	–
5-HT_7	Gs Activate adenylyl cyclase Increase cAMP	Hippocampus, GIT	Smooth muscle contraction	–	–

Abbreviations: 5-HT, 5-hydroxytryptamine; CSF, cerebrospinal fluid; CTZ; chemoreceptor trigger zone; GIT, gastrointestinal tract; NTS, nucleus tractus solitarius.

peripherally as well as in the CNS. Peripheral action within GIT (smooth muscles, sensory cells, and myenteric plexus) leads to peristalsis and secretion, and ACh release with contraction of lower esophageal sphincter. Drugs that act as 5-HT_4 agonists are used as prokinetic drugs.

Research has found that 5-HT_5 receptors are related with cognition and circadian rhythms. 5-HT_6 receptors are linked with cognition and motor control. The 5-HT_7 receptors are under scrutiny for depression. One of the findings shows clozapine (atypical antipsychotic) to have high affinity for 5-HT_6 and 5-HT_7 receptors in addition to being 5-$HT_{2A/2C}$ antagonist.

Pathophysiological Role and Pharmacological Action of 5-HT

5-HT is a neuromodulator and neurotransmitter with potent depolarizing action. It has variable actions on different organ systems (**Table 42.2**).

Drugs Acting on 5-HT (Serotonin) System

Drugs that decrease and increase the concentration of 5-HT are listed in **Table 42.3** and **Table 42.4**, respectively.

Table 42.2 A summary of pharmacological action of serotonin

Organ system	Physiological functions	Role in pathological conditions	Pharmacological applications
CNS	Act as neuromodulators and neurotransmitter Serotonergic axons are projected throughout the brain and spinal cord; thus, they mediate multiple functions such as regulation of sleep, temperature, cognition, behavior, appetite, mood, and thought as well as sensory and motor perception	Based on experimental models, it is confirmed that serotonin plays a role in pathogenesis of depression, psychosis, anxiety, aggression, and other behavioral disorders In migraine, 5-$HT_{1D/1B}$ mediated proinflammatory reaction	Nonselective 5-HT agonists promote onset time of sleep and prolongs total duration of sleep. Clinical trial suggests that 5-$HT_{2A/2C}$ antagonist drug ritanserin leads to increase slow-wave sleep 5-HT_{2C} receptor agonism leads to satiety and decrease food consumption, so lorcaserin was used for weight loss 5-$HT_{1D/1B}$ agonists, i.e., "triptans," are used in acute attack of migraine
CVS	Blood vessels such as renal, splanchnic, pulmonary, and cerebral are constricted that may be reverted, owing to release of endothelial NO and prostaglandin synthesis	Effect of 5-HT on blood pressure: triple response, which is early sharp fall followed by brief rise and prolonged fall in BP	5-HT agonist leads to stimulation of isolated heart by direct as well as NE release; but no therapeutic application
GIT	It is synthesized and stored in enterochromaffin cells of gut mucosa. It regulates peristalsis and emesis	It controls emetic response and is used for diagnosis of "carcinoid syndrome"	5-HT_3 antagonists, i.e., "setrons" such as ondansetron, are used as antiemetic agents
Platelets	Platelets have the ability to uptake, store, and release 5-HT. Upon endothelial injury, platelets secondarily release 5-HT along with other platelet-aggregating substances. If injury is deeper, 5-HT leads to vasoconstriction effect and helps in hemostasis	May lead to acute vasospastic episodes in larger arteries, leading to Raynaud's phenomena, variant angina, or hypertension	5-HT_2 receptor antagonist such as ketanserin may have potential role in prophylaxis of these vasospastic episodes but there is no therapeutic success to date. Recently, 5-HT_{2A} and 5-HT_{2B} antagonist sarpogrelate has shown convincing results for treatment of variant angina
Inflammation	5-HT serves as proinflammatory mediator in acute inflammatory conditions	Correlation between higher expression of 5-HT_{2A} receptor and acute airway inflammation such as asthma has triggered interest in further research	Additional research is needed for action of 5-HT on inflammation before establishment of any therapeutic use

Abbreviations: 5-HT, 5-hydroxytryptamine; BP, blood pressure; CNS, central nervous system; NE, norepinephrine.

Table 42.3 Drugs that decrease concentration of 5-HT

Mode of action	Drug name	Therapeutic use
Inhibition of synthesis of 5-HT: inhibition of enzyme tryptophan hydroxylase which greatly reduce synthesis of 5-HT	PCPA Parachloroamphetemine	Can be useful for treatment of carcinoid syndrome but not preferred because of high toxicity
Deletion of storage of 5-HT: blockade of 5-HT and Na uptake into storage vesicle by inhibition of VMAT2 leads to deletion of monoamines	Reserpine	Hypertension and psychosis. But because of high tendency of suicidal ideation and depression, not used currently
Destruction of 5-HT neurons	5,6-dihydroxytryptamine	Under research

Abbreviations: 5-HT, 5-hydroxytryptamine; PCPA, p-chlorophenylalanine; VMAT2, vesicular monoamine transporter 2.

5-HT Agonist and 5-HT Partial Agonist Drugs

Serotonin receptor agonists and partial agonists act via different types of receptor subfamily. They have variable chemical structure and different action on different subtypes of receptors. 5-HT agonist drugs are therapeutically used in migraine and anxiety and as prokinetics. Some of the other drugs are undergoing research for their role in depression and schizophrenia.

Triptans

See the later part of this chapter for details.

Table 42.4 Drugs that increase concentration of 5-HT

Mode of action	Drug name	Therapeutic use
Increase synthesis of 5-HT	Tryptophan	No clinical use (used only in animals for experimental purpose)
Inhibition of enzymatic degradation of 5-HT: Monoamine oxidase (MAO) inhibitor increases 5-HT level by inhibiting degradation of 5-HT	Tranylcypromine (nonselective MAO inhibitor) Clorgyline (selective MAO-A inhibitor)	With availability of better drugs, MAO inhibitors are seldom used as antidepressants
Increase release of 5-HT: these drugs cause release of 5-HT from serotonergic nerve terminals	Fenfluramine Dexfenfluramine	In management of obesity as anorexiant but banned owing to toxicity
Blockage of reuptake: TCA inhibits reuptake of both 5-HT and Na, while SSRI inhibits only 5-HT reuptake	TCA: imipramine SSRI: fluoxetine, sertraline	SSRIs are first choice of drugs in depression, anxiety, phobias, posttraumatic disorder, and obsessive compulsive disorder

Abbreviations: 5-HT, 5-hydroxytryptamine; SSRIs, selective serotonin reuptake inhibitors; TCA, tricyclic antidepressant.

Azapirones

Drugs such as buspirone and gepirone act as 5-HT_{1A} partial agonists. Unlike benzodiazepine, they relieve anxiety without producing sedation. They are now being studied for the treatment of depression.

Prokinetics

Cisapride and its newer congeners are found to hasten gastric emptying and relieve nausea and emesis related to gastroesophageal reflux disease (GERD). They are selective 5-HT_4 receptor agonists at enterochromaffin cells of gastric mucosa.

D-Lysergic Acid Diethyl Amide (LSD)

This is an ergot alkaloid and nonselective 5-HT agonist with potent hallucinogenic effect. Current theory says that LSD leads to 5-HT_{2A} receptor–mediated sensory distortion, especially visual. For details, refer to the section "Ergot Alkaloids" in this chapter.

Adverse Drug Reactions of Serotonin Agonists

Side effects of triptans are mentioned in detail in the last section of this chapter.

Azapirone group of drugs leads to nausea, headache, dizziness, tinnitus, and, rarely, palpitation. Although patients on buspirone remain alert, still those who are operating machine or vehicles should be cautioned. The recommended dose is 5 to 15 mg orally once to three times a day.

Commonly used gastric prokinetic agents such as metoclopramide are well-tolerated but sedation, dizziness, loose stools, and muscle dystonia are possible, whereas long-term use of metoclopramide can cause gynecomastia, galactorrhea, and parkinsonism. Metoclopramide is secreted in milk and therefore it should be prescribed wisely in lactating mothers. The recommended dose of metoclopramide is 10 mg orally and 0.3 to 2 mg/kg slow IV/IM. Other prokinetic drugs such as cisapride and mosapride are now banned because of QT prolongation and cardiac arrhythmias. Newer 5-HT_4 agonists such as itopride are unlikely to produce cardiac arrhythmias; however, itopride has side effects such as diarrhea, headache, galactorrhea, and gynecomastia. It is available in 50-mg tablet form.

5-HT Antagonist Drugs

Majority of 5-HT antagonist drugs have additional antihistaminic, anticholinergic, or dopaminergic-blocking action. Hence, these are nonspecific drugs. However, well-established "setron" group of drugs such as ondansetron and granisetron have only 5-HT_3 antagonistic action, and one of the new drugs, which is 5-HT_{2A} and 5-HT_{2B} antagonist, also solely acts on serotonin receptor.

Main features of the specific and nonspecific antagonists are emphasized in **Table 42.5**.

Cyproheptadine

It has antihistaminic and anticholinergic action in addition to 5-HT_{2A} receptor–blocking property. Because of its H1 antihistaminic action, it was used to increase weight in children as it increases appetite. Its main action as anti-5-HT is utilized for controlling carcinoid and postgastrectomy dumping syndrome as well as treatment of priapism/orgasmic delay due to some drugs such as fluoxetine (5-HT uptake inhibitors). Side effects such as weight gain, dry mouth, and drowsiness are seen with it.

Sarpogrelate

This drug has been found to have antithrombotic effect because of its 5-HT_2 receptor–blocking action. It also leads to inhibition of vascular contraction. It is proposed to be used for peripheral vascular diseases, coronary heart disease, chronic vascular occlusion, and thrombotic diseases. It has been shown that sarpogrelate inhibits platelet aggregation and plasminogen activation in stable angina pectoris patients, which suggest its beneficial role as adjuvant for such patients. This drug got approval in Japan.

Table 42.5 Serotonergic receptor antagonist drugs

Drug name	Receptor antagonist	Mechanism of action	Therapeutic uses
Cyproheptadine Ketanserin Risperidone	5-HT_{2A}	Inhibition of neuronal excitation at cerebral cortex; additional H_1 antihistaminic and anticholinergic action Inhibition of platelet aggregation and contraction of smooth muscle; additional H_1 and dopaminergic-blocking activity Antagonist at cerebral cortex; additional D_2 antagonist	Control of intestinal manifestation of carcinoid and postgastrectomy dumping syndrome In children (off-label use) to promote appetite for weigh gain Antihypertensive However, because of availability of newer efficacious drugs, it did not gain popularity Antipsychotic to ameliorate negative symptoms of schizophrenia
Sarpogrelate	5-HT_{2A} and 5-HT_{2B}	Inhibition of platelets aggregation	Tested for atherosclerosis, Raynaud's disease, coronary artery disease, angina pectoris, Buerger's disease
Methysergide Clozapine	5-$HT_{2A/2C}$	Antagonist at vascular and visceral smooth muscles Antagonist at basal ganglia and substantia nigra; additional DA antagonist action	Migraine prophylaxis Carcinoid and postgastrectomy dumping syndrome; not presently used as it causes pulmonary, endocardial and abdominal fibrosis Efficacious antipsychotic in resistant cases of schizophrenia
"Setrons": Ondansetron Granisetron Palonosetron	5-HT_3	Antagonist at enterochromaffin cells of gastric smooth muscle	Potent antiemetic Prophylaxis use in chemotherapy or radiotherapy drug–induced vomiting

Abbreviation: 5-HT, 5-hydroxytryptamine.

Adverse Effects and Contraindication of Serotonin Antagonists

Cyproheptadine may lead to side effects such as dry mouth, drowsiness, confusion, ataxia, and weight gain. As it has a sedative effect, it should be avoided if operating machinery or driving vehicles. The recommended dose of cyproheptadine is 4 mg orally. Side effects of ketanserin are related to its vasoconstriction action. Methysergide is also now abandoned from use because of its pulmonary, endocrinal, and abdominal fibrosis.

Both clozapine and risperidone are used as antipsychotic agents. Clozapine's major concerns are its tendency to cause agranulocytosis (0.8%) and other blood dyscrasias, weight gain, hyperglycemia, and hyperlipidemia. Other side effects are sedation, tachycardia, urinary incontinence, and seizures (at high doses). Risperidone has fewer side effects than clozapine; however, it can cause postural hypotension, agitation, weight gain, seizures, and extrapyramidal symptoms. Caution is needed in the elderly because of the risk of stroke by risperidone.

Setrons are generally well-tolerated. Common side effects are headache, dizziness, abdominal discomfort, and mild constipation. Some patients may experience bradycardia, hypotension, and allergic reactions when setrons are administered intravenously. For hyperemesis gravidarum, ondansetron can be used with caution. The recommended dose of ondansetron is 4 or 8 mg orally twice a day for 3 to 5 days and 8 mg IV by slow injection over 15 to 30 minutes before chemotherapy, followed by two similar doses 4 hours apart.

Serotonin Syndrome

It is a life-threatening syndrome that is precipitated by the overuse of serotonergic drugs. Most commonly, it is mediated by postsynaptic 5-HT_{1A} and 5-HT_2 receptor overactivation of central and peripheral serotonergic system. This syndrome shows combination of autonomic and neuromuscular hyperactivity as well as mental status changes. Many drug combinations can also cause serotonin syndrome.

List of Drugs Causing Serotonin Syndrome

Drugs that inhibit serotonin uptake and metabolism, those drugs that increase release or synthesis of 5-HT, or 5-HT receptor agonists are the culprits.

1. Amphetamine–weight loss drug.
2. L-tryptophan–from diet.
3. Mirtazapine–antidepressant.
4. Dextromethorphan–cold remedy.
5. Buspirone–anxiolytics.
6. Triptans–antimigraine.
7. LSD–drug of abuse.
8. Lithium–mood stabilizer.
9. Metoclopramide–prokinetic drug.
10. CYP450 inhibitors such as:
    a. Fluoxetine, sertraline–CYP2D6 inhibitor.
    b. Ritonavir, ciprofloxacin–CYP3A4.
    c. Fluconazole–CYP2C19.

Management

Discontinuation of the causative agent, application of cooling measures, and stabilization of vital signs form the mainstay of therapy. Benzodiazepines (diazepam) is given if the patient has agitation, fever, and tachycardia. If not controlled, serotonin antagonist (cyproheptadine) is employed. If the condition is worse, admission of the patient into an intensive care unit must be considered.

Ergot Alkaloids

Ergot is derived from a fungus named *Claviceps purpurea*, which grows on rye and millets in damp atmosphere. Ergot alkaloids are chemically intricate compounds. Because of the complexity of its action, its therapeutic uses are limited. It has partial agonist or antagonistic action on serotonergic, dopaminergic, and adrenergic receptors. All ergot alkaloids are derivatives of tetracyclic compound 6-methylergoline.

Ergotism

Accidental consumption of ergot alkaloid–contaminated grains leads to poisoning known as ergotism. In ergot poisoning, gangrene of fingers and toes (due to vasoconstriction), hallucination, dementia, abortion in pregnant women, and, in some cases, convulsion can occur.

Classification

Natural Ergot Alkaloids

They are derived from lysergic acid–containing tetracyclic indole compound.

1. Amine alkaloids: ergometrine (ergonovine)—oxytocic in action and used clinically.
2. Amino acid alkaloids: ergotamine, ergotoxine—vasoconstrictor as well as α-adrenergic blocker/partial agonist action; ergotamine is used clinically, while ergotoxine is not.

Semisynthetic Derivatives

Clinically Used

1. Methylergometrine: oxytocic.
2. Dihydroergotamine (DHE), dihydroergotoxine (codergocrine): antiadrenergic, cerebroactive.
3. Bromocriptine: dopaminergic D_2 agonist—to control secretion of prolactin.
4. Methysergide: mainly has anti-5-HT action; rarely used for prophylaxis of migraine.

Not Used Clinically

1. D-lysergic acid.
2. D-lysergic acid ethylamide (often abused due to its hallucinogenic property).
3. Ergostine.
4. Ergotoxine.

Mechanism of Action

Mainly all ergot alkaloids act as agonist, partial agonist, or antagonist at different serotonergic, adrenergic, and dopaminergic receptors in a tissue-specific manner.

Clinically useful drugs and their receptor-mediated actions are mentioned in **Table 42.6**.

Pharmacological Action

Smooth Muscles

Vascular Smooth Muscles

Most blood vessels are constricted due to partial agonistic action on α-adrenergic and serotonergic receptors, resulting in a rise of blood pressure (BP).

Uterine Smooth Muscles

Contraction of uterus occurs due to agonistic/partial agonistic action on 5-HT_2 and α-adrenergic receptors. It acts as an uterotonic, which depends on gestational status, and is more predominant at full-term pregnant uterus.

GIT Smooth Muscles

Gastric motility suppression leads to nausea and vomiting due to 5-HT and dopamine action.

CNS

LSD, a synthetic derivative, causes hallucination via presynaptic and postsynaptic 5-HT_2 receptor agonist action. Higher doses lead to ergotism. 5-HT receptor–mediated action leads to vasoconstriction of cerebral blood vessels. This action is used for management of acute attack of

Table 42.6 Clinically useful ergot derivatives and its receptor-mediated action

Drug	Receptor
Ergotamine	Partial agonist and antagonist at 5-HT_1 and 5-HT_2 receptor and adrenergic receptors (blood vessels); no action on dopaminergic receptors
Dihydroergotamine	Partial agonist and antagonist at 5-HT_1 and 5-HT_2 receptor; more α-receptor-blocking property, less potent vasoconstrictor action
Dihydroergotoxine (codergocrine)	Partial agonist and antagonist at 5-HT receptors; more potent α-blocker
Bromocriptine	Agonist/partial agonist at D_2 receptor; weak α-blocker
Ergometrine/methylergometrine	Weak antagonist/partial agonist 5-HT and α-adrenergic receptors; weak agonist at dopaminergic receptor

Abbreviation: 5-HT, 5-hydroxytryptamine.

migraine. However, it has potent emetic action via CTZ and vomiting center stimulation, which can augment nausea and vomiting of migraine. Dopamine agonistic action–mediated extrapyramidal effects and control of prolactin release have been seen. No other predominant systemic action has been observed.

Pharmacokinetic

Oral bioavailability of the amino acid ergot alkaloids is variable and low because of high first-pass metabolism. Bioavailability may be higher with sublingual and rectal routes, but absorption is still erratic. Derivatives such as bromocriptine are well-absorbed orally. They are metabolized in the liver and excreted by the bile. They have short half-life (2 hours) but, because of sequestration of ergotamine in tissues, its effect persists for 24 hours. Bioavailability of ergotamine and DHE can be enhanced by coadministration of caffeine (as it increases the rate of absorption and peak plasma concentration). Ergot alkaloids can effectively cross the blood–brain barrier.

Therapeutic Uses of Ergot Alkaloids

1. Migraine: in acute attack of migraine, ergotamine and DHE are useful. Methysergide is useful in prophylaxis of migraine.
2. Postpartum hemorrhage: ergometrine and methylergometrine are less toxic and more efficacious than ergotamine.
3. Hyperprolactinemia: dopamine agonist bromocriptine is useful.
4. Parkinson's disease: bromocriptine is useful.
5. Acromegaly: bromocriptine reduces growth hormone secretion.
6. Dementia: dihydroergotoxine may prove useful for senile dementia and Alzheimer's disease.
7. Carcinoid syndrome: 5-HT2 antagonist methysergide is used.

Adverse Drug Reaction

Nausea and vomiting can occur with all ergot alkaloids. Diarrhea and hallucination occur with methysergide. Other nonspecific adverse drug reactions are muscle cramps, weakness, and paresthesia. Some patients experience chest pain due to vasoconstriction.

Contraindication

Ergot alkaloids should not be prescribed in the following conditions:

1. Ischemic heart disease.
2. Hypertension.
3. Peripheral vascular disease.
4. Sepsis.
5. Pregnant and lactating mother.
6. Liver and kidney disease.

Precaution

Ergot alkaloids should not be used with or within 24 hours of use of any type of vasoconstrictor agents and triptan group of drugs.

Ergot Toxicity

A daily dose of 10 mg or more of ergotamine usually leads to toxicity. Mostly, it is found in patients taking it chronically for migraine. Vasospastic complications may occur in some patients even with normal doses.

Symptoms

Mild intoxication leads to nausea and vomiting, which may progress to serious poisoning because of vasoconstriction. In extremities, paresthesia, pain, pallor, loss of pulse in hand and feet (typical feature), and gangrene can occur. Other symptoms are myocardial infarction, coronary ischemia, visual impairment, stroke, psychosis, convulsion, and coma.

Treatment

First and foremost, sodium nitroprusside as IV infusion or nitroglycerine must be started till vasoconstriction is present. The major concern is to maintain circulation; along with this, symptomatic treatment should be provided as per the patient's condition.

Triptans

Migraine is known to mankind for ages; however, drugs specific for migraine management were not developed until the latter half of the twentieth century. Triptans were the first group of drugs designed specifically for migraine. Sumatriptan, the prototype triptan, got marketing approval in 1992 in the United States. After that, many new members were added in this group. The main advantage of newer triptans is better pharmacokinetic profile than sumatriptan. The triptans are indole derivatives.

Pharmacology and Mechanism of Action

The efficacy of triptans in reliving acute attack of migraine supports the hypothesis that 5-HT_1 receptor subfamily is involved in migraine pathology. Triptans have selective vasoconstricting property at the intracranial but not at the extracerebral blood vessels. They act potently at 5-HT_{1D} and 5-HT_{1B} receptors, and similar to serotonin, bind on trigeminal nerve endings along with blood vessels. The result is a decrease in the release of numerous nociceptive peptides such as calcitonin gene-related peptide (CGRP) and substance P, thereby relieving migraine headache and its associated symptoms (**Fig. 42.2a, b**).

Triptans have a low or no affinity for other subtypes of 5-HT receptors, a_1-, a_2-, and β-adrenergic, dopaminergic, cholinergic, and benzodiazepine receptors, which explains its minimal side effect profile. Unlike ergot derivatives, triptans can decrease rather than exacerbate the nausea and vomiting related with migraine.

Pharmacokinetics

Sumatriptan has shorter half-life and low bioavailability (15%) when given orally as compared to newer congeners.

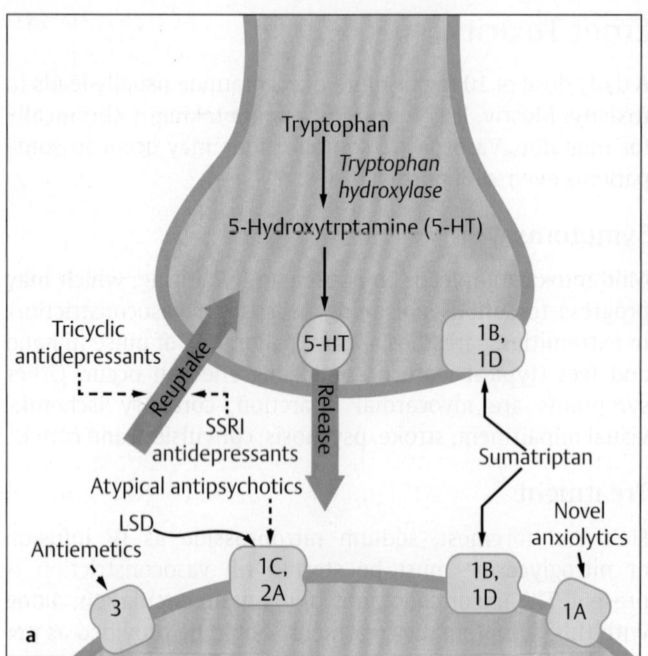

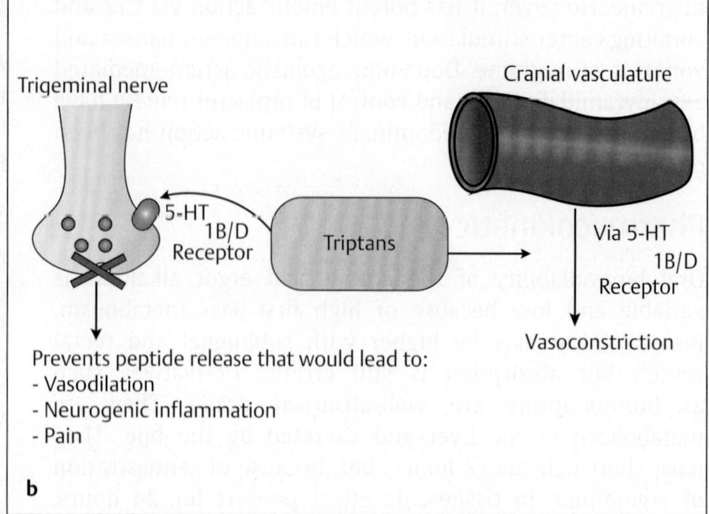

Fig. 42.2 **(a)** Drugs acting on 5-HT subreceptors. **(b)** Mechanism of action of triptans.

Table 42.7 Pharmacokinetics of triptans

Drug name	Formulation	Time to onset (h)	Dose (mg)	Half-life (h)
Almotriptan	Oral tablets	2.6	6.25–12.5	3.3
Eletriptan	Oral tablets	2	20–40	4
Frovatriptan	Oral tablets	3	2.5	27
Naratriptan	Oral tablets	2	1–2.5	5.5
Rizatriptan	Oral tablets	1–3	5–10	2
Sumatriptan	Oral tablets	1.5	25–100	2
	Nasal spray	1–1.5	20	
	Subcutaneous	0.25	6	
	Rectal suppository	–	25	
Zolmitriptan	Oral tablets			2.8

However, sumatriptan is also available for subcutaneous, rectal, and nasal administration. Sumatriptan is absorbed rapidly and completely after subcutaneous injection. Time to onset of action and half-life are variable within the class (**Table 42.7**).

Triptans are rapidly metabolized by MAO-A isoenzyme, and metabolites are excreted in the urine. It can be noted that, in contrast to other triptans, naratriptan and frovatriptan have longer half-life, thus reducing the chances of headache recurrence. For other triptans, the duration of action is shorter than the period of headache; therefore, multiple doses may be needed. However, maximum safe daily dose limit may prove to be a setback.

Therapeutic Uses of Triptans

Triptans are the most popular class of drugs to abort moderate-to-severe episodes of acute migraine. Owing to their selective action and efficacy, they are preferred over ergot alkaloids. A significant advantage is its ability to suppress nausea and vomiting, which may be the result of migraine itself. However, triptans are expensive and thus must be used wisely. While all the triptans are effective in acute management, frovatriptan is also used in chronic prophylaxis of migraine.

Adverse Drug Reactions

Triptan are usually well-tolerated. Minor dose-related side effects include dizziness, weakness, tightness in head and chest, feeling of heat, and paresthesia in extremities, especially common after a subcutaneous injection. Pain and irritation at injection site after subcutaneous injection and bitter taste after nasal use of sumatriptan are expected. Serious side effects occur due to vasoconstricting property of triptans, which can produce coronary vasospasm, leading to chest pain, bradycardia, and risk of myocardial infarction. Seizures and hypersensitivity reactions are rare.

Contraindications

Triptans are contraindicated in those with a history of coronary artery disease, peripheral vascular disease, or stroke. Naratriptan and eletriptan are contraindicated in patients with severe hepatic or renal impairment. Zolmitriptan is contraindicated in patients with Wolff–Parkinson–White syndrome. All triptans are contraindicated in patients with near-term prior exposure to ergot alkaloids or other 5-HT agonists.

Clinical Types of Headache

Any painful sensation located in the head, neck, or jaw is referred to as headache. While the etiology of headache is diverse, it is important from a clinical point to view to judge whether it is a primary headache disorder, where there is no identifiable cause, or it is a sign of an underlying more serious disease. Out of the many causes of headache outlined by the International Headache Society's International Classification of Headache Disorders, three main primary headache syndromes, namely, migraine, cluster, and tension headache, are noteworthy. Important secondary causes include neurological conditions, such as intracranial tumors or bleed, infection (meningitis), temporal arteritis, and glaucoma (**Fig. 42.3**). It is imperative to carefully consider and rule out any serious neurological disease before making diagnosis of primary headache syndrome. Please note that migraine is essentially a clinical diagnosis and there are at present no laboratory or imaging modalities available to confirm this diagnosis.

One should attempt to start investigating headache by taking a detailed clinical history and complete neurological examination to arrive at a differential diagnosis. The key point in history-taking is to ascertain the number of such episodes. Primary headaches are often recurrent. However, if it is a first-time headache, especially when severe (often described as "the worst headache of my life" and/or "thunderclap") and rapidly peaking, it strongly suggests serious underlying pathology such as subarachnoid hemorrhage. Headache with fever and neck stiffness can lead one toward meningitis as a likely cause. Patients with intracranial neoplasms usually report symptoms such as deep-seated, dull, pain interfering with sleep, often with emesis. As reported in the literature, headaches associated with posterior fossa brain tumor are induced by coughing, lifting, or bending. In patients with acute angle closure glaucoma, headaches usually occur after other ocular symptoms such as red eyes and eye pain. Finally, investigations such as computed tomography (CT) scan and cerebrospinal fluid examination must be used with clinical acumen.

Often, patients present with recurrent and troublesome headache, and it is difficult to classify it into any of the three primary headache categories. However, each headache syndrome has some peculiarities, which we should keep in mind. Remember, migraine headache is the most common of them.

Cluster headaches are far more common in middle-aged men. It begins without warning and is characteristically described as agonizing, unilateral, and periorbital pain that rapidly peaks in intensity. The attacks last from 30 minutes to 3 hours and occur multiple times in a day for some weeks. Red eyes, watering from eyes and nose, nasal stuffiness, nausea, and sensitivity to alcohol are frequently accompanying clinical features. Tension-type headaches are largely reported as tight, bandlike headaches occurring

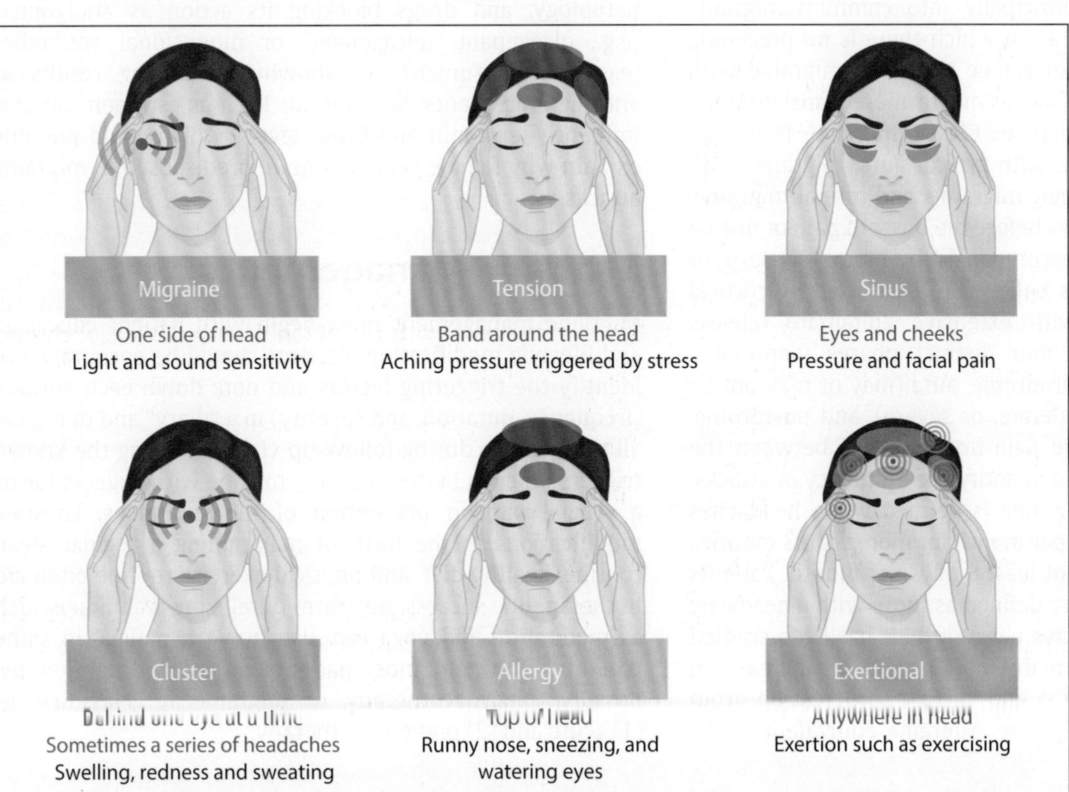

Fig. 42.3 Clinical types of headache.

on both sides, often associated with tightness of the neck muscles. Mostly, the pain builds up gradually and can persist for days without aggravating factors.

Migraine affects approximately 10 to 20% of the western population, with a higher female predominance. The prevalence of this chronic neurological disease peaks between 25 and 55 years of age, that is, during the most productive years of life. Thus, migraine can significantly impair the ability to function in academics and in social settings.

Migraine is notorious for presenting with varied manifestations. The attacks are characterized by headache, often accompanied by nausea and/or vomiting, with other varying neurologic dysfunctions. Typically, headache is described as pulsatile or throbbing in nature, often localized to one side of the head and worsened by slight movement. Other associated features could be photophobia (increased sensitivity to light) and phonophobia (increased sensitivity to sound). Usually, each episode lasts for 4 to 72 hours. Careful observation by patients can often identify a trigger(s). Triggers could be environmental such as exposure to alcohol or certain foods (such as chocolate, cheese, monosodium glutamate), physiological (changes in hormonal levels during a menstrual cycle, hunger, or irregular sleep patterns), or psychological. A genetic predisposition has also been argued (e.g., multiple genes have been shown in heritance of familial hemiplegic migraine). When a typical trigger is identified, migraine is a probable diagnosis and it helps rule out other primary headache syndromes.

Migraine Headache (PH1.16, IM17.11, IM17.12, IM17.14)

Migraine is classified principally into common migraine (or migraine without aura), in which there is no preceding focal neurologic deficit, or classic migraine (migraine with aura). Aura is usually defined as one or more transient, fully reversible neurological deficits. Classic migraine is further subdivided into migraine with typical aura, migraine with brain stem aura, hemiplegic migraine, and retinal migraine. Aura can begin a few hours before the onset of pain or during the attack and is often accompanied by motor, sensory, or visual symptoms. Aura is believed to be caused by cortical spreading depression with extensive glutamate release. Many times, there are four distinct phases identifiable during an acute attack: prodrome, aura (may or may not be present), pain (mild, moderate, or severe), and postdrome. Since patients experience pain-free intervals between the episodes, it is necessary to quantify the frequency of attacks. Recurrent or chronic migraine is defined when headaches occur on at least 15 days per month for more than 3 months, with clinical features on at least 8 days per month. Patients with episodic migraine are defined as those with a headache burden of less than 15 days per month. It has been studied that suboptimal acute treatment leads to an increase in migraine-related disability and disease progression from episodic to recurrent migraine. Migraine equivalent is the term used when there are localized neurologic symptoms without the classic complaints of headache and/or emesis and nausea.

Pathophysiology of Migraine

Although migraine is known to mankind for a long time, its etiology is still not fully understood. There are three main hypotheses that have gained consideration in the pathophysiology of migraine. The first is the "vascular theory," which proposes that dilatation of intracranial extracerebral vascular system is the sole etiological factor. The second is the "neuronal theory," which suggests that migraine is triggered by a cortical spreading depression. The third and currently acceptable theory is the "trigeminovascular theory," which postulates that migraine is triggered by inflammation of trigeminal nerves and vessels around trigeminal ganglion cells.

Modern imaging techniques are still finding clues to how an attack is triggered. It could be owing to cortical spreading depression or high activity of hypothalamic area. Anyhow, once the reaction is "triggered," there occurs fluctuation in neuronal activity, leading to activation of the trigeminovascular system in the meninges. Upon activation, the trigeminal afferent can release various vasoactive peptides (especially CGRP), producing an inflammatory response that probably causes head pain. Simultaneously, a decrease in the levels of neurotransmitters such as serotonin (serotonin receptors have been found on the trigeminal nerve and cranial vessels) is also observed. These vasoactive and neuropeptides work together to deliver the nociceptive information to the central neurons in the brain stem that, in turn, relay the pain signals (**Fig. 42.4a, b**). In the recent times, CGRP has received considerable importance in migraine pathology, and drugs blocking its action as antagonists (e.g., olcegepant, telcagepant) or monoclonal antibodies (e.g., fremanezumab) are showing promising results as antimigraine agents. Sex steroids such as estrogen can also influence serotonin and CGRP levels, which could possibly explain why female gender is more predisposed to migraine attacks.

Migraine Management

Migraine management must begin with patient education and lifestyle modification. Patients should be encouraged to identify the triggering factors and note down each episode (frequency, duration, and severity) in a "diary" and to review all such details during follow-up visits. Avoiding the known triggers or, even better, learning to cope with triggers forms a crucial part in prevention of future attacks. Lifestyle modifications in the form of maintaining a regular sleep routine, healthy diet, and physical exercise routine often aid in therapeutic success. Any form of relaxing techniques such as meditation and yoga can also prove beneficial in some patients. However, most patients do need drug therapy. Broadly, pharmacotherapy of migraine be classified as (1) acute and (2) preventive therapy.

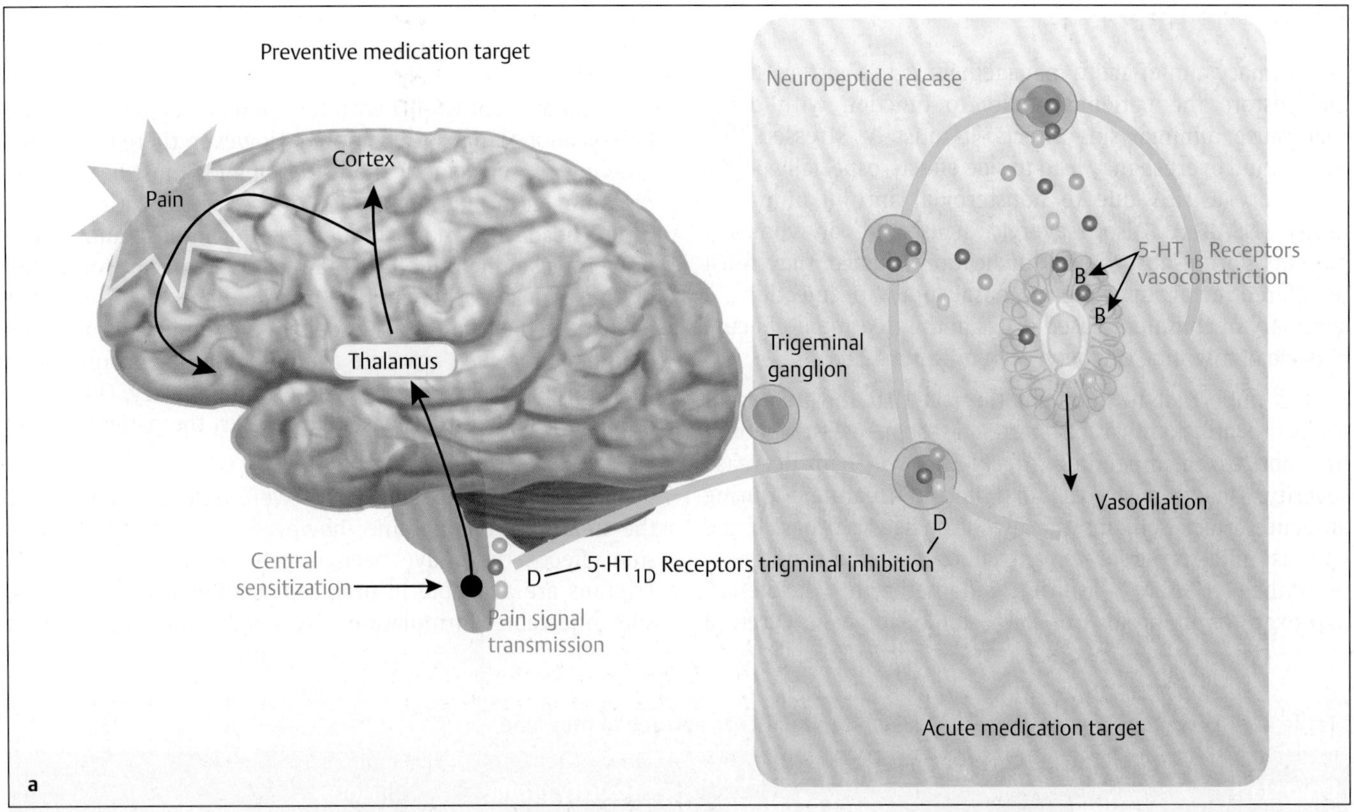

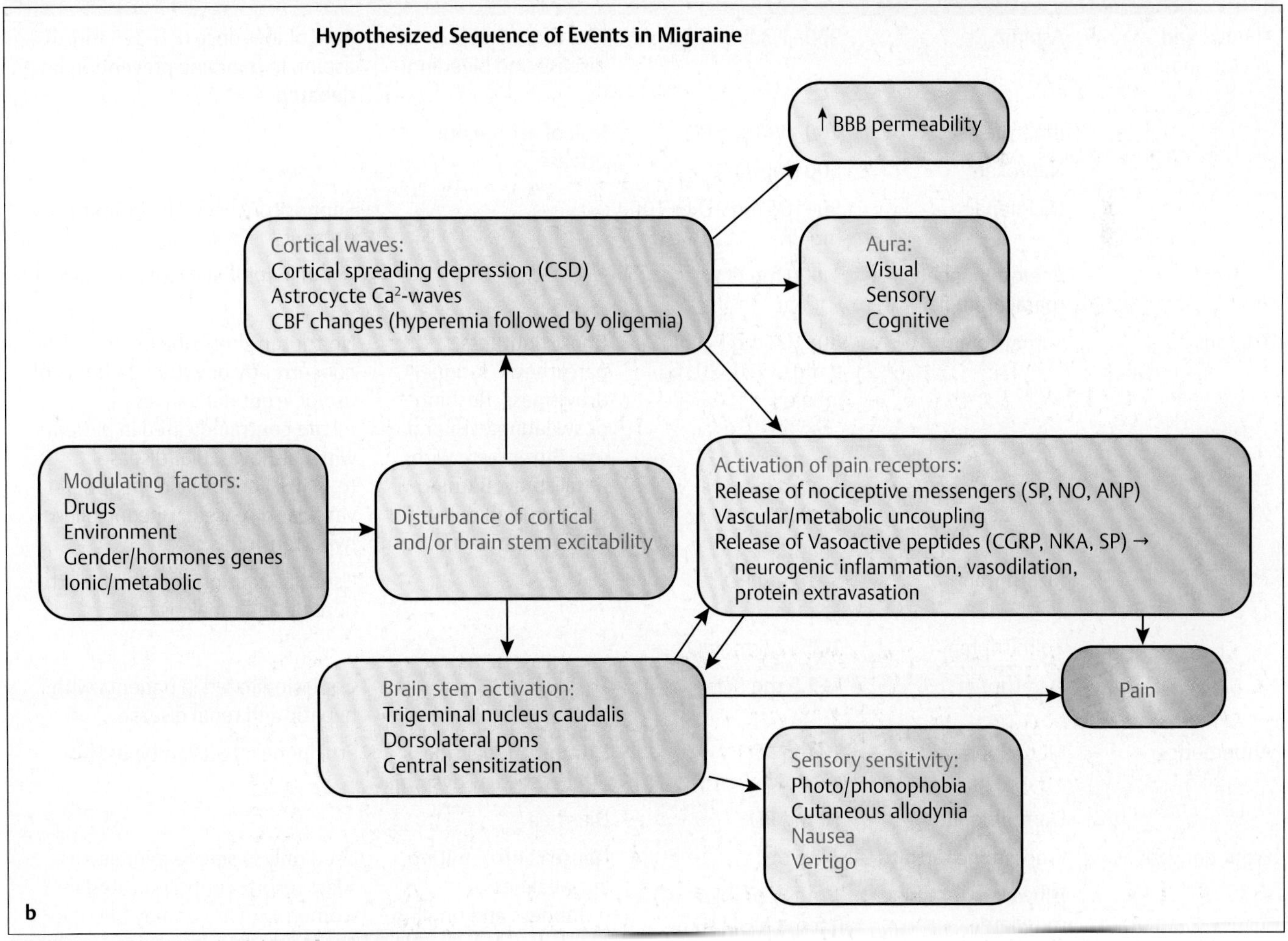

Fig. 42.4 (a, b) Pathophysiology of migraine.

Acute Treatment

The primary aim of acute management is to abort an attack and restore the patient's ability to function with drugs that cause minimal side effects. It must be stressed that medication overuse may lead to side effects, especially peptic ulcers or gastritis due to nonsteroidal anti-inflammatory drugs (NSAIDs). Also, severely nauseated or vomiting patients do not absorb oral medications; hence, they must be offered rectal suppositories, nasal sprays, or injections. A summary of commonly used drugs in the treatment of acute episode of migraine can been seen in **Table 42.8**.

It is important to highlight the fact that the treatment for acute attack must be started as soon as the patient first notices an impending attack. This will help decrease severity. Unanimously, the first line of treatment during an acute attack remains the use of analgesic drugs. If the pain is mild-to-moderate, a trial of over-the-counter or prescribed NSAIDs (aspirin, indomethacin, diclofenac, naproxen, or ibuprofen) or paracetamol is given. Often, a combination of high dose of aspirin with paracetamol with/without caffeine is found useful. If the pain is moderate-to-severe or the patient experiences side effects to it, then a combination of NSAID with low-potency opioids (codeine or oxycodone) may be attempted. However, there has been a growing consensus that the use of opioids must be strongly discouraged in migraine in lieu of the fact that it can make future headaches more frequent and/or intense and render preventives unhelpful. If the pain is severe or not controlled by these measures, one of the migraine-specific drugs must be instituted without further delay. As a thumb rule, patients who have received an acute agent should be encouraged to treat three attacks with it to determine efficacy. Only if no relief is provided in at least two attacks, the patient should be switched to another acute agent.

In the past, ergot derivatives were extensively used for the treatment of migraine; however, owing to their many side effects, they have been largely replaced by triptans. Triptans are available in oral, self-dissolving tablets, nasal, and injectable formulations. A fixed dose combination

Table 42.8 Commonly used drugs in the treatment of acute episode of migraine

Drug class	Generic name of drug	Dose taken at the onset of attack	Toxicity profile	Notes
NSAIDs and acetaminophen	Aspirin	900–1,300 mg PO	Risk of acid-peptic disease and bleeding	Role of low-dose (81–325 mg/d) aspirin in migraine prevention is debated
	Ibuprofen	200–400 mg PO	Risk of acid-peptic disease	
	Naproxen	500 mg PO		
	Diclofenac	50–100 mg PO or 100 mg PR		Suppository useful if vomiting is present
	Acetaminophen (paracetamol)	1,000 mg PO		Avoid in patients with liver disease
Triptans	Sumatriptan	50–100 mg PO or 6 mg SC 10–20 mg inhaled	Chest tightness, paresthesia, fatigue, drowsiness, flushing or sweating with oral use. Bitter taste with nasal spray. Burning, stinging, and pain after subcutaneous injection	No triptan should be used concurrently or within 24 hours of use of ergot derivatives All are contraindicated in patients with cardiovascular disease (e.g., IHD or stroke or peripheral vascular disease or uncontrolled hypertension)
	Rizatriptan	5–10 mg PO		Use with caution in patients with hepatic and renal disease
	Zolmitriptan	1.25–2.5 mg PO		
	Naratriptan	1–2.5 mg PO		Contraindicated in patients with hepatic and renal disease
Antiemetics	Metoclopramide	10 mg PO	Extrapyramidal side effects such as dystonia	Prokinetic effect can be useful
	Domperidone	10 mg PO	Diarrhea	
Ergot derivatives	Ergotamine tartrate	2 mg SL	Nausea and vomiting, leg weakness, numbness and tingling, coronary vasospasm	Used only in severe migraine as a last resort; contraindicated in women who are or may become pregnant
	Dihydroergotamine mesylate	1 mg IV or IM or SC; 0.5 mg nasal spray		

Abbreviations: IHD, ischemic heart disease; IM, intramuscular; IV, intravenous; NSAIDs, nonsteroidal anti-inflammatory drugs; PO, per oral; PR, per rectal; SC, subcutaneous; SL, sublingual.

of sumatriptan with naproxen is also marketed in some countries. Many patients also suffer from GI symptoms such as nausea and vomiting during an attack. Antiemetic drugs such as metoclopramide or domperidone and/or ondansetron should be offered to them.

Preventive Therapy

These drugs are used when migraine headaches occur frequently and/or are debilitating. The goal of preventive therapy is to reduce the attack frequency, severity, duration, and disability. Preventive treatments can be used occasionally in situations where exposure to a triggering factor is unavoidable or in most patients for long term. Hardly, if any, drugs that are available in the market today for prevention were designed specifically for migraine. Also, the efficacy and safety of these oral preventive treatments are questionable.

On the basis of current research findings, the American Headache Association, in its latest guidelines of 2019, has suggested preventive therapies for migraine. The following drugs have established efficacy in migraine prevention—antiepileptic drugs such as valproate sodium and topiramate, β-blockers such as metoprolol, propranolol, and timolol, triptans such as frovatriptan and onabotulinum toxin A, antidepressants such as amitriptyline and venlafaxine, and β-blockers such as atenolol and nadolol are probably effective, while angiotensin-converting enzyme inhibitors (lisinopril), α-agonists (clonidine, guanfacine), antiepileptic drugs (carbamazepine), β-blockers (nebivolol or pindolol), antihistamines (cyproheptadine), and angiotensin receptor blockers (candesartan) are possibly effective. **Table 42.9** mentions drugs commonly used in preventive therapies.

It might be optimal to begin with low doses of oral medicine and gradually increase the dose until the desired response or the maximum allowed dose is reached with least adverse effects. It might be better to combine preventive drugs from different drug classes, especially when the desired response is not adequate with single agent or adverse effects are concerning.

The severity, frequency, and characteristics of migraine vary considerably between patients and even within the same patient over time. Therefore, optimizing the treatment for a patient remains challenging. The current best standard practice is to make individualized treatment plans considering factors such as patient preference, the frequency and severity of attacks, history of other comorbid diseases (e.g., ischemic heart disease or peripheral vascular disease), reproductive status of the patient (pregnant, lactating, or plans to conceive), prior treatment response, and the use of concomitant medications. To individualize therapy for every patient, a trial-and-error approach may be needed before finalizing the treatment.

As mentioned previously, currently many drugs targeting CGRP are under clinical trials for use as antimigraine therapy. To name a few, other migraine-specific drugs in the pipeline are targeting glutaminergic pathway, neuroinflammatory pathways (e.g., substance P/neurokinin-1), or neuropeptides (e.g., orexin). It is interesting to note that fewer neuromodulation strategies such as transcranial magnetic stimulation, supraorbital nerve stimulation, and transcutaneous vagal nerve stimulation are also under trial for migraine management.

In summary, for treatment of acute episode, NSAIDs such as aspirin, ibuprofen, or paracetamol are first-line agents. For those patients who are still symptomatic, triptans such as sumatriptan is an effective second-line therapy. In addition, antiemetic drugs such as metoclopramide or domperidone, or less potent morphine derivatives (e.g., codeine), may be needed. Ergot alkaloids are reserved only for severe attack when earlier mentioned therapies fail, albeit with caution. For prevention, many prescription medicines are used, e.g., propranolol and metoprolol (β-blockers), antiepileptics (e.g., valproate and topiramate), antidepressants such as amitriptyline, and SSRIs (e.g., fluoxetine).

Table 42.9 Commonly used drugs in prevention of migraine

Drug class	Generic name of drug	Dosing schedule[a]	Toxicity
β-blockers	Propranolol	Up to 80 mg twice daily	Nightmares, erectile dysfunction, exercise intolerance
Antiepileptics	Valproate sodium	500 mg twice a day	Liver toxicity, weight gain, tremor, teratogenicity
	Topiramate	Up to 100 mg/day	Cognitive impairment, paresthesia, precipitates glaucoma, and renal stones
Triptans	Frovatriptan	2.5 mg twice a day	Like triptans
Antidepressants	Amitriptyline	Up to 1 mg/day	Constipation, dry eyes and mouth, drowsiness, weight gain; drug interactions with SSRIs
	Venlafaxine	75–150 mg/day in extended-release form	Psychiatric symptoms, serotonin syndrome
Angiotensin receptor blocker	Candesartan	16–32 mg/day	Postural hypotension: regular monitoring of serum electrolytes is necessary
Calcium channel blocker	Flunarizine	5–15 mg/day	Weight gain and drowsiness, psychiatric symptoms

Abbreviation: SSRI, selective serotonin reuptake inhibitor.
[a]All doses are per oral.

Multiple Choice Questions

1. Serotonin is synthesized from which of the following?

A. Tyrosine.
B. L-Tryptophan.
C. Glutamine.
D. Dopamine.

Answer: B

5-HT synthesis is a two-step process. It is synthesized from the amino acid L-tryptophan. Tryptophan is converted into 5-hydroxytryptophan with the help of hydroxylase, which in turn undergoes decarboxylation by decarboxylase enzyme and gives rise to 5-hydroxytryptamine.

2. The neurotransmitter serotonin plays a role in:

A. Migraine headache.
B. Anxiety and temperature regulation.
C. Depression.
D. All of the above.

Answer: D

Raphe nuclei within the brainstem is a major locus of 5-HT neurons. Multiple functions such as sensory and motor activity, regulation of temperature, pain, behavior, mood, appetite, and sexual behavior are carried out by 5-HT receptors. 5-HT$_{1D/1B}$ receptor agonists such as triptans are used as antimigraine drugs, while 5-HT$_{1A}$ partial agonists azapirones are antianxiety drugs. According to a hypothesis, depression is caused by depletion of 5-HT and/or NA neurotransmitters within the limbic system of the brain. Thus, the agents that increase concentration of 5-HT and/or NA are employed as antidepressant drugs.

3. Carcinoid syndrome in the gastrointestinal tract involves overproduction and release of serotonin. Which of the following effects is/are thereby observed?

A. Diarrhea.
B. Constipation.
C. Irritation.
D. None of the above.

Answer: A

Major pool of 5-HT is stored and released from enterochromaffin cells of the gastric mucosa. It plays a major role in regulation of peristalsis of gastric and intestinal smooth muscle.

4. Which subtype of 5-HT (serotonin) receptor is involved in the vomiting reflex?

A. 5-HT$_{2A}$.
B. 5-HT$_3$.
C. 5-HT$_4$.
D. Both B and C.

Answer: D

Mechanical stretching via vagal response or food leads to the release of 5-HT, which regulates local GI functions. 5-HT$_3$ receptor stimulation (at GIT as well as at CNS level) results in emesis, so 5-HT$_3$ antagonists, i.e., "setron" group of drugs such as ondansetron and granisetron, have been developed as antiemetics, while 5-HT$_4$ agonists, also known as prokinetic drugs, inhibit release of 5-HT and increase ACh, ultimately promoting gastric emptying. Therefore, prokinetics are used to control symptoms in GERD.

5. Which of the following is/are a characteristic(s) of serotonin?

A. Major pool of 5-HT in humans is found within enterochromaffin cells of GIT.
B. It is a neuromodulator in brain as well as in spinal cord.
C. It is stored in serotonergic nerve endings and platelets, utilizing an active serotonin transport system known as SERT.
D. All of the above are true.

Answer: D

5-HT is a neuromodulator and neurotransmitter with potent depolarizing action. It has variable action on different organ systems, and it is expressed in the brain as well as in the spinal cord. 5-HT is stored within the storage granules and released. 5-HT action is terminated mainly by reuptake via an amine pump serotonin transporter (SERT), which is Na$^+$-dependent carrier present at membrane of platelets and serotonergic nerve endings. The free form of 5-HT is not present in circulation. Platelets that lack nucleus cannot synthesize 5-HT, but they acquire it while passing through the intestinal blood vessels. SERT pump is inhibited by selective serotonin reuptake inhibitors (SSRIs) and tricyclic antidepressants (TCAs). Major pool of 5-HT is stored and released from enterochromaffin cells of gastric mucosa. It plays a major role in regulation of peristalsis.

6. Which of the following serotonin receptor antagonist with additional antimuscarinic action is used to treat carcinoid syndrome?

A. Cimetidine.
B. Cyproheptadine.
C. Methysergide.
D. Ketanserin.

Answer: B

Cyproheptadine is a 5-HT$_{2A}$ antagonist with additional H1 antihistaminic and anticholinergic actions. It is used in carcinoid syndrome.

7. What is the rationale behind coadministering ergotamine and caffeine?

A. The combination decreases side effects of ergotamine.
B. Rate of absorption and peak plasma concentration of ergotamine increase.
C. To enhance the effect of ergotamine in the presence of food.
D. None of the above.

Answer: B

Oral absorption of ergotamine without caffeine is delayed and incomplete. This combination is used in acute attack of migraine. Patients suffering from migraine already have gastric stasis, which could further reduce absorption of ergotamine. It is

found that the rate of absorption and peak plasma concentration of ergotamine increase with addition of caffeine, and this combination can be considered as rational.

8. Why ergometrine is used over ergotamine in management of postpartum hemorrhage?

A. It is less toxic and more efficacious than ergotamine.
B. It has more potent action on α-adrenergic receptors.
C. Both of the above statements are true.
D. None of the above statements are true.

Answer: A

Ergometrine and methylergometrine, followed by ergotamine, are more efficacious and have a high specificity for uterine action. Other ergot alkaloids do not have any uterotonic action. Ergometrine has weak antagonistic and partial agonistic activity on serotonin and α-adrenergic receptors as compared to ergotamine.

9. Which of the following is a true statement?

A. Migraine headache is a diagnosis of exclusion.
B. Cluster headache has high incidence in females.
C. Tension-type headache is often throbbing in nature.
D. All the headaches have serious underlying pathology.

Answer: A

Migraine is essentially a clinical diagnosis and there are at present no laboratory or imaging modalities available to confirm this diagnosis. Also, migraine is the most common primary headache disorder.

10. Which of the following is a true statement?

A. Serotonin antagonists are useful in the treatment of migraine.
B. Triptans are used in acute attack of migraine only when NSAIDs fail.
C. Ergotamine is the first-line drug for treatment of acute attack of migraine.
D. Lasmiditan is approved for migraine prophylaxis.

Answer: B

Triptans, though very efficacious, are reserved for moderate-to-severe migraine episodes, i.e., when NSAIDs fail. 5-HT agonists at 1B/1D receptors are used in migraine (and not the antagonists).

11. Which of the following is not a contraindication for sumatriptan?

A. History of myocardial infarction.
B. Recent use of ergotamine.
C. Presence of liver disease.
D. History of peripheral vascular disease.

Answer: C

Sumatriptan is contraindicated in patients with a history of coronary artery disease, peripheral vascular disease, or stroke. Additionally, all triptans are to be avoided within 24 hours of use of ergot derivatives.

12. Ergot alkaloids act via multiple receptors. Which of the below-mentioned action is useful in migraine?

A. Adrenergic.
B. Cholinergic.
C. Serotonergic.
D. Dopaminergic.

Answer: C

Mainly, all ergot alkaloids act as agonist or partial agonist or antagonist at different serotonergic, adrenergic, and dopaminergic receptors. However, its action at serotonergic receptors on extracerebral blood vessels is useful in migraine.

13. Which of the following drugs used for migraine prophylaxis provides maximum benefit?

A. Propranolol.
B. Methysergide.
C. Candesartan.
D. Carbamazepine.

Answer: A

The American Headache Association, in its latest guidelines of 2019, has suggested preventive therapies for migraine. The following drugs have established efficacy in migraine prevention: antiepileptic drugs such as valproate sodium and topiramate, β-blockers such as metoprolol, propranolol, and timolol, triptans such as frovatriptan and onabotulinum toxin A, antidepressants such as amitriptyline and venlafaxine, and β-blockers such as atenolol and nadolol are probably effective.

Chapter 43 Eicosanoids–Prostaglandins, Thromboxanes, and Leukotrienes

Vishalkumar K. Vadgama

PH1.16: Describe mechanism/s of action, types, doses, side effects, indications, and contraindications of the drugs which act by modulating autacoids.

Learning Objectives

- Prostaglandins.
- Thromboxane.
- Leukotrienes.
- Platelet-activating factor.
- Serotonin.

Introduction

The word "autacoids" is derived from the Greek language, where *autos* means self, and *acos* means a medicinal agent or remedy. The term autacoids was coined by Sir Edward Albert Sharpey-Schafer. He described an autacoid as a specific organic substance formed by the cells of one organ and passed from them into the circulating fluid to produce effects upon other organs similar to those produced by drugs. This concept was later refined and autacoids are now described as biological factors which act like local hormones, have a brief duration of action, and act near the site of synthesis.

Autacoids can be classified as shown in **Fig. 43.1**.

Prostaglandins (PG), leukotrienes (LT), platelet-activating factor (PAF), and serotonin (5HT) will be discussed in the current chapter.

Prostaglandins

Prostaglandins are derived from arachidonic acid by the action of phospholipase A2 and cyclooxygenases (**Fig. 43.2**). Among different functional types of prostaglandins, PGE1, PGE2, PGI2, and PGF2α are the pharmacologically important ones to remember. Each of these prostaglandins, with significant characteristics, act by way of specific receptors (**Table 43.1**).

Actions of Prostaglandins on Human Body

Reproductive System

Prostaglandins are important functional regulators of reproductive track. They moderate menstruation, parturition, expulsion of placenta, and postpartum hemorrhage.

At the end of each ovarian cycle, there is reduction of estrogen and, predominantly progesterone. Low levels of these sex hormones lead to vasospasm of tortuous blood vessels of the mucosal layers of endometrium, leading to onset of menstrual bleeding. Vasospasm of these vessels are mediated by loss of dilator stimuli with the help of low levels of estrogen and progesterone as well as the release of a vasoconstrictor stimuli–vasoconstrictor type of prostaglandins, which are synthesized in excess due to low levels of estrogen and progesterone.

Prostaglandins make cervical mucus less viscid around the ovulation period. In addition, prostaglandins trigger reverse peristaltic contractions in the uterus and fallopian tubes. Both of these actions of prostaglandins improves cervical penetration and transport of sperms to the ovaries to aid fertilization of ova.

Fetal adrenal glands produce copious amounts of cortisol near term, which is involved in the fetal lung maturation of extrauterine life. In addition, cortisol also promotes corticotropin-releasing hormone (CRH), oxytocin, and prostaglandins (especially, PGE2) synthesis. CRH and prostaglandins both upregulate each other's synthesis. Finally, at term, due to increased levels of CRH, there is upsurge in prostaglandins synthesis, especially PGF2α and PGE2 by fetal membranes and decidua. Elevated levels of PGE2 and PGF2α aid in onset of labor and subsequent parturition processes. Additionally, PGE2 appears to be involved in the physiologic softening of the cervix at term. Owing to these, PGE2 has been used to induce labor, while PGF2α is used to control postpartum hemorrhage.

Prostaglandins also play important role in male sexual functions. PGE1 along with other chemical transmitters from

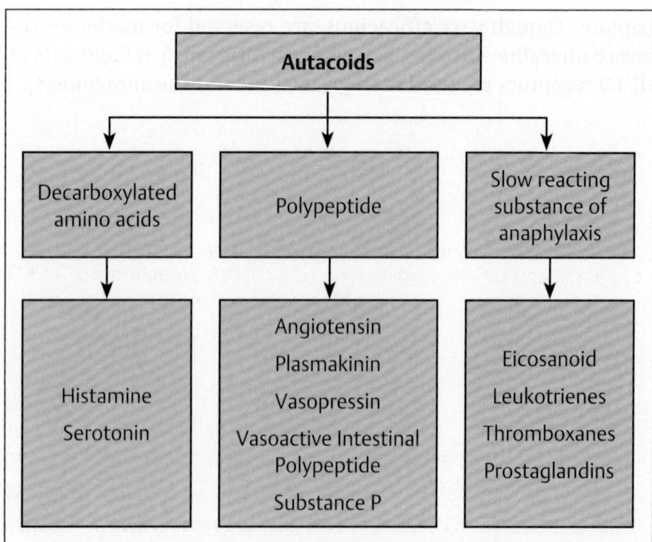

Fig. 43.1 Classification of autacoids.

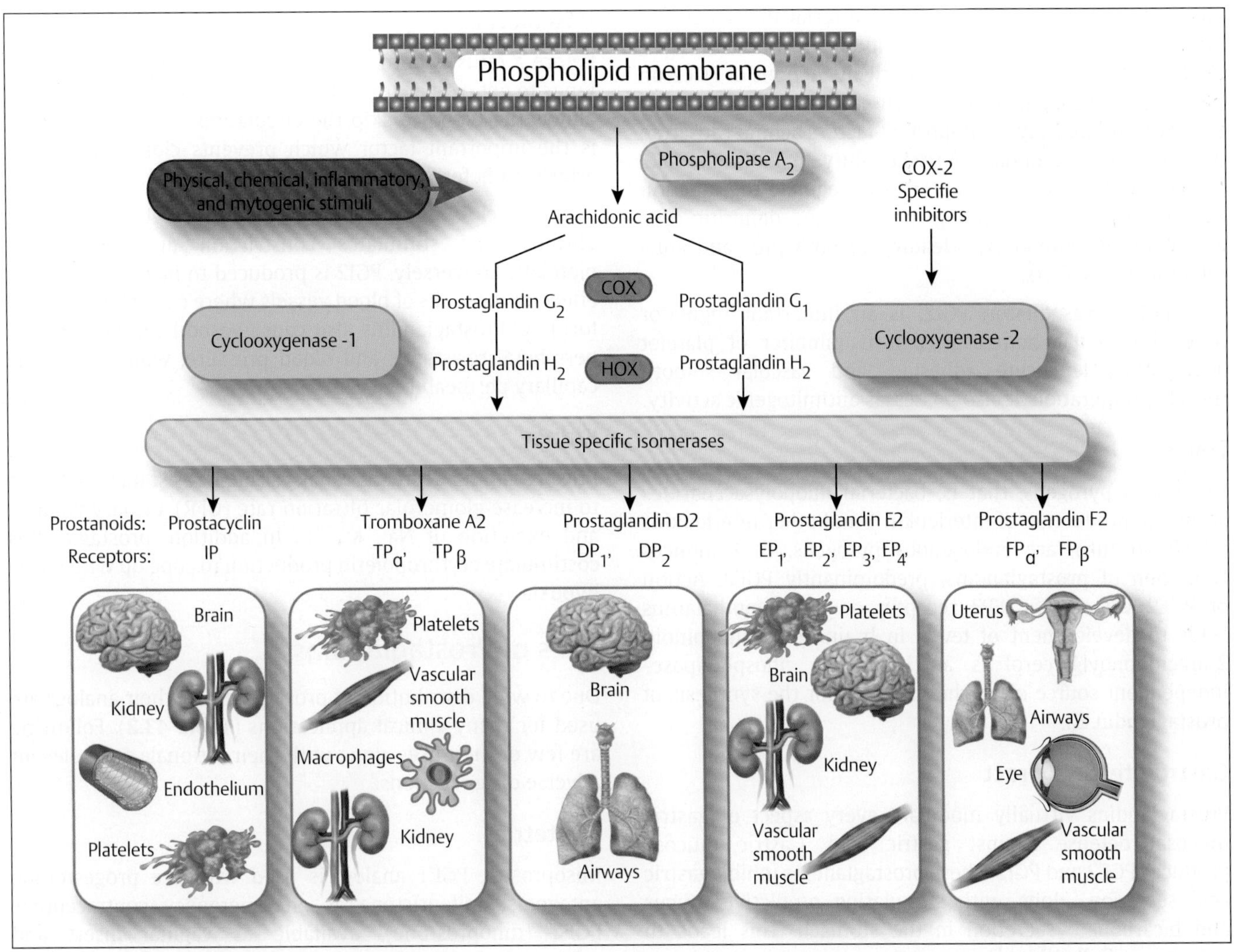

Fig. 43.2 Synthesis and functions of prostaglandins.

Table 43.1 Characteristics of prostaglandin receptors

Receptors	Primary activating PGs	Type of G protein	Subsequent signaling pathways upon receptor activation
EP_1	PGE1, PGE2	Gq alpha subunit	Stimulates PLC, IP3, PKC, ERK, and CREB
EP_2	PGE1, PGE2	Gs alpha subunit	Stimulates AC, raises cAMP, stimulates beta catenin and glycogen synthase kinase 3
EP_3	PGE1, PGE2	Gi & G12 subunit	Inhibits AC, decreases cAMP, stimulates PLC & IP3, raises Ca^{2+}
EP_4	PGE1, PGE2	Gs alpha subunit	Stimulates AC, PKA, PI3K, AKT, ERK, and CREB; raises cAMP
FP	PGF2a	Gq alpha subunit	Stimulates PLC, IP3, & PKC; raises Ca^{2+}
IP	PGI2, PGE1, PGE2, PGF2a	Gs alpha subunit	Stimulates AC & PKA; raises cAMP

Abbreviations: AC, adenyl cyclase; AKT, protein kinase B; CREB, cAMP response element-binding protein; ERK, extracellular signal-regulated kinase; IP3, inositol trisphosphate; PI3K, phosphoinositide 3-kinase; PKA, phosphokinase A; PKC, phosphokinase C; PLC, phospholipase C.

the corporeal cavernous nerve terminals is released upon sexual stimulation. This results in relaxation of corporeal smooth muscles, leading to dilatation of the arterioles and arteries by increased blood flow. This expands sinusoids and compresses subtunical venular plexuses and emissary veins of tunica which, in turn, reduces the venous outflow to a minimum. Ultimately, increased arterial blood flow and reduced venous outflow increases intracavernous pressure, raising the penis from the dependent position to the erect state. In addition, prostaglandins are also involved in regulation of spermatogenesis, sperm maturation, and transport.

Inflammation

Prostaglandins, especially PGE2, are involved in all processes culminating in the classic signs of inflammation: redness, swelling, and pain. PGE2-mediated arterial dilatation and increased microvascular permeability of the inflamed tissue lead to redness and edema, respectively. Actions of PGE2 on peripheral sensory neurons, spinal cord, and brain lead to pain perception. They are important factors behind causation of hyperalgesia secondary to tissue injury. In addition, PGE2, binding to different EP receptors, can regulate the function of many cell types including macrophages, dendritic cells and T and B lymphocytes, leading to both pro- and anti-inflammatory effects.

A potent vasodilator, PGI2, is an important regulator of cardiovascular homeostasis. It is inhibitor of platelet aggregation, leukocyte adhesion, and vascular smooth muscle proliferation. It also possesses antimitogenic activity.

Fever

Exogenous pyrogens, that is, bacterial lipopolysaccharides stimulate production of interleukin 1 and other interleukins which, in turn, are endogenous pyrogens. IL 1 induces formation of prostaglandins, predominantly PGE2. Action of PGE2 via specific EP3 receptor on the hypothalamus leads to development of fever. In brain, endocannabinoid 2-arachidonoylglycerol is an important, phospholipase-independent source of arachidonic acid for the synthesis of prostaglandin E2.

Gastrointestinal Tract

Prostaglandins virtually modulate every aspect of gastric mucosal defense against gastric acid. Gastric mucosa produces PGE2 and PGI2. These prostaglandins inhibit gastric acid secretion, along with stimulating protective mucus and bicarbonate secretion in the stomach. This leads to formation of alkaline pH microenvironment in mucoid cap, covering damaged gastric epithelium and preventing further damage. Being vasodilator, PGE2 and PGI2 increase gastric mucosal blood flow by acting on EP2/EP4 and IP receptors, respectively. This helps in repair and regeneration of gastric mucosa, preventing stomach digesting itself.

Vasculature

Before a fetus is born, its blood does not need to go to the lungs to get oxygenated. The ductus arteriosus is a hole that allows the blood to skip the circulation to the lungs. PGE2 is the important factor which prevents closure of ductus arteriosus before birth of baby.

Blood clots form when a blood vessel is damaged. Thromboxane stimulates constriction and clotting of platelets. Conversely, PGI2 is produced to have the opposite effect on the walls of blood vessels where clots should not be forming. Prostaglandins also cause vasodilatation, decrease peripheral resistance and blood pressure, while enhancing capillary permeability.

Kidney

Prostaglandins decrease renal vascular resistance and tend to increase glomerular filtration rate (GFR), urinary volume, and excretion of Na^+, K^+, Cl^-. In addition, prostaglandins costimulate erythropoietin production to cope up with tissue hypoxia.

Uses of Prostaglandins

Due to wide distribution of prostaglandins, their analogs are used for many clinical applications (**Table 43.2**). Following are few of their uses along with their rationale and relevant adverse drug reactions.

Obstetrics

Misoprostol, PGE1 analog, is used with the progesterone antagonist mifepristone as an emergency contraceptive. PGE2 (dinoprostone), available as vaginal insert and endocervical gel, softens the cervix at term and is used for the same before induction of labor with oxytocin. As both PGE2 and PGF2α elicit strong uterine contractions, they have been used as abortifacients in the second trimester of pregnancy. These uterine contractions are not interrupted by in-between relaxations. Hence, although these can

Table 43.2 Uses of prostaglandins

Drug	Preparation	Use
Dinoprostone	Vaginal tab/gel	Induction of labor
		Mid-term abortion
Dinoprost	Intra-amniotic inj	Mid-term abortion
Carboprost	IM, Intra-amniotic inj	Mid-term abortion
		Control of PPH
Gemeprost	Vaginal pessary	Cervical priming in early pregnancy
Alprostadil	IV infusion, IV inj	Maintenance of a patent ductus arteriosus in neonates
	Intra-cavernosal inj	Erectile dysfunction
Misoprostol	Oral	Abortion & Peptic ulcer
Enoprostil		Peptic ulcer
Epoprostenol	IV infusion	Pulmonary hypertension
Latanoprostol	Topical	Glaucoma
Iloprost	IM	Dec. Infarct size, when given IM after MI

induce labor at term, they are not routinely used for the same, as they are commonly associated with adverse fetal (fetal acidosis) and maternal outcomes (nausea, vomiting, diarrhea, stomach, or abdominal pain).

Pediatrics

PGE1, a potent vasodilator, is used as a continuous infusion to maintain patency of the ductus arteriosus in infants with certain cardiac anomalies like transposition of the great vessels until surgical correction is carried out.

Pulmonary Hypertension and Dialysis

Prostacyclin (PGI2) is indicated (as epoprostenol) in treatment of pulmonary hypertension when other vasodilators like calcium channel blockers, phosphodiesterase inhibitors, and endothelin receptor blockers have failed. PGI2, owing to antiaggregatory activity, is used to prevent platelet aggregation and thrombosis in patients on dialysis. Use of PGI2 is associated with certain adverse effects like agitation, anxiety, chest pain, hypotension, flushing, headache, nervousness, nausea, and vomiting. Other side effects include abdominal pain, bradycardia, and dizziness.

Peptic Ulcer Associated with NSAID Use

Misoprostol is considered as most appropriate drug for the prevention or treatment of peptic ulcers in patients who are on high doses of nonsteroidal anti-inflammatory drugs (NSAIDs) for prolonged duration. Most frequent GI adverse effects with use of misoprostol are diarrhea and abdominal pain. Additionally, spotting, cramps, hypermenorrhea, and dysmenorrhea may be observed in few female patients.

Urology

PGE1 (as alprostadil) is indicated for the treatment of male impotence. It is to be given through intracavernosal injection or as a urethral suppository. The most common adverse reaction is penile pain, which is observed in ≥ 10% patients, followed by prolonged erection, penile fibrosis, and injection site hematoma. It rarely causes testicular pain, scrotal edema, hematuria, pelvic pain, hypotension, vasodilation, vasovagal reaction, diaphoresis, and rash.

Ophthalmology

Latanoprost, a PGF2α derivative, increases the uveoscleral outflow of aqueous humor. It is considered as first-line treatment for the topical treatment of glaucoma. Bimatoprost, travoprost, and unoprostone are similar drugs. Local conjunctival hyperemia, eyelash changes like increased length, thickness, pigmentation, and number of lashes; eyelid skin darkening; intraocular inflammation (iritis/uveitis); iris pigmentation changes; and macular edema including cystoid macular edema are important adverse drug reactions following latanoprost or similar drugs' use.

Antagonists and Inhibitors of Prostaglandins (Fig. 43.3)

Effects of various prostaglandins many a time culminate or aggravate various pathological conditions; hence, inhibition of their actions can be utilized as effective measure to control many disease states. This can be achieved by the following measures:

Uteroglobulin and gravidin are pregnancy-induced protein inhibitors of PLA2. Their physiological/pharmacological role has yet not been established, but they may be involved in the mediation of progesterone-controlled uterine quiescence.

Corticosteroids are lipid-soluble agents. They enter target cells to bind with glucocorticoid receptors (GR) in the cytoplasm. This steroid-GR complex then translocates into the nucleus to interact with specific regulatory elements of target genes. This either increases or infrequently decreases transcription of target genes, resulting in up or down regulation of these gene products. One of the upregulated factors is lipocortin, a direct inhibitor of phospholipase A2, while downregulation of AP-1 and NF-κB is an important pathway for anti-inflammatory effects of corticosteroids. Corticosteroids have broad anti-inflammatory activity, and hence they are of immense value in treatment of many chronic inflammatory disorders like asthma, chronic obstructive pulmonary disease, sarcoidosis, atopic dermatitis, rheumatoid arthritis, systemic lupus erythematosus (SLE), etc., yet prolonged moderate-to-high dose corticosteroid therapy is associated with varied adverse effects like osteoporosis, hypertension, diabetes, weight gain, increased vulnerability to infection, cataracts and glaucoma, and skin changes.

To avoid grievous, and many a time unavoidable adverse drug reactions of long-term corticosteroid therapy, NSAIDs were invented. Cyclooxygenase enzymes carry out successive steps in the synthesis of thromboxane, prostaglandins, and prostacyclin. Hence, if cyclooxygenase enzyme is inhibited, formation of proinflammatory factors can be halted. The same is achieved by NSAIDs. Cyclooxygenase enzymes comes in two forms, COX 1 and COX 2; the former is a constitutive enzyme, while the latter is an inducible form. As the name suggests, inducible COX 2 is induced at inflammation site by various proinflammatory factors or factors notifying tissue injury. Hence, it is preferable to inhibit COX 2 selectively to reduce or inhibit inflammation. Most of the currently available NSAIDs, that is, aspirin, ibuprofen, and naproxen are nonselective inhibitors of both COX-1 and COX-2. While meloxicam is a preferential COX-2 inhibitor, and etoricoxib is the most selective COX-2 inhibitor, NSAIDs are used for control of fever, inflammation, pain of arthritis and backache, common cold, headaches, dysmenorrhea, joint or bone injuries, sprains, strains, muscle or joint complaints, and toothache.

Thromboxane

Thromboxane A2 (TxA2) is a metabolite of arachidonic acid generated by the sequential action of three enzymes–phospholipase A2, COX-1/COX-2, and TxA2 synthase. COX-1 is a constitutive enzyme present in most cells, while COX-2 is a readily inducible enzyme. TxA2 is synthesized in platelets, macrophages, neutrophils, and endothelial cells (Fig. 43.4). As the name suggests, thromboxane A2 plays a significant role in thrombosis or stoppage of bleeding at

Anti-inflammatory agents

Glucocorticoids (Corticosteroids)
Betamethasone, Cortisone, Dexamethasone, Hydrocortisone, Methylprednisolone, Prednisolone, Prednisone, Triamcinolone

Membrane phospholipids

Prostaglandin H_2

Arachidonic acid

NF-κB (⊖) IκB (⊕)

Endoperoxide synthesis (Cyclooxygenase)

Leukotriene synthesis (5-Lipoxygenase)

Zileuton

Leukotriene receptor antagonists

Montelukast
Zafirlukast

5- Lipoxygenase

COX-2 ONLY: Celecoxib

COX-1, COX-2: Aspirin (irreversible), Other NSAIDs (reversible), Diclofenac, Ketorolac, Ibuprofen, Naproxen, Indomethacin

COX-2

COX-1

5- HPETE

Cyclic endoperoxides

Leukotrienes

Prostacyclin

Prostaglandins

Thromboxane

LTC_4 LTD_4 LTB_4: ↑ Bronchial tone

LTB_4: ↑ Neutrophil chemotaxis

PGI_2: ↓ Platelet aggregation, ↓ Vascular tone — Epoprostenol

PGE_1: ↓ Vascular tone — Alprostadil

PGE_2: ↓ Vascular tone — Dinoprostone

$PGE_{2\alpha}$: ↓ Vascular tone — Carboprost

TXA_2: ↑ Platelet aggregation, ↑ Vascular tone

LTB_4 is a neutrophil chemotactic agent.
PGI_2 inhibits platelet aggregation and promotes vasodilation.

Neutrophils arrive "B4" others.
Platelet-Gathering Inhibitor.

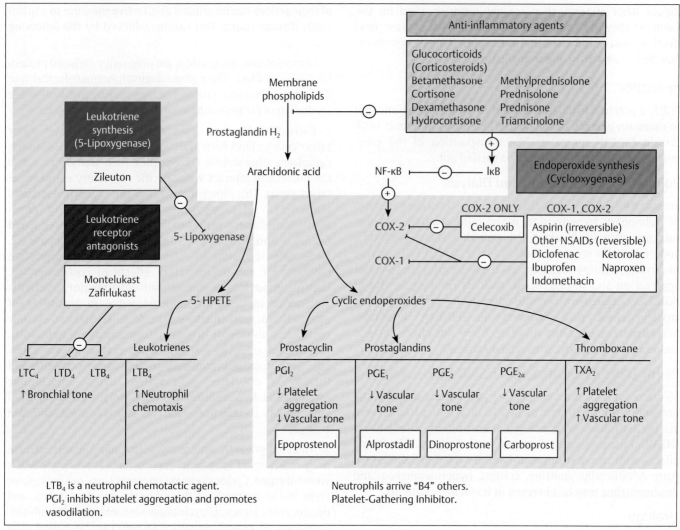

Fig. 43.3 Antagonists and inhibitors of prostaglandins.

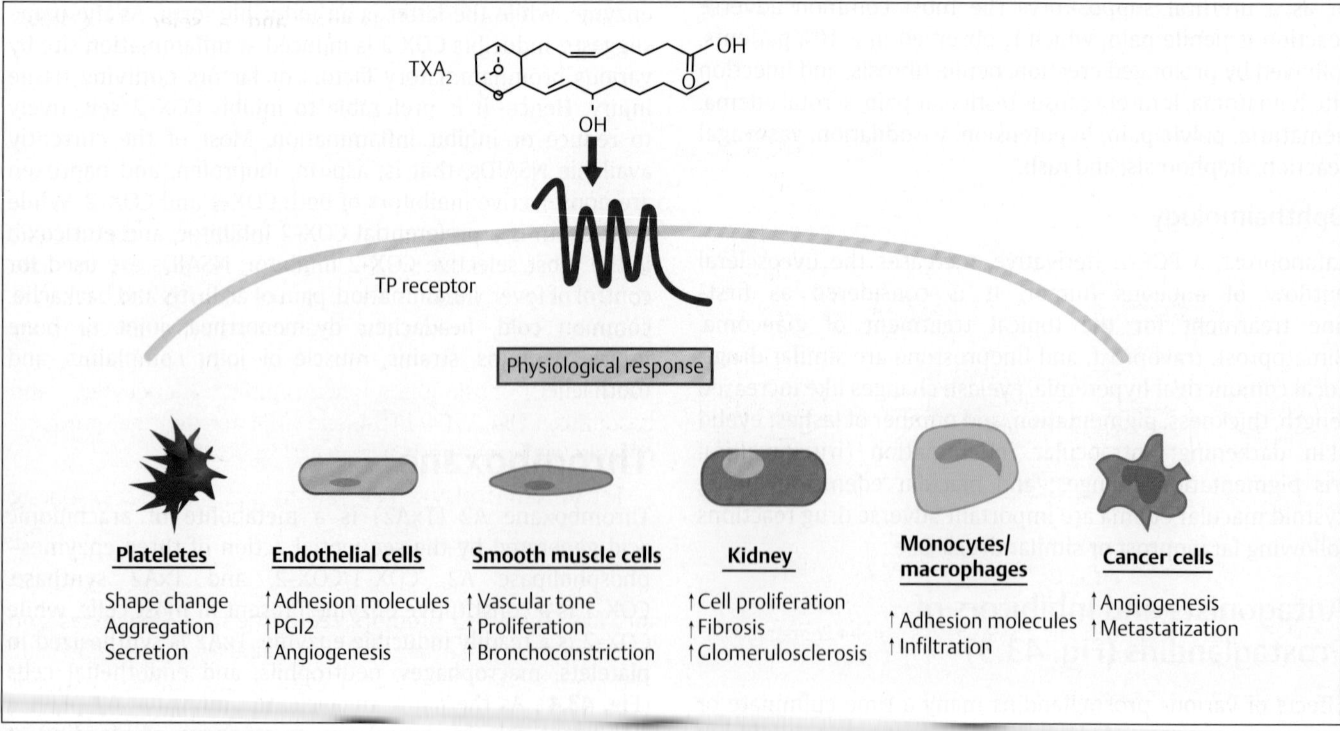

Fig. 43.4 Actions of thromboxane.

times of tissue injury and inflammation. It achieves this chiefly with the help of two mechanisms. First, it activates platelets and causes platelet aggregation. Second, TxA2 is a potent vasoconstrictor. Both these actions are additive in nature with regard to preventing blood loss following injury. To counterbalance TxA2's thrombotic and vasoconstrictor properties, PGI2 is released from endothelial cells, which possesses powerful vasodilator and platelet antiaggregator activities. Normally, these two act in balance, maintaining hemostasis (**Fig. 43.5**). Yet, in some pathological conditions, this balance is lost, and one of them, usually TxA2, becomes overpowering. This becomes precipitating factor for many cardiovascular disorders like atherosclerosis, myocardial infarction, and stroke.

Antagonists and Inhibitors of Thromboxane

Normally, thromboxane A2 is produced in very minute quantity by human body. However rarely, this goes haywire and PGI2 becomes unable to balance out the effects of TxA2, producing undesirable actions primarily on the cardiovascular system. To prevent subsequent morbidity and mortality, it becomes necessary to decrease/block actions of TxA2. The same can be achieved with the help of the following modalities:

COX Inhibitor

Aspirin is the most commonly used drug for prevention of cardiovascular thrombotic events. It is classified under NSAIDs and works by inhibiting both COX-1 and COX-2 irreversibly. Relatively low doses of aspirin are utilized for its antiplatelet action. Its effects and respective mechanisms of action vary in accordance with dose– low doses (typically 75 to 81 mg/day) are sufficient to irreversibly inhibit cyclooxygenase COX-1, primarily in the platelets, while passing through portal circulation. This effect selectively inhibits platelet generation of thromboxane A2, resulting in an antithrombotic effect lasting up to 7 days after last dose. Even low dose of aspirin is not completely devoid of side effects. Some of the common side effects are allergy and GI bleeding, while stroke caused by a burst blood vessel is one of the most dreadful. One of the early signs of aspirin toxicity is tinnitus, usually observed after use of high doses for prolonged time.

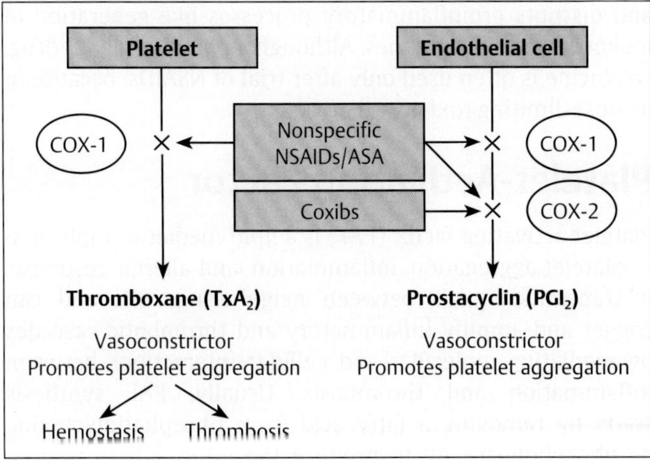

Fig. 43.5 Differing actions of prostacyclin and thromboxane.

Inhibitors of Thromboxane Synthase (TXS)

The inhibitors of TXS prevent the conversion of PGH2 to TXA2. These drugs reduce TXA2 synthesis, mainly in platelets, and may improve TXA2-mediated thrombosis formation and related disorders. Inhibition of TXS inhibitors divert PGH2 to the production of other prostaglandins, that is, PGI2 and others. PGI2 possesses the ability to inhibit platelet aggregation induced by all inducers including TxA2. Hence, theoretically, these agents have advantage over aspirin. Several TXS inhibitors are available like dazoxiben, dazmagrel, pirmagrel, and ozagrel. Their clinical evaluation revealed that they are of little help in prevention of cardiovascular accidents, because of incomplete inhibition of production of TxA2. Hence, they are very less commonly used nowadays.

Dual TXS Inhibition/Thromboxane Prostanoid (TP) Antagonism

Ridogrel is one such drug having dual actions like TXA2 inhibition with additional TP antagonist properties. It has been shown to limit myocardial infarction (MI) size after mechanical coronary occlusion and reperfusion. Although ridogrel failed to offer any advantage over aspirin in a large clinical trial, it was more effective in preventing new ischemic events. Another similar drug is picotamide.

TP Antagonists

Terutroban is an orally active, selective thromboxane prostanoid antagonist. Although, in clinical trials, it was not found to be superior to aspirin, terutroban was found be better at secondary prevention of acute thrombotic complications. Terutroban does not have affinity toward other prostanoid receptors; thus, it does not antagonize antivasoconstrictive effects of PGI2 and PGD2.

Dual COXIB/TP Antagonists

Certain NSAIDs like diclofenac and a selective COXIB–lumiracoxib possess weak competitive antagonistic activity at the TP receptor. However, because of its weak TP antagonist activity, these drugs are not for clinical use.

Leukotrienes

Leukotrienes are another set of eicosanoid inflammatory mediators produced by the oxidation of arachidonic acid and eicosapentaenoic acid with the help of the enzyme 5-lipoxygenase. Leukotrienes are synthesized predominantly in leukocytes and other immunocompetent cells, including mast cells, eosinophils, neutrophils, monocytes, and basophils. LTB4, LTC4, LTD4, and LTE4 are the final products of leukotriene synthesis pathway (**Fig. 43.6**).

Leukotrienes play a key role in many illnesses; among them, asthma is the most prominent. Leukotrienes, especially LTC4 and LTD4, facilitate smooth muscle proliferation and constriction of the bronchioles, leading to narrowing of the airways. They also promote recruitment of leukocytes and subsequent release of cytokines, leading to inflammation and hypersensitivity of the airways. By facilitating the mucus production, they further make the airways narrow. All these factors in combination leads to development of many of the classical characteristics of asthma. Because of this, people suffering from severe asthma have been reported to benefit from antileukotriene therapy.

Interestingly, chronic inflammation, where elevated levels of leukotrienes are present, is known to promote cancerous transformation. Leukotrienes also facilitate upregulation of Bcl-2, a protein which inhibits cell apoptosis and increases survival of the cells. Henceforth, chronic inflammation seen in inflammatory bowel disease (IBD) is associated with increased occurrence of colorectal adenocarcinoma, and correspondingly, many leukemias and lymphomas, esophageal, breast, and skin cancers have upregulated functioning of Bcl-2. Antileukotriene therapies are found to have beneficial role in these malignancies, as these malignancies have been shown to produce elevated levels of leukotrienes synthesis machinery.

Few acquired pathological conditions, that is, HIV, malnutrition, and induced low leukotriene activity (achieved by use of leukotriene receptor blockers or 5LOX inhibitors, i.e., MK 886) are associated with increased incidence of reactivation of pulmonary tuberculosis, conforming leukotriene's role in acquired innate immune responses.

Leukotrienes facilitate both attraction of macrophages and their differentiation into foam cells. Foam cells are one of the important building blocks of atheromatous plaque. Interestingly, atherosclerotic vascular lesions contain 5-lipooxygenase, FLAP, and other distal enzymes essential for synthesis of leukotrienes, and their levels are well-correlated with severity of the atherosclerotic disease. Hence, it is observed that elevated levels of leukotrienes are found to have increased risk of stroke and myocardial infarction.

Antagonists and Inhibitors of Leukotrienes (Figs. 43.6 and 43.7)

Leukotriene activity can be reduced or terminated by two ways: either by blocking the synthesis of them or by blocking their receptors. Similar to NSAIDs, which inhibit COX enzyme and production of prostaglandins, zileuton is a specific inhibitor of 5-lipoxygenase and thus inhibits leukotriene (LTB4, LTC4, LTD4, and LTE4) formation. Leukotrienes are substances that induce numerous biological effects, including augmentation of neutrophil and eosinophil migration, neutrophil and monocyte aggregation, leukocyte adhesion, increased capillary permeability, and smooth muscle contraction. These effects contribute to inflammation, edema, mucus secretion, and bronchoconstriction in the airways of asthmatic patients. Hence, by inhibiting production of various leukotrienes and their effects on respiratory track, zileuton is indicated for the prophylaxis and chronic treatment of asthma in adults and children 12 years of age and older, but not for termination of acute attack. Animal studies reported increased incidence of liver, kidney, and vascular tumors in 2-year study. Common adverse effects of zileuton are headache, pain, and asthenia.

The cysteinyl leukotrienes (LTC4, LTD4, and LTE4) are products of arachidonic acid metabolism and are released from various cells, including mast cells and eosinophils. These eicosanoids bind to cysteinyl leukotriene (CysLT) receptors. The CysLT type-1 (CysLT1) receptor is found in the human airway—on airway smooth muscle cells and airway macrophages, and on other proinflammatory cells including eosinophils and certain myeloid stem cells. In asthma, leukotriene-mediated effects include airway edema, smooth muscle contraction, and altered cellular activity associated with the inflammatory process, while CysLTs are released from the nasal mucosa after allergen exposure in allergic rhinitis. Montelukast and zafirlukast are orally active compounds that bind with high affinity and selectivity to the CysLT1 receptor, inhibiting actions of LTD4 at the CysLT1 receptor without any agonist activity. Hence, these drugs are used in the management of chronic asthma and allergic rhinitis. Montelukast is also approved for the treatment of exercise-induced asthma. Taken once daily, it can help prevent symptoms that accompany exercise. Rarely, analgesic doses of aspirin produce overproduction of 15 lipoxygenase-derived arachidonic acid metabolites, namely, 15-hydroxyicosatetraenoic acid and eoxins by the eosinophils. These metabolites precipitate acute attack of asthma in susceptible persons. As zafirlukast and montelukast, block cysLTC4 and D4 receptors, they prevent the actions of abnormal metabolites, namely, 15-hydroxyicosatetraenoic acid and eoxins. Thus, zafirlukast and montelukast can be used for the treatment of aspirin-induced asthma. Use of montelukast and zafirlukast is associated with adverse drug reactions like headache, dyspepsia, pain, asthenia, and elevation of liver enzymes.

Gout is a painful, chronic, relapsing-remitting inflammatory condition, mainly affecting joints of the body. Acute attack of gout predominantly involves hyperplasia and infiltration of joint cavity by inflammatory cells. Acute trauma, illness, excess alcohol intake, or drugs may alter serum uric acid levels, which gets diffused into the synovial fluid and cavity. Increased concentration of urate in the tissues, especially in joints, leads to formation of monosodium urate crystals from preformed deposits within the joint. This, in turn, is responsible for cellular infiltration and inflammation, leading to immensely limiting joint movements and severe pain. As acute attack of gout is associated with inflammation, NSAIDs are first-line therapy for acute gout. In addition, colchicine, a novel drug, acts by modulating pro- and anti-inflammatory pathways associated with gout. It prevents formation of microtubule assembly and disrupts proinflammatory processes like generation of leukotrienes and cytokines. Although a potent antigout drug, colchicine is often used only after trial of NSAIDs, because of its dose-limiting toxicity– diarrhea.

Platelet-Activating Factor

Platelet activating factor (PAF) is a lipid mediator implicated in platelet aggregation, inflammation, and allergic response. It transmits signals between neighboring cells and can trigger and amplify inflammatory and thrombotic cascades by mediating molecular and cellular interactions between inflammation and thrombosis. Usually, PAF synthesis starts by removing a fatty acid from phosphatidylcholine by phospholipase A2 to produce the intermediate lyso-PC (LPC). Subsequently, acetyl group is attached to it by LPC

Cell membrane phospholipids
Steroids inhibit
Phospholipases
COOH
CH_3
Arachidonic acid
Other Lipoxygenases
HPETEs
HETEs
COX-1 and COX-2 inhibitors, aspirin, indomethacin inhibit
Cyclooxygenase
5-Lipoxygenase
Postaglandin G_2(PGG_2)
Postaglandin H_2(PGH_2)
5-HPETE
5-HPETE
Chemotaxis
Leukotriene B_4
Leukotriene receptor antagonists inhibit
Leukotriene A_4(LTA_4)
Prostacyclin PGI_2
Causes vasodilation inhibits platelet aggregation
Leukotriene G_4(LTC_4)
Leukotriene D_4(LTD_4)
Leukotriene E_4(LTE_4)
Bronchospasm increased vascular permeability
Thromboxane A_2 TXA_2
Causes vasoconstriction, promotes platelet aggregation
12-Lipoxygenase
PGD_2 PGD_2
Causes vasodilation, increased vascular permeability
Lipoxin A_4(LXA_4)
Lipoxin B_4(LXB_4)
Inhibition of inflammation

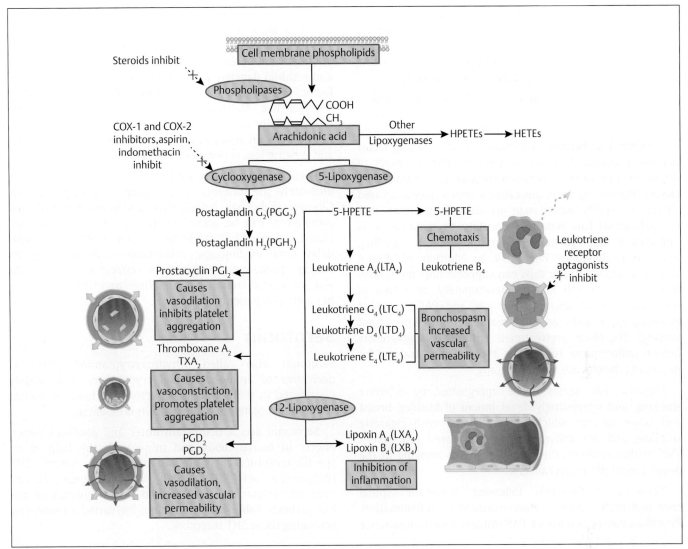

Fig. 43.6 Drugs acting on prostaglandin and leukotriene pathways.

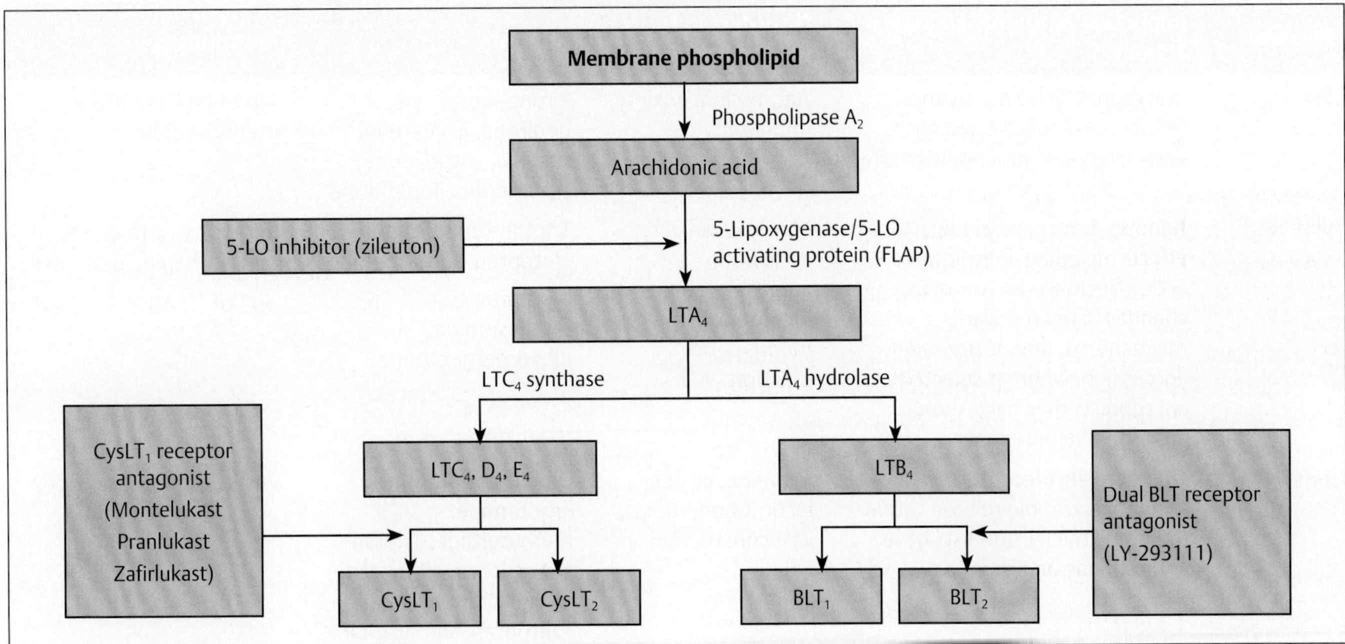

Fig. 43.7 Antagonists and inhibitors of leukotrienes.

acetyltransferase in order to produce PAF. Main source of PAF is leukocytes due to their ability to generate large amounts of PAF. Yet, PAF can also be generated by both endothelial cells and platelets, which is consistent with the platelet-activating capacity of PAF, in addition to other cells of the body.

Activation of PAF receptors (PAF-R) has been linked with degranulation of inflammatory cells and secretion of interleukins and other proinflammatory mediators. Henceforth, PAF becomes an important determining factor of chronic inflammation and anaphylaxis. PAF also plays an important role in cell migration through proinflammatory factors. Interestingly, certain cancers which have increased ability to rapidly metastasize are difficult to treat, that is, melanoma. This notorious capacity to metastasize is imparted at least partially by proinflammatory signaling, which is mediated by PAF/PAF-R. In addition, PAF/PAF-R activation among tumor cells can suppress host immunity-mediated tumor cell killing. Unfortunately, as a tool of protection, tumor cells produce PAF and PAF-like lipids following exposure to radiation treatment for their persistent survival. Therefore, pretreatment with PAF-R antagonists before radiotherapy represents a promising strategy for improving the efficacy of radiotherapy.

Likewise, PAF seems to be upregulated by cigarette smoking, and interestingly development of bladder, breast and other cancers which are associated with cigarette smoking and are known to have increased PAF levels. This further confirms the role of cigarette smoking in the development of various cancers.

Neuronal dysfunction, following traumatic spinal cord and brain injuries, is accompanied by inflammation. Proinflammatory activity of PAF imparts much importance here, as it changes cellular adhesion and alters permeability of blood–brain barrier (BBB)-enhancing chemotaxis. This cellular infiltration and subsequent neuronal damage are important determining factors in deciding CNS recovery and residual damage. In addition, being a proinflammatory factor, PAF is also a key mediator of neurodegenerative diseases like Alzheimer's disease. Hence, blocking PAF/PAF-R activity improves chances of positive outcome after traumatic brain injury as well as decreases cognitive decline and synapse loss in dementia animal models.

Renal mesangial cells are source of glomerular PAF and, ultimately, the sufferers of its disproportionate production. Glomerular damage, culminating in glomerulosclerosis and proteinuria, can be accredited to mesangial cell damage. Hence, actions of PAF can be suppressed in order to prevent/delay renal dysfunction; remarkably, vitamin D and its analog– paricalcitol inhibited PAF effects in human cells and decreased renal inflammation and dysfunction in hemodialysis patients.

Serotonin

Serotonin, also called 5-hydroxytryptamine (5HT), is derivative of amino acid and tryptophan. It is widely distributed in the body and its activity in brain, intestinal tissue, blood platelets, and mast cells is essential.

Serotonin acts a neurotransmitter and produces varied effects in human body and mind with the help of its specific receptors. There are various types of serotonin/5HT receptors, namely, $5HT_1$ to $5HT_7$, which are widely distributed throughout most tissue and organ systems of the human body. **Table 43.3** enumerates the varied responses by activating these 5HT receptors.

Table 43.3 Summary of serotonin receptors, actions, agonists, antagonists, and their uses

Receptor	Important patho/physiological actions	Disorders in focus for treatment	Agonists	Antagonists
5HT1A	Presynaptic 5HT1A activation reduces 5HT release and exerts antianxiety and procognitive effects	Aggression, anxiety, impulsivity	Pirone–buspirone, gepirone, ipsapirone, urapidil, vortioxetine, ziprasidone, iloperidone	Alprenolol, nebivolol, methysergide
5HT1B	Agonists have several behavioral effects including antimigraine action, increased locomotion, changes in brain reward mechanisms, and decreased aggression, whereas selective antagonists may have some procognitive potential	Migraine, anxiety, addiction, aggression, learning, locomotion, memory, mood, penile erection	Triptan– zolmitriptan, eletriptan, sumatriptan Ergotamine, methysergide, dihydroergotamine	Ketanserin, ritanserin, methiothepin, asenapine
5HT1D	These are autoreceptors that regulate serotonin release within the raphe nuclei, agonists have antimigraine activity	Migraine, anxiety, locomotion, mood, vasoconstriction	Dihydroergotamine, ergotamine, methysergide, Triptan–almotriptan, eletriptan, frovatriptan, naratriptan, rizatriptan, sumatriptan, zolmitriptan	Vortioxetine, ziprasidone

(Continued)

Table 43.3 (*Continued*) **Summary of serotonin receptors, actions, agonists, antagonists, and their uses**

Receptor	Important patho/physiological actions	Disorders in focus for treatment	Agonists	Antagonists
5HT1F	Like 5HT1B receptors, 5HT1F is expressed in trigeminal ganglion and vestibular nuclei and has a high affinity for triptan drugs that are used for the treatment of migraine	Migraine, vasoconstriction	Lasmiditan, Triptan–naratriptan, eletriptan	-
5HT2A	Agonists produce psychotomimetic effects (most famously LSD), and therefore high affinity 5-HT2A receptor antagonists are used as antipsychotic medications	Addiction, anxiety, appetite, cognition, imagination, learning, memory, mood, perception, sexual behavior, sleep	Lisuride, LSD, mescaline, psilocybin	Antipsychotics– clozapine, olanzapine, quetiapine, risperidone, ziprasidone, aripiprazole, haloperidol, iloperidone mirtazapine, ketanserin, mianserin, pimavanserin, ritanserin, pizotifen
5HT2B	Sparsely expressed in CNS, but are heavily expressed in liver, kidney, heart and stomach fundus; affects cardiac function and anxiety	Anxiety, appetite, GI motility, sleep	MDMA, fenfluramine, norfenfluramine, methylphenidate	Asenapine, methysergide
5HT2C	Few atypical antipsychotics are 5HT2C receptor agonist and inverse agonist; agonists also display antianxiety, appetite-reducing. and antipsychotic drug actions.	Appetite suppression, GI motility, mood, locomotion, penile erection, sexual behavior, sleep, thermoregulation	Aripiprazole, ergonovine, lorcaserin, trazodone	Antipsychotic– asenapine, clozapine, haloperidol, iloperidone, mirtazapine, mianserin, eltoprazine
5HT3	Activation of the 5-HT3 receptor facilitates dopamine, GABA and 5-HT release, and inhibits acetylcholine release in the cortex mediated via GABAergic interneurons; antagonists alleviate nausea and vomiting, resulting from anticancer chemo- and radiotherapy and also postoperative emesis, particularly evident following procedures involving the abdomen, as well as have some symptomatic beneficial role in IBS	Nausea, emesis, GI motility, learning, memory	Quipazine	Antiemetics– alosetron, dolasetron, ondansetron, granisetron, tropisetron. Clozapine, memantine, metoclopramide, mirtazapine, vortioxetine
5HT4	5-HT4 receptor agonists increase peristaltic motility of GI tract	Appetite, GI motility, neuroprotection	Dazopride, mosapride, prucalopride, renzapride, metoclopramide A gastroprokinetic, cisapride and tegaserod, developed for IBS-c was withdrawn due to CVS side effects, which was consistent with the expression of 5-HT4 receptors in atria	Piboserod

(Continued)

Table 43.3 (*Continued*) Summary of serotonin receptors, actions, agonists, antagonists, and their uses

Receptor	Important patho/physiological actions	Disorders in focus for treatment	Agonists	Antagonists
5HT5A	5HT5A receptor has also been implicated in the regulation of rodent circadian rhythm; antagonists improve locomotion and exploratory behavior	Locomotion, sleep	Ergotamine valerenic acid	Asenapine, ritanserin dimebolin
5HT6	Antagonists reduce anxiety and also demonstrate antidepressant action; antagonists are also promising agents for cognitive enhancement and possibly weight loss	Anxiety, cognition, learning, memory, mood	-	Asenapine, mianserin, clozapine, quetiapine, olanzapine
5HT7	Implicated in affective behavior, circadian rhythmicity, vasodilation and fear learning; antagonists may produce fast antidepressant effects	Anxiety, memory, mood, sleep, thermoregulation	Aripiprazole	Amitriptyline, imipramine, vortioxetine Asenapine, haloperidol, iloperidone, olanzapine, risperidone Ketanserin, ritanserin, metergoline

Abbreviations: CNS, central nervous system; CVS, cyclic vomiting syndrome; GI, gastrointestinal; IBS, inflammatory bowel syndrome; LSD, lysergic acid diethylamide.

Multiple Choice Questions

1. A 13-year-old woman complains of an itchy, runny nose during the fall season. She says she experienced similar symptoms around the same time last year. Her family history is significant for hay fever in her mother. Which of the following would be the best choice to treat this patient?

A. Aspirin.
B. Epinephrine.
C. Montelukast.
D. Naproxen.
E. Terbutaline.

Answer: C

This patient's presentation and history suggest that seasonal allergies are causing her symptoms. Allergy symptoms are the result of mediators released because of a type 1 hypersensitivity reaction, in which an allergen simultaneously binds two IgE molecules on a mast cell's surface. This simultaneous binding initially causes mast cell degranulation, releasing histamine, and leads to the later conversion of arachidonic acid to leukotrienes. Montelukast is a leukotriene receptor inhibitor and would be the most useful of the drugs listed to treat this patient.

2. A 6-year-old boy is brought to his primary care physician with a history of hay fever and asthma. He usually has two to three attacks per week. For symptom control, he uses an albuterol inhaler, but his parents would like to try something more. They would like him to take something that would lessen the amount of attacks he has. Although corticosteroids would probably work best for prophylaxis, they are contraindicated in children. He is instead given montelukast. How does montelukast work?

A. Blocks leukotriene receptors.
B. Blocks muscarinic acetylcholine receptors.
C. Inhibits COX-1 and COX-2.
D. Inhibits COX-2 only.
E. Inhibits lipoxygenase.

Answer: A

Arachidonic acid is the precursor for the eicosanoids such as prostaglandins and leukotrienes. First, phospholipase A2 cleaves cell membrane phospholipids to release arachidonic acid. Arachidonic acid can then be converted into prostaglandins by cyclooxygenase (inhibited by aspirin and celecoxib) or into leukotrienes by lipoxygenase (inhibited by zileuton). Prostaglandins are drivers of inflammation. Leukotrienes cause bronchoconstriction, mucus production, and increased vessel permeability, leading to the symptoms of asthma. Montelukast works by preventing leukotrienes from binding to their receptors.

3. You have been monitoring a 62-year-old man who is a retired small business owner over the past year and have noted a slowly changing intraocular pressure bilaterally. You have started him on latanoprost to treat his open-angle glaucoma. How does latanoprost affect intraocular pressure?

A. Lowers pressure by decreasing aqueous humor secretion.
B. Lowers pressure by decreasing aqueous humor synthesis.
C. Lowers pressure by increasing aqueous humor outflow.
D. Raises pressure by decreasing aqueous humor outflow.
E. Raises pressure by increasing aqueous humor secretion.

Answer: C

Glaucoma usually involves an increase in intraocular pressure (IOP). Latanoprost, a PGF2α analog, decreases intraocular pressure by increasing uveoscleral outflow of aqueous humor.

4. A 28-year-old woman presents to the emergency department in an acute asthma exacerbation. Her asthma developed in her 20s after she had recurrent upper respiratory infections. She was doing well, but she twisted her ankle yesterday and was taking aspirin to reduce inflammation. She is diagnosed with aspirin-induced asthma. What is the most appropriate long-term treatment for her condition?

A. Albuterol.
B. Cromolyn.
C. Ipratropium.
D. Theophylline.
E. Zafirlukast.

Answer: E

The first-line treatment of aspirin-induced asthma is desensitization to aspirin. The next treatment options are steroids or leukotriene inhibitors. Zafirlukast blocks leukotriene receptors and is used in the treatment of aspirin-induced asthma.

5. A 19-year-old man presents to the emergency room with a broken ankle after a fall. He is given hydrocodone for the pain and, soon after, his stomach becomes upset. He has vomited once. The patient is given ondansetron to treat his nausea. What is the mechanism of action of ondansetron?

A. 5-HT3 antagonist.
B. D2-receptor antagonist.
C. H2-receptor inhibitor.
D. Serotonin-norepinephrine reuptake inhibitor.
E. Substance P antagonist.

Answer: A

The mechanism of action of ondansetron is the antagonism of the 5-HT3 receptor. This blocks serotonin activation of the vomiting center in the medulla, thus producing its antiemetic effect.

6. A 37-year-old woman with mild arthritis presents to the clinic for follow-up. She states that she is doing much better because of doubling her dose of ibuprofen. Some days, she even triples her dose throughout the day. The physician warns the patient about peptic ulcers and bleeding from taking too much ibuprofen. She is offered alternatives, but the patient refuses because the ibuprofen works so well. What is the most appropriate therapy for this patient to prevent peptic ulcers?

A. Bismuth.
B. Famotidine.
C. Lansoprazole.
D. Misoprostol.
E. Pirenzepine.

Answer: D

Misoprostol is a synthetic prostaglandin E1 used for the treatment of nonsteroidal anti-inflammatory drug (NSAID)-induced peptic ulcers. Misoprostol inhibits gastric acid secretion from parietal cells at higher doses. At low doses, it increases the production and secretion of gastric mucus.

7. A 23-year-old woman presents to the emergency department with a headache. Her headaches began on the right frontal side and radiated to the back of the right side of her head. She has vomited twice. She has photophobia and phonophobia. She usually takes sumatriptan as her headache begins, but she has none left. What is the mechanism of action of sumatriptan?

A. 5-HT1A agonist.
B. 5-HT1A antagonist.
C. 5-HT1B/1D agonist.
D. 5-HT1B antagonist.
E. 5-HT3 agonist.

Answer: C

Sumatriptan is a 5-HT1B/1D agonist. This causes vasoconstriction of cerebral arteries that are thought to be inflamed during a migraine. It also decreases the activity of the trigeminal nerve, which is proposed to be the cause of some of the pain during migraines.

8. A 72-year-old woman presents to her primary care physician with vision loss over the past year. She has noticed painless loss of her peripheral vision. Her peripheral vision has become darker. She is diagnosed with open-angle glaucoma and started on medication. She returns in 1 month and says her vision has improved, but now her blue eyes turned brown. What was the most likely medication given to treat her glaucoma?

A. Acetazolamide.
B. Epinephrine.
C. Latanoprost.
D. Pilocarpine.
E. Physostigmine.

Answer: C

Latanoprost is a prostaglandin F2a analog that increases the outflow of aqueous humor from the eye. A side effect of latanoprost is causing darkening of the iris, which the patient exhibits with her blue eyes turning brown.

9. A 31-year-old woman presents to the clinic for follow-up of her abdominal pain. The pain has been occurring for a couple of years but has worsened recently. She is often constipated and then will have periods of diarrhea. Her pain does usually improve after a bowel movement. After multiple negative tests, the diagnosis of constipation-predominant irritable bowel syndrome (IBS) is made. Which of the following is an appropriate treatment for this patient?

A. Infliximab.
B. Metoclopramide.
C. Ondansetron.

D. Sulfasalazine.

E. Tegaserod.

Answer: E

Tegaserod is a 5-HT4 serotonin receptor agonist used in the treatment of constipation-predominant IBS. The 5-HT4 receptor is thought to help control GI motility; therefore, being an agonist will increase GI motility and prevent constipation.

10. A 53-year-old man spends his mornings outside gardening. He frequently develops tension headaches, and the only medication he keeps at home is aspirin. After taking two regular-sized aspirin tablets almost daily for a few weeks, which of the following side effects is he most at risk for?

A. Angina.

B. Insomnia.

C. Hypercoagulability.

D. Nephrolithiasis.

E. Tinnitus.

Answer: E

Aspirin or acetylsalicylic acid is an anti-inflammatory salicylate. Its primary therapeutic effects are caused by its ability to inhibit cyclooxygenase (COX) enzymes in order to prevent production of proinflammatory prostaglandins and platelet aggregation factors. Chronic use of high doses of salicylates such as aspirin, however, can lead to salicylate toxicity. Often, some of the primary symptoms of salicylate toxicity are tinnitus and hearing loss. These usually resolve with cessation of aspirin therapy.

Chapter 44 Nonsteroidal Anti-Inflammatory Drugs (NSAIDs)

Satish Eknath Bahekar

PH1.16: Describe mechanism/s of action, types, doses, side effects, indications, and contraindications of the drugs which act by modulating autacoids, including: antihistamines, 5-HT modulating drugs, NSAIDs, drugs for gout, antirheumatic drugs, and drugs for migraine.

Learning Objectives

- Nonselective COX inhibitors.
- Preferential COX-2 inhibitors.
- Selective COX-2 inhibitors.
- Analgesic-antipyretic with poor anti-inflammatory action.
- Choice of NSAIDs.
- Topical NSAIDs and analgesic combinations.

Introduction

NSAIDs are the cornerstone of the management of diseases involving pain, fever, and inflammation. These physiological phenomenon are very closely and directly associated with specific group of chemical substances named "autacoids," which are released in response to a variety of stimuli (chemical, mechanical, etc.), act quickly in immediate environment, and after a short period of action, get degraded.

Among these, eicosanoids are a chemically diverse family derived from arachidonic acid. It has multiple bioactivities associated with pain, fever, and inflammation.

Physiology of Eicosanoid Metabolism

Eicosanoids are involved in multiple metabolic pathways, which play a role in inflammation and cellular signaling, majorly that of arachidonic acid **(Fig. 44.1)**.

Arachidonic acid is a common precursor of inflammatory pathways obtained from the essential fatty acid precursor linoleic acid (released from inflammatory source). In the cell, it is esterified to membrane phospholipids and released by enzyme phospholipase A2, which hydrolyzes the acetyl ester bond (this is the first and overall rate limiting step in the generation of eicosanoids). Phospholipase A2 is present in two isoforms, namely, membrane bound (*secretory*) or soluble (*cytoplasmic*).

Arachidonic acid then undergoes different pathways, leading to the formation of variety of eicosanoids. The major pathways are cyclooxygenase pathway, lipooxygenase pathway, and epoxygenase pathway. The cyclooxygenase pathway leads to the formation of prostaglandins, prostacyclines, and thromboxane. The lipooxygenase pathway leads to the formation of leukotriene and lipoxins. The epoxygenase pathway leads to the formation of epoxyeicosatrienoic acids.

Cyclooxygenases (COX)

These are also known as prostaglandin H synthetase, which are glycosylated, homodimeric, and membrane-bound, heme-containing enzymes which are ubiquitous in humans. There are two major isoforms, namely, COX-1 and COX-2, which differ in cellular, genetic, physiologic, pathologic, and pharmacological profiles.

Each cyclooxygenase catalyzes two essential reactions.

1. First, oxygen-dependent cyclization of arachidonic acid, which leads to the formation of prostaglandin G_2 (PGG_2).

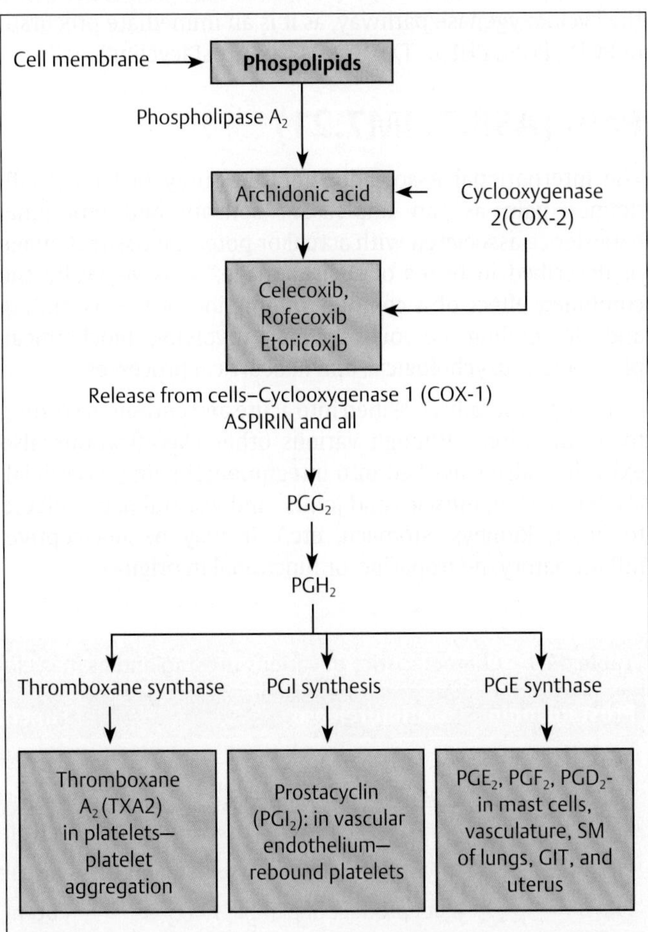

Fig. 44.1 Schematic of prostaglandin synthesis and sites of actions of nonsteroidal anti-inflammatory drugs (NSAIDs) (lipooxygenase pathway omitted).

2. Second, peroxidation which leads to the reduction of PGG_2–formation of PGH_2.

Ultimately, COX-1 and COX-2 produce different sets of eicosanoid products that are involved in different pathways and functions.

COX-1: constitutively expressed; function in housekeeping and physiological functions like vascular homeostasis, maintenance of renal and gastrointestinal (GI) blood flow, renal functions, intestinal mucosal proliferation, platelet functions, antithrombogenesis, etc.

COX-2: inducible; as needed or for specialized functions like inflammation, fever, pain, transduction of painful stimuli in spinal cord, mitogenesis in GI epithelium, renal adaptation to stress, ovulation, placentation, uterine contractions, etc.

COX-3: This is a putative isoform of cyclooxygenase, which may be the product of same gene as COX-1 but with different protein characteristics. It is primarily expressed in central nervous system (CNS; site of action of acetaminophen).

Prostaglandins

These are a large family of structurally similar compounds having individual potent and specific biological functions (**Table 44.1**). Three major subseries among them are PG_1, PG_2, and PG_3.

Among all these, PGH_2 represent the common element in the cyclooxygenase pathway, as it is an immediate precursor of PGD_2, PGE_2, $PHF_2\alpha$, TXA_2, and PGI_2 (prostacyclins).

Pain (AS8.3, IM7.21)

The International Association for the Study of Pain (IASP) defines pain as "an unpleasant sensory and emotional experience associated with actual or potential tissue damage or described in terms of such damage." It is generally the combined effect of a complex interaction of the ascending and descending nervous systems involving biochemical, physiologic, psychological, and neocortical processes.

Pain is generally classified into acute and chronic according to its duration, although various other classifications also exist. It is also classified into integumental pain (superficial, related to skin, muscles and joints) and visceral pain (related to heart, kidneys, stomach, etc.). It may be nociceptive, inflammatory, neuropathic, or functional in origin.

It is postulated that free nerve endings get sensitized by different proinflammatory autacoids like prostaglandins, bradykinin, cytokines, histamine, 5-HT, interleukins (IL_1 & IL_8), etc. Alongside these, neuropeptides like substance-P and calcitonin gene-related peptides (CGRP) are also involved in the development of pain. The most important prostaglandins involved in pain pathophysiology seem to be PGE2, which also modulates edema that is commonly associated with inflammatory pain.

Fever

Fever is one of the most common presenting symptoms encountered by physicians in clinical practice. It is commonly associated with other symptoms like chills, rigor, body ache, generalized weakness, headache, anorexia, etc. The most important physiological organ involved in the control of normal body temperature is hypothalamus. Hypothalamic set point maintains the balance between heat production and heat loss. In fever-producing conditions like infections, tissue damage, inflammations, etc. this set point get elevated, which results in hyperpyrexia. As with pain, the most important prostaglandins involved in fever pathophysiology seem to be PGE2, which also elevate the body temperature by disturbing the hypothalamic thermostatic set point.

Nonsteroidal Anti-Inflammatory Drugs (NSAIDs)

NSAIDs are the drugs which are commonly used for the treatment of the diseases associated with pain, fever, and inflammation. In general, these have analgesic, antipyretic, and anti-inflammatory properties, although individual agents have variations in these properties. NSAIDs are more commonly used in the treatment of integumental type of pain. These drugs are also known as nonopioid or non-narcotic analgesics to differentiate them from opioids or narcotics which are much more potent analgesics. These drugs possess some common characteristics such as the following:

- Nonsteroidal in nature.
- Have analgesic, anti-inflammatory, and antipyretic actions (e.g., paracetamol).
- No CNS or respiratory depression.
- No dependence.

Table 44.1 Characteristics of various prostaglandins in cyclooxygenase pathway

Prostaglandin	Location/release	Functions
PGD2	Mast cells, neurons	Bronchoconstriction, sleep control function, role in Alzheimer's disease
PGE2	Mast cells, macrophages	Vasodilation, bronchoconstriction, cytoprotection, fever, inflammatory cell activation, mucus production and possibly erectile dysfunction
PHF2a	Smooth muscles of vessels and uterus	Vascular tone, bronchoconstriction, reproductive function (abortifacient)
TXA2	Chief product of platelets	Potent vasoconstriction, promoter of platelet adhesion and aggregation
PGI2	Vascular endothelium	Vasodilation, venodilation, inhibition of platelet adhesion and aggregation

Platelets express TXA_2 but, no PGI_2, while vascular endothelium [illegible] balance [illegible] two is absolutely essential in regulation of thrombogenesis and systemic blood pressure. Imbalance can lead to thrombosis, hypertension, ischaemia, coagulopathy, myocardial infarction, stroke etc.

- Act by inhibiting prostaglandins (e.g., nimusulide and nefopam).
- Produces dose-dependent uricosuric action.

Classification

NSAIDs are basically classified according to their specificity in inhibiting the different types of COX enzymes.

A. Nonselective COX inhibitors (traditional)

a. Salicylates: aspirin.
b. Propionic acid derivatives: ibuprofen, ketoprofen.
c. Fenamates: mephenemic acid.
d. Enolic acid derivatives: piroxicam, tenoxicam.
e. Acetic acid derivatives: ketorolac, indomethacin, nabumetone.
f. Pyrazolone derivatives: phenylbutazone, oxyphenbutazone.

B. Preferential COX-2 inhibitors: nimusulide, aceclofenac, diclofenac.

C. Selective COX-2 inhibitors: elecoxib, rofecoxib, etoricoxib, parecoxib.

D. Analgesic-antipyretic with poor anti-inflammatory action:

a. Paraaminophenol derivatives: paracetamol (acetaminophen).
b. Pyrazolone derivatives: metamizol (dipyrone), propyphenazone.
c. Benzoxazocine derivative: nefopam.

Nonselective COX Inhibitors

Nonselective COX inhibitors are commonly utilized, as they are efficacious treatments for pain and inflammation. These agents have a toxicity profile with side effects generally affecting the gastrointestinal tract (GIT), heart, and kidneys. However, they constitute a chemically varied group of drugs. NSAIDs are unified by a common mechanism of action, that is, they inhibit the enzyme COX. This also accounts for much of their side effects. The enzyme is present in at least two isoforms. COX-1 produces prostaglandins with physiological functions. COX-2 is induced by inflammation and its physiologic role is currently unclear. Traditional NSAIDs like diclofenac, ibuprofen, and naproxen are nonselective COX inhibitors, blocking the production of both physiologic and inflammatory prostaglandins.

Aspirin (Prototype)

Aspirin is a prototype agent for nonsteroidal anti-inflammatory group of drugs. Aspirin gets rapidly converted into salicylic acid in the body. Aspirin inhibits both COX-1 and COX-2 enzymes in the inflammatory cascade, thereby inhibiting the inflammatory prostaglandins and bring about analgesic, anti-inflammatory, and antipyretic actions.

Pharmacological Effects of Aspirin and Its Therapeutics Uses with Doses

Analgesic Action

- Aspirin inhibits prostaglandins synthesis and blocks pain-sensitizing mechanism caused due to inflammatory mediators like bradykinin, interleukins, TNF-α, etc. This ultimately relieves the integumental pain associated with inflammation and tissue injury, but it is not useful in visceral type of pain.
- It also acts at the subcortical level and increases pain threshold.
- Effective dose: 300 to 600 mg every 6 to 8 hours.

Used in

- Headache, backache, toothache.
- Muscle pain, myalgias, neuralgias.
- Pain of rheumatoid arthritis.
- Cancer metastasis pain.
- Dysmenorrhea.

Antipyretic Action

- Aspirin decreases the temperature in fever but not at normal body temperature.
- It inhibits both COX-1 and COX-2 enzymes—decreases prostaglandin secretion in hypothalamus and resets the hypothalamic thermostat; once it returns to normal, sweating and cutaneous vasodilatation decrease fever.
- Effective dose: 75 to 100 mg/kg/ day in divided doses.
- Useful in fever of any origin.

Anti-Inflammatory Action

- Aspirin inhibits two most important prostaglandins responsible for inflammation, that is, PGE_2 and PGI_2. This decreases vasodilatation and edema.
- It also stabilizes leucocyte lysosomal membrane and prevents the spread of infection.
- Effective dose: 75 to 100 mg/kg/ day in divided doses.
- Used in acute rheumatic fever, rheumatoid arthritis, osteoarthritis, etc.

Inhibition of Platelet Aggregation

- TXA_2 enhances platelet aggregation and PGI_2 increases platelet aggregation.
- On normal therapeutic doses, aspirin inhibits both TXA_2 and PGI_2, but at low doses (75–100 mg), it irreversibly inhibits TXA_2 production only by inhibiting COX-1 for the total life span of platelets (7 days)—platelets lack nucleus and hence they cannot synthesize new COX-platelet aggregation is inhibited for this time period.
- But, at this dose, PGI_2 has no effect because of widespread distribution.
- Can be useful in lowering the risk of reinfarction in postmyocardial infarction or stroke patients.
- It can also be used in the treatment of transient ischemic attacks, deep venous thrombosis (DVT), or pulmonary embolism (PE).

Dysmenorrhea

Aspirin decreases PGE_2 and PGI_2, prevents intermittent myometrial ischemia, and reduces cramps.

Closure of Ductus Arteriosus

- During fetal circulation, ductus arteriosus is kept patent by PGE_2 and PGI_2. Their synthesis switches off at time of birth, which brings about the closure of ductus arteriosus.
- If this process fails at birth, aspirin is administered, which inhibits the synthesis of PGE_2 and PGI_2 and brings about the closure of ductus arteriosus.

Miscellaneous Uses

- Colonic and rectal cancers.
- Pre-eclampsia.
- Alzheimer's disease.
- Familial colonial polyposis.
- Niacin-induced cutaneous pruritis and rash.
- Slowing down of cataract progression.
- Pregnancy-induced hypertension.

Adverse Effects

Gastric Mucosal Damage

- Aspirin inhibits PGE2 and PGI2, which also causes nullification of their gastroprotective effects like decrease in the gastric acid secretion, stimulation of mucus secretion, and increase in the bicarbonate secretion.
- This results in clinical features like nausea, vomiting, epigastric pain, dyspepsia, and gastric bleeding.
- Note: Aspirin, being a weakly acidic drug, remains unionized in acidic gastric juice. It enter gastric mucosal cells by passive diffusion; once inside of alkaline medium, it ionizes and gets trapped in the gastric mucosal cells, leading to increased gastric toxicity.

Effect on Respiration and Acid-Base Balance

This effect is dose-dependent

- At normal therapeutic dose: mild uncoupling of oxidative phosphorylation, leading to mild increase in oxygen consumption and CO_2 production–normal pCO2 and acid-base balance.
- Plasma levels 400 to 500 mg/mL: direct stimulation of respiratory center, leading to decrease in pCO2 levels and causing hyperapnea and respiratory alkalosis– salicylism, which is marked by headache, vertigo, tinnitus, nausea, and vomiting.

  Treated with acidifying agents like ascorbic acid or ammonium chloride along with intravenous (IV) fluids.
- Plasma levels 500 mg to 1 mg/mL: medullary depression and respiratory depression, leading to excessive decrease in pCO2 levels as well as decrease in bicarbonate levels–respiratory acidosis.
- Plasma levels over 1 mg/mL: In acidic pH, aspirin is released to salicylic acid, levels of H_3PO_4 and H_2SO_4 are increased and carbohydrates and fat metabolism get deranged, leading to accumulation of lactic acid, pyruvic acid, acetoacetic acid, etc.–metabolic acidosis marked by loss of vision, renal failure, respiratory failure, vascular collapse, dehydration, convulsions, coma, and death.

Increase in Bleeding Tendency

On long-term use, there is a decrease in the prothrombin levels, and increase in prothrombin time (PT), which increases the bleeding tendency. It should be stopped 1 week before surgery and is contraindicated in hemophilia patients.

Hypersensitivity

Rash, rhinitis, bronchial asthma, angioneurotic edema, etc.

Effect on Uric Acid Secretion

At high dose, it increases uric acid secretion–precipitation of gouty arthritis.

Renal Effects

On chronic consumption, there is analgesic nephropathy–chronic nephritis and renal papillary necrosis.

In patients afflicted with congestive heart failure (CHF), hepatic cirrhosis, and renal disease, there is acute but reversible renal insufficiency.

Rey's Syndrome

In children suffering from viral fever, administering aspirin leads to liver damage and hepatic encephalopathy. It is contraindicated in children below 12 years of age.

Endocrine Effects

Large doses stimulate adrenal cortex through an effect on hypothalamus and plasma adrenocorticosteroid levels. Also, it decreases thyroid uptake of iodine, leading to goiter.

Local Irritating Effects

Can cause irritation to skin and destroy epithelial cells (can be used as keratolytic for warts, corns, etc.).

Drug Interactions

Aspirin has many important clinically useful as well as harmful drug interactions by virtue of its pharmacokinetic and pharmacodynamics properties.

Pharmacokinetic Interactions

1. By inhibiting the metabolism through plasma protein binding, aspirin leads to the toxicity of some drugs like oral anticoagulants (increase in bleeding tendency), sulfonylureas (hypoglycemia) phenytoin, etc.
2. Aspirin reduces the renal excretion of some administered drugs like methotrexate, digoxin, lithium, etc., which lead to their toxicity.

Pharmacodynamic Interactions

1. Decreases the pharmacological effects of some drugs like furosemide and thiazide diuretics (reduce diuresis), and spironolactone (reduces potassium conservation property), when coadministered with aspirin.
2. Some drugs, when administered with aspirin, increase their adverse effects by virtue of pharmacodynamics interactions, for example, alcohol (increases risk of GI bleeding), cyclosporine (increases nephrotoxicity), corticosteroids (increases risk of GI bleeding), etc.

Preferential COX-2 Inhibitors

This group contain agents like nimusulide, diclofenac sodium, and aceclofenac. These are the NSAIDs which act by specifically inhibiting only COX-2 enzymes and have no inhibitory action on the rest of COX enzymes. Like other NSAIDs, these also block the formation of prostaglandins, thereby reducing pain and inflammation.

Nimusulide

It is relatively weak inhibitor of prostaglandin synthesis. It exerts anti-inflammatory activity by some other mechanisms like reduced generation of superoxide by neutrophils, inhibition of platelet activating factor, TNFα release, free radical scavenging, and inhibition of metalloproteinase activity in cartilage.

Because of the specificity for COX-2 activity, as opposed to COX-1, it has little effect on gastric mucosa and platelet function, leading to fewer side effects in the regard. Thus, it has relatively minor effect on platelet function or loss of gastric cytoprotection, which is mainly associated with COX-1 activity. It has a rapid onset of action (t1/2 of 2–5 hours) and used primarily used for short-lasting inflammatory conditions as in sports injuries, dental surgeries, bursitis, low backache, osteoarthritis, fever, etc. Country-wise variations regarding its use are there' it is used in adults in 100 mg twice daily dose for less than 15 days.

Nimusulide is completely absorbed by oral route, 99% plasma-bound, extensively metabolized, and excretion occurs mainly through urine. It is generally well-tolerated, but side effects can include GI (heart burn, nausea, loose motions, epigastric pain), headache, dizziness, somnolence, peripheral edema, and dermatological (rash and pruritis).

However, it has some serious concerns like fulminant hepatic failure and hence has been withdrawn in many countries like Spain, Singapore, Turkey, and Ireland. Its use in pediatric population is also banned in India, Israel, and Portugal. It is not marketed in countries like USA, UK, Canada, and Australia. Despite these, it is valuable in certain patients such as asthmatics and those who develop bronchospasm because of aspirin or other NSAIDs.

Diclofenac Sodium

This is one of the most commonly used NSAIDs in routine clinical practice. It is most commonly used to treat pain and certain inflammatory diseases like gout. As with other NSAIDs, the primary mechanism responsible for its analgesic, antipyretic, and anti-inflammatory action is inhibition of prostaglandin synthesis by inhibition of the transiently expressed cycloxygenase-2 (COX-2). As it spares COX-1, it does not exert antiplatelet activity. It also exhibits bacteriostatic activity by inhibiting bacterial DNA synthesis. This is supported by the fact that it reduces neutrophil chemotaxis and superoxide production at inflammatory sites. Besides the COX inhibition, there are some molecular targets where this drug acts, which possibly contributes to its analgesic activity like voltage-dependent sodium channels blockade, blockade of acid-sensing ion channels, and opening of positive allosteric modulation of KCNQ- and BK-potassium channels, leading to hyperpolarization of the cell membrane.

Diclofenac sodium is well-absorbed by oral route, 99% plasma-bound, metabolized, and excretion occurs through urine and bile. It produces side effects like nausea, epigastric pain, headache, dizziness, and rashes. However, gastric bleeding and ulceration are less. But nevertheless, it can increase risk of heart attack and stroke. Also, it has a propensity of elevation of serum aminotransferases although reversibly; rarely, it causes kidney damage too.

The major clinical indications of diclofenac are painful and inflammatory conditions like musculoskeletal complaints, especially arthritis, rheumatoid arthritis, polymyositis, dermatomyositis, osteoarthritis, dental pain, temporomandibular joint (TMJ) pain, spondylarthritis, ankylosing spondylitis, gout attacks, and pain management in cases of kidney stones and gallstones. It can be useful in acute attack of migraine too. It is very commonly used in the mild-to-moderate postoperative or posttraumatic pain, in particular associated with inflammation. It is also very effective against dysmenorrhea and endometriosis. In topical forms, it can be useful for osteoarthritis but not for other types of long-term musculoskeletal pain.

Selective COX-2 Inhibitors

This group contains agents like celecoxib, rofecoxib, valdecoxib, etoricoxib, parecoxib, etc. These are sulfonic acid derivatives which have 100 times greater selectivity to COX-2 than COX-1. However, these possess comparable analgesic, antipyretic, and anti-inflammatory activities as compared to traditional NSAIDs. Because of lack of COX-1 inhibition, they do not possess antiplatelet action.

Primarily, these drugs are useful in the treatment of osteoarthritis, acute pain in adults, rheumatoid arthritis, and primary dysmenorrhea. However, these should be used only in those patients who are at high risk of peptic ulceration, perforation, and gastric bleeding. Moreover, these should be implied in lowest possible dose for shortest period of time. Among these drugs, only celecoxib is an approved drug in United States. It is the only Food and Drugs Administration (FDA)-approved selective COX-2 inhibitor. Rofecoxib was withdrawn in 2004 due to its association with increased risk of myocardial infarction (MI) and stroke. Later on, in 2005, valdecoxib was also withdrawn.

Various reasons are postulated behind these adverse effects with coxibs, but the main reason is increased thrombogenicity with their prolonged use. This may be due to prolonged inhibition of vascular COX-2 in endothelial cells, which ultimately leads to decreased PGI2 formation. Additionally, coxibs causes problems in wound healing, angiogenesis, and resolution of inflammation.

These drugs should be avoided in the patients with the history of ischemic heart diseases, cardiac failure, hypertension, or cerebrovascular diseases. **Table 44.2** compares and contrasts selective COX-2 inhibitors with nonselective COX inhibitors.

Analgesic-Antipyretic with Poor Anti-Inflammatory Action

These drugs, especially paracetamol, are part of the class of drugs known as "aniline analgesics"; it is the only such drug still in use today. It is not considered an NSAID because it does not exhibit significant anti-inflammatory activity (it is a weak COX inhibitor). This is despite the evidence that paracetamol and NSAIDs have some similar pharmacological activity.

Paracetamol (Acetaminophen)

Paracetamol is deethylated active metabolite of phenacetin, which was an extensively used analgesic and antipyretic

Table 44.2 Comparison between selective COX-2 inhibitors with nonselective COX inhibitors

Features	Activity	Selective COX-2 inhibitors	Nonselective COX inhibitors
Comparing features	Analgesic activity	Present	Present
	Antipyretic activity	Present	Present
	Anti-inflammatory activity	Present	Present
	Renal salt and water retention	Present	Present
	Labor delay or prolongation	Present	Present
Contrasting features	Antiplatelet activity	Absent	Present
	Gastric mucosal damage	Absent	Present
	Aspirin-induced airway hyperactivity	Absent	Present
	Closure of ductus arteriosus	Questionable	Present
	Reye syndrome in children as side effect	Absent	Present

earlier (banned now). It is classified as NSAID but technically is not NSAID because it has negligible anti-inflammatory activity compared with others. This is because it is a very weak inhibitor of COX enzyme, particularly in the peripheral tissues but more active on the COX enzyme in the brain. This is may be due to absence of peroxides at the site of inflammation in the brain, which are commonly generated in periphery in the presence of which paracetamol cannot inhibit COX. It is another postulation that paracetamol inhibits another type of COX enzyme, that is, CO-3 which also accounts for its analgesic-antipyretic activity. Paracetamol is a very potent and promptly acting antipyretic agent with weak peripheral anti-inflammatory action. Like aspirin, it also raises pain threshold to exert central analgesic action. But in contrast with aspirin, it does not stimulate respiration or affect acid-base balance, does not interfere with cellular metabolism, cardiovascular functions are unaffected, and gastric erosion, bleeding, and irritation are also much less. Additionally, it has no effect on platelet functions, clotting factors, or uric acid levels.

It is very commonly used over-the-counter drug worldwide for various indications. Most common among these are for mild-to-moderate pains like mild migraine, headache, myalgia, musculoskeletal pain, dysmenorrhea, etc. It is one of the most commonly used and effective antipyretics for fever of any origin in all age groups. Particularly, it is indicated in patients allergic to aspirin, hemophiliacs, have peptic ulcer, or are asthmatic. It has very less drug interactions too.

Paracetamol is absorbed well orally, very less protein bound, and gets distributed uniformly across all body compartments. It is metabolized mainly by the process of glucuronic acid and sulfate conjugation, conjugated easily, and excreted in urine. Plasma half-life is around 2 to 3 hours.

Adverse Effects

In therapeutic dosages, paracetamol is a very safe drug with very few and minor side effects like nausea or skin rashes. In very rare cases, mild but reversible increase in hepatic enzymes can occur. However, when the drug is taken in excessive dosages than normally indicated, symptoms of acute poisoning occur as mentioned below.

Acute Paracetamol Poisoning (PE14.4)

It more commonly occurs in children than adults, as children have relatively lower glucuronide conjugation ability. Adults can also suffer from this problem, particularly those with compromised hepatic functions or in chronic alcoholics. If a large dose more than 150 mg/kg or more than 10 gm in adults is taken, risk of acute and serious toxicity increases. If dose exceeds 250 mg/kg, it can prove fatal many times.

To start with, early manifestations appear in the form of nausea, vomiting, and abdominal pain. On palpation, liver tenderness can be elicited. However, initially consciousness remains intact. After 10 to 12 hours, hepatic necrosis, renal tubular necrosis, and hypoglycemia can deteriorate the consciousness, and patient can go to comatic condition. If not treated at this level, fulminant hepatitis and death are likely complications.

Mechanism of Toxicity and Treatment

- Paracetamol undergoes metabolism by two pathways—major pathway is glucuronide or sulfate conjugation, and minor pathway is Cyt P 450 pathway.
- Both pathways lead to synthesis of toxic metabolite–N-acetyl-P-bebzoquinoimine (NAPQI).
- Normally, N-acetyl-P-bebzoquinoimine undergoes glutathione conjugation and gets eliminated from the body.
- However, in case of toxicity, this toxic metabolite forms the covalent bond with hepatic and renal cellular proteins and leads to necrosis and death of these cells.
- Treatment should be started within 16 hours with vomiting induction, gastric lavage, and activated charcoal.
- Specific antidote for paracetamol poisoning is either N-acetylcysteine (IV) or methionine (PO), which bring about glutathione conjugation of the toxic metabolite and produce the N-acetylcysteine or methionine conjugates that get excreted from the body.

Choice of NSAIDs in Different Clinical Conditions (Table 44.3)

It is of no doubt that NSAIDs are very important group of drugs in pain management because of the integrated role of the COX pathway in the generation of inflammation

Table 44.3 Choice of NSAIDs in different clinical conditions

Clinical scenario/Age/ Concurrent diseases	Preferable agent/s
Gastric diseases/gastric intolerance	Selective cyclooxygenase-2 inhibitors or paracetamol
Mild-to-moderate pain with little inflammation	Paracetamol or low-dose ibuprofen
Acute pain: musculoskeletal, injury, osteoarthritis	Aspirin, propionic acid derivatives; preferential COX inhibitors like diclofenac or nimusulide; paracetamol
Postoperative pain/acute but short-lasting pain	Propionic acid derivatives; ketorolac; preferential COX inhibitors like diclofenac or nimusulide
Asthmatics/aspirin sensitive patients/allergic to other NSAIDs	COX-2 inhibitors, nimusulide
Hypertensives/heart attack or stroke patients	Aspirin, propionic acid derivatives
Rheumatoid arthritis (exacerbation)/Ankylosing spondylitis (exacerbation)/gout (acute)/rheumatic fever (acute)	Aspirin (high dose), indomethacin, piroxicam, naproxen
Pediatric patients	Paracetamol
Pregnancy and lactating ladies	Paracetamol, low-dose aspirin
Elderly patients	Selected NSAID agent lowest possible dose for shortest period

Abbreviation: NSAID, nonsteroidal anti-inflammatory drug.

and pain. Both traditional NSAIDs and selective COX inhibitors have their own pharmacological profiles, leading to varied indications and side effects too. It is very clear that while prescribing the NSAIDs to the patients, it is of utmost importance to keep the related adverse effects of the individual agent, as these definitely affect the clinical outcome in most cases. This is because all these agents individually differ in effectivity as well as adverse effects too. So, no single drug is superior or inferior to other and choice is exclusively empirical.

There are many factors which should be keep in mind while prescribing the specific NSAID like the nature of pain (acute, chronic mild, moderate, and severe), etiology of pain, association of inflammation, etc. Along with these, patient-related factors are also important in this aspect like age, associated diseases, pregnancy or lactating phase, concurrent drug therapies, etc. Along with these, other important factors are like affordability, compliance, past experience, individual preference, etc. In the context of availability of large number of NSAIDs for clinical use, a few guidelines can be adopted for the finalization of the best suitable option for individuals.

Topical NSAIDs

There are many NSAIDs available in clinical practice in topical formulations. However, their use for pain relief has always been a controversial subject in analgesic practice. There is no doubt regarding their safety as compared to that of orally administered NSAIDs, but it is always in terms of efficacy. Topical NSAIDs are applied over painful muscles and joints in the form of gels, creams, sprays, or plasters. These penetrate the skin, tissues, or joints, and reduce pain in the tissue. Because of the nonsystemic administration, their plasma levels are very much lower than with the same drug taken by oral or injectable route. Obviously, this minimizes the risk of harmful effects, particularly gastric effects because of minimal systemic involvement. Over the years, common indications of topical NSAIDs are sports injuries, osteoarthritis, muscle sprains, backache, spondylitis, other mild painful conditions, etc. It is very common practice to use these drugs in combination with oral NSAIDs, particularly in mild-to-moderate osteoarthritic pain conditions.

Many reports on clinical efficacy of topical NSAIDs are variable. On the basis of measurement of tissue concentrations and systemic blood of these drugs, it is evident that these have very slow systemic absorption. Additionally, these concentrations are more up to the level of dermis only and thereafter decrease in deeper tissues and blood. There is marked variation in the muscles and joints, depending on the type of formulation, site of application, etc.

Despite all these, it is always postulated that these formulations are particularly useful in short-lasting musculoskeletal pain, especially with agents like diclofenac and ketoprofen. So, the value of topical NSAIDs cannot be neglected even in lesser conditions. NSAIDs available in topical formulations are diclofenac, ibuprofen, nimusulide, piroxicam, ketoprofen, flurbiprofen, naproxen, etc.

Analgesics Combinations

It is an ancient practice adopted by physicians to combine various drugs in order to achieve extraordinary results than using single drug for the clinical entity. In pain management, many analgesic combinations are tried over the years, and many of them are found effective as well. As with any other drugs, analgesic combinations are most effective when the individual agents act through different analgesic mechanisms and act synergistically. With this type of combination, broader spectrum of analgesic activity can be achieved by reduced adverse drug reactions. However, combining analgesics with different mechanisms of action can also provide better analgesic actions. With analgesic combination, one can achieve the benefits in terms of tolerability, efficacy, and less adverse effects of the individual drugs. The doses of individual drugs are minimized leading to reduction in overall adverse effects with comparable analgesia. To achieve sustained and long-term benefits, short-acting and long-acting agents can be combined to achieve good results in terms of shorter onset and longer duration of analgesia. These types of combinations can prove clinically useful in the patients of chronic diseases like hypertension, CHF, diabetes, HIV, asthma, dyslipidemia, coronary artery disease, etc.

In this context, many analgesic combinations are available in clinical practice. The most commonly used combination is of paracetamol and aspirin, which is an excellent example of additive combination. Paracetamol can be combined with other NSAIDs to achieve additional analgesic effect like diclofenac, ibugesic, etc. The other commonly available analgesic combination is of codeine with aspirin or paracetamol, which is also additive.

Despite all of these discussions, in general, these combinations are mostly misused and of irrational nature. In view of this, the fixed dose combinations of analgesics with hypnotics, sedatives, and anxiolytics are banned in India. NSAIDs like oxyphenbutazone, phenylbutazone, or metamizol are banned for fixed dose combinations with any other drugs.

Multiple Choice Questions

1. A 68-year-old man suffers from myocardial infarction (MI). He is admitted to the cardiac intensive care unit and is prescribed aspirin and β-blocker. A catheterization procedure is scheduled. Explain why the patient is being given aspirin and not another nonsteroidal anti-inflammatory drug (NSAID). What is the best answer to this question?

A. Aspirin inhibits both COX-1 and COX-2 enzymes.

B. Aspirin has much greater antithrombotic activity.

C. Aspirin is a weak acid.

D. Aspirin is excreted by the kidneys.

Answer: B

Aspirin has a much greater antithrombotic activity than other NSAIDs; hence, it is used for the prevention of MI in patients with a history of cardiovascular diseases like MI, angina, or cardiac surgery. The rest of the options are correct in relation to aspirin. Aspirin nonselectively inhibits COX-1 and COX-2. Aspirin is a weak acid and is excreted by the kidneys; however, these are not the reasons why aspirin is preferred over other NSAIDs in the setting of prevention of MI.

2. Acute paracetamol toxicity mainly affects?

A. Kidney.

B. Brain.

C. Liver.

D. Heart.

Answer: C

Acute paracetamol toxicity mainly affects liver and kidney, but the former is mainly affected in the form of hepatitis.

3. Which of the following is an example of selective COX-2 inhibitor?

A. Nimesulide.

B. Celecoxib.

C. Rofecoxib.

D. Valdecoxib.

Answer: A

Nimesulide is an example of preferential COX-2 inhibitor.

4. Which of the following is a pharmacotherapeutic option/s in the treatment of acute paracetamol poisoning?

A. N-acetyl cysteine (orally).

B. Methionine (intravenously).

C. Activated charcoal.

D. All the above.

Answer: C

Activated charcoal is used in this condition.

5. Nonsteroidal anti-inflammatory drug (NSAID) agent of choice in pregnant women is?

A. Aspirin.

B. Paracetamol.

C. Nimusulide.

D. Both a and b are correct.

Answer: B

6. Which of the following statements regarding paracetamol is correct?

A. It has analgesic, antipyretic, and anti-inflammatory actions.

B. It is absolutely contraindicated in pregnant women.

C. It inhibits cyclooxygenase-3 (COX-3) in central nervous system (CNS).

D. It has very good antiplatelet activity.

Answer: C

7. Which of the following selective COX-2 inhibitors has approval status?

A. Valdecoxib.

B. Rofecoxib.

C. Etoricoxib.

D. Celecoxib.

Answer: D

Celecoxib is approved in the United States.

8. Because of which adverse effects aspirin is strongly avoided in children below 12 years age group?

A. Hypersensitivity.

B. Hepatic encephalopathy.

C. Renal effects.

D. Local irritation effects.

Answer: B

Aspirin therapy in children below 12 years age group having viral infections lead to Reye syndrome, a rare form of hepatic encephalopathy.

9. Which of the following drug interactions of aspirin is pharmacokinetically mediated?

A. Spironolactone-reduction on potassium conservation.
B. Alcohol-increase in gastrointestinal (GI) bleeding.
C. Cyclosporin-risk of nephrotoxicity.
D. Sulfonylureas-hypoglycemia.

Answer: D

10. Which of the following is not a common characteristic shared by NSAIDs?

A. These are nonsteroidal in nature.
B. These do not produce dependence.
C. These act by inhibiting prostaglandin synthesis exclusively.
D. These produce dose-dependent uricosuric actions.

Answer: C

Nimusulide and nefopam are exceptions to this; these act by other mechanisms too.

Chapter 45 Rheumatoid Arthritis and Gout

Suneha Sikha

PH1.16: Describe the mechanism/s of action, types, doses, side effects, indications, and contraindications of antirheumatic drugs.

Learning Objectives

- Rheumatoid arthritis.
- Immunomodulators.
- Immunosuppressants.
- Tumor necrosis factor (TNF) inhibitors.
- Interleukin-1 (IL-1) antagonists.
- Glucocorticoids.
- Gout.
- Nonsteroidal anti-inflammatory drugs (NSAIDs) used in acute gouty arthritis.
- Colchicine.
- Xanthine oxidase inhibitors.
- Uricosuric agents.

Rheumatoid Arthritis (IM7.22, IM7.23, IM7.24)

Rheumatoid arthritis (RA) is an autoimmune disorder involving chronic and progressive joint inflammation. It mainly affects multiple small joints of the hands and feet. RA affects approximately 1% of the population. Its signs and symptoms are as follows:

1. Warm, swollen, and painful joints.
2. Symmetrical joint swelling.
3. Morning stiffness (at least for 1 hour).
4. Joint deformity.
5. Immobility.
6. Fever and fatigue.
7. Loss of appetite and loss of weight.

Rheumatoid factor (RF) and anti–cyclic citrullinated peptide (anti-CCP) are the antibodies occurring in the blood of patients with RA. High levels (more than 20 IU/mL) of RF occur in RA. Presence of RF and anti-CCP in combination with signs and symptoms can play an important role in the diagnosis of RA. There are two types of RA:

1. Palindromic rheumatism: It is a rare type of RA involving recurrent, self-resolving inflammatory attacks in and around the joints.
2. Juvenile idiopathic arthritis (JIA): It is a type of RA of unknown etiology, which occurs in children under 16 years of age. It is characterized by swollen and painful joints, with functional limitation for at least 6 weeks. It is also associated with growth disturbances.

Etiopathogenesis of RA

The exact cause of RA is not known. However, it appears to be an autoimmune disorder that targets multiple joints. Synovium is the major site of inflammation. Many cytokines such as interleukin-1 (IL-1), interleukin-6 (IL-6), and tumor necrosis factor-α (TNF-α) have been found in the rheumatoid synovium. If this synovitis is left untreated, it results in irreversible damage of adjacent cartilage and bone. Genetic and environmental factors may increase the risk of RA.

Inflammatory process in RA involves the activation of lymphocytes, particularly T cells and B cells. Activated T cells produce T cell–derived cytokines (IL-1 and TNF-α). Activated B cells produce proinflammatory cytokine (IL-6). These cytokines are the major regulatory molecules of the immune and inflammatory systems. They are chemotactic for neutrocytes. Lysosomal enzymes secreted by these inflammatory cells will damage cartilage and gradually destroy bone. This inflammatory process produces prostaglandins (PGs) causing vasodilation as well as pain. C-reactive protein (CRP) is also released into the blood stream. CRP is a marker of inflammation.

Goals of Drug Therapy in RA

The main goal of drug therapy in RA is to put the disease in remission.

1. **Immediate goals**:
   a. Decrease joint pain and swelling.
   b. Preserve or enhance joint function.
2. **Long-term goals**:
   a. Slow or stop the joint damage.
   b. Prevent disability.

Antirheumatic Drugs

Nonsteroidal anti-inflammatory drugs (NSAIDs) are also used in management of RA (**Fig. 45.1**). Antirheumatic drugs are classified into disease-modifying antirheumatic drugs (DMARDs) and adjuvant drugs (**Fig. 45.2**).

The drugs used to treat RA are:

1. NSAIDs.
2. DMARDs.
3. Adjuvant drugs.

NSAIDs

They are used as first-line drugs for RA. Symptomatic relief can be attained through the use of NSAIDs in mild RA. They are used to treat pain, inflammation, morning stiffness, and immobility. NSAIDs used in RA are cyclooxygenase-2 (COX-2) inhibitors.

Disease-Modifying Antirheumatic Drugs (DMARDs)

DMARDs induce alteration of underlying disease rather than treating the symptoms. Hence, they are used to slow down the disease progression. These are also known as slow-acting antirheumatic drugs (SAARDs). The onset of benefit with SAARDs can be seen after using them regularly for a few months.

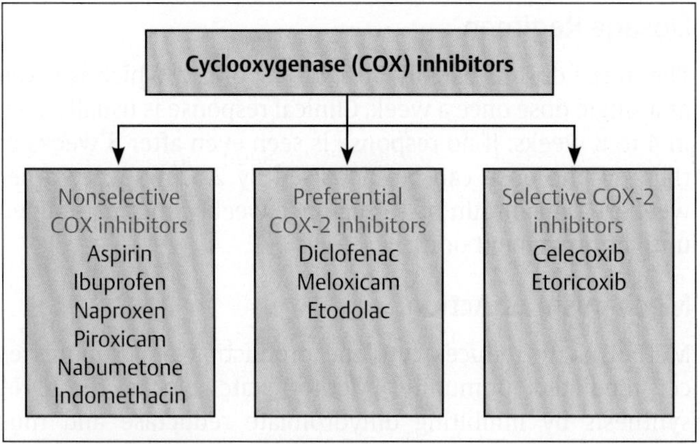

Fig. 45.1 Nonsteroidal anti-inflammatory drugs (NSAIDs) used in rheumatoid arthritis.

Adjuvant Drugs

Adjuvant drugs are used temporarily along with DMARDs. They are used to enhance the activity of DMARDs. Glucocorticoids are the adjuvant drugs used in RA.

Immunomodulators (PH1.50)

Chloroquine (CQ): Aralen

Dosage Regimen

The recommended dose is 150 mg (base) per day. Lifetime cumulative dose is limited to 460 g in order to reduce the risk of retinal toxicity.

Hydroxychloroquine (HCQ): Plaquenil

Dosage Regimen

The recommended dose is 400 mg/day for 4 to 6 weeks, followed by maintenance dose of 200 mg/day. Lifetime cumulative dose is limited to 1,000 g in order to reduce the risk of retinal toxicity.

Antirheumatic drugs

Disease-modifying antirheumatic drugs (DMARDs)

Adjuvant drugs

Conventional synthetic DMARDs (csDMARDs)

Biological DMARDs (bDMARDs)

Glucocorticoids
Prednisone
Prednisolone
Dexamethasone

Immunosuppressants

Dihyrofolate reductase inhibitor
Methotrexate

Purine synthesis inhibitor
Azathioprine

Calcineurin inhibitor
Cyclosporine

Other immunomodulators

Tyrosine kinase inhibitor
Tofacitinib

Chloroquine/
Hydroxychloroquine

Sulfasalazine

Leflunomide

TNF-α inhibitors
Etanercept
Infliximab
Adalimumab

IL-1 antagonist
Anakinra

IL-6 receptor antagonist
Tocilizumab

T cell activation inhibitor
Abatacept

Anti B-lymphocyte antibody
Rituximab

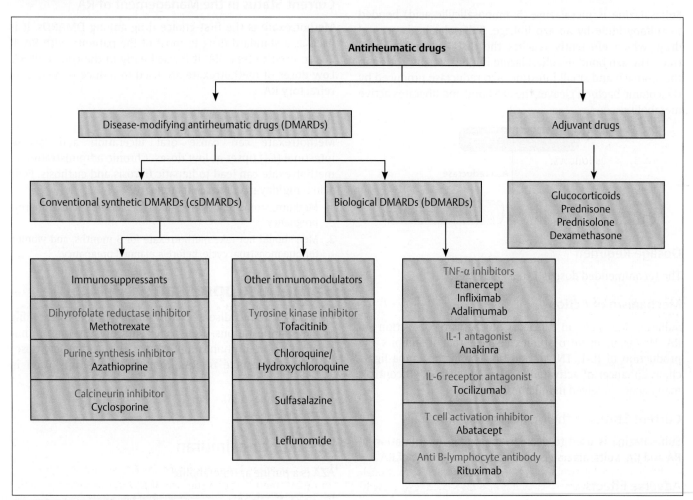

Fig. 45.2 Types of antirheumatic drugs.

Mechanism of Action

CQ/HCQ can reduce monocyte IL-1 and consequently inhibit B-lymphocytes. They can interfere with antigen processing. They stabilize lysosomes and act as free radical scavengers.

Current Status in the Management of RA

CQ/HCQ can induce remission in most of the patients with RA on long-term use of 3 to 6 months. They are used in mild RA, in which only one or few joints are affected. They are also used along with methotrexate or sulfasalazine.

Adverse Effects

CQ/HCQ can accumulate in melanin-rich tissues due to their prolonged use in RA. Accumulation of CQ can cause a toxic lesion on the retina called "bull's-eye" maculopathy, which results in decreased visual acuity. HCQ accumulation causes retinal damage and corneal opacity. HCQ causes reversible and less ocular toxicity when compared to CQ. Hence, HCQ is preferred over CQ. CQ/HCQ can also cause rash, gray hair, irritable bowel syndrome, myopathy, and neuropathy. Patients receiving chronic CQ/HCQ therapy should have periodic eye examinations to reduce the risk of retinal toxicity.

Sulfasalazine

Sulfasalazine is mesalazine (5-aminosalicylic acid) bonded to sulfapyridine by an azo linkage. Sulfasalazine is an oral drug, which efficiently reaches the distal gastrointestinal tract. The azo bond in sulfasalazine inhibits its absorption in the stomach and small intestine. Azo reductase produced by the colonic bacteria cleaves the azo bond and liberates active metabolites.

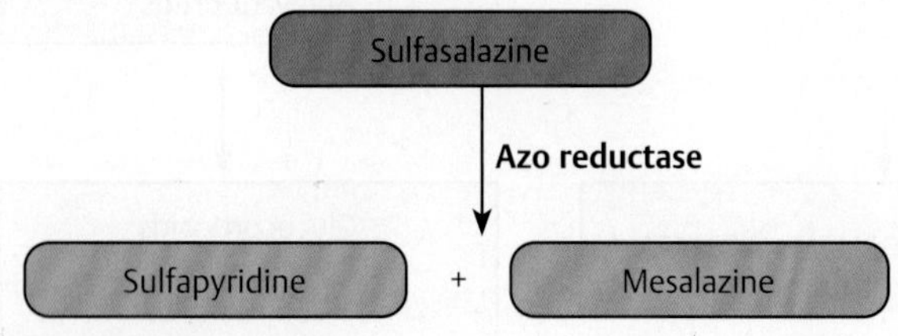

Dosage Regimen

The recommended dose is 1 to 2 g/day.

Mechanism of Action

Sulfasalazine has an unclear mechanism of action in RA. However, in vitro studies suggest that it inhibits the production of IL-1, TNF-α, and nuclear factor kappa-light-chain-enhancer of activated B cells (NF-κB). NF-κB controls many genes involved in inflammation.

Current Status in the Management of RA

Sulfasalazine is used to decrease pain and inflammation in RA and JIA. Sulfasalazine is used early in the course of RA.

Adverse Effects

Sulfasalazine causes dose-related adverse effects including headache, nausea, and fatigue. Dose reduction or medication with meals can decrease such type of adverse effects. Sulfasalazine can cause rash, fever, Stevens–Johnson syndrome, hepatitis, pneumonitis, hemolytic anemia, and bone marrow suppression. It also causes neutropenia or thrombocytopenia in most of the patients. Decreased sperm count occurs while taking sulfasalazine.

Methotrexate: Rheumatrex

Methotrexate is a folate antagonist. It is a potent immunosuppressant with anti-inflammatory property.

Dosage Regimen

The initial dose is usually 5 to 7.5 mg orally, which is taken as a single dose once a week. Clinical response is usually seen in 4 to 8 weeks. If no response is seen even after 8 weeks of therapy, the dose can be increased by 2.5 mg every other week to a maximum of 15 mg once weekly and maintained until improvement occurs.

Mechanism of Action

Methotrexate reduces cytokine production and suppresses cell-mediated immunity. Methotrexate blocks the DNA synthesis by inhibiting dihydrofolate reductase and thus causes cell death.

Current Status in the Management of RA

Methotrexate is the first-choice drug among DMARDs. It is used as a standard drug in most of the patients with RA. It is also used to treat JIA. It is used early in the course of RA. Low doses of methotrexate are used to induce remission in refractory RA.

Adverse Effects

Methotrexate can cause oral ulceration and gastrointestinal (GI) upset at low doses. Chronic administration of methotrexate can lead to hepatic fibrosis and cirrhosis. Folic acid 5 mg/day may reduce its toxicity.

1. Methotrexate is teratogenic, and it should not be used during pregnancy.
2. Men should not take methotrexate for 3 months, and women for one menstrual cycle, before a planned pregnancy.

Immunosuppressants (PH1.50)

RA is a systemic disease with serious vision-threatening ocular manifestations. Hence, it requires systemic immunosuppression. Immunosuppressants are used at low doses early in the course of RA. Immunosuppressants used in RA are:

1. Azathioprine (AZA).
2. Cyclosporine.

Azathioprine: Imuran

AZA is a purine antimetabolite.

Dosage Regimen

The recommended dose is 1 mg/kg/day.

Mechanism of Action

AZA primarily suppresses cell-mediated immunity. It inhibits purine synthesis and thus reduces the production of DNA and RNA needed for the synthesis of white blood cell.

Current Status in the Management of RA

It is used to treat progressive RA.

Adverse Effects

The main adverse effect of AZA is bone marrow suppression, which includes leucopenia (common), thrombocytopenia (less common), and anemia (uncommon). AZA also causes hepatotoxicity, alopecia, GI toxicity, pancreatitis, and high risk of neoplasia. AZA can increase the vulnerability to infections, particularly varicella and herpes simplex viruses.

Cyclosporine

It is a calcineurin inhibitor.

Mechanism of Action

Cyclosporine mainly suppresses cell-mediated immunity. It also causes the suppression of humoral immunity, but it acts more effectively against the mechanisms of T cell–mediated immunity. Nuclear factor of activated T cell cytoplasmic (NFATc) is activated by calcineurin through dephosphorylation. This activated NFATc translocates into nucleus and forms a complex with nuclear components, essential to activate T cells completely, along with the transactivation of IL-2 and other lymphokine genes. Cyclosporine binds with cyclophilin to form a complex. Cyclophilin is a cytoplasmic receptor protein found in target cells. The cyclosporine/cyclophilin complex binds with calcineurin. Thus, the T cell activation is inhibited by the cyclosporine.

Current Status in the Management of RA

Cyclosporine is used to treat patients with severe RA who do not respond to methotrexate. It is also used along with methotrexate by monitoring both drug levels carefully, as cyclosporine has a narrow therapeutic window.

Pharmacokinetics

Oral bioavailability of cyclosporine is 20 to 50%. In the circulation, 50% is bound to erythrocytes, 10% to leucocytes, and 40% to lipoproteins in the plasma. It is almost completely metabolized.

Adverse Effects

Cyclosporine mainly causes nephrotoxicity and hypertension. Nephrotoxicity results in cessation or modification of cyclosporine therapy. Other frequent adverse effects include tremors, hirsutism, hyperlipidemia, and gum hyperplasia.

TNF Inhibitors

In patients with RA, the joints have increased levels of TNF-α. TNF-α is a proinflammatory cytokine, which is secreted by activated macrophages and other immune cells. It activates $TNFR_1$ and $TNFR_2$ receptors found on T cell surface and macrophage surface. TNF inhibitors can neutralize TNF-α and inhibit the activation of TNF receptors. Thus, TNF inhibitors mainly suppress the functions of T cells and macrophages. TNF-α inhibitors used in RA are:

1. Etanercept.
2. Infliximab.
3. Adalimumab.

Etanercept: Enbrel

It is a fusion protein of a human TNF-α receptor and Fc portion of human immunoglobulin G1 (IgG1).

Mechanism of Action

Etanercept inhibits the activation of TNF receptors by binding to TNF-α.

Current Status in the Management of RA

Etanercept is used to treat RA and polyarticular JIA. It is most commonly used along with methotrexate to treat patients who are unresponsive to methotrexate alone.

Adverse Effects

Etanercept causes reactions at injection site, which include erythema, itching, pain, and swelling.

Infliximab: Remicade

It is a chimeric monoclonal antibody.

Dosage Regimen

Intravenous (IV) infusion every 4 to 8 weeks is recommended.

Mechanism of Action

Infliximab binds to TNF-α and inhibits the activation of TNF receptors.

Current Status in the Management of RA

Infliximab is used to treat refractory RA. It can be used along with methotrexate to treat patients who are unresponsive to methotrexate monotherapy. This combination therapy increases the response and reduces the formation of antibodies against infliximab.

Adverse Effects

Acute reaction caused by infliximab infusion involves fever, chills, urticaria, bronchospasm, and anaphylaxis. It can cause increased susceptibility to respiratory infections. It can worsen congestive heart failure.

Adalimumab: Humira

It is a recombinant human IgG1 monoclonal antibody.

Mechanism of Action

Adalimumab binds to TNF-α and inhibits the activation of TNF receptors.

Current Status in the Management of RA

Adalimumab is used to treat RA and JIA. Use of adalimumab in combination with methotrexate increases the response and reduces the formation of antibodies.

Adverse Effects

Adalimumab can cause injection site reaction and respiratory infections.

IL-1 Antagonists

Patients with active inflammation have increased levels of IL-1 in their plasma. IL-1 is a proinflammatory cytokine. An IL-1 antagonist used in RA is anakinra.

Anakinra: Kineret

It is a recombinant human IL-1 receptor antagonist.

Mechanism of Action

Anakinra competes with IL-1 to bind with the receptor and blocks the activity of IL-1.

Current Status in the Management of RA

Anakinra is used to treat refractory RA. It is used in patients who do not respond to other DMARDs. It is also used in combination with methotrexate and TNF-α inhibitors to improve its efficacy.

Adverse Effects

Anakinra mainly causes local reactions as well as chest infections.

Glucocorticoids

Synthetic glucocorticoids are used regularly due to their immunosuppressive as well as anti-inflammatory properties. They can be used at any stage of RA in combination with first- or second-line drugs. Commonly used glucocorticoids in RA are:

1. Prednisone.
2. Prednisolone.
3. Dexamethasone.

Dosage Regimen

Oral glucocorticoids produce dramatic symptomatic relief, which lasts as long as they are used. Prednisolone is started in the dose of 1 mg/kg/day, and then decreased gradually to a maintenance dose of 7.5 mg/day. The small maintenance dose may be continued as needed.

Mechanism of Action

Glucocorticoids negatively regulate the genes for COX-2 and inflammatory cytokines. They decrease the levels of IL-1. They inhibit NF-κB activation, T cell proliferation, and cytotoxic T lymphocyte activation. They also inhibit the functions of neutrophils and monocytes. Their protein interactions suppress the expression of genes that encode many cytokines and enzymes, such as collagenase and stromelysin. These cytokines and enzymes are mainly responsible for joint destruction in inflammatory arthritis. Thus, the negative effects on gene expression contribute to the anti-inflammatory and immunosuppressive effects of the glucocorticoids.

Current Status in the Management of RA

Glucocorticoids provide rapid relief within hours of therapy. Hence, short-term use of glucocorticoids is generally recommended for quick control of inflammation. High doses can be started and decreased gradually, based on the size and number of joints involved. Glucocorticoids are injected intra-articularly if only a few joints are involved.

Adverse Effects

Glucocorticoids on long-term use cause adrenal suppression. They can cause increased blood glucose levels, increased weight, and increased risk of infections. They can also cause hypertension, cushingoid habitus, osteoporosis, glaucoma, cataracts, depression, anxiety, and psychosis.

Principles of Management of RA (Fig. 45.3)

Diagnostic Confirmation

High levels (more than 20 IU/mL) of RF occur in the blood of patients with RA. Presence of RF and anti-CCP in combination with signs and symptoms can play an important role in the diagnosis of RA. Other diagnostic evaluations include physical examination and X-ray.

Nonpharmacological Treatment

RA is a chronic disease, which needs supportive therapy along with drug therapy.

1. Physiotherapy.
2. Occupational therapy.
3. Use of firm mattress.
4. Recumbent position.
5. Physical and mental rest.
6. Splinting of affected joints.
7. Use of warm baths and hot packs.
8. Immobilization of inflamed joints for 4 weeks, followed by active exercises.
9. Treatment of comorbid states such as osteoporosis, cardiovascular (CV) disorders, and depression.

Surgery

When drugs cannot control the severe joint pain in RA, surgery can be done to restore the joint function. The most common surgeries are:

1. **Joint replacement:** The most common joints replaced are knees and hips.

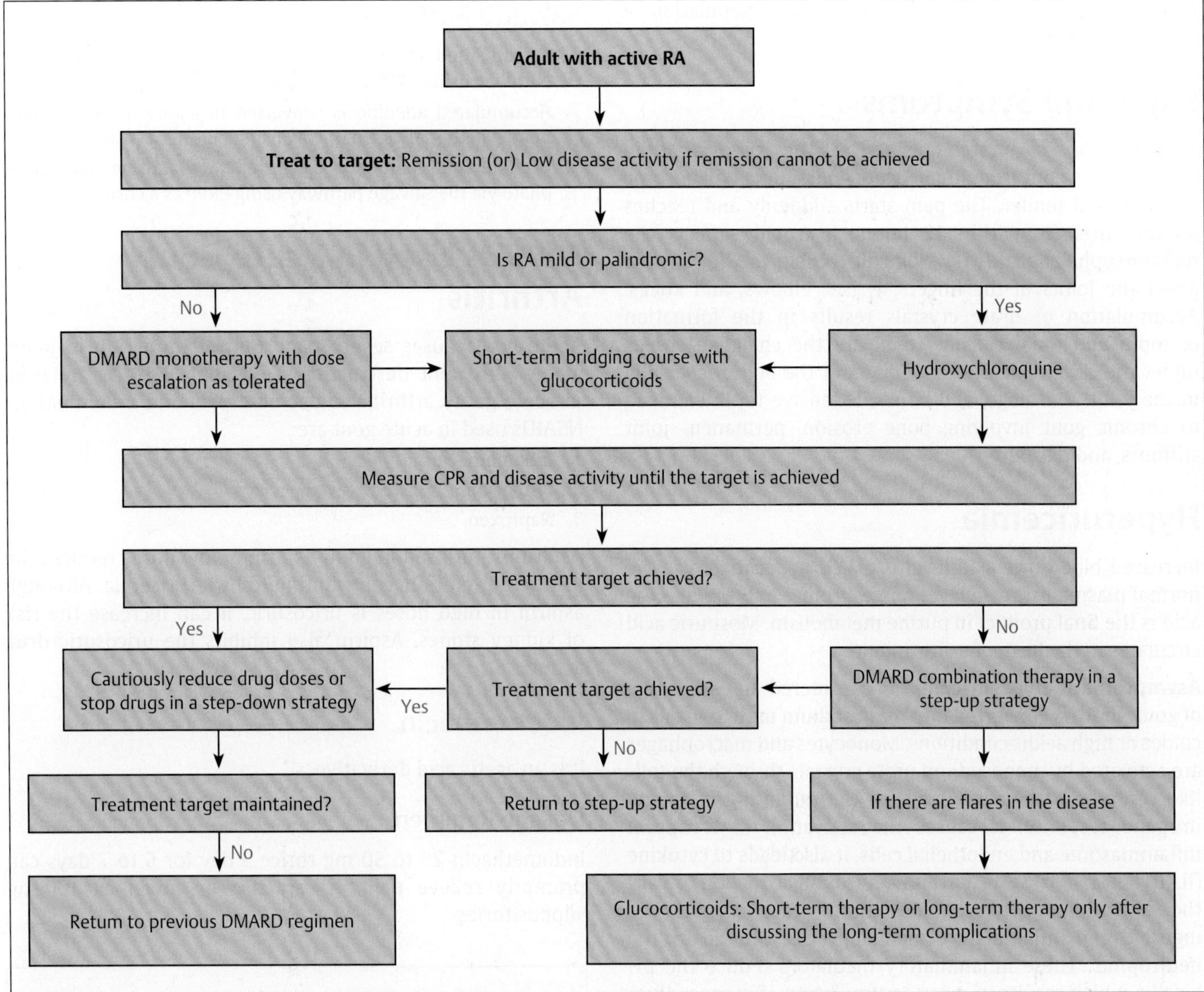

Fig. 45.3 Management of RA. DMARD, Disease-modifying anti-rheumatic drug; RA, rheumatoid arthritis.

2. **Synovectomy:** The synovial tissue surrounding the affected joint is removed.
3. **Arthrodesis:** Joint fusion is done to relieve intractable joint pain.

Combination Therapy in RA

Indications

1. Combination therapy is used when monotherapy is no longer effective.
2. Sometimes, combination therapy is used to minimize the adverse effects.
3. Combination therapy is used because it is well tolerated when compared to monotherapy.

Dual Therapy

Methotrexate in combination with other DMARDs is used in patients with RA who are unresponsive to methotrexate monotherapy. A popular dual therapy used to treat RA is methotrexate–sulfasalazine. Other methotrexate combinations used in RA are:

1. Methotrexate–CQ.
2. Methotrexate–cyclosporine.
3. Methotrexate–AZA.
4. Methotrexate–leflunomide.
5. Methotrexate–adalimumab.
6. Methotrexate–infliximab.
7. Methotrexate–etanercept.
8. Methotrexate–doxycycline.

Triple Therapy

Triple DMARD therapy is more effective than monotherapy and dual therapy. A popular triple therapy used to treat RA is methotrexate–sulfasalazine–hydroxychloroquine.

Gout

Gout is a type of arthritis arising from the urate crystal accumulation in the joints. It is characterized by severe pain and inflammation in joints. Obesity, high purine diet (meat and fish), and excess alcohol consumption are the main risk factors of gout. Older men are mostly affected by gout. Gout was historically referred to as “the disease of kings” or “rich man's disease." Gout affects 3% of the adult population of western countries.

Signs and Symptoms

Accumulation of urate crystals in the synovial fluid differentiates gout from RA. In acute gout, joints will become red, hot, and tender. The pain starts suddenly and reaches its full intensity within 12 hours. It usually affects the metatarsophalangeal (MTP) joint of the big toe. It can also affect the joints of the fingers, wrists, elbows, and knees. Accumulation of urate crystals results in the formation of tophi and renal calculi. Tophi are the chalklike stones under the skin, which form throughout the body, especially in the joints, cartilage, and bones. Extensive tophi can lead to chronic gout involving bone erosion, permanent joint stiffness, and disability.

Hyperuricemia

Increased blood uric acid level is called hyperuricemia. The normal plasma uric acid level ranges from 2 to 6 mg/dL. Uric acid is the final product in purine metabolism. Most uric acid circulates in the form of urate anion.

Asymptomatic hyperuricemia is considered an early stage of gout. Urate is converted into monosodium urate crystals in colder or high acidic conditions. Monocytes and macrophages are activated by monosodium urate crystals through the toll-like receptor pathway. It leads to the mounting of innate immune response. It causes the activation of cryopyrin inflammasome and endothelial cells. It also leads to cytokine (IL-1β and TNF-α) secretion and neutrophil attraction toward the inflammatory site. Monosodium urate crystals are ingested and inflammatory mediators are secreted by the neutrophils. These inflammatory mediators reduce the pH locally, which results in more accumulation of monosodium urate. It leads to acute attack of gouty arthritis involving sudden and severe inflammation in joints. In acute gout, the MTP joint of the big toe is mostly affected.

Long-standing hyperuricemia results in the formation of tophi and renal calculi. Tophi are the chalklike stones under the skin, which form throughout the body, especially in the joints, cartilage, and bones. Extensive tophi can lead to chronic gout involving bone erosion, permanent joint stiffness, and disability.

Purine Metabolism (Fig. 45.4)

1. Purines (adenine and guanine) are the derivatives of the nucleotide inosine monophosphate (IMP).
2. IMP is a derivative of de novo synthesis that involves phosphoribosyl pyrophosphate (PRPP).
3. Hypoxanthine, xanthine, and uric acid are the purine derivatives involved in purine metabolism. The main enzyme responsible for the purine metabolism is xanthine oxidase.
4. Xanthine oxidase converts hypoxanthine to xanthine. In xanthine oxidase–deficient patients, xanthine is formed from guanine.
5. Xanthine oxidase also converts xanthine into uric acid.
6. Uric acid is the final product in purine metabolism.

Salvage Pathway

1. Accumulated hypoxanthine is converted to IMP via the salvage pathway using PRPP as a cosubstrate.
2. Accumulated adenine is converted to adenosine monophosphate via the salvage pathway using PRPP as a cosubstrate.
3. Accumulated guanine is converted to guanosine monophosphate via the salvage pathway using PRPP as a cosubstrate.

NSAIDs Used in Acute Gouty Arthritis

Acute gout causes severe pain and inflammation in joints along with joint destruction. Traditional NSAIDs are used in acute gouty arthritis to decrease pain and inflammation. NSAIDs used in acute gout are:

1. Indomethacin.
2. Piroxicam.
3. Naproxen.

Aspirin is not used in gout. Aspirin in low doses reduces the uric acid excretion, contributing to hyperuricemia. Although aspirin in high doses is uricosuric, it can increase the risk of kidney stones. Aspirin also inhibits the uricosuric drug action.

Indomethacin

It is an acetic acid derivative.

Dosage Regimen

Indomethacin 25 to 50 mg thrice a day for 5 to 7 days can promptly relieve pain. It can also be given as 100-mg suppositories.

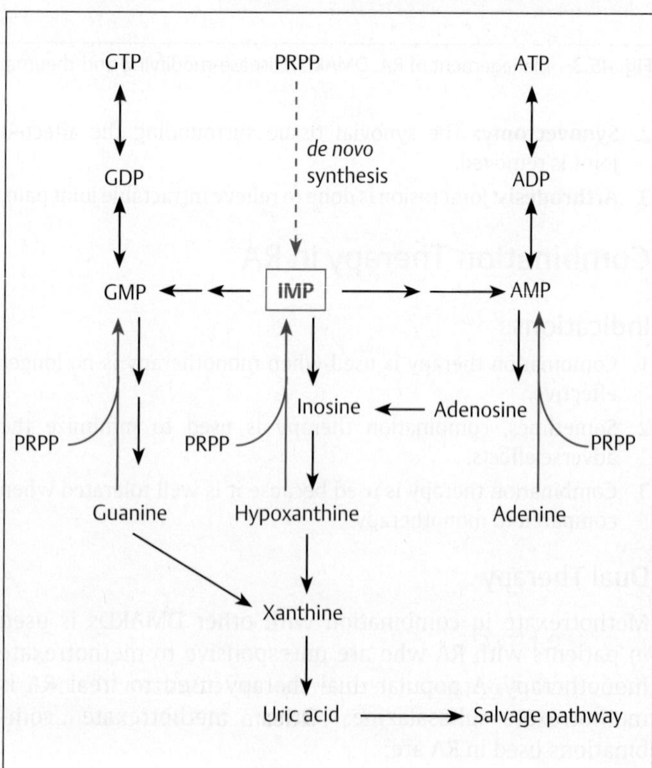

Fig. 45.4 Purine metabolism.

Role in Acute Attack of Gouty Arthritis

Indomethacin is used in acute attack of gouty arthritis due to its potent anti-inflammatory activity. It is effective in relieving pain, swelling, and tenderness of the joints.

Mechanism of Action

Indomethacin nonselectively inhibits the COX enzyme. The motility of polymorphonuclear leukocytes and neutrophils is also inhibited by indomethacin. Indomethacin inhibits PG synthesis as well.

Adverse Effects

Indomethacin causes GI toxicity, which includes gastric irritation, nausea, anorexia, diarrhea, and gastric bleeding. The most frequent central nervous system (CNS) effect occurring from long-term use of indomethacin is severe frontal headache. Other CNS adverse effects include dizziness, vertigo, light-headedness, and mental confusion. Indomethacin can cause seizures, depression, psychosis, hallucinations, and suicide. Indomethacin can also cause hematopoietic reactions such as neutropenia, thrombocytopenia, and aplastic anemia.

Piroxicam: Feldene

Piroxicam is an enolic acid derivative.

Dosage Regimen

The usual daily dose is 20 mg.

Therapeutic Use

It is used to treat acute gout. It is a long-acting, potent NSAID.

Pharmacokinetics

The onset of action of piroxicam is slow, and the attainment of steady state is delayed. It is rapidly and completely absorbed.

Role in Acute Attack of Gouty Arthritis

Piroxicam is used in the treatment of acute attack of gouty arthritis due to its potent anti-inflammatory and analgesic activities. It decreases the concentration of PGs in synovial fluid. It decreases leucocyte chemotaxis. It inhibits the activation of neutrophils.

Mechanism of Action

Piroxicam can inhibit inflammation in many ways. Piroxicam nonselectively and reversibly inhibits the COX enzyme. It decreases the synovial fluid PG levels. It decreases leucocyte chemotaxis. It inhibits the activation of neutrophils.

Adverse Effects

High doses of piroxicam frequently cause ulcers and bleeding in GI tract. Low doses of piroxicam are less ulcerogenic. Other adverse effects include rashes, pruritus, edema, and reversible azotemia.

Naproxen: Aleve

Naproxen is a propionic acid derivative.

Dosage Regimen

Initial dose of 750 mg is recommended, followed by 250 mg every 8 hours till the attack declines.

Therapeutic Use

It is used to treat acute gout.

Role in Acute Attack of Gouty Arthritis

Naproxen is used in the treatment of acute attack of gouty arthritis due to its potent anti-inflammatory activity. Naproxen prominently inhibits the leukocyte function. It may have slightly better efficacy in providing analgesia.

Mechanism of Action

Naproxen nonselectively inhibits the COX enzyme. Leucocyte migration is inhibited by naproxen.

Adverse Effects

Naproxen causes a typical and slightly severe upper GI toxicity. CNS toxicity includes drowsiness, headache, dizziness, sweating, fatigue, depression, and ototoxicity. Naproxen causes pruritus and a variety of skin problems. It can also cause jaundice, angioedema, thrombocytopenia, agranulocytosis, and impairment of renal function.

Analgesic Nephropathy

High risk of analgesic nephropathy can be caused due to the chronic use of NSAID combinations in high doses. Analgesic nephropathy is characterized by renal failure progression, which occurs slowly with decreased renal tubule concentrating ability and sterile pyuria. Risk of analgesic nephropathy can also be enhanced by frequent urinary tract infections. Discontinuation of NSAIDs after the recognition of analgesic nephropathy may result in the recovery of renal function.

Risk Factors Associated with NSAIDs

1. Prevalence of serious adverse effects of NSAIDs increases with age. Hence, caution should be taken while choosing dose for elderly patients. In elderly patients, "start low and go slow" approach is more effective while prescribing NSAIDs.
2. NSAIDs can aggravate peptic ulcer disease. Oral NSAIDs can irritate the gastric mucosa and cause ulcers. Due to this local irritation, acid diffuses back into the mucosal layer of GI tract and damages the tissues.
3. Kidney function can be worsened by NSAIDs, especially in patients with renal disease, cardiac disease, and cirrhosis.
4. NSAIDs' labeling includes a black box warning with cardiovascular risks. NSAIDs should not be used after a recent coronary artery bypass graft surgery.
5. Seizure threshold is reduced by NSAIDs.

Colchicine

Colchicine is an alkaloid obtained from *Colchicum autumnale*.

Pharmacological Basis

Colchicine is the oldest available drug used to treat acute gout. Colchicine effectively treats acute gout and prevents recurrent gout.

Mechanism of Action

Colchicine inhibits microtubule formation. In affected joints, monosodium urate crystals are coated by either anti-IgG antibodies or lipoprotein containing apolipoprotein. Then, they are ingested by granulocytes. These granulocytes then release a glycoprotein, which increases neutrophil infiltration into the joint. Colchicine binds to tubulin, depolymerizes microtubules in the granulocytes, and interferes with the mitotic spindles. It results in decreased neutrophil migration into the inflamed area. Thus, it prevents the intra-articular release of inflammatory mediators by neutrophils. It also inhibits the mast-cell release of histamine.

Pharmacokinetics

Oral absorption of colchicine is variable. Colchicine is 50% protein-bound and accumulates in the kidney, liver, and spleen. It undergoes enterohepatic circulation. Urinary excretion is only 10 to 20%. Its plasma $t_{1/2}$ is 9 hours. Patients with hepatic or renal damage should not use colchicine.

Indications

Colchicine is used in the treatment of acute gouty arthritis and in the prevention of recurrent gout. It is also used to prevent attacks of familial Mediterranean fever.

Treatment of Acute Gout Using Colchicine

Colchicine can control an acute attack of gout due to its fast action. It is administered orally in a single dose of 1.2 mg, followed by 0.6 mg after an hour. Pain, swelling, and redness decrease within 12 hours and disappear within 48 to 72 hours. Colchicine is used intravenously in the treatment of acute gouty arthritis when other medications are ineffective, when the patient is not able to take medications orally, or when rapid therapeutic intervention is required. Therapy should not be repeated within 4 days to prevent cumulative toxicity.

The response to colchicine is specific to gout. Hence, colchicine therapeutic trial may be used as a diagnostic tool in differentiating gouty arthritis from other forms of arthritis. Colchicine is valuable in patients with heart failure, as it does not cause fluid retention. It can also be given to patients receiving anticoagulants.

Prevention of Recurrent Gout Using Colchicine

Colchicine is mainly indicated to prevent the recurrent gout. Prophylactic administration of 0.6 mg twice daily for 6 months can reduce the frequency of attacks in patients having three or more attacks in a year. Long-term use of colchicine in small doses is better tolerated than NSAIDs.

Adverse Effects

Colchicine mostly causes nausea, vomiting, diarrhea, and abdominal pain. As soon as these adverse effects are observed, colchicine administration should be withdrawn.

Colchicine Toxicity

Accumulation of colchicine in the intestine is responsible for toxicity. Colchicine should not be administered within 7 days to prevent the cumulative toxicity.

Acute colchicine toxicity can cause:

1. Ascending paralysis of the CNS.
2. Hemorrhagic gastropathy.

Colchicine toxicity due to chronic use can cause:

1. Proteinuria, hematuria, and acute tubular necrosis.
2. Disseminated intravascular coagulation.
3. Bone marrow suppression.
4. Proximal myopathy.
5. Gouty nephropathy.
6. Thrombocytopenia.
7. Agranulocytosis.
8. Azoospermia.

Xanthine Oxidase Inhibitors

1. Allopurinol.
2. Febuxostat.

Allopurinol: Zyloprim

Allopurinol is 4-hydroxypyrazolo-(3,4-d)pyrimidine.

Dosage Regimen

The initial dose of allopurinol is 100 mg per day. Serum uric acid levels are monitored after 2 weeks of allopurinol administration. The dose can be increased gradually every 2 weeks till the level of serum uric acid falls below 6 mg%. The maximum approved dose is 800 mg/day. A single dose is preferred as the half-life of the active metabolite, oxypurinol, is about 20 hours. In chronic renal failure, the dose of allopurinol should be reduced in the same proportion as glomerular filtration rate (GFR).

Therapeutic Use

Allopurinol is mainly used for the long-term treatment and prevention of gout. It is used to control hyperuricemia. It can be used in patients with tophi, uric acid renal calculi, and renal failure. Allopurinol may be combined with uricosuric drugs. Secondary hyperuricemia occurs following the use of cytotoxic drugs in the treatment of leukemia and lymphoma. Hence, allopurinol is started before starting chemotherapy. Initiation of allopurinol therapy during an acute attack of gout can cause high risk of gout flares.

Mechanism of Action

Allopurinol is a xanthine oxidase inhibitor (XOI). It prevents uric acid synthesis by inhibiting xanthine oxidase enzyme. Due to the inhibition of xanthine oxidase, both the synthesis of xanthine from hypoxanthine and the synthesis of uric acid from xanthine are inhibited (**Fig. 45.5**).

Allopurinol is a competitive inhibitor of xanthine oxidase at low concentrations. However, it noncompetitively inhibits the xanthine oxidase at high concentrations. Xanthine oxidase metabolizes allopurinol. The primary metabolite of allopurinol is alloxanthine. Alloxanthine is also known as oxypurinol and is a noncompetitive XOI. Most of the pharmacological activity of allopurinol is exerted by alloxanthine, as it is persistent in tissues for a long time.

Adverse Effects

Most of the patients can tolerate allopurinol. Allopurinol mostly precipitates an acute flare of gout. It is due to the decreasing of urate, which leads to the shedding of urate crystals from articular cartilage into the joint space and results in acute inflammation.

Allopurinol also causes hypersensitivity reactions that can occur after months or years of treatment with it. It causes pruritic, erythematous, or maculopapular eruption. It rarely causes toxic epidermal necrolysis or Stevens–Johnson syndrome. Stevens–Johnson syndrome can be fatal, and it can occur only within the first 2 months of allopurinol therapy. In most of the patients, rash may occur before the occurrence of severe hypersensitivity reactions. Hence, allopurinol should be discontinued in patients who develop a rash.

Allopurinol also causes fever, malaise, and myalgias. These effects are more frequent in patients with renal impairment. Rare reactions caused by allopurinol include transient leukopenia or leukocytosis and eosinophilia. If these reactions occur, treatment with allopurinol may need to be discontinued. Allopurinol can also cause hepatomegaly, progressive renal insufficiency, and elevated levels of transaminases in plasma.

Drug Interactions

Allopurinol can interact with many drugs. **Table 45.1** includes a list of important drug interactions of allopurinol.

Febuxostat: Uloric

Febuxostat is a nonpurine analog of allopurinol.

Dosage Regimen

Febuxostat is orally active. The maximum daily dose is 80 mg.

Therapeutic Use

Febuxostat is used in the treatment of gout. It is well tolerated and can be used in patients with allopurinol intolerance. It is also used in patients allergic to allopurinol.

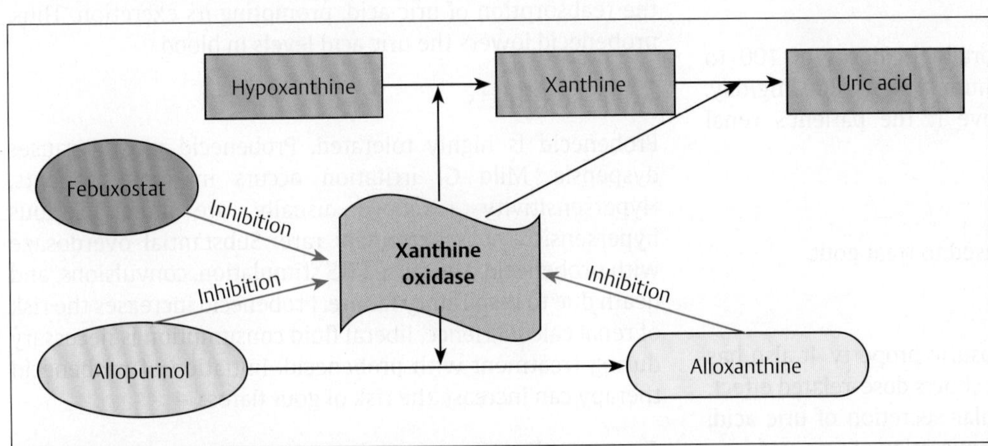

Fig. 45.5 Mechanism of action of xanthine oxidase inhibitor (XOI).

Table 45.1 List of important drug interactions of allopurinol

Interacting drugs	Outcomes
6-Mercaptopurine (6-MP)	Enzymatic inactivation of 6-MP is inhibited. Hence, the dose of 6-MP should be decreased to one-third
Azathioprine (AZA)	Enzymatic inactivation of AZA is inhibited. Hence, the dose of AZA should be decreased to one-third
Probenecid	$t_{1/2}$ of probenecid is increased, which leads to increased uricosuric effect of probenecid $t_{1/2}$ of alloxanthine is decreased, which leads to increased clearance of alloxanthine, resulting in the increased dose requirements of allopurinol
Warfarin	Metabolism of warfarin is inhibited, making it more potent
Ampicillin	Risk of skin rashes is increased
Cyclosporine	Metabolism of cyclosporine is decreased, which leads to increase in blood concentrations
Cyclophosphamide	Risk of bone marrow suppression is increased
Thiazide diuretic	Hypersensitivity reactions can occur in patients with compromised renal function
Theophylline	Accumulation of 1-methylxanthine (active metabolite of theophylline) is increased

Pharmacokinetics

Febuxostat is mainly metabolized in the liver. Mild-to-moderate renal insufficiency does not alter its serum uric acid–lowering ability.

Mechanism of Action

Febuxostat is an XOI. It inhibits purine metabolism by inhibiting the enzyme, xanthine oxidase. Thus, it reduces the uric acid levels.

Adverse Effects

Febuxostat can cause liver function abnormalities, headache, nausea, and Steven–Johnson syndrome.

Uricosuric Agents

Uricosuric agents enhance the uric acid excretion by preventing its reabsorption through organic anion transporters. The drugs that come under uricosuric agents are:

1. Probenecid.
2. Sulfinpyrazone.
3. Benzbromarone.

Sulfinpyrazone

It is a sulfoxide derivative of phenylbutazone.

Dosage Regimen

Sulfinpyrazone is administered orally in doses of 100 to 200 mg thrice a day. The maximum dose is 600 mg/day. Sulfinpyrazone becomes ineffective if the patient's renal function is impaired.

Therapeutic Use

Sulfinpyrazone is less commonly used to treat gout.

Mechanism of Action

Sulfinpyrazone has a marked uricosuric property. It also has some anti-inflammatory activity. It shows dose-related effect. In low doses, it prevents the tubular secretion of uric acid, while in high doses it promotes the excretion of uric acid.

Adverse Effects

Sulfinpyrazone causes vomiting, upper abdominal discomfort, and skin rashes. It can cause bone marrow depression. It inhibits platelet aggregation.

Benzbromarone

It is a benzofuran compound.

Therapeutic Use

Benzbromarone is less commonly used to treat gout.

Mechanism of Action

Benzbromarone shows potent uricosuric activity. It is effective even when the GFR is reduced to 25 to 50% of normal.

Probenecid: Probalan

Probenecid is a uricosuric agent.

Therapeutic Use

Probenecid is used in the treatment of gout and hyperuricemia due to its uricosuric property. Low doses of probenecid decrease the distal tubular secretion of uric acid. However, high therapeutic doses of probenecid increase the excretion of uric acid by blocking tubular reabsorption. After treatment for some months, the serum uric acid may return to its normal levels together with considerable mobilization of gouty tophi.

Dosage Regimen

Probenecid is given orally. It is given initially in doses of 0.5 g once daily, gradually increasing to three times daily.

Mechanism of Action

Probenecid competitively inhibits the active transport of organic acids by organic anion transporting polypeptides (OATPs) at all sites, mainly in the renal tubules. Active transport results in large reabsorption of uric acid. Only 1/10th of the filtered uric acid is eliminated through urine. The main transporter responsible for the uric acid reabsorption is urate transporter 1 (URAT-1) URAT-1 belongs to the OATP family. Therefore, probenecid blocks the reabsorption of uric acid, promoting its excretion. Thus, probenecid lowers the uric acid levels in blood.

Adverse Effects

Probenecid is highly tolerated. Probenecid mostly causes dyspepsia. Mild GI irritation occurs in some patients. Hypersensitivity reactions usually are mild. Serious hypersensitivity is extremely rare. Substantial overdosage with probenecid can cause CNS stimulation, convulsions, and death due to respiratory failure. Probenecid increases the risk of renal calculi. Hence, liberal fluid consumption is necessary during treatment with probenecid. Initiation of probenecid therapy can increase the risk of gout flares.

Contraindications

Probenecid is contraindicated in patients having:

1. Known probenecid allergy.
2. A history of peptic ulcer.
3. Creatinine clearance of <50 mL/minute.
4. Overproduction of uric acid.
5. Nephrolithiasis.

Treatment of Acute Gouty Arthritis (Fig. 45.6)

Diagnostic Confirmation

The diagnostic confirmation of acute gouty arthritis is mainly done by synovial fluid test. The synovial fluid from the affected joint is collected for evaluation. Acute gout is

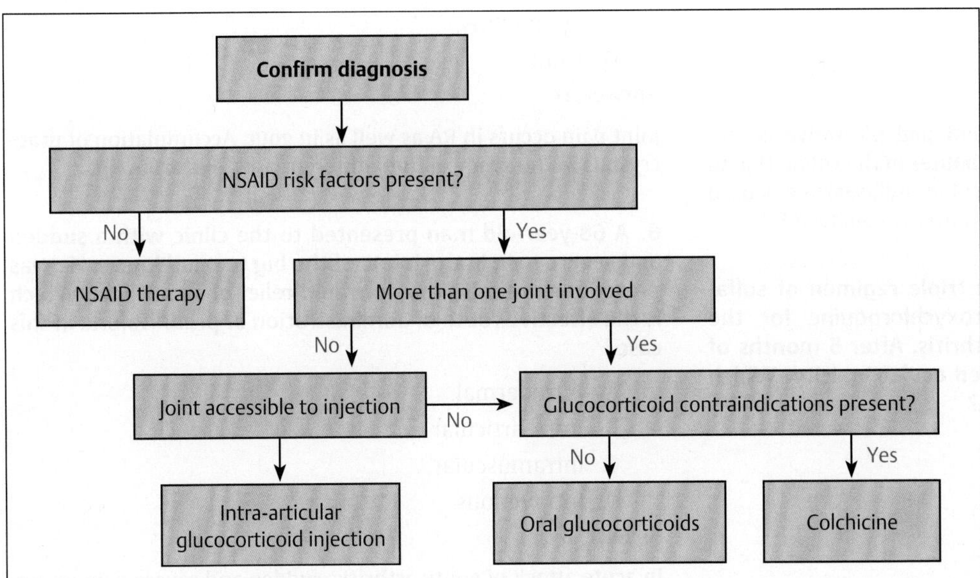

Fig. 45.6 Treatment of acute gout.

diagnosed by the presence of monosodium urate crystals in the synovial fluid. Synovial fluid test is considered as a gold standard test for the diagnosis of acute gout. Other diagnostic evaluations include blood test to measure the serum urate levels, physical examination, and X-ray.

Nonpharmacological Treatment

1. Control of comorbid conditions such as obesity, metabolic syndrome, hypertension, hyperlipidemia, diabetes, and chronic kidney disease.
2. Lifestyle changes such as regular exercise and weight reduction.
3. Regular consumption of cereals, pulses, fruits, vegetables, nuts, and low-fat milk.
4. Avoid consumption of high-purine diet such as meat and fish.
5. Minimize consumption of fatty food.
6. Cessation of smoking and alcohol consumption.

The symptoms can be reduced by the application of ice on the affected area and by taking rest.

Drugs Therapy

The drugs used to treat acute gouty arthritis are:

1. NSAIDs.
2. Glucocorticoids.
3. Colchicine.

Uric Acid Nephrolithiasis

Uric acid nephrolithiasis is the development of uric acid calculi in the kidney. Long-standing hyperuricemia causes uric acid nephrolithiasis. It subsequently leads to acute uric acid nephropathy.

Risk Factors

1. Low-urine volume.
2. Acidic urine.
3. Hyperuricosuria.

Treatment

Dietary Therapy

1. Scheduled fluid to increase urine output.
2. Dietary purine restriction.
3. Dietary protein restriction.

Urine Alkalinization

Alkalinization of urine is done by the administration of IV sodium bicarbonate. It is done to maintain the urine pH level > 7. It increases the solubility of uric acid. However, there should be adequate urine flow around the calculi. Allopurinol is used to reduce the overproduction of uric acid.

Multiple Choice Questions

1. A 12-year-old girl is presented to the clinic with swelling and stiffness in the joints of her hands. She is diagnosed with rheumatoid arthritis. The following drugs can be used for the treatment except:

A. Methotrexate.
B. Sulfasalazine.
C. Azathioprine.
D. Adalimumab.

Answer: C

Rheumatoid arthritis occurring in children is called juvenile idiopathic arthritis (JIA). Azathioprine is not used in JIA.

2. A 58-year-old woman with a 3-month history of rheumatoid arthritis was presented to the clinic with lower abdominal pain and bloody diarrhea. Colonoscopy revealed ulcerative lesions. Which of the following antirheumatic drugs can be used to treat her symptoms?

A. Azathioprine.
B. Sulfasalazine.

C. Cyclosporine.

D. Methotrexate.

Answer: B

Colonoscopy indicates that the patient had ulcerative colitis. Sulfasalazine liberates its active metabolites in the colon. Due to its anti-inflammatory activity in the colon, sulfasalazine is used to treat ulcerative colitis. It is used in the early course of RA.

3. A patient is being treated with triple regimen of sulfasalazine, methotrexate, and hydroxychloroquine for the treatment of active rheumatoid arthritis. After 5 months of triple therapy, the patient developed ocular toxicity. Which of the following might be the cause?

A. Sulfasalazine.

B. Methotrexate.

C. Hydroxychloroquine.

D. All of the above.

Answer: C

Hydroxychloroquine on long-term use can cause ocular toxicity.

4. A 60-year-old woman complained of stiffness in both her knees and wrists, which lasts for more than 1 hour every morning. Which of the following class of drugs can be used as a treatment?

A. Cyclooxygenase inhibitors.

B. Xanthine oxidase inhibitors.

C. Uricosuric agents.

D. Microtubule inhibitors.

Answer: A

Morning stiffness that lasts for more than 1 hour indicates rheumatoid arthritis. Symmetrical joint swelling is also seen in RA. Nonsteroidal anti-inflammatory drugs (NSAIDs) such as cyclooxygenase inhibitors are used to treat both RA and gout.

5. A 63-year-old man presented to the clinic with severe and frequent attacks of joint pains in wrists, elbows, knees, and ankles. Synovial fluid test revealed the presence of urate crystals. Which can be the most likely diagnosis in this case?

A. Rheumatoid arthritis.

B. Osteoarthritis.

C. Spondylitis.

D. Gout.

Answer: D

Joint pain occurs in RA as well as in gout. Accumulation of urate crystals in the synovial fluid differentiates gout from RA.

6. A 68-year-old man presented to the clinic with a sudden and severe pain in the joints of the big toe and knees. He was prescribed prednisolone for rapid relief of symptoms. Which is the effective route of administration of prednisolone in this case?

A. Intradermal.

B. Intra-articular.

C. Intramuscular.

D. Intravenous.

Answer: B

In acute attack of gouty arthritis, sudden and severe pain occurs in the joints, especially in the big toe joint. Glucocorticoids are used to provide rapid relief in acute gouty arthritis. They are injected intra-articularly if only a few joints are involved.

7. A 70-year-old man complained of extremely painful and swollen right foot. Blood tests showed excess uric acid levels. Which of the following NSAIDs is not a drug of choice in this case?

A. Indomethacin.

B. Piroxicam.

C. Aspirin.

D. Naproxen.

Answer: C

Painful swelling of specific joint and presence of excess uric acid in blood indicate gout. Aspirin is not to be used in gout, as it can contribute to hyperuricemia in low doses and kidney stones in high doses.

Part VII

Drugs Used in Respiratory System

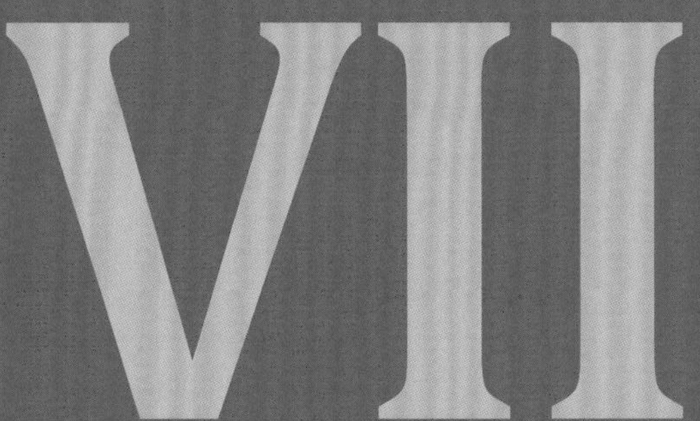

Chapter 46

Pharmacotherapy of Bronchial Asthma

Farhana Dutta Majumder

PH1.32: Describe the mechanism of action, types, doses, side effects, indications, and contraindications of the drugs used in bronchial asthma and chronic obstructive pulmonary disorder (COPD).

Learning Objectives

- Bronchodilators.
- Leukotriene receptor antagonist.
- Mast cell stabilizer.
- Corticosteroids.
- Status asthmaticus.

Introduction

Asthma is a frequent disease and ranges in severity from a very mild, sporadic wheeze to acute, life-threatening airway closure. It commonly manifests in childhood and is accompanied with other symptoms of atopy like eczema and hay fever. It is a very regular childhood disorder causing hospital admissions and rising health care costs. The important characteristic is airway hyperresponsiveness, which may be precipitated due to numerous factors. If not managed quickly, asthma has a high mortality.

Pathophysiology

Earlier it was thought that asthma was due to bronchospasm, and treatment involved relieving bronchospasm by bronchodilator. In 1980, researchers demonstrated a major advance in the understanding of asthma as a heterogeneous disorder, which is characterized by airway obstruction, airway inflammation, airway hyperresponsiveness, and airway modelling. Various risk factors which could be associated with asthma are viral respiratory tract infections in infancy, environmental exposure (aeroallergens, pollution, and tobacco smoke), lifestyle (living on a farm, diet and antibiotic use), comorbid conditions (atopic dermatitis, obesity), occupational exposure, and also genetic factors. Exacerbation factors are allergens, infections, exercise, nonsteroidal anti-inflammation drugs (NSAIDs), gastroesophageal reflux, psychosocial factors, etc.

Cellular Mechanism of Asthma

Acute phase of asthma is mainly due to allergic inflammation. Allergic inflammation occurs mainly due to CD4 + T-helper 2 (Th2) lymphocytes which secrete interleukin (IL)-4, IL-5, and IL-13. This type of pattern of inflammation is called type 2 (T2) asthma. Eosinophils are also an important characteristic feature of allergic inflammation. Families of cytokines and chemokines (e.g., IL-5, RANTES, and eotaxin) recruit eosinophils to the airways of asthmatic patients and cause persistent inflammations.

Molecular Mechanism of Asthma

Studies in recent years also shows that Th9 cells play an important role in inflammation. Cytokines such as IL-21 and tumor necrosis factor-α (TNF-α) promote differentiation and proliferation through TNFR2-STAT5 signaling pathway and NF-κB signaling pathway of Th9 cells. Th9 cells in some studies show that it secretes IL-9 and could promote the expression of various chemokines in bronchial epithelial cells, such as eosinophils and mast cells and aggravated respiratory inflammation.

Classification of Drugs for Bronchial Asthma (CT2.16)

1. **Bronchodilators**
   a. **β_2-sympathomimetics**
      i. Short-acting beta-agonists (SABA)—albuterol (salbutamol), levalbuterol, metaproterenol, terbutaline, pirbuterol, enoterol, tulobuterol, and rimiterol.
      ii. Long-acting beta-agonist (LABA)—salmeterol, formoterol, and arformoterol.
      iii. Ultralong-acting beta-agonist–indacaterol, vilanterol, and olodaterol.
   b. **Methylxanthines**
      Theophylline, aminophylline, hydroxyethyl theophylline, doxophylline.
   c. **Anticholinergics**
      Ipratropium, tiotropium.
2. **Leukotriene receptor antagonist**
   Montelukast, zafirlukast.
3. **Mast cell stabilizer**
   Sodium cromoglycate.
4. **Corticosteroids**
   a. Systemic corticosteroids–prednisolone, hydrocortisone, dexamethasone.
   b. Inhaled corticosteroids–beclomethasone dipropionate, budesonide, fluticasone, mometasone, and ciclesonide.

Bronchodilators

β_2-Sympathomimetics (β_2-Adrenergic Agonist)

Short-Acting Beta-Agonists (SABA)

Inhaled SABA are the drugs of choice for acute severe asthma. Inhalation through pressurized metered dose inhaler (pMDIs) or dry powder inhalers (DPIs) are more convenient, rapid onset, and without systemic side effects. The bronchoprotective effect of SABA can be seen within minutes and its duration last for 4 to 6 hours. Even though SABA is considered as the drug of choice for quick relief of asthma, recent guidelines on global strategy for asthma management and prevention, updated by Global Initiative for Asthma (GINA) 2019, does not recommend SABA as a monotherapy because of misuse by the subjects in various countries. It has provided a guideline to use step-up and step-down therapy for asthma subjects, for example, albuterol (salbutamol), levalbuterol, metaproterenol, terbutaline, pirbuterol, enoterol, tulobuterol, and rimiterol.

Long-Acting Beta-Agonist (LABA)

In asthma and COPD therapy, salmeterol, formoterol, and arformoterol showed significant improvement. Inhaled LABA is used as an add-on drug along with leukotriene receptor antagonists, slow-release theophylline, or tiotropium for the treatment of asthma. Duration of action of these drugs is more than 12 hours.

Ultra LABA

Indacaterol was approved by the Food and Drugs Administration (FDA) in 2011 for maintenance therapy in COPD patients. It is a rapid-acting drug because of its rapid absorption. Indacaterol is delivered by inhalation as a dry powder. Other drugs included in this group are vilanterol and olodaterol. Duration of action is more than 24 hours for these drugs.

Mechanism of Action of β_2–Agonist

β_2-agonist binds to the β_2-receptor located in various airway smooth muscle cells. It inhibits the release of bronchoconstrictor mediators from inflammatory cells and bronchoconstrictor neurotransmitters from airway nerves via various mechanisms—(1) prevents release of mediators from isolated human lung mast cells via β_2-receptors; (2) prevents microvascular leakage, which causes bronchial mucosal edema after exposure to mediators such as histamine, LTD_4, and prostaglandin D_2; (3) mucociliary clearance is enhanced across the airway epithelium by increasing the mucus secretion from submucosal glands and ion transport; and (4) in the presynaptic β_2-receptors, β_2-agonist reduces neurotransmission.

Salbutamol

Duration of Action

Inhaled salbutamol produces bronchodilation within 5 minutes and lasts for 2 to 4 hours; oral salbutamol acts for 4 to 6 hours, and its bioavailability is 50%.

Side Effects

Muscle tremor (dose-related), palpitation, restlessness. nervousness, throat irritation (inhaled salbutamol), ankle edema, and hypokalemia are observed.

Dose

A total of 2 to 4 mg orally; 0.25 mg intravenously (IV)/ subcutaneously (SC) slowly at a rate of 5 to 10 µg /minute; 0.5 mg intramuscularly (IM)/SC every 4 hours; 100 to 200 µg by inhalation.

Oral β_2-agonist drugs are used for severe asthma patients as alternatives or adjuvant medications or in patients who cannot correctly use inhalers.

Terbutaline

Duration of Action

Inhaled terbutaline produces bronchodilation within 5 minutes and last for 4 to 6 hours, whereas oral terbutaline acts for 6 hours.

Dose

Oral dose range is from 1.25 to 5.0 mg every 6 hours. MDI dose of terbutaline is 200 µg/puff, and the usual dosage is two puffs every 4 to 6 hours. In hospitalized patients, SC terbutaline dose is 0.01 mg/kg/dose (maximum 0.25 mg) SC every 20 minutes for three doses, as necessary. IV terbutaline is given in severe cases—0.1 to 10 µg/kg/min as a continuous infusion prepared in 0.9% normal solution.

Bambuterol

Dose

Single evening dose of 10–20 mg oral, used in nocturnal asthma and in chronic cases.

Salmeterol

Dose

25 g MDI 2 puffs twice daily; severe cases 4 puffs twice daily.

Formoterol

Dose

12 to 24 µg by inhalation twice daily.

Methylxanthines

Methylxanthines are alkaloids that can be found in naturally occurring substances such as tea, coffee, and chocolate.

Methylxanthines are weak bronchodilators but extensively used in developing countries in the treatment of asthma and COPD because it is inexpensive. However, methylxanthines are found to be more effective when used as an add-on therapy with inhaled β_2-agonist and inhaled corticosteroids in patients with severe asthma and COPD.

Mechanism of Action

There are various mechanisms of action of methylxanthines which have been proposed:

Inhibition of Phosphodiesterase (PDE)

Isoenzymes of PDE families such as PDE3, PDE4, and PDE5 have been identified in bronchial smooth muscles. Theophylline is a nonselective PDE inhibitor which eventually results in elevation of cellular cyclic adenosine monophosphate (cAMP) and cyclic guanosine monophosphate (GMP). The rise in intracellular cAMP stimulates large-conductance, voltage-gated, Ca^{2+}-activated K^+ channels in the cell membrane of bronchial smooth muscles, which leads to cell hyperpolarization and muscle relaxation.

Adenosine Receptor Antagonism

Adenosine releases histamine and leukotrienes from mast cells, which results in hyperresponsiveness of airways in asthma patients. Antagonism of A1, A2, and A3 adenosine receptor by theophylline may relieve from bronchoconstriction. Because of adenosine receptor antagonism, other pharmacological action occurs like (i) stimulation of central nervous system (CNS), causing improvement of mental performance and alertness; (ii) Stimulation of the heart which increases the force of myocardial contraction. This increases the heart rate but decreases the rate by vagal stimulation. Usually, tachycardia is common with theophylline. (iii) In kidney, it reduces tubular Na^+ reabsorption, which leads to natriuresis and diuresis.

Interleukin-10 Release

IL-10 is thought to have anti-inflammatory effect. Studies have seen that in asthma patients, there is reduction of IL-10, and theophylline therapy has increased the level of IL-10.

Effects on Gene Transcription

Theophylline reduces the expression of inflammatory genes in asthma and COPD by preventing the translocation of the proinflammatory transcription factor nuclear factor (NF)-κB into the nucleus. These effects are seen in higher concentrations of theophylline.

Effect on Kinase

Theophylline directly inhibits phosphoinositide 3-kinases δ subtype enzyme, which is responsible for oxidative stress.

Effects on Apoptosis

In vitro studies shows that theophylline promotes apoptosis in neutrophils. Theophylline also induces apoptosis of eosinophils, which is seen to be associated with a reduction in the antiapoptotic protein Bcl-2.

Histone Deacetylase Activation

Studies shows that in COPD cells, there is reduction of HDAC2 activity and expression. Theophylline at a concentration of 10^{-6} M restores HDAC2 activity. Due to selective inhibition of phosphoinositide-3-kinase-δ (PI3K-δ) by theophylline, there is an increase in reactive oxygen species (ROS) and nitric oxide, resulting in formation of peroxynitrite radicals and inhibition of the HDAC2 activity. Theophylline reduces the formation of peroxynitrite, thus increasing the HDAC2 activity in asthma and COPD patients.

Theophylline

Pharmacokinetics

Therapeutic range of theophylline is 5 to 15 mg/L (nonbronchodilator effects can be seen in < 10 mg/L). For children, one half the adult dose is given. Theophylline is rapidly and completely absorbed, but there are large interindividual variances in clearance because of difference in hepatic metabolism.

Factors Affecting Increased Clearance

When theophylline is administered along with CYP1A2 enzyme induction drugs such as rifampicin, barbiturates, and ethanol, while smoking tobacco and marijuana, and consuming diets such as high-protein, low-carbohydrate, or including barbecued meat.

Factors Affecting Decreased Clearance

When theophylline is administered along with CYP inhibition drugs (cimetidine, erythromycin, ciprofloxacin, allopurinol, fluvoxamine, zileuton, zafirlukast), in disease conditions such as congestive heart failure, liver disease, pneumonia, viral infection and vaccination, while consuming high-carbohydrate diet, and in old age.

Dose

Oral dose is 100 to 300 mg TDS (15 mg/kg/day). Since fast-release (FR) tablets produce high peak and low trough plasma, only sustained-release (SR) tablets or capsules, which produce effective blood levels for 12 to 24 hours, are used.

Side Effects

Nausea and vomiting, headache, gastric discomfort, diuresis, behavioral disturbances, cardiac arrhythmias, epileptic seizures.

Aminophylline

Dose

IV infusion in 5% glucose in a dose of 6 mg/kg is given over 20 to 30 minutes, followed by a maintenance dose of 0.5 to 1 mg/kg per hour, not exceeding 25 mg/min. For acute exacerbations of asthma and COPD, nowadays, nebulized β_2-agonists are more preferred than IV aminophylline.

Hydroxyethyl Theophylline

Dose

250 mg oral/IM/IV.

Doxophylline

A long-acting oral methylxanthine.

Dose

Oral dose for adult is 400 mg once or twice daily and children is 12 mg/kg/day.

Anticholinergic Drugs

Two centuries back, asthma was treated with *Datura stramonium* (jimson weed), a plant from the nightshade family. Later, this plant was purified, and alkaloid atropine was used as a treatment of asthma. Ipratropium bromide and its congener were developed later due to significant side effects of atropine.

Mechanism of Action

Acetylcholine (ACh) released from cholinergic parasympathetic nerves act directly on airway smooth muscle and induce smooth muscle contraction (bronchoconstriction). Currently, it is seen that functional role for muscarinic receptors exists only for M_1, M_2, and M_3 receptors, and are target for muscarinic receptor antagonists for the treatment of asthma and COPD.

In the lungs, ACh causes bronchoconstriction. M_2 receptors antagonized $G\alpha_s$-induced relaxation, contributing to smooth muscle contraction. M_3 receptors are responsible for both vagal and exogenous ACh-induced mucin secretion. ACh induces release of leukotriene B_4 and other factors from alveolar macrophages and also induces inflammations. Air remodeling causes measurable changes in the airway structure, which is an important pathological condition in asthma and COPD patients. ACh enhances smooth muscle cell proliferation by inducing platelet-derived growth factor and epidermal growth factor.

In COPD patients, muscarinic antagonists increase airflow by blocking the cholinergic receptor M_3 present in the smooth muscles of the airway. In asthmatic patients, not only do muscarinic antagonists block the M_3 receptor and increase the airflow, but they also block reflex bronchoconstriction mediated by the vagus nerves. Currently, anticholinergics are used through inhalation for treating asthma and COPD patients.

Side Effects of Anticholinergics

Inhaled anticholinergic drugs are generally well-tolerated by the patients. After cessation of the treatment, increase in airway responsiveness has been seen in some patients. Viscous mucus, unpleasant bitter taste of inhaled ipratropium, glaucoma in elderly patients due to a direct effect of the nebulized drug on the eye, and paradoxical bronchoconstriction with ipratropium bromide (this can be largely explained by the use of a nebulizer and the effects of the hypotonic nebulizer solution and benzalkonium chloride and ethylene diamine tetra-acetic acid [EDTA]) are some of the side effects of anticholinergics.

Ipratropium Bromide

It is a short-acting quaternary ammonium derivative of atropine. It is a second-line bronchodilator (first-line is β_2-agonist). Ipratropium is a nonselective muscarinic antagonist like atropine, but unlike atropine, it does not cross the blood-brain barrier (BBB) and is poorly absorbed from the gastrointestinal tract (GIT). When administered as aerosol, it is better absorbed and the mechanism, may be due to uptake by organic cation/carnitine transporters (OCTN1 and OCTN2) in airway epithelium. In case of severe exacerbations of asthma or COPD, combination of inhaled ipratropium with β_2-agonists are preferred, as they produce a longer lasting bronchodilatation. Nebulized ipratropium mixed with salbutamol is employed in refractory asthma.

Dose

Inhalation of 2 to 4 puffs every 6 hours. Peak bronchodilation within 60 to 90 minutes of inhalation.

Tiotropium Bromide

It is also a longer acting quaternary ammonium like ipratropium, with a much higher affinity towards muscarinic receptors.

Dose

1 rotacap once a day.

Bronchodilators under Development

Magnesium Sulfate ($MgSO_4$)

A 2016 Cochrane review of three randomized control trials found that treatment with IV magnesium sulfate reduces the symptoms of acute asthma exacerbations. Magnesium sulfate was given to patients who were ineffective to inhaled short-acting bronchodilators and corticosteroids. Magnesium sulfate was found effective, as it mediates bronchodilation.

Potassium Channel Openers

Locally released bronchoconstrictors such as ACh, leukotriene D4, endothelin, and histamine, activate Gq/11-coupled receptors on airway smooth muscle cells. This results in elevation of cytosolic calcium concentration ($[Ca^{2+}]$ cyt), leading to airway smooth muscle cell contraction. Voltage-gated sensitive Ca^{2+} channels are opposed by K^+ channels which prevent airway smooth muscle cell contractions, for example, cromakalim or levcromakalim.

Vasoactive Intestinal Polypeptide (VIP) Analogs

VIP analogs lead to in vitro bronchodilation of human airway smooth muscle cells but is not that effective in vivo. The reason being the former's fast metabolism and vasodilator side effects.

Bitter Taste Receptor Agonists

Bitter taste receptors (TAS2R) are G protein-coupled receptors (GPCRs) that are expressed in airway smooth muscle and mediate bronchodilation in response to agonists, such as quinine and chloroquine.

Leukotriene Receptor Antagonist

Cysteinyl leukotrienes (cys-LTs) are produced in eosinophils, basophils, mast cells, macrophages, and myeloid dendritic cells. cys-LTs are potent bronchoconstrictor and leukotriene antagonists which inhibit airway inflammation. Montelukast and zafirlukast are two cys-LTs receptor antagonists established for the treatment of asthma.

Montelukast

Mechanism of Action

Montelukast acts by blocking the action of leukotriene D4 (and secondary ligands, leukotrienes C4 and E4) on the Cys-LT1 receptor in the lungs and bronchial tubes by binding to it.

Pharmacokinetics

It is well-absorbed orally, binds to high-plasma protein, and is metabolized by CYP2C9 and CYP3A4. The plasma $t_{1/2}$ of montelukast is 3 to 6 hours.

Dose

Oral dose for adults is 10 mg once a day; children 2 to 5 years 4 mg once a day, 6 to 14 years 5 mg once a day to be taken in the evening.

Side Effects

Mostly well-tolerated. Common symptoms include headache and GI symptoms. Other symptoms include hypersensitivity reactions, sleep disorders, drowsiness, increased bleeding tendency, hallucination, and possible mood changes and suicidal thoughts, Churg–Strauss syndrome (vasculitis with eosinophilia) has been reported rarely.

Zafirlukast

Mechanism of Action

Zafirlukast blocks leukotriene synthesis by inhibiting 5-lipoxygenase, an enzyme of the eicosanoid synthesis pathway.

Pharmacokinetics

Well-absorbed orally, metabolized by CYP2C9, and bound by high-plasma protein. The plasma $t_{1/2}$ of zafirlukast is 8 to 12 hours.

Dose

Oral dose for adult is 20 mg BD, for children 5 to 11 years dose is 10 mg twice a day. It is mainly used as a complementary therapy in adults in addition to inhaled corticosteroids (ICSs) if they alone do not bring the desired effect.

Side Effect

Hepatotoxicity

Mast Cell Stabilizer

Mechanism of Action

Sodium cromoglycate, derivative of khellin, which was an Egyptian herbal remedy. Later, a structurally related drug nedocromil sodium was added to cromoglycates. In 2010, Laura Jenkins and her colleagues from United Kingdom and Yuhua Yang and his colleagues from San Francisco demonstrated various potential therapeutic mechanisms of cromoglycate, which modulate the GPCR and activate an endogenous anti-inflammatory system.

Sodium Cromoglycate

Use

Bronchial asthma, allergic rhinitis, allergic conjunctivitis.

Dose

Poor oral absorption. So, delivered as an aerosol through MDI in asthma. 2 puffs 4 times daily. For allergic conjunctivitis, one drop (2% and 4%) in each eye four times daily.

Side Effects

Minimal systemic toxicity because of poor oral absorption. With powdered inhalation—bronchospasm, throat irritation, and cough occur in some patients.

Corticosteroids

In 1956, the first corticosteroid was used for the treatment of acute asthma exacerbation. Later, corticosteroids were developed with less mineralocorticoid activity, such as prednisone, and those that have no mineralocorticoid activity, such as dexamethasone. In 1972, Clark TJ showed that inhaled corticosteroids were more effective in the management of asthma than systemic steroids and with less side effects. Oral corticosteroids remain the mainstay of treatment of several other pulmonary diseases, such as sarcoidosis, interstitial lung diseases, and pulmonary eosinophilic syndromes.

In vitro and in vivo experiments show that steroids potentiate the effects of β-agonists on bronchial smooth muscle and prevent and reverse β-receptor desensitization in airways. Corticosteroids also increase the transcription of the β_2 receptor gene in human lung in vitro and in the respiratory mucosa in vivo. It increases the stability of its messenger ribonucleic acid (RNA) and prevents or reverses uncoupling of β_2 receptors to Gs.

Mechanism of Action

Evidence suggested that airway structural cells (e.g., epithelial cells, smooth muscle, endothelial cells, and fibroblasts) are the major source of inflammatory mediators, such as lipid mediators, inflammatory peptides, cytokines, chemokines, inflammatory enzymes, adhesion molecules, and growth factors. The expression of these proinflammatory mediators is regulated by genetic transcription through nuclear factor kappa-beta (NF-kβ), activating protein-1 (AP-1), nuclear factor activated T-cell (NF-AT), signals of transcription activators and transducers (STATs). These proinflammatory mediators activate the intrinsic histone acetyltransferase (HAT) activity. Cytosolic glucocorticoid receptors bind to the corticosteroids, forming a receptor-ligand complex, which translocates to the nucleus and inhibits the HAT activity, leading to the suppression of activated inflammation.

Systemic Corticosteroids

Systemic therapy includes corticosteroids such as hydrocortisone, dexamethasone, prednisolone, prednisone, and methylprednisolone. Prednisone and prednisolone are the most commonly used oral steroids. Methylprednisolone is IV administered. These drugs are restored to following conditions:

Severe Chronic Asthma

Frequent recurrences of asthma, with increasing severity, or patients not responding to bronchodilators and ICSs.

Dose

Prednisolone 20 to 60 mg (or equivalent) daily. If good control of asthma is seen in the patient, then reduction of drug after 1 to 2 weeks and finally shifting to ICS.

Status Asthmaticus or Acute Asthma Exacerbation

High dose of a rapidly acting IV glucocorticosteroid (generally acts in 6–24 hours) could be started if asthma attack is not responding to intensive bronchodilator therapy. IV dose could be shifted to oral therapy after normalization for 5 to 7 days and then discontinued after tapering.

COPD

Some patients of COPD during an exacerbation might benefit with a short course of oral glucocorticoid for 1 to 3 weeks.

Pharmacokinetics

Corticosteroids are well-absorbed by oral route. Water soluble esters, for example, are hydrocortisone hemisuccinate and dexamethasone sod. Phosphate can be given IV or IM. Insoluble esters, for example, hydrocortisone acetate and triamcinolone acetonide cannot be IV administered but are slowly absorbed from IM site and produce more prolonged effects.

Hydrocortisone undergoes high first-pass metabolism. As much as 90% of hydrocortisone binds to plasma protein, cortisol-binding globulin (CBG), and albumin. Corticosteroids are metabolized by hepatic microsomal enzymes. Plasma $t_{1/2}$ of hydrocortisone is 1.5 hours.

Side Effects

Long-term oral corticosteroid therapy may cause fluid retention, increased appetite, weight gain, osteoporosis, capillary fragility, hypertension, peptic ulceration, diabetes, cataracts, and psychosis.

Inhaled Corticosteroids (ICSs)

Inhaled Corticosteroids in Asthma

Beclomethasone dipropionate, budesonide, fluticasone, mometasone, and ciclesonide are numerous ICSs which are currently available. ICSs are recommended as first-line therapy (should be included in step 1 management of asthma) for patients who required β_2-agonist inhaler to control asthma symptoms, which exacerbate more than twice a week. Both adult and children are effective with these drugs in mild, moderate, and severe asthma. ICSs reduce the frequency of asthma attack, decrease the use of β_2-agonist, and improve lung function.

Dose

Starting with 100 to 200 g twice a day and then titrate the dose upward every 3 to 5 days till 400 µg four times a day. It is seen that ICS has no further benefit beyond 400 µg. After 4 to 7 days of instituting ICS, peak effect can be seen. Benefits of ICS persists for a few weeks after discontinuation.

Inhaled Corticosteroids in COPD

In COPD patients, corticosteroids do not seem to have significant anti-inflammatory effect. For severe cases of COPD with frequent exacerbations patients, only high dose of ICSs are beneficial.

Side Effects

The most common side effects are hoarseness of voice, dysphonia, sore throat, and asymptomatic or symptomatic oropharyngeal candidiasis.

Based on various studies and clinical comparability, Global Initiative for Asthma, 2019 has updated low, medium and high dose of ICS which is shown in **Table 46.1**.

Anti-IgE Antibody

Mechanism of Action

Omalizumab is a humanized monoclonal antibody against immunoglobulin E (IgE). The mechanism of omalizumab established after research shows a complex interaction of genetic and environment exposure such as allergen. This exposure was thought to occur during infancy and childhood. Omalizumab binds to the constant region of circulating IgE molecule and prevents free IgE from interacting with the high- and low-affinity IgE receptors (FcεRI and FcεRII).

Dose

Dosage is selected depending upon serum IgE level of the asthmatic patient. A total of 75 to 375 mg by SC injection every 2 or 4 weeks.

Patient Awareness

1. Inhaler training skill.
2. Even if symptoms are infrequent, patients should be encouraged to use controller medications (drugs use to reduce airway inflammation and control symptoms and risks of exacerbation).

Table 46.1 Treatment strategies for control of asthma and reduction of risk (according to Global Initiative for Asthma, 2019)

Presenting symptoms	Steps	Treatment strategy
Asthmatic symptoms with less than twice a month in adult patient and no exacerbation risk factor Children 6–11 years	1	▪ Preferred controller option: along with SABA, low-dose ICS ▪ Preferred controller option: along with SABA low-dose ICS
Step up—Despite good adherence to asthmatic drugs, patients' symptoms are not controlled Children 6–11 years	2	▪ Preferred controller option: regular low dose ICS ▪ Other controller options: leukotriene receptor antagonist ▪ Preferred controller option: regular low-dose ICS Step down: Once there is good control over asthma, patient's minimum effective dose needs to be found out to control both symptoms and exacerbations
Step up—Patient's symptoms are not controlled with low-dose ICS Children 6–11 years	3	▪ Preferred controller option: low dose ICS + LABA or medium-dose ICS ▪ Other controller options: low-dose ICS + leukotriene receptor antagonist ▪ Preferred controller option: medium-dose ICS or low-dose ICS + LABA Step down: Once there is good control over asthma, patient's minimum effective dose needs to be found out to control both symptoms and exacerbations
Step up—Patient's asthma symptoms are not controlled by low-dose ICS + LABA Children 6–11 years		▪ Preferred controller option: medium-dose ICS + LABA ▪ Refer for expert advice ▪ Other controller options: High-dose ICS + LABA for patients > 6 years with history of exacerbations, add-on therapy of tiotropium mist inhaler, or add-on leukotriene receptor antagonist ▪ Preferred controller option: medium dose ICS + LABA and refer for expert advice Step down: Once there is good control over asthma, patient's minimum effective dose needs to be found out to control both symptoms and exacerbations
Step up—Patient (both adult and children 5–11 years) is uncontrolled despite step 4 treatment	5	▪ Preferred controller option: High-dose ICS + LABA, assessed for contributory factors leading to severity of symptoms, referred to an expert for assessing severe asthma phenotype, add-on therapy of tiotropium mist inhaler for patients > 6 years with history of exacerbations, SC omalizumab anti-IgE ▪ Other controller options: low dose oral corticosteroids

Abbreviations: IgE, immunoglobulin E; ICS, inhaled corticosteroid; LABA, long-acting β_2-agonist; SABA, short-acting β-agonist; SC, subcutaneous.

3. Training in self-monitoring of asthma symptoms to control and minimize symptoms and risks of exacerbation.
4. Awareness regarding modifiable risk factors such as smoking, low-lung function.
5. Awareness regarding nonpharmacological strategies such as cessation of smoking, breathing exercises, avoidance of occupational exposures and medications that aggravate asthma, healthy diet, avoidance of indoor allergens, emotional stress.

Status Asthmaticus

Status asthmaticus is an extreme form of asthma exacerbation despite GINA 2019 step 4 and 5 treatment. It is a medical emergency.

Management

This is according to the guidelines of GINA 2019

- Required hospitalization and ICU for the patient.
- Confirm the diagnosis (asthma or differential diagnosis).
  - If asthma, patient should be considered for referral to a specialist or severe asthma clinic.
- Look for factors contributing to symptoms and exacerbation.
  - Incorrect inhaler techniques, suboptimal adherence, comorbidities, modifiable risk factors and triggers, regular or overuse of SABA, anxiety, depression and socioeconomic problems, medicine side effects.
- Optimize management.
  - Asthma self-management education.

- Optimized inhaled controller medications.
  - Suitable inhaler for the patient.
  - Switch to ICS-formoterol (beclomethasone-formoterol or budesonide-formoterol) if there is a history of exacerbation.
- Treatment of comorbidities (anxiety and depression, obesity, chronic rhinosinusitis, gastroesophageal reflux disease [GERD], COPD, cardiac diseases, obstructive sleep apnea) and modifiable risk factors (smoking, environmental exposure to allergens, medications such as beta-blockers, aspirin, and other NSAIDs).
- Nonpharmacological therapy (cessation of smoking, physical activity, breathing exercise, healthy diet, weight reduction).
- Consider adding nonbiologic medication to medium/high dose ICSs such as LABA, leukotriene receptor antagonist, tiotropium (anticholinergics).
- Consider a trial of high dose ICS if not already attempted.
- Assess the response of the drugs and other intervention. If asthma is controlled, then try to do step down, and if still not controlled, then consider the next criteria.
- Type 2 or nontype 2 inflammatory phenotype of the patient should be assessed. Type 2 inflammation is characterized by cytokines such as IL-4, IL-5, and IL-13. Biomarkers are eosinophils, sputum eosinophils, and FeNO. If the patient is type 2 phenotype:
  - Maintenance of oral corticosteroids.
  - Consider adding type 2 targeted biologics along with high ICS + LABA.

    For example, anti-IgE—omalizumab SC.
    - Anti-IL5—mepolizumab subcutaneously, reslizumab IV.
    - Anti-ILR—benralizumab SC.
    - Anti-IL4—dupilumab SC.
- If the patient does not show any type 2 inflammation
  - Additional investigations such as high-resolution chest X-ray and bronchoscopy can be considered.
  - Add-on treatment of nonbiologicals can be tried.

    For example, anticholinergic (tiotropium), leukotriene modifiers (montelukast, zafirlukast), low-dose macrolide.

    Review the patient every 3 to 6 months.

Multiple Choice Questions

1. Which drug is considered as ultralong-acting β_2-agonist?

A. Arformoterol.
B. Levalbuterol.
C. Indacaterol.
D. Salmeterol.

Answer: C

Indacaterol was approved by FDA in 2011 for maintenance therapy in chronic obstructive pulmonary disorder (COPD) patients. It is a rapid-acting drug because of its rapid absorption. Indacaterol is delivered by inhalation as a dry powder. Other drugs included in this group are vilanterol and olodaterol. Duration of action is more than 24 hours for these drugs.

2. A 35-year-old woman from a low socioeconomic background and with a known case of asthma now shows symptoms of tuberculosis. She is on theophylline tablets for treatment of asthma. Which antitubercular drug will increase the clearance of theophylline?

A. Isoniazid.
B. Ethambutol.
C. Pyrazinamide.
D. Rifampicin.

Answer: D

When theophylline is administered along with CYP1A2 enzyme induction drugs such as rifampicin, barbiturates, and ethanol, while smoking tobacco and marijuana, and consuming diets such as high-protein, low-carbohydrate, or including barbecued meat.

3. A 25-year-old patient is using a salbutamol inhaler for management of the acute episodes of asthma and develops symptoms that he attributes to salbutamol. Which of the following is *not* a recognized action of salbutamol?

A. Diuretic effect.
B. Positive inotropic effect.
C. Skeletal muscle tremor.
D. Smooth muscle relaxation.
E. Tachycardia.

Answer: A

Salbutamol is a β_2-agonist; however, in moderate to high doses it causes β_1 cardiac effects along with β_2-mediated smooth and skeletal muscle effects. It does not have a diuretic effect.

4. Omalizumab inhibits:

A. IgM.
B. IgE.
C. IgG.
D. IgA.

Answer: B

Omalizumab is a humanized monoclonal antibody against immunoglobulin E (IgE). The mechanism of omalizumab established after research shows a complex interaction of genetic and environment exposure such as allergen. This exposure was thought to occur during infancy and childhood. Omalizumab binds to the constant region of circulating IgE molecule and prevents free IgE from interacting with the high- and low-affinity IgE receptors (FcεRI and FcεRII).

5. Churg–Strauss syndrome is a side effect of:

A. Montelukast.
B. Budesonide.
C. Formoterol.
D. Tiotropium.

Answer: A

Churg–Strauss syndrome, that is, vasculitis with eosinophilia has been reported with montelukast.

6. A 67-year-old woman is admitted in the emergency department with fever for 2 days, dyspnea, and increase in

cough with green sputum production. She was diagnosed with chronic obstructive pulmonary disorder (COPD) 2 years ago. She used albuterol several times yesterday but there was no relief of dyspnea. 6 months ago, she did a spirometry which showed a forced expiratory volume (FEV_1) of 48%. She is taking tiotropium and albuterol as needed.

On physical examination, her temperature is 102.0 °F, blood pressure is 124/80 mm Hg, pulse rate is 118/min, and respiration rate is 30/min. Oxygen saturation is 82% breathing ambient air. Pulmonary examination reveals bilateral diffuse expiratory wheezing.

The patient is hospitalized. Treatment started with albuterol nebulizer and 2 L of oxygen by nasal canula. Along with short-acting bronchodilator and oxygen therapy, what other appropriate treatment would you like to start?

A. Azithromycin and prednisolone.
B. Clarithromycin and fluticasone.
C. Doxycycline and salmeterol.
D. Erythromycin and romflumilast.

Answer: A

The patient has acute exacerbation of COPD. One of the most common causes of acute exacerbation of COPD is bacterial or viral infections. Along with oxygen therapy and short-acting beta agonist, antibiotics and systemic glucocorticosteroids are also indicated.

7. A 25-year-old patient is admitted to the emergency department following seizures caused due to an overdose of a medication he has been consuming. He had developed insomnia after taking it. Which of the following is a direct bronchodilator commonly prescribed for asthmatics orally which can lead to insomnia and seizures?

A. Cromolyn.
B. Ipratropium.
C. Prednisone.
D. Salmeterol.
E. Theophylline.

Answer: E

Theophylline is a bronchodilator that is active by the oral route. It leads to insomnia in therapeutic doses and seizures on overdose.

8. Following a successful management of an acute attack of asthma, the patient was referred to the OPD to follow-up. Which of the following is *not* an established prophylactic strategy for asthma?

A. Avoidance of antigen exposure.
B. Blockade of histamine receptors.
C. Blockade of leukotriene receptors.
D. IgE antibody blockade.
E. Inhibition of phospholipase A_2.

Answer: B

Histamine does not have an important cause in asthma, and antihistaminic drugs are least used. Antigen avoidance is well-recognized. Inhibition of leukotriene receptors with montelukast, suppression of phospholipase with corticosteroids, and inhibition of mediator release with the immunoglobulin E (IgE) antibody are also beneficial.

9. A 55-year-old patient is a past smoker with ischemic heart disease and severe chronic obstructive pulmonary disease (COPD) associated with regular symptoms of bronchospasm. The bronchodilator beneficial for COPD and least possible to cause cardiac arrhythmia is:

A. Cromolyn.
B. Ipratropium.
C. Metoprolol.
D. Prednisone.

Answer: B

Ipratropium is the bronchodilator that is most likely to be useful in COPD without causing arrhythmias. Tiotropium is similar.

Chapter 47 Drugs for Treatment of Cough

Farhana Dutta Majumder

PH1.33 Describe the mechanism of action, types, doses, side effects, indications, and contraindications of the drugs used in cough (antitussive, expectorants, mucolytics).

Learning Objectives

- Cough reflex pathway.
- Classification.
- Treatment for common cold.

Introduction

Normally, cough is an essential mechanism to expel respiratory secretions and foreign bodies from the air passage. But it becomes alarming when cough becomes a consequence of aspiration, inhalation of some irritants, pathogens, accumulated secretions, postnasal drip, inflammation, and mediators associated with inflammation.

Cough Reflex Pathway

It has been observed from animal studies that cough reflex mechanism can be peripheral or central. Peripheral cough reflex is controlled by a subset of bronchopulmonary unmyelinated C-fibers and mechanically sensitive cough receptors. C-fiber nociceptors have their terminals in and around the mucosal surface of the airways. They are sensitive to bradykinin, activators of ion channels, and transient receptor potential vanilloid 1 (TRPV1) (e.g., capsaicin and protons). Prostaglandin E2, nicotine, adenosine, and serotonin are some of the other inflammatory mediators and irritants that activate bronchopulmonary C-fibers. Mechanically sensitive cough receptors are embedded beneath the epithelium of large airways, and these receptors are insensitive to chemical mediators. These receptors are sensitive to punctate mechanical stimuli delivered to the mucosal surface (**Fig. 47.1**).

Central cough mechanism model proposes that vagal afferent fibers enter the brain stem via the nucleus tractus solitarius (NTS) and activate the central cough pattern generator, a collection of neurons that generate respiratory rhythm in the ventral respiratory group in the brain stem (**Fig. 47.2**).

Classification, Etiology, and Management

The etiology of a cough is a subjective classification, established mainly on the duration of a cough. If a cough is present for less than 3 weeks, it is labelled as acute. If a cough is present for 3 to 8 weeks, it is labelled as subacute. If a cough is present for more than 8 weeks, it is labelled as chronic.

Most cases of acute cough ought to be treated empirically, and treatment should emphasize on symptomatic assistance. This comprises supportive methods of over-the-counter (OTC) cough and cold medicines, although several OTC antihistamine-decongestant medications have been demonstrated to provide no clinical benefit over placebo. Cough suppressants could be utilized to reduce the cough by blunting the cough reflex, and expectorants could be used when excessive mucous secretions are ascertained to be the primary issue to increase mucus clearance. It is essential to remember that coughing is a basic defense mechanism

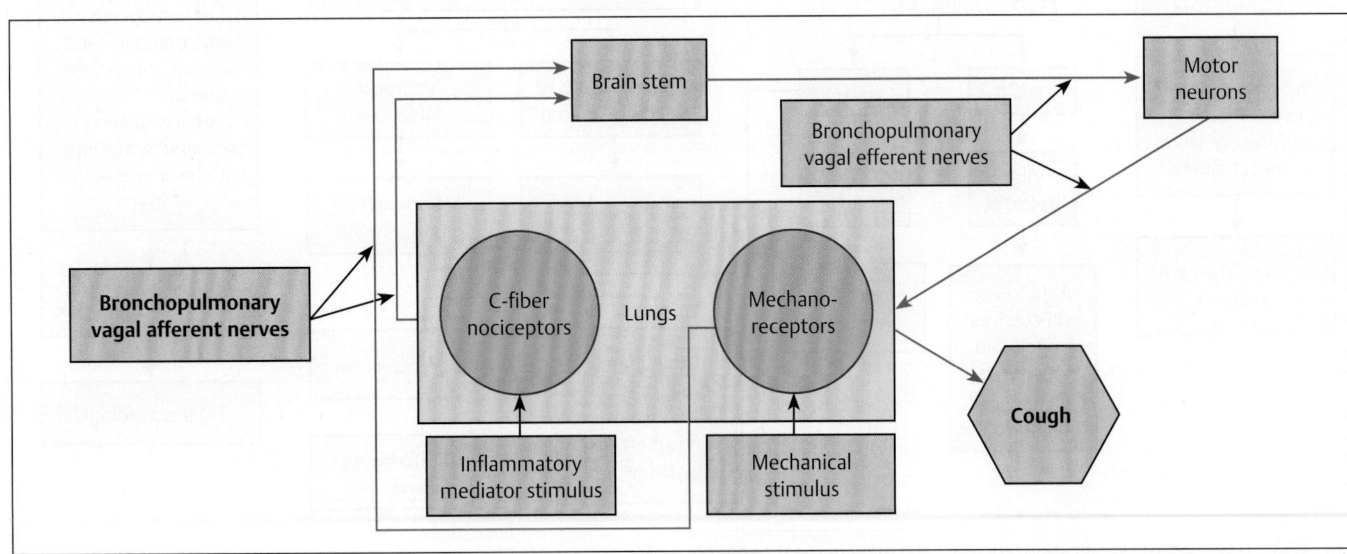

Fig. 47.1 Schematic diagram of peripheral cough reflex.

and participates in a significant part of the body's immune systems. Consequently, reducing the cough reflex could lead to negative influences on the recovery time of illness. **Fig. 47.3** mentions the classification and management of cough.

Classification

Drugs that act in the central nervous system (CNS) to inhibit cough are referred to as centrally acting, and this labelling is dependent primarily on evidence derived from animal models. This classification may comprise drugs that act at both peripheral and central sites subsequent to their systemic administration. These drugs are meant to decrease the frequency and/or intensity of coughing due to disorders of any etiology. **Fig. 47.4** shows the classification of drugs.

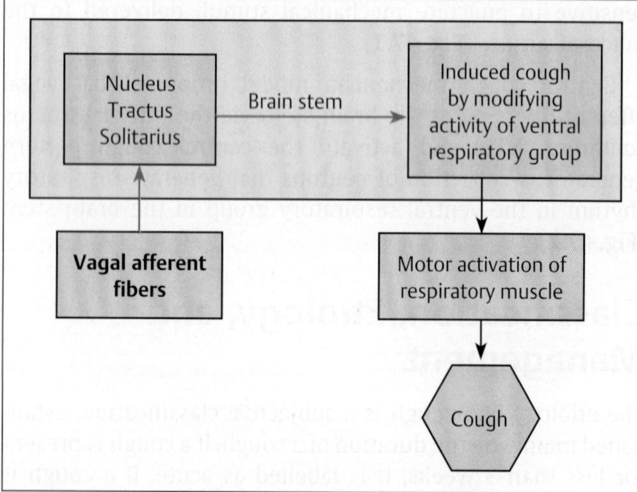

Fig. 47.2 Schematic diagram of central cough reflex.

Antitussive

Centrally Acting Antitussives

Opioids

Codeine, pholcodine, and ethylmorphine are synthetic opioid analgesics but are less potent than morphine. Morphine is not suitable as antitussive because of its liability to become dependence. Among these, codeine is considered as a standard antitussive. Various studies explained that codeine is sensitive to opioid receptor μ (mu). μ opioid receptors are present in the NTS, and codeine acts as an agonist in suppressing the cough center.

Side Effects

One of the side effects of opioids is constipation; at higher doses, they are likely to cause respiratory depression in children.

Contraindications

They are contraindicated in those who are hypersensitive to opioids, asthmatic, and patients with respiratory reserve.

Cough
Acute (< 3 weeks)
Subacute (3–8 weeks)
Chronic (> 8 weeks)
Life-threatening conditions
Non-life-threatening conditions
History of hemoptysis, environmental and occupational factors
Life-threatening conditions, history of hemoptysis, environmental and occupational factors, smoker > 45 years with a new cough, systemic symptoms with fever and weight loss
Pneumonia, severe exacerbation of asthma or COPD, heart failure
URTI
LRTI
Postinfectious or life-threatening
Non-post infectious
Evaluate the case and treat
Viral, bacterial
Pertussis
Treat accordingly
Workup for chronic cough
Further investigtions
Antibiotics, anti-tussives, expectorant, mucolytics, pharyngeal demulcent
Appropriate antibiotics
TB in endemic areas or high-risk group-antitubercular drugs
Acute bronchiectasis
Treat underlying cause
Treat accordingly

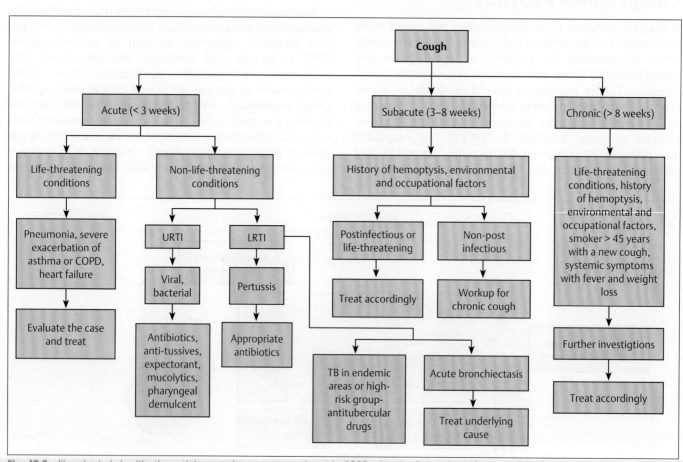

Fig. 47.3 Flowchart of classification, etiology, and management of cough. COPD, chronic obstructive pulmonary disease; URTI, upper respiratory tract infections; LRTI, lower respiratory tract infections.

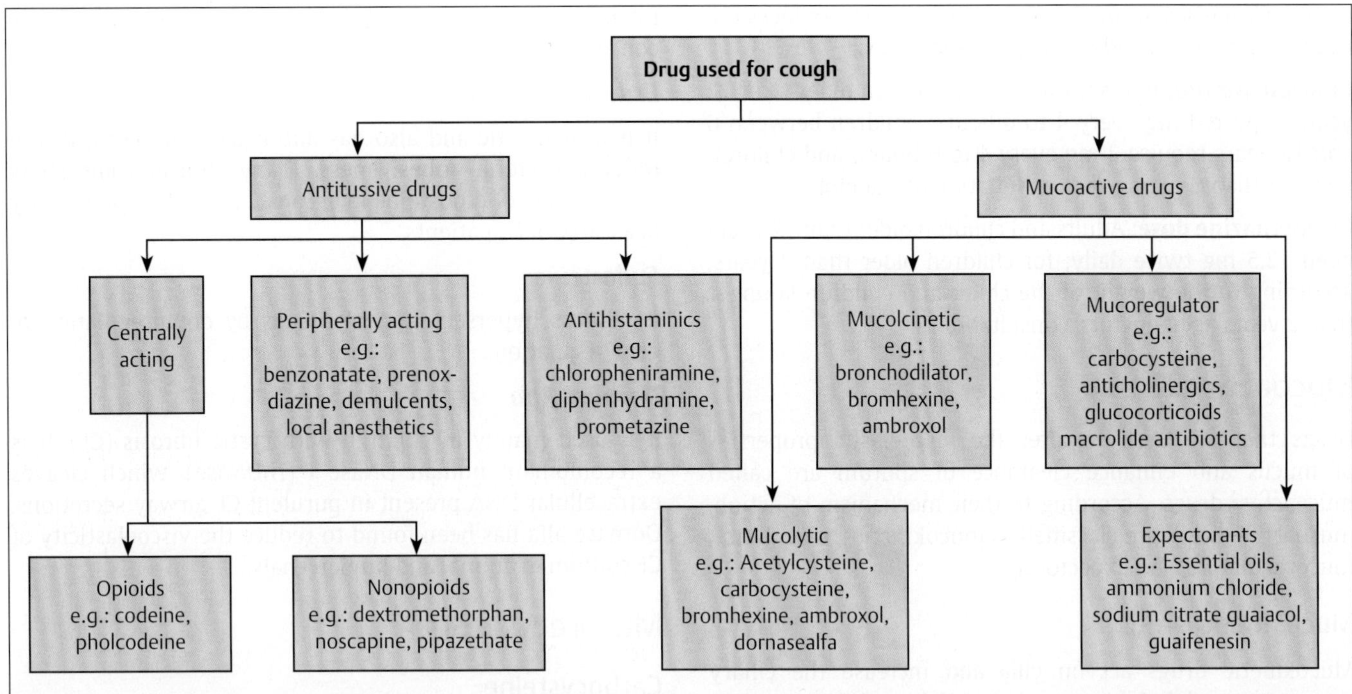

Fig. 47.4 Classification of drugs use in cough.

Dose

1. **Codeine:** Adult and children older than 12 years can have 15 to 30 mg three to four times daily. It is contraindicated in children younger than 12 years. In the elderly, dose adjustment is required if there is renal or hepatic function impairment.
2. Pholcodine and ethylmorphine are closely related to codeine. They are use as antitussives.
   a. **Pholcodine:** Adults and children older than 12 years, 5 mL two times; in children between 6 and 12 years, 5 mL once not more than 5 days; and in the elderly, dose reduction is not required.
   b. **Ethylmorphine:** 10 to 30 mg thrice daily.

Nonopioids

Dextromethorphan, a nonopioid antitussive, inhibits G protein-coupled inwardly rectifying K^+ channel (GIRK) and antagonizes the 5-HT hyperpolarization in the CNS.

Dose

In adults, the recommended dose is 10 to 20 mg; in children between 6 and 12 years, it is 5 to 10 mg; and in children younger than 6 years, it is not advisable.

Side Effects

Blurred vision, confusion, dizziness, nausea, and vomiting.

Drug Interaction

Monoamine oxidase (MAO) inhibitors such as isocarboxazid, selegiline, and rasagiline.

Noscapine is a nonopioid alkaloid that acts on sigma opioid receptor to elicit the central effect of antitussive.

Dose: Adults, 15 to 30 mg; children between 2 and 6 years, 7.5 mg; children between 6 and 12 years, 15 mg.

Side effects: Nausea, headache, and tremors.

Peripherally Acting Antitussives

Benzonatate

It is an antitussive that has a structure similar to local anesthetics such as procaine and tetracaine. It acts as an antitussive by anesthetizing the pulmonary stretch receptors.

Dose

Adult dose is 100 to 200 mg.

Side Effects

Nausea, dizziness, headache, sedation, somnolence, and, in some cases, numbness of the tongue.

Prenoxdiazine

It is a peripherally acting cough suppressant that inhibits the pulmonary stretch receptors.

Dose

Adult dose is 100 to 200 mg.

Pharyngeal Demulcents

It acts as a protective coating over the sensory receptor of pharynx. Examples include honey, licorice, and syrup vasaka. It is more effective in dry cough.

Local Anesthetics

Lidocaine, benzocaine, hexylcaine, hydrochloride, and tetracaine are used to inhibit the cough reflex before bronchoscopy or bronchography.

Antihistamines

Antihistamines, mainly first generations such as *chlorpheniramine* and *promethazine*, are commonly used as antitussives. These drugs reduce the cholinergic transmission of nerve impulses in cough reflex, which, in turn, reduces the frequency of cough and dries up the secretions.

Chlorpheniramine dose: Adults and children older than 12 years require 4 mg every 4 to 6 hours; children between 6 and 12 years require 2 mg every 4 to 6 hours; and children younger than 6 years need consultation of a doctor.

Promethazine dose: Adults and children older than 12 years need 12.5 mg twice daily; for children older than 2 years, according to the weight of the child; and children younger than 2 years need doctors' consultation.

Mucoactive Drugs

Drugs that are used to alter the viscoelastic properties of mucus and enhance clearance of sputum are called mucoactive drugs. According to their mechanism of action, mucoactive drugs are classified as mucokinetics, mucolytics, mucoregulators, and expectorants.

Mucokinetic Drugs

Mucokinetic drugs act on cilia and increase the ciliary movement and help in expulsion of bronchial secretion. Mucokinetic medication includes bronchodilators, bromhexine, and ambroxol.

Bronchodilators

Some studies claim that it relieves cough in individuals with bronchoconstriction. However, there is controversy regarding the activity of β_2-adrenergic agonist on clearance of mucus from the ciliary cells.

Bromhexine

It increases mucus production, sputum quality and quantity, ciliary activity, and expulsion of mucus.

Dose

Adults, 8 mg thrice daily; children between 5 and 10 years, 4 mg thrice daily; children between 2 and 5 years, 4 mg twice daily; and children younger than 2 years, not recommended.

Ambroxol

It is thought to stimulate surfactant and mucous secretion and also helps in promoting normalization of mucous viscosity in viscid secretions.

Dose

Adults, 15 to 30 mg thrice daily.

Side Effects

Rhinorrhea and lacrimation, nausea, gastric irritation, and hypersensitivity.

Mucolytics

Mucolytics are agents that alter the chemical characteristics of mucus and decrease its viscosity. Hence, they facilitate removal of mucus by coughing or ciliary action.

N-Acetylcysteine

When administered as aerosol, it cleaves the mucin disulfide bonds and reduces viscosity. *N*-acetylcysteine also decreases inflammation by reducing lysozyme and lactoferrin concentrations in smokers.

Erdosteine

It is a mucolytic and also has antioxidant property. It also reduces bacteria adhesiveness. Many clinical trials show effectiveness of erdosteine in chronic obstructive pulmonary disease (COPD) patients.

Fudosteine

It reduces hypersecretion of mucus by downregulation of gene regulation.

Dornase Alfa

It is used mainly in children with cystic fibrosis (CF). It is a recombinant human DNase I (rhDNase), which cleaves extracellular DNA present in purulent CF airway secretions. Dornase alfa has been found to reduce the viscoelasticity of CF sputum in animal and human trials.

Mucoregulators

Carbocysteine

It reduces inflammation by reducing infiltration of neutrophil into the airway lumen and decreasing the levels of interleukin (IL-8, IL-6) and cytokine. This drug is mainly used in COPD. Carbocysteine also has the ability to restore the viscoelastic properties of mucus.

Anticholinergic Agents

Agents such as atropine, ipratropium, scopolamine, glycopyrrolate, and tiotropium reduce glandular output and sputum volume. This action is mediated by M_3 receptor expressed on submucosal airway cells.

Glucocorticoids

It is an anti-inflammatory agent used mainly in patients with asthma and COPD. It is seen that glucocorticoids enhance mucociliary clearance.

Macrolide Antibiotics

These are azithromycin, clarithromycin, and erythromycin. These antibiotics reduce sputum production.

Expectorants

Hypertonic Saline

Saline, urea, or ascorbic acid has been thought to induce ciliary motility, proteolysis, and mucous liquefactions as well as improve lung function of CF patients. Nebulized hypertonic saline has proved to be effective in clinical trials.

Iodine-Containing Compounds

Domiodol and iodinated glycerol in chronic bronchitis reduce chest discomfort and act as antitussive agents.

Guaifenesin (Glyceryl Guaiacolate)

It is a plant product mainly recommended in symptomatic treatment of cough to enhance bronchial secretion.

Ion Channel Modifiers

They are uridine triphosphate and adenosine triphosphate, which regulate ion transport through P2Y2 purinergic receptors that increase intracellular calcium and are also thought to enhance mucociliary clearance.

Fixed-Dose Combinations of Drugs

When two or more drugs are combined together in a fixed ratio in a single dosage form, it is known as a fixed-dose combination (FDC). FDCs are accepted only when the combination dosage has proven advantage over single compound administered separately. In India, the Central Drugs Standard Control Organisation (CDSCO) is the National Regulatory Authority (NRA) that ensures safety, efficacy, and quality of the medical product manufactured, imported, and distributed in the country.

1. Ambroxol HCl 30 mg + guaiphenesin 200 mg tablet for cough and congestion.
2. Desloratadine (2.5 mg) + ambroxol (30 mg) + guaiphenesin (50 mg) + menthol 1 mg/5 mL syrup for productive cough.
3. Levocetirizine 5 mg + ambroxol hydrochloride sustained release (75 mg) tablet for productive cough.
4. Dextromethorphan HBr 10 mg + chlorpheniramine maleate 2 mg/5 mL syrup for relief of cough due to throat irritation, sneezing, and running nose.

Treatment for Common Cold

Common cold is upper respiratory tract infection caused most commonly by rhinovirus. This is a self-limiting viral infection, which involves nose, sinuses, pharynx, and larynx. Usually, viruses are transmitted through sneezing, coughing, or nose blowing. Symptoms generally last for 7 to 10 days but may also persist for 3 weeks. Symptoms include sore throat, rhinitis, rhinorrhea, cough, and malaise. Various studies have shown the benefit of different therapies in common cold in children (**Table 47.1**).

Therapy Not Effective for Treatment of Common Cold

1. **Antibiotics:** From nine Cochrane data base systemic reviews, it was seen that antibiotics do not make any difference in symptoms of common cold.
2. **Antihistamines:** From 32 Cochrane data base systemic reviews, it was observed that antihistamines and placebo have same effects.
3. **Codeine:** According to the American College of Chest Physician, codeine is not recommended in common cold.

Nasal Decongestants for Common Cold

Nasal decongestants are drugs that help in relieving congestion of nasal mucosa. Drugs are available for both systemic and topical use. They are sympathomimetic drugs that cause local vasoconstriction and eventually reduce congestion and edema of nasal mucosa. Among the sympathomimetic drugs, imidazoles (e.g., naphazoline, oxymetazoline, xylometazoline) and catecholamine derivatives (epinephrine, ephedrine, phenylephrine) are used locally for application in nose. Since nasal decongestants are available OTC, many people self-medicate and misuse the drug. Prolonged use of nasal decongestant can cause serious adverse effects such as rebound congestion, rhinitis medicamentosa, and ophthalmic adverse effects such as dry eyes, corneal edema, and cataracts, which can be seen after using xylometazoline.

Table 47.1 List of therapies that may be effective for children in the treatment of common cold

Therapy	Dosing	Duration of therapy
Acetylcysteine	Variable dose according to age	Variable; can be continued for up to 28 days
Corticosteroids for wheezing	Budesonide 1,600 µg by MDI with nebulizer	Until asymptomatic for 24 hours
	Beclomethasone 2,250 µg daily by MDI	5 days
Honey (buckwheat)	2.5 mL, 5 mL, 10 mL according to age; not recommended below 12 months of age	Single night-time dose
Nasal irrigation with saline	3 to 9 mL per nostril	Up to 3 weeks
Vapor rub	5 mL, 10 mL	Once
Zinc sulfate	10–15 mL syrup per 5 mL	10 days
Prophylaxis		
• Probiotics	1 g (1 × 1,010 CFU) mixed with 120 mL of 1% milk twice daily	6 months
• Vitamin C	0.2 to 2 g daily	2 weeks to 9 months

Abbreviations: CFU, colony-forming unit; MDI, metered dose inhaler.

Multiple Choice Questions

1. An 18-year-old boy came to OPD and complained of dry cough with no sputum, headache, body pain, and fever for 2 days. He has no history of smoking. What will be your advice to the patient?

A. Give him a course of antibiotics.

B. Give him paracetamol tablets for fever and ask him to drink plenty of fluids and take rest.

C. Advise him to revisit OPD if the cough does not go off within 3 weeks or it becomes productive.

D. Both B and C.

Answer: D

2. A 50-year-old man who has been suffering from dry cough for the last 3 months comes to medicine OPD. He recently observed shortness of breath and red blood spots on his handkerchief while coughing. He has a 20-year history of smoking. What advice you will give to the patient?

A. Ask the patient to stop smoking.

B. Refer the patient immediately to a chest physician for further investigation.

C. Both A and B.

D. Send the patient back home after prescribing antibiotics and cough suppressants.

Answer: C

Part VIII

Drugs Acting on Blood and Blood-forming Organs

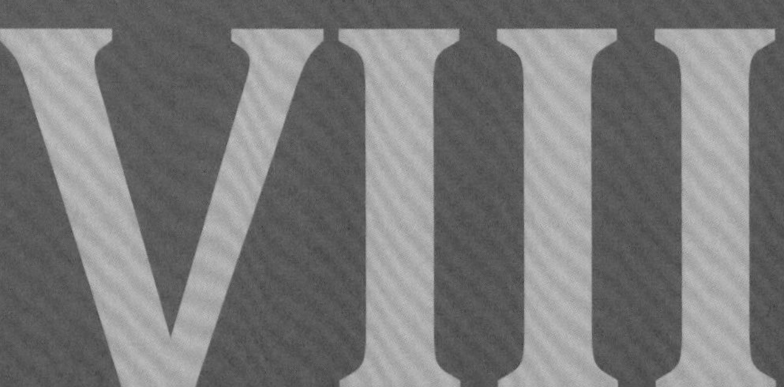

Chapter 48 Hematinics and Treatment of Anemia

Shikha Jaiswal Shivhare

PH1.35:Describe the mechanism/s of action, types, doses, side effects, indications and contraindications of drugs used in hematological disorders like:

1. Drugs used in anemias

2. Colony Stimulating factors

Learning Objectives

- Hematopoiesis.
- Anemia and its types: iron deficiency, megaloblastic, pernicious.
- Iron: requirements, role, sources, formulations (oral & parenteral).
- Erythropoietin.
- Vitamin B_{12}.
- Folic acid.

Hematopoiesis

Hematopoiesis is continuous replacement of mature blood cells by bone marrow. Erythrocyte production in anemia can increase 20-fold. Leucocyte production in systemic infection increases many folds, while in state of thrombocytopenia, platelet production increases 10- to 20-fold. For organized functioning, hematopoietic machinery needs some exogenous nutrients (hematinics) like iron, vitamin B_{12}, folic acid, and certain endogenous factors like granulocyte-macrophage colony-stimulating factors (GM-CSF), granulocyte colony-stimulating factors (G-CSF), erythropoietin, thrombopoietin, and interleukin 1 and 11. In addition to exogenous and endogenous factors, there are certain accessory hematinics which are required for normal hematopoiesis, which include copper, cobalt, and manganese.

Anemia

Anemia is reduced oxygen-carrying capacity of the blood due to reduction of hemoglobin content or red blood cell (RBC) volume below the range value in healthy individuals.

Causes of Anemia

Table 48.1 mentions the causes of anemia.

Pathophysiology

1. Deficiency of substance—Exogenous substance deficiency like iron deficiency leads to iron deficiency anemia (microcytic hypochromic anemia), vitamin B_{12} and folic acid deficiency leads to megaloblastic anemia (macrocytic hypochromic anemia). Intrinsic factor deficiency leads to pernicious anemia.
2. Genetic abnormalities—Heme chain abnormality leads to sickle cell disease, and defect in globin leads to thalassemia.
3. Excess loss of blood like in helminthic infestation or in chronic disease like peptic ulcer, colon cancer, and malabsorption syndromes can lead to microcytic hypochromic anemia.
4. Excessive hemolysis is seen with various drugs like antimalarials and in G6PD-deficient persons.
5. Drug induced like cytotoxic drugs, chloramphenicol, methotrexate, phenytoin, phenobarbitone, and biguanides.

Types of Anemia

1. Microcytic hypochromic anemia—characterized by small RBC size with low hemoglobin content and usually caused by iron deficiency.
2. Macrocytic hyperchromic anemias or megaloblastic anemia—characterized by large nucleated primitive RBCs with increasingly pigmented blood smear and usually caused due to deficiency of vitamin B_{12} and/or folic acid.
3. Normocytic normochromic anemia—characterized by normal-sized RBC, with no to slight hypochromia usually seen in chronic diseases/inflammation.

Iron

Iron is essential for hematopoiesis. One of the most common causes of anemia is iron deficiency.

Role of Iron

It is an essential component of hemoglobin, myoglobin, heme enzymes like cytochromes, catalases, peroxidase,

Table 48.1 Causes of anemia

Nutrition	Genetic hemoglobin disorder	Infectious disease	Others
Iron deficiency	Thalassemia	Helminthic infestation	Drug induced
Folic acid deficiency	Sickle cell disease	Malaria	Excess blood loss
Vitamin B_{12} deficiency	G6PD deficiency	Tuberculosis	
Protein energy malnutrition	Ovalocytosis	AIDS	
		Malabsorption disorders	

metalloflavoprotein enzymes like xanthine oxidase and α-glycerophosphate oxidase, and mitochondrial enzymes α-glycerophosphate oxidase. Iron is also important for normal functioning of brain. Iron deficiency leads to learning and behaviour problems in children.

Sources of Iron

Animal sources—oyster, meat, liver, egg yolk, chicken, and fish.

Plant sources—wheat germs, dry fruits, spinach, dried beans, apple, banana, jaggery, milk and milk products, beet root, etc.

The daily requirement of iron differs with age and is mentioned in **Table 48.2.**

Iron Content in Body

In a normal adult male of 70 kg, the iron content is 55 mg/kg (4 gm), while in females, it is about 40 mg/kg. Two-third of it is in form of hemoglobin. About one-sixth of iron is in storage form and is utilized for synthesis of hemoglobin. The remaining amount is present in myoglobin and iron-containing enzymes.

Iron Absorption

The Indian daily diet contains 10 to 20 mg of iron. It is actively absorbed in ferrous form in duodenum, proximal jejunum, and in little amount from distal part of small intestine. On an average, 10% of dietary iron is absorbed, but in cases of deficiency, it may increase to 20% to 30%. Heme iron present in meat is absorbed as such but inorganic or nonheme iron is absorbed after getting reduced to ferrous form. There are two iron transporters in the small intestine's mucosal cells that function for iron absorption. DMT1 (divalent metal transporter1) carries ferrous iron into mucosal cells. Ferroportin (FP) transporter transports iron released from heme across the basolateral membrane. Iron is stored in intestine mucosal cell as a water-soluble complex, ferritin (central core of ferric oxide covered with apoferritin), that is, there is a mucosal barrier, and excess iron is not transported from mucosal cells and remains stored there. The mucosal store of ferritin is only for 2 to 4 days (life span of mucosal cells) and lost when mucosal cells are shed. When iron stores are low or body requirement is high, then the iron absorbed is immediately transported from the mucosal cells to the bone marrow for hemopoiesis. On the other hand, when stores are high or body requirement is low, the newly absorbed iron is converted to ferritin in order to be stored in mucosal cell.

Table 48.2 Daily requirement

Subject	Iron requirement (mg/kg)
Infant	67
Child	22
Adolescent male	21
Adolescent female	20
Adult male	13
Adult female	21
2nd & 3rd trimester of pregnancy	80
Menstruating women	15

Factors Altering Iron Absorption

1. Iron absorption is increased by ascorbic acid, succinic acid, and cysteine. These facilitate conversion of ferric to ferrous.
2. Antacids (alkali) make iron insoluble, thus hampering its absorption.
3. Phosphates, phytates, coffee, tea, and presence of other food in stomach hinder iron absorption.
4. Tetracyclines hinder iron absorption.

Iron Deficiency Anemia (PE13.5)

The causes for iron deficiency anemia are as follows:

1. Inadequate dietary intake of iron (nutritional iron deficiency).
2. Blood loss (from gastrointestinal tract [GIT], during childbirth, menorrhagia, etc.).
3. Prematurity, intrauterine growth restriction (IUGR) babies.
4. Failure to fulfill increase demand during pregnancy, menstruation.

Treatment

Oral iron therapy is treatment of choice. In case of failure to response, parenteral iron therapy is given.

Iron Preparations (IM9.14)

See **Table 48.3**.

Oral Iron

Iron is preferably given through oral route. Inexpensive ferrous salts have high-iron content and are better absorbed than ferric salts, especially at higher doses.

1. Ferrous sulfate is the cheapest preparation. It often produces metallic taste.
2. Tasteless ferrous fumarate has 33% iron and is less water-soluble than ferrous sulfate.
3. Carbonyl iron: It is high purity fine powder form of iron produced by decomposition of iron pentacarbonyl. It is absorbed

Table 48.3 Different types of iron preparations

Oral	Parenteral
Ferrous sulfate	Iron dextran (IM, IV)
Ferrous gluconate	Iron sodium gluconate (IV)
Ferrous fumarate	Ferrous sucrose (IV)
Ferrous succinate	Ferric carboxy maltose (IV)
Ferrous aminoate	Iron sorbitol (IM)
Carbonyl iron	Iron sorbitol-citric acid (IM)
Ferric ammonium citrate	
Ferric glycerophosphate	
Ferric hydroxy polymaltose	

Abbreviations: IM, intramuscular; IV, intravenous.

from intestine for a long time and has good gastric tolerance. Its bioavailability is three-fourth of ferrous sulfate.

4. Ferrous succinate has 35% iron, ferrous gluconate has 12% iron, ferric ammonium citrate has 20% iron, ferrous aminoate has 10% iron; ferric glycerophosphate and ferric hydroxy polymaltose are better absorbed and tolerated due to their lower iron content. Generally, these are more expensive.

The elemental iron content per dose should be taken into consideration while prescribing iron therapy. Expensive sustained release preparations are irrational because most of the iron is absorbed in upper intestine, and these preparations release iron in lower part of intestine. The bioavailability of such preparation is variable.

A total of 200 mg elemental iron is given daily in three divided doses for 6 months for best therapeutic results. In infants and children, therapeutic dose is 3 to 5 mg/kg body wt/day. Prophylactic dose is 30 mg/day. Optimum response to therapy is a rise in hemoglobin (Hb) level by 0.5 to 1 g/dL per week.

Adverse Effects

Nausea, vomiting, metallic taste, heart burn, epigastric discomfort, bloating, abdominal colic, staining of teeth, constipation, and loose motions. Initiating therapy at low dose and gradually increasing to the optimum dose reduces development of tolerance.

Parenteral Iron

Parenteral iron therapy should be used cautiously because of serious adverse effect by this route. It should be given if there is failure of oral iron therapy, malabsorption, inflammatory bowel disease, noncompliance to oral iron, and chronic bleeding.

$$\text{Iron requirement (mg)} = 4.4 \times \text{body weight (kg)} \times \text{Hb deficit (g/dL)}$$

This formula is used to calculate iron required for replenishment of stores. Parenteral therapy replenishes store quickly.

Parenteral Administration

Intramuscular (IM) Administration

Deep IM injection is given in upper outer quadrant of gluteus major by Z track technique after sensitivity test. In this technique, the skin is displaced laterally before the injection, and this is practiced to prevent discoloration of skin and scar at the site of injection.

Intravenous (IV) and Subcutaneous (SC) Administration

Iron dextran and iron sorbitol citric acid have been used for about 50 years, while ferrous sucrose and ferric carboxy maltose are being used over the past few years. Newer formulations have less adverse effects and are safe to use.

1. Iron sorbitol

   It is low-molecular weight (mol wt < 500) complex of iron sorbitol citric acid. It rapidly provides iron in blood via IM route, as it does not bound locally in muscular tissue. It binds with transferrin and may saturate it; about 30% iron which is unbound is excreted in urine, imparting black color to urine due to formation of iron sulphide. Injection is painful.

2. Iron dextran

   It is a colloidal solution of ferric oxyhydroxide polymerized with dextran. It is a dark brown viscous liquid. It is given by both IM and IV route. IV availability is 100%. Sensitivity test with 0.25 to 0.5 mL is done ½ hour to 1 hour before administering it as IV infusion is recommended.

3. Iron sodium gluconate

   It is used by IV route and incidence of hypersensitivity is far much less than iron dextran.

4. Iron sucrose

   It is given by IV route. It shows minimal hypersensitivity, but on chronic use, it can damage renal tubules.

5. Ferric carboxy maltose

   It is a macromolecule iron complex that contains ferric hydroxide core and a carbohydrate shell. It provides controlled delivery of iron to reticoendothelial system (bone marrow, liver, spleen). It is administered by IV route up to a dose of 1000 mg (maximum in a week). It is not given by IM or SC route due to local irritation and permanent skin discoloration. It causes rapid rise in hemoglobin in iron deficiency anemia. The common side effects are pain at injection site, rashes, headache, and abdominal discomfort. It is not used in children < 14 years of age. Dose is 100 mg IV daily or 1000 mg IV infusion in 100 mL of normal saline over 10 to 20 minutes every week.

Adverse Effects

1. Local–IM administration causes pain, pigmentation, and sterile abscess at the site of injection.
2. Systemic–headache, joint pain, fever, dyspnea, palpitation, chest pain, metallic taste, and anaphylaxis
3. Toxic effects–
   a. Acute iron poisoning–It is common in children after accidental ingestion of large dose (>60 mg/kg). Symptoms are vomiting, pain in abdomen, hematemesis, loose motions, lethargy, dehydration, cyanosis, acidosis, convulsions, shock, cardiovascular collapse, and death in 6 to 36 hours. Symptoms are outcome of hemorrhage, inflammation in GIT, hepatic necrosis, and brain damage. Treatment aims at prevention of further absorption of iron from gut by inducing vomiting or gastric lavage with sodium bicarbonate, egg-yolk and milk, preventing further absorption.

      Desferrioxamine is the drug of choice (DOC) and life-saving. It is given 50 mg/kg IM or 20 mg/kg IV route till serum iron falls below 300 mcg/dL. Alternatives are DTPA and calcium edetate. Exchange transfusion may be required in case of renal damage. Supportive measures include acidosis correction, oxygen inhalation, blood pressure (BP) maintenance by IV fluids, and control of convulsions by diazepam.

   b. Chronic iron toxicity (hemochromatosis and hemosiderosis)–This damages pancreas and causes bronze diabetes, as skin develops dark bronze or gray tone due to excess iron. Treatment is intermittent phlebotomy in which repeated venesection is performed every week. Desferrioxamine by parenteral route can also be used if needed. Deferiprone is given in cases of chronic iron overload.

Interactions

1. Iron forms chelating compound with tetracycline, fluoroquinolones, penicillamine, methyldopa, levodopa, and carbidopa.
2. Stable complexes with thyroxine, captopril, and bisphosphonates.

Such interactions can be minimized if iron is administered at a gap of 3 hours with the above agents.

Megaloblastic Anemia

Megaloblastic anemia is characterized by macrocytic red blood cells and erythroid precursors, which show nuclear dysmaturity. Common causes are deficiency of vitamin B_{12} (cobalamin) and folic acid. A study has estimated the incidence of folate deficiency is 6.8%, that of vitamin B_{12} is 32%, and combined deficiency is 20% in north India.

Megaloblastic changes affect all hematopoietic cell lines with resultant anemia, thrombocytopenia, and leucopenia. DNA synthesis is impaired because of lack of methyl tetrahydrofolate (a folic acid derivative). Vitamin B_{12} plays an important role as a cofactor in this reaction, which is necessary for DNA base synthesis.

Role of Vitamin B_{12}

Active coenzyme of vitamin B_{12} are deoxyadenosylcobalamin (DAB_{12}) and methyl-cobalamin (methyl B_{12}).

1. Vitamin B_{12} is essential to convert homocysteine to methionine. Methionine is required as a methyl group donor in many metabolic reactions and for protein synthesis. This reaction also causes formation of tetrahydrofolate (THFA) from methyl THFA. In vitamin B_{12} deficiency, methyl THFA is trapped as a result of which number of one-carbon transfer reactions suffer.
2. Defective one carbon transfer affect purine and pyrimidine synthesis and unavailability of thymidylate for DNA production.
3. Malonic acid–Succinic acid is an important step in propionic acid metabolism. It is needed in synthesis of phospholipids and myelin. This step is responsible for demyelination seen in vitamin B_{12} deficiency.
4. Vitamin B_{12} is needed for cell growth and multiplication.

Role of Folic Acid

Folic acid is ris converted to DHFA, which in turn is converted to THFA by folate reductase and dihydrofolate reductase, respectively. THFA mediates a number of one-carbon transfer reactions like:

1. Conversion of homocysteine to methionine.
2. Thymidylate generation, an essential constituent of DNA.
3. Conversion of serine to glycine, which is utilized in thymidylate synthesis.
4. Synthesis of purine.
5. Histidine metabolism.

Sources

It is only synthesized by microorganisms; humans' gut flora can produce vitamin B_{12} but is not capable to absorb it.

Plant source–legumes.

Animal source–liver, kidney, marine fish, egg yellow, meat, and cottage cheese.

Daily Requirement (Table 48.4)

Table 48.4 Daily requirement of vitamin B_{12} and folic acid

Vitamin B_{12}	Folic acid
1–3 mg/day in adults	0.1–0.2 mg/day in adults
3–5 mg/day in pregnancy and lactation	0.8 mg/day in pregnancy and lactation

Causes of Megaloblastic Anemia (Table 48.5)

Table 48.5 Causes of megaloblastic anemia

Folic acid deficiency	Vitamin B_{12} deficiency
Decreased ingestion	Decreased ingestion
Impaired absorption like in celiac disease, malabsorption states, phenytoin, phenobarbitone	Impaired absorption like in intrinsic intestinal disease, intestinal parasites, Giardia infection, intrinsic factor deficiency, failure to release vitamin B_{12} from proteins, proton pump inhibitors
Impaired utilization like by drugs interfering with metabolism—methotrexate, trimethoprim, pyrimethamine, azathioprine	Impaired utilization like in orotic aciduria, prolonged parenteral nutrition, hemodialysis, autoimmune disorders, drugs interfering with cobalamin metabolism like metformin, neomycin, 6-mercaptopurines, 6-thioguanine, azathioprine, hydroxyurea, cytarabine, arabinoside, zidovudine, 5-flurouracil
Increased requirement like in infancy, hyperthyroidism, chronic hemolytic diseases	Maternal vitamin B_{12} deficiency in lactating mothers
Inborn error of metabolism—congenital malabsorption of folic acid, deficiency of dihydrofolate reductase, deficiency of N5-methyltetrahydrofolate homocysteine methyltransferase	Congenital intrinsic factor deficiency, deficiency of transcobalamin 1 and 2, cobalamin malabsorption due to defect in intestinal receptors, methyl malonic aciduria, homocystinuria

Clinical Manifestation

a. Anemia, jaundice, anorexia, irritability, and easy fatigability.
b. Glossitis, stomatitis, hyperpigmentation of skin over knuckles and terminal phalanges, and enlargement of liver and spleen (30–40% cases).
c. Neurological—subacute combined degeneration of spinal cord, peripheral neuritis, and diminished position and vibration sense. Late effects are paresthesias, depressed stretch reflex, hallucinations, changes of mood, and poor memory.

Treatment

Treatment depends on underlying cause. If the cause is not identified, therapeutic doses of folate (1–5 mg/day) and vitamin B_{12} (1000 mg) are administered. Only folate therapy may correct anemia but will not correct cobalamin deficiency-associated neurological disorder and result in progression of neuropsychiatric symptoms. So, for vitamin B_{12} deficiency correction, we give injections of vitamin B_{12} in therapeutic dose as described above. A decrease in mean corpuscular volume (MCV), reticulocytosis, and higher platelet and neutrophil count is observed within few days of therapy.

Folate deficiency, due to dietary insufficiency or due to increased demand, is treated by folate supplementation. Folate deficiency due to antifolate medication is treated by eliminating the implicating agent and supplementation of folic acid. A dose of 1 to 5 mg/day is recommended for 3 to 4 weeks.

The formulations of vitamin B_{12} preparation are as follows:

1. Cyanocobalamin 35 mg/5 mL.
2. Hydroxocobalamin 500 mg, 1000 mg injection.

In India, both oral and injectable preparation are available. Hydroxocobalamin is preferred for parenteral administration.

Prophylactic dose—3 to 10 mg/day.

Therapeutic dose—hydroxocobalamin 1 mg IM/SC injection daily for 2 weeks, followed by 1 mg every month for maintenance lifelong. If neurological manifestation is present, then in maintenance phase, injection is given once a week or once in 2 weeks for about 6 months followed by once a month for lifelong.

Methylcobalamin is the active coenzyme form of vitamin B_{12}. It is required for synthesis of methionine and S-adenosyl methionine. Both are needed for integrity of myelin. A total of 1.5 mg/day is given for correction of neurological defects in diabetics, alcoholics, and other forms of neuropathy.

Pernicious Anemia

It is an autoimmune disorder due to genetic deficiency of intrinsic factor of castle or destruction of intrinsic factor by autoantibodies against gastric parietal cells, which are responsible for synthesis of intrinsic factor. Intrinsic factor combines with vitamin B_{12} and forms IF-B_{12} complex, which binds with IF receptor in ileum enterocyte. In enterocytes, it liberates cobalamin, which then converts to methylcobalamin. So, in pernicious anemia, the dietary vitamin B_{12} is not absorbed, leading to its severe deficiency. It cannot be corrected by oral use of vitamin B_{12}; thus, it is given by parenteral route, either SC or IM. IV route is avoided because of risk of anaphylactic reaction and formation of antibodies against transcobalamin-vitamin B_{12} complex.

In pernicious anemia, vitamin B_{12} (1000 mg) should be given IM daily for 2 weeks, then weekly, till hemogram is normal, and then monthly for life.

Erythropoietin

Erythropoietin (EPO) is a sialoglycoprotein hormone which is produced by the kidney's peritubular cells. It is essential for normal erythropoiesis. Anemia and hypoxia are two triggers for erythropoietin release by kidneys. EPO acts on erythroid marrow cells, stimulates colony-forming cells of erythroid series, and induces erythroblast maturation and hemoglobin formation. It also releases reticulocytes in circulation and induces erythropoiesis in dose-dependent manner.

Epoetin α and β are forms of recombinant human erythropoietin. They are administered by SC or IV route. They have $t_{1/2}$ of 6 to 10 hours, and their actions remain for several days.

Use

In anemia of chronic renal disease which is due to low levels of erythropoietin. It is given to only symptomatic patients with Hb < 8 g/dL. It is also used for correction of anemia in AIDS patients, cancer chemotherapy patients, and preoperatively in presumptive autologous transfusion during surgery.

Dose

A total of 25 to 100 U/kg SC or IV three times a week (max. 600 U/kg/week) raises hematocrit and reduces need of blood transfusion, hence improves quality of life. Target hematocrit is 30% to 36% and Hb 10 to 11 g/dL. Trials have found higher mortality if Hb is raised to > 13.5 g/dL. Concurrent parenteral/oral iron therapy is required for optimum response in patients with low-iron stores.

Darbepoetin is a modified erythropoietin that has $t_{1/2}$ > 24 hours and can be administered once every 2 to 4 weeks.

Adverse Effects

Sudden increase in hematocrit, blood viscosity, and peripheral vascular resistance. There is increase in tendency of clot formation, hypertensive episodes, thromboembolic phenomenon, and rarely seizures can occur. There are flu-like symptoms in some patients.

Multiple Choice Questions

1. A young pregnant woman in second trimester comes for anemia evaluation. She had normal hemoglobin (Hb) before conception. Peripheral smear showed macrocytic anemia. Iron studies showed high-transferrin level. serum vitamin B_{12} was normal. She is suffering from?

A. Vitamin B_{12} deficiency
B. Folic acid deficiency.

C. Intrinsic factor deficiency.

D. Iron deficiency.

Answer: B

Folic acid deficiency or vitamin B_{12} deficiency can lead to megaloblastic anemia but she has normal B_{12} level, so likely diagnosis is folic acid deficiency.

2. What is the treatment of microcytic, hypochromic anemia during pregnancy?

A. Inj. erythropoietin.

B. Tab. ferrous sulfate.

C. Tab. folic acid.

D. Green leafy vegetables.

Answer: B

Iron deficiency anemia is the most common cause of microcytic hypochromic anemia during pregnancy. It is treated by ferrous sulfate supplementation.

3. A case of acute iron poisoning presents with?

A. Dizziness, hypertension, and cerebral hemorrhage.

B. Hyperthermia, delirium, and coma.

C. Hypotension, cardiac arrhythmias, and seizures.

D. Necrotizing gastroenteritis, shock, and metabolic acidosis.

Answer:. D

Acute iron poisoning causes direct corrosive gastrointestinal injuries. Fluid loss from gut leads to shock and cellular dysfunction which, in turn, leads to metabolic acidosis.

4. How will you manage a case of acute iron poisoning?

A. Oral deferasirox.

B. Activated charcoal.

C. Parenteral deferoxamine.

D. Parenteral dantrolene.

Answer: C

Oral deferasirox is effective for chronic iron toxicity.

5. Tumor removal surgery done in a patient of carcinoma stomach. Postoperatively, patient develops megaloblastic anemia. Cause of his anemia is A and is treated by B. What are A and B?

A. A = intrinsic factor; B = folic acid.

B. A = intrinsic factor; B = vitamin B_{12}.

C. A = extrinsic factor; B = parenteral iron.

D. A = extrinsic factor; B = granulocyte-macrophage colony-stimulating factors (GM-CSF).

Answer: B

Resection surgery of stomach leads to loss of intrinsic factor and the patient develops vitamin B_{12} deficiency.

6. A 10-year-old boy is suffering from anemia due to chronic renal insufficiency and is treated by?

A. Granulocyte colony-stimulating factors (G-CSF).

B. Granulocyte-macrophage colony-stimulating factors (GM-CSF).

C. Erythropoietin.

D. Ferrous sulfate.

Answer: C

The kidney produces erythropoietin; patients with chronic renal insufficiency often require exogenous erythropoietin to avoid chronic anemia.

7. Which of the following is administered to pregnant women prophylactically to prevent neural tube defects in fetus?

A. Riboflavin.

B. Iron.

C. Vitamin B_{12}.

D. Folic acid.

Answer: D

Folate deficiency has been implicated in neural tube defects like spina bifida, encephalocele, and anencephaly. Daily dose of 400 to 500 µg folic acid before, during, and after pregnancy till breastfeeding is recommended. If there is history of neural tube defects, then 4 mg/d is recommended.

8. Therapy with folinic acid is used to treat anemia associated with?

A. Antituberculosis drugs isoniazid and pyrazinamide.

B. Antiparkinsonian drug levodopa.

C. Methotrexate therapy.

D. Anticancer agent carboplatin.

Answer: C

Folinic acid or leucovorin calcium is a derivative of tetrahydrofolic acid. Its use lies in circumventing the inhibition of dihydrofolate reductase as a part of high-dose methotrexate therapy. It is also used to counteract toxicity of folate antagonist like pyrimethamine or trimethoprim.

9. Deficiency of folic acid is characterized by?

A. Microcytic, hypochromic anemia.

B. Megaloblastic anemia.

C. Sickle cell anemia.

D. Red cell aplasia.

Answer: B

Megaloblastic anemia is early sign of folic acid and vitamin B_{12} deficiency. It is characterized by macrocytic anemia, polysegmented neutrophils, and megakaryocytes.

Chapter 49

Coagulants and Anticoagulants

Tejus A.

PH1.25: Describe the mechanism/s of action, types, doses, side effects, indications, and contraindications of the drugs acting on blood, such as anticoagulants, antiplatelets, fibrinolytics, and plasma expanders.

Learning Objectives

- Coagulants and anticoagulants.
- Vitamin K.
- Heparin.
- Low-molecular weight heparin (LMWH).
- Warfarin.
- Direct factor Xa inhibitors.

Physiology of Blood Hemostasis

Hemostasis is a complex physiological process involved in the maintenance of normal blood flow. It relies on an established subtle balance between prothrombotic and anticoagulant mechanisms, predominantly involving the endothelial cells, platelets, coagulation factors, and inhibitors of coagulation and fibrinolysis. Endothelial cells provide a barrier against subendothelium, and secrete various factors like nitric oxide, von Willebrand factor (vWf), prostacyclin, endothelin, heparin, and phospholipids, which modulate vascular contractility, reactivity of platelets, coagulation, and fibrinolysis. In contrast to endothelial cells, the subendothelial layer of vessel wall, due to its contents like collagen, vWf, laminin, thrombospondin, and vitonectin, is highly thrombogenic.

Platelets play a vital role by forming the initial hemostatic plug (primary hemostasis) involving platelet adhesion, secretion, and aggregation. In the scenario of injury to vessel wall, vWf in subendothelium bridges with glycoprotein complex Ib (GPIb), a surface receptor on platelets (platelet adhesion). This is followed by degranulation of platelets consisting of alpha granules, which contain fibrinogen, coagulation factors V, VII, P-selectin, platelet-derived growth factor (PDGF), tumor growth factor-α (TGF-α), and delta granules, which contain calcium, histamine, serotonin, adenosine triphosphate (ATP), adenosine diphosphate (ADP), and epinephrine (platelet secretion). The activated platelets (platelet activation) secrete thromboxane A2 (TXA2) which, along with ADP, further aggregate the platelets, leading to the formation of platelet plug (platelet aggregation), which helps to initially seal the bleeding vessel wall.

The activated platelets secrete phospholipids which, along with calcium, provide a template for further steps involving coagulation factors. The factors involved in the coagulation cascade are precursors of proteolytic enzymes called zymogens, each of which, on activation, cleaves another zymogen to produce its activation form, named with check suffix "a" after roman numeral for clotting factors. The various factors involved in coagulation cascade include factor I (fibrinogen), factor II (prothrombin), factor III (tissue factor), factor IV (calcium), factor V (proacclerin/labile factor), factor VI (unassigned), factor VII (stable factor/proconvertin), factor VIII (antihemophilic factor A), factor IX (antihemophilic factor B/Christmas factor), factor X (Stuart–Prower factor), factor XI (plasma thromboplastin antecedent), factor XII (Hageman factor), factor XIII (fibrin-stabilizing factor), factor XIV (prekallikrein/F-Fletcher), factor XV (high molecular weight kininogen–Fitzgerald [HMWK/F]), factor XVI (vWf), factor XVII (antithrombin III), factor XVIII (heparin cofactor II), factor XIX (protein C), and factor XX (protein S).

All factors except factor III, IV, and VIII are produced by the liver. The coagulation factors are also classified as belonging to the fibrinogen family (factors I, V, VIII, and XIII), vitamin K-dependent proteins (factors II, VII, IX, and X), and contact family (factors XI, XII, HMWK, and prekallikrein). Traditionally, coagulation cascade is divided into extrinsic and intrinsic pathways. In extrinsic pathway, coagulation cascade starts with injury to vessel wall, leading to exposure of tissue factor (TF) in the subendothelium, which, along with calcium and factor VIIa, activates factor X to Xa (common pathway) being regulated by tissue factor pathway inhibitor (TFPI). The factor V present in platelets, released on platelet activation, is activated by thrombin to factor Va, which binds to Xa and forms a complex (prothrombinase complex). This complex activates prothrombin (factor II) to thrombin (IIa), which further amplifies its self-production by activating factors IX and VIII (**Fig. 49.1**). This explains why the deficiency of factors XII and XI produce mild bleeding disorders in comparison to deficiency of factor VIII (hemophilia A) and factor IX (hemophilia B). Extrinsic and intrinsic pathways are not parallel pathways of coagulation, because although the extrinsic pathway begins the cascade of coagulation, its further amplification is dependent on activation of intrinsic pathway of coagulation (**Fig. 49.1**).

The intrinsic pathway begins in vitro on contact of contact family factors with glass/kaolin and in vivo with any valves/devices, leading to activation of factor XII to XIIa. Further activated factor XIIa converts factor XI to XIIa, which further converts factor IX to IXa. The factor VIII bound to vWF in platelets is released free into circulation and activated to factor VIIIa by thrombin. The factor VIIIa serves as a receptor for factor IXa, which, along with calcium and anionic phospholipids, converts factor X to factor Xa (common pathway), further activating prothrombin to thrombin. Thrombin activates fibrinogen to fibrin monomers (soluble) and further produces fibrin polymers (insoluble). The factor XIII, activated by thrombin, plays a crucial role by cross-linking fibrin polymers into platelet plug (secondary

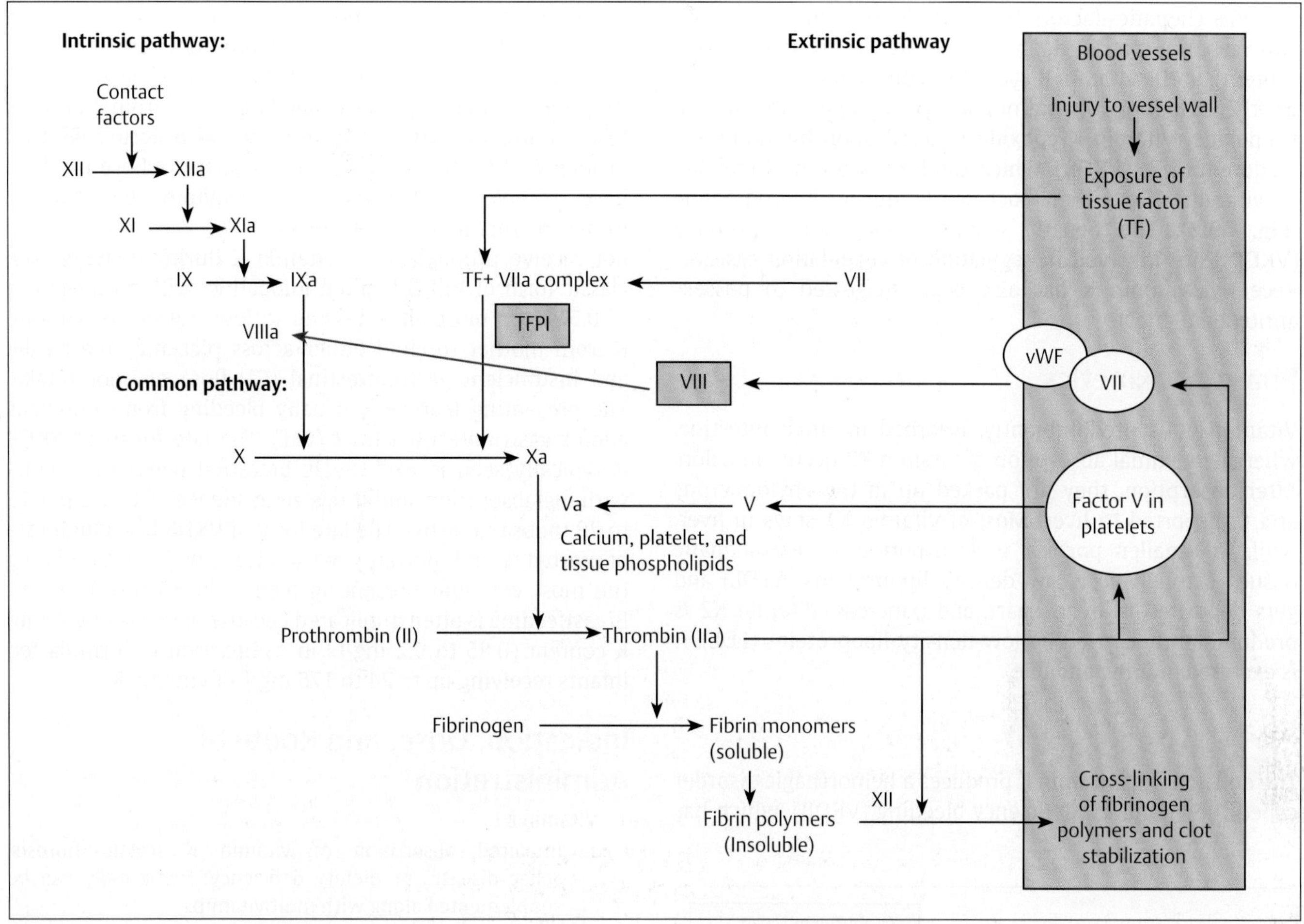

Fig. 49.1 Coagulation cascade. TFPI, tissue factor pathway inhibitor.

hemostasis), leading to stabilization of clot. The naturally occurring anticoagulants include antithrombin, TFPI, protein C, and protein Z, which regulate the delicate balance, thereby maintaining fluidity of blood.

Coagulants

Coagulants are the substances which promote or produce coagulation themselves and act as an aid in hemorrhagic disorders.

1. Vitamin K:
   a. Natural origin (lipid soluble):
      i. Vitamin K1: phylloquinone.
      ii. Vitamin K2: menaquinones (MK).
   b. Synthetic origin: vitamin K3
      i. Lipid soluble: Menadione, acetomenaphthone, menadiol.
      ii. Water soluble: Menadione sodium bisulfate (trihydrate), menadione sodium phosphate.
2. Others: fibrinogen, desmopressin, prothrombin complex concentrates, tranexamic acid, aminocaproic acid (epsilon-aminocaproic acid).

Vitamin K

Vitamin K belongs to a family of fat-soluble compounds playing a crucial role in maintaining blood fluid homeostasis. It was identified in 1936, when chickens that were fed with a low-fat diet developed severe bleeding. After analyzing lipid portion of the diet, a novel antihemorrhagic factor was identified and was named vitamin K, which coincided with the first letter of "koagulation," a German word. There are three types of vitamin K, namely, vitamin K1 (phylloquinone), vitamin K2 (menaquinones–MK) occurring naturally, and synthetic origin vitamin K3 (menadione). All three types share the common structure of menadione (2-methyl-1, 4-naphthoquinone), with variable phytyl side chain comprising four prenyl units at 3-position for vitamin K1. It is the most common dietary vitamin K, which is predominantly found in green leafy vegetables and fruits like avocado, kiwi, and grapes.

Vitamin K2 is synthesized by the bacteria in human gut, especially large intestine. Its primary dietary sources are dairy products, meat, and fermented foods. The World Health Organization (WHO) recommends a dietary intake of 65 µg/day for males and 55 µg/day for females. Vitamin K1 deficiency has hardly been noted due to its presence in diet, whereas K2 supplementation is advisable.

Physiological Actions

The most vital role of vitamin K is it acts as a cofactor for gamma-glutamylcarboxylase (GGCX), which catalyzes the carboxylation of glutamate residues of vitamin K-dependent proteins (hepatic—factors II, VII, IX, X, protein C, S, Z, and extrahepatic—matrix gla proteins, osteocalcin and gla-rich protein). In the vitamin K cycle, this conversion is dependent on the oxidation of vitamin K hydroquinone to vitamin K epoxide. Vitamin K epoxide is acted upon by vitamin K oxidoreductase (VKOR), which catalyzes vitamin K epoxide to vitamin K and then back to vitamin K hydroquinone (**Fig. 49.2**). The hepatic vitamin K-dependent proteins (VKDPs) are involved in regulation of coagulation cascade. Recently, vitamin K has also been suggested to possess antioxidant effects.

Pharmacokinetics

Vitamin K1 is predominantly absorbed in small intestine, whereas maximal absorption of vitamin K2 occurs in colon. After absorption, they are packed up in the chylomicrons and transported to liver. Most of vitamin K1 stays in liver, while a smaller portion is transported to extrahepatic tissues through very low density lipoproteins (VLDL) and gets deposited in liver, heart, and pancreas. Vitamin K2 is predominantly carried by low-density lipoproteins (LDL). It is excreted in urine and bile.

Vitamin K Deficiency

The deficiency of vitamin K produces a hemorrhagic disorder called the vitamin K deficiency bleeding (VKDB), which has replaced the earlier terminology of hemorrhagic disorder of newborn (HDN). VKDB is classified into three forms, namely, early (occurring within the first 24 hours of birth), classic (between 24 hours to 7 days), and late forms (from 2nd week to 6 months of birth). Early form of VKDB occurs with an incidence of 6 to 12% in high risk neonates whose mothers have received carbamazepine, phenytoin, barbiturates, isoniazid, rifampicin, cephalosporins or warfarin, and did not receive prophylaxis of vitamin K during delivery. The classic form of VKDB is often idiopathic, with an incidence of 0.5%. It is most often related to low transfer of vitamin K from mother to child either across placenta/breast milk and insufficient gastrointestinal (GI) flora or poor intake. The presenting feature is usually bleeding from umbilicus and/or gastrointestinal tract (GIT). The late forms of VKDB is typically seen in exclusively breastfed newborns/infants with malabsorption, and it has an incidence of 1 case per 15 to 20 thousand births. The late form of VKDB has a high rate of morbidity and mortality, with intracranial bleeding being the most common presenting feature in 30 to 60% cases. Breastfeeding is often implicated because of its lower vitamin K content (0.85 to 9.2 mg/L) in comparison to formula fed infants receiving up to 24 to 175 mg/L of vitamin K.

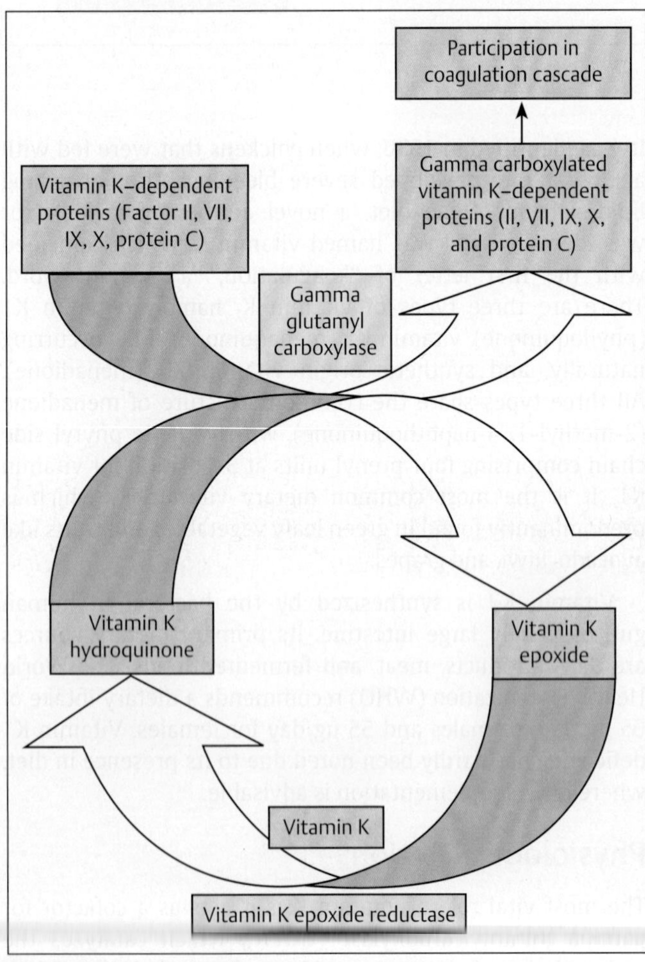

Fig. 49.2 Vitamin K cycle.

Indication, Dose, and Route of Administration

1. Vitamin K1:
   a. Impaired absorption of vitamin K (cystic fibrosis, celiac disease) or dietary deficiency: 5 mg daily can be supplemented along with multivitamins.
   b. Pregnancy:
      i. On anticonvulsant drugs: 10 mg intramuscularly (IM) daily for 2 to 7 days and 10 mg orally daily from 36 weeks (always avoid vitamin K3 for this purpose, because it causes oxidative damage and hemolysis).
      ii. Factor VII deficiency in megaloblastic anemia.
      iii. After bariatric surgery, in order to avoid severe anemia, low-birth weight, and congenital anomalies.
      iv. To improve prothrombin and partial thromboplastin activity in neonates, hence reducing the severity of intraventricular hemorrhages.
   c. VKDB: There is insufficient evidence to support the vitamin K supplementation. It improves:
      i. Early form: recommended to administer vitamin K to at-risk pregnant mothers.
      ii. Classic and late form: single IM injection (400 µg for neonates with birth weight < 2.5 kg and 1 mg for > 2.5 kg). An oral dose of 2 mg with first feed followed by two doses at 4th to 6th and 6th to 8th weeks of age can be administered for children whose parents refuse IM injection.
   d. Reversal of warfarin-induced bleeding.
   e. May reduce the risk of fracture due to osteopenia and osteoporosis (5 mg daily).
   f. In combination with vitamin D, it delays the vascular calcifications, deteriorating elasticity of arteries.
   g. May reduce the overall risk and mortality from coronary heart disease.
   h. Improves insulin sensitivity.
   i. May improve cognitive function and benefit elderly with Alzheimer's disease.

2. Vitamin K2
   a. May reduce hip, vertebral, and nonvertebral fractures (45–90 mg/day).
   b. Prevention of deaths from cirrhosis and hepatocellular carcinoma: trials carried out at a dose of 45 or 90 mg/day.
   c. Vitamin K2-7 (MK-7) capsules 200 µg once daily for 12 weeks has been shown to provide symptomatic improvement in peripheral neuropathy due to vitamin B12 deficiency and type 2 diabetes mellitus.

Adverse effects include injection site pain, flushing, altered taste sensations, rarely dizziness, hypotension, and cyanosis. It can also cause anaphylactoid reaction with intravenous (IV)/IM administration, but studies suggest that it is the solubilizer that is the reason for such a reaction.

Other Coagulants

1. Fibrinogen: The normal level of fibrinogen is about 200 to 400 mg/dL, but it can be much more during the third trimester pregnancy. It is often used to manage bleeding in perioperative cardiac surgical patients.
2. Desmopressin: It is V2 receptor analogue of arginine vasopressin, which acts by releasing stores of vWF from endothelium and plays a key role in coagulation cascade. Often used to control bleeding (0.3 µg/kg intravenous infusion over 15 to 30 min) in mild hemophilia A and von Willebrand disease.
3. Prothrombin complex concentrates: It contains variable concentrations of coagulants (factors II, VII, IX, and X), anticoagulants (proteins C, S, and Z), thrombin, and heparin. It is often used for the emergent reversal of vitamin K and nonvitamin K oral anticoagulants.
4. Recombinant activated factor VIIa: A dose of 90 to 120 µg/kg is often used for hemophilias and Glanzman's thrombasthenia. Its use is often followed by thromboembolic complications.

Local Hemostatics (Styptics)

Local hemostatics are substances which help in control of bleeding from a local site of bleeding. An ideal local hemostatic must be effective, safe for administration, including its metabolites, and affordable. They are broadly classified as passive and active hemostatic agents (**Table 49.1**). The passive agents act by providing a template which adheres itself to bleeding site and activates the extrinsic pathway of coagulation. Active agents can themselves initiate the cascade of coagulation.

Use of Styptics

Passive Hemostatic Agents

Collagen-Based Products

They are obtained from bovine tendon/dermal collagen. On administration, they attract platelets into their fibrous mass and form a platelet plug, followed by degranulation of platelets, activation of clotting factors, and initiation of coagulation cascade. They are applied in a dry form to the site of moderate-to-severe capillary/venous/small arterial bleedings. It is contraindicated in those with known hypersensitivity reactions and produce adverse reactions including inflammation, formation of adhesions and abscess formation. The absorbable collagen hemostat sponge (Helistat) is obtained from bovine tendons and has the unique capacity of high absorption and can hold fluid much more than its own weight.

Cellulose-Based Products

1. Surgicel (oxidized regenerated cellulose): obtained from alpha cellulose of plants and is available as a meshwork. It can absorb blood 7 to 10 times its own weight and produces mechanical pressure to achieve hemostasis. Adverse effects include delayed wound healing, granulomas, burning sensations, and neurological complications.
2. ActCel and Gelitacel: It can expand 3 to 4 times its size on contact with blood and converts itself into a gel, followed by biodegradation within 1 to 2 weeks.

Gelatin-Based Products (Gelfoam)

It is most commonly used for the control of minor bleeding and obtained from gelatin of purified pork skin. It can absorb 40 times its weight of blood and can expand up to 200% its volume. Adverse effects include formation of hematoma, abscess formation, infections, granulomas, fibrosis, and toxic shock syndrome.

Polysaccharide Hemispheres

It is obtained from vegetable starch.

Table 49.1 Difference between passive and active hemostatic agents

Passive hemostatic agents	Active hemostatic agents
Provide a matrix which attaches to bleeding site and activates the extrinsic pathway of coagulation	They possess biological activity and can participate directly in coagulation pathway
Useful only in those with an intact coagulation cascade	Can themselves activate coagulation cascade
They are available for use immediately and are preferred as first-line agents	Often used in combination with passive agents
Requires no special preparation or storage facilities	Needs special preparation/storage regulations
Relatively inexpensive, minimum quantities needed	Relatively more expensive
a. Collagen-based products b. Cellulose based c. Gelatine based d. Polysaccharides	a. Thrombin b. Flowable hemostatic agents

Active Hemostatic Agents

Thrombin

It is obtained from bovine/human plasma/recombinant DNA technology. It is used as a dry powder and applied topically often in combination with gelatin sponges. It has a faster onset of action by converting fibrinogen to fibrin and is used for moderate-to-severe bleeding. It is contraindicated in bleeding from large vessels, as it can cause fatal extensive intravascular thrombus formation.

Flowable Hemostatic Agent (FloSeal)

It is composed of bovine-derived granules of gelatin that are coated with thrombin. It carries risk of transmitting viral infections and is contraindicated in those allergic to bovine products. Adverse effects include arrhythmias, thrombosis, atrial fibrillation, hypotension, edema, and pleural effusion.

Sealants

They act as barriers to the flow of liquids, including fibrin sealants, polyethylene glycol sealants, albumin with glutaraldehyde, and cyanoacrylate.

Other Hemostatic Agent

1. **Aprotinin:** It is a broad-spectrum serine protease (plasmin, protein C, trypsin, chymotrypsin, kallikrein, and thrombin) inhibitor approved for reducing blood transfusion in patients undergoing coronary artery bypasses grafting (CABG) with cardiopulmonary bypass.
2. **Chitosan-based products:** Chitosan is a polysaccharide obtained from deacetylation of chitin and is used in surgical hemostatic dressings. Although its mechanism is unclear, it is postulated that its positive charge promotes adhesion of erythrocytes, adsorbs fibrinogen, and promotes wound healing.
3. Polysaccharide-based hemostats (poly-N-acetyl glucosamine-based, and QuiKclot contains zeolites and porous aminosilicates as adsorbents).
4. Tannic acid is often used as a natural polymer anticoagulant in treating wastewater.
5. Lysine analogs: epsilon-aminocaproic acid.
6. Bone hemostats: bone wax, ostene.
7. **Sclerosing agents:** These are used for treatment of varicose veins, and telangiectasia includes the following:
   a. Detergents: polidocanol (0.25–1%), sodium tetradecyl sulfate (0.1%), sodium morrhuate, and ethanolamine oleate. They act by desquamating the endothelial cells, interfering with their cell membrane lipids, and initiating coagulation. For the treatment of varicose veins, detergents are combined with carbon dioxide/oxygen/room air to produce foam (1–3%); with a volume of 6 to 10 mL injected, it induces inflammation and obliteration of veins.
   b. Hyperosmolar or hypertonic agents: includes hypertonic saline (11.7–23.4%), hypertonic dextrose (up to 75%), and sodium salicylate. They act by dehydrating the endothelial cells.
   c. Chemical irritants: Glycerine (72%) acts as a caustic on vessel wall; it can be diluted with lidocaine (1%) with or without epinephrine.
   d. ClariVein is developed for treatment of large varicose veins. It uses mechanical rotating dispersion wire to mill and disperse sclerosing agents onto the vessel wall.

Anticoagulants

Anticoagulants are the drugs which prevent the coagulation of blood and are used in various coagulation disorders (**Fig. 49.2**).

Anticoagulants acting in vitro to preserve the analytical samples include heparin, citrate, and ethylene-diaminotetra acetic acid.

Heparin

Heparin (Greek word "hepar") was discovered more than 100 years ago by Jay Mclean and William Howell in 1916 from canine liver cells. It is a polysaccharide found on surface of various mammalian cells and in the extracellular matrix. It is involved in embryonic development, blood coagulation, infections, and inflammatory responses. Although dog liver and bovine lung/liver was used initially for wide-scale manufacturing purpose, it is the porcine intestine which is used as a primary source. It has a heterogenous structure with a molecular weight ranging from 3,000 to 30,000 Daltons (~ 45 saccharide units) and is also called as unfractionated heparin (UFH).

Mechanism of Action

Heparin is considered as an indirectly acting anticoagulant, as it works only on binding to antithrombin (AT), an endogenous vitamin K independent 50 kDa glycoprotein anticoagulant from liver. AT exhibits a broad spectrum but a weak anticoagulant action in vivo by inhibiting thrombin, factors Xa, IXa, and weakly inhibiting factors VIIa, XIa, XIIa, plasmin, kallikrien, and trypsin. Together with protein C, it plays a vital role in inhibiting coagulation cascade.

Pharmacological Actions

The main reason for AT being a weak inhibitor is due to the fact that its active loop at the center is folded into its structure, to be activated only on formation of a complex between intermediate proteinases, pentasaccharide sequence of heparin, and AT. This activation occurs in two steps, initial binding of three monosaccharide units leading to a conformational change in AT, exposing its active loop at the center, and in the next step, this activated confirmation of AT is stabilized. This activated AT binds to protease, forming a complex, and inactivation occurs, followed by release of heparin, which is available for the next reaction. The above-mentioned mechanism is sufficient for inhibition of factors Xa, IXa, and VIIa, whereas inhibition of thrombin requires additional 13 saccharide chain of heparin, so that it provides a scaffold for binding to both AT and thrombin. A direct interaction between factor VIIa and heparin has also been noted, which is predominantly calcium-mediated.

Pharmacokinetics

The preferred route for administration of UFH is IV, followed by subcutaneous (SC) routes due to better bioavailability. On entering the systemic circulation, it binds to plasma proteins. UFH is cleared from the body predominantly by depolymerization at therapeutic doses, with a half-life of 1 to 2 hours (can be as long as 8 hours, depending on the dose). At higher doses, renal clearance sets in, which is nonsaturable, selective clearance of larger molecular weight chains of UFH, leading to enhanced anticoagulation effect.

Adverse Effects

1. Bleeding: Heparin increases risk of bleeding by interfering with normal coagulation mechanisms, but it is also influenced by various risk factors like dose, duration, indication, procedure, and contraindications. The prevalence of bleeding has shown wide variation ranging from 0.6 to 14%, depending on trial, where most of them exclude high-risk patients. The anticoagulant effect is monitored by daily measurement of activated partial thromboplastin time (aPTT) levels, as it is considered a useful tool for assessing anticoagulation of medications acting through intrinsic and common pathway.
2. Heparin-induced thrombocytopenia (HIT): It is the most common nonbleeding adverse effect of heparin, with a prevalence of 2.6%. There are two types HIT, type I and type II (**Table 49.2**).
3. Skin necrosis: often presents as painful plaques with well-defined margins, which are erythematous and can undergo necrosis. Various mechanism suspected include thrombocytopenia-induced, immune-mediated aggregation of platelets or formation of antigen antibody-mediated thrombosis of cutaneous blood vessels, leading to necrosis. Prompt discontinuation often reverses the reaction.
4. Osteoporosis: Long-term administration of heparin often binds to osteoprotegerin (OPG) and prevents interaction with RANK ligand, leading to activation of osteoclasts.
5. Others:
   a. Alopecia.
   b. Elevated liver enzymes.
   c. Hyperkalemia.

Contraindications

1. Thrombocytopenia (platelet count < 1,00,000/mm).
2. Active, uncontrolled bleeding (except disseminated intravascular coagulation).
3. History of heparin-induced thrombocytopenia.
4. Those who cannot undergo routine monitoring.

Uses

1. Anticoagulant:
   a. Treatment of deep venous thrombosis (DVT) and pulmonary embolism (PE). Although LMWHs are standard of therapy, UFH is preferred in those with high risk of bleeding, as the anticoagulant effect can be easily stopped by terminating heparin infusion and the availability of a reversal agent–protamine sulfate. Loading dose: 80 units/kg or maximum 4,000 units bolus IV, followed by continuous IV infusions of 18 units/kg/hr with a target international normalized ratio (INR) of 1.5 to 2.5 times of control (anti-Xa levels: 0.3–0.7 units/mL) for at least 5 days till the effect of oral anticoagulants take effect. The aPTT has to be measured every 6 hours and dose can be titrated based on the results. The treatment is continued for 3 months and to continue the prophylaxis further is based on the bleeding risk of an individual.

      In pregnancy, UFHs and LMWH are anticoagulants of choice, as they minimally cross the placental barrier.
   b. Acute coronary syndrome (ACS): ST segment elevated myocardial infarction (STEMI) and as adjunct to fibrinolytic therapy. Started with a bolus dose of 60 units/kg (maximum of 4,000 units), followed by a maintenance infusion of 12 units/kg per hour (maximum of 1,000 units). The target aPTT is 1.5 to 2.0 times the control (Anti-Xa levels: 0.2–0.5 units/mL).
   c. Percutaneous coronary intervention (PCI): 50 to 70 U/kg IV bolus along with glycoprotein (GP) IIb/IIIa receptor antagonists, with a therapeutic activated clotting time (ACT). The dose is 70 to 100 U/kg bolus without GP IIb/IIIa antagonists.
   d. Bridge therapy for atrial fibrillation: 60 to 80 units/kg IV boluses with a target aPTT range of 50 to 70 seconds.
   e. Prophylaxis of venous thromboembolism (VTE):
      i. Medically ill/surgical population: 5,000 units subcutaneously every 8 to 12 hours.
      ii. Pregnancy: 7,500 to 15,000 units SC every 12 hours.
   f. To maintain patency of circuit for continuous renal replacement therapy (CRRT) in those with contraindication to the use of citrate.
   g. Catheter patency: 10 units/mL (<10 kg) and 10 to 100 units/mL (>10 kg) instill sufficient volume.
2. Nonanticoagulant uses:
   a. Anti-inflammatory effects: In animal models, it is found to inhibit hyper-responsiveness of bronchus and inhibits leukocyte accumulation, thereby providing protection during ischemia-reperfusion injury.
   b. Cancer: Apart from benefitting from prophylaxis of VTE, heparin is found to reduce metastasis in animal models of carcinoma, probably due to its anti-inflammatory effect by inhibiting accumulation of fibrin around tumor cells. Other suggested mechanisms include inhibition of heparinase, selectins, and TFPI.
   c. Wound healing and tissue repair, especially in patients with burns.

Table 49.2 Difference between type I and II HIT

Type I	Type II
More common	Less common
Mild thrombocytopenia	Severe thrombocytopenia
Faster onset	Delayed onset (usually after 4 days of initiation of treatment)
Cessation of heparin not needed	Cessation needed
Not autoimmune related	Immune related

Abbreviation: HIT, heparin-induced thrombocytopenia.

d. Shortens the induction of labor probably by modulating mediators of inflammation like IL-8 and cytokines.

Low Molecular Weight Heparin (LMWH)

Various LMWHs include enoxaparin, dalteparin, tinzaparin, reviparin, nadroparin, parnaparin, ardeparin, certoparin, and bemiparin.

Mechanism of Action

In order to overcome the most adverse effects with UFH, heparin was depolymerized chemically/enzymatically to produce heparin with one third of its molecular weight (1,000 to 10,000 kDa). These are known as LMWHs, which have reduced ability to inhibit factor II, as it does not provide a scaffold to bind AT and thrombin together, but retains its ability to inhibit factor Xa similarly to heparin. The ratio of factor Xa to factor II inhibition ranges between 2 to 4:1 for LMWH, whereas it is 1:1 for heparin (**Fig. 49.3**).

Uses (As per Table 49.3)

Differentiate between Heparin and LMWH (Table 49.4)

Fondaparinux

Mechanism of Action

Similar to UFH and LMWH, fondaparinux acts indirectly through AT potentiation by almost 300 times to inhibit factor Xa, further blocking the coagulation cascade. It is also known as pentasaccharide anticoagulant, because it is made up of pentasaccharide units, the active sequence of UFH and LMWH. Due to its small molecular size, it cannot bind thrombin; hence, it acts as a selective factor Xa inhibitor (**Fig. 49.4**).

Advantages over unfractionated heparin:

1. 15 times higher affinity to AT in comparison to UFH.

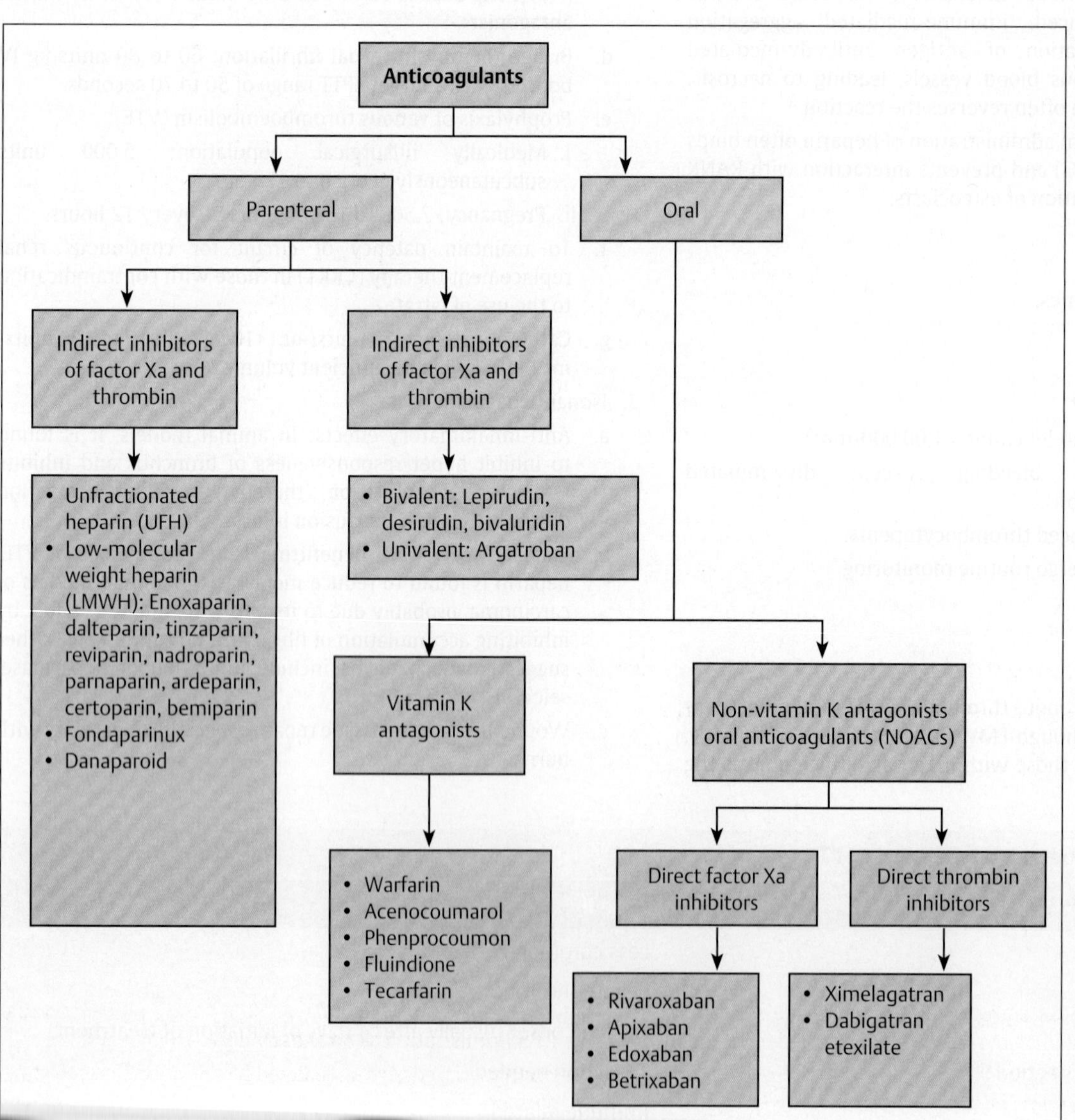

Fig. 49.3 Classification of anticoagulants.

Table 49.3 Uses of LMWHs

LMWH	Indication with dose
Enoxaparin: Approved in 1993 by US FDA, it is obtained by benzylation of UFH, followed by alkaline hydrolysis. Molecular weight 4,500 kDa BA: 90 to 92% $t_{1/2}$: 4.5 hours	▪ Prophylaxis of DVT postabdominal surgery/medically ill patients: 40 mg SC once daily (up to 12–14 days) ▪ Prophylaxis of DVT post knee/hip replacement: 30 mg SC every 12 hours up to 14 days ▪ Treatment of DVT ± PE: 1 mg/kg SC every 12 hours up to 17 days ▪ STEMI: 30 mg IV bolus followed by 1 mg/kg along with fibrinolytic (tenecteplase) and then 1 mg/kg SC every 12 hours for at least 8 days ▪ Unstable angina and non-Q wave MI: 1 mg/kg SC every 12 hours with aspirin ▪ Prophylaxis/bridge therapy for AF/cardioversion: 1 mg/kg SC every 12 hours or 1.5 mg/kg SC/day
Dalteparin: obtained from depolymerization using nitrous acid. BA: 87% $t_{1/2}$: 3 to 5 hours	▪ Prophylaxis of DVT: ◦ Medical ill patients: 5,000 IU SC once daily ◦ Abdominal surgery: 2,500 IU SC, followed by 2,500 IU SC after 12 hours and then 5,000 IU SC once daily ◦ Hip replacement: 2,500 IU SC 4 to 8 hours after surgery and then 5,000 IU SC once daily ▪ Unstable angina and non-Q wave MI: 120 IU SC every 12 hours with aspirin
Tinzaparin: obtained after heparinase digestion by UFH, molecular weight: 6,500 kDa, BA: 87%, $t_{1/2}$: 3.4 hours.	Used only for prophylaxis of DVT without PE at dose of 175 IU/kg once a day.

Abbreviations: AF, atrial fibrillation; DVT, deep vein thrombosis; IV, intravenous; LMWH, low-molecular weight heparin; MI, myocardial infarction; PE, pulmonary embolism; SC, subcutaneous; STEMI, ST elevation myocardial infarction; UFH, unfractionated heparin; US FDA, United States Food and Drug Administration.

Table 49.4 Difference between UFH and LMWH

UFH	LMWH
Anti-Xa: Anti IIa activity = 1:1	Anti Xa: Anti IIa activity = 2 to 4:1
Less SC bioavailability (30%)	Enhanced SC bioavailability (90–100%)
Administered intravenous, hence self-administration not possible	Self-administration possible
Unpredictable dose response relationship	Predictable dose response relationship: due to lesser interaction with plasma proteins other than anticoagulant plasma proteins, macrophages and endothelial cells
Minimal renal excretion; hence, no dose adjustment needed	Dose-dependent clearance by kidneys—accumulates in patients with severe renal failure (needs dose modifications/monitoring with anti-Xa levels)
Relatively shorter half-life (1–2 hours), can extend up to 8 hours, depending on the dose	Longer plasma half-life (4–7 hours)
Dose titrated based on anticoagulant response	Fixed doses
Bleeding: No statistical difference noted between UFH and LMWH	
Higher incidence of HIT (up to 5%)	Lesser incidence of HIT (1/10th in comparison to UFH) < 1%
More risk of osteoporosis on prolonged treatment	Lesser frequency of osteoporosis due to lesser binding with osteoblasts
Rapid and complete reversal by protamine	Partial reversal (protamine reverses 100% of antifactor IIa activity but only 60% of antifactor Xa activity)

Abbreviations: HIT, heparin-induced thrombocytopenia; LMWH, low-molecular weight heparin; UFH, unfractionated heparin.

2. Does not inhibit other plasma proteins; hence, it has less inter- and intraindividual variability in coagulation achieved, making laboratory monitoring unnecessary.
3. As it does not bind to platelets or PF4, it does not cause HIT and poses lesser risk of osteoporosis.
4. Administered SC with 100% bioavailability and a $t_{1/2}$ of 17 hours make its administration as once daily dose.
5. Excreted through kidneys unchanged has no significant food or drug interaction.

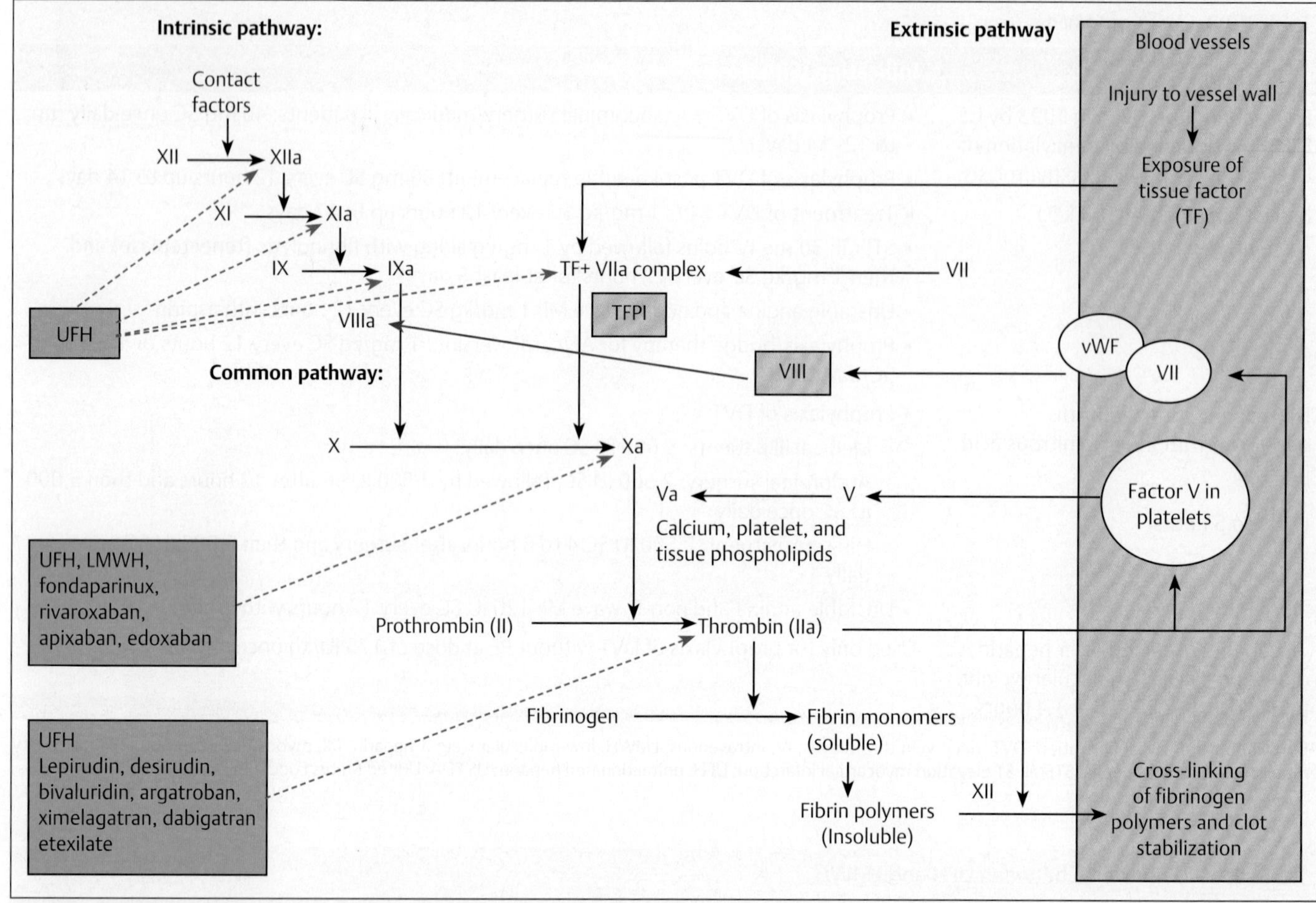

Fig. 49.4 Summary of mechanism of action of various anticoagulants.

Indications

1. ACS with or without ST segment elevation: 2.5 mg SC once daily.
2. PCI.
3. DVT and PE.
4. As an alternate for UFH/LMWH hypersensitivity.

Adverse Effects

Bleeding complications, anemia, insomnia, hypokalemia, hypotension, dizziness, increased drainage of wounds, confusion, hematoma, and purpura.

Contraindications

Hypersensitivity, creatinine clearance < 30 mL/min.

Limitations

Parenteral administration, no reversal agents.

Idraparinux

Second-generation, long-acting—80 hours, idrabiotaparinux—idraparinux covalently binds to biotin, water-soluble B-complex vitamin. Its anticoagulant effect can be reversed with avidin infusion.

Danaparoid

It is a heparinoid, a mixture of heparan sulfate (84%), dermatan sulfate (12%), and chondritin sulfate (4%). It is used in HIT to augment AT anticoagulant action with antifactor Xa to IIa ratio of 22:1. It also inhibits thrombin by potentiating heparin cofactor II. It has 100% SC BA, $t_{1/2}$ = 25 hours, undergoes renal excretion, and has no interference with platelet function. There is no need of laboratory monitoring (antifactor Xa assay) and there is no antidote.

Heparin Antagonists

Protamine Sulfate

It is the only Food and Drugs Administration (FDA)-approved drug to reverse the anticoagulation induced by UFH, which can be used during dialysis, acute ischemic strokes, and various invasive surgeries. Originally isolated from the sperm of salmon fish, it is being currently being produced by recombinant DNA technology. The positively charged cationic peptides of protamine strongly antagonize anionic heparin by forming aggregates, neutralizing it within 5 minutes. A total of 1 to 1.5 mg of protamine is used to neutralize 100 units of heparin, and the required dose is administered as an IV infusion slowly over 10 to 15 minutes. A prior test dose is always administered to rule out anaphylactic response seen in 0.06 to 10.6% cases. Treatment of anaphylaxis due to protamine includes methylprednisolone, antihistamines, vasopressin, salbutamol, norepinephrine, fluids, glucagon, and echocardiography. Other adverse effects include pulmonary hypertension and renal and hepatic abnormalities. It is generally administered through a peripheral vein rather than central line due to the increased risk of hypotension.

Other Less Toxic Alternatives (Not Approved)

Universal heparin reversal agent (UHRA), low-molecular weight protamine (LMWP), 40 kDa dextrans (Dex40), glycidyltrimethylammonium chloride (GTMAC3), andexanet alfa, and ciraparantag.

Direct Parenteral Thrombin Inhibitors

Table 49.5 lists outs parenteral direct thrombin inhibitors.

Thrombin inhibition was a well-recognized strategy to achieve anticoagulation. In the late 1800s, hirudin, the first direct thrombin inhibitor, was isolated from *Hirudo medicinalis*, a medicinal leech. But due to issues related to its purification techniques and availability, it was overtaken by the introduction of heparin as an anticoagulant.

1. Bivalent: lepirudin, bivaluridin.
2. Univalent: argatroban.

Table 49.5 Parenteral DTIs

DTI, mechanism of action & advantages (Fig. 49.3)	Indication and dose	Adverse effects and disadvantages
Bivalent parenteral DTIs		
Lepirudin: The first DTI is a recombinant version of hirudin. Irreversibly binds to thrombin at a ratio of 1:1, but at 10 times less affinity in comparison to hirudin. Plasma $t_{1/2}$ 80 minutes post IV or SC administration Needs monitoring by aPTT	HIT: 0.4 mg/kg bolus ® 0.15 mg/kg/hr IV/SC (Readjustment in renal failure)	a. Bleeding b. Antihirudin antibodies (40% cases) c. Anaphylaxis rarely d. Narrow therapeutic window e. No specific antidote
Desirudin: Similar to hirudin Fixed dose used subcutaneously $t_{1/2}$: 2 hours No dose calculations based on weight. No routine lab monitoring of aPTT except in cases with creatinine clearance < 30 mL/min.	DVT posttotal hip replacement and HIT: 15 mg twice daily	Bleeding
Bivaluridin: Synthetic bivalent DTI, 800 times lesser affinity to thrombin than hirudin (less risk of bleeding) Reversible thrombin inhibition Faster onset of action $t_{1/2}$: 25 min Elimination: 80% (proteolytic cleavage & hepatic), 20% (renal)—dose adjustment in renal insufficiency Monitoring with ACT = 365 ± 100 seconds	Alternative to heparin in HIT patients with or without thrombosis undergoing PCI: 0.75 mg/kg IV bolus, followed by 1.75 mg/kg/hr for 4 hours	Bleeding
Univalent parenteral DTIs		
Argatroban: Synthetic, noncovalent, and reversible inhibition of active site of thrombin $t_{1/2}$: 45 min Elimination: biliary (dose adjustment in hepatic impairment) Monitoring: aPTT = 1.5 to 3 times from baseline, prolongs PT & INR	HIT Anticoagulation in patients with h/o HIT/ at risk of HIT undergoing PCI 2 µg/kg/min IV infusion	Coadministration with warfarin discontinued if INR > 4

Abbreviations: ACT, activated clotting time; aPTT, activated partial thromboplastin time; DTI, direct thrombin inhibitor; DVT, deep vein thrombosis; HIT, heparin-induced thrombocytopenia; INR, international normalized ratio; IV, intravenous; PCI, percutaneous coronary intervention; PT, prothrombin time; SC, subcutaneous.

Oral Anticoagulants

1. Vitamin K antagonists: warfarin, acenocoumarol, phenprocoumon, fluindione, tecarfarin.
2. Nonvitamin K antagonist:
   a. Direct factor Xa inhibitors: rivaroxaban, apixaban, edoxaban, betrixaban.
   b. Direct thrombin inhibitors: ximelagatran, dabigatran etexilate.

Warfarin

Chemically warfarin is (RS), available as an equal racemic mixture of (R) and (S) enantiomers, with the (S) enantiomer being 5 times more potent than (R) enantiomer.

Warfarin is a vitamin K antagonist, which acts by inhibiting the cyclical conversion of vitamin k epoxide to vitamin K hydroquinone by inhibiting the enzyme vitamin K epoxide reductase (**Fig. 49.2**). This conversion is essential for the gamma carboxylation of clotting factors like factors II, VII, IX, X, and their further participation in maintaining blood homeostasis. It is also involved in the gamma carboxylation of endogenous anticoagulants like protein C and S. The mechanism clearly underlines the fact that when warfarin administration is started, further formation of clotting factors is inhibited but has no effect on the already gamma carboxylated clotting factors in circulation. Hence, there is a delay in the onset of anticoagulant effect of warfarin by 2 to 7 days after administration, as pre-existing factors II ($t_{1/2}$–48 to 60 hours), VII ($t_{1/2}$–1.5 to 6 hrs), IX ($t_{1/2}$–20 to 24 hours) and X ($t_{1/2}$–24 to 48 hours) are eliminated from circulation. Warfarin paradoxically has a procoagulant effect initially, as the protein C inhibited by it has a short half-life of 1.5 to 6 hours and is the first to disappear from circulation. This procoagulant effect of warfarin gets exaggerated in individuals to protein C deficiency.

Pharmacokinetics

After oral administration, warfarin is absorbed rapidly from upper GIT with a bioavailability of 79 to 100%. Upon entering the systemic circulation, it is largely bound to plasma proteins (99%), predominantly albumin and alpha-1 acid glycoproteins. Being highly plasma protein bound, it has a low volume of distribution of 0.14 L/kg. The more potent (S) enantiomer is metabolized by the cytochrome enzyme CYP2C9 in liver to 7-hydroxywarfarin. The (R) enantiomer is metabolized predominantly by CYP1A2. The metabolites are inactive, eliminated through kidneys (92%) predominantly, and to a lesser extent in bile with a half-life of 20 to 60 hours. Vitamin K epoxide reductase complex 1 (VKORC1) mediates pharmacodynamic effects of warfarin.

Indications of Warfarin at Various INR

Table 49.6 mentions indications of warfarin with target INR levels.

Adverse Effects

1. Bleeding: Warfarin, due to its influence of environmental factors and drug interactions, has a narrow therapeutic index. It increases risk of major bleeding by 0.3 to 0.5% per year and risk of most severe hemorrhage (intracranial) by 0.2%. Management varies depending on INR values and presence or absence of bleeding (see chapter on vitamin K for details).
2. Purple toe syndrome: It is a rare adverse effect seen with warfarin use, occurring after 3 to 8 weeks of use and affecting 1 in 5,000 patients. The risk increases to 5% in those with protein C deficiency. It is characterized by the appearance of purple lesions over the toes, often bilateral and blanch on pressure. The pathogenesis was believed to be due to toxic insult to capillaries, leading to dilation and increased vascular permeability, but the new theory suggests it to be due to cholesterol microemboli or bleeding into atherosclerotic plaques. Replacing warfarin with other anticoagulants is the treatment of choice. Although it is reported with other anticoagulants but not with apixaban.
3. Skin necrosis: As warfarin inhibits protein C initially before clotting factors, it might induce paradoxical hypercoagulability, producing microthrombi in cutaneous and subcutaneous venules, leading to plaques over breasts, abdomen, buttocks, thighs and calves, and ultimately producing skin necrosis. It occurs very rarely after 3 to 5 days, with an incidence of 1 in 10,000 patients treated with warfarin. Treatment includes warfarin withdrawal, UFH/LMWH being started, and then warfarin can be reintroduced later. Occasionally, protein C concentrates/vitamin K/prostacyclins are also used. Large necrosis requires skin grafting.
4. Calciphylaxis: It is an ischemic necrosis resulting from calcification of arterioles (due to inhibition of vitamin K-dependent matrix Gla protein), followed by thrombosis (due to inhibition of proteins C and S).
5. Others: Nausea, vomiting, pain abdomen, flatulence and altered taste sensations.

Table 49.6 Indications of warfarin with target INR levels

Indication	Dose	Range of INR (target INR)
Treatment of venous thrombosis and pulmonary embolism	2.5 to 10 mg once per day (start with <5 mg/day in debilitated patients, congestive heart failure, liver disease, recent surgery)	2.0–3.0 (2.5)
AF		2.0–3.0 (2.5)
After MI		2.0–3.0 (2.5)
Prosthetic heart valves in both atrial and mitral positions	2.5 to 5 mg every 24 hours	2.5–3.5 (3.0)

Abbreviations: AF, atrial fibrillation; DTI, direct thrombin inhibitor; INR, international normalized ratio; MI, myocardial infarction.

Contraindications

Hypersensitivity, hemorrhagic tendencies, pregnancy (fetal warfarin syndrome), and malignant hypertension (increased risk of hemorrhagic stroke).

Factors Affecting the Warfarin Anticoagulant Effect

Factors Enhancing

1. Drug interactions:
   a. Inhibition CYP2C9 leading to decreased hepatic metabolism of warfarin which, in turn, lead to enhanced anticoagulant effect, prolonged INR and increasing risk of bleeding on coadministration of amiodarone, verapamil, fluconazole, fluvastatin, metronidazole, trimethoprim-sulfamethoxazole, and zafirlukast.
   b. Metabolic enzyme inhibition = cimetidine, ciprofloxacin, erythromycin, fluvoxamine, isoniazid, and itraconazole.
   c. Thyroid hormone (↑ metabolism of vitamin K).
   d. Aspirin (Antiplatelet effect).
2. Lower body mass index (BMI) → unstable anticoagulation.
3. Age > 50 years (evidence not conclusive).

Factors Decreasing

1. Higher BMI (studies suggest BMI > 27 producing poor anticoagulation) due to altered pharmacokinetics.
2. Diabetes, heart failure (HF), h/o stroke, peripheral arterial disease, MI (hypertension [HTN] no effect).
3. Females (higher risk of stroke from atrial fibrillation [AF] irrespective of warfarin use).
4. Lower adherence.
5. Drug interactions: Induction of cytochrome enzymes leading to increased metabolism of warfarin: barbiturates, carbamazepine, and rifampicin. Propylthiouracil decreases vitamin K metabolism, decreasing the effect of warfarin and glibenclamide.

Drug Interaction between Warfarin and Cephalosporins

Third-generation cephalosporins eradicates the gut microbes, producing vitamin K2, leading to less antagonism of warfarin and also possesses a direct inhibition of vitamin K epoxide reductase.

Drug Interactions of Warfarin with Salicylates, Sulphonamides, Phenytoin, Barbiturates, and Oral Contraceptives

Salicylates

Nonsteroidal anti-inflammatory drugs (NSAIDs): increased risk of bleeding due to injury to GI mucosa and also its antiplatelet effect.

Sulphonamides

Sulfamethoxazole is indicted for inhibiting metabolism of (S) warfarin and also displaces protein bound warfarin, elevating INR and increasing the risk of bleeding.

Phenytoin

The interaction between warfarin and phenytoin is highly variable and unpredictable. Phenytoin can induce various cytochrome enzymes, leading to increased metabolism of warfarin. But this interaction might not affect blood levels of warfarin because of the interaction at the plasma protein binding, and can also potentiate half-life of phenytoin. Both of them are also known to possess intrinsic metabolizing capabilities.

Barbiturates

Being an enzyme inducer, it reduces anticoagulant effect of warfarin by inducing its metabolism through hepatic microsomal enzymes.

Oral Contraceptives

1. Tibolone: enhanced anticoagulant effect (androgenic component of tibolone reduces factor VIIa and other vitamin K-dependent coagulation factors).
2. Combined pills: decreased anticoagulant effect (contrarily few reports suggest enhanced effectiveness). Hence, close monitoring of INR is suggested during their use.
3. Progesterone only pills (emergency pills): enhanced anticoagulation.

Direct Factor Xa Inhibitors

Razaxaban, rivaroxaban, apixaban, and edoxaban.

Mechanism of Action of Direct Factor Xa Inhibitors

The interest in factor X as a target for anticoagulation stems from LMWHs, which inhibited factor Xa predominantly in comparison to UFH, and this was reconfirmed by fondaparinux, which was a more specific factor Xa inhibitor in comparison to thrombin inhibition. In the late 1980s, a few natural compounds like antistatin from Mexican leech *Haementeria officinalis* and tick anticoagulant peptides were used to inhibit factor Xa, but most of them were indirectly acting. Hence, selective factor Xa inhibitors like rivaroxaban and apixaban, small molecules and direct and reversible inhibitors of activated factor X (Xa), were synthesized. They act at the confluence of both intrinsic and extrinsic pathways of coagulation cascade factor Xa, thereby not only blocking the amplification of thrombin downstream but also successfully blocking coagulation (**Fig. 49.3**). It has no antiplatelet effect and provides predictable coagulation blockade, as they exhibit linear pharmacokinetics. These properties make their use more user friendly as no monitoring is required.

Uses of Direct Factor Xa Inhibitors

Razaxaban

It was the first oral factor Xa inhibitor to be tested for clinical use. However, its development was stopped in 2005, when phase II trial suggested higher bleeding in comparison to enoxaparin.

Rivaroxaban

It is the first oral selective factor Xa inhibitor approved for clinical use in the European Union (EU) in October 2008 and by US FDA in November 2011. It is approved for use in patients of nonvalvular AF as a prophylaxis for stroke and systemic embolism. It inhibits factor Xa in circulation as well as those bound within prothrombinase complex. The adverse effects include bleeding; other nonhemorrhagic adverse effects are seen very rarely like drug-induced liver injury, immunological side effects including toxic skin eruptions, cutaneous vasculitis, rash, anaphylaxis/anaphylactic shock, and hair loss.

Indications with Dose

1. Nonvalvular AF: 20 mg once daily (15 mg if creatinine clearance less than 50 mL/min) once daily with evening meal.
2. Chronic coronary artery disease/peripheral arterial disease to reduce incidence of cardiovascular events: 2.5 mg twice daily ± food along with aspirin.
3. Treatment of DVT and PE: Start with 15 mg twice daily for 3 weeks and then 20 mg once daily with food.
4. Prophylaxis of DVT and PE: 10 mg once daily for 5 weeks postsurgery.
5. Prophylaxis of DVT after hip replacement: 10 mg once daily for 5 weeks postsurgery.
6. Prophylaxis of DVT after knee replacement: 10 mg once daily for 12 days.
7. Prophylaxis of VTE in acutely ill medical patients: 10 mg once daily for 31 to 39 days ± food.

Apixaban

It is a selective and reversible factor Xa inhibitor, which inhibits both free and bound Xa. It has a half-life of 12 hours and demonstrates predictable pharmacokinetics. Hence, it is administered twice daily with no requirement of laboratory monitoring. It is eliminated in bile, mostly with renal elimination, contributing to only 27%. The most common adverse effect is bleeding seen in 1 to 10% cases, with severe bleeding in less than 3% cases. Other less common adverse effects include nausea, anemia and, rarely, hypersensitivity reactions.

Uses

1. Prophylaxis of stroke in patients with nonvalvular AF: 5 mg twice a day (Dose is reduced to 2.5 mg if the patient has two of the following: > 80 years old, serum creatinine ≥ 1.5 mg/dL or body weight ≤ 60 kg).
2. Prophylaxis of VTE posthip/knee surgery: 2.5 mg twice daily beginning 12 to 24 hours postsurgery and then continued for 35 days (hip replacement) and 12 days (knee replacement).
3. Treatment of DVT and PE: 10 mg twice daily for 7 days and then 5 mg twice daily.
4. Prophylaxis for recurrent DVT/PE: 2.5 mg twice daily.

Edoxaban

It is a selective factor Xa inhibitor which inhibits free factor Xa, thereby reducing thrombin generation and decreasing thrombus formation. Although it prolongs PT, aPTT and INR, the changes are small to necessitate routine monitoring.

Uses

1. Prophylaxis for stroke and systemic embolism in patients of nonvalvular AF: 60 mg once daily (Reduced dose if creatinine clearance 15 to 50 mL/min and is contraindicated if creatinine clearance > 95 mL/min).
2. Treatment of DVT and PE: 60 mg once daily (Reduce the dose to 30 mg if creatinine clearance 15 to 50 mL/min or body weight ≤ 60 kg or there is use of p-glycoprotein inhibitors like verapamil, quinidine, dronedarone and ketoconazole).

Betrixaban

It is the latest factor Xa inhibitor approved by US FDA in 2017 for the prophylaxis of VTE. It is started with 160 mg once daily with food, followed by 80 mg once daily for 35 to 42 days.

Oral Direct Thrombin Inhibitors

Table 49.7 lists outs the oral direct thrombin inhibitors.

Mechanism of Action of Direct Thrombin Inhibitors (DTIs)

The activated factor Xa activates prothrombin (factor II) to thrombin which, in turn, converts fibrinogen to soluble fibrin and then to insoluble fibrin. Fibrin stimulates platelet activation, leading to clot formation. Thrombin overall plays a crucial role in thrombus generation by activating factors V, VIII, and XII, leading to exponential increase in its generation and also activates factor XIII, which plays a crucial role in cross-linking of fibrin and stabilization of clot. Thrombin has three domains: an active site, exosite 1 which binds to most substrates of thrombin (fibrinogen, PAR1 and protein C), leading to stabilization of sodium binding site, which allosterically activates active site, and exosite 2, which acts as a heparin-binding domain. The classification of direct thrombin inhibitors is based on their binding characteristic to thrombin, those binding to both active site and exosite 1 are called bivalent DTIs, and those binding only to active site are called univalent DTIs.

Table 49.7 Oral DTIs

DTI, mechanism of action & advantages	Indication and dose	Adverse effects and disadvantages
Oral univalent DTIs		
Ximelagatran: first oral direct thrombin inhibitor prodrug of melagatran	Prevention of VTE postorthopedic surgeries	Hepatotoxicity if used > 35 days Removed from market
Dabigatran etexilate: prodrug of dabigatran-specific, potent, reversible thrombin inhibitor, converted to active form through two intermediates in hepatocytes Rapid onset of action Consistently absorbed in acidic environment (newer formulation contains small pellets with core of tartaric acid coated with dabigatran etexilate to enhance absorption) $t_{1/2}$: 12 to 14 hours, Vd = 60 to 70 L No food/drug interactions, no interaction cytochrome P450 enzymes Broad therapeutic window Administered in a fixed dose No hepatotoxicity Monitoring: ECT, diluted thrombin time assay	• Prophylaxis of VTE post hip/knee replacement surgery 150 mg/220 mg once daily • AF	A/E: dyspepsia potential drug interactions with quinidine, rifampicin, amiodarone, verapamil

Abbreviations: AF, atrial fibrillation; DI, direct thrombin inhibitor; ECT, electroconvulsive therapy; VTE, venous thromboembolism.

Table 49.8 Advantages of NOACs over warfarin

Warfarin	Nonvitamin K oral anticoagulants
Less predictable anticoagulant effect due to unpredictable pharmacokinetics	More predictable anticoagulation
Individualized dose	Fixed doses, except those in hepatic/renal insufficiency
Indirect action: Inhibits activation of vitamin K–dependent coagulation factors	Direct action: Inactivates factor Xa or IIa
Significant drug–drug and drug–food interactions	Lesser interactions
Routine laboratory monitoring of INR	Laboratory monitoring not needed
Narrow therapeutic window	Relatively wider therapeutic window
Longer half-life	Shorter half-life
Always initiated along with LMWH for faster onset of anticoagulation	Need not initiate LMWH concurrently

Abbreviations: INR, international normalized ratio; LMWH, low-molecular weight heparin; NOAC, new oral anticoagulant.

Advantages of New Oral Anticoagulants (NOACs) over Warfarin

Table 49.8 mentions advantages of NOACs over warfarin.

Choice of Anticoagulant for Various Clinical Conditions

Table 49.9 mentions the criteria for choosing anticoagulants.

Table 49.9 Guide for selection of anticoagulant

Indication	Anticoagulant of choice
Treatment of acute VTE	
PE, unstable hemodynamically	Thrombolysis (treatment of choice) UFH preferred over other parenteral anticoagulants/NOACs
Altered renal function	UFH LMWH with monitoring by antifactor Xa activity Fondaparinux and NOACs accumulate (usually not preferred; if used, dose reduction is suggested)
Pregnant women	LMWH (continued for at least 6 weeks postdelivery) Vitamin K antagonists are contraindicated NOACs under investigation
Elderly	NOACs preferred over vitamin K antagonist: rivaroxaban dabigatran etexilate (at reduced doses 110 mg)
Prevention of recurrence of VTE	Start with LMWH/fondaparinux + vitamin K antagonists/NOACs In case of malignancy, LMWH is preferred over warfarin
Acute treatment of ACS	Fondaparinux (first choice)/LMWH/UFH (as adjunct to antiplatelet therapy)
Patients of ACS undergoing PCI	▪ UFH/LMWH (preferred) during catheterization ▪ Bivaluridin (short half-life, effective, reduced risk of bleeding), increased risk of acute stent thrombosis
Prophylaxis of valvular thrombosis and embolism in cases of mitral valvular stenosis with mechanical valves (Note: Biprosthetic tissue valves are less thrombogenic and may not warrant anticoagulation except for presence of arrhythmias)	▪ Vitamin K antagonist/NOACs ▪ In pregnancy: o In initial 6 to 12 weeks, LMWH is preferred (shift from warfarin to LMWH if on warfarin before pregnancy) o 12 to 38 weeks: shift to warfarin (maximum evidence of efficacy and safety) o Last 2 weeks of pregnancy: switch back to LMWH

Abbreviations: ACS, acute coronary syndrome; LMWH, low-molecular weight heparin; NOAC, new oral anticoagulant; PCI, percutaneous coronary intervention; PE, pulmonary embolism; UFH, unfractionated heparin; VTE, venous thromboembolism.

Multiple Choice Questions

1. A 60-year-old woman with a known case of deep venous thrombosis (DVT) has been placed on warfarin 5 mg once daily. She presents to your clinic after 5 weeks of warfarin with purple lesions over the bilateral toes that blanch on pressure. What would be your most likely action?

A. Continue warfarin and reassure the patient.
B. Stop warfarin, switch over to low-molecular weight heparin (LMWH).
C. Stop warfarin, switch over to apixaban.
D. Stop warfarin, switch over to bivaluridin.

Answer: C

The signs and symptoms in this case, like purple lesions over toes bilaterally, which blanch on pressure 5 weeks after starting warfarin is suggestive of purple toe syndrome. It mandates removal of warfarin and starting another anticoagulant. It is better to start apixaban, as other anticoagulants have been shown to cause similar symptoms.

2. A 40-year-old man who presented with deep venous thrombosis (DVT) and pulmonary embolism (PE) was started on UFH 4,000 units intravenous (IV) bolus followed by 1,000 units IV infusions every 6 hours. Next morning, you notice his blood platelets falling to 1,20,000 cells/cumm from 3,00,000 cells/cumm. What shall be your next line of action?

A. Stop heparin infusions.
B. Stop heparin and start low-molecular weight heparin (LMWH).
C. Stop heparin and start bivaluridin.
D. Do not stop heparin, monitor the patient.

Answer: D

The signs are suggestive of heparin-induced thrombocytopenia (HIT). But early onset within 24 hours and mild thrombocytopenia are suggestive of more common type I HIT. As it is not autoimmune related, no cessation of heparin therapy needed. But as the platelets are low, closely monitor the patient and act accordingly. Bivaluridin is the drug of choice for HIT (type II) in which replacement of heparin is warranted.

3. A 50-year-old man on warfarin treatment for his deep venous thrombosis (DVT) visits your outpatient department. An international normalized ratio (INR) of 6 is reported in his evaluation, but no signs of bleeding are observed. What will be your plan of action?

A. Continue treatment, reassure.
B. Stop few doses of warfarin and revaluate INR.

C. Start injection vitamin K 1 to 2 mg.

D. Stop warfarin, start low-molecular weight heparin (LMWH).

Answer: B

The patient with his INR of 9.0 and no bleeding necessitates only withholding one or two doses of warfarin, with frequent monitoring of INR.

4. A 55-year-old man with a known case of deep venous thrombosis (DVT) of proximal thigh on warfarin 5 mg once daily. He is diagnosed as a case of inguinal hernia, and after evaluation, you decide to take him for surgery next week (found to have low bleeding risk and low risk of thromboembolism). During investigation a day prior to surgery, his international normalized ratio (INR) is 3. What would be your course of management?

A. Take him up for surgery.

B. Add heparin bridge therapy before surgery.

C. Add 2.5 mg vitamin K1.

D. None of the above.

Answer: C

The patient has a low risk of bleeding during surgery and also has a low risk of thromboembolism. As his INR is more on the day of surgery, it is better to add oral vitamin K and induce reversal of anticoagulation before starting surgery to minimize bleeding during surgery.

5. A 60-year-old man presents to your clinic with pain over limbs. On evaluation, he was diagnosed as a case of deep venous thrombosis (DVT) proximal veins and was admitted in the ward. UFH 4,000 units' bolus intravenous (IV) was given, followed by 1,000 units per hour infusions with an international normalized ratio (INR) of 2.5 and activated partial thromboplastin time (aPTT) measurement every 6 hours. Next morning, you receive a call that he has developed acute ischemic stroke. What should be your line of management for his anticoagulation?

A. Continue heparin infusions.

B. Stop heparin infusions.

C. Stop heparin infusions and start reversal with protamine.

D. Any of the above.

Answer: C

The patient has developed acute ischemic stroke, and continuing heparin infusions carries high risk of intracerebral bleed; hence, stopping heparin infusions is essential. Although the half-life of heparin is short, reversal of unfractionated heparin (UFH) effects might take time, therefore reversal of anticoagulant effect with Protamine is indicated.

6. A 25-year-old woman undergoing 32nd week of gestation, reports to the hospital with pain over the calf over the past 1 week. Ultrasound color Doppler points to a deep venous thrombosis (DVT) and treating physician decides to start on anticoagulant prophylaxis for embolisms. What will be the anticoagulant of choice?

A. Low-molecular weight heparin (LMWH).

B. Fondaparinux.

C. Warfarin.

D. Dabigatran.

Answer: A

The patient has been diagnosed with DVT during pregnancy, hence she has to be started on anticoagulant prophylaxis for prevention of embolism. In pregnancy, UFH/LMWH are preferred choices, as they cross placental barrier minimally.

7. A 60-year-old man suffered from idiopathic pulmonary embolism a week ago, admitted in your hospital, where he was treated with heparin and warfarin. He was discharged from hospital with warfarin 5 mg once daily dose and his international normalized ratio (INR) was 2.5. Two days later, he visits your hospital for evaluation follow-up. Although his vitals were stable, his INR was 1.3. What would be your line of management in him?

A. Continue warfarin at the same dose.

B. Increase the dose of warfarin.

C. Increase the dose of warfarin and add low-molecular weight heparin (LMWH).

D. Any of the above.

Answer: C

The patient has been discharged after idiopathic pulmonary embolism; however, suboptimal anticoagulation often can precipitate a recurrence of pulmonary embolism (PE). Hence, although the choice of anticoagulants appears appropriate, INR of 1.3 is low. Therefore, apart from increasing the dose of warfarin, it is vital to add LMWH, as increased dose of warfarin will take time for its effect to set in.

8. A 50-year-old man presents to the emergency department of your hospital with complaints of leg pain and swelling over his right lower extremity. He has no history of venous thrombosis and his vitals are stable. Color Doppler confirmed deep venous thrombosis (DVT) of proximal veins in thigh and he was admitted. What would be ideal management in his case?

A. Low-molecular weight heparin (LMWH) for at least 3 days with concurrent warfarin therapy and an international normalized ratio (INR) of 2 or higher.

B. LMWH for at least 5 days and start warfarin on day 5 while withdrawing LMWH with an INR of 2 or higher.

C. LMWH for at least 3 days and start warfarin on day 3 while withdrawing LMWH with an INR of 2 or higher.

D. LMWH for at least 5 days with concurrent warfarin therapy and an INR of 2 or higher.

Answer: D

The patient was diagnosed with DVT, and therefore he needs coverage with anticoagulants for preventing embolism. As long-term prophylaxis is needed, vitamin K antagonists can be started, but the onset of warfarin action is delayed due to the need for elimination of already activated clotting factors (II, VII, IX, and X). Hence, it is essential to provide coverage with parenteral anticoagulants (LMWH preferred over unfractionated heparin [UFH]) concurrently until warfarin takes over action.

9. A 45-year-old woman has undergone hysterectomy for her cervical carcinoma. She has no history of bleeding or deep vein thrombosis (DVT). Her vitals are stable with

mild edema over her lower limbs and normal prothrombin time, activated partial thromboplastin time (aPTT) and international normalized ratio (INR). What would be next line of management?

A. Early mobilization + elastic stockings + pain killers.
B. Early mobilization + elastic stockings + pain killers + low-molecular weight heparin (LMWH) for 5 weeks.
C. Early mobilization + elastic stockings + pain killers + warfarin for 3 months.
D. Any of the above.

Answer: B

In cases of malignancy, there is a high risk of developing deep vein thrombosis (DVT) which can progress to systemic embolism. Hence, it is always preferred to start anticoagulant prophylaxis, preferably LMWH.

10. A 60-year-old woman was receiving warfarin 5 mg once daily for 5 years. She visits emergency department with fever and burning micturition. She was admitted and started on injection ceftriaxone 1 g. After 3 days, her international normalized ratio (INR) was 10.5 but had no bleeding. What would be line of management?

A. Stop ceftriaxone, start alternate antibiotic.
B. Stop few doses of warfarin.
C. Add vitamin K1 2.5 mg orally.
D. All of the above.

Answer: D

The patient was on chronic warfarin treatment and was started on ceftriaxone, a third-generation cephalosporin for her urinary tract infection (UTI). Third-generation cephalosporins and warfarin share a drug reaction, as cephalosporins inhibit gut microbes, producing vitamin K2, and may also possess a direct anticoagulant effect, which enhances anticoagulant action. Although her international normalized ratio (INR) is high, still she has no signs and symptoms of bleeding; therefore, apart from stopping cephalosporins and stopping warfarin, it is wise to add vitamin K1 to reverse warfarin anticoagulation and INR.

11. An elderly man, 74-year-old, a known case of atrial fibrillation (AF) on warfarin therapy for past 5 years. He is diagnosed as a case of carcinoma of the colon and is being taken up for surgical resection (moderate bleeding risk during procedure and high risk of thromboembolism). His renal function is deranged with a creatinine clearance of 30 mL/kg/min. What according to you must be his anticoagulant cover during time of surgery to prevent bleeding intraoperatively?

A. Continue warfarin treatment.
B. Bridge therapy with unfractionated heparin (UFH), last dose 6 hours before surgery.
C. Bridge therapy with low-molecular weight heparin (LMWH), last dose 24 hours before surgery.
D. Postpone surgery for 6 months.

Answer: B

As the individual carries a high risk of thromboembolism, bridging therapy is mandated. As his renal function is impaired, UFH is the anticoagulant of choice for bridging therapy after stopping warfarin 5 days before surgery.

12. A 65-year-old woman is scheduled to undergo hip replacement surgery. She has a history of developing severe thrombocytopenia with prior use of heparin. What would be the anticoagulant of choice in her postop to prevent risk of deep vein thrombosis (DVT) and thromboembolism?

A. Unfractionated heparin (UHF).
B. Low-molecular weight heparin (LMWH).
C. Fondaparinux.
D. Bivaluridin.

Answer: D

The patient undergoing hip replacement surgery needs anticoagulant prophylaxis postoperatively to prevent DVT and embolisms. She has a history of developing heparin-induced thrombocytopenia (HIT); therefore, the anticoagulant of choice in her will be bivaluridin.

13. A 70-year-old man with diabetes on warfarin prophylaxis for embolism and atrial fibrillation (AF) visits your clinic. After evaluation, you decide to shift him from warfarin to dabigatran etexilate. His international normalized ratio (INR) value is 3.5. What would be the ideal scenario for shifting him to dabigatran from warfarin?

A. Stop warfarin, start dabigatran immediately.
B. Start dabigatran, withdraw warfarin after 48 hours.
C. Stop warfarin, start dabigatran after 48 hours.
D. Any of the above.

Answer: C

The decision to replace warfarin to dabigatran appears suitable, as his INR is higher than the targeted INR of 2 to 3. Hence, it is better to omit few doses of warfarin and restart dabigatran, so as to obtain desired anticoagulation without the risk of bleeding.

14. A 40-year-old woman has undergone knee replacement surgery, and you decide to start anticoagulant prophylaxis with new oral anticoagulants (NOACs). She is a known case of gastric ulcer and is on proton pump inhibitors. Which NOAC is not the preferred choice in this case?

A. Dabigatran.
B. Rivaroxaban.
C. Apixaban.
D. Edoxaban.

Answer: A

The patient is a known case of gastric ulcer and is on proton pump inhibitors. Dabigatran is known to cause dyspepsia and also needs acidic environment for better absorption. Hence, it is better to avoid dabigatran in her case.

Chapter 50 Drugs Used in Dyslipidemias

Shraddha M. Pore

PH1.31: Describe the mechanisms of action, types, doses, side effects, indications, and contraindications of the drugs used in the management of dyslipidemias.

Learning Objectives

- Drugs used in dyslipidemias.
- Principles of low-density lipoprotein- cholesterol (LDL-C) lowering therapy.

Introduction

Lipids are important components of human body. Besides acting as energy source, lipids perform various structural and functional roles. Poorly soluble lipids (triglycerides, cholesterol, fat-soluble vitamins) are transported within body fluids (plasma lymph, interstitial fluid) with the help of lipoproteins.

Lipoproteins are large macromolecular complexes of lipids (free and esterified cholesterol, triglycerides [TGs], and phospholipids) and proteins (apolipoproteins or apoproteins). The core of lipoproteins consists of hydrophobic lipids (cholesterol esters and triglycerides), which are surrounded by a hydrophilic shell composed of water-soluble lipids (phospholipids and free cholesterol) and apolipoproteins (apo-A1, apo-A2, apo-A5, apo-B100, apo-B48, apo-CI, apo-CII, apo-CIII, apo-E, apo-A). Apolipoproteins provide structural stability and may act as ligands or cofactors for lipoprotein metabolism. Mutations in lipoproteins or lipoprotein receptors are linked to familial dyslipidemias and premature death due to accelerated atherosclerosis.

Based on relative density, lipoproteins are divided into five major classes: chylomicrons, very low-density lipoproteins (VLDL), intermediate-density lipoprotein (IDL), low-density lipoprotein (LDL), and high-density lipoprotein (HDL). Chylomicrons and VLDLs are rich in TGs, while LDL is rich in cholesterol.

Chylomicrons transport dietary TGs and cholesterol from intestine to thoracic duct and then to systemic circulation. Absorption of intestinal cholesterol is mediated by Niemann–Pick C1-like 1 protein. Incorporation of lipids into chylomicrons requires action of microsomal TGs transfer protein (MTP). In circulation, TGs in chylomicron are hydrolyzed on endothelial surface of capillaries of tissues, synthesizing lipoprotein lipase (LPL) (adipose tissue, heart, skeletal muscle, and lactating breast tissue) to release free fatty acids (FFAs), which are taken up and used by adjacent tissues. Removal of TGs from chylomicrons lead to formation of chylomicron remnants, which are cleared by liver through apo-E mediated endocytosis via LDL receptors or LDL receptor-related protein.

Liver synthesizes TG-rich VLDL particles during fasting. Synthesis of VLDL requires action of MTP. Circulating VLDL is hydrolyzed by LPL, leading to formation of IDL. Liver removes 40 to 60% of IDL by receptor-mediated endocytosis. Remainder of IDL is further hydrolyzed by hepatic lipase (HL) to form LDL. About two third of plasma cholesterol is contained in LDL. Liver removes most of plasma LDL from circulation through LDL-receptors (LDL-Rs). Familial hypercholesterolemia, characterized by high LDL-C levels and increased risk of premature coronary heart disease (CHD), results from mutation in LDL-R. Proprotein convertase subtilisin/kexin type 9 (PCSK9) is a hepatic protease that binds with LDL-R and promotes its degradation. Inhibition of PCSK9 increases number of LDL-Rs on hepatocytes.

LDL is highly atherogenic, and lowering LDL-C level is an important therapeutic strategy to protect from atherosclerotic cardiovascular diseases (ASCVDs). Considering importance of LDL-R-mediated removal of LDL in circulation, increasing expression or activity of hepatic LDL-R constitutes most effective pharmacological means to reduce plasma LDL-C levels.

Low HDL levels is an independent risk factor for CHD. The protective effect of HDL is supposed to be due to its role in reverse cholesterol transport, that is, from peripheral cells to liver and intestine. Lipoprotein-A (LP [a]) is similar to LDL but contains additional lipoprotein apo (a). Lp (a) is considered to be atherogenic.

Dyslipidemias are disorders of lipoprotein metabolism which lead to increase or decrease in specific lipids or lipoproteins. Because lipid screening is commonly performed, dyslipidemias are commonly encountered in clinical practice. Genetic disorders as well as secondary causes (obesity, diabetes, insulin resistance, metabolic syndrome, hypothyroidism, nephrotic syndrome and certain drugs such estrogen, glucocorticoids, thiazides, thiazolidinediones) can lead to dyslipidemias. Dyslipidemias increase the risk of ASCVDs such as CHD, cerebrovascular disease, and peripheral vascular disease. Drug therapy with cholesterol-lowering agents significantly reduces clinical complications of ASCVD. Patients with markedly elevated levels of TGs require pharmacological therapy to reduce risk of acute pancreatitis.

Drugs Used in Dyslipidemias (IM2.18)

- **Drugs used in hypercholesterolemia (raised LDL-C levels)**
    - **Inhibitors of 3-hydroxy-3-methylglutaryl coenzyme A (HMG-CoA) reductase (statins).**
        - Simvastatin, atorvastatin, lovastatin, pravastatin, rosuvastatin, fluvastatin.

- **Inhibitors of cholesterol absorption.**
  - Ezetimibe.
- **Bile acid sequestrants (bile acid-binding resins).**
  - Cholestyramine, colestipol, colesevelam.
- **PCSK9 inhibitors**
  - Alirocumab, evolocumab.

- **Drugs used in hypertriglyceridemia**
  - **Fibric acid derivatives (fibrates)**
    - Clofibrate, gemfibrozil, fenofibrate, bezafibrate.
  - **Omega 3 fatty acids (fish oils)**
    - Eicosapentaenenoic acid (EPA), docasahexaenoic acid (DHA).
- **Drugs used in hypertriglyceridemia and hypercholesterolemia**
  - Niacin (nicotinic acid).

Inhibitors of HMG-CoA Reductase (Statins)

Statins are most commonly used drugs to lower LDL-C levels and constitute one of the most effective strategies to prevent ASCVD complications.

Mechanism of Action

Statins are competitive inhibitors of HMG-CoA reductase which carry out the early and rate limiting step in cholesterol biosynthesis. Inhibition of HMG-CoA leads to decreased hepatic cholesterol content and increased expression of LDL-R on hepatocytes which, in turn, enhances uptake of circulating LDL by liver and lowering of plasma LDL-C levels. An additional mechanism suggested for LDL-lowering effect of statins is increased uptake of LDL precursors VLDL and IDL and decreased VLDL production secondary to reduced hepatic cholesterol content.

Therapeutic Effects

Effect on LDL-C

The primary therapeutic effect of statins is lowering plasma LDL-C levels in a dose-dependent manner, with approximately 60% reduction in LDL levels along with high-intensity regimen. Each doubling of dose leads to approximate 6% further reduction in LDL-C levels. Maximal effect of statins is achieved in 7 to 10 days. Almost all patients with raised LDL-C respond favorably to statins. But in patients with dysfunctional LDL-R in homozygous familial hypercholesterolemia, response to statins is attenuated. Different statins vary with respect to potency and maximal LDL-C-lowering effect. Consequently, the agent and dose used depend on intensity of effect desired (described later in chapter).

Effects on Triglycerides

Statins reduce TGs in a dose-dependent manner, especially in patients with TG level > 250 mg/dL. The magnitude (percent reduction) of this effect is similar to LDL-C-lowering effect. The underlying mechanism is considered to be decreased VLDL production by liver.

Effect on HDL-C

Statins cause moderate increase (5–10%) in HDL-C levels, irrespective of the dose or statin used. The mechanism of this effect is not known.

Pleiotropic Effects of Statins

Use of statins lead to plaque stabilization. Statins also show antiproliferative, antiplatelet, and antioxidant properties. Such cholesterol independent effects of statins are termed as pleiotropic effects. Whether these pleiotropic effects contribute to beneficial effects of statins in preventing ASCVD is not precisely known. Much of the beneficial effects of statins are attributed to its LDL-C-lowering effects.

Pharmacokinetics

Statins are given orally. The absorption varies from 30 to 85%. Simvastatin and lovastatin are prodrugs which are transformed to active β-hydroxy acid form in the liver. There is extreme hepatic uptake of all statins during first pass, primarily mediated through organic anion transporter (OATP 1B).

The pharmacokinetic differences in statins have important clinical implications with regard to safety, drug interactions, and clinical use. Lovastatin, pravastatin, simvastatin, and fluvastatin have short half-life (1–3 hours), while atorvastatin, rosuvastatin, and pitavastatin have long half-lives (17–20 hours). Since hepatic cholesterol synthesis is maximal between midnight and 2 am, the statins with $t_{1/2}$ of 4 h and less should be taken in the evening, while statins with longer half-lives (atorvastatin and rosuvastatin) can be taken at other times of the day.

Clearance of statins takes place primarily by liver and gastrointestinal tract (GIT). Renal clearance of statins is generally low, with atorvastatin having very low renal clearance (can be used in patients with significant renal dysfunction). Simvastatin, lovastatin, and atorvastatin are metabolized by CYP3A4 enzyme. Inhibitors of CYP3A4 (ketoconazole, itraconazole, erythromycin, clarithromycin, HIV protease inhibitors, amiodarone, diltiazem, verapamil and cyclosporine, and grapefruit juice) increase plasma levels and hence toxicity (myopathy) of these statins.

Other statins metabolized by CYP2C9, mainly fluvastatin, rosuvastatin and pitavastatin (to minimal extent) or statins not undergoing CYP metabolism (pravastatin) are not associated with clinically important drug-drug interactions.

Therapeutic Uses

Statins are drugs of choice for primary and secondary prevention of ASCVD, which is discussed later in the chapter.

Adverse Effects

Statin therapy is usually well-tolerated and safe.

Myopathy

Myopathy is the most frequent adverse effect of statin therapy that often results in nonadherence. The risk is increased by higher dose and higher plasma concentration.

Subjective myalgias (with normal creatinine kinase [CK] level) are reported frequently (5–20%). Statin-associated myalgias are usually bilateral, occur after initiation of statin, and resolve after discontinuation of statins. The predisposing factors include advanced age (> 80 years), low body mass index (BMI), concomitant use of certain drugs (refer pharmacokinetics), Asian ancestry, excess alcohol, high levels of physical activity, trauma, and comorbidities (HIV, renal, liver, thyroid, and preexisting myopathy).

In case of statin-induced muscle symptoms, statin should be discontinued until symptoms resolve. The therapy can often be reinstituted with reduced dose or alternative agent or alternative dosing regimen while monitoring for recurrent symptoms. Measurement of CK is recommended in case of severe symptoms and presence of objective muscle weakness.

Myopathy with objective muscle weakness and significantly raised CK levels (myositis) are rare but require prompt discontinuation of statin. Rhabdomyolysis (CK > 10 times upper limit of normal [ULN], myoglobinuria, renal injury) is very rare and requires immediate medical attention. The patients who experience rhabdomyolysis may need to discontinue statin use indefinitely.

Statin-induced autoimmune myopathy is characterized by presence of HMG-CoA reductase antibodies, and persistent CK elevation is a rare disorder that requires statin cessation.

The most common drugs involved in statin interaction are gemfibrozil, cyclosporine, digoxin, warfarin, macrolide antibiotics, and azole antifungals. Occasionally, HIV protease inhibitors, amiodarone, nefazodone and, rarely, niacin are reported to increase risk of statin myopathy. Gemfibrozil inhibits glucuronidation, leading to nearly doubling of plasma concentration of statin.

Other Adverse Effects

Rarely, statins can cause serious hepatotoxicity. The current guidelines recommend measuring baseline liver function before initiation of statin therapy; routine monitoring is not advocated. Liver enzymes should be measured in patients with symptoms suggestive of hepatotoxicity. Statins modestly increase the risk of new-onset diabetes in individuals with predisposing risk factors. The underlying mechanism is not clear, but it appears that statins unmask diabetes in susceptible individuals. Statins are contraindicated in pregnancy and lactation.

Inhibitors of Cholesterol Absorption (Ezetimibe)

Inhibitors of cholesterol absorption are used in combination with statin therapy to achieve further reduction in LDL-C levels.

Mechanism of Action

Ezetimibe inhibits transport protein NPC1L1, which is highly expressed in proximal jejunum and plays a crucial role in intestinal cholesterol absorption. Cholesterol in intestine is derived from diet (nearly 25%) and bile acids (nearly 75%). Consequently, ezetimibe can lower cholesterol absorption, even from low cholesterol diet. Inhibition of absorption of cholesterol from intestine decreases cholesterol content in chylomicrons and causes compensatory increase in cholesterol synthesis in liver. This ultimately leads to increased expression of LDL receptors and enhances clearance of LDL from plasma. The compensatory increase in cholesterol synthesis, induced by ezetimibe, can be inhibited by statins. Thus, ezetimibe is more effective when used in combination with statins. Additionally, ezetimibe reduces atherogenesis through direct effect. This is a consequence of lowered cholesterol content in chylomicron remnants, which are highly atherogenic.

Effects on Plasma Lipids

Ezetimibe shows modest LDL-lowering effect. When used in combination with statins, it causes further reduction of 15 to 20% in LDL-C, which is equivalent to three titrations of statin dose (e.g., adding ezetimibe is equivalent to increasing atorvastatin from 10 to 80 mg per day).

Pharmacokinetics

Following absorption, ezetimibe is rapidly glucuronidated in intestinal epithelium. It then enters enterohepatic circulation, which makes it long-acting. It is mostly excreted in feces; hence, dose adjustment is not needed in renal impairment. As it is not metabolized by CYP system, drug interactions is not an important concern with ezetimibe.

Therapeutic Use

Ezetimibe is used as 10 milligram tablet taken anytime of the day with or without food as an adjunct to statin and other hypolipidemic agents, except bile acids, which inhibits its absorption. Use of ezetimibe with low-dose statin greatly potentiates effects of statins. When used with maximal dose of potent statin (rosuvastatin 40 mg), it helps to achieve LDL-C goal in majority of patients. Monotherapy with ezetimibe has limited role in statin-intolerant patients.

Adverse Drug Reactions

Ezetimibe is devoid of serious adverse effects. Rarely, it can cause allergic reactions. As statins are contraindicated in pregnancy, fixed-dose combination (FDC) of statin and ezetimibe too is contraindicated.

Bile Acid Sequestrants (Bile Acid-Binding Resins)

Bile acid sequestrants are not as effective as statins in lowering LDL-C, but are safest as these are not absorbed.

Mechanism of Action

Bile acid sequestrants are highly positively charged and bind with bile acids, which are negatively charged. The complex so formed is excreted in feces. Normally, more than 95% of bile acids are reabsorbed in intestine. Loss of bile acids causes reduction in pool of bile acids and leads to enhanced bile acid synthesis from liver. As cholesterol is used up for synthesis of bile acids, cholesterol content in hepatocytes is reduced, ultimately leading to increased LDL receptor expression and enhanced LDL clearance. Along with increased LDL-R expression, there is upregulation of HMG CoA reductase, which partially offsets LDL-C-lowering effect of resins. Therefore, inhibition of HMG-CoA reductase by concomitant use statins substantially improves effectiveness of resins.

Effects on Plasma Lipids

Bile acid sequestrants cause dose-dependent reduction in LDL-C levels (12–18%). Addition of bile acid sequestrants to statins lead to further reduction in LDL-C level by 10 to 25%. When used in combination with ezetimibe, further reductions of 10 to 20% can be achieved compared to use of either agent alone. The effect of bile acid sequestrants on TG level varies. In patients with normal TG level, its level may rise transiently, but in patients with higher baseline plasma TG, the effect may be substantial and use of bile acid sequestrants is contraindicated when TG level > 400 mg/dL. The bile acid sequestrants cause small increase (3–9%) in HDL levels.

Effects on Plasma Glucose

Bile acid sequestrants, in particular colesevelam, have been shown to reduce fasting glucose levels and HbA1c levels (reduction of 0.5–1%) when used in combination with standard glucose-lowering therapy.

Pharmacokinetics

Bile acid sequestrants are neither absorbed nor modified by digestive juices, producing localized effects in intestine. But these can interfere with intestinal absorption of many drugs such as thiazides, furosemide, propranolol l-thyroxine, digoxin, warfarin, statins, ezetimibe, fibrates, and fat-soluble vitamins. Colesevelam does not appear to reduce absorption of statins, ezetimibe, and fenofibrate. To prevent these interactions, bile acid sequestrants should be administered 1 hour before or 3 to 4 hours after meals.

Preparations and Therapeutic Uses

Cholestyramine (4 g/dose) and colestipol (5 g/dose) are available as powder that is mixed with water or juice or crushed ice in blender and drunk as slurry twice daily before meals. Colestipol is also available as tablets (1 g). Colesevelam is available as powder (3.75 g per packet) and tablets (0.625 g per tablet). The maximum dose of cholestyramine is 24 g, that of colestipol is 30 g, and colesevelam is 4.375 g. The dose is increased after several weeks as tolerated. Generally, patients do not take more than two doses twice a day. Bile acid sequestrants are used as second-line agents in statin-intolerant patients. These drugs also can be used in combination with statin and ezetimibe to achieve greater reductions in LDL-C levels. Colesevelam is used to improve glycemic control in type 2 diabetes in combination with standard therapy.

Adverse Drug Reactions

Although bile acid sequestrants are not absorbed systematically, adherence to therapy is often poor because of unacceptable GI effects, limiting clinical utility of these agents. Gritty sensation from drinking slurry, dyspepsia, bloating, abdominal discomfort, constipation, and aggravation of hemorrhoids are commonly seen. Moreover, many patients find it difficult to take powder that does not dissolve or swallow tablets that are bit too large. GI adverse effects can be reduced by slow upward titration of dose, suspending powder for several hours in liquid before drinking (reduces gritty sensation), and increasing hydration and fiber (reduces constipation). Among bile acid sequestrants, colesevelam appears to be better tolerated. Colesevelam is available as hard capsule, and it absorbs water and forms soft-gelatinous mass, which is claimed to reduce GI irritation.

In patients with high TG levels, bile acid sequestrants may worsen hypertriglyceridemia. Since these agents are administered as chloride salts, rarely hyperchloremic acidosis can occur. The intestinal absorption of many drugs is reduced by bile acid sequestrants (refer pharmacokinetics). The important contraindications include intestinal obstruction, preexisting gastrointestinal conditions, and TG levels > 400mg/dL. Cholestyramine and colestipol are safe during pregnancy; safety of colesevelam in pediatric patients and pregnant women is not known.

PCSK9 Inhibitors

Alirocumab and evolocumab are humanized monoclonal antibodies that inhibit PCSK9 protein. PCSK9 is a protease that binds with LDL-R and promotes its degradation. Inhibition of PCSK9 increases number of LDL-Rs on hepatocytes. These agents show remarkable LDL-C-lowering ability in dose-dependent manner (70% when used as monotherapy and 60% when used with statins). In distinction to statins and bile acid sequestrants, PCSK9 inhibitors also reduce Lp (a) levels by 25 to 30%. PCSK9 inhibitors are used as an adjunct to diet and maximally tolerated statin therapy in patients of familial hypercholesterolemia or patients with clinical ASCVD. The risk of myopathy does not appear to be increased. These are administered as subcutaneous (SC) injection once every 2 weeks. Injection site reactions (pain, itching, redness, tenderness) are most common adverse effects. Use of these agents is associated with slightly increased risk of infections (nasopharyngitis, urinary tract infection, upper respiratory tract infections). Higher cost is major limitation to widespread use of these agents.

Fibric Acid Derivatives (Fibrates)

Fibrates constitute important therapy for raised TG levels.

Mechanism of Action

Fibrates interact with peroxisome proliferator-activated receptor (PPAR)-α receptor, a nuclear hormone receptor that is highly expressed in liver and other tissues involved in fatty acid metabolism. The altered gene transcription resulting from binding of fibrates to PPAR-α receptors leads to various effects such as increased fatty acid oxidation, increased LPL synthesis, increased VLDL clearance. Increased expression of apo-AI and apo-A II leads to increase in HDL levels

Effects on Plasma Lipids

Primary therapeutic effect of fibrates is reduction in plasma TG levels. Fasting plasma TG levels decrease by 25 to 50%. The magnitude of this effect depends on baseline TG levels in such a way that patients with highly elevated baseline TGs show greater reduction. Fibrates cause modest effect on HDL levels (5–20%). LDL levels decrease slightly or remain unchanged.

Other Effects

Fibrates show antithrombotic effect, possibly, mediated through platelet inhibition.

Pharmacokinetics

Fibrates are rapidly and efficiently absorbed when taken with meal. Absorption is lower on empty stomach. Peak concentrations are achieved in 1 to 4 hours. Fibrates are highly protein bound (to albumin). Plasma $t_{1/2}$ varies within the group (gemfibrozil 1.1 hours, fenofibrate 20 hours). Fibrates are widely distributed in body fluids, and concentration in liver, kidney, and intestine exceeds plasma level. These are transferred across placenta. Fibrates are excreted primarily as glucuronide conjugates, and excretion is impaired in renal failure.

Therapeutic Uses

Lifestyle modifications (avoiding alcohol, reducing dietary fat, reducing intake of simple carbohydrates, exercise, and weight loss) are first-line therapy for patients with hypertriglyceridemia. But despite these interventions, many patients (especially with TGs > 500 mg/dL) require pharmacological treatment to reduce the risk of acute pancreatitis.

Fibrates are drugs of choice to treat type III hyperlipoproteinemia (dysbetalipoproteinemia). These patients show dramatic lowering of TGs and cholesterol with fibrates; tuberoeruptive and palmer xanthomas may regress. Fibrates are also preferred in chylomicronemia syndrome and other conditions leading to severe hypertriglyceridemia. Gemfibrozil is available as 300 mg capsules; the dose in adults is 600 mg twice a day, taken 30 minutes before food. Fenofibrate tablets (67 mg, 200 mg) is administered at a dose of 67 mg twice or thrice a day or 200 mg once daily with food.

Use of fibrates with statins does not cause any further reduction in ASCVD and hence is not recommended.

Adverse Effects

Fibrates are generally well-tolerated. GI adverse effects are seen in about 5% cases. Rash, urticaria, hair loss, myalgias, headache, impotency, and anemia are infrequent. Minor increases in liver transaminases and alkaline phosphatases may occur. Clofibrate, fenofibrate, and bezafibrate potentiate action of warfarin, while gemfibrozil increases risk of statin myopathy (refer statins). All fibrates alter composition of bile by increasing cholesterol concentration and can lead to gallstone formation. Fibrates are contraindicated in renal dysfunction, hepatic dysfunction, children, and pregnant women.

Niacin (Nicotinic Acid)

Niacin was the first drug approved for clinical use in dyslipidemias. It belongs to group of B-complex vitamins. It functions as vitamin after conversion to nicotinamide adenine dinucleotide (NAD) or nicotinamide adenine dinucleotide phosphate (NADP), while only niacin in larger doses exhibits hypolipidemic effect.

Mechanism of Action

Lipid-lowering effect of niacin is mediated through multiple mechanisms. In adipose tissues, niacin inhibits hormone sensitive lipase, leading to decreased lipolysis, decreased free fatty acids delivery to liver, and reduced TG synthesis. In liver, niacin reduces synthesis of fatty acids and reduces their esterification, which leads to reduction in VLDL output. Activity of lipoprotein lipase is enhanced, leading to increased clearance of TGs from chylomicrons and VLDL. Niacin also decreases clearance of HDL, leading to increased levels of HDL.

Effects on Plasma Lipids

TG level decreases by 35 to 50%. Thus, niacin at a dose of 2 to 6 g/day is as effective as fibrates and statins in lowering plasma TGs. Maximum effect is seen in 4 to 7 days. Niacin at a dose of 4.5 to 6 g/day causes reduction in LDL levels by 25%, which takes 3 to 6 weeks to manifest. Niacin is most effective for increasing HDL levels, which is raised by 30 to 40%, although the effect is less in patients with HDL < 35 mg/dL. Niacin also decreases Lp (a) levels significantly.

Pharmacokinetics

Niacin is completely absorbed when given orally. Plasma half-life is 60 minutes. It is metabolized by liver through conjugation and amidation. Toxic intermediate metabolites formed during amidation are implicated in hepatotoxicity.

Therapeutic Uses

Niacin is the only lipid-lowering agent that exhibits salutary effects on overall lipid profile. Unfortunately, tolerability to niacin is poor. Although it can be used in hypertriglyceridemia and hypercholesterolemia, other agents with better safety profile are preferred.

Adverse Effects

Flushing and dyspepsia limit compliance to niacin therapy. It tends to be more intense on initiation of therapy and with increments in dose. Tolerance develops with continued treatment. Flushing is also increased by alcohol and hot beverages. Flushing and itching is mediated through prostaglandins and can be minimized by prior treatment with aspirin. Other cutaneous adverse effects include rashes, acanthosis nigricans, and dry skin.

Concomitant use with statins increases risk of myopathy but does not further reduce risk of ASCVD (**Box 50.1**). Hence, combination therapy is not recommended. Niacin (especially extended-release [ER] formulations) in doses greater than 2 g has been linked to hepatotoxicity. GI adverse effects include

Box 50.1 Risk factors for ASCVD

- Age (male > 45 years of age or female > 55 years of age)
- Family history of premature CHD in first-degree relative
- Current cigarette smoking (smoking within the preceding 30 days)
- Hypertension (systolic blood pressure ≥ 140, diastolic pressure ≥ 90 or use of antihypertensive medication)
- Low HDL-C (< 40 mg/dL for males and < 50 mg/dL for women)
- Obesity (BMI > 25 kg/m²) and waist circumference > 40 inches (men) or > 35 inches (women)
- Type 2 diabetes mellitus (considered as high risk or very high risk)

Table 50.1 Statin therapy on the basis of LDL-C reductions achieved with daily dosing

Type of statin therapy Characteristic	High intensity	Moderate intensity	Low intensity
Reduction in LDL-C	≥ 50%	30% to < 50%	< 30%
Statin used and its daily dose	Atorvastatin 40–80 mg Rosuvastatin 20–40 mg	Atorvastatin 10–20 mg Fluvastatin 40 mg twice daily Lovastatin 40 mg Pitavastatin 2–4 mg Pravastatin 40–80 mg Rosuvastatin 5–10 mg Simvastatin 20–40 mg	Fluvastatin 20–40 mg Lovastatin 20 mg Pitavastatin 1 mg Pravastatin 10–20 mg Simvastatin 10 mg

Abbreviation: LDL-C, low-density lipoprotein-cholesterol.

nausea, vomiting, and diarrhea. Niacin is contraindicated in peptic ulcer. Other adverse effects are hyperglycemia (caution required in diabetes), increased uric acid levels and precipitation of gout, atrial tachycardia and atrial fibrillation in elderly patients and, rarely, toxic amblyopia and toxic maculopathy. Niacin is contraindicated in pregnant women, as it associated with birth defects in experimental animals.

Omega 3 Fatty Acid Ethyl Esters (Fish Oil)

Omega 3 fatty acid especially EPA and DHA ethyl esters are used in adult patients with severe hypertriglyceridemia as an adjunct to diet in the dose of 3 to 4 g per day. These drugs show modest effect on TG levels (reduction up to 25%). The underlying mechanism is decreased production and secretion of VLDL by liver. LDL-C levels are generally not changed but may increase in patients with TG level > 500 mg/dL. Fish oil also contains omega 3 fatty acids. Various fish oil products are available over the counter and as prescription products. The dose and formulation of these products vary considerably and need to be chosen carefully. Some fish oil preparations may increase LDL cholesterol levels in patients with severe hypertriglyceridemia. Addition of omega 3 fatty acids to statins is not advocated, as no extra benefit is derived from such combination in preventing ASCVD. The main adverse effects are nausea, fishy burps, arthralgias, raised LDL levels, and increased bleeding time.

Principles of LDL-C Lowering Therapy

There is compelling evidence from many clinical trials that lowering LDL-C levels substantially reduces risk of CVDs, including myocardial infarction, stroke, and total mortality. Pharmacotherapy for hypercholesterolemia is indicated when lifestyle modifications are inadequate. Appropriate management of other modifiable risk factors is also important. Statins are first-line drugs for secondary and primary prevention of ASCVDs. Clinical ASCVD includes acute coronary syndrome (ACS), history of myocardial infarction, stable and unstable angina, coronary or other revascularization, transient ischemic attacks, history of cerebrovascular disease, stroke, transient ischaemic attacks, and peripheral vascular disease including aortic aneurysm. In general, the LDL-C goal recommended for preventing ASCVD is < 100 mg/dL, while in patients with very high risk (history of ASCVD or diabetes with multiple risk factors or end organ damage), the recommended goal is < 70 mg/dL. The choice and dose of statin depends on LDL-C goal, as depicted in **Table 50.1**. Ezetimibe and /or PCSK9 inhibitors can be added if maximally tolerated dose of statin is inadequate to achieve desirable LDL-C goal. Primary prevention using low-to-moderate intensity statin therapy is recommended for patients 40 through 75 years of age with LDL 70 to 189 mg/dL.

The decision to start preventive therapy in these patients should be based on calculation of 10 year risk for CVD using pooled cohort equation. Patients with risk of more than > 7.5% merit consideration for statin therapy, irrespective of LDL level.

Multiple Choice Questions

1. A 55-year-old male, a current smoker with history of type 2 diabetes mellitus (DM) since past 10 years, has lipid profile as given below:

Low-density lipoprotein-cholesterol (LDL-C): 198 mg/dL.

High-density lipoprotein-cholesterol (HDL-C): 32 mg/dL.

Triglycerides (TG): 180 mg/dL.

Which of the following lipid lowering regimen is the most appropriate for the above patient?

A. Atorvastatin 40 mg once daily.
B. Gemfibrozil 600 mg twice daily.
C. Nicotinic acid 2 g twice daily.
D. Ezetimibe 10 mg once daily.

Answer: A

This patient has high risk of atherosclerotic cardiovascular diseases (ASCVDs) as he is diabetic and is a current smoker. LDL goal is <100 mg/dL; he would require high-intensity statin therapy with atorvastatin, which lowers LDL-C level > 50%.

2. Mrs. AH is a 60-year-old female. She has history of type 2 diabetes mellitus (DM) and hypertension since last 8 years. She exercises regularly and leads a physically active life. She was receiving following treatment till last month:

Tab metformin 500 mg twice daily.

Tab amlodipine 5 mg once daily.

Tab losartan 50 mg once daily.

Tab atorvastatin 10 mg once daily.

As her low-density lipoprotein-cholesterol (LDL-C) level was found to be higher than goal, therefore her dose of atorvastatin was raised from 10 mg to 20 mg since last month. Now, she is experiencing tenderness, soreness, and pain in both lower limbs since last few days. The creatinine kinase (CK) levels are mildly elevated and her liver function tests are within normal limits. What should be further course of action in this patient?

A. Replace metformin with glimepiride.
B. Replace amlodipine with metoprolol.
C. Keep the doses of atorvastatin unchanged.
D. Stop atorvastatin; monitor and review after few days.

Answer: D

Myalgia in this patient appears to be statin-related, as it has started after increasing dose of atorvastatin, is bilateral, and patient has mildly elevated CK levels. Moreover, two risk factors for statin-induced myopathy are present in this patient, namely, female sex and physical activity.

3. Which of the following drugs can be prescribed in a pregnant female with hypercholesterolemia?

A. Atorvastatin.
B. Fixed dose combination of atorvastatin and ezetimibe.
C. Colestipol.
D. Niacin 2 g once daily.

Answer: C

Statins and niacin are contraindicated during pregnancy; colestipol is not absorbed and is not known to cause fetal harm.

4. A 50-year-old patient, with body mass index (BMI) 30, history of type 2 diabetes mellitus (DM) and hypertension since 7 years, had undergone percutaneous coronary artery catheterization 3 years back. On routine examination, his blood report was found to be:

Total cholesterol: 200 mg/dL.

Low-density lipoprotein-cholesterol (LDL-C): 120 mg/dL.

High-density lipoprotein-cholesterol (HDL-C): 30 mg/dL.

Triglycerides (TGs): 200 mg/dL.

He has already been taking rosuvastatin 40 mg once daily for his high-cholesterol levels. Which of the following drugs would you like to add to this patient's prescription to control his LDL-C levels further, considering efficacy, safety, and patient acceptability?

A. Tab gemfibrozil 300 mg once daily.
B. Tab ezetimibe 10 mg once daily.
C. Tab nicotinic acid 500 mg thrice daily.
D. Tab cholestyramine 4 g thrice daily.

Answer: B

Ezetimibe which potentiates action of statins. Gemfibrozil and nicotinic acid increase risk of myopathy, while cholestyramine is poorly tolerated by many patients.

5. Which of the following drugs/drug class is preferred to reduce highly raised triglyceride (TG) levels in patients with type III hyperlipoproteinemia (dysbetalipoproteinemia)?

A. Bile acid sequestrants.
B. Fibrates.
C. Nicotinic acid.
D. Ezetimibe.

Answer: B

Fibrates are drugs of choice in type II hyperlipoproteinemia.

6. Which of the following classes of drugs is associated with increased risk of gallstones formation?

A. Statins.

B. Bile acid-binding resins.

C. Fibric acid derivatives (fibrates).

D. Niacin.

Answer: C

7. Gemfibrozil, the drug most commonly associated with statin-induced myopathy, leads to increased plasma concentration of statins by which of the following mechanism?

A. Inhibiting hepatic uptake and glucuronidation of statins.

B. Inhibiting renal excretion of statins.

C. Causing displacement from plasma protein-binding sites.

D. Facilitating intestinal absorption of statins.

Answer: A

Inhibiting hepatic uptake and glucuronidation of statins.

Part IX

Drugs Affecting Gastrointestinal System

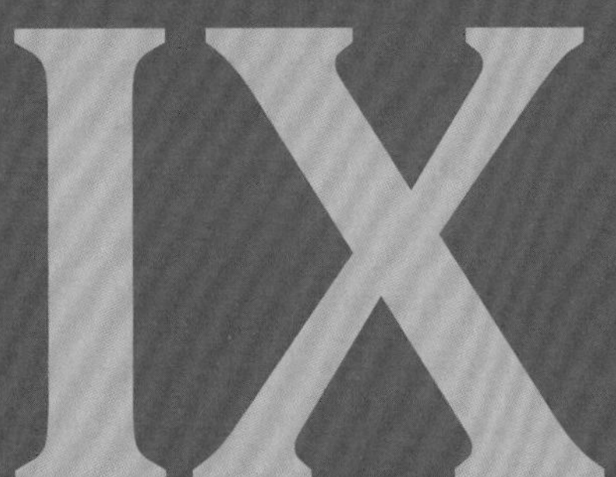

Chapter 51 Antiplatelet and Thrombolytic Drugs

Upinder Kaur and Sankha Shubhra Chakrabarti

PH1.25 Describe the mechanism/s of action, types, doses, side effects, indications, and contraindications of the drugs acting on blood, such as anticoagulants, antiplatelets, fibrinolytics, and plasma expanders.

Learning Objectives

- Antiplatelet drugs.
- Fibrinolytic drugs.

Antiplatelet Drugs (PH1.25)

These drugs inhibit platelet activation or platelet aggregation and therefore interfere with thrombus formation. As shown in **Fig. 51.1**, thromboxane A2 (TXA2), generated by the cyclooxygenase-1 (COX-1) pathway, and adenosine diphosphate (ADP) activate platelets and result in the overexpression of glycoprotein IIb–IIIa (GPIIb–IIIa) receptors. These receptors mediate platelet aggregation in association with fibrinogen and von Willebrand factor (vWF), resulting in the formation of thrombus.

Classification

As shown in **Fig. 51.1**, antiplatelet drugs can be classified as:

- COX or TXA2 synthesis inhibitors.
- ADP receptor blockers.
- Protease-activated receptor 1 (PAR1) receptor blockers.
- GP–IIb-IIIa inhibitors.
- Others: e.g., phosphodiesterase inhibitors, prostacyclin (PGI2) analogs.

Aspirin

Aspirin belongs to the class of nonsteroidal anti-inflammatory drugs (NSAIDs) and exerts antiplatelet action when given at the low dose of 75 to 300 mg/day. Aspirin acetylates and irreversibly inhibits COX-1 enzyme responsible for the generation of TXA2. Since platelets lack genetic material for protein synthesis, new generation of TXA2 does not occur until fresh platelets are formed. Thus, the action of aspirin lasts for at least 7 days. By also inhibiting COX-2, aspirin inhibits the generation of PGI2, a vasodilator and inhibitor of platelet aggregation. As PGI2 can be generated from endothelial cells which are nucleated, its synthesis is not affected much by aspirin, and the overall action of aspirin at low dose remains antiplatelet aggregatory.

Adverse Effects

The main adverse effect of aspirin is bleeding. Aspirin, by blunting the synthesis of constitutive prostaglandins such as PGE2, exerts a cytotoxic effect over the gastric mucosa, and this can result in gastritis and peptic ulcers. In fact, gastrointestinal bleeding due to aspirin is an important cause of hospital admission in the elderly. Gastric side effects can occur even with doses as low as 40 mg/day. Thus, no dose of aspirin is completely safe for the gastric environment. Aspirin use is not advisable in patients with peptic ulcer disease. Other rare but serious adverse effects include hypersensitivity reactions such as urticaria, sneezing, rashes, and anaphylaxislike reactions.

Aspirin at present is advised for secondary prevention of cardiovascular disease (CVD), that is, in patients who have suffered an attack of myocardial infarction (MI), unstable angina, or stroke. The dose of aspirin for acute coronary syndrome (ACS) is 300 mg loading dose given by oral route, followed by a maintenance dose of 75 mg/day. Aspirin is combined with clopidogrel and the two antiplatelet drugs are continued for at least 1 year in patients with ST-elevation myocardial infarction (STEMI)/non-ST-elevation myocardial infarction (NSTEMI). Because of the risk of cerebral and gastrointestinal bleed, its use for primary prevention of CVD in otherwise healthy individuals younger than 70 years is not recommended. Aspirin is used for primary prevention only if additional risk factors such as diabetes, coronary artery disease, and dyslipidemia are present, and that too on case-by-case basis.

Other Uses of Aspirin

Aspirin in high doses (3–5 g/day) is used as an anti-inflammatory drug of choice in acute rheumatic fever.

The drug is used for the prevention of preeclampsia and perinatal mortality in women with a history of preeclampsia. The drug is given at the dose of 75 to 100 mg/day from the 12th to 14th week of gestation.

Aspirin is used for the prevention of flushing induced by niacin, a hypolipidemic drug. The drug is also given for the prevention of colonic polyp and colorectal carcinoma in at-risk individuals.

Drug Interactions and Contraindications

Aspirin displaces certain drugs from plasma proteins. These include sulfonylureas, phenytoin, warfarin, methotrexate, and naproxen. Thus, the unbound fraction of these drugs increases, and this can result in toxicity.

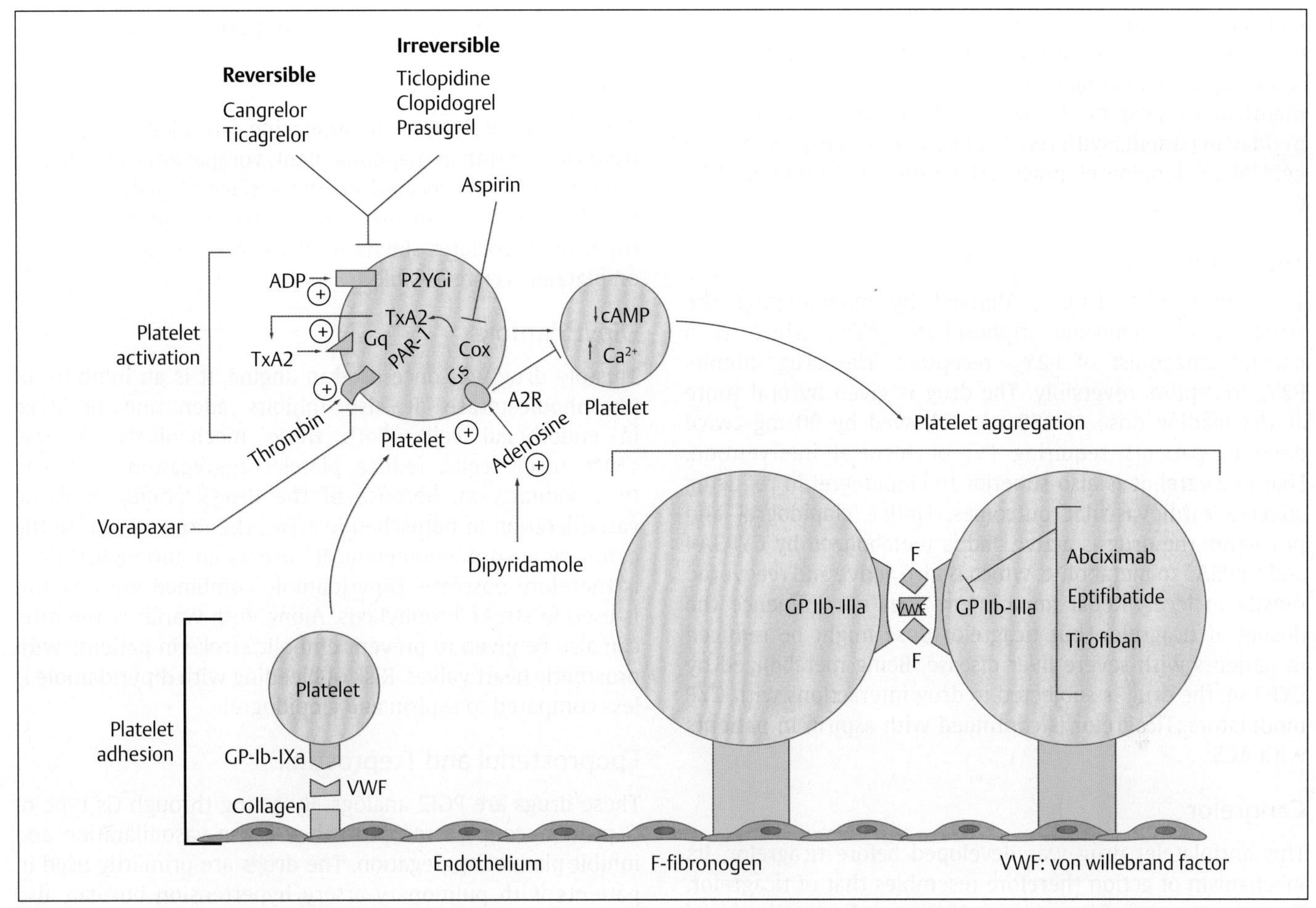

Fig. 51.1 Classes of antiplatelet agents based on their sites of action. (The image is provided courtesy of Dr. Ritwick Mondal, IPGMER, Kolkata.)

Aspirin interferes with the action of diuretics and probenecid. Ibuprofen should be given at a gap of 40 minutes to 1 hour after aspirin use, as it interferes with the antiplatelet action of aspirin.

The drug should be avoided in patients with bleeding tendencies, viral fever, uncontrolled hypertension, and peptic ulcers. Some asthmatic patients with no history of atopy are sensitive to aspirin. Use of aspirin in such patients can produce lacrimation, rhinorrhea, sneezing, and even an acute asthmatic attack. Aspirin thus should be used cautiously in patients with a history of asthma.

Patients with variant angina are hypersensitive to aspirin and therefore aspirin should be avoided in such patients.

Aspirin is stopped 7 days before major surgery.

ADP Receptor Blockers

Clopidogrel

This antiplatelet drug interferes with the action of ADP by blocking its receptors $P2Y_{12}/P2Y_{AC}$ irreversibly. Inhibition of these receptors decreases cyclic adenosine monophosphate (cAMP) inside platelets and also decreases the surface expression of GPIIb–IIIa receptors, resulting in the inhibition of platelet aggregation. Clopidogrel is a prodrug that requires activation by the cytochrome enzyme CYP2C19. Genetic polymorphisms of CYP2C19 and drugs inhibiting CYP2C19 such as omeprazole can therefore interfere with the antiplatelet action of clopidogrel. Rabeprazole and pantoprazole are relatively safe. However, proton-pump inhibitors in general and omeprazole in particular should be avoided concomitantly with clopidogrel. The combination of clopidogrel and aspirin is superior to aspirin alone in reducing adverse cardiovascular outcomes in patients with ACS. Risk of bleeding, however, increases when the two drugs are given together.

Prasugrel

Like clopidogrel, prasugrel is also a prodrug and is activated by carboxylesterase into thiolactone form. Thiolactone is activated by CYP3A5 and CYP2B6 to active form that inhibits the ADP receptor $P2Y_{AC}$ irreversibly. Prasugrel has rapid onset of action and predictable pharmacokinetics. The drug is superior to clopidogrel in reducing adverse cardiovascular outcomes in patients with ACS, and combined with aspirin, it is given in patients requiring percutaneous coronary intervention (PCI). The drug is particularly beneficial in diabetic patients requiring PCI. It is not given in patients with a history of stroke or transient ischemic attack (TIA) because of increased risk of intracranial bleeds. Dosing schedule of prasugrel is loading dose of 60 mg orally, followed by a maintenance dose of 10 mg/day. The latter is reduced to 5 mg/day in patients with renal failure and weight less than 60 kg. Unlike clopidogrel, prasugrel action is not influenced by CYP2C19 status.

Ticagrelor

This antiplatelet drug is derived by manipulating the structure of adenosine triphosphate (ATP), which is a natural antagonist of $P2Y_{AC}$ receptors. The drug inhibits $P2Y_{AC}$ receptors reversibly. The drug is given by oral route at the loading dose of 180 mg, followed by 90 mg twice daily in patients requiring PCI or medical intervention. Like prasugrel, it is also superior to clopidogrel in reducing adverse cardiovascular outcomes. Unlike clopidogrel and prasugrel, the drug is active and is metabolized by CYP3A4 and CYP3A5 to metabolite, which is also active and recovered mostly in feces. Renal impairment does not influence the dosing of ticagrelor, but ticagrelor dose might be reduced in patients with severe liver disease. Being metabolized by CYP3A4, the drug is subjected to drug interactions with CYP modulators. Ticagrelor is continued with aspirin in patients with ACS.

Cangrelor

This antiplatelet drug was developed before ticagrelor. Its mechanism of action therefore resembles that of ticagrelor. The requirement of intravenous (IV) route limits the use of this drug. It may be given in patients needing PCI.

Anti-GPIIb–IIIa Integrin: Abciximab, Eptifibatide, and Tirofiban

These drugs are generally given in patients requiring PCI. They are available as IV preparations and given as bolus, followed by infusion for up to 3 days. Heparin is administered along with them and antiplatelet drugs are also continued.

Abciximab

It is a chimeric monoclonal antibody. Its plasma $t_{1/2}$ is 20 to 25 minutes, but platelet $t_{1/2}$ is long. Hence, the action of the drug lasts up to 24 hours. It is nonspecific for GPIIb–IIIa. Binding of abciximab to platelets exposes certain neoantigens on their surface, resulting in the generation of antiplatelet antibodies. This causes thrombocytopenia. Arrhythmias and bradycardia are also reported with abciximab.

Eptifibatide

This is a heptapeptide-based drug having the KGD amino acid sequence that inhibits the binding of fibrinogen and vWF to GPIIb–IIIa receptor.

Tirofiban

It is a nonpeptide drug and a RGD sequence mimic that also inhibits GPIIb-IIIa-mediated platelet aggregation. Thrombocytopenia risk with eptifibatide and tirofiban is less compared to abciximab.

Other Drugs with Antiplatelet Action

Vorapaxar

A synthetic derivative of himbacine, an alkaloid obtained from the Australian magnolia plant, vorapaxar is a reversible inhibitor of PAR1 located on the surface of platelets. Since the elimination $t_{1/2}$ of the drug is long (around 8 days) and the drug dissociates slowly from its receptor, its final effect on platelets is irreversible.

Dipyridamole

This old drug was once used in angina. It is an inhibitor of phosphodiesterase. It also inhibits adenosine reuptake in endothelial cells. Both these mechanisms increase cAMP inside cells, reduce platelet aggregation, and lead to vasodilatation. Because of the drug's ability to cause vasodilatation in nonischemic areas, the drug can cause the coronary steal phenomenon. Its use as an antianginal drug is therefore obsolete. Dipyridamole combined with aspirin is used in stroke prophylaxis. Along with warfarin, the drug can also be given to prevent embolic stroke in patients with prosthetic heart valves. Risk of bleeding with dipyridamole is less compared to aspirin and clopidogrel.

Epoprostenol and Treprostinil

These drugs are PGI2 analogs. By acting through Gs type of G protein–coupled receptor, they cause vasodilatation and inhibit platelet aggregation. The drugs are primarily used in patients with pulmonary artery hypertension but can also be used for their antiplatelet action in patients requiring dialysis to maintain the patency of atrioventricular shunts in whom heparin is contraindicated. They can also reduce the requirement of heparin in dialysis patients. Main adverse effects are hypotension, flushing, headache, and jaw pain. Risk of bleeding is less but not nil. The drugs can cause bleeding from esophageal varices. Epoprostenol is given by IV route and treprostinil by subcutaneous or IV routes.

Heparin

Mainly used as an anticoagulant, heparin in high doses has additional antiplatelet action.

Nonsteroidal Anti-Inflammatory Drugs (NSAIDs) Other Than Aspirin

All NSAIDs are antiplatelet drugs but, unlike aspirin, they cause reversible inhibition of COX. Hence, they are not preferred in ischemic CVDs.

Daltroban and Sultroban

These TXA2 receptor antagonists are of limited use.

Dazoxiben

This oral TXA2 synthase inhibitor is also of limited use in peripheral arterial disease.

Uses

- MI (NSTEMI and STEMI).
- Unstable angina.

- Stable angina.
- Peripheral artery disease (PAD).
- Stroke and TIA.
- Dialysis patients—to maintain patency of shunts if heparin is contraindicated.
- Patients with atrial fibrillation, in order to prevent stroke (if anticoagulants cannot be given).
- Patients with prosthetic heart valves, in order to prevent stroke.

Fibrinolytics (PH1.25)

These drugs form the cornerstone of medical therapy in STEMI. By activating plasminogen and degrading fibrin, the drugs dissolve clots and restore arterial blood flow.

Fibrinolytic Drugs

Streptokinase

Obtained from streptococci and *Escherichia coli*, streptokinase activates tissue plasminogen activator (t-PA) and generates plasmin from plasminogen. Plasmin then degrades fibrin to fibrin degradation products. Since streptokinase is not specific for clot-bound plasminogen, plasmin is also generated in circulation and this can degrade fibrin and fibrinogen, resulting in increased risk of bleeding. Other than bleeding, hypersensitivity reactions, transient arrhythmias, and hypotension are also observed with the use of streptokinase. The drug is not given a second time if a patient has received the drug ≥ 4 days back and less than 1 year back. This is because of the appearance of neutralizing antibodies.

Anistreplase

Anistreplase is acylated plasminogen–streptokinase activator complex. Being acylated, it is protected from hydrolysis by intrinsic plasmin inhibitors and has a long $t_{1/2}$ of 80 to 100 minutes. Like streptokinase, hypotension and allergic reactions are common with anistreplase.

Urokinase

Urokinase is increased in the body at sites of inflammation and is present in the urine. Commercially obtained from cultured kidney cells, urokinase also activates plasminogen activators such as streptokinase. Its use for MI and PAD is now supplanted by other better thrombolytics.

Recombinant t-PA and Derivatives

Alteplase, reteplase, and tenecteplase.

Alteplase

It is a recombinant t-PA produced from *E. coli*. Its $t_{1/2}$ is 4 to 8 minutes. Hence, it is given as an infusion following a bolus dose.

- Dose in MI: 15 mg IV bolus, then 50 mg over 30 minutes, and 35 mg over 60 minutes.
- Dose in pulmonary embolism: 100 mg IV over 2 hours.
- Dose in stroke: 0.9 mg/kg, first 10% as IV bolus, remaining 90% over 1 hour.

Reteplase

It is a glycosylated version of t-PA. Compared to alteplase, its binding to fibrin is weak. The drug is given as two boluses, a dose of 18 mg (10 unit) each over 2 to 3 minutes and separated by a gap of 30 minutes. Its $t_{1/2}$ is 13 to 15 minutes.

Tenecteplase

It is a long-acting recombinant t-PA with initial $t_{1/2}$ of 20 to 25 minutes and elimination $t_{1/2}$ of 90 to 130 minutes. Compared to alteplase, it is more specific toward fibrin-bound plasminogen and more resistant to PAI inhibition. Intracranial bleed risk with tenecteplase is similar to alteplase, while other sites' bleed risk is less. The drug is given as a single IV bolus dose of 0.5 mg/kg over 10 seconds.

Desmoteplase

It is obtained from the saliva of vampire bats and has a $t_{1/2}$ of 4 hours.

Uses

- STEMI.
- Stroke.
- Deep venous thrombosis and pulmonary embolism.
- PAD.

Contraindications

- Any intracranial bleed.
- Past history of ischemic stroke in the last 3 months.
- Major head or face trauma in the last 3 months.
- History of major surgery in the past 3 weeks.
- Uncontrolled hypertension (systolic blood pressure > 180 mm Hg, diastolic blood pressure > 110 mm Hg).
- Intracranial vascular abnormality or neoplasm.
- Aortic dissection.
- Active bleed (other than menses).
- Use of anticoagulants.
- Pregnancy.

Multiple Choice Questions

1. All of these are fibrinolytics except:

A. Streptokinase.
B. Alteplase.
C. α-glucosidase.
D. Reteplase.

Answer: C

α-Glucosidase is an enzyme involved in carbohydrate digestion.

2. A 66-year-old diabetic man with a known history of coronary artery disease is admitted with a chief complaint of chest pain and sweating. Cardiac markers were elevated but ECG showed nonspecific ischemic changes. A plan of giving medical therapy was made. The patient is going to receive all the following medicines except:

A. Aspirin.
B. Heparin.

C. Clopidogrel.

D. Prasugrel.

Answer: D

This seems to be a case of NSTEMI. The antiplatelet drug prasugrel is generally given to patients with ACS requiring PCI.

3. In the above scenario, if urgent PCI is planned, then the patient is going to be managed by all except:

A. Aspirin.

B. Heparin.

C. Alteplase.

D. Prasugrel.

Answer: C

In NSTEMI, the blood flow is present but limited by stenosis. Thrombolytics must be avoided in NSTEMI as there is no clear benefit of their use.

4. Eptifibatide is:

A. Anti-P2Y antibody.

B. Anti-GPIIb IIIa peptide.

C. Anti-IL-5 peptide.

D. Anti-GPIIb IIIa antibody.

Answer: B

Eptifibatide is a heptapeptide-based drug having the KGD amino acid sequence that inhibits the binding of fibrinogen and vWF to GPIIb–IIIa receptor.

5. Clopidogrel works by which of the following mechanism?

A. Reversible inhibitor of P2Y.

B. Reversible inhibitor of P2X.

C. Irreversible inhibitor of PAR1.

D. Irreversible inhibitor of P2Y.

Answer: D

Clopidogrel is irreversible inhibitor of P2Y12 receptor on platelets.

Chapter 52 Drug Therapy of Peptic Ulcer and Gastroesophageal Reflux Disease

Harpinder Kaur, Phulen Sarma, Bikash Medhi, and Chandra Das

PH1.34: Describe the mechanism/s of action, types, doses, side effects, indications, and contraindications of the drugs used in the following:

1. **Acid peptic disease and gastroesophageal reflux disease**
2. **Antiemetics and prokinetics**
3. **Antidiarrheals**
4. **Laxatives**
5. **Inflammatory bowel disease**
6. **Irritable bowel disorders and biliary and pancreatic diseases**

Learning Objectives

- Peptic ulcer.
- H2-receptor antagonists.
- Proton-pump inhibitors.
- Prostaglandin analog.
- Antacids.
- Mucosal protective drugs.
- Potassium-competitive acid blockers.
- Anti–*Helicobacter pylori* drugs.
- Gastroesophageal reflux disease.

Introduction (MI3.6)

Acid peptic disorders comprise gastroesophageal reflux, gastric or duodenal ulcers, and injury of mucosa associated with stress. In such disorders, gastric acid and pepsin play an important role but are mostly not sufficient to cause pathogenesis. In normal circumstances, the damage induced by acid and pepsin is prevented by intrinsic defense mechanisms. In the absence of barrier to reflux of gastric constituents into the esophagus, dyspepsia and/or erosive esophagitis may occur. The treatment of these disorders involves reducing gastric acidity, improving lower sphincter of esophagus, or stimulating motility of esophagus. The gastric mucosa is defended by mucus and bicarbonate, disruption of which can lead to peptic ulcers. The treatment of ulcers involves decreasing gastric acidity, increasing mucosal protection, or treating infection by *Helicobacter pylori*, which plays a crucial part in the pathogenesis of peptic ulcers.

Physiology of Acid Secretion

Secretion of gastric acid is regulated in such a way that it increases the benefits and reduces the harmful effects. Acid has several beneficial effects, which include killing ingested microbes, relative sterilizing of the stomach as well as the small intestine, modulating the gut microbiota, assisting in digestion of proteins, facilitating the absorption of nonheme iron, vitamin B_{12}, and calcium, and enhancing bioavailability of some medicines. Secretion of gastric acid is an intricate and continuous process regulated by neuronal (which involves acetylcholine [ACh]), paracrine (which involves histamine), and endocrine (which involves gastrin) components. End point of this process is secretion of H^+ by H^+ K^+ ATPase (proton pump) present on the canalicular surface of parietal cells when activated by ACh, histamine, or gastrin. Gastrin (CCK2), histamine, and ACh (M3) receptors are present on parietal cells, while enterochromaffinlike (ECL) cells present nearby parietal cells contain gastrin and ACh receptors. ECL cells are the main source for release of histamine. The action of gastrin and ACh is, to a large extent, indirect through release of histamine from paracrine ECL cells; therefore, histamine has a dominant role to play in acid secretion. Histamine binds to H2 receptors and stimulates acid secretion by proton pump via activating the Gs-adenylyl cyclase-cyclic AMP-PKA pathway, while ACh and gastrin bind to M3 and CCK2 receptors, respectively, and stimulate acid secretion by increasing cytosolic calcium via G_q-phospholipase C-IP3-DAG pathway. Hydrogen ions present inside the cell are traded for potassium ions across the membrane of parietal cells by the proton pump, and this generates a large ion gradient, with pH inside cells of around 7.3 and an intracanalicular pH of around 0.8. The process of acid secretion is depicted in **Fig. 52.1**.

Central nervous system (CNS) stimulates secretion of acid via the vagal nerve's dorsal motor nucleus, the solitary tract nucleus, and the hypothalamus. Efferent fibers that originate in the dorsal motor nuclei reach the stomach by means of the vagus nerve to synapse with enteric nervous system (ENS) ganglion cells. The muscarinic M1 receptor is present on the ganglion cells of the intramural plexus and mediates vagal responses. The muscarinic receptor present on the parietal cells is of M3 subtype. The CNS mainly modulates ENS activity via ACh released from postganglionic vagal fibers, stimulating secretion of acid from stomach in response to food's smell, sight, taste, or expectation. Direct acid secretion by ACh is stimulated through M3 receptors and has an indirect effect on the parietal cells by increasing histamine and gastrin release from the ECL cells and G cells, respectively. Histamine is a paracrine mediator that diffuses from ECL cells to proximate parietal cells and activates H2 receptors. Gastrin is secreted from the G cells present in the antrum. It is a potent inducer of acid secretion and has trophic effects on the ECL cells. Gastrin release is stimulated

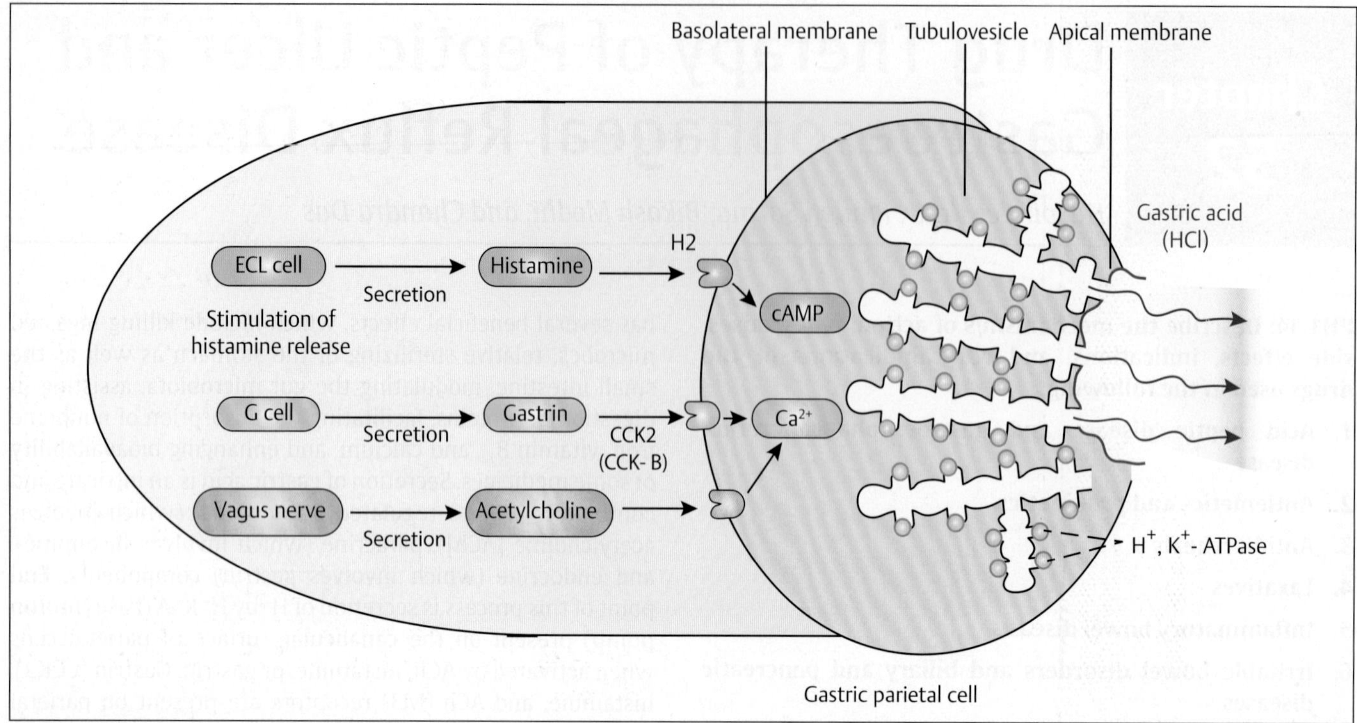

Fig. 52.1 Physiological regulation of gastric acid secretion. The diagram represents the interactions between enterochromaffin-like cell, which releases histamine, and parietal cell, which releases H^+. ACh, acetylcholine; CCK2, cholecystokinin receptor; EP3, prostaglandin receptor; H, histamine receptor; M, muscarinic receptor; PG, prostaglandin.

by activation of CNS, local distension, and chemical components of stomach contents (amino acids and proteins present in food are the main activators). Gastrin-releasing peptide stimulates release and formation of gastrin. Stomach pH also regulates release of gastrin; increased acidity inhibits gastrin and vice versa.

Somatostatin is an inhibitory peptide released from the antral D cells; it inhibits gastric acid secretion. Somatostatin is released when the pH of gastric lumen is greater than 3, and it inhibits release of gastrin in a negative feedback loop. The cells that produce somatostatin are reduced in *H. pylori*–infected patients, which may contribute to increased production of gastrin.

Defenses against Acid

Strong defense mechanisms are present for protection of the esophagus and the stomach from highly acidic environment in the lumen of the stomach. A lower esophageal sphincter (LES) checks that the acidic contents of the stomach do not reflux back into the esophagus and is the main defense system of esophagus. The defense mechanisms of the stomach include secretion of a mucus layer, production of which is triggered by prostaglandins E2 and I2, and these prostaglandins also have a direct effect on inhibition of gastric acid by opposing cyclic adenosine monophosphate (cAMP) generation in parietal cells. Gastric mucus is soluble on secretion; however, it rapidly forms an insoluble gel that covers gastric mucosal surface, slows the diffusion of ions, and protects the mucosa from damage by pepsin. Therefore, drugs that inhibit the formation of prostaglandins reduce mucus secretion and increase chances of acid peptic disease development. Another mucosal defense is bicarbonate ions secretion by superficial epithelial cells of the stomach, which neutralize acid in the mucosal cells and create a pH gradient ranging from 7 at the surface of mucosa to 1 to 2 in the lumen of the stomach. These defense mechanisms of the stomach require proper mucosal blood flow, because gastric mucosa has high metabolic activity and requires proper oxygen. Moreover, mucus and tight junctions of epithelial cells control back diffusion of acid and pepsin. Blood transports bicarbonate as well as important nutrients to cells present on the surface. Damaged epithelium is restored by the process of restitution in which gland neck cells migrate to seal small erosions and intact epithelium is established again.

Peptic Ulcer (IM15.15)

An ulcer is a localized and circumscribed necrosis of the wall of the intestine that extends beneath the level of muscularis mucosae. Lesions that do not extend to this depth are known as erosions. Peptic ulcers (gastric and duodenal) occur as a consequence of lack of balance between the hostile (acid, pepsin, bile) and the protective (secretion of mucus and bicarbonate, prostaglandins, blood flow, nitric oxide, mucosal cells' innate resistance) mechanisms of the gastrointestinal tract (GIT). In earlier days, acid hypersecretion was considered to be the only important factor causing peptic ulcers. However, the role of acid was overemphasized. Acid secretion is commonly normal or less in the case of gastric ulcers, while in the case of duodenal ulcers it is more in 50% of the individuals and normal in the remaining. Injury in the case of gastric ulcers is due to weak mucosal defence and less production of bicarbonate. Infection due to *H. pylori* and use of nonsteroidal anti-inflammatory drugs (NSAIDs) are the two main reasons behind occurrence of ulcers. Use of serotonin reuptake inhibitors can also lead to ulcers. Other factors that can lead to development of ulcers are Zollinger–Ellison syndrome (ZES), anastomosis ulcer after subtotal gastric resection, and tumors. ZES is described as hypersecretion of gastrin from gastrinomas, which results in refractory peptic ulcers in the upper GIT. Individuals having ulcers can be asymptomatic or have the following symptoms: pain in upper stomach, nausea, retching, feeling of fullness, and bleeding characterized by melena or vomit. Esophagogastroduodenoscopy (upper endoscopy) is usually used for diagnosis of ulcers.

H. pylori are microaerophilic gram-negative bacteria that can cause gastritis, peptic ulcer, and malignant diseases. They are classified by the World Health Organization (WHO) as group I carcinogen leading to gastric adenocarcinoma. Colonization of the stomach by *H. pylori* is accompanied by inflammation of the stomach; however, only a few individuals harboring *H. pylori* progress to peptic ulceration, while the rest remain asymptomatic. It attaches itself underneath the mucus and produces ammonia due to its high urease activity, which helps the bacteria to endure the acidic gastric environment. *H. pylori* may increase acid secretion in individuals with duodenal ulcers and decreases the acid secretion in gastric ulcer or cancer patients. Its infection can cause reduced somatostatin production, which leads to reduced inhibition of gastrin production, causing increased production of acid. Patients with *H. pylori* infection who have reduced acid secretion are prone to developing gastric cancer because of reduction in vitamin C absorption as well as enhanced growth of salivary and intestinal bacteria inside the stomach.

NSAIDs can lead to bleeding, perforation, and ulceration of GIT. Effects of NSAIDs are mediated through reduced production of prostaglandins due to inhibition of cyclooxygenase-1 (COX-1) and through topical effects that play a part in the initial processes of injury. The direct effects are mediated through mitochondrial dysfunction. Impairment of barrier function of intestine allows gram-negative bacteria to invade the mucosa, which, in coordination with endogenous molecules, trigger inflammatory cascades leading to ulceration.

Peptic ulcer disease is a chronic condition, and relapse occurs within 1 year in most of the cases that do not receive prophylactic acid suppression. As *H. pylori* plays a significant role in pathogenesis of peptic ulcers, relapse can be prevented by its elimination from the stomach.

Approaches for Peptic Ulcer Treatment (Fig. 52.2)

1. H2-receptor antagonists (H2RAs): ranitidine, nizatidine, famotidine, roxatidine.
2. Proton-pump inhibitors (PPIs): omeprazole, pantoprazole, lansoprazole, rabeprazole, esomeprazole, dexlansoprazole.
3. Prostaglandin analog: misoprostol.
4. Antacids: sodium bicarbonate, calcium carbonate, aluminum hydroxide, magnesium hydroxide.
5. Mucosal protective agents: sucralfate, bismuth compounds.
6. Potassium-competitive acid blocker: vonoprazan.
7. Other drugs: pirenzepine, telenzepine, carbenoxolone, rebamipide.
8. Anti–H. pylori drugs: amoxicillin, clarithromycin, tetracycline, levofloxacin metronidazole, tinidazole, bismuth compounds.

H2-Receptor Antagonists

H2RAs are reversible and competitive inhibitors of parietal cell H2 receptors. They are extremely selective for H2

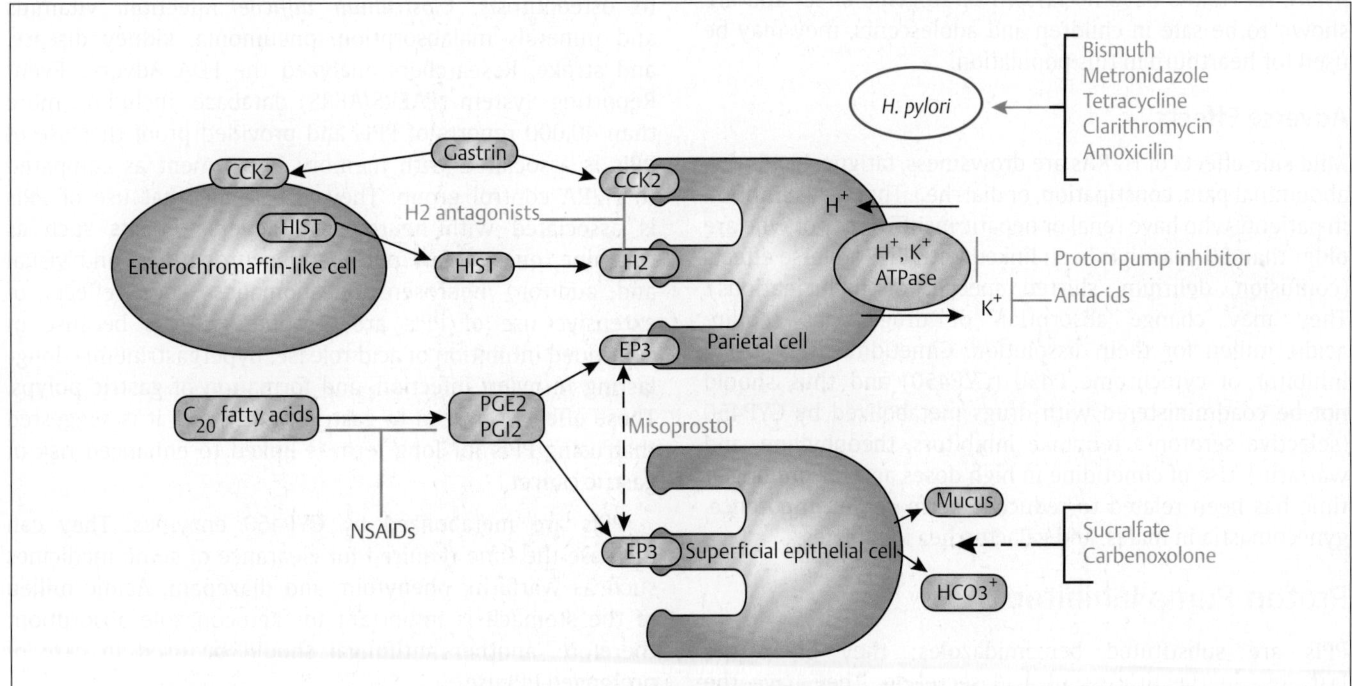

Fig. 52.2 Approaches for peptic ulcer treatment. PGE2, prostaglandin E2₂; PGI2, prostaglandin I2; CCK2, cholecystokinin receptor.

receptors and have no effect on H1 and H3 receptors. They also decrease the volume of acid secreted from the stomach as well as pepsin concentration. They are effective in reducing the amount of acid released on stimulation by gastrin and ACh in addition to that by histamine. First, histamine secreted by ECL cells as a result of gastrin or vagal stimulation is prohibited from binding to H2 receptors on parietal cells; in addition, there is reduced acid secretion through direct parietal cell stimulation by gastrin or ACh when H2 receptors are blocked. H2RAs predominantly prevent basal acid secretion; that is why they are effective in inhibiting night-time acid secretion, which is mostly dependent on histamine. However, they do not have much effect on acid secretion stimulated by meals, which is triggered by gastrin, Ach, and histamine. They inhibit more than 90% of night-time acid and simply 60 to 80% of acid secretion during daytime. Evening dose of H2RAs is suitable for the treatment of most cases of duodenal ulcers, as nocturnal acidity is an important factor in such ulcers. H2RAs generally vary in their pharmacokinetics and tendency to result in drug interactions. The first H2RA to be introduced in the mid-1970s was cimetidine. The potency of these drugs is less than that of PPIs.

The shortcomings of this class of drugs are their short duration of action (4–8 hours) and the fact that they lose their acid-inhibiting potency on prolonged use (within 2 weeks of daily dosage) because of tachyphylaxis.

Indications

H2RAs are used for short periods of time in manageable gastroesophageal reflux disease (GERD) therapy, gastric or duodenal ulcers, gastric hypersecretion, and for slight-to-sporadic heartburn or dyspepsia (Food and Drug Administration [FDA]–approved indications). They may also be used for prophylaxis of stress ulcers, esophagitis, gastritis, GI hemorrhage, or urticaria. They are also occasionally incorporated in multidrug regimen for eradication of *H. pylori*. As H2RAs have no known teratogenic effect and are shown to be safe in children and adolescents, they may be used for heartburn in this population.

Adverse Effects

Mild side effects of H2RAs are drowsiness, fatigue, headache, abdominal pain, constipation, or diarrhea. Their consumption in patients who have renal or hepatic insufficiency or who are older than 50 years has been linked with CNS adverse effects (confusion, delirium, slurred speech, or hallucinations). They may change absorption of drugs that require acidic milieu for their dissolution. Cimetidine is a strong inhibitor of cytochrome P450 (CYP450) and thus should not be coadministered with drugs metabolized by CYP450 (selective serotonin reuptake inhibitors, theophylline, and warfarin). Use of cimetidine in high doses and for prolonged time has been related to reduced sperm count, impotence, gynecomastia in males, and galactorrhea in females.

Proton-Pump Inhibitors

PPIs are substituted benzimidazoles; they block the last step in the process of acid secretion. They have the maximum potency as compared to other categories and are the most widely used drugs. They are effective despite other stimulating factors. The drugs in this category are prodrugs, and they are activated in the acidic milieu. After they are absorbed and reach systemic circulation, diffusion of prodrug into the gastric parietal cells takes place, and it is accumulated in the acidic secretory canaliculi, where it is converted into its active form, tetracycline sulfonamide, by proton-catalyzed reaction. The drug is trapped, and back diffusion across the canalicular membrane is not possible. The active form attaches covalently to sulfhydryl groups of cysteine and irreversibly inhibits the proton pump. The acid secretion starts again when fresh molecules of pump are produced and placed in the luminal membrane. They suppress both basal and meal-stimulated release of acid and their effect lasts for about 16 to 18 hours. Moreover, they do not develop tolerance because of lack of receptor inhibition. PPIs should be taken half an hour prior to meals because they require acidic pH for their activation. Omeprazole was the first PPI to be introduced in 1989.

Indications

PPIs are prescribed extensively and are regarded as safe for over-the-counter use. They are used for the management of GERD, peptic ulcer disease, prophylaxis of stress ulcers, *H. pylori* infection, protection in case of chronic use of NSAIDs, upper GIT bleeding, dyspepsia, erosive esophagitis, and ZES.

Adverse Effects

Common adverse drug reactions (ADRs) of this class of drugs noticed in clinical trials were flatulence, nausea, vomiting, diarrhea, and headache. Severe ADRs were difficulty in breathing, rash, swelling of face, and tightness of throat. Some studies have potentially associated prolonged use of PPIs with greater risk of fractures related to osteoporosis, *Clostridium difficile* infection, vitamins and minerals malabsorption, pneumonia, kidney disease, and stroke. Researchers analyzed the FDA Adverse Event Reporting System (FAERS/AERS) database, including more than 40,000 reports of PPIs and provided proof that use of PPIs is associated with memory impairment as compared to H2RA control group. They also found that use of PPIs is associated with neurological adverse effects such as migraine, quite a few peripheral neuropathies, and visual and auditory neurosensory anomalies. Local effects of extensive use of PPIs are atrophic gastritis because of continued inhibition of acid release, hypergastrinemia, long-lasting *H. pylori* infection, and formation of gastric polyps. These effects can lead to gastric cancer, and it is suggested that using PPIs for long term is linked to enhanced risk of gastric cancer.

PPIs are metabolized by CYP450 enzymes. They can increase the time required for clearance of some medicines such as warfarin, phenytoin, and diazepam. Acidic milieu of the stomach is important for ketoconazole absorption; therefore, another antifungal should be used in case of prolonged PPI use.

Prostaglandin Analog

A synthetic analog of PGE1, that is, misoprostol, is also utilized in some cases. It inhibits the release of gastric acid (reduces cAMP generation stimulated by histamine after binding to receptors for prostaglandins [EP3] present on parietal cells) and pepsin and also enhances the resistance of the gastric mucosa. It is useful in bleeding small intestinal ulcers that are induced by NSAIDs, but its protection is inadequate; hence, it is used in combination with other drugs. It has a half-life that is less than half an hour and thus administration is required three to four times a day. Its side effects (cramping, abdominal pain, and diarrhea) limit its use. Misoprostol is contraindicated during pregnancy because it stimulates contractions of uterus.

Antacids

Antacids were the first drugs that were used widely for management of peptic ulcers until the discovery of PPIs. Antacids decrease the acid that reaches duodenum by neutralization of acid present in the stomach; however, they are associated with regular acid rebound after their intake and therefore large amounts of these are required. Milliequivalent of acid-neutralizing capacity, which is described by means of the amount of 1N HCl, stated in mEq, and which can be brought to pH 3.5 in 15 minutes, is used to express relative efficacy of antacid preparations. According to requirements of FDA, antacids ought to have neutralizing capacity of no less than 5 mEq per dose. Antacids have therapeutic use in heartburn symptoms in GERD, duodenal ulcers, gastric ulcers, stress gastritis, and nonnuclear dyspepsia.

Sodium bicarbonate leads to the production of carbon dioxide plus sodium chloride after it reacts with hydrochloric acid of the stomach. As sodium bicarbonate is soluble in water to a great extent, it is absorbed rapidly from the stomach and thus the alkali and sodium can present a risk to individuals who have cardiac or renal failure. Calcium carbonate is not as soluble as sodium bicarbonate and forms carbon dioxide and calcium chloride on reaction with HCl. Calcium can cause rebound secretion of acid, requiring more frequent administration. Carbon dioxide released from antacids containing either bicarbonate or carbonate can lead to distention of stomach, belching, nausea, and flatulence. Antacids that contain magnesium hydroxide and aluminum hydroxide react at slow speed with acid to produce magnesium chloride or aluminum chloride plus water. These antacids do not cause belching and metabolic alkalosis. Combinations containing magnesium (fast-reacting) and aluminum (fast-reacting) are preferred for balanced neutralizing capacity and to reduce the effect on bowel function because unabsorbed salts of magnesium can result in osmotic diarrhea and salts of aluminum in constipation. Patients who have renal insufficiency should be warned against prolonged use of these antacids because absorption and excretion of magnesium and aluminum take place via the kidneys. All antacids can have an effect on absorption of other medicines due to drug binding, alteration of its dissolution, or solubility (mainly weakly acidic and basic drugs) by increasing gastric pH. Thus, antacids are not to be administered in a period of 2 hours of administration of fluoroquinolones, tetracyclines, iron, and itraconazole.

Mucosal Protective Drugs

Sucralfate

Sucralfate is basic aluminum salt of sucrose octasulfate. It has a local mucosal protective effect and inhibits pepsin activity. Sucralfate goes through extensive cross-linking at pH less than 4 and yields a polymer that is viscous and sticky and sticks to epithelial cells and ulcer craters. It remains bound for until 6 hours when one dose is administered. It may also stimulate production of prostaglandins as well as epidermal growth factor. A total of 1 g of sucralfate is administered four times every day 1 hour before meals on an empty stomach. It decreases the chances of upper GIT bleed in terminally ill hospitalized patients when given in the form of slurry through nasogastric tube. However, it is not as efficacious as H2RAs given intravenously. It is also utilized for prophylaxis of bleeding linked to stress. It does not have any systemic side effects as it is not absorbed. Aluminum salt can cause constipation in few patients. It can impair the absorption of other drugs by binding to them.

Bismuth Compounds

Bismuth subcitrate potassium and bismuth subsalicylate are the two bismuth compounds that can be used. To counter acid and pepsin, bismuth creates a protective layer around ulcers and erosions. It may trigger secretion of mucus, bicarbonate, and prostaglandin, too. Bismuth subsalicylate decreases the frequency and liquidity of stool in the case of acute infectious diarrhea because salicylate inhibits secretion of intestinal prostaglandin and chloride. It is beneficial in prevention and treatment of traveler's diarrhea, because it has direct antimicrobial effects and it binds enterotoxins. Compounds of bismuth also possess direct antimicrobial action against *H. pylori* and are utilized in drug regimens for eradication of the bacterium. Bismuth-containing formulations are very safe. They cause blackening of stool and tongue (liquid formulations), which is harmless. They are not to be used for long term and in the case of renal inadequacy. Higher doses of bismuth subsalicylate can cause salicylate toxicity.

Potassium-Competitive Acid Blockers

Vonoprazan was introduced in Japan and is available only in the Japanese market for the management of acid-related disorders. It is a potassium-competitive acid inhibitor, which blocks H^+, K^+-ATPase in parietal cells at the last step of the acid-secretory process. Vonoprazan differs from PPIs because it inhibits the proton pump in a K^+ competitive and reversible manner, and does not need an acidic environment for its activation. Moreover, its onset of action is rapid, and it controls intragastric acidity for long time. It was observed that vonoprazan (10 and 20 mg) is not inferior to lansoprazole when used to prevent reappearance of ulcers in Japanese patients on NSAIDs or those who needed aspirin for protection of their cerebrovascular or cardiovascular system.

It is well-tolerated, has a comparable safety profile, and has no new safety concerns. Moreover, 5 weeks of vonoprazan therapy significantly reduced postendoscopic submucosal dissection bleeding as compared to 8 weeks of therapy with PPIs. Likewise, it was revealed that vonoprazan is better than esomeprazole and rabeprazole for scarring artificial ulcers. It is used at a dose of 20 mg twice daily in eradication treatments.

Other Drugs

Antagonists of muscarinic M1 receptors (pirenzepine and telenzepine) are able to decrease the basal acid production to almost half. They act via suppression of acid produced on neuronal stimulation of M1 receptors present on intramural ganglia. Pirenzepine is a tricyclic antimuscarinic agent, which was developed in West Germany. It is very hydrophilic and has poor blood–brain barrier permeability. It is effective in the dose of 100 to 150 mg/day. Telenzepine is more potent as compared to pirenzepine. As their effectiveness is less as compared to other drugs and they have unwanted anticholinergic adverse effects, they are seldom used nowadays. Pirenzepine is also associated with risk of blood disorders.

Carbenoxolone, a synthetic triterpenoid derivative of glycyrrhizic acid from the root of licorice, has shown beneficial effect in gastric as well as duodenal ulcers. It has anti-inflammatory, antiulcer, and hypoglycemic properties. It is supposed to act via increasing secretion and production of mucus and changing its chemical composition. It is believed to increase the life-time of epithelial cells of the stomach, reduce unusually high cell shedding rate, and have antipeptic action against pepsin. Cytoprotective activity of carbenoxolone is also attributed to its ability to increase PGF1a and PGE2. However, carbenoxolone results in retention of sodium and hypokalemia because of its marked mineralocorticoidlike activity on metabolism of electrolytes.

Rebamipide is a mucosal protective agent that can be used for prevention of gastric ulcers, particularly in patients having less acid secretion. It is reported to act as a scavenger of hydroxyl radicals, suppressor of production of superoxide radicals from activated neutrophils, and an enhancer of PGE2 and PGI2. Rebamipide also inhibits the inflammatory cascade caused by infection due to *H. pylori* and improves gastritis, and may play a role to prevent ulcers caused by NSAIDs because of increase in blood flow and decrease in free radicals.

Anti–*H. pylori* Drugs

Infection by *H. pylori* can be diagnosed by invasive methods such as those demanding endoscopy and biopsy (e.g., histological analysis, culture, and urease test) and by noninvasive methods, which consist of urea breath test, serology, urine/blood, or antigen detection in stool specimen. PPI in combination with two antibiotics has been effective in the management of *H. pylori* infection. The bacterium enters replicative phase at a pH of 6 to 7 and changes to a coccoid form resistant to antibiotics at a pH of 3 to 6. Therefore, increasing intragastric pH by PPIs when an antibiotic-based therapy is administered appears important. But increased resistance to the effective antibiotics poses great risk to the management of *H. pylori* infection and also makes mass eradication impractical. Recurrence of *H. pylori* infection is also a major concern in its management in addition to increase in antibiotic resistance. Recurrence can be due to recrudescence (recurrence of the original strain that was temporarily suppressed and not detected after treatment) or reinfection (new strain infection after effective eradication). Recrudescence is due to the failure of eradication regimen, and reinfection is due to new infection after successful eradication.

American College of Gastroenterology (ACG) Clinical Guideline for Management of Infection by *H. pylori*

First-line treatment strategies:

1. Any prior exposure to antibiotics should be considered while choosing the regimen for treatment.
2. Clarithromycin triple therapy (PPI + clarithromycin + amoxicillin/metronidazole) for a 14-day period in areas with clarithromycin resistance less than15% and in patients who had not taken macrolides earlier due to some reason.
3. Bismuth quadruple therapy (PPI + bismuth + tetracycline + nitroimidazole) for a 10- to 14-day period particularly in patients who had prior exposure to macrolide or are allergic to penicillin.
4. Concomitant treatment with PPI + clarithromycin + amoxicillin + nitroimidazole for a period of 10 to 14 days.
5. Sequential treatment with PPI + amoxicillin for a 5- to 7-day period, followed by PPI + clarithromycin + nitroimidazole for a period of 5 to 7 days.
6. Hybrid treatment with PPI + amoxicillin for a 7-day period, followed by PPI + amoxicillin + clarithromycin + nitroimidazole for a period of 7 days.
7. Levofloxacin triple therapy with PPI + levofloxacin + amoxicillin for a period of 10 to 14 days.
8. Fluoroquinolone sequential treatment with PPI + amoxicillin for a period of 5 to 7 days, followed by PPI + fluoroquinolone + nitroimidazole for a period of 5 to 7 days.

A number of combinations of PPI, clarithromycin, and amoxicillin are approved by the FDA. The FDA has not given approval to the combination of PPI with clarithromycin and metronidazole. Similarly, the FDA has not given approval to PPI, bismuth, tetracycline, and metronidazole if prescribed individually. However, it has approved Pylera, which is a product consisting of combination of bismuth subcitrate, tetracycline, and metronidazole combined with a PPI, for a period of 10 days.

The first-line treatment strategies for management of *H. pylori* are given in **Table 52.1**.

Options for salvage therapy after the failure of first-line therapy are as follows:

1. In patients who have persistent infection, antibiotics previously taken by the patient should be avoided. Suitable salvage regimen is to be selected based on the data of local antimicrobial resistance as well as patient's prior use of antibiotics.

Table 52.1 First-line treatment strategies for *H. pylori* infection

Regimen	Drugs	Dose	Frequency of dosage
Clarithromycin triple	PPI	Standard dose or double dose	Twice daily
	Clarithromycin	500 mg	
	Amoxicillin/metronidazole	1 g/500 mg thrice daily	
Bismuth quadruple	PPI	Standard dose	Twice daily
	Bismuth subcitrate/subsalicylate	120–300 mg/300 mg	Four times daily
	Tetracycline	500 mg	Four times daily
	Metronidazole	250–500 mg	Four times daily (250) Three to four times daily (500)
Concomitant	PPI	Standard dose	Twice daily
	Clarithromycin	500 mg	
	Amoxicillin	1 g	
	Nitroimidazole (metronidazole or tinidazole)	500 mg	
Sequential	PPI + amoxicillin	Standard dose + 1 g	Twice daily
	PPI + clarithromycin + nitroimidazole	Standard dose + 500 mg + 500 mg	Twice daily
Hybrid	PPI + amoxicillin	Standard dose + 1 g	Twice daily
	PPI + amoxicillin + clarithromycin, nitroimidazole	Standard dose + 1 g + 500 mg + 500 mg	Twice daily
Levofloxacin triple	PPI	Standard dose	Twice daily
	Levofloxacin	500 mg	Once daily
	Amoxicillin	1 g	Twice daily
Levofloxacin sequential	PPI + amoxicillin	Standard or double dose + 1 g	Twice daily
	PPI + amoxicillin + levofloxacin + nitroimidazole	Standard or double dose + 1 g + 500 mg once a day + 500 mg	Twice daily
Load	Levofloxacin	250 mg	Once daily
	PPI	Double dose	Once daily
	Nitazoxanide	500 mg	Twice daily
	Doxycycline	100 mg	Once daily

Abbreviation: PPI, proton-pump inhibitor.

2. Bismuth quadruple or levofloxacin salvage therapy is favored in case an individual had taken a first-line therapy consisting of clarithromycin.
3. Salvage regimes consisting of clarithromycin or levofloxacin are preferred in case an individual had taken bismuth quadruple therapy as a first-line treatment.

The subsequent therapies can be used as salvage treatment:

1. Bismuth quadruple therapy for a period of 14 days: recommended salvage therapy.
2. Levofloxacin triple regimen for a period of 14 days: recommended salvage therapy.
3. Concomitant therapy for 10 to 14 days period: suggested salvage therapy.
4. Clarithromycin triple therapy is not to be used as a salvage therapy.
5. Rifabutin triple regime (PPI + amoxicillin + rifabutin) for a period of 10 days: suggested salvage therapy.
6. High-dose dual therapy (PPI + amoxicillin) for a period of 14 days: suggested salvage therapy.

The options for salvage therapy are given in **Table 52.2.**

Management of Peptic Ulcer Disease

1. *H. pylori* eradication treatment for *H. pylori*–positive individuals.
2. In individuals on NSAIDs and having peptic ulcer disease, discontinue NSAIDs if feasible. Propose standard dose of PPI (**Table 52.3**) or H2RA for a period of 8 weeks. If the individual is having *H. pylori* infection, propose subsequent eradication treatment.
3. Periodic endoscopy (6–8 weeks after starting treatment) in individuals having gastric ulcers and infection with *H. pylori.*
4. *H. pylori* retesting (6–8 weeks after starting treatment) in individuals having peptic ulcers and infection with *H. pylori.*

Table 52.2 Salvage therapy for *H. pylori* infection

Regimen	Drugs	Dose	Frequency of dosage
Bismuth quadruple	PPI	Standard dose	Twice daily
	Bismuth subcitrate/subsalicylate	120–300 mg/300 mg	Four times daily
	Tetracycline	500 mg	Four times daily
	Metronidazole	500 mg	Three or four times daily
Levofloxacin triple	PPI	Standard dose	Twice daily
	Levofloxacin	500 mg	Once daily
	Amoxicillin	1 g	Twice daily
Concomitant	PPI	Standard dose	Twice daily
	Clarithromycin	500 mg	Twice daily
	Amoxicillin	1 g	Twice daily
	Nitroimidazole	500 mg	Two or three times daily
Rifabutin triple	PPI	Standard dose	Twice daily
	Rifabutin	300 mg	Once daily
	Amoxicillin	1 g	Twice daily
High-dose dual	PPI	Standard to double dose	Three or four times daily
	Amoxicillin	1 g thrice daily or 750 mg four times daily	Three or four times daily

Abbreviation: PPI, proton-pump inhibitor.

Table 52.3 Standard and double dose of PPIs

PPI	Standard dosage	Double dosage
Esomeprazole	20 mg once daily	40 mg once daily
Lansoprazole	30 mg once daily	30 mg twice daily
Omeprazole	20 mg once daily	40 mg once daily
Pantoprazole	40 mg once daily	40 mg twice daily
Rabeprazole	20 mg once daily	20 mg twice daily

Abbreviation: PPI, proton-pump inhibitor.

5. Standard dose of PPI (**Table 52.3**) or H2RA for a period of 4 to 8 weeks in individuals who neither are *H. pylori*–positive nor are on NSAIDs.
6. In individuals who are continuing NSAIDs even after ulcer healing, possible damage that the NSAIDs could cause should be discussed. The requirement for the usage of NSAIDs should be reviewed. Dose reduction, paracetamol replacement, alternative NSAID, and ibuprofen low dosage (1.2 g/day) should be considered.
7. For high-risk individuals (prior ulcers) or for those who require continuation of NSAIDs, an NSAID that is selective for COX-2 with a PPI should be considered.
8. In individuals in whom the ulcer is not healed, check for nonadherence, failure to identify *H. pylori* infection, unintended usage of NSAIDs, another drug that can cause ulcers, and ZES and Crohn's disease.
9. On recurrence of symptoms post first treatment, give PPI at possible minimum dose for controlling symptoms or individual management of symptoms based on the need.
10. If reaction to a PPI is not adequate, give treatment with H2RA.

Dose of PPIs is mentioned in **Table 52.3** and **Table 52.4**.

Gastroesophageal Reflux Disease

GERD results from reflux of stomach's acidic contents into the esophagus when LES is relaxed and causes bothersome symptoms or esophageal damage. It is mainly thought to be the result of modifications in LES, which can be caused by various factors such as transitory relaxations of LES, hypotensive LES, or anatomic disorder of the gastroesophageal junction (hiatal hernia, obesity, and reduced abdominal length). Aspects such as changes in esophageal peristalsis, delay in gastric emptying, hyposalivation, gastrinomas, and hypersensitivity to gastric acid can also lead to the development of GERD. Environmental factors such as being overweight/obese, improper dietary habits, absence of regular physical activity, consumption of alcohol or coffee, and smoking also contribute to the development of GERD. The most commonly seen symptoms of GERD include heartburn, which worsens on lying down or eating, feeling of food coming back up into the mouth, sore throat, cough, asthma, pain in chest, sensation of a lump in the throat, nausea or vomiting, pain on swallowing, and

Table 52.4 Dose of PPIs for severe esophagitis

PPI	Standard dosage	Double dosage
Esomeprazole	40 mg once daily	40 mg twice daily
Lansoprazole	30 mg once daily	30 mg twice daily
Omeprazole	40 mg once daily	40 mg twice daily
Pantoprazole	40 mg once daily	40 mg twice daily
Rabeprazole	20 mg once daily	20 mg twice daily

Abbreviation: PPI, proton-pump inhibitor.

frequent burping. Phenotypic presentations of GERD include erosive esophagitis, nonerosive reflux disease, and Barrett's esophagus. One-tenth of the individuals have Barrett's esophagus in which the metaplastic columnar epithelium replaces the stratified squamous epithelium of distal esophagus, which can lead to the development of esophageal adenocarcinoma. First-line therapy of GERD should consist of dietary and lifestyle modifications.

Severity of GERD can be categorized into three stages. Stage I consists of periodic simple heartburn, frequently in situation of recognized triggering factor. It is not normally the main trouble and there are fewer than two to three episodes every week with no other symptoms. Stage II consists of frequent symptoms, with or without esophagitis, and there are more than two to three episodes every week. Stage III is characterized by chronic, relentless symptoms; immediate relapse when therapy is stopped; and complications of esophagus such as Barrett's metaplasia.

Guidelines for Management of GERD

1. Individuals who are overweight or had recent weight gain are recommended to lose weight.
2. Elevating bed's head and not having food 2 to 3 hours before going to bed are recommended to individuals with nocturnal GERD.
3. Routine total elimination of foods triggering reflux (such as caffeine, alcohol, chocolate, acidic and/or spicy foods) is not recommended for GERD therapy. In a set of guidelines on diagnosing and managing GERD, the American College of Gastroenterology state that they do not recommend eliminating trigger foods because the dietary connection is not straightforward.
4. Eight-week PPI therapy is the preferred treatment to relieve symptoms as well as heal erosive esophagitis with no significant difference in effectiveness of different PPIs.
5. Traditional PPIs having delayed release should be given 30 to 60 minutes prior to meals for maximum control of pH, while the latest PPIs may offer flexibility in dosing in relation to timings of meal.
6. Treatment with PPIs is to be started at one time daily dosing prior to the first meal of the day.
7. Patients who do not respond to PPIs are to be referred for assessment.
8. In individuals who do not show full response to treatment with PPI, increasing the dose to two times a day or substituting with another PPI may afford further symptom relief.
9. Maintenance PPI therapy is to be given in patients in whom symptoms persist after discontinuation of PPI and in patients who have complications such as erosive esophagitis and Barrett's esophagus. Patients requiring long-term PPI therapy should be given lowest effective dose, comprising on-demand or intermittent therapy.
10. H2RAs can be used for maintenance treatment in individuals who do not have erosive disease if they experience relief from heartburn. Bedtime H2RA can be combined with daytime PPI in certain patients with objective evidence of reflux during night if required; however, it may lead to development of tachyphylaxis after use for several weeks.
11. Treatment for GERD except acid expression, consisting of prokinetic therapy and/or baclofen, is not to be used in patients without diagnostic assessment.
12. Sucralfate has no role in the nonpregnant patient with GERD.
13. PPIs, if clinically indicated, are safe in pregnant patients.

Multiple Choice Questions

1. A 30-year-old unmarried woman with rheumatoid arthritis on frequent diclofenac use also suffered from frequent acid peptic disease for which she is taking drug X for a long time. She now presented with a history of galactorrhea. Identify drug X which was used for the treatment of acid peptic disease:

A. Pantoprazole.
B. Omeprazole.
C. Famotidine.
D. Cimetidine.

Answer: D

NSAIDs, which are frequently used pain killers, cause acid peptic diseases for which drugs such as H2 blocker or PPI are prescribed to the patients. Cimetidine inhibits binding of dihydrotestosterone to androgen receptors, inhibits metabolism of estradiol, and increases serum prolactin levels. When used long term or in high doses, it may cause gynecomastia or impotence in men and galactorrhea in women.

2. A 65-year-old man with type 2 diabetes mellitus and coronary artery disease, recently treated with drug-eluting stent on dual antiplatelet therapy with clopidogrel and aspirin, was prescribed some proton-pump inhibitor (PPI) for acid peptic disease; now, the patient has again presented with chest pain, and the coronary angiogram revealed stent thrombosis. Which of the following drugs may be the possible drug causing stent thrombosis?

A. Antacid gel.
B. Sucralfate.

C. Famotidine.

D. Omeprazole.

Answer: D

Clopidogrel is a prodrug and needs activation by hepatic P450 CYP2c19 isoenzyme, which is also involved in metabolism of PPIs such as omeprazole, esomeprazole, lansoprazole, and dexlansoprazole. Therefore, these drugs can reduce clopidogrel activation, ultimately leading to stent thrombosis.

3. A patient with atrial fibrillation on warfarin, digoxin, and calcium channel blocker is now having dry cough and chest discomfort. Upper GI endoscopy revealed gastroesophageal reflux. Which one of the following should be the preferred drug for the patient?

A. Omeprazole.

B. Esomeprazole.

C. Cimetidine.

D. Famotidine.

Answer: D

PPIs such as omeprazole, esomeprazole, and H2 blocker cimetidine have drug interaction with the metabolism (through interaction with CYP2C9/10 and CYP2C19) of warfarin, digoxin, and calcium channel antagonist. Therefore, these agents should be avoided in patients with cardiac diseases.

4. A patient of hypertension and chronic kidney disease is having recurrent peptic ulcer disease. Which of the following should be avoided?

A. H2 blocker.

B. PPI.

C. Metronidazole.

D. Sucralfate.

Answer: D

Sucralfate is a salt of sucrose complexed to sulfated aluminum hydroxide. A small amount of aluminum is absorbed from sucralfate, so it should not be used for prolonged period in a patient with renal insufficiency.

5. A 35-year-old woman is on nonsteroidal anti-inflammatory drugs (NSAIDs) for recurrent join pain. She has a history of previous peptic ulcer. She has come for advice regarding pregnancy. Which of the following should be stopped immediately?

A. NSAIDs.

B. PPI.

C. Sucralfate.

D. Misoprostol.

Answer: D

Misoprostol, a prostaglandin analogue, binds to uterine smooth muscle and causes contraction, which may cause abortion.

Chapter 53

Pharmacotherapy of Nausea and Vomiting

Arulmozhi S. and Saieswari Natesan

PH1.34: Describe the mechanism/s of action, types, doses, side effects, indications, and contraindications of the drugs used in the following:

1. **Acid peptic disease and gastroesophageal reflux disease**
2. **Antiemetics and prokinetics**
3. **Antidiarrheals**
4. **Laxatives**
5. **Inflammatory bowel disease**
6. **Irritable bowel disorders and biliary and pancreatic diseases**

Learning Objectives

- Physiology of vomiting.
- Antidopaminergics.
- 5-HT_3 antagonists.
- Antihistamines.
- Antimuscarinics.
- Glucocorticoids.
- Substance P antagonists.

Nausea and Vomiting

Vomiting is a response generated by our system to expel toxic or irritant materials from the stomach and intestine. By definition, nausea is an unpleasant sensation preceding vomiting, and vomiting is forceful expulsion of gastric contents through the mouth. Nausea and vomiting can occur as a side effect of several drugs, as a result of bacterial and viral infections, during motion sickness and pregnancy, and during the course of various diseases.

Phases of Vomiting

1. Pre-ejection.
2. Retching.
3. Ejection.

In pre-ejection phase, the gastric muscles undergo relaxation and retroperistalsis. Retching involves contraction of abdominal, intercostal, and diaphragmatic muscles against a closed glottis. The last phase, ejection, is characterized by intense contraction of abdominal muscles and relaxation of upper esophageal sphincter.

Physiology of Vomiting

Let us take a closer look at the mechanisms leading to phases of vomiting.

Irritation in gastrointestinal (GI) areas, bacterial or viral infections, chemotherapeutic agents, or other miscellaneous drugs can stimulate enterochromaffin cells, present in the lining of the stomach to release 5-HT3. This leads to activation of the vagus nerve that sends signals to the chemoreceptor trigger zone (CTZ) via solitary tract nucleus (STN) and eventually vomiting center (VC) in the brain, resulting in vomiting reflex. STN also has the capability to directly activate the VC. Various neurotransmitters such as serotonin, dopamine, acetylcholine, substance P, and histamine are involved in this pathway and their receptors are enlisted in **Fig. 53.1**. Drugs that enter blood stream from GI tract (GIT) or those injected via intravenous (IV) route can directly act on CTZ, as it is unprotected by blood–brain barrier (BBB). Apart from this, even episodes of pain, unpleasant smells, repulsive or revolting sights, and fear can activate VC through higher centers or various areas of cerebral cortex. The vestibular apparatus in the ear along with the cerebellum plays a vital role in maintaining the body balance. Have you ever noticed people vomiting after riding a bus or adventure rides in an amusement park? This is due to disturbances in the body equilibrium, which is detected by vestibular apparatus located in the inner ear. Eventually, it stimulates the VC, through vestibular nuclei and cerebellum, by means of neurotransmitter serotonin (**Fig. 53.1**).

The physiological mechanism of nausea is unclear. It may occur along with vomiting or separately. It is easier to treat vomiting than nausea, as many antiemetics have shown poor response to nausea.

Principles of Pharmacotherapy of Nausea and Vomiting

1. Prevention of the episode of nausea and vomiting if possible, for example, prevention of postoperative and motion sickness–induced vomiting.
2. The cause of nausea or vomiting should be treated, if possible, appropriately.
3. The presumed receptor involved should be aimed at.
4. Use of combinations of medications if necessary.
5. Nonoral routes should also be considered.
6. Environmental measures (odor, taste) should be adjusted.

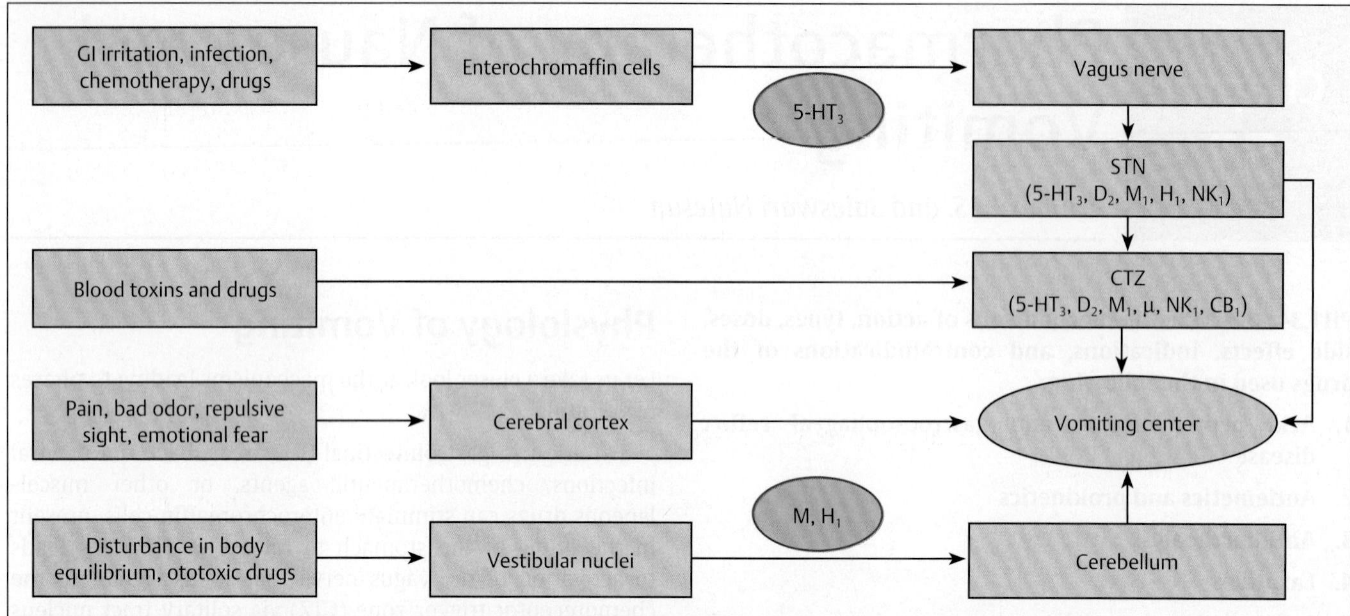

Fig. 53.1 Illustration of pathways and mechanisms facilitating emetic response. 5-HT_3, 5-hydroxytryptamine 3 receptor; μ, opioid receptor; CB1, cannabinoid 1 receptor; CTZ, chemoreceptor trigger zone; D_2, dopamine 2 receptor; GI, gastrointestinal; H_1, histamine 1 receptor; M, muscarinic receptor; NK_1, neurokinin 1 receptor; STN, solitary tract nucleus.

Table 53.1 Classification of antiemetics, their mechanism of action, and drugs

Class	MOA	Examples/drugs
Antidopaminergics (dopamine antagonists)	Block D2 receptors in CTZ and/or GI tract	Chlorpromazine, prochlorperazine, phenothiazine, metoclopramide, domperidone
5-HT_3 antagonists	Block 5-HT_3 receptors in CTZ and GI tract	Ondansetron, granisetron, palonosetron
Antihistamines	Block H_1 receptors in the CNS (can cause sedation) and vestibular afferents	Cinnarizine, cyclizine, dimenhydrinate, diphenhydramine promethazine
Antimuscarinics	Actions on M receptors in vestibular apparatus and possibly in other areas	Hyoscine, dicyclomine
Glucocorticoids	Antiemetic effects due to their anti-inflammatory effects (suppression of prostaglandin production)	Dexamethasone
Substance P antagonists	Blocks NK_1 receptors in CTZ and STN	Aprepitant

Abbreviations: 5-HT_3, 5-hydroxytryptamine 3 receptor; CNS, central nervous system; CTZ, chemoreceptor trigger zone; D_2, dopamine 2 receptor; GI, gastrointestinal; H_1, histamine 1 receptor; M, muscarinic receptor; MOA, mechanism of action; NK_1, neurokinin 1 receptor; STN, solitary tract nucleus.

7. Correction of fluids and electrolyte balance.
8. Correction of metabolic disturbances such as acidosis and alkalosis.
9. Prevention of serious complications of severe vomiting.

Classification of Antiemetics

There are various antiemetic agents developed based on the understanding of physiological mechanisms in vomiting. The classes and their details are illustrated in **Table 53.1**.

Antidopaminergics

Antipsychotic

Antipsychotic phenothiazines such as chlorpromazine, prochlorperazine, and trifluoperazine are found to be effective in cancer chemotherapy, radiation therapy, opioids, and drug-induced and postoperative nausea and vomiting (PONV). Apart from this, they also help in alleviating vomiting as a result of diseases such as gastroenteritis, migraine, and liver disease. Common adverse effects include sedation, hypotension, dystonia, and tardive dyskinesia.

Chlorpromazine

Chlorpromazine can be administered via oral, IV, and intramuscular (IM) routes.

They antagonize D_2 receptors in the CTZ and also exert blocking effects on histamine and muscarinic receptors. It shows strong antiadrenergic and weaker peripheral anticholinergic activity.

Pharmacokinetics

It is readily absorbed from GIT, but its bioavailability is affected due to first pass metabolism. It has a half-life of approximately 30 hours. It is metabolized in the liver and kidney by CYP2D6, CYP1A2, and CYP3A4, and is excreted in urine.

Dose

The recommended dose is 25 mg; route: IM (if the vomiting does not stop, 25–50 mg dose is administered every 3–4 hours until vomiting stops).

Interactions

Potentially fatal effects can be observed when administered with sedatives, hypnotics, antihistamines, general anesthetics, opioids, and alcohol due to additive depressant effect.

Adverse Effects

Sedation, dry mouth, agitation, coma, dyspnea, irregularities in heartbeat, low blood pressure, etc.

Prokinetics

These drugs increase the propulsive motility of GIT, thereby speeding up gastric emptying. The most commonly used drugs in this category are metoclopramide and domperidone (**Fig. 53.2**).

Metoclopramide

It is closely related to phenothiazine group. It acts as an antagonist of D_2 receptor in CTZ and 5-HT_3 receptors present on STN and CTZ, thereby suppressing vomiting reflex. Metoclopramide-induced increased gastric motility is due to increase in acetylcholine (ACh) released by myenteric motor neurons. This is attributed to 5-HT_4 receptor agonism and D_2 receptor antagonism produced by the drug. 5-HT_4 receptor is present on primary afferent neurons (PANs) of the enteric nervous system (ENS).

Gastrointestinal Tract

Metoclopramide has more pronounced effect on upper GIT as it speeds up gastric emptying by increasing gastric peristalsis and relaxing pylorus and initial part of duodenum. It increases intestinal motility to some extent but has no significant action on motility of colon and gastric secretions.

Central Nervous System

It acts on CTZ and STN by blocking dopamine and serotonergic receptors. Its administration has also shown to augment prolactin secretion and extrapyramidal effects.

Pharmacokinetics

When administered orally, the onset of action is within 30 minutes to 1 hour, and is within 10 and 2 minutes after IM and IV injections, respectively. Half-life ranges between 3 and 6 hours; it undergoes partial conjugation in the liver and is excreted in urine within 24 hours. It can cross BBB and placenta, and is secreted in milk.

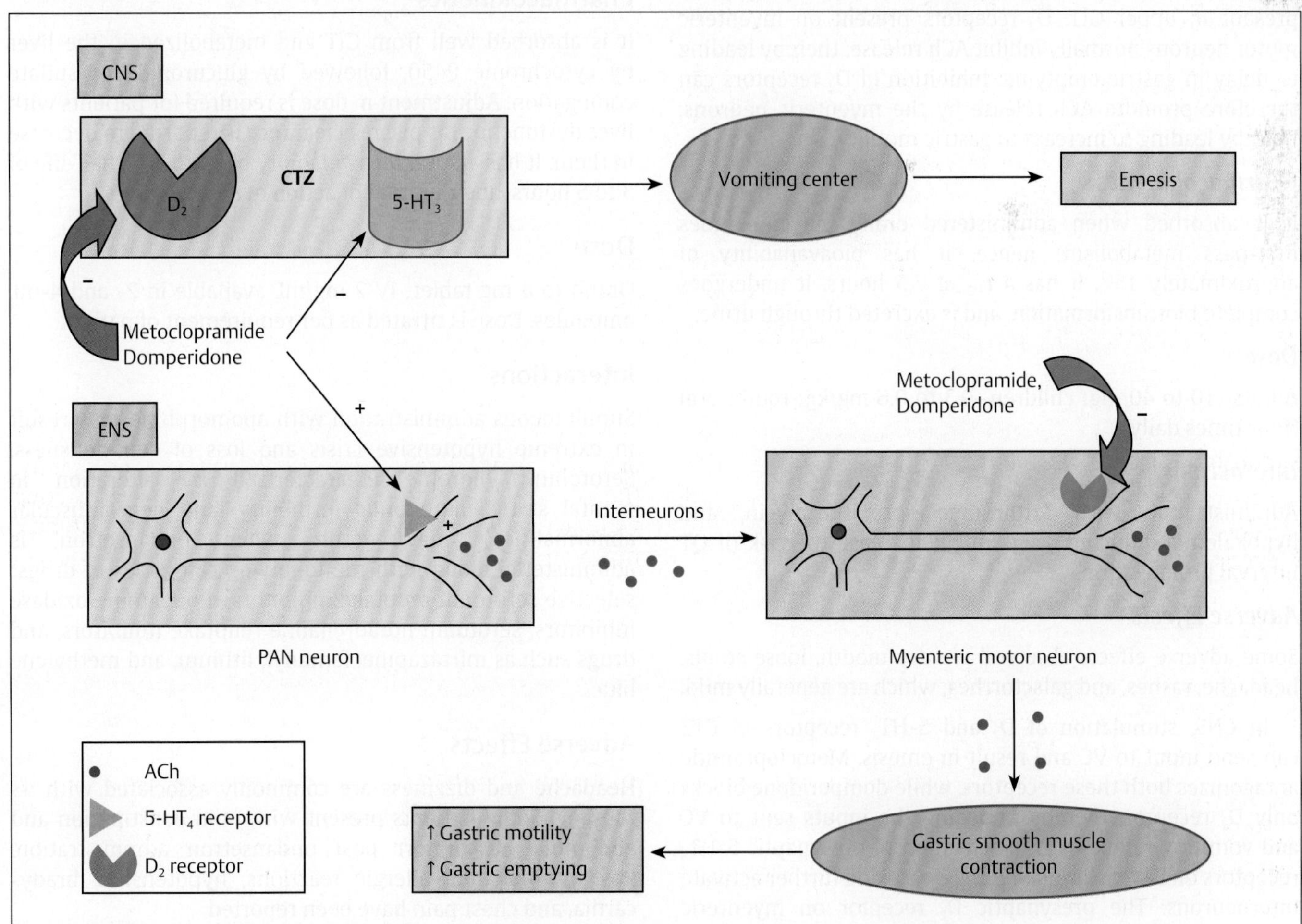

Fig. 53.2 Schematic diagram illustrating mechanism of action of prokinetics. 5-HT_3, 5-hydroxytryptamine 3 receptor; ACh, acetylcholine; CNS, central nervous system; CTZ, chemoreceptor trigger zone; D_2, dopamine 2 receptor; ENS, enteric nervous system; PANs, primary afferent neurons.

Dose

Adults—10 mg; children—0.2 to 0.5 mg/kg; route—oral (four times daily)/IM.

Interactions

As it facilitates gastric emptying, it has been observed to increase the absorption of drugs such as aspirin and diazepam and decrease the absorption of digoxin (by reducing its residence time). It has also been found to decrease the bioavailability of cimetidine.

Adverse Effects

Adverse effects include sedation, disorders of movements, especially in children and women, spasmodic torticollis (involuntary twisting of neck), galactorrhea, and disorders of menstruation (due to prolactin release). No harmful effects are reported on its administration during pregnancy. However, as it is secreted in milk in small amounts, the nursing infant can develop dystonia, myoclonus, and loose stools.

Domperidone

It antagonizes D_2 receptor. It shows poor BBB crossing but can exert effect on CTZ (as it is not protected by BBB). Due to its poor bioavailability in CNS, the extrapyramidal adverse effects as those seen with metoclopramide are reduced. Its prokinetic action is based on blockade of D_2 receptors present in upper GIT. D_2 receptors present on myenteric motor neurons normally inhibit ACh release, thereby leading to delay in gastric emptying. Inhibition of D_2 receptors can therefore promote ACh release by the myenteric neurons, thereby leading to increase in gastric motility.

Pharmacokinetics

It is absorbed when administered orally but undergoes first-pass metabolism; hence, it has bioavailability of approximately 15%. It has a $t_{1/2}$ of 7.5 hours. It undergoes complete biotransformation, and is excreted through urine.

Dose

Adults—10 to 40 mg; children—0.3 to 0.6 mg/kg; route: oral (four times daily).

Interactions

Administration with azithromycin, roxithromycin, and hypokalemia-inducing drugs might increase the risk of QT interval prolongation.

Adverse Effects

Some adverse effects observed are dry mouth, loose stools, headache, rashes, and galactorrhea, which are generally mild.

In CNS, stimulation of D_2 and 5-HT_3 receptors in CTZ can send input to VC and result in emesis. Metoclopramide antagonizes both these receptors, while domperidone blocks only D_2 receptor, thereby impeding the inputs sent to VC and vomiting reflex. In ENS, activation of presynaptic 5-HT_4 receptors on PANs stimulate ACh release and further activate interneurons. The presynaptic D_2 receptor on myenteric motor neuron blocks the ACh release, thereby leading to slowing of gastric motility due to relaxation of gastric smooth muscle. Metoclopramide acts as 5-HT_4 receptor agonist, while both metoclopramide and domperidone antagonize D_2 receptor, thereby promoting ACh release. This stimulates gastric smooth muscle contraction, leading to increased gastric motility and emptying.

Anti-5-HT_3 Drugs

These drugs act as antagonists on 5-HT_3 receptors in CTZ and are found to be more effective against postoperative vomiting, chemotherapy-induced nausea and vomiting (CINV), and hyperemesis in pregnancy. They can be administered orally or intravenously. Drugs falling in this category are ondansetron, granisetron, and palonosetron.

Ondansetron

Ondansetron blocks the depolarizing (activating) effects of serotonin in GIT on 5-HT_3 receptors in vagal afferents as well as in the STN and CTZ, thereby leading to suppression of vomiting reflex. It is commonly used for treating PONV, chemotherapy and radiation therapy, and disease- or other drug-induced vomiting. It is not very effective against vomiting associated with motion sickness.

Pharmacokinetics

It is absorbed well from GIT and metabolized in the liver by cytochrome P450, followed by glucuronide or sulfate conjugation. Adjustment in dose is required for patients with liver dysfunction, as plasma clearance is reported to decrease in them. It has an oral bioavailability of 60 to 70%, half-life of 3 to 5 hours, and duration of action of 8 to 12 hours.

Dose

Oral 4 to 8 mg tablet; IV 2 mg/mL available in 2- and 4-mL ampoules. Dose is titrated as per requirement of patient.

Interactions

Simultaneous administration with apomorphine may result in extreme hypotensive crisis and loss of consciousness. Serotonin syndrome (characterized by alteration in mental status, autonomic instability, and neuromuscular abnormalities) may result when ondansetron is administered along with the following categories of drugs: selective serotonin reuptake inhibitors, monoamine oxidase inhibitors, serotonin noradrenaline reuptake inhibitors, and drugs such as mirtazapine, fentanyl, lithium, and methylene blue.

Adverse Effects

Headache and dizziness are commonly associated with its therapy. Some patients present with mild constipation and abdominal discomfort post ondansetron administration. Post IV injection, allergic reactions, hypotension, bradycardia, and chest pain have been reported.

Antihistaminics

Drugs belonging to this category, including cinnarizine, cyclizine, promethazine, diphenhydramine, dimenhydrinate, etc., act on histamine receptor H_1 as antagonists. Antihistaminics act on the H_1 receptors located in the vestibular afferents, thereby preventing transmission of signal to the VC (**Fig. 53.3**). They are commonly used for nausea and vomiting arising from motion sickness; some are used to treat morning sickness during pregnancy and PONV. This category of drugs is also used by NASA to treat motion sickness arising in space. Drowsiness and sedation are common side effects of these drugs.

Promethazine and Dimenhydrinate

Due to their action on the vestibular afferents, they are widely used to treat motion sickness. Promethazine is also used to treat morning sickness in pregnant women. They are also known to have anticholinergic properties in the CNS; hence, if administered along with metoclopramide, they can suppress its extrapyramidal side effects and accentuate its antiemetic action. Promethazine is also reported to have a weak inhibitory effect on central dopaminergic receptors. These two drugs in combination with diphenhydramine are used to treat CINV.

Adverse Effects

Drowsiness and sedation are chief unwanted effects.

Antimuscarinics

These drugs are muscarinic receptor antagonists and are principally used to treat vomiting associated with motion sickness (**Fig. 53.3**). They have no effect on chemotherapy-induced vomiting.

Scopolamine

It is principally administered for both prophylaxis and treatment of vomiting associated with motion sickness via oral route or as transdermal patch. Its action is based on blocking cholinergic receptors present in the pathway connecting vestibular apparatus and VC.

Pharmacokinetics

It is rapidly absorbed from GIT and has a half-life of 4.5 hours. The drug and its metabolites are excreted in urine.

Dose

The recommended dose is 0.2 to 0.4 mg; route—oral, IM, or transdermal patch (1.5 mg) can deliver drug over 3 days. When applied behind the pinna, it has shown to suppress motion sickness, while showing only mild side effects.

Interactions

Drugs with anticholinergic effects (e.g., antihistamines, amantadine) may augment the effects of scopolamine. It may affect the absorption of other oral medications due to its ability to delay gastric emptying.

Adverse Effects

Dry mouth, blurred vision, and drowsiness are commonly observed. Sedation is lesser than antihistamines, as it shows poor BBB penetration.

In motion sickness, disturbances in body equilibrium send signals to cerebellum through H_1 and M receptors in vestibular afferents. This activates VC and results in emesis. Antihistaminics and antimuscarinics are commonly prescribed for treating nausea and vomiting associated with

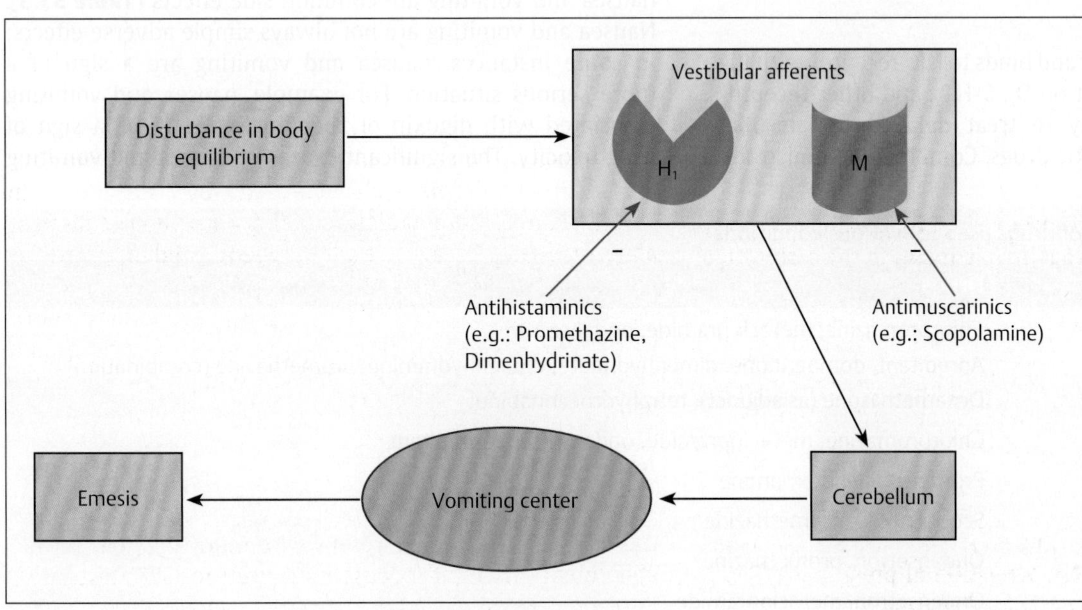

Fig. 53.3 Illustration of mechanism of action of drugs used for motion sickness. H_1, histamine 1 receptor; M, muscarinic receptor.

motion sickness. They act by blocking H_1 and M receptors in vestibular afferents.

Glucocorticoids

Dexamethasone

It is used as an adjunct therapy against CINV. The possible mechanism of action is thought to be due to suppression of peritumoral inflammation and prostaglandin production, which forms its basis for anti-inflammatory action. It is frequently administered in combination with ondansetron, phenothiazine, or aprepitant.

Dose

The recommended dose is 8 to 20 mg; route: IV.

Interactions

It might augment anticoagulant effect of warfarin and renal clearance of salicylates. It can also enhance hypokalemic effects of diuretics (loop, thiazide, acetazolamide).

Adverse Effects

Suppression of immune responses to infection or injury, osteoporosis, muscle wasting, and hyperglycemia are some adverse effects observed.

Substance P Antagonists

Substance P is released by gastrointestinal vagal afferents due to emetogenic drugs given as part of chemotherapy or other stimuli. This results in activation of NK_1 receptors in the CTZ and STN, thereby stimulating the VC. Therefore, antagonists have been developed against NK_1 receptors to be used as antiemetics.

Aprepitant

It is a selective antagonist and binds to NK_1 receptor with high affinity. It has little effect on D_2, 5-HT_3, and other receptors. It is administered orally to treat delayed or late-phase emesis caused by cytotoxic drugs. Combined administration of aprepitant with ondansetron and dexamethasone has shown enhanced antiemetic efficacy in cisplatin-based chemotherapy (highly emetogenic). A prodrug of aprepitant has been developed and is called fosaprepitant. It can be administered via IV route.

Pharmacokinetics

It is absorbed well orally with a $t_{1/2}$ of 9 to 13 hours and can also cross BBB. It is metabolized by liver enzyme CYP3A4, and the metabolites undergo excretion in feces (via bile) and urine.

Interactions

Drugs that induce or inhibit enzyme CYP3A4 can possibly interact with aprepitant. Doses of drugs such as dexamethasone and warfarin need to be decreased when administered along with it. Drugs such as cisapride, which can elongate Q-T interval, should not be administered along with aprepitant.

Dose

For CINV: 125 mg is administered before chemotherapy, followed by 80 mg each on days 2 and 3 orally along with IV administration of ondansetron and dexamethasone. For PONV: single oral dose of 40 mg is administered before surgery.

Adverse Effects

Weakness, fatigue, flatulence, and increase in liver enzymes.

Table 53.2 summarizes the different antiemetic drugs used for various conditions.

Drugs-Induced Vomiting

Among the drug-induced gastrointestinal adverse effects, nausea and vomiting are common side effects (**Table 53.3**). Nausea and vomiting are not always simple adverse effects; in some instances, nausea and vomiting are a sign of a more serious situation. For example, nausea and vomiting associated with digoxin or theophylline may be a sign of drug toxicity. The significant causes of nausea and vomiting

Table 53.2 A summary of drugs used for various conditions

Conditions	Drugs
CINV	Chlorpromazine, metoclopramide, ondansetron Aprepitant, domperidone, dimenhydrinate, diphenhydramine, promethazine (combination) Dexamethasone (as adjunct), tetrahydrocannabinol
PONV	Chlorpromazine, metoclopramide, ondansetron, aprepitant
Morning sickness	Promethazine, doxylamine
Motion sickness	Scopolamine, promethazine
Gastrohepatic disorders	Ondansetron, promethazine
Uremia	Ondansetron, metoclopramide
Radiation sickness	Ondansetron, chlorpromazine, prochlorperazine, trifluoperazine
Gastroparesis	Metoclopramide, cisapride, domperidone

Abbreviations: CINV, chemotherapy-induced nausea and vomiting; PONV, postoperative nausea and vomiting.

Table 53.3 Drugs inducing vomiting as adverse effects at therapeutic doses

Class	Drugs
Cardiovascular drugs	Digoxin, calcium channel blockers, β blockers, antiarrhythmics (drug toxicity)
Dopaminergics	L-Dopa, bromocriptine (dopamine-mediated)
Analgesics	NSAIDs (gastric irritation)
Neurological	Anticonvulsants
Antibiotics	Tetracycline, sulfonamides, acyclovir, erythromycin
Chemotherapeutic agents	Severe: cisplatin, dacarbazine, nitrogen mustard Moderate: etoposide, methotrexate, cytarabine Mild: fluorouracil, vinblastine, tamoxifen
Miscellaneous drugs	Oral contraceptives, estrogen

Abbreviation: NSAID, nonsteroidal anti-inflammatory drug.

include iatrogenic causes, toxicity, infectious causes, GI disorders, and CNS or psychiatric conditions. Among iatrogenic causes, chemotherapeutic agents are the most well known. Infectious and toxic causes are usually self-limiting and include viral gastroenteritis as well as bacteria and their toxins. There are several mechanisms by which drugs may cause nausea. Some agents cause GI mucosal irritation or ulceration (e.g., nonsteroidal anti-inflammatory [NSAIDs], doxycycline). Other agents activate the CTZ (levodopa) of the area postrema via dopaminergic receptors, the specific neural pathways by which nausea is triggered. CNS or psychiatric causes include increases in intracranial pressure, migraine, and emotional or physical stressors.

Multiple Choice Questions

1. A 38-year-old industrial worker injured his right leg while on the job. His medical history includes poorly controlled type 2 diabetes mellitus. He now presents with cellulitis in his right leg for which he is given empiric IV vancomycin. He also complains of nausea for which he is given an antiemetic. Which of the following antiemetics is also an antihistamine?

A. Droperidol.
B. Famotidine.
C. Loratadine.
D. Ondansetron.
E. Promethazine.

Answer: E

There are many drugs that act on different receptor types and can decrease nausea. Promethazine is a phenothiazinelike chlorpromazine but has a much lower affinity for dopamine receptors and as such is not used as a neuroleptic. Its primary action is to antagonize H1 receptors, although its antiemetic properties appear to be related to its central anticholinergic effects.

2. A 65-year-old man with early-onset Alzheimer's disease is under primary care. Consideration is made to begin the therapy with an anticholinesterase inhibitor. The patient and his family are made aware of such side effects as nausea, vomiting, diarrhea, and muscle cramps. The mechanism of action of these effects likely involves which of the following?

A. Adrenergic transmission.
B. Cholinergic transmission.
C. Purine metabolism impairment.
D. Transaminase enzyme elevation.
E. Uremia.

Answer: B

Common adverse effects of anticholinesterase inhibitors to treat Alzheimer's disease include nausea, diarrhea, vomiting, anorexia, tremors, bradycardia, and muscle cramps, all of which are predicted by the actions of the drugs to enhance cholinergic neurotransmission.

3. A 22-year-old woman with diabetes complains of daily nausea and occasional vomiting. She has observed that eating small amounts of food at a time helps decrease the frequency of vomiting. She is diagnosed with diabetic gastroparesis and started on metoclopramide. What is a side effect of metoclopramide?

A. Dry mouth.
B. Gynecomastia.
C. Headache.
D. Increased risk of abortion.
E. Tardive dyskinesia.

Answer: E

Metoclopramide is a D_2-receptor antagonist. Because of the inhibition of dopamine, Parkinsonlike symptoms can occur, such as tardive dyskinesia. Tardive dyskinesia is most common in young adults who are on metoclopramide for more than 3 months.

4. A 61-year-old woman is experiencing dizziness when looking up or rapidly changing the position of her head, often accompanied by nausea and vomiting. These episodes severely limit her ability to work and function normally. Suggest the medication to best help control her symptoms.

A. Amlodipine.
B. Meclizine.

C. Midodrine.

D. Mirtazapine.

E. Ondansetron.

Answer: B

This patient's symptoms are consistent with positional vertigo. Vertigo is characterized by a sensation of dizziness and, as in this case, may be accompanied by nausea and vomiting. Meclizine is an anti-H_1 antihistamine and anticholinergic drug used to treat vertigo. Although the mechanism is not completely understood, meclizine is reported to decrease signals from the labyrinth and vestibule of the ear.

5. A 29-year-old woman presents to the emergency room with a broken ankle after a fall. She is administered with hydrocodone for the pain and, soon after, her stomach becomes upset and she vomited once. The patient is given ondansetron to treat her nausea. What is the mechanism of action of ondansetron?

A. 5-HT_3 antagonist.

B. D_2-receptor antagonist.

C. H_2-receptor inhibitor.

D. Serotonin-norepinephrine reuptake inhibitor.

E. Substance P antagonist.

Answer: A

The mechanism of action of ondansetron is the antagonism of the 5-HT_3 receptor. This blocks serotonin activation of the vomiting center in the medulla, thus producing its antiemetic effect.

6. A 51-year-old woman with acute myelogenous leukemia is on weekly intravenous infusion of chemotherapeutic agents. Upon completion of each cycle, she develops severe nausea and vomiting. A pharmacologic agent is administered intravenously, which seems to decrease nausea in this patient. This agent might have a mechanism of action at which of the following receptors?

A. Histaminic receptor.

B. Cholinergic receptor.

C. 5-HT_3 receptor.

D. Dopamine receptor.

Answer: C

Antagonists at the 5-HT_3 receptor agents such as ondansetron are highly effective in the treatment of chemotherapy-associated nausea and vomiting. These agents inhibit receptors for 5-HT_3 in the area postrema, which will prevent nausea and vomiting and might have an added effect by reducing peripheral sensation of pain.

7. A 28-year-old woman is planning to take a 7-day cruise. She has never been on a ship before and fears developing motion sickness. She has been prescribed scopolamine transdermal patch. When is the best time for her to place the patch to maximize drug efficacy?

A. After nausea first begins.

B. After nausea occurs for 2 hours.

C. After vomiting occurs.

D. Prior to the onset of symptoms.

Answer: D

Although similar to atropine, therapeutic use of scopolamine is limited to prevention of motion sickness (for which it is particularly effective) and to blocking short-term memory. As with all such drugs used for motion sickness, it is much more effective prophylactically than for treating motion sickness once it occurs. The amnesic action of scopolamine makes it an important adjunct drug in anesthetic procedures.

8. A 15-year-old girl complains of nausea and vomiting whenever she is on a long road trip. She is expected to be on another such trip, so she wants medication to decrease her nausea. The physician prescribes an antinausea drug with anticholinergic activity. Which of the following drugs is this?

A. Dimenhydrinate.

B. Droperidol.

C. Marijuana.

D. Ondansetron.

Answer: A

This girl's complaint is most consistent with motion sickness. This is a sensation that occurs when visual stimuli do not comply with information from the vestibular system of the inner ear. Dimenhydrinate can be used to interrupt signals from the vestibule, in order to prevent the disagreement between visual and vestibular inputs. Although the mechanism is not completely clear, it has been proposed that the anticholinergic activity possessed by dimenhydrinate blocks signals from the vestibule.

9. A 72-year-old man with debilitating Parkinson's disease is currently taking levodopa with carbidopa. One week after initiation of treatment, the patient complains of anorexia, nausea, and vomiting. What is the most likely explanation for these findings?

A. Drug toxicity.

B. Idiosyncratic drug reaction.

C. Stimulation of the chemoreceptor trigger zone.

D. Underlying infection.

Answer: C

One of the adverse effects of carbidopa is nausea and vomiting, which is due to stimulation of the chemoreceptor trigger zone of the medulla. This is not a drug toxicity nor is it an unexpected idiosyncratic drug reaction.

10. A 16-year-old girl with primary dysmenorrhea, abnormal menses, and pelvic pain consults her physician. The physician begins therapy with oral estradiol. Which of the following is the most common adverse effect for this patient to be aware of?

A. Vomiting.

B. Breast discharge.

C. Diarrhea.

D. Nausea.

Answer: D

Nausea and breast tenderness are among the most common adverse effects of estrogen therapy. Postmenopausal uterine bleeding can occur. In addition, the risk of thromboembolic events, myocardial infarction, and breast and endometrial cancer is increased with use of estrogen therapy.

Chapter 54

Drug Treatment of Diarrhea

Vetriselvan Subramaniyan, Neeraj Kumar Fuloria, Shivkanya Fuloria, and Iswar Hazarika

PH1.34: Describe the mechanism/s of action, types, doses, side effects, indications, and contraindications of the drugs used in the following:

1. **Acid peptic disease and gastroesophageal reflux disease**
2. **Antiemetics and prokinetics**
3. **Antidiarrheals**
4. **Laxatives**
5. **Inflammatory bowel disease**
6. **Irritable bowel disorders and biliary and pancreatic diseases**

Learning Objectives

- Drug treatment of diarrhea.

Introduction

Diarrhea is passing loose, watery stools three or more times a day. Stools in diarrhea contain more water than normal. Therefore, they are often termed as loose or watery stools. Patients with diarrhea eat less and they have less ability to absorb nutrition. Diarrhea can be caused by viruses, bacteria, protozoa, or helminths. Diarrhea that is transmitted from the stool of one individual to another is termed fecal–oral transmission. Diarrhea can be of the following two types:

1. Acute diarrhea—lasts for 1 or 2 days.
2. Chronic diarrhea—lasts for at least 4 weeks:
   a. Secretory diarrhea.
   b. Osmotic diarrhea.
   c. Inflammatory diarrhea.
   d. Hypermotoric diarrhea.

Etiology

Common causes of acute and chronic diarrhea are food poisoning, bacterial infection (*Escherichia coli*, *Shigella*, *Salmonella*, *Campylobacter*, *Yersinia*), viral infection (*Rotavirus*), and protozoal infections (*Entamoeba*, *Giardia lamblia*).

Signs and symptoms of diarrhea include mild stomach pain, crampy pain in the abdomen, vomiting, high temperature, and headache.

Dehydration

Dehydration is caused due to the disturbance in the water balance, wherein more fluid is lost from the body than is absorbed, resulting in reduction of blood volume.

During diarrhea, more water and salt pass into the bowel from the body, causing loss of a large amount of salt and water from the body. This results in dehydration.

Dehydration is caused mainly because of two reasons—inadequate water intake and excessive fluid loss.

Prevention of Dehydration

Drinking an ample amount of fluid at the early onset of diarrhea can prevent dehydration. Taking homemade fluids such as gruel, soup, or rice water, increasing the frequency of breastfeeding, and giving milk feeds prepared with twice the usual amount of water are recommended to increase the water intake. Different homemade fluids or solutions can be used depending on the following:

1. Local traditions for diarrhea treatment.
2. Ease of use of a suitable food-based solution.
3. Accessibility of people to health services.
4. Availability of sugar and salt.
5. Availability of oral rehydration salts (ORS).

Treatment for Dehydration

Fluid replacement using ORS solution is the best treatment option for diarrhea.

Pathophysiology of Diarrhea

In the mature cells lining the villous tips of ileum and colon, Na^+/K^+ATPase-mediated salt absorption takes place. With the help of Na^+/glucose cotransporter in the ileum, Na^+ gets absorbed. Each Na^+ is transported along with a glucose molecule, which helps in the absorption of water. Inhibition of Na^+/K^+ATPase and structural damage to the mucosal cells result in the inhibition of water absorption, thereby causing diarrhea. At the molecular level, any stimuli that enhance cyclic adenosine monophosphate (cAMP) or cyclic guanosine monophosphate (cGMP) inhibit absorption of NaCl in villus cells and promote secretion in crypt cells, which results in net loss of salt and water (**Fig. 54.1**). Many bacterial toxins such as cholera toxin, *Staphylococcus aureus*, and *Salmonella* activate adenylyl cyclase, which produces more cAMP, thereby promoting the secretion. The concurrent inhibition of absorption results in the loss of water and salt.

Drug Treatment of Diarrhea (IM6.13, IM16.16, PE24.5, PE24.8)

Principles of diarrhea treatment include: (1) fluid and electrolyte replacement, (2) specific therapy to treat the cause, and (3) antimotility and antisecretory agents.

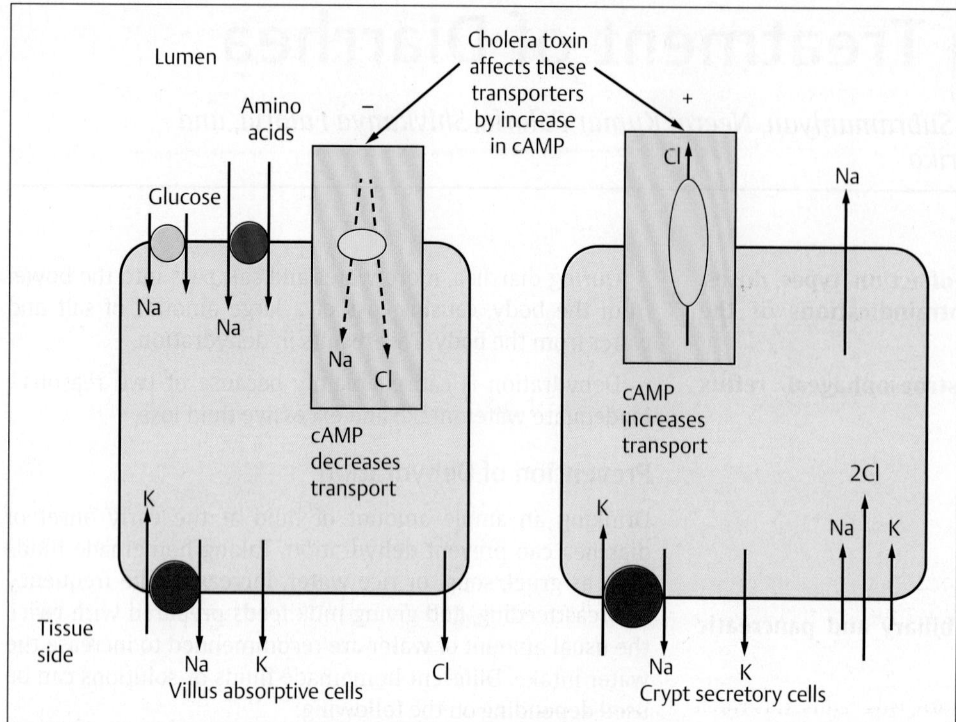

Fig. 54.1 Pathophysiology of diarrhea.

Fluid and Electrolyte Replacement

It is life-saving in infants, since death is usually due to dehydration.

Oral Rehydration Salts (ORS) Solution

It is an inexpensive, simple, safe, and life-saving formulation. The World Health Organization (WHO) formula for the same is as follows: NaCl, 2.6 g; KCl, 1.5 g; Na citrate, 2.9 g; glucose, 13.5 g; and water, 1 L. Glucose and citrate increase Na absorption in ileum, and citrate is more stable than bicarbonate. Homemade ORS is prepared by using 5 g table salt (one pinch) along with 20 g sugar. Dissolve both in 1 L of boiled and cooled water. Super ORS is an improved ORS formulation with additional amino acids for better Na absorption. However, they are expensive. Rice-based ORS (40–50 g/L) provides glucose and amino acids and is cheap; hence, it is preferred in developing countries. Wheat, maize, or potato can be used as an alternative to rice. For severe dehydration, intravenous fluids are used. ORS is also used in heat stroke, burns, and after trauma/surgery.

Dose

1. Children under 24 months: 50 to 100 mL after each loose stool (approximately 500 mL daily).
2. Children from 2 to 10 years: 100 to 200 mL after each loose stool (approximately 1000 m: daily).
3. Children over 10 years and adults: 200 to 400 mL after each loose stool (approximately 2000 mL daily).

Specific Therapy

The cause of diarrhea includes viral, bacterial, or protozoal infection. Viral cause is usually self-limiting, and hence no antibiotics are required.

Mild bacterial diarrhea, too, is self-limiting. For diarrhea due to typhoid, cholera, or amoebic dysentery, treat the specific cause with the following:

1. *Campylobacter jejuni*–ciprofloxacin 500 mg twice daily for 5 days.
2. *E. coli*–ciprofloxacin 500 mg twice daily for 5 days.
3. *Entamoeba histolytica*–metronidazole 400 mg twice daily for 5 days, followed by diloxanide furoate 500 mg thrice daily for 7 days. *G. lamblia*–metronidazole 200 mg thrice daily for 5 days.
4. *Salmonella*–ciprofloxacin 500 mg twice daily for 10 days.
5. *Shigella*–ciprofloxacin 500 mg twice daily for 5 days.
6. *Vibrio cholera*–doxycycline 100 mg twice daily for 5 days.

Antimotility, Antisecretory Agents, and Adsorbents

They offer only symptomatic relief in noninfective diarrhea.

Adsorbents

These include pectin, kaolin, chalk, and activated charcoal. Pectin is sourced from apples, whereas kaolin is hydrated magnesium and aluminum silicate. They adsorb intestinal microorganisms and toxins, and coat them. They are not absorbed and hence do not have systemic side effects. These agents decrease the absorption of concurrent medications; hence, a 2-hour interval should be present between their administration.

Antimotility Agents

Antimotility agents should be avoided in infective diarrheas, since they increase systemic invasion and may lead to intestinal perforation. These agents slow down clearance of pathogens and can cause toxic megacolon. Antimotility agents include the following.

Codeine

It is a natural opium alkaloid that stimulates opioid receptors in gastrointestinal (GI) smooth muscles. Hence, it reduces GI peristalsis and decreases secretions. It is used for symptomatic treatment of diarrhea.

Diphenoxylate

It is structurally similar to pethidine; however, it is a very potent antidiarrheal having an abuse liability in high doses. Hence, it is combined with atropine to discourage abuse, since atropine will cause side effects. Adverse drug reactions (ADRs) include paralytic ileus, respiratory depression, and toxic megacolon in children. Hence, it is contraindicated in children. Therefore, it is banned in many countries.

Loperamide

This is an analog of opiate, which acts on μ-receptors in GI tract. It has selective GI action; hence, it has less action on the central nervous system (since there is no crossing of the blood–brain barrier). It is a powerful antidiarrheal, which reduces GI motility and increases anal sphincter tone. It decreases secretion induced by *E. coli* and cholera toxin. However, it is less sedating and less addicting; thus, it is most commonly used in acute, chronic, and travelers' diarrhea. The onset of action is 1 to 2 hours, and its duration of action is 12 to 18 hours. It is contraindicated in children younger than 4 years, as it can lead to paralytic ileus, toxic megacolon, and abdominal distension.

Antisecretory Agents

Racecadotril

Racecadotril is a prodrug that is converted to its active metabolite thiorphan, which inhibits enkephalinase in gut and peripheral tissues. Thus, it reduces degradation of enkephalins (μ/δ agonist) and decreases intestinal secretions. Enkephalins are GI neurotransmitters, which have antisecretory properties; hence, it corrects hyper-secretion of water and electrolytes. However, there is no change in intestinal motility. It has a quick onset and is used in symptomatic treatment of secretory diarrhea. It is used only for short duration, not more than 7 days. It can be used in children. ADRs include flatulence, nausea, and drowsiness.

Octreotide

It is a synthetic analogue of somatostatin. Somatostatin decreases GI motility and secretions of gastrin, secretin, cholecystokinin, growth hormone, insulin, glucagon, 5-hydroxytryptamine, pancreatic polypeptide, and vaso-active intestinal peptide.

Octreotide is a long-acting formulation; hence, it is given subcutaneously. It is used in the following cases: GI tumor-causing diarrhea, diarrhea due to vagotomy, dumping syndrome, and AIDS.

Antispasmodics

These include atropine derivatives such as propantheline and dicyclomine.

Drotaverine

It is related to papaverine, which is a direct smooth muscle relaxant. It is also an analgesic, which inhibits phosphodiesterase enzymes (PDE); hence, it increases cAMP/cGMP, causing relaxation. It uses include renal, intestinal, biliary colic, and irritable bowel syndrome. ADRs comprise dizziness, flushing, and constipation.

Clonidine

It is an antisecretory and antimotility agent used as in diarrhea due to opioid withdrawal and diarrhea due to diabetic autonomic neuropathy. ADRs include hypotension and mental depression.

Probiotics

These include *Lactobacillus acidophilus* and *Lactobacillus sporogenes*, which colonize the intestine and increase growth of commensal saprophytic flora. It alters gut pH, thus inhibiting the growth of pathogenic organisms in the gut. It is also used in antibiotic-associated diarrhea. It is available as tablets and powders. Home-based probiotics include curds/butter milk. They are inexpensive alternatives to synthetic probiotics.

Multiple Choice Questions

1. Mrs. Rajina Thomas, a 29-year-old woman, was admitted with acute diarrhea, abdominal pain, fever, mucus, and blood in stools. After laboratory investigation, she was diagnosed with *Shigella enteritis*. Which of the following drugs will be suitable for Mrs. Rajina?

A. Atovaquone.
B. Gentamicin.
C. Ciprofloxacin.
D. Streptomycin.

Answer: C

Ciprofloxacin and azithromycin are two recommended oral antibiotics. A study reported that ciprofloxacin, ceftriaxone, or pivmecillinam effectively cleared *Shigella* pathogens in 96% of cases (95% confidence interval, 88–99).

2. Mr. John, a 33-year-old patient, presented with acute diarrhea and abdominal pain. He was prescribed an opioid drug. Which of the following drugs is likely to be prescribed?

A. Kaolin pectin.
B. Loperamide.
C. Attapulgite.
D. Atropine.

Answer: B

Loperamide is a drug of choice to treat diarrhea (runny poo). Loperamide can help in the treatment of irritable bowel syndrome or short-term diarrhea. It is also used for longer lasting diarrhea from bowel problems such as ulcerative colitis, short bowel syndrome, and Crohn's disease.

3. A 22-year-old man has been treated with bismuth subsalicylate. Which of the following conditions has he been treated for?

A. Chronic diarrhea.

B. Constipation.

C. Travelers' diarrhea.

D. Anticipatory nausea.

Answer: C.

Two tablets of bismuth subsalicylate four times daily (2.1 g/day) is a safe and effective way to reduce the occurrence of travelers' diarrhea among persons who are at risk for up to 3 weeks.

Chapter 55

Drug Treatment for Constipation and IBD

Prasan R. Bhandari

PH1.34: Describe the mechanism/s of action, types, doses, side effects, indications, and contraindications of the drugs used in the following:

1. **Acid peptic disease and gastroesophageal reflux disease**
2. **Antiemetics and prokinetics**
3. **Antidiarrheals**
4. **Laxatives**
5. **Inflammatory bowel disease**
6. **Irritable bowel disorders and biliary and pancreatic diseases**

Learning Objective

- Laxatives.
- Treatment of irritable bowel syndrome.
- Inflammatory bowel diseases.

Laxatives

Laxatives facilitate evacuation of formed stools, and they have a mild action. Purgatives/cathartics cause evacuation of watery stools, and they have a powerful action. However, these terms are used interchangeably. Carminatives, on the other hand, promote expulsion of gases from the gut.

Classification (Based on the Mechanism of Action)

Bulk-forming dietary fibers include bran, methylcellulose, husk, *isphagula* (*isabgol*), agar, platango seeds.

1. Osmotic purgatives:
   a. Magnesium sulfate, magnesium hydroxide, magnesium citrate, sodium phosphate, sodium sulfate, sodium phosphate, sodium sulfate, sodium potassium tartrate, lactulose, sorbitol, polyethylene glycol (PEG).
2. Stimulant or irritant purgatives:
   a. Phenolphthalein, bisacodyl, castor oil, sodium picosulfate.
   b. Anthraquinone derivatives—senna, cascara sagrada.

Stool softeners—docusate sodium (DOSS), liquid paraffin (emollients/stool-wetting agents)

3. Miscellaneous:
   a. 5HT4 agonists—prucalopride, cisapride.
   b. Opioid antagonists—methylnaltrexone, alvimopan.
   c. Chloride channel activator—lubiprostone.

The mechanisms of action of laxatives are given in **Fig. 55.1**.

Bulk Laxatives

These are dietary fibers which consist of cell walls and other parts of fruits and vegetables. These are indigestible, hydrophilic vegetable substances which absorb water, swell up, and increase the bulk of stools. They increase the volume, and decrease the viscosity of intestinal contents. They form large, soft, and solid stools. This causes mechanical distention, thus stimulating peristalsis and promoting defecation. Their onset of action is around 1 to 3 days. These agents are helpful in irritable bowel syndrome symptoms like both constipation and diarrhea. Sufficient water intake along with these agents is important to prevent intestinal obstruction. It is recommended to avoid these in patients with gastrointestinal (GI) obstruction. Additionally, these agents interfere with absorption of many drugs.

1. Bran—residue of flour of cereals contains 40% fiber.
2. *Isphaghula*, platango seeds (psyllium):
   a. Contains natural mucilage.
   b. Forms gelatinous mass with water.
   c. More palatable than bran.
3. Methylcellulose:
   a. Semisynthetic derivative of cellulose.
4. Agar:
   a. Mucilaginous substance from marine algae.
   b. Contains hemicellulose.

Stool Softeners

Docusate sodium (dioctyl sodium sulphosuccinate or DOSS)

It is an anion detergent which reduces the surface tension of intestinal contents. Hence, there is accumulation of fluid and fat in feces, which softens stools. Its onset too is 1 to 3 days. It increases the absorption of many drugs. It increases the absorption of liquid paraffin; hence, they are not given together. It is given orally or as retention enema. Since it is bitter, it can cause nausea and abdominal pain.

Liquid Paraffin

It is a mineral oil and is therefore unpalatable. Chemically, it is inert and not digested. Since it has a lubricant action, it helps in smooth evacuation of feces. It is useful in cardiac patients, because it avoids straining while passing stools. Adverse drug reactions like lipoid pneumonia occur due to its aspiration into lungs; hence, avoid giving it at bedtime and in lying down position.

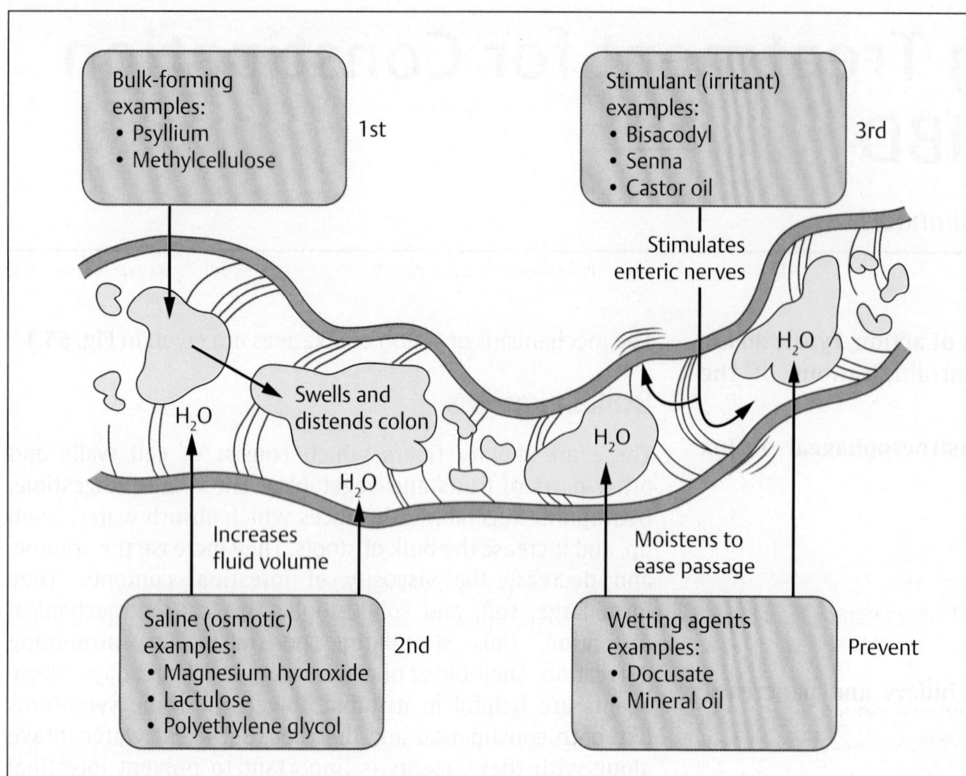

Fig. 55.1 Mechanisms of action of laxatives.

Malabsorption of fat-soluble vitamins A, D, E, and K and leakage of fecal matter from anus causes soiling of undergarments. Intestinal paraffinomas can occur since they can get absorbed into intestines.

Stimulant Purgatives

These agents have direct action on GI mucosa and neurons. They increase PGs and cAMP in the enteric cells. Additionally, they inhibit Na^+ K^+ ATPase activity in intestinal mucosa, thereby increasing secretion of water and electrolytes and stimulating peristalsis. They act primarily on colon and produce semifluid stools. Long-term use can lead to atonic colon. High dose can cause fluid/electrolyte imbalances. It is contraindicated during pregnancy as it can cause reflex stimulation of the uterus.

Anthraquinones

Bacteria liberate active anthraquinones in the intestines which stimulate myenteric plexus in colon. The onset of action is approximately 6 to 7 hours; hence, it is given at bedtime, so the effect is seen in the morning. Since it is secreted in milk, it is contraindicated during lactation. Its long-term use can lead to discoloration of urine and melanotic (black) pigmentation of colon. Cascara sagrada and senna are its examples sourced from plants.

Phenolphthalein

It is an indicator and was discovered accidentally. The site of its action is the large intestine, with an onset of 6 to 8 hours. It produces soft, semiliquid stools and also produces griping (cramps). It undergoes enterohepatic circulation, which prolongs its duration of action. Adverse drug reactions include pink color skin lesions, cardiac toxicity, and colic.

Bisacodyl

It is similar to phenolphthalein which is activated in bowel by esterases. This agent stimulates colon with an onset of 6 to 8 hours; hence, it is administered at bedtime as an oral tablet (enteric coated) or rectal suppository. The rectal suppository acts within 15 to 30 minutes. It is one of the popular agents for the management of constipation. The adverse drug reactions are local inflammation and irritation (proctitis). Anal soreness occurs due to leakage of contents, hence not used for 10 days at a time. It is used to empty bowel before endoscopy, surgery, or radiological investigations.

Sodium Picosulfate

It is similar to bisacodyl and is activated by colonic bacteria. It is used orally at bedtime since onset is after 6 to 8 hours.

Castor Oil

This agent is metabolized in upper intestine to ricinoleic acid. This metabolite is a local irritant; hence, it stimulates intestinal motility. It is one of the most powerful and oldest agents used in the management of constipation. However, it causes cramps, so is not used frequently.

Osmotic Purgatives

These are powerful and fast-acting agents. They are solutes that are not absorbed and are retained in the intestinal lumen. Since they osmotically retain water, the intestinal contents increase. Magnesium salts release cholecystokinin also, hence they distend the bowel, which stimulates peristalsis, and assists evacuation of the stools. Evacuation of fluid stools is seen within 1 to 3 hours. These agents include:

1. Nonabsorbable salts:
   a. Saline purgatives like Mg hydroxide (milk of magnesia).
   b. Mg sulfate (Epsom salt), Na phosphate, Na sulfate, Na K tartrate (Rochelle's salt).
2. Nonabsorbable sugars–lactulose, sorbitol, glycerin.
3. PEG.

Avoid using these in children and those afflicted with renal failure, since they can cause central nervous system (CNS)/ cardiovascular (CVS) depression. Na salts are to be avoided in cardiac patients, due to the risk of water retention and aggravation of the situation.

Lactulose (IM5.16)

It is a synthetic disaccharide of fructose and galactose which is not absorbed. Colonic bacteria convert it to lactic, acetic acids, and short chain fatty acids which exert osmotic effect. It also inhibits growth of colonic ammonia-producing bacteria, thereby reducing absorption of ammonia by decreasing pH and thus lowering blood ammonia levels. Hence, it is used in hepatic coma, since ammonia worsens coma. Sorbitol is similar to lactulose, whereas lactitol is similar to lactulose, but more palatable. Glycerin is used as rectal suppository or enema.

Polyethylene Glycol (PEG)

It is a nonabsorbable sugar. A balanced isotonic solution is given with PEG. This avoids electrolyte disturbances. It is used in cleaning bowel before endoscopy. A total of 3 to 4 liters is given over 2 hours. PEG powder and water are used for chronic constipation. There is no flatulence or abdominal cramps on administering PEG.

Miscellaneous

5HT4 Receptor Agonist

They have a prokinetic action. It is used in severe chronic constipation, when not responding to other laxatives, for example, prucalopride and cisapride.

Chloride Channel Activator

It is a derivative of prostanoic acid which opens chloride channels in small intestine, thereby causing secretion of chloride-rich fluid. This stimulates intestinal motility, in 24 hours. It is used in chronic constipation and irritable bowel syndrome, for example, lubiprostone.

Opioid Antagonists

There is no crossing of blood-brain barrier (BBB); hence, it does not antagonize analgesic effect of opioids. It is used in opioid-induced constipation (in coma and terminally ill patients). Methylnaltrexone is given subcutaneously once in 2 days. Alvimopan is given orally in patients of postoperative ileus. It should be used short-term (1 week), as it can cause CVS toxicity, for example, methylnaltrexone and alvimopan block opioid receptors in gastrointestinal tract (GIT).

Use of Laxatives/Purgatives

- Acute functional constipation–bulk laxatives.
- Avoid straining at stools (CVS patients, eye surgery, hernia)–bulk laxatives/docusates.
- Hepatic coma (to reduce blood ammonia)–lactulose.
- Preoperative (GI surgery, radiology investigation)–osmotic purgatives/bisacodyl.
- Following anthelmintics to expel worms–osmotic purgatives.
- Drug poisoning elimination from gut–osmotic purgatives.
- Constipation in children/pregnancy–lactulose.

Contraindications

It is contraindicated in intestinal obstruction and undiagnosed acute abdomen.

Drugs Causing Constipation

- Opioids.
- Anticholinergics.
- Iron.
- Calcium channel blockers.
- Tricyclic antidepressants–due to anticholinergic action.
- Antihistamines–due to anticholinergic action.

Laxative Abuse

It occurs due to stimulant laxatives. It causes loss of electrolytes, loss of calcium, malabsorption, and irritable bowel syndrome. Clear patient's misconception of bowel habits to prevent it. The normal variations in bowel motions are generally between 3 per day and 2 per week.

Nonpharmacological Measures

These include fiber-rich diet, adequate fluid intake, and regular physical activity. Laxatives/purgatives must be used only if above measures fail.

Treatment of Irritable Bowel Syndrome (PH1.34)

This disorder has no specific cause and is manifested as abnormal bowel functions like diarrhea/constipation and abdominal pain. The cause could include stress, food allergy, emotional disturbances, and lack of dietary fiber. The management for constipation symptoms includes *ispaghula* (dietary fiber), whereas for diarrhea it is administration of loperamide. For anxiety component, benzodiazepines or newer antidepressants are recommended.

Alosetron

It is a selective 5HT3 receptor antagonist which inhibits reflex activation of GI smooth muscle. Hence, it decreases colonic motility. It is used in women with IBS prominent diarrhea unresponsive to other drugs. Adverse drug reactions comprise constipation and colitis.

Tegaserod

It is a partial 5HT4 agonist which increases gastric emptying and increases chloride secretion in colon. It is recommended for IBS prominent constipation. Its adverse drug reactions are diarrhea and a 10-fold increase risk of heart attacks and stroke. This is due to the inhibition of 5HT1B. Hence, it has been withdrawn in many countries.

Mebeverine

It is a reserpine derivative which possess antispasmodic activity. It is also a direct GI relaxant and indirectly reduces colonic hypermotility. It decreases Na^+ ion permeability of smooth muscle and also decreases K^+ ion efflux of smooth muscle. It is used in IBS and dysentery. The adverse drug reactions include dizziness, constipation, and gastritis. No anticholinergic side effects are seen.

Other Antispasmodics

Dicyclomine and drotaverine are also used.

Inflammatory Bowel Diseases (IBD) (PH1.34, IM16.16)

It comprises ulcerative colitis and Crohn's disease which is manifested as diarrhea, bleeding, abdominal discomfort, anemia, and weight loss. The drugs used to manage IBD are as follows:

- Aminosalicylates–sulphasalazine, mesalamine.
- Glucocorticoids–prednisolone, budesonide.
- Immunosuppressants–azathloprine, methotrexate, 6-mercaptopurine (6-MP).
- Biological response modifiers–antitumor necrosis factor (TNF) therapy, anti-integrin therapy.

Aminosalicylates

It is a prodrug. Colonic bacteria break it down to liberate two components, that is, 5-aminosalicylate (5-ASA) and sulfapyridine (**Fig. 55.2**). 5-ASA acts locally as anti-inflammatory, whereas sulfapyridine is absorbed systemically. Hence, it produces side effects such as diarrhea, allergy, megaloblastic anemia and, rarely, Stevens–Johnson syndrome.

Mesalamine

It is 5-ASA, which is well-tolerated and has minor side effects. It is given as either delayed release capsules, pH-dependent tablets, retention enema, or suppository.

Olsalazine

It is made up of two molecules of 5-ASA with azo link. Colonic bacteria split the two molecules. Since it has poor absorption, it has less side effects.

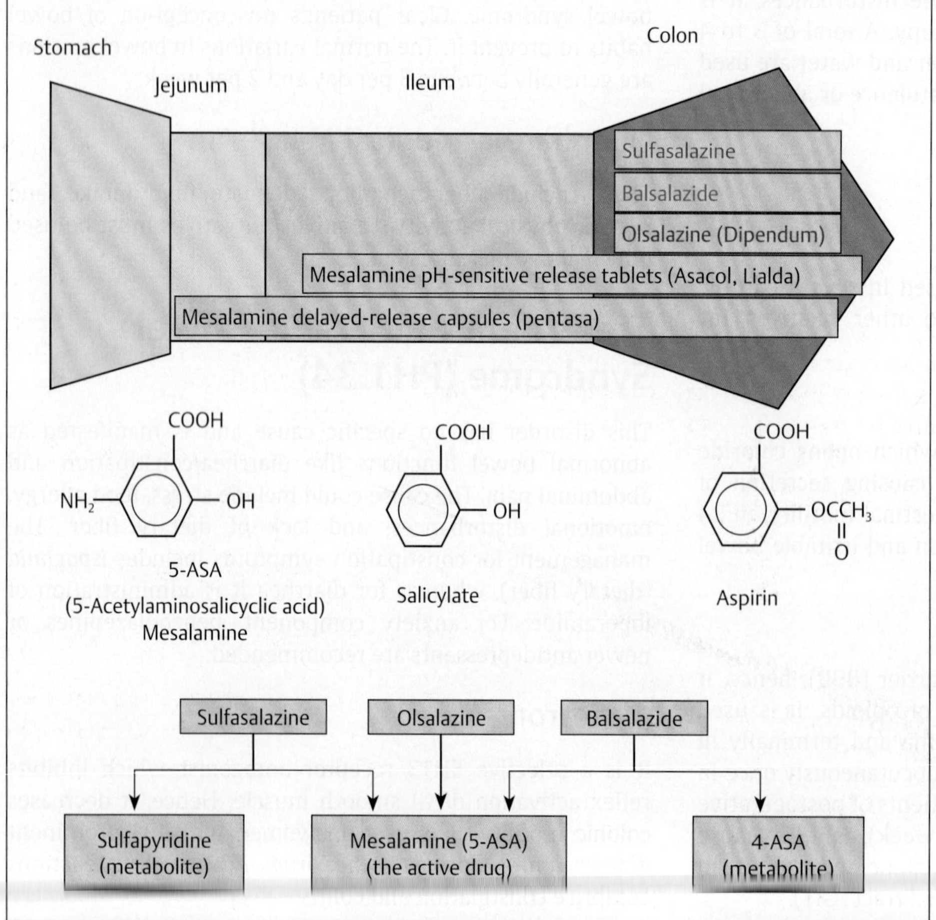

Fig. 55.2 Mechanism of aminosalicylates

Balsalazide

It contains mesalamine and an inert carrier, which is split into 5-ASA and released into the colon. It is used in mild-to-moderate IBD.

Glucocorticoids

Prednisolone (oral), methylprednisolone (oral, parenteral), hydrocortisone (enema, suppository), and budesonide (oral) are used for short-term in moderate-to-severe IBD. IBD of distal bowel (distal ileum and colon) is managed with oral therapy, whereas IBD of sigmoid colon or rectum is controlled by retention enema. Long-term therapy is recommended for steroid-dependent IBD.

Immunosuppressants

It is used for induction and maintenance of remission in active IBD, steroid-dependent IBD, and steroid-unresponsive IBD, for example, azathioprine, methotrexate, and 6-MP.

Biological Response Modifiers

Antitumor Necrosis Factors (Anti-TNF) Therapy

As TNF is proinflammatory in IBD, these agents are monoclonal antibodies to TNF. Its use includes moderate-to-severe IBD unresponsive to other therapies. Adverse drug reactions comprise high cost and increased infection risk, for example, infliximab.

Anti-Integrin Therapy

Integrins are adhesion molecules on leukocyte surface. They bind to other adhesion molecules on vascular endothelium. These agents are monoclonal antibodies to integrins which bind integrins on inflammatory cells; hence, block their migration and inflammatory process. It is used in Crohn's disease unresponsive to other therapies. Adverse drug reactions are increased susceptibility to infections and not being cost-effective, for example, natalizumab.

Multiple Choice Questions

1. A 75-year-old man with several medical complications develops worsening constipation during his hospitalization for lower extremity cellulitis. The physician chooses to give a laxative. Which of the following is a suitable choice and why?

A. Psyllium, since it is a bulk-forming laxative good for chronic constipation.
B. An osmotic agent, like senna, that is given rectally.
C. A stool softener such as methyl cellulose that inhibits water reabsorption.
D. A salt-containing osmotic agent; for example, docusate, which is beneficial in preventing constipation.

Answer: A

Psyllium and methylcellulose are bulk-forming agents good for chronic constipation.

2. A patient, who is administered verapamil for hypertension and angina, develops constipation. Which of the following is an osmotic laxative that may be used to manage the patient's constipation?

A. Aluminum hydroxide.
B. Diphenoxylate.
C. Magnesium hydroxide.
D. Metoclopramide.

Answer: C

A laxative which mildly stimulates the gut would be the best fit in a patient taking a smooth muscle relaxant drug such as verapamil. By retaining water in the intestine, magnesium hydroxide offers added bulk and stimulates increased contractions.

3. A 40-year-old woman has irritable bowel syndrome with diarrhea, which is not responsive to conventional therapies. Regardless of the minor risk of severe constipation and ischemic colitis, the patient decides to initiate therapy with alosetron. Alosetron has which of the following receptor actions?

A. 5-HT3 receptor antagonist.
B. 5-HT4 receptor agonist.
C. D2 receptor antagonist.
D. Muscarinic receptor antagonist.

Answer: A

Serotonin plays the main regulatory role in the enteric nervous system, and the powerful 5-HT3 receptor antagonist alosetron has displayed efficacy in handling women with irritable bowel syndrome that is accompanied by diarrhea.

4. A drug that is useful in angina but causes constipation, edema, and increased cardiac size is:

A. Atenolol
B. Hydralazine
C. Isosorbide dinitrate
D. Verapamil

Answer: D

Verapamil (and diltiazem) is beneficial for prophylaxis of both effort and vasospastic angina. Calcium blockers decrease cardiac work and oxygen demand. They also cause constipation and, occasionally, peripheral edema, which is not associated with heart failure.

Part X
Chemotherapy

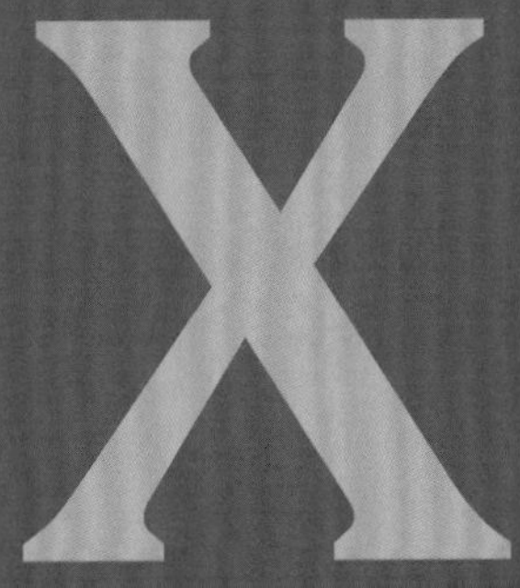

Chapter 56 General Considerations

Shruti Chandra

PH1.42: Describe general principles of chemotherapy.

Learning Objectives

- Classification of antimicrobial agents.
- Adverse effects of antimicrobial agents.
- Type of bacterial resistance.
- General principal of chemotherapy.
- Combined use of antimicrobials.
- Use of antimicrobials for prophylaxis of infections.

Introduction

The introduction of antimicrobial drugs in therapeutics made a drastic and remarkable change in the treatment of various diseases. These drugs not only palliate but also cure many infectious diseases. In developing countries, where infective diseases predominate, antimicrobials gain a lot of importance. Antimicrobials are the most commonly used as well as misused drugs.

Evolution of Antibiotics

In the past, many chemicals were used: for example, for intestinal worm, male fern was used by the ancient Greeks and *Chenopodium* was used by the Aztecs; for boils, moldy curd was used by the Chinese; for leprosy, chaulmoogra oil was used by the Hindus; for syphilis, mercury was used by Paracelsus in the 16th century; and for malaria, cinchona bark was used in Europe in the 17th century.

Later on, in the 19th century, it came to be known that microbes are causes of diseases. Paul Ehrlich (1854–1915), a German scientist, developed arsenicals, arsphenamine in 1906, and neoarsphenamine in 1909 for syphilis, that is, the first cure for syphilis, and coined the term chemotherapy. He was considered the father of chemotherapy.

Subsequently, Gerhard Domagk (1895–1964), a bacteriologist and pathologist, in 1935 developed the first sulfonamide, a brick-red dye prontosil (effective against streptococcal infection). Prontosil is converted into the active metabolite sulfanilamide. Sulfanilamide was introduced in 1936 and was found to be dramatically effective for puerperal sepsis, meningitis, and pneumonia. Sulfanilamide was the first molecule to be introduced in modern chemotherapy (marketed in 1938). The Nobel Prize was given to Domagk (1939) for his discovery. Alexander Fleming in 1928 noticed that a substance produced by penicillium mold destroyed the staphylococcus on culture plate and named it penicillin. In 1939, H. W. Florey, a professor of pathology, and E. B. Chain investigated the substances produced by microorganisms as antibiotics. An antibiotic is a substance that is obtained from one microorganism and proves fatal for other microorganisms in dilute solution, that is, low concentration. Louis Pasteur in 1877 showed the process of antibiosis. The term *antibiotic* was coined by Waksman. Chain and Florey prepared penicillin, and in 1941, it was introduced for clinical use. Fleming, Chain, and Florey were awarded the Nobel Prize for their discovery. Subsequently, Waksman and his coworkers obtained streptomycin from *Streptomyces griseus* (actinomycetes). The discovery of streptomycin led to a series of isolation of antibiotics from actinomycetes, and soon erythromycin, tetracycline, and chloramphenicol were isolated. For the discoveries of antibiotics that entirely changed the scenario for the treatment of infections, Waksman also received the Nobel Prize. Later on, when the chemical structure of antibiotics became known, successful attempts have been made to chemically synthesize newer antimicrobial agents (AMAs), including semisynthetic derivatives of older antibiotics.

Terminology

Chemotherapy

When the treatment of systemic infections is done with specific drugs that selectively suppress/kill the causative pathogen, it is called chemotherapy. The drug used does not significantly affect the host. The treatment of cancer with drugs is also termed *chemotherapy*.

Antibiotics (IM3.12, IM3.13)

Antibiotics are usually derived from one microorganism. They usually act on another organism to suppress the growth of a selected pathogen or kill it. The concentration required is often very low. Certain other substances that are formed by organisms and needed in high concentrations (ethanol, lactic acid) are not called antibiotics. Antibodies that inhibit microorganisms also do not fall in this category.

Antimicrobial Agent

It is a large group containing all natural, semisynthetic, and synthetic agents that attenuate microorganisms. Thus, it is better to use the term *antimicrobial agent*, which also includes antibiotics.

Classification of Antimicrobial Agents

Antimicrobial drugs can be classified on the basis of many characteristics:

- **On the basis of activity against organism:**
  - Antibacterial: penicillins, aminoglycosides, erythromycin, fluoroquinolones, etc.

- Antifungal: griseofulvin, amphotericin B, ketoconazole, etc.
- Antiviral: acyclovir, amantadine, zidovudine, etc.
- Antiprotozoal: chloroquine, pyrimethamine, metronidazole, diloxanide, etc.
- Anthelmintic: mebendazole, pyrantel, niclosamide, diethylcarbamazine, etc.

- **On the basis of chemical structure:**
  - Sulfonamides and related drugs: sulfadiazine and others, sulfones (dapsone [DDS]), *para*-aminosalicylic acid.
  - Diaminopyrimidines: trimethoprim, pyrimethamine.
  - Quinolones: nalidixic acid, norfloxacin, ciprofloxacin, prulifloxacin, etc.
  - β-lactam antibiotics: penicillins, cephalosporins, monobactams, carbapenems.
  - Tetracyclines: oxytetracycline, doxycycline, etc.
  - Nitrobenzene derivative: chloramphenicol.
  - Aminoglycosides: streptomycin, gentamicin, amikacin, neomycin, etc.
  - Macrolide antibiotics: erythromycin, clarithromycin, azithromycin, etc.
  - Lincosamide antibiotics: lincomycin, clindamycin.
  - Glycopeptide antibiotics: vancomycin, teicoplanin.
  - Oxazolidinone: linezolid.
  - Polypeptide antibiotics: polymyxin B, colistin, bacitracin, tyrothricin.
  - Nitrofuran derivatives: nitrofurantoin, furazolidone.
  - Nitroimidazoles: metronidazole, tinidazole, etc.
  - Nicotinic acid derivatives: isoniazid, pyrazinamide, ethionamide.
  - Polyene antibiotics: nystatin, amphotericin B, hamycin.
  - Azole derivatives: miconazole, clotrimazole, ketoconazole, fluconazole.
  - Others: rifampin, spectinomycin, sodium fusidate, cycloserine, viomycin, ethambutol, clofazimine, griseofulvin.

- **On the basis of mechanism of actions** (**Fig. 56.1**):
  - Cell wall synthesis inhibitor: penicillin, cephalosporin.
  - Alteration in cell membrane permeability: nystatin, amphotericin B, polymyxin.
  - Protein synthesis inhibitors:
    - Misreading of m-RNA code and change in permeability: streptomycin, gentamicin.
    - Others: tetracyclines, chloramphenicol, erythromycin.
  - Interfere with nucleic acid metabolism:
    - DNA synthesis: zidovudine, idoxuridine.
    - DNA gyrase inhibitor: 4-FQ (ciprofloxacin).
    - RNA synthesis: rifampicin.
    - Indirectly: sulfonamides, trimethoprim.

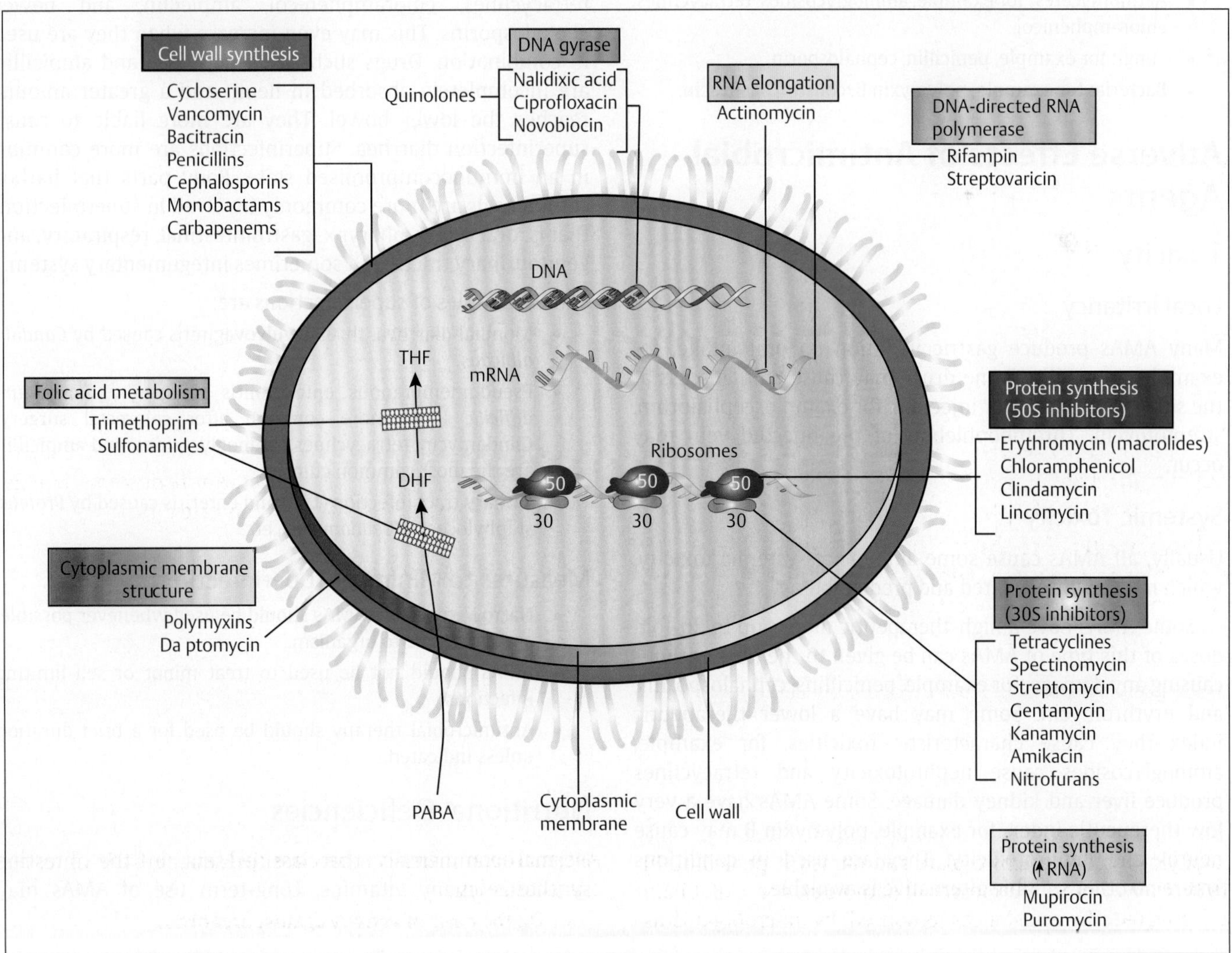

Fig. 56.1 Classes of antimicrobial agents based on their mechanism of action.

- Miscellaneous.
  - Affecting microtubules and/or microfilaments: benzimidazole (albendazole, anthelminthic).
  - Muscle fiber: piperazine, ivermectin, pyrantel.
- **On the basis of spectrum of activity:**
  - Narrow-spectrum—act on selected bacteria: penicillin G, streptomycin.
  - Broad-spectrum—act on group of bacteria: chloramphenicol and tetracycline.
  - Extended spectrum: ampicillin, amoxicillin, ciprofloxacin.
- **On the basis of type of action:**
  - Bacteriostatic—which inhibit the growth of pathogen: sulfonamides, tetracyclines, clindamycin, linezolid, ethambutol, erythromycin, chloramphenicol.
  - Bactericidal—which kills the causative pathogen: penicillins, cephalosporins, vancomycin, polypeptides, fluoroquinolones, aminoglycosides, rifampin, metronidazole, isoniazid, cotrimoxazole, pyrazinamide.

Some bacteriostatic drugs may behave as cidal at higher concentrations, such as erythromycin and nitrofurantoin. Some cidal drugs such as cotrimoxazole and streptomycin may behave as static under certain situations.

Natural Sources of Antibiotics

- Actinomycetes: for example, aminoglycosides, tetracyclines, chloramphenicol.
- Fungi: for example, penicillin, cephalosporin.
- Bacteria: for example, polymyxin B, colistin, bacitracin.

Adverse Effects of Antimicrobial Agents

Toxicity

Local Irritancy

Many AMAs produce gastric irritation on oral intake, for example, ampicillin. Some drugs may cause pain/abscess at the site of intramuscular injection, for example, cephalothin, streptomycin. Thrombophlebitis of the injected vein may occur.

Systemic Toxicity

Usually, all AMAs cause some amount of systemic toxicity, which may be dose-related and predictable.

Some AMAs have a high-therapeutic index—up to 20-fold doses of this type of AMAs can be given to the host without causing any damage, for example, penicillins, cephalosporins, and erythromycin. Some may have a lower therapeutic index—they cause characteristic toxicities, for example, aminoglycosides cause nephrotoxicity and tetracyclines produce liver and kidney damage. Some AMAs have a very low therapeutic index, for example, polymyxin B may cause neuro- and nephrotoxicity. They are used in conditions where no other suitable alternative is available.

Hypersensitivity/Allergic Reactions

In normal course, hypersensitivity reactions cannot be predicted and are usually not related to dose. They may be caused by all AMAs. The most common AMAs causing hypersensitivity reactions are penicillins, cephalosporins, sulfonamides, fluoroquinolones, etc.

Drawback with the Use of Antimicrobial Agents

Superinfection/Suprainfection/ Opportunistic Infection

When we use AMAs for the treatment of one infection, there may be appearance of a new infection, called superinfection. This is due to changes in the normal commensals of the host's body. Normal microbial flora of the body releases a substance called bacteriocin, which inhibits pathogenic organism. Due to alteration in normal microbial flora, even nonpathogenic organisms, for example, *Candida*, may cause disease. Stronger the AMA to suppress the flora, more will be the chances of superinfection. Broad/extended-spectrum antibiotics are more commonly involved in causation of superinfection as they are stronger. Some examples are tetracyclines, chloramphenicol, ampicillin, and newer cephalosporins. This may even increase when they are used in combination. Drugs such as tetracyclines and ampicillin are incompletely absorbed in ileum and a greater amount reaches the lower bowel. They are more liable to cause superinfection diarrhea. Superinfections are more common in an immunocompromised state. Body parts that harbor commensals are more commonly involved in superinfection, that is, oral cavity, pharynx, gastrointestinal, respiratory, and genitourinary tracts, and sometimes integumentary system.

Some examples of superinfections are:

- Monilial diarrhea, thrush, vulvovaginitis caused by *Candida albicans*.
- Pseudomembranous enterocolitis caused by *Clostridium difficile*. It is more common after colorectal surgery. Clindamycin, tetracyclines, aminoglycosides, and ampicillin are the most common culprits.
- Urinary tract infection (UTI) and enteritis caused by *Proteus*, staphylococci, *Pseudomonas*, etc.

Measures to Minimize Superinfections

- Narrow-spectrum AMAs should be used whenever possible, as it is specific to organism.
- AMAs should not be used to treat minor or self-limiting infections.
- Antimicrobial therapy should be used for a brief duration unless indicated.

Nutritional Deficiencies

Normal commensals that are present in the intestine synthesize many vitamins. Long-term use of AMAs may alter intestinal flora, which may lead to vitamin deficiencies. Neomycin is an aminoglycoside that causes structural abnormalities in the intestinal mucosa, which may result in steatorrhea and malabsorption syndrome.

Masking of an Infection

Sometimes, brief duration of AMA is given to treat one infection, as it completely eradicates one organism. However, if there is another microorganism that is simultaneously present in the patient's body, it will only be suppressed. This incompletely suppressed infection will be hidden initially, but later it will appear again in a severe form. For examples:

- Syphilis may appear later when penicillin is given to treat gonorrhea if both the infections are simultaneously present.
- Tuberculosis may be hidden by injection of streptomycin used for a minor respiratory infection.

Drug Resistance (CT1.4, MI1.6)

When a pathogen does not respond to a particular antimicrobial agent, for which it was sensitive earlier, the condition is known as drug resistance.

Type of Bacterial Resistance

Natural Resistance

Some microbes do not have a metabolic process or target site where a certain drug acts; that is why, they are always resistant to certain AMAs, for example, penicillin does not affect gram-negative bacilli, metronidazole does not suppress aerobic organisms, and aminoglycoside antibiotics do not inhibit anaerobic bacteria.

Acquired Resistance

Sometimes an organism acquires resistance to an AMA for which it was sensitive earlier. This may stand true for any organism and is a major clinical problem. The development of drug resistance may be because of the microorganism or the drug. Some bacteria such as staphylococci, coliforms, and tubercle bacilli acquire resistance very rapidly. Some bacteria do not acquire resistance to AMA in spite of using it for a long time, such as *Streptococcus pyogenes* and spirochete against penicillin. Gonococci develop resistance to sulfonamides very quickly, but they develop slow and low-grade resistance to penicillin.

Mechanism of Drug Resistance (Fig. 56.2)

Mutation

It is an alteration in the structure of chromosomal DNA, which may occur spontaneously or randomly among microorganisms. Higher concentration of AMA will be required to inhibit the same microorganism if it contains mutant cells. These mutant cells grow selectively when sensitive cells are killed by AMA. After sometime, a sensitive organism is replaced by a mutant one that is resistant to AMA. This process is termed as vertical transfer of resistance. The speed of vertical transfer is usually low and the severity is also less. It may be of two types:

- One step: Mutation and resistance may develop in one step, which emerges rapidly, for example, enterococci to streptomycin. One-step mutation is a mutation in a single gene, which usually causes high level of resistance.
- Multistep: If a number of gene modifications are involved, it is called multistep mutation. In multistep mutation, sensitivity decreases gradually, for example, resistance to erythromycin, tetracyclines, and chloramphenicol.

Infectious Drug Resistance (Gene Transfer)

There may be transfer of a gene from one bacterium to other bacterium. This is called horizontal transfer of resistance. This mechanism causes rapid development of resistance. Resistance to multiple drugs is usually acquired by this process. The spread of resistance from one organism to another occurs via the ways discussed in the following.

Conjugation

It refers to the passage of resistance genes or extra-chromosomal DNA by direct sexual contact. This happens by the formation of a connection or sex pili, which act as a bridge between the two organisms. This process is called

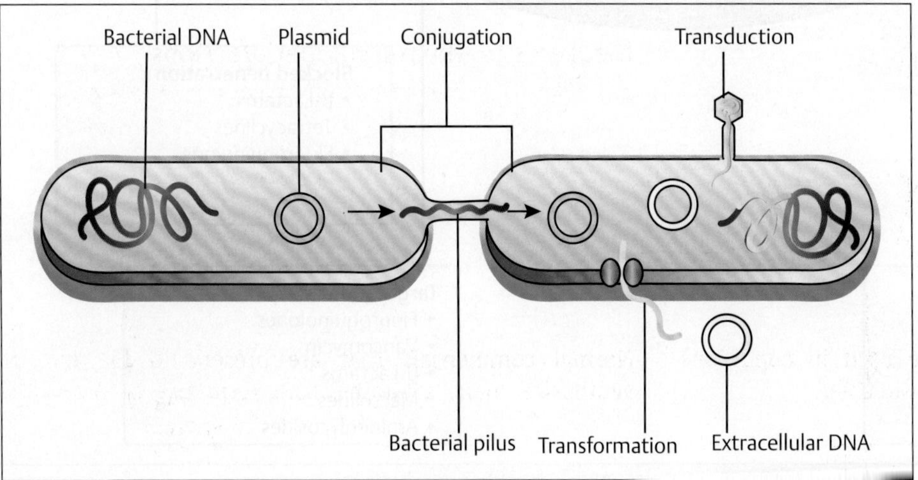

Fig. 56.2 Mechanism of drug resistance.

conjugation. This is common in several gram-negative bacilli. The most common site for conjugation is colon. The presence of "resistance transfer factor" is mandatory for the transfer of resistant genes. Some examples of this mechanism are:

- *Salmonella typhi*—chloramphenicol resistance.
- *Escherichia coli*—streptomycin resistance.

Transduction

Direct incorporation of gene carrying resistance through specific bacteriophage is called transduction. Bacteriophage takes up the R factor from one bacterium and delivers it to another bacterium that it infects. Few examples of this mechanism include resistance to penicillin, erythromycin, and chloramphenicol.

Transformation

The resistance-carrying DNA is released by resistant bacterium inside the medium directly, and this is taken up by another sensitive organism. Thus, it also shows resistance to the particular drug. Certain pneumococci develop resistance to penicillin by this mechanism.

Organisms that are resistant survive, and their number gradually increases. Now, AMA can only kill sensitive strain and not the resistant ones. There could be mechanisms by which resistant organisms exhibit their resistance, discussed in the following (**Fig. 56.3**).

Impermeable to Drugs

The drug is not able to enter the organism or is thrown out.

- Loss of porin channel: The concentration of antibiotic that is required to kill any organism is not achieved inside the bacteria due to loss of porin channels by the resistant strains. For example, in gram-negative bacteria that show resistance to aminoglycosides and tetracyclines, concentration of these antibiotics has been found very low than in the sensitive ones.
- Efflux protein: Some resistant bacteria express efflux proteins in the cell membrane, which throw out the drug by using energy, for example, tetracyclines. Concentration of drug inside the organism falls. This is plasmid-mediated and inducible. Also, inadequate concentration of chloroquine is achieved in resistant *Plasmodium falciparum* malaria.

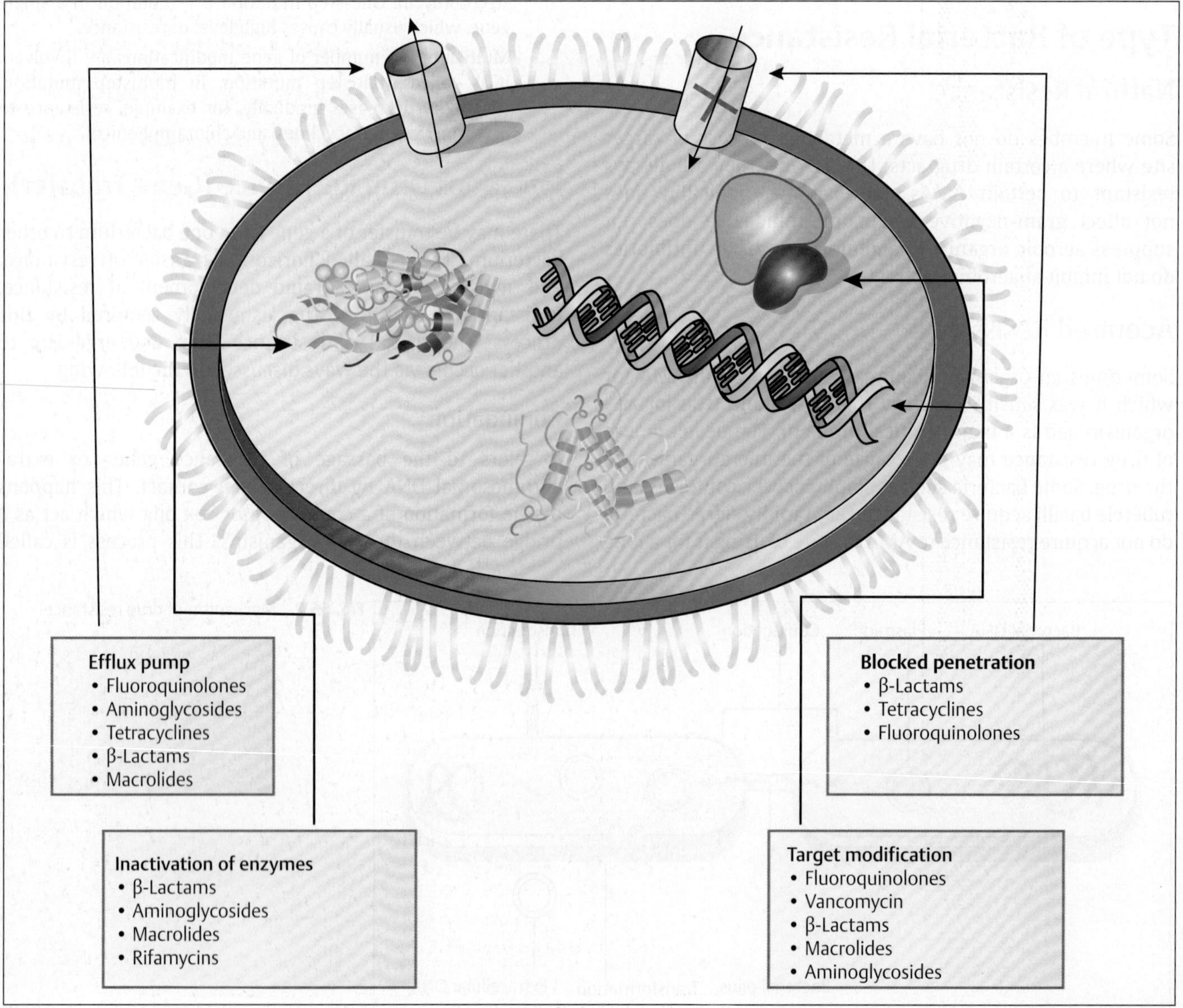

Fig. 56.3 Mechanism by which resistant organisms exhibit their resistance.

Tolerant to the Drug

- By developing altered penicillin-binding proteins, penicillin-resistant pneumococcal strains become resistant to penicillin.
- Fluoroquinolone and macrolide resistance is exhibited by mutational target site modification.
- Synthesis of RNA polymerase enzyme that does not bind rifampin by resistant *Staphylococcus aureus* and *E. coli*.

Destroying the Drug

The resistant organisms release an enzyme that inactivates/break the chemical structure of the drug, for example:

- Bacteria such as staphylococci and gonococci release β-lactamase, which inactivate penicillin G by breaking its β-lactam ring.
- Gram-negative bacilli synthesize various enzymes that are involved in chemical alteration of drugs, for example, aminoglycoside. It may result in ineffectiveness of the drug. These processes may be acetylation, phosphorylation, etc.
- *E. coli* and *S. typhi* destroy chloramphenicol by releasing acetyl transferase.

Cross-Resistance

Cross-resistance is a phenomenon in which a microorganism that is resistant to one drug is also resistant to another drug. Chemically or mechanically related drugs usually show this phenomenon, for example, if an organism possesses resistance to one sulfonamide, it means it will most likely show resistance to all other sulfonamides. In the same way, if an organism is resistant to one tetracycline, it may show no responsiveness to all other related drugs. This type of cross-resistance is usually complete. This may not be true for all classes of drugs: if an organism is resistant to one aminoglycoside, it may be sensitive to another aminoglycoside, for example, pathogens that are resistant to gentamicin are usually sensitive to amikacin. Partial cross-resistance is another phenomenon that is seen in unrelated drug classes sometimes, for example, tetracyclines and chloramphenicol, erythromycin and lincomycin.

How to Prevent Development of Drug Resistance

Measures to stop development of drug resistance are very important in clinical practice.

Certain things that can be done are as follows:

- Prolong, inadequate, and indiscriminate use of AMAs should be avoided. The selection pressure will be minimized and resistant strains will spread less. If infection is acute and localized, symptom-determined shorter courses of AMAs should be given.
- AMAs that are rapidly acting and act on selected (narrow-spectrum) organisms should be preferred whenever possible. When it is not possible to select a specific one, only then a broad-spectrum drug should be used.
- If there is a requirement of prolonged therapy, combination of AMAs should be used, for example, tuberculosis, subacute bacterial endocarditis (SABE), HIV-AIDS.
- Notorious organisms known for developing resistance should be treated aggressively, for example, *S. aureus*, *E. coli*, *Mycobacterium tuberculosis*, *Proteus*, etc., are known to acquire fast resistance. These must be treated intensively and aggressively.

General Principles of Chemotherapy

Clinical Diagnosis

Presumptive clinical diagnosis should be made first. This helps in choosing the suitable AMA.

Selection of Best Drugs

The use of AMA in a particular condition is a very important decision because improper use may lead to resistance. While choosing the drug, the following factors should be kept in mind.

Factors Related to Causative Organism

AMAs are usually effective against few and selective organisms. Treatment should be rational as per the diagnosis. Before starting AMA, definitive bacteriological diagnosis is required but bacteriological testing takes time. Also, it is expensive. Proper collection of suitable sample for correct bacterial diagnosis is important. This process may be challenging sometimes. In such situations, use of empirical therapy is recommended. It is important to know the following points beforehand:

- Prevalence of infection.
- Sensitivity pattern.
- Resistance pattern.

On the basis of these points, the choice of AMAs should be made.

Clinical Diagnosis

Sometimes, clinical diagnosis itself tells about the right choice of antibiotics. For example, in diseases such as syphilis, diphtheria, tetanus, plague, cholera, trachoma, thrush, tuberculosis, lobar pneumonia, leprosy, amoebiasis, herpes simplex, etc., infecting organisms and its sensitivity pattern are well known.

Causative Organism Can Be Guessed

For some infections, for example, tonsillitis, otitis media, boils, vaginitis, and urethritis, the most appropriate specific AMA should be guessed on the basis of clinical features and local experience about the type of organism and its sensitivity pattern.

Based on Bacteriological/Diagnostic Examination

In certain infections, for example, bronchopneumonia, empyema, meningitis, osteomyelitis, UTI, wound infection, etc., it is difficult to guess the organism. In these situations, an AMA should be selected on the basis of culture and sensitivity tests or other suitable diagnostic tests, for example, antigen/antibody tests, PCR (polymerase chain reaction), etc. The following situations may arise.

Not Possible to Conduct Bacteriological Diagnosis

In this situation, empirical therapy that covers all possible [illegible] organisms should be started. A broad-spectrum drug, such as fluoroquinolone or tetracycline, or a combination, such as gentamicin–cephalosporin, can be used. In the case of suspicion of anaerobes, metronidazole or clindamycin, which has coverage of anaerobes, should be added. On the basis of clinical response, treatment should be modified.

Possible to Conduct Bacteriological Diagnosis and Immediate Treatment Is Necessary

In cases of serious/life-threatening infections, such as meningitis and septicemias, treatment should not be delayed. A sample for bacteriological examination should be collected beforehand. Once bacteriological diagnosis is obtained, treatment should be modified accordingly.

Possible to Conduct Bacteriological Diagnosis and Treatment Is Not Urgent

The physician should wait for bacteriological diagnosis and then start definitive therapy according to the sensitivity of pathogen, for example, chronic UTI.

Culture and Sensitivity Testing

The method utilized for bacteriological diagnosis is disk-agar diffusion method. This method utilizes culture plate, which has standardized concentrations of various AMAs on the basis of attained plasma concentrations. This testing should be used as guide, as there may be differences in the activity of AMAs in vitro and in vivo. Thus, doctors should use their clinical judgment while using the reports. There are few concepts about AMA that help us to understand their activity. They are as follows.

Minimum Inhibitory Concentration (MIC)

Microwell culture plates with serial dilutions of the AMAs are used to determine MIC. Minimum concentration of an antimicrobial that inhibit the growth of a pathogen after 24 hours' incubation is known as MIC. The disk-diffusion method can also be used for this purpose. It provides a quantitative measurement of the inhibitory action of an antibiotic and its MIC. This is more informative but not used routinely.

Minimum Bactericidal Concentration (MBC)

MBC is the concentration of the antibiotic that kills 99.9% of the bacteria. It is estimated by subculturing the pathogen from tubes with no visible growth. There will be no growth if the organism is killed. However, growth will be seen on subculture (antibiotic-free) if it is only inhibited. If the drug is bactericidal, the difference between MIC and MBC is minimal, while a large difference indicates that the drug is bacteriostatic. MBC is not used to guide selection of antibiotics in clinical practice.

Postantibiotic Effect (PAE)

Once an organism is placed in an antibiotic-free medium after a brief exposure to AMA, it starts growing again but there is a time gap. This time gap period before reattainment of growth is known as "postantibiotic effect" (PAE). This depends on the antibiotic as well as the organism. It is the time needed for regaining the logarithmic growth. The in vivo PAEs are generally much longer than the in vitro PAEs. Some AMAs such as fluoroquinolones, aminoglycosides, and rifampin show a long and dose-dependent PAE.

Factors Related to AMA

When multiple AMAs are available to treat an infection, the choice of suitable drug depends on properties of the drug. These special properties are discussed in the following text.

Antibacterial Spectrum

A narrow-spectrum antibiotic that acts specifically on the causative organism should be preferred. The reason behind this is that it does not disturb the normal microbial flora of the body. Also, it is more effective than the broad-spectrum drug. However, if empirical therapy is to be given, a broad-spectrum drug should be used, as it will help to cover all suspected pathogens.

Type of Action

A bactericidal drug is preferred over bacteriostatic drugs. It directly kills the bacteria at the site of infection; also, its action is fast. This property is especially helpful in acute serious infections. A bacteriostatic drug only inhibits the growth of bacteria, so there are chances of resumption of growth of organism when the drug's concentration falls below MIC. In conditions such as impaired host defense, life-threatening infections, hidden infections (SABE), or typhoidlike infections, bactericidal drugs should always be preferred.

Sensitivity of the Organism

Sensitivity toward a particular antibiotic should always be kept in mind while choosing the drug. This should be determined on the basis of MIC values of different AMAs toward one organism. Also, PAE should be kept in mind.

Relative Toxicity

Preference should be given to antibiotic that shows minimal toxicity, for example, β-lactam antibiotics are less toxic than aminoglycoside. In the same way, erythromycin can be used over clindamycin.

Pharmacokinetic Property of the Drug

Drugs should reach the site of action for their effectiveness; also, sufficient concentration should be present for sufficient length of time. Their pharmacokinetic properties decide their behavior inside the body, which may be as follows:

- Antibiotics are usually prescribed at 2 to 4 half-life intervals, so that they can maintain therapeutic concentrations. There are certain drugs that produce "concentration-dependent killing," where the ratio of peak concentration to the MIC decides the killing behavior of the drug, for example, aminoglycosides, fluoroquinolones, and metronidazole. Single daily dose of gentamicin shows better response than divided doses of two to three portions, when daily dose remains the same. On the other hand, some drugs show "time-dependent killing," where duration of time above which the concentration of AMA remains more than the MIC decides the action of the drug, for example, β-lactams, glycopeptides, and macrolides. In this case, daily dose should be prescribed in divided doses, as it facilitates the action of the drug. While prescribing, it should be kept in mind that the entire organism should be killed, which can be achieved by proper division of doses.

- Good penetrability at the site of infection is very important. A drug with high penetrability achieves high concentration at the site of infection. That is why, its effect will be more. For example, fluoroquinolones are more effective in treating infections of soft tissues, lungs, prostate, joints, etc., as it attains high concentration in these tissues due to good penetration capability. In cases of meningitis, cefuroxime, ceftriaxone, chloramphenicol, and ciprofloxacin are used, as these attain high cerebrospinal fluid concentration.

Route of Administration

The preferred route of administration is the oral route. Mostly, AMAs can be given by any route. Certain drugs can be given by parenteral route only, such as aminoglycosides, penicillin G, ticarcillin, many cephalosporins, and vancomycin. The oral route is preferred for mild-to-moderate infections, while serious infections, such as meningitis and septicemias, are usually treated by a parenteral antibiotic.

Evidence of Clinical Efficacy

Drugs that have proven efficacy on comparative clinical trial are preferred. The trial results determine their dosage regimen and duration of treatment.

Cost of the Drug

Drugs with lower cost should be preferred unless there is more benefit in using high-cost drugs.

Factors Related to Consumer

Age

Certain AMAs may affect adversely in extreme of ages, for example, tetracyclines are avoided in children younger than 6 years. They get deposited in the developing teeth and bone of the child and produce discoloration of teeth. It also reduces the strength of the bone. Chloramphenicol should not be used in neonates. The process of conjugation of the drugs in the liver and excretion from the kidney is immature in the newborn. If large doses are given, neonates develop gray baby syndrome. Sulfonamides can cause kernicterus in the neonate, as it displaces bilirubin from protein-binding sites.

Hepatic Function

Some drugs should be avoided in poor hepatic function, for example, pefloxacin, moxifloxacin, erythromycin, etc. Dose reduction may be required for isoniazid, rifampicin, and clindamycin.

Renal Function

Some of the AMAs should be given carefully if patients' kidney function is impaired, for example, tetracyclines and cephaloridine. The dose should be reduced if it is very necessary to use, for example, aminoglycosides and amphotericin B (see **Box 56.1**).

Local Factors

Response to an antibiotic is affected by the local site condition.

- Presence of pus: Sulfonamides and aminoglycosides show decreased efficacy in the presence of pus and secretions. Drainage of the abscess is necessary for the action of antibiotics. This process reduces the number of the infecting organism. It also leads to suppression of anaerobes by exposure to oxygen. Now, the drug can easily diffuse inside the abscess.
- Presence of foreign body: It is difficult to treat infections in the presence of catheters, implants, and prosthesis. Bacteria form a biofilm around them and their growth becomes very slow if they come in contact with a foreign body. They become less vulnerable to the antibiotic.
- Anaerobic environment: This reduces transport of antibiotic, for example, aminoglycoside.

Previous Exposure to Drug

If the patient is already taking a certain drug, history about allergy and effectiveness should be obtained, for example, tetracycline should be used in a patient with syphilis if he/she is allergic to penicillin.

Immunocompromised Patients

Immune system of a patient plays an important role in fighting with infection, especially if bacteriostatic drug is used. If the patient has normal host defense, a bacteriostatic

Box 56.1 Drugs requiring dose alterations in hepatic dysfunction
Examples of AMAs that need dose reduction in hepatic dysfunction
Clindamycin, isoniazid, rifampicin, chloramphenicol, metronidazole
Example of AMAs avoided in hepatic dysfunction
Erythromycin, moxifloxacin, pefloxacin, pyrazinamide
Examples of AMA whose dose needs to be reduced in renal failure
Mild failure: acyclovir, aminoglycosides, amphotericin B, ethambutol, vancomycin
Severe failure: carbenicillin, cefotaxime, ciprofloxacin, cotrimoxazole, gemifloxacin, metronidazole, norfloxacin
Examples of AMAs to be avoided in renal dysfunction
Tetracycline (except doxycycline), nalidixic acid
Nitrofurantoin, cephaloridine, cephalothin
Examples of AMAs safe in renal function
Cephalexin, cefaclor, cefoperazone, ceftriaxone
Pefloxacin, moxifloxacin
Dicloxacillin, azithromycin
Erythromycin, azithromycin
Doxycycline, chloramphenicol

drug can easily cure the infection, but in cases of impaired host defense, for example, AIDS and neutropenia, aggressive treatment with bactericidal drug is required. If cell-mediated immunity is hampered in a patient, for example, AIDS, infections by intracellular pathogens are more likely to occur, while in neutropenic patients pyogenic infections are more common.

Pregnancy

Usually, all AMAs pose risk to the pregnant woman as well as to the fetus. That is why, they should be better avoided. Some AMAs such as penicillin, many cephalosporins, and erythromycin are safe in pregnancy. Tetracyclines should not be used in pregnancy, as it carries risk of acute yellow atrophy of the liver, pancreatitis, and kidney damage in the mother. Also, teeth and bone deformities can be induced in the unborn child. Aminoglycoside is an ototoxic drug, and it may damage ear in fetus. Metronidazole has mutagenic potential, so it should be used cautiously during pregnancy.

Genetic Factors

Glucose-6-phosphate dehydrogenase (G6PD) deficiency is a condition in which red blood cells break down when the body is exposed to certain drugs or the stress of infection. It is hereditary. Some AMAs may cause hemolysis in G6PD-deficient patient, for example, primaquine, nitrofurantoin, sulfonamides, chloramphenicol, and fluoroquinolones.

Combined Use of Antimicrobials

Usually, treatment with one antibiotic is sufficient for majority of infections. However, more than one antibiotic may be required for certain situations. The purpose of using antimicrobial combinations may be as follows.

To Prevent Development of Drug Resistance

Two or more AMAs are used together for chronic infections that need prolonged therapy. It has been seen that very few organisms show resistance to the combination of AMAs even if they show resistance to the drugs separately. This strategy is used in many infections such as tuberculosis, leprosy, HIV, *Helicobacter pylori*, and malaria. Acute and short-lived infections usually do not follow this, because resistance rarely develops during such a short course of treatment.

To Obtain Synergistic Effect (IM17.13)

Each antimicrobial has a specific effect on a selected pathogen.

- Combination of two bacteriostatic drugs: Synergistic effect is obtained when two bacteriostatic drugs are used together, for example, trimethoprim and sulfamethoxazole used in UTI, typhoid, etc.; together, they become bactericidal.
- Combination of two bactericidal drugs: Usually additive action is obtained. Synergistic action may be seen if an organism is sensitive to both the prescribed drugs. Few examples are as follows:
  - Enterococcal SABE: Here penicillin/ampicillin + streptomycin/gentamicin or vancomycin + gentamicin is given. In this combination, penicillins inhibit cell wall synthesis, which increases entry of the aminoglycoside inside the bacteria.
  - *Pseudomonas* infection: Ticarcillin + gentamicin is used. This combination is particularly used in neutropenic patients.
  - *Pseudomonas*-infected prosthesis: Ceftazidime + ciprofloxacin combination is used in orthopaedics.
  - Tuberculosis: Rifampin + isoniazid is a well-known combination used in tuberculosis.
- A bactericidal and a bacteriostatic drug combination: This combination may behave as synergistic or antagonistic, which depends on the organism:
  - When the pathogen shows high sensitivity to the cidal drug: Bacteriostatic drug inhibits the multiplication of bacteria, while bactericidal drug kills fast-growing bacteria. This will result in apparent antagonism. The response of the combination is equal to the bacteriostatic drug given alone. For example:
    - Pneumococcal meningitis: Penicillin + tetracycline/chloramphenicol is used in this case because the sensitivity to penicillin is very high. However, mortality is more with this combination than penicillin alone in these patients, as they together exert antagonistic action.
    - Group A streptococcal infection: Penicillin + erythromycin.
    - *E. coli*: Nalidixic acid + nitrofurantoin.
  - If the organism shows low sensitivity towards cidal drug, synergism may be seen, for example:
    - Penicillin + sulfonamide for actinomycosis.
    - Streptomycin + tetracycline for brucellosis.
    - Streptomycin + chloramphenicol for *Klebsiella pneumonia* infection.
    - Rifampin + dapsone in leprosy.

Synergistic combinations should be preferably used to cure tough infections. Full doses of individual drugs should be given for optimum synergism.

Role of MIC

When two different antibiotics are used together, they may show various effects such as synergism (supra-additive effect), additive action, or antagonism. This depends on the drug pair as well as the causative pathogen. These effects are exerted on the basis of MIC of the two drugs. The MIC of one or both the drugs may be decreased in presence of one another. For example:

- Synergism: when MIC of each drug is reduced to 25% or less.
- Additive: when MIC of each drug is reduced by 25 to 50%.
- Antagonism: When MIC is decreased by more than 50% for each AMA.

Thus, it can be concluded that a synergistic drug sensitizes the organism to the action of the other drug of the combination. That is why, the combination is more effective and faster in killing the organisms. There may be prolongation of PAE with the synergistic combination, for example, β-lactams with an aminoglycoside.

To Broaden the Spectrum of Antimicrobial Action

For the Treatment of Mixed Infection

Mixed infection usually comprises aerobic and anaerobic organisms. Both are sensitive to different drugs. Examples of mixed infection are peritonitis, certain UTIs, brain abscesses, bronchiectasis, diabetic foot, bedsores, gynecological infections, etc. In such infections, the use of multiple AMAs is required to cover the possible causative organism. Bacteriological diagnosis and sensitivity pattern of the organism should be kept in mind while prescribing the drug. Full doses of the drug should be used for better coverage. For anaerobes, clindamycin or metronidazole are good options. It may happen that a single drug may cover all the causative pathogens.

For the Treatment of Severe Infections

For a serious or life-threatening infection, it is important to treat aggressively. Various drugs that cover different organisms should be used in combination; for example:

- Penicillin (for gram-positive) + gentamicin (for gram-negative).
- Cephalosporin or erythromycin (for gram-positive) + an aminoglycoside (for gram-negative) ± metronidazole or clindamycin (for anaerobes).

Combination like these may be started as empirical therapy if bacterial diagnosis is not known. The use of rational combination of drug increases the chances of cure. After confirmation of the causative pathogen, one should switch to definitive therapy. It is always better to avoid combinations if the right diagnosis is not known.

Topical

Usually, topical infections are caused by more than one organism, which is why more than one AMAs are used to cover the spectrum, for example, bacitracin, neomycin, polymyxin B.

Problems with the Use of Antimicrobial Combinations

- There are more chances of superinfections as normal flora of the body is suppressed more.
- Combination may pose more toxicity.
- Development of resistance may trigger if inadequate doses are used.
- Cost of therapy may be increased.

Use of Antimicrobials for Prophylaxis of Infections

AMAs are useful for the prophylaxis of infection. Prophylaxis is defined as prevention of establishment of an infection or suppression of contacted infection before its clinical manifestation. Prophylaxis may not be always effective. If the organism is susceptible to a drug, it can be used against infection specifically. The prophylactic use of antibiotics is divided into the following.

Prophylaxis against Specific Infection (IM1.27, IM17.13)

When the organism is highly sensitive, the drug of choice is clear-cut. This is especially targeted against specific organisms:

- Rheumatic fever: It is caused by group A streptococci, which are known to cause recurrences. Here, benzathine penicillin is used as prophylaxis.
- Tuberculosis: Isoniazid is used for prophylaxis of tuberculosis. It is used in exposed individuals, HIV positive, or other susceptible contacts.
- *Mycobacterium avium* complex: HIV/AIDS patients with low CD4 count are more prone to catch this infection. Azithromycin or clarithromycin can be used to protect them.
- HIV infection: There are chances of exposure of health care workers to blood by needle stick injury. Prophylaxis is needed in such cases. Drug used for this purpose is a combination of tenofovir + emtricitabine ± lopinavir/atazanavir. The newborn of HIV-positive mother has to be given tenofovir + lamivudine + efavirenz. After delivery, the neonate should be given syrup nevirapine for 6 weeks.
- Meningococcal meningitis: Rifampin/ciprofloxacin/ceftriaxone are used for prophylaxis of contacted patients.
- Gonorrhea/syphilis: Ampicillin/ceftriaxone is used for this purpose.
- Recurrent genital herpes simplex: If the number of recurrences is more than four in a year, acyclovir prophylaxis should be used.
- Malaria: Mefloquine or doxycycline is used for prophylaxis of malaria. This is usually required for individuals who travel in endemic areas, where transmission rates are very high.
- Influenza A2 or H1N1 (swine flu): Oseltamivir is used for contacts during epidemics.
- Cholera: Tetracycline prophylaxis is used for individuals who come in contact with clinically active cases.
- Whooping cough: Erythromycin or azithromycin can be used for prophylaxis if a nonimmunized child comes in contact with a clinical case.
- Plague: In case of an outbreak or epidemic, mass prophylaxis with doxycycline is used for contacts.
- *Pneumocystis jiroveci* pneumonia: Cotrimoxazole is used for prophylaxis of transplant recipients on immunosuppressants/leukemia or AIDS patients.

Prevention of Infection in Patients with High Risk

Sometimes AMAs are used for high-risk patients, discussed in the following.

Immunocompromised Patients

Immunity is compromised in those who are taking corticosteroids for long term, cancer patients on chemotherapy, and organ transplantation candidates on immunomodulators. In these patients, prevention from serious/opportunistic infections becomes necessary.

Penicillin or cephalosporin ± an aminoglycoside or fluoroquinolone is used to prevent pneumonias and septicemia. However, chances of superinfections are more with aggressive therapy.

Various Procedures

Tooth extraction, tonsillectomy, and endoscopies may damage the mucosa at the site of the procedure, which results in disturbance in commensal bacteria. It may also result in bacteremia. Sometimes, serious infections such as endocarditis may develop because of this, especially in patients with valvular defects. Thus, prophylaxis with amoxicillin or clindamycin is used in these patients few hours before and few hours after the procedure to prevent these complications.

Catheterization or Instrumentation

There is an increased risk of UTI following minor procedures such as urinary catheterization. Prophylaxis with cotrimoxazole or norfloxacin is used to decrease the risk of UTI. Special protection and care are needed in patients with heart valve lesions. Ampicillin, gentamicin, or vancomycin is used for this purpose during catheterization in these patients.

Patients with Anomaly of the Tract

Recurrent UTI is common in patients with defective anatomy. In these patients, prophylaxis with cotrimoxazole or nitrofurantoin is generally used.

Acute exacerbation is common in chronic obstructive lung disease/chronic bronchitis–like conditions. Ampicillin/doxycycline/ciprofloxacin is used for prevention.

Prophylaxis of General Infections

Giving prophylaxis for some general conditions is common in clinical practice but this should be discouraged, as specificity is lacking in most cases. For example:

- Secondary bacterial infections are common in patients with viral respiratory tract infections. To prevent these secondary bacterial infections, prophylaxis with antibacterial should be given.
- In unconscious patients, rates of pneumonias are very high due to aspiration.
- Patients on ventilators are given protections from respiratory infections by using antibiotics.
- Prolonged or instrumental delivery increases the risk of infection in newborns. Both mother and child are covered through prophylaxis.

Prophylaxis in Surgery

Surgical site infection (SSI) includes superficial incision infections (e.g., stitch abscess), deep incision infection (of soft tissue), and organ/space infection.

Indication of Prophylaxis

Surgical prophylaxis is necessary to decrease the incidence of SSI with maintenance of normal microbial flora of the host body. Surgical wounds are classified into four classes by Centers for Disease Control and Prevention (CDC), according to which drugs for prophylaxis are selected. The classification is as follows:

- **Class I/clean**: An uninfected operative wound in which no inflammation is encountered and the respiratory, alimentary, genital, or uninfected urinary tract is not entered (e.g., mastectomy).
- **Class II/clean-contaminated**: An operative wound in which the respiratory, alimentary, genital, or urinary tract is entered with minimal contamination. There is no evidence of infection or major break in sterile technique (e.g., tonsillectomy, hysterectomy).
- **Class III/contaminated**: Open, fresh, accidental wounds, major breaks in sterile technique, uncontrolled spillage from the gastrointestinal tract, and incisions in which acute, nonpurulent inflammation is encountered (e.g., hemorrhoidectomy).
- **Class IV/dirty-infected**: Open, traumatic, dirty wounds, traumatic visceral perforation, and acute inflammation with pus in the field (e.g., chronic wound debridement).

Measure to Minimize SSI

During surgery, bacterial contamination of the surgical site is the most common cause of wound infection. The operating surgeon is responsible for preventing the wound infection, which could be achieved by careful handling of instruments and tissues. There are certain measures that may help reduce SSI, such as:

- The entire instrument should be properly decontaminated and sterilized.
- Cross-infection should be avoided by taking proper measures such as antiseptic/disinfectant.
- Best possible/good surgical technique should be used. This helps in minimizing tissue damage.

Guidelines for SSI

- After extensive and prolonged surgeries, prophylaxis becomes necessary. When the duration of surgery is more than 2 hours, the rate of incidence of postoperative infection is higher.
- Prophylaxis becomes mandatory for surgeries in which prosthesis is used. When prosthesis is inserted into the bone or soft tissue, there are chances of more growth of bacteria; also, risk of resistance is high.
- Prophylaxis is necessary if comorbidities are present, such as diabetes, corticosteroid intake, and other immunocompromised states. Infants, elderly, and malnourished individuals should also be given prophylaxis.
- Prophylaxis is recommended when tissue handling during the surgery is extensive.
- Use of electrocautery also warrants prophylactic prevention, as the damage is comparatively more.

Selection of AMA for Prophylaxis

It is challenging to select the drug, dose, timing, and duration of treatment for prophylaxis. The following points should be kept in mind while choosing the AMA for prophylaxis:

- Antibiotics should not be started prematurely.

- It should not be continued beyond the time when bacteria have access to the surgical wound. Peak level of drug should match the clot formation of surgical wound.
- In case of prolonged surgery, the AMA may be repeated intravenously (IV) during the procedure.
- In case of contaminated and dirty surgery, administration of the AMA is recommended after 4 hours. It should be continued for 5 days.

Antimicrobial drugs that are commonly used for surgical prophylaxis are as follows:

- **Oral (single dose given 1 hour before procedure):**
  - Amoxicillin 2 g (50 mg/kg).
  - Cephalexin 2 g (50 mg/kg).
  - Cefadroxil 2 g (50 mg/kg).
- **For patients allergic to penicillin:**
  - Clindamycin 600 mg (20 mg/kg).
  - Azithromycin 500 mg (15 mg/kg).
  - Clarithromycin 500 mg (15 mg/kg).
- **Parenteral (single injection just before procedure):**
  - Ampicillin 2 g (50 mg/kg) intramuscularly (IM)/IV.
  - Cefazolin 1 g (25 mg/kg) IV.
  - Vancomycin 1 g (20 mg/kg) IV (in methicillin-resistant *Staphylococcus aureus* [MRSA] prevalent areas and/or penicillin-allergic patients).
  - Clindamycin 600 mg (20 mg/kg) IV (for penicillin-allergic patients) for gut and biliary surgery.
  - Cefuroxime 1.5 g (30 mg/kg) IV + metronidazole 0.5 g (10 mg/kg) IV.
  - Gentamicin 160 mg (3 mg/kg) IV + metronidazole 0.5 g (10 mg/kg) IV.
- **Dirty contaminated wounds (including roadside accidents):** The antimicrobial regimens are generally administered for 5 days in case of contaminated dirty wounds: are:
  - Cefazolin 1 g IV 8 hourly + vancomycin 1 g IV 12 hourly.
  - Cefoxitin 1 g IV 6 hourly/ceftizoxime 1 g IV 12 hourly.
  - Clindamycin 0.6 g IV 8 hourly + gentamicin 80 mg IV 8 hourly.
  - Ampicillin 2 g IV 6 hourly/vancomycin 1 g IV 12 hourly + gentamicin 80 mg IV 8 hourly + metronidazole 0.5 g IV 8 hourly.
  - Amoxicillin 1 g + clavulanate 0.2 g IV 12 hourly.

Failure of Antimicrobial Therapy

Clinically, it can be judged whether an antimicrobial therapy is successful or not by looking at the symptoms and signs. Microbiologically, the effectiveness of an antimicrobial therapy can be determined by assessing its capability to eradicate the infecting organism. For an antimicrobial therapy to be successful, the drug should reach in right concentration the site of action. Selection of right AMA with adequate dose and frequency of administration is very important.

Sometimes, it may not be possible for AMAs to completely cure an infection. Sometimes, even it may cause relapse. If response to AMA is not adequate, there is a need for reviewing the therapy.

There are certain factors that are responsible for failure of antimicrobial therapy:

- **Drug-related:**
  - Faulty selection of drug, dose, route, or duration of treatment.
  - Development of resistance.
  - Drug interactions.
  - Use of bacteriostatic agent in immunocompromised individual.
- **Physician-related:**
  - Treatment started very late.
  - Necessary adjuvant measures were not taken, for example, drainage of abscesses, empyema, removal of renal stones, foreign body removal, etc.
  - Uncontrolled diabetes or hypertension.
  - Treatment is given in certain conditions where it is not indicated, for example, untreatable (viral) infections or other causes of fever (malignancy, collagen diseases).
- **Patient-related:** Poor host defense as in leukemias, neutropenia, and other causes, especially if a bacteriostatic AMA is used.
- **Organism-related:**
  - Infecting organisms present behind barriers such as vegetation on heart valves (SABE), inside the eyeball, blood–brain barrier.
  - Presence of dormant or altered organisms (the "persisters"), which later give rise to a relapse.

Multiple Choice Questions

1. Time-dependent killing (TDK) and prolonged post-antibiotic effect are seen with:

A. Fluoroquinolones.

B. β-lactam antibiotics.

C. Clindamycin.

D. Erythromycin.

Answer: B

Killing activity is shown by cidal drugs only. β-lactams and fluoroquinolones are cidal among the options. Time-dependent killing (TDK) is shown by β-lactam antibiotics.

2. All of the following drugs are bactericidal except:

A. Isoniazid.

B. Tigecycline.

C. Daptomycin.

D. Ciprofloxacin.

Answer: B

Tigecycline is a newer drug in the class "glycylcyclines." Its mechanism of action and most properties are similar to tetracyclines. However, it is resistant to efflux pump (major mechanism of resistance to tetracyclines). Most protein

synthesis–inhibiting drugs (including tetracyclines and tigecycline) are bacteriostatic except aminoglycosides

3. Drug resistance transmitting factor present in bacteria is:

A. Plasmid.
B. Chromosome.
C. Introns.
D. Centromere.

Answer: A

Plasmids contain extrachromosomal DNAs that help in transferring the genes responsible for multiple drug resistance among bacteria. These are therefore involved in horizontal transfer of resistance. As it is not due to penicillinase, β-lactamase inhibitors such as clavulanic acid cannot reverse this resistance.

4. True statement regarding the development of drug resistance in MRSA is:

A. It results due to penicillinase enzyme production.
B. It occurs due to change in penicillin-binding proteins.
C. It is chromosome-mediated.
D. It is treated with amoxicillin + clavulanic acid.

Answer: B

Methicillin resistance occurs due to altered penicillin-binding proteins; thus, no penicillin (in fact no β-lactam antibiotic) is useful against methicillin-resistant *Staphylococcus aureus* (MRSA) infections.

5. Drug inactivation by enzymes is the main mode of resistance to:

A. Aminoglycosides.
B. Quinolones.
C. Rifamycins.
D. Glycopeptides.

Answer: A

Most important mechanism of resistance for aminoglycosides is inactivation of drug by various enzymes. Resistance to quinolones is due to altered DNA gyrase, to rifamycin is due to mutation in gene *rpoB*, reducing its ability for the target, and for glycopeptides like vancomycin due to reduced affinity for target site.

6. Which of the following antibiotics acts by inhibiting cell wall synthesis?

A. Cefepime.
B. Aminoglycosides.
C. Erythromycin.
D. Doxycycline.

Answer: A

Cefepime is a β-lactam antibiotic, which acts by inhibiting cell wall synthesis.

7. Which antibiotic acts by inhibiting protein synthesis?

A. Cefotetan.
B. Doxycycline.
C. Ciprofloxacin.
D. Oxacillin.

Answer: B

Doxycycline is a tetracycline that acts by inhibiting protein synthesis.

8. Which of the following drugs requires dose adjustment in renal failure?

A. Cefoperazone.
B. Doxycycline.
C. Streptomycin.
D. Rifampicin.

Answer: C

Streptomycin is an aminoglycoside and requires dose adjustment in renal failure.

9. An antimicrobial agent that acts by inhibition of cell wall synthesis is:

A. Erythromycin.
B. Tetracycline.
C. Lomefloxacin.
D. Cefepime.

Answer: D

Cephalosporins inhibit cell wall synthesis by inhibiting enzyme transpeptidase involved in cross-linking of peptidoglycan layer.

10. All of the following antibacterial agents act by inhibiting cell wall synthesis except:

A. Carbapenems.
B. Monobactams.
C. Cephalosporins.
D. Nitrofurantoin.

Answer: D

Cephalosporins, carbapenems, and monobactam are bacterial cell wall inhibitors, while reactive intermediates of nitrofurantoin inactivate/alter bacterial ribosomal proteins.

11. A patient after operation developed septicemia. He was given a combination of two drugs empirically. There was no improvement even after 10 days of antibiotics therapy. On being investigated, it was found that the combination of antibiotics that was prescribed was mutually antagonistic in action. Which of the following is the most likely combination that was given?

A. Amikacin, vancomycin.
B. Gentamicin, cephalexin.
C. Chloramphenicol, ampicillin.
D. Piperacillin, ciprofloxacin.

Answer: C

Combination of a bactericidal (ampicillin) and a bacteriostatic drug (chloramphenicol) is usually antagonistic in nature. This is because cidal drugs are usually acting on a fast-multiplying organisms, whereas static drugs decrease this multiplication.

12. All of the following drugs act on cell membrane except:

A. Nystatin.
B. Griseofulvin.
C. Amphotericin B.
D. Polymyxin B.

Answer: B

Griseofulvin acts by affecting mitosis but the exact mechanism is not known.

13. Bacitracin acts on:

A. Cell wall.
B. Cell membrane.
C. Nucleic acid.
D. Ribosome.

Answer: A

Bacitracin acts by inhibiting the synthesis of cell wall.

14. All of the following combinations of drugs show antimicrobial synergism except:

A. Penicillin + streptomycin in SABE.
B. Ampicillin + tetracycline in endocarditis.
C. Sulfamethoxazole + trimethoprim in UTI.
D. Amphotericin B + flucytosine in cryptococcal meningitis.

Answer: B

The combination of ampicillin + tetracycline does not show antimicrobial synergism in endocarditis. When organism is highly sensitive to the cidal drug, response to the combination is equal to the static drug given alone (apparent antagonism) as observed in above combination.

15. All of the following antibiotics act by interfering with cell wall formation except:

A. Ceftriaxone.
B. Vancomycin.
C. Cycloserine.
D. Clindamycin.

Answer: D

Clindamycin acts by inhibiting the protein synthesis.

16. The persistent suppression of bacterial growth that may occur after limited exposure to some antimicrobial drug is called:

A. Time-dependent killing
B. Postantibiotic effect.
C. Concentration-dependent killing.
D. Sequential blockade.

Answer: B

Postantibiotic effect is the lag in resumption of bacterial growth after limited exposure to antibiotics.

17. Which of the following is not an established antimicrobial drug synergism at clinical level?

A. Amphotericin B and flucytosine in cryptococcal meningitis.
B. Carbenicillin and gentamicin in pseudomonal infections.
C. Penicillin and tetracycline in bacterial meningitis.
D. Trimethoprim and sulfamethoxazole in coliform infections.

Answer: C

Combination of a bacteriostatic and a bactericidal drug in most cases is antagonistic. Bactericidal drugs act on fast-multiplying organisms, whereas bacteriostatic drugs inhibit the growth. Here, penicillins are bactericidal, whereas tetracyclines are bacteriostatic.

18. Which of the following drugs is not excreted in bile?

A. Erythromycin.
B. Ampicillin.
C. Rifampicin.
D. Gentamicin.

Answer: D

Gentamicin is an aminoglycoside and is excreted via renal route.

19. Multiple drug resistance is transferred through:

A. Transduction.
B. Transformation.
C. Conjugation.
D. Mutation.

Answer: C

Multiple drug resistance is transferred through plasmids, mostly by conjugation.

20. The most common mechanism for transfer of resistance in Staphylococcus aureus is:

A. Conjugation.
B. Transduction.
C. Transformation.
D. Mutation.

Answer: B

Transduction is particularly important in transfer of resistance among staphylococci.

21. Elaboration of inactivating enzymes is an important mechanism of drug resistance among all of these antibiotics except:

A. Quinolones.
B. Penicillin.
C. Chloramphenicol.
D. Aminoglycosides.

Answer: A

Resistance to fluoroquinolones is mediated by mutation in DNA gyrase.

22. Pneumococcal resistance to penicillin G is mainly acquired by:

A. Conjugation.

B. Transduction.

C. Transformation.

D. All of the above.

Answer: C

Acquisition of antibiotic resistance by transduction is common in staphylococcal.

23. A bactericidal drug would be preferred over a bacteriostatic drug in a patient with:

A. Neutropenia.

B. Cirrhosis.

C. Pneumonia.

D. Heart disease.

Answer: A

Bactericidal drugs kill the bacteria, whereas bacteriostatic drugs only inhibit bacterial growth. Bacteriostatic activity is adequate for the treatment of most infections, while bactericidal activity may be necessary for cure in patients with altered immune systems such as neutropenia, HIV, and other immunosuppressive conditions.

24. Which of the following antibiotic acts by inhibiting cell wall synthesis?

A. Chloramphenicol.

B. Gentamicin.

C. Erythromycin.

D. Penicillin.

Answer: D

Penicillin is a cell wall inhibitor. Chloramphenicol and erythromycin inhibit protein synthesis while gentamicin causes misreading of m-RNA.

25. Superinfection is common in:

A. Narrow-spectrum antibiotics.

B. Immunocompromised host.

C. Low-spectrum antibiotics.

D. Nutritional deficiency.

Answer: B

Superinfection is appearance of new infection as a result of antimicrobial therapy. It is common with the use of broad-spectrum antibiotics and immunocompromised host.

Chapter 57

Sulfonamides and Cotrimoxazole

Prasan R. Bhandari

Learning Objectives

- Sulfonamides.
- Trimethoprim.
- Cotrimoxazole.

History

Way back in the early decades of the 20th century, scientists, notably Domagk, in Farben industries, and Bayer Pharmaceuticals, synthesized azo dyes, primarily prontosil. He demonstrated that it was effective in the treatment of murine (mice) streptococcal infections. Although prontosil was not effective in vitro, in vivo its hydrolysis in tissues liberated a compound called sulfanilamide (para-aminobenzene sulfonamide). Similarly, in 1933, Foerster demonstrated that administration of prontosil cured an infant suffering from staphylococcal septicemia. For his scientific contribution in the field of chemotherapy, Domagk was conferred a Nobel Prize in Medicine. These compounds proved to reduce morbidity associated with infectious diseases. In 1956, trimethoprim was developed. Subsequently, a fixed-drug combination of sulfonamide and trimethoprim was introduced as fixed-dose combination (FDC) to take advantage of the sequential inhibition of the essential folic acid metabolic pathway.

However, the discovery of penicillin by Alexander Fleming and other antimicrobial agents later on diminished the utilization of these individual folate inhibitors from clinical practice. Nevertheless, the FDC continues to be utilized in the present era as well.

Sulfonamides

They are classified based on their elimination into:

1. Short-acting ($t_{1/2}$ < 8 hours)—sulfadiazine, sulfisoxazole, sulfacetamide.
2. Medium-acting ($t_{1/2}$ < 16 hours)—sulfamethoxazole.
3. Long-acting ($t_{1/2}$ < 17–48 hours)—sulfadoxine, sulfamethopyrazine.
4. Poor oral absorption, hence active in bowel—sulfasalazine.
5. Topical—silver sulfadiazine, mafenide, sulfacetamide.

Mechanism of Action

The one-carbon molecules transfer reactions necessary for the synthesis of thymidine and purines primarily utilize folic acid as its coenzyme. Notably, animal cells are to synthesize FA; however, it can absorb it from the diet. Humans, too, do not produce FA but obtain it from the diet. Bacteria, protozoa, Pneumocystis jirovecii (P. carinii) and certain fungi too cannot take FA from the environment. They depend on cellular components like para-aminobenzoic acid (PABA) to produce FA.

The important chemical component in the Sulfonamide is the SO $2NH_2$group (**Fig. 57.1**), which is necessary for its action. Even furosemide and bumetanide (diuretics) and dapsone (antileprotic) have a similar chemical structure.

Sulfonamides are structural analogs of PABA (**Fig. 57.1**), hence it competitively inhibits the enzyme dihydropteroate synthetase. This enzyme catalyzes the initial step in folate synthesis (**Fig. 57.2**). Furthermore, sulfonamides could be incorporated within the folate derivatives, thereby interfering with the vital carbon-transfer reactions. Due to the depletion of folate, the DNA, RNA, and protein synthesis is affected, leading to the suppression of the cell growth. The animal cells are not affected, as it does not have the enzyme dihydropteroate reductase. Hence, these are bacteriostatic in nature, and its efficacy is reduced by PABA (i.e., presence of pus).

Spectrum of Activity

Sulfonamides had a wide spectrum of activity during their initial use. These included Gram-positive and negative bacteria, chlamydia, certain nontubercular mycobacteria, Nocardia, plasmodia, and some fungi. Rickettsia, mycoplasma, and treponemes are resistant. Certain strains

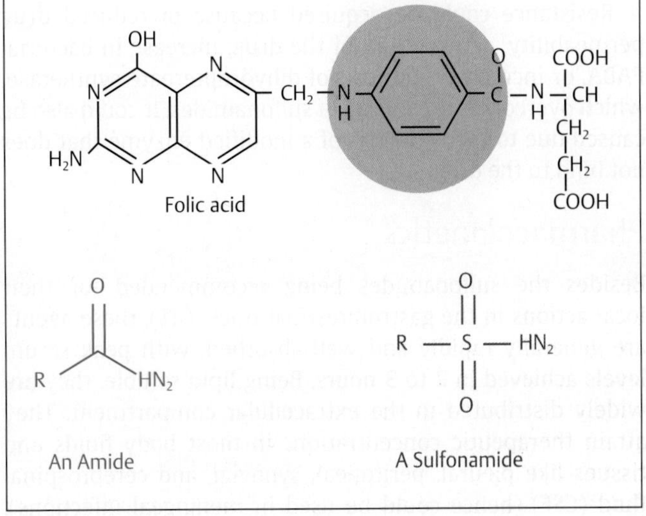

Sulfanilamide

p-aminobenzoic acid

Folic acid

An Amide

A Sulfonamide

Fig. 57.1 Chemical structure of sulfonamide.

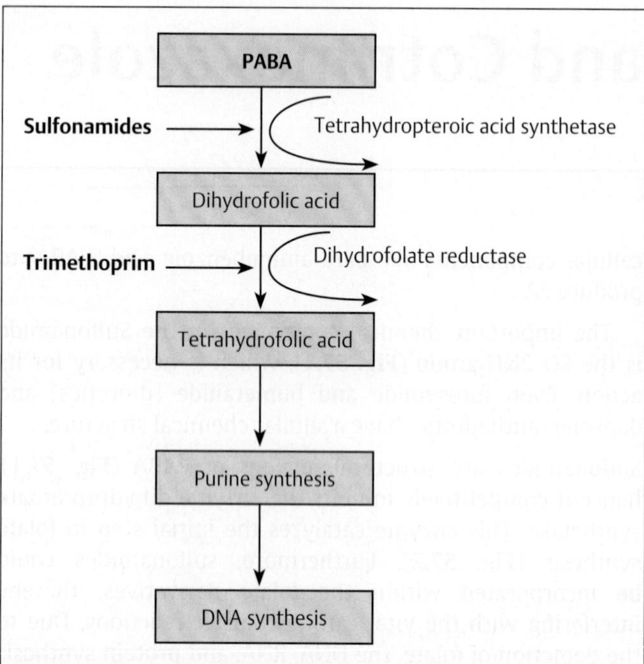

Fig. 57.2 Mechanism of action—sequential inhibition of enzymes by sulfonamides and trimethoprim. PABA, para-aminobenzoic acid.

of Listeria monocytogenes are sensitive. Methicillin-resistant staphylococcus aureus (MRSA) may be vulnerable. Enterococci and Pseudomonas aeruginosa are resistant like most anaerobes. However, frequent use and misuse of the agents had caused the development of resistant strains, thereby reducing its efficacy and utility. As mentioned earlier, they are primarily bacteriostatic in nature, hence necessitating the presence of an active cellular and humoral immunity to eradicate the infection.

Mechanisms of Resistance

Resistance is initiated either by random mutation or by transfer of resistance by plasmids. The acquired resistance is usually permanent. However, there is no cross-resistance seen with other classes of antimicrobial agents, but cross-resistance is observed among the sulfonamides.

Resistance could be acquired because of reduced drug permeability, active efflux of the drug, increase in bacterial PABA, or increased synthesis of dihydropteroate synthetase, which overcomes the effects of sulfonamides. It could also be caused due to the synthesis of a modified enzyme that does not bind to the drug.

Pharmacokinetics

Besides the sulfonamides being recommended for their local actions in the gastrointestinal tract (GIT), these agents are generally rapidly and well-absorbed, with peak serum levels achieved in 2 to 3 hours. Being lipid soluble, they are widely distributed in the extracellular compartment. They attain therapeutic concentrations in most body fluids and tissues like pleural, peritoneal, synovial, and cerebrospinal fluid (CSF) (hence could be used in meningeal infections). It even reaches the anterior chamber of the eye, crosses the placenta, and reaches the fetal blood and amniotic fluid. They are secreted in human milk in minute concentrations. Thus, breastfeeding and sulfonamide use is compatible, not posing as significant risk to the healthy term neonate. However, breastfeeding is not recommended to preterm infants or those who have G6PD deficiency. All sulfonamides achieve a high-urinary concentration. The protein binding varies from 50 to 90%. The highly protein-bound agents could displace other compounds, for example, bilirubin from their protein-bound sites. In newborn infants, this could lead to increased levels of free (unbound) bilirubin causing "Kernicterus." These drugs are primarily metabolized in the liver by acetylation to a variable extent with every agent. The elimination of sulfonamides is primarily renal via glomerular filtration and tubular secretion. Hence, potentially toxic metabolites may accumulate in patients of renal dysfunction, necessitating adjustments in dose and dosing interval, based on the creatinine clearance. The older agents may precipitate in acidic urine, leading to the deposits of crystals and causing crystalluria. This could lead to urinary obstruction. Drinking lots of water and alkalinization of urine could prevent it.

Adverse Reactions

Crystalluria

It is because of the poor solubility/insolubility of the sulfonamide or its metabolite in acidic urine. The chances are less with soluble agents like sulfisoxazole. The incidence can be minimized/prevented by maintaining the urine output to at least 1200 mL in adults. These agents solubility can be increased by alkalinizing the urine. The risk of crystalluria is more in dehydrated patients with AIDS, where sulfadiazine is given in toxoplasma encephalitis. It is manifested as hematuria, oliguria, or anuria.

Blood Dyscrasias

They could be fatal in nature; however, they are rare. These include acute hemolytic anemia (frequently seen in patients with G6PD deficiency). Other rare reactions include agranulocytosis (seen with sulfadiazine, recovery is natural with supportive case requiring weeks to months). Aplastic anemia, which is reversible, is frequent in patients having limited bone marrow reserve (e.g., AIDS or patients on myelosuppressive treatments).

Hypersensitivity Reactions

Milder reactions include simple rashes or urticaria. Serious reactions comprise Stevens–Johnson syndrome or exfoliative dermatitis. Rare ones include serum sickness, drug fever, photosensitivity reactions, or polyarteritis nodosa. Hepatitis too may occur. These reactions are usually seen in the first week of treatment, although they may occur early in previously sensitized persons.

Reactions in Fetus and Neonates

Due to its high plasma protein binding, sulfonamides displace bilirubin from their binding sites. This increases the free concentration of bilirubin, leading to hyperbilirubinemia. This is especially seen in premature and newborn infants. Due to their ill-developed blood–brain barrier (BBB), the free bilirubin crosses it and gets deposited in the basal ganglia and subthalamic nuclei. This encephalopathy is termed kernicterus. This is the rationale for their contraindication in pregnant and lactating women (since sulfonamides cross-placental barrier and are also secreted in milk).

Drug Interaction, Precautions, and Contraindications

Sulfonamides are contraindicated in patients with hypersensitivity to this group of drugs, G6PD deficiency, hepatorenal disorders, blood dyscrasias, and pregnancy. Salicylates, indomethacin, and probenecid increase the concentration of sulfonamides by displacing them from protein-binding sites. Sulfonamides increase the levels of phenytoin, warfarin, and methotrexate by displacing them from their protein-binding sites. The renal elimination of methotrexate is also inhibited, thereby increasing its blood concentration and consequently its toxicity. Hence, dose adjustments/caution may be required in such cases.

Sulfonamides commonly cause rash, so to remember adverse effects of sulfonamides, one must know ABC of RASH.

A – Aplastic anemia

B – Bilirubin displacement (kernicterus)

C – Crystalluria

R – Rash (MC side effect)

A – Acetylation

S - SLE

H – Hemolysis in G-6-PD

Individual Agents

Sulfisoxazole

Compared to other older sulfonamides, this agent has lesser chances of renal toxicity like hematuria and crystalluria, because of its high solubility in the urine.

However, all sulfonamides must be cautiously administered in patients with kidney dysfunction. It has rapid absorption and excretion; hence, it is short-acting.

Sulfamethoxazole

It is only available as an FDC along with trimethoprim. It is structurally similar to sulfisoxazole; however, sulfamethoxazole has a slower absorption and excretion compared to it. It is metabolized by acetylation, and the insoluble metabolite could lead to crystalluria. The possibility of crystalluria could be reduced by ensuring a urine output of at least 1,200 mL in adults and an equivalent amount in children. Administration of sodium bicarbonate to alkalinize the urine too can decrease the chances of crystalluria. The FDC is administered orally for treating urinary as well as systemic infections. Intravenous (IV) FDC preparations are recommended for patients unable to take the drug orally.

Sulfadiazine

It is the drug of choice (DOC) of patients afflicted with toxoplasmosis along with pyrimethamine.

Sulfadoxine

It has duration of action ranging from 7 to 9 days.It is recommended for the prevention and treatment of chloroquine-resistant P. falciparum malaria along with pyrimethamine (500 mg sulfadoxine + 25 mg pyrimethamine as Fansidar). It is also efficacious in mefloquine-resistant malaria. Additionally, it could be beneficial for P. jirovecii pneumonia and toxoplasmosis. The possibility of developing Stevens–Johnson syndrome is higher with this agent. Sulfadoxine is not beneficial for acute infection, since its plasma concentration is subtherapeutic.

Sulfasalazine

Since its oral absorption is relatively poor (around 30%), it primarily has local action on the GIT. Due to this reason, it is used in the management of inflammatory bowel disease (IBD) and ulcerative colitis of mild-to-moderate severity. It is broken down to sulfapyridine and 5-aminosalicylic acid (5-ASA, mesalamine) by the colonic bacteria. Sulfapyridine is the active compound that is absorbed and excreted in the urine. This agent is the component responsible for toxicity. This component is beneficial for patients afflicted with rheumatoid arthritis, whereas 5-ASA produces local anti-inflammatory action; hence, it is beneficial for IBD. The important adverse effects seen with this drug include reversible infertility in males, agranulocytosis, acute hemolytic anemia in patients with G6PD deficiency, and Heinz body anemia.

Silver Sulfadiazine

It demonstrates high activity against Pseudomonas, a common organism seen in patients of burns. The silver is slowly liberated topically, which inhibits the pathogens. It reduces the colonization of pathogens and infection in patients with burns. Hence, the topical formulation is the DOC in wounds because of burns. However, it should not be used to treat deeper infections.

Sulfacetamide

It is a derivative of sulfanilamide. It has a very high aqueous solubility (around 90 times of sulfadiazine) and its sodium salt is used primarily for the treatment of ocular infections. It is a nonirritant even if concentrated solution is used. However, patients sensitive to sulfonamides can develop sensitization; hence, its use is discouraged in such patients. Due to these properties, it is used in the treatment of susceptible ocular infections like trachoma. The other sulfonamides have poor aqueous solubility and their aqueous solution is alkaline and is an irritant to the eyes; thus, it is not suitable for ocular use.

Mafenide

It inhibits the microbial colonization and infection in burns by a wide array of Gram-positive and negative bacteria on topical application. It can be rapidly absorbed from the burn surface, and peak concentration is attained in 4 hours. It can cause pain/burning sensation at the site of application. Occasionally, superinfection with Candida species could occur. Its metabolite inhibits carbonic anhydrase enzyme in kidneys; hence, the urine becomes alkaline. Metabolic acidosis and compensatory tachypnea (hyperventilation) limit its use. The topical application of the cream should be subsequent to cleansing and debridement of the wound. Application of 1 to 2 mm thickness once or twice daily should be continued till the grafting is performed. Established deep infection should not be treated with this agent.

Current Therapeutic Status/Uses

The availability of less toxic antimicrobial agents and the emergence of pathogens resistant to sulfonamides have reduced the clinical utility of these agents. However, the combination of sulfonamides and trimethoprim continues to be a part of the therapeutic armamentarium of the clinicians. For the treatment of other infections, sulfonamides are used in combination with other drugs as mentioned below:

1. Used as cotrimoxazole (as discussed later).
2. Combination with other drugs:
   a. Sulfadiazine + pyrimethamine: toxoplasmosis chorio-retinitis, active toxoplasmosis, and acute attack of malaria. Folic acid is also added.
   b. Sulfadoxine + pyrimethamine: treatment of chloroquine-resistant malaria.
3. Specific use: sulfasalazine for IBD and rheumatoid arthritis.
4. Topical use:
   a. Ocular preparation of sulfacetamide is used for chlamydial eye infections, that is, trachoma and inclusion conjunctivitis. The simultaneous systemic use of sulfonamides or tetracyclines enhances its efficacy.
   b. Silver sulfadiazine or mafenide is applied topically for prevention and treatment of burns infection.
5. Urinary tract infection (UTI): Sulfisoxazole attains bactericidal concentrations in the urine; hence, it may be used for acute uncomplicated UTI due to susceptible Gram-negative organisms (especially *E. coli*) sensitive to sulfonamides. However, they are not suitable for complicated upper UTIs. Cotrimoxazole, trimethoprim, ampicillin, or quinolone are however preferred.
6. Nocardiosis: Sulfisoxazole or sulfadiazine could be administered in such patients. However, cotrimoxazole is the drug of choice. Alternatively, a sulfonamide along with erythromycin, ampicillin, or an aminoglycoside may be used following culture and sensitivity test.
7. Miscellaneous:
   a. Streptococcal pharyngitis and rheumatic fever as an alternative to penicillin—allergic patients.
   b. Alternative to tetracyclines and erythromycin in other chlamydial infections like lymphogranuloma venereum and pneumonia.

Trimethoprim

Mechanism of Action

It is a diaminopyridine and has actions similar to that of pyrimethamine (antimalarial), that is, it competitively inhibits the enzyme dihydrofolate reductase (DHFR) responsible for converting dihydrofolate (folic acid) to tetrahydrofolate (folinic acid). Folinic acid is the immediate precursor of the one-carbon transfer cofactors essential for the DNA, RNA, and protein synthesis. The affinity of trimethoprim for human DHFR is 20,000 to 60,000 times less than the bacterial DHFR. This leads to its selective toxicity against the bacterial only, without majorly affecting the human cells.

Resistance

It is possible if there is overproduction of DHFR or reduced affinity for the drug. Other mechanisms of resistance include reduced permeability or active efflux of the drug. If thymine-dependent mutants with decreased folic acid requirements are selected and also leads to resistance.

Pharmacokinetics

It is almost completely absorbed following oral administration. Peak concentration is achieved in 1 to 4 hours. Because of its high-lipid solubility, it has a high volume of distribution and thus penetrates well in prostatic tissues as well as CSF. It is primarily excreted from the kidneys in unchanged form.

Spectrum of Activity

They have wide spectrum of activity like sulfonamides. However, its activity against Nocardia, clostridia, Neisseria, and brucella is less than that of sulfonamides.

Clinical Indications

Presently, the clinical utility of trimethoprim has declined as a single drug. However, it still finds use in patients for prophylaxis and treatment of uncomplicated UTI, prostatitis (due to its high concentration), and respiratory infections caused due to susceptible organisms.

Adverse Effects

Trimethoprim may still bind to human DHFR, and lead to megaloblastic anemia, leukopenia, and thrombocytopenia, although this incidence is rare. These effects, however, can be reversed by the administration of folinic acid, without impairing the antimicrobial efficacy of trimethoprim.

Cotrimoxazole

It is a combination of trimethoprim and sulfamethoxazole. Although there are other agents which are combined with sulfonamides, this is most commonly used.

Mechanism of Action

The individual agents sequentially block the bacterial synthesis of folinic acid in two steps; hence, having a synergistic effect (separately both sulfamethoxazole and trimethoprim are bacteriostatic, whereas the combination is bactericidal). Sulfamethoxazole is a structural analog of PABA and competes with PABA to suppress the formation of dihydrofolic acid, a step essential for the synthesis of tetrahydrofolic acid. Sulfamethoxazole attaches to the enzyme dihydropteroate synthetase, which catalyzes this step. Similarly, trimethoprim inhibits bacterial more than human enzyme DHFR, reducing the synthesis of tetrahydrofolic acid. Decreased concentration of tetrahydrofolic acid inhibits thymidine formation and thus the later steps of DNA production. Hence, even a minute concentration of thymidine can reverse the activity of this combination (e.g., in pus). Because human cells utilize preformed folic acid, sulfonamides do not affect the human cells. Likewise, trimethoprim is highly selective for the bacterial rather than human cells; hence, human cells are not affected at therapeutic levels.

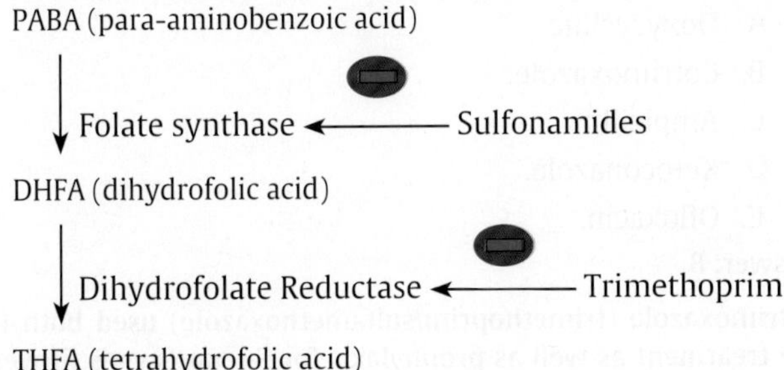

Pharmacology

The maximum synergistic activity is observed when trimethoprim-sulfamethoxazole plasma concentration ratio is 1:20. This ratio is attained in the plasma by combining these individual agents in the ratio of 1:5 (trimethoprim 80 mg + sulfamethoxazole 400 mg). This is because of the difference in the pharmacokinetics of the individual drugs. Trimethoprim is rapidly and totally absorbed but has large volume of distribution and thus concentrated in many tissues. Bioavailability of both drugs is nearly 85%. The plasma protein binding of trimethoprim is 40%, whereas that of sulfamethoxazole is 65%. Additionally, trimethoprim is more lipophilic then sulfomethoxazole. The half-life of both compounds is approximately 10 to 12 hours. Dose should be adjusted inpatients with reduced renal function. This is a rational FDC. It reduces the minimum inhibitory concentration (MIC) of both agents, widens the spectrum, and decreases the incidence of resistance.

Spectrum of Activity

This combination is more efficacious against a broad spectrum of aerobic Gram-positive and Gram-negative bacteria, P. jirovecii and certain protozoa, as compared to individual components. Examples include S. typhi, MRSA, P. jirovecii, Nocardia, Klebsiella, and Yersinia enterocolitica. Certain microorganisms that are acquired nosocomially or seen in immunodeficient patients too are inhibited by the combination sensitivity pattern which varies from one area to another.

Resistance

Because of the frequent use of this FDC, resistance has emerged in most species throughout the world. However, the development of resistance to FDC is slow as compared to individual agents. The mechanisms include:

1. Decreased permeability to the drugs.
2. Target enzyme with reduced affinity for drugs.
3. Acquisition of plasmids with genes encoding drug-resistant enzymes.
4. Active efflux of the drug.

Clinical Indications

1. Pneumocystis jirovecii (carinii) pneumonia: This organism frequently causes infection, that is, severe pneumonia in patients afflicted with AIDS. It is the DOC for the prophylaxis as well as treatment. It is also very efficacious in other Gram-positive and Gram-negative infections in patients afflicted with AIDS. The dose generally preferred is one double strength (DS) tablet 4 to 6times in a day. In certain conditions, IV cotrimoxazole may be used.
2. Typhoid: The current DOC is ciprofloxacin. However, this FDC could be used as an economical option.
3. Urinary tract infection (UTI): Generally beneficial only in complicated lower UTI which is caused by *E. Coli*. It can also be recommended as a prophylaxis in patients with recurring UTI in lower doses. Single dose treatment of 4 tablets can be used for acute cystitis.
4. GIT infections: It is comparable in efficacy to fluoroquinolones (FQs) for treating travelers' diarrhea (bacillary dysentery) caused by *E. coli* and Shigella. It is also effective in treating diarrhea caused because of Salmonella and Campylobacter jejuni. It has less efficacy in diarrhea due to cholera. However, it is the DOC for Y. enterocolitica.
5. Respiratory infections: It is beneficial in pneumonia caused by Streptococcus pneumoniae and *H. influenzae*. Likewise, it is used both for infections of upper and lower respiratory tract like otitis media and chronic bronchitis.
6. Miscellaneous (as alternative)
   - Nocardiosis: commonly encountered in AIDS patients. This FDC is the DOC.
   - For Burkholderia cepacia (Pseudomonas) and Stenotrophomonas (Xanthomonas maltophilia), it is the DOC.
   - Chancroid (*H. ducreyi*): As an option to other drugs like azithromycin, erythromycin, ceftriaxone, or ciprofloxacin.
   - Brucellosis: Alternative to the DOC, that is, doxycycline +gentamicin.

- Granuloma inguinale (Calymmatobacterium granulomatis): Alternative to the DOC, that is, tetracycline.
- Listeriosis: Alternative to the DOC, that is, amoxicillin + gentamicin.
- Bubonic plague, Enterobacter, citrobacter, serratia–as alternative.
- Intestinal parasites–cyclospora and Isospora.

Dosage & Administration

- Oral single strength (SS) tablet–80 mg trimethoprim + 400 mg sulfamethoxazole.
- Oral double strength (DS) tablet–160 mg trimethoprim + 860 mg sulfamethoxazole.
- Oral suspension–40 mg trimethoprim + 200 mg sulfamethoxazole per 5 mL.
- IV–80 mg trimethoprim + 400 mg sulfamethoxazole/5 mL.

Adverse Reactions & Precautions

They are generally well-tolerated; however, the chances are more and severe in HIV-infected patients. It is managed by stopping the drug. The more common reactions include nausea vomiting, rash and pruritus, and acute hemolytic anemia in patients with G6PD deficiency. Certain life-threatening reactions can occur in HIV-infected patients and older adults, including Stevens–Johnson syndrome, exfoliative dermatitis, toxic epidermal necrolysis (TEN), and hyperkalemia, especially in patients on angiotensin-converting enzyme inhibitor (ACEI), angiotensin receptor blocker (ARB), and spironolactone, and can lead to sudden death. Precautions should be taken in folate-deficient patients, where it can lead to megaloblastic anemia (pregnancy, chronic hemolytic anemia). This is because trimethoprim weakly inhibits enzyme DHFR essential for folate recycling.

The efficacy of the FDC can be reduced by folic acid and folinic acid (leucovorin). Patients with allergy to sulfonamides should not be administered this FDC. Avoid the use of this combination during pregnancy and lactation. They can increase the risk of neural tube defects and kernicterus in neonates. It can also lead to acute hemolysis in infants with G6PD deficiency. This risk is more if the infant is jaundiced, premature, or ill.

Drug Interactions

This FDC can interact with many drugs, necessitating the dose adjustment and frequent monitoring of therapy. These include rifampicin, oral hypoglycemics, oral anticoagulants, phenytoin, dapsone, cyclosporine and, possibly, ACEI/ ARB.

Multiple Choice Questions

1. A 45-year-old woman has symptoms of intermittent diarrhea associated with lower abdominal cramping and recurrent rectal bleeding. On examination, the patient looked well-nourished and with normal blood pressure. There was moderate abdominal pain and tenderness. The only medication the patient is on is loperamide for diarrhea. There is mucosal edema, friability, and some pus seen in sigmoidoscopy. Investigations reveal mild anemia and reduced serum albumin. Stool examination does not demonstrate signs of either bacterial, amebic, or cytomegalovirus involvement. The best-suited drug to use is:

A. Ciprofloxacin.
B. Azithromycin.
C. Albendazole.
D. Sulfasalazine.
E. Cotrimoxazole.

Answer: D

Since there is no clear evidence of a definite microbial cause for the colitis, a drug that reduces inflammation is recommended. Sulfasalazine has significant anti-inflammatory property, and its oral administration causes symptomatic improvement in ulcerative colitis. It is also beneficial due to its anti-inflammatory effects in rheumatoid arthritis.

2. A 50-year-old man with HIV arrives in the casualty complaining of breathlessness. Investigations show a CD4+ count of 150 along with hypoxia in arterial blood gas. There is bilateral interstitial infiltrates seen in chest X-ray. The likely diagnosis is Pneumocystis jirovecii pneumonia, which is confirmed by bronchoscopy and silver staining of bronchial washings. The most appropriate medicine would be:

A. Doxycycline.
B. Cotrimoxazole.
C. Ampicillin.
D. Ketoconazole.
E. Ofloxacin.

Answer: B

Cotrimoxazole (trimethoprim/sulfamethoxazole) used both for the treatment as well as prophylaxis for Pneumocystis jirovecii pneumonia. Azithromycin too is beneficial in Mycobacterium avium intracellulare (MAC complex).

3. A 30-year-old woman has symptoms of urinary frequency, urgency, and dysuria. Urine examination reveals bacteria and white blood cells; hence, she is administered cotrimoxazole as empiric treatment. A couple of days later she complains of fever and blisters around, and inside, her mouth and nose. The most probable cause could be:

A. Herpes zoster infection.
B. Aphthous stomatitis.
C. Red man syndrome.
D. Steven–Johnson syndrome.

Answer: D

Steven–Johnson syndrome is a type of erythema multi-forme, which is infrequently linked with sulfonamide use. Manifestations include fever and a red or purple rash that spreads. The rash is usually tender and may result in blisters on mucous membranes like mouth, nose, and genital areas.

4. A 35-year-old AIDS patient is to be treated for chemoprophylaxis for Pneumocystis pneumonia (PCP) and cerebral toxoplasmosis. The most suited medication for the prevention of both PCP and cerebral toxoplasmosis would be:

A. Ciprofloxacin.
B. Trimethoprim-sulfamethoxazole.
C. Erythromycin.
D. Quinine.
E. Flucytosine.

Answer: B

Trimethoprim–sulfamethoxazole daily or three times a week has proved to prevent both PCP and toxoplasmosis in AIDS patients.

5. A 5-day-old baby has developed sulfonamide-induced kernicterus. The most probable mechanism involved would be:

A. Displacement of bilirubin from binding sites on plasma proteins.
B. Underdeveloped bilirubin hepatic conjugation and metabolism.
C. Physiological jaundice because of destruction of fetal red cells.
D. Liver congestion and cholestasis due to the pregnancy.
E. Primary hepatic cirrhosis.

Answer: A

Sulfonamides compete for bilirubin protein binding sites and enhance fetal blood levels of unconjugated bilirubin. Free/unbound bilirubin crosses the ill-formed blood–brain barrier (BBB) in the neonate and gets deposited in the basal ganglia and subthalamic nuclei, causing kernicterus, a toxic encephalopathy.

6. An 8-year-old boy was prescribed a 7-day course of trimethoprim-sulfamethoxazole for external otitis. The mechanism of action of the sulfonamides is:

A. Selective inhibition of incorporation of para-aminobenzoic acid (PABA) into human cell folic acid synthesis.
B. Competitive inhibition of incorporation of PABA into microbial folic acid.
C. Inhibition of transpeptidation reaction in bacterial cell wall synthesis.
D. Inhibition of DNA gyrases.
E. Inhibition of bacterial ribosomes

Answer: B

Humans cannot synthesize folic acid; diet is their major source. Sulfonamides selectively suppress microbially synthesized folic acid. Incorporation of PABA into microbial folic acid is competitively inhibited by sulfonamides. The trimethoprim-sulfamethoxazole combination is synergistic because it acts at different steps in microbial folic acid synthesis. All sulfonamides are bacteriostatic.

7. A 65-year-old male patient suffering from Pneumocystis jirovecii pneumonia is put on high-dose cotrimoxazole (trimethoprim-sulfamethoxazole therapy for 3 weeks. The treating physician should be cautious of which of the following adverse reactions?

A. Bone marrow toxicity.
B. Megaloblastic anemia.
C. Uremia.
D. All of the above

Answer: D

An elderly patient given long-term high-dose trimethoprim-sulfamethoxazole has a high chances of developing all of the mentioned adverse reactions including bone marrow toxicity, and megaloblastic anemia can occur in patients with marginal folate levels. Uremia can occur in patients with impaired renal function.

8. A 55-year-old male patient has been prescribed long-term trimethoprim-sulfamethoxazole for the treatment of his recurrent prostatitis. His renal parameters are normal. His treating physician should advise him about the possibility of:

A. Uremia; hence, dialysis.
B. Crystalluria; hence, acidify the urine and decrease fluid intake.
C. Crystalluria; hence, increase fluid intake and alkalinize the urine.
D. Uremia; hence, alkalinize the urine.

Answer: C

The patients being administered long-term trimethoprim-sulfamethoxazole have a high incidence of developing crystalluria. This is frequent with compounds like sulfamethoxazole, which are primarily acetylated in liver, and its inactive metabolite is insoluble in urine; hence, causing precipitation of crystals in urine. This can be minimized by increasing the fluid intake to a minimum of 1,200 mL. Alkalinization of urine rather than acidification will prevent the formation as well as enhance the excretion of crystals. Since the renal parameters are within normal range, there is less chances of developing uremia.

9. A newborn neonate has developed ophthalmia neonatorum. The treating physician would prefer which of the following:

A. Mafenide.
B. Sulfacetamide.
C. Sulfasalazine.
D. Sulfomethoxazole.

Answer: B

Sulfacetamide sodium is a highly soluble compound, yielding neutral solution which does not irritate the eyes on topical application. Hence, it is used in this case as well as other susceptible bacteria and chlamydia oculogenitalis.

10. A 30-year-old patient suffering from burn injury would most likely be prescribed the topical antibiotic to prevent infection from pseudomonas is:

A. Sulfasalazine.

B. Sulfacetamide.

C. Silver sulfadiazine.

D. Sulfadoxine.

Answer: D

Silver sulfadiazine used topically as 1% cream is active against a variety of bacteria and fungi even those resistant to other sulfonamides, for example, pseudomonas. The silver ions too possess antimicrobial properties. It is most effective for preventing burn infection of burnt surfaces and chronic ulcers. However, it is not beneficial for treating established infection.

Chapter 58 Fluoroquinolones

Shweta Sinha

Learning Objectives

- First-generation fluoroquinolones.
- Second-generation fluoroquinolones.
- Third-generation fluoroquinolones.
- Fourth-generation fluoroquinolones.

Introduction

Before the discovery of quinolones in the 1960s, antibiotics were majorly sourced from natural products, such as plants and animals, or isolated directly from microorganism cultures themselves. Quinolones are unusual among antimicrobials in that they were not isolated from living organisms, but were rather synthesized by chemists. The first quinolone, nalidixic acid, was derived from the antimalarial drug chloroquine. George Lesher (the acknowledged discoverer) and his coworkers at Sterling Drugs (now part of Sanofi) are known for reporting the antibacterial activities of this class of drugs in the 1960s. Later on, various agents were obtained through side chain and nuclear manipulation.

Classification

The development of different fluoroquinolones is depicted in generational terms, with each generation having either antimicrobial spectra or similar characteristics. First-generation agents are highly active against aerobic gram-negative bacteria but are less active against aerobic gram-positive bacteria or anaerobes. The prototypical compound of the quinolones, nalidixic acid of this class, was brought into clinical practice in 1962 to cure uncomplicated urinary tract infections (UTIs). Second-generation agents provide enhanced activity against gram-negative bacteria and moderately enhanced activity against gram-positive bacteria. These fluoroquinolones are known for having fluorine atom at position C-6, and because of fluorine inclusion, quinolones are often termed "fluoroquinolones." Third-generation agents possess more prominent potency against gram-positive bacteria, specifically, pneumococci, and also have better activity against anaerobes. Fourth-generation fluoroquinolones have superior coverage against pneumococci and anaerobes (**Table 58.1**).

First Generation

The first-generation agents are the oldest and least used quinolones, which include nalidixic and cinoxacin acid. Both are highly susceptible toward bacterial resistance because of frequent dosing requirement as compared to newer quinolones. Also, these are not advised to be taken by population having poor renal function.

Table 58.1 Fluoroquinolones for clinical use

Generation	Drugs	Antimicrobial spectrum	Clinical indications
First generation	Nalidixic acid Cinoxacin (not in use)	Gram-negative organism (except *Pseudomonas* species)	Uncomplicated UTIs
Second generation	Norfloxacin (Noroxin) Enoxacin (Penetrex) Ciprofloxacin (Cipro) Lomefloxacin (not in use) Ofloxacin (Floxin)	Gram-negative organisms (including *Pseudomonas* species), some gram-positive organisms (including *Staphylococcus aureus* but not *Streptococcus pneumoniae*), and some atypical pathogens	Uncomplicated and complicated UTIs and pyelonephritis, sexually transmitted diseases, prostatitis, skin, and soft-tissue infections
Third generation	Levofloxacin (Levaquin) Sparfloxacin (not in use) Gatifloxacin (not in use) Grepafloxacin (not in use) Moxifloxacin (Avelox)	Similar to second-generation plus extended activity against gram-positive coverage (penicillin-sensitive and penicillin-resistant *S. pneumonia*) and on atypical pathogens	Acute aggravation of chronic bronchitis, community-acquired pneumonia
Fourth generation	Trovafloxacin (not in use) Gemifloxacin (Factive)	Same as for third-generation agents plus broad anaerobic coverage	Same as for first-, second-, and third-generation agents (excluding complicated UTIs and pyelonephritis) plus intra- abdominal infections, nosocomial pneumonia, pelvic infections

Abbreviation: UTIs, urinary tract infections.

Second Generation

The second-generation quinolones, such as norfloxacin, enoxacin, lomefloxacin, ciprofloxacin, and ofloxacin, have improved activity against gram-negative and some gram-positive bacteria as well as on atypical pathogen. These agents have wide range of clinical applications as compared with first-generation agents. These are mostly used to treat complicated UTIs and pyelonephritis, sexually transmitted diseases, selected pneumonias, and skin infections. Among the second-generation agents, ciprofloxacin is highly effective against *Pseudomonas aeruginosa*, and ofloxacin has potent activity against *Chlamydia trachomatis*. Both ciprofloxacin and ofloxacin are extensively used because of their broad range of FDA-labelled indications and their ease of accessibility in both intravenous and oral formulations.

The second-generation agents are not recommended as the first-line treatment for lower respiratory tract infections and acute sinusitis, as *Streptococcus pneumoniae* can easily acquire resistance to these agents.

Third Generation

The third-generation quinolones have even more broad activity against gram-positive bacteria, specifically penicillin-sensitive and penicillin-resistant *S. pneumoniae*, and atypical pathogens such as *Mycoplasma pneumoniae* and *Chlamydia pneumoniae*. Currently, these include levofloxacin, gatifloxacin, moxifloxacin, and sparfloxacin. The third-generation quinolones have also expanded gram-negative coverage; however, comparatively, they are not as much active as ciprofloxacin on *Pseudomonas* species. Due to broad antimicrobial spectrum, these quinolones are used primarily in the treatment of community-acquired pneumonia, acute exacerbations of chronic bronchitis, and acute sinusitis, which are FDA-labeled indications. Gatifloxacin is also indicated for use in UTIs and gonorrhea.

Fourth Generation

The fourth-generation quinolones are same as the third-generation quinolones but have expanded anaerobic coverage. This includes gemifloxacin, an oral fluoroquinolone antibiotic, which is used currently in the treatment of less severe respiratory tract infections. Gemifloxacin was approved for use in 2003 in the United States, but it is as commonly prescribed as ciprofloxacin and levofloxacin. Gemifloxacin is rarely linked to acute liver injury. Current indications of gemifloxacin are limited to acute exacerbations of chronic bronchitis and community-acquired pneumonia.

Mechanism of Action

Fluoroquinolones display their activity by hindering the action of two enzymes that are involved in the process of bacterial DNA synthesis. These enzymes are DNA topoisomerases I (DNA gyrase) and IV, which are usually not present in human cells but are major constituents of DNA replication in bacterial cell. This feature of fluoroquinolones enables them to be more particular and bactericidal. DNA topoisomerases are known for segregating the two DNA strands from each other, cleaving the strand to insert another strand of DNA and finally resealing the prior segregated strands. These agents associate with the enzyme-bound DNA complex (i.e., DNA gyrase or topoisomerase IV with bacterial DNA), which results in conformational alterations that hinder the enzyme activity required for normal functioning. This newly formed complex then stops the sequential events of DNA replication process at the replication fork, thereby hindering normal DNA synthesis, which immediately results in bacterial cell death. More specifically, in case of gram-negative bacteria, DNA gyrase is the main target for fluoroquinolones activity, whereas fluoroquinolones act typically at topoisomerase IV in gram-positive bacteria.

Mechanism of Resistance

There are two mechanisms by which fluoroquinolones develop resistance: (1) modification in the drug target enzymes and (2) modification in the permeation of the drug to reach its target. Modification in the drug target enzymes can occur due to either mutations in DNA gyrase or mutations in topoisomerase IV. However, the comparative effect of these mutations is found to be different in the process of owning resistance among distinct bacterial types. Generally, DNA gyrase is considered the primary target of quinolones in gram-negative species and topoisomerase IV the chief target in gram-positives, with exceptions. Out of these, the most prevalent mechanisms that lead to fluoroquinolone resistance are: (1) reduction in the affinity of enzymes DNA gyrase and topoisomerase IV to fluoroquinolones, which occur due to chromosomal mutation, and (2) heightened expression gene-regulating endogenous multidrug resistance pumps. The action of plasmid-mediated quinolone resistance determinants, like *qnr* genes, continues to increase. The phenotype of these genes usually reveals a low-grade resistance toward fluoroquinolones; however, it also contributes to escalate fluoroquinolone resistance mechanisms, which lead to further high-level resistance.

Pharmacokinetics

Fluoroquinolones have rapid oral absorption (except norfloxacin, 35–70%), reaching peak serum concentrations in 1 to 2 hours. Fluoroquinolones depict huge volume of distribution, which ranges from 1 to < 4 L/kg, with wide distribution in all tissues and body fluids. Their concentration in blood and urine is markedly greater than the minimum inhibitory concentrations for distinct bacterial pathogens. Fluoroquinolones are chiefly absorbed in the duodenum and the proximal jejunum and do not depend on acidic or alkaline pH, and are absorbed to the same extent with or without meal. The extended long half-lives enable dosing at interval of 12 to 24 hours. Due to superior bioavailability, oral dosing is often preferred over parenteral administration. After administration, they are thoroughly disseminated in body fluids and are mostly accumulated in the lungs, prostate, and bile. The newer fluoroquinolones depict adequate oral absorption to get optimum bactericidal activity for systemic infections. Oral absorption of fluoroquinolones decreases when they are given along with polyvalent cations (calcium, aluminum, zinc magnesium, and iron preparations).

Fluoroquinolones have mostly low protein binding (14–45%). The protein binding of ciprofloxacin, ofloxacin, levofloxacin, and gatifloxacin is 10 to 25%. Newer fluoroquinolones such trovafloxacin (65–70%), gemifloxacin (60%), and moxifloxacin (40–50%) have higher protein binding. Fluoroquinolones are mainly metabolized in the liver and get excreted in the urine. However, moxifloxacin is found to be primarily eliminated in the bile.

Spectrum of Activity

Fluoroquinolones have broad spectrum of bactericidal effect, showing concentration-dependent hindrance in bacteria replication. Fluoroquinolones act efficiently against Enterobacteriaceae and various gram-negative bacteria such as *Haemophilus influenzae*, *Neisseria meningitides*, *Neisseria gonorrhoeae*, and *Moraxella catarrhalis*. They also act on methicillin-susceptible *Staphylococcus aureus* and *Staphylococcus epidermidis*. The earlier quinolones (norfloxacin, ciprofloxacin, ofloxacin) are less effective on several streptococcal species, such as *S. pneumoniae*, *Streptococcus pyogenes*, and viridans streptococci. These agents also show moderate-to-poor effect on *Enterococcus* and are inactive against most anaerobic bacteria. Levofloxacin has prominent activity against gram-positive bacteria as well as against atypical organisms as compared to ciprofloxacin. Both the agents also possess activity against gram-negative pathogens including *P. aeruginosa*. The newer quinolones (gatifloxacin, moxifloxacin, and gemifloxacin) are even more effective against gram-positive and atypical organisms in contrast to levofloxacin. However, these agents are less active as compared with levofloxacin and ciprofloxacin against *P. aeruginosa*.

Clinical Uses

Genitourinary Infections

Fluoroquinolones, particularly ciprofloxacin and levofloxacin, are extremely useful in treating complicated UTIs and pyelonephritis.

Respiratory Tract Infections

Fluoroquinolones are widely used to treat sinusitis, bronchitis, community-acquired and nosocomial pneumonia, and complicated cystic fibrosis. These agents are found either superior or equivalent in its efficacy to other antimicrobial agents such as β-lactams or combination of β-lactam/macrolide.

Prostatitis

Fluoroquinolones are efficacious for prostatitis treatment, mainly because of their excellent ability to penetrate into prostatic tissue. Agents such as ciprofloxacin, ofloxacin, and levofloxacin are effective in the treatment of severe bacterial prostatitis caused by Enterobacteriaceae, and the success rate is approximately 60 to 80% in 4 to 6 weeks. These are considerable treatment options to trimethoprim–sulfamethoxazole. However, there is difficulty in eradicating infections due to enterococci and *P. aeruginosa*.

Gastroenteritis

Fluoroquinolones such as norfloxacin and ciprofloxacin are often used to treat travelers' diarrhea and found to be comparatively similar in action to trimethoprim–sulfamethoxazole. Norfloxacin is also comparatively better than doxycycline and trimethoprim–sulfamethoxazole for the treatment of *Vibrio cholerae* infection. Ofloxacin and ciprofloxacin are mostly recommended for enteric typhoid fever.

Skin and Soft-Tissue Infections

Most fluoroquinolones have restricted activity against gram-positive organisms, and thus they are not recommended as the first choice for any skin and soft-tissue infections. However, quinolones and antibiotics together in combination can be used for the treatment of diabetic foot, a polymicrobial infection. Fluoroquinolones such as moxifloxacin are often opted over ciprofloxacin for this condition due to their enhanced gram-positive activity.

Osteomyelitis

Fluoroquinolones such as ofloxacin and ciprofloxacin are effectively used for osteomyelitis treatment, which is caused by gram-negative organisms, with a 70 to 80% cure rate within a short span of time. These antibiotics are also used to treat osteomyelitis due to *S. aureus* with a higher dose range. Ofloxacin/rifampin combination is used in infected hip prostheses in a rare case.

Intra-abdominal Infections

Intravenous moxifloxacin or intravenous levofloxacin or ciprofloxacin combined with metronidazole is used for a variety of intra-abdominal and hepatobiliary infections.

Mycobacterial Infections

Fluoroquinolones are mostly preferred as second-line treatment option over most recommended drugs because of their potential to easily develop resistance. Moxifloxacin (single daily 400 mg dose) and levofloxacin (single daily 500–750 mg dose) are well-tolerated and cost-effective medication with good activity against *Mycobacterium tuberculosis*. Also, they are used most often with various antimycobacterial agents in the treatment of pulmonary disease caused by distinct atypical mycobacterium (*Mycobacterium chelonae* and *Mycobacterium fortuitum*).

Conjunctivitis

FDA has approved the topical application of fluoroquinolones such as ciprofloxacin, besifloxacin, gatifloxacin, ofloxacin, levofloxacin, and moxifloxacin for conjunctivitis in children younger than 12 months and adults. Ophthalmic solution of norfloxacin, ofloxacin, ciprofloxacin, and moxifloxacin are used successfully for the treatment of conjunctivitis and keratitis, mainly caused by *P. aeruginosa*, *S. aureus*, *S. pneumoniae*, and *H. influenzae*. Gonococcal conjunctivitis can also be effectively treated by giving a single systemic norfloxacin (1,200 mg) dose.

Choice of Fluoroquinolones

Fluoroquinolones, namely, ciprofloxacin, norfloxacin, ofloxacin, levofloxacin, and moxifloxacin are used most frequently, as they show a broad spectrum of antibacterial activity and desirable pharmacokinetic parameters. However, several newer fluoroquinolones have been discontinued mainly because of their toxicity issues. These agents are trovafloxacin (severe hepatotoxicity), grepafloxacin (cardiac toxicity), gatifloxacin (hypo- and hyperglycemia), temafloxacin (hemolytic anemia, hypoglycemia, hepatotoxicity, coagulopathy, acute renal failure), and enoxacin, lomefloxacin, and sparfloxacin.

Norfloxacin

Norfloxacin mostly acts on gram-negative organisms (including *Pseudomonas* species) and is generally less active than ciprofloxacin. Norfloxacin is mainly used in uncomplicated or acute UTI, chronic or complicated UTI, gastroenteritis, gonococcal and nongonococcal urethritis, and prostatitis. The half-life is approximately 4 hours (400 mg oral dose). Bioavailability is approximately 70%, and it has fast absorption. However, absorption slightly gets delayed when it is given along with food. It is metabolized and almost 30% (oral dose) is excreted in the urine in its original form. Norfloxacin is not recommended for respiratory and other systemic infections (specifically in cases of gram-positive cocci).

Ciprofloxacin

Ciprofloxacin is the most active form among the second-generation fluoroquinolones, which act effectively against both gram-positive and gram-negative bacteria, and also the first choice against *P. aeruginosa*. Ciprofloxacin is used as a treatment option in a variety of infections, especially against gram-negative organisms. These mainly include complicated UTI, skin and bone infections, sexually transmitted diseases (chancroid and gonorrhea), lower respiratory tract infections, gastrointestinal infections (multiresistant pathogens), febrile neutropenia, intra-abdominal infections, and malignant external otitis. Ciprofloxacin is comparatively more effective than aminoglycosides and trimethoprim–sulfamethoxazole for the treatment of complicated UTI in 7- to 10-day courses. It is also the rarest broad-spectrum agent that is accessible in both oral and intravenous formulations. Ciprofloxacin is reported to have same efficacy as fleroxacin, ceftriaxone, and ceftazidime and higher than that of imipenem–cilastatin in pneumonia patients (especially nosocomial). The main target of ciprofloxacin is bacterial DNA gyrase. Adverse events linked with ciprofloxacin intake are usually not very serious, involving nutritional disorders or gastrointestinal tract, metabolic, or central nervous system (CNS) problem. Therefore, ciprofloxacin is mostly recommended to continue despite these effects. Ciprofloxacin is primarily metabolized by CYP1A2. It is mainly excreted unchanged in the feces and urine; however, traces of metabolites have also been detected. The half-life is approximately 4 hours and oral bioavailability is of 70 to 80%.

Levofloxacin

Levofloxacin is an optically active L-isomer of ofloxacin. Levofloxacin depicts its activity against a wide range of gram-positive, gram-negative, and other atypical organisms such as *Legionella pneumophila*, *C. pneumoniae*, and *M. pneumoniae*. Levofloxacin is quickly assimilated after oral intake, having peak plasma concentrations within 1 to 2 hours. The bioavailability (~99%) is equivalent in different formulations (tablet and intravenous) of levofloxacin. Levofloxacin is used in the treatment of complicated UTI, acute pyelonephritis, acute bacterial sinusitis, and community-acquired pneumonia. Ophthalmic solution of levofloxacin (0.5%) is also used to treat conjunctivitis. Clinically adverse effects with levofloxacin, such as symptomatic hypo- and hyperglycemia, have been seen in diabetes mellitus patients who are on hypoglycemic agents/insulin. Levofloxacin has not been recommended in infants due to its toxic effect on the developing joints. Breastfeeding should be avoided for at least 4 to 6 hours after taking levofloxacin dose by the nursing mother to decrease drug exposure to the infant.

Moxifloxacin

Moxifloxacin, like other fluoroquinolones, is recommended to treat infections caused by both gram-positive and gram-negative bacteria, and has comparatively better activity than ciprofloxacin. It can also act on *C. trachomatis*. Among other fluoroquinolones, it has a high potency against *M. tuberculosis*. Moxifloxacin acts particularly on the topoisomerase IV bacterial enzyme. The bioavailability is approximately 90%, showing good absorption from the gastrointestinal tract after oral intake. The half-life is approximately 11.5 to 15.6 hours (single dose, oral, 400 mg). Moxifloxacin is mostly given for the treatment of sinusitis, bronchitis, pneumonias, and otitis media, and its action is comparable to β-lactam antibiotics. It is not recommended for UTI. Moxifloxacin is usually well tolerated, and most of the adverse events are related to the CNS (mild headache, dizziness) or gastrointestinal tract (constipation, abdominal pain, nausea, diarrhea, vomiting, taste alteration, vaginitis). Caution is warranted while it is used in patients who have electrolyte imbalance (hypomagnesemia, hypokalemia, or hypocalcemia), those who are on starvation or liquid protein fast diets, abnormal QT_c intervals, and previous/current history of coronary artery disease or arrhythmias.

Adverse Effects

Glucose Levels Alteration

Fluoroquinolone causes either hypo- or hyperglycemia. The reason behind this alteration is still unknown. Gatifloxacin (not in use now) causes most serious effect. Levofloxacin and ciprofloxacin were found least associated with significant dysglycemia.

CNS Effects

CNS adverse effects include mood swing, insomnia, mild headache, dizziness, and drowsiness, which are observed in less than 5% of the population who are on fluoroquinolone medication. Seizures are rare and mostly occur at higher doses. Nonsteroidal anti-inflammatory drugs given concomitantly with fluoroquinolones were found to elevate CNS stimulatory effect and hence are not recommended in patients with CNS disorder.

QT_c Prolongation

Few quinolones were discontinued mainly due to extensive QT_c prolongation. This situation can produce torsades de pointes, a less common but possibly lethal ventricular tachycardia. Least prolongation of QT_c interval has been seen mainly in levofloxacin and ciprofloxacin.

Hepatotoxicity

Some fluoroquinolones such as ofloxacin, levofloxacin, and moxifloxacin have shown rare evidence of hepatotoxicity. Hepatotoxicity may range from asymptomatic increase in hepatic enzymes to, occasionally, clinical jaundice.

Phototoxicity

Fluoroquinolones lead to photosensitivity, which can be observed as hyperpigmentation, erythema, desquamation, and edema. The symptom vanishes within a few weeks after withdrawal of the drug causing the symptom. This adverse effect is related to dosages and is not related to patient's age.

Allergic Reactions

Almost all fluoroquinolones cause pruritus and rashes to some extent. Levofloxacin, gatifloxacin, and moxifloxacin are found to cause rash in almost 1% of patients, whereas gemifloxacin causes rashes in approximately 4.8% of patients.

Peripheral Neuropathy

It can arise soon after drug intake and sometimes get permanent. Fluoroquinolones are not advisable further if symptoms (such as numbness, pain, tingling burning, weakness, loss of sensation) appear on its use; otherwise, it may lead to irreversible damage.

Tendinopathy

Tendinopathy is a rare side effect of fluoroquinolones; however, a black box caution has been recently added to fluoroquinolones. Clinically, it may extend from mild tendinitis to overt tendon disruption in which the "Achilles tendon" is the main affected site. Patients with degenerative diseases, diabetes, or renal failure or those on steroid medications are at higher risk.

Clostridium difficile–Associated Diarrhea

Fluoroquinolones may lead to *Clostridium difficile*–associated diarrhea (pseudomembranous colitis), particularly caused by hypervirulent *C. difficile* ribotype 027.

Contraindications

Clinically, fluoroquinolones are contraindicated due to suspected toxicities in some groups of population, which include elder and pediatric patients as well as pregnant and breastfeeding women. The potential of fluoroquinolones for aortic disruption and dissection side effects is a cause of concern among old-aged patients, where there are chances of hemorrhage or even death.

Drug Interaction

Drugs that contain metal ions (such as antacids having sucralfate and ferrous sulfate, magnesium, and aluminum, aluminum hydroxide, and sulfate sucrose complex) are found to interact with most newer fluoroquinolones. These drugs lead to bioavailability reduction from about 85 to 35% of concomitantly administered fluoroquinolones. This interaction is supposed to be mediated via chelation of metal cations with the fluoroquinolones, which results in the formation of insoluble drug–cationic complexes. This complex reduces the absorption and hence bioavailability of the agents. Therefore, it is suggested to take these fluoroquinolones at least 2 hours before taking any drugs having metal ions. Several drugs in the fluoroquinolone class of antibiotics (ciprofloxacin or norfloxacin) are known to interfere with the metabolism of theophylline, where blood theophylline concentrations double. Caution should be exercised while prescribing quinolones and theophylline together, especially in the elderly. Some fluoroquinolones antagonize the association of GABA with both the sodium-dependent (presynaptic) and the sodium-independent (postsynaptic) GABA receptors, and competitively displace GABA from the GABA receptors. Administration of ciprofloxacin together with warfarin leads to aggravated anticoagulation, especially in higher age group patients. This occurs due to reduction in metabolism of warfarin. A potentially toxic interaction of ciprofloxacin and tizanidine has been observed. This is given for relaxation from muscle pain linked with muscle tension or spasticity. Interaction between these drugs leads to exaggerated CNS effects and drastic fall in blood pressure. This may happen due to reduced liver metabolism of tizanidine. Now, this combination is contraindicated.

Multiple Choice Question

1. A 66-year-old man develops renal failure. Which of the following drugs requires a major adjustment in dosage?

A. Levofloxacin.
B. Ceftriaxone.
C. Amphotericin B.
D. Clindamycin.
E. Ampicillin.

Answer: A

Most of the fluoroquinolones are renally excreted and therefore require dose adjustment in renal failure. Exceptions are moxifloxacin and pefloxacin, which are metabolized by the liver.

Chapter 59A Penicillin

Shantanu R. Joshi

Learning Objectives

- Mechanism of action of penicillin.
- Narrow-spectrum penicillins.
- Broad-spectrum penicillins.
- Beta-lactamase inhibitors.
- Carbapenems.

History

In 1928, Alexander Fleming, a microbiologist, while doing some experiments noticed that one of the molds prevented the growth of bacteria in culture plates. The mold was of Penicillium notatum; hence, he gave the name "Penicillin" to that antibacterial substance. Today, penicillin is commercially obtained from high-yielding Penicillium chrysogenum.

In 1940s at Oxford University, well-organized research under Florey, Chain, and Abraham resulted in the production of penicillin in the form of few milligrams sufficient to treat only one person with a single dose. Later, with the developments in synthesis process, a significant amount of penicillin was possible to produce. In 1942, clinical trials were organized at Yale University and Mayo Clinic involving 200 patients with a mix of streptococcal and staphylococcal infections. The results were so amazing that the surgeon general of the U.S. Army authorized the clinical trial of penicillin in military hospital. This became a part of routine treatment of U.S. military services during World War II.

Chemistry Side Chain R Beta-lactam Ring Thiazoline Ring

The basic structure of penicillin consists of two important rings 1. beta-lactam ring and 2. thiazoline ring (**Fig. 59A.1**).

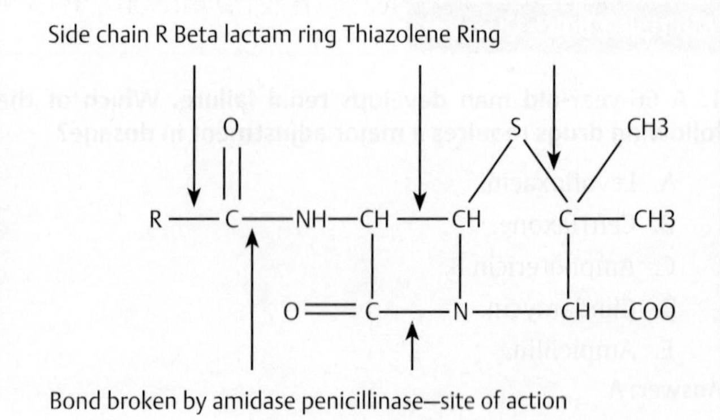

Side chain R Beta lactam ring Thiazolene Ring

Bond broken by amidase penicillinase—site of action

Fig. 59A.1 Basic structure of penicillin molecule.

For biological activity of penicillin, beta-lactam ring is a must. The side chain of penicillin molecule determines the pharmacological properties of the specific penicillin. It also defines its antimicrobial activity.

Mechanism of Action of Penicillin

The bacterial cytoplasm is hyperosmolar and tends to absorb water from outside. This leads to swelling and bursting of bacteria. However, the bacteria is surrounded by cell wall. This cell wall is made up of peptidoglycan, which is rigid and does not allow bacteria to swell and burst. It is actually a polymer of disaccharides; the two disaccharides repeat, namely, N-acetyl-glucosamine and N-acetyl-muramic acid. They are attached to peptide side chains, which are cross-linked, providing considerable strength to cell wall (**Fig. 59A.2**).

In peptide linkage of N-acetyl muramic acid, the D-alanine residue is attached to the L-Lysine residue of the next peptide linkage of N-acetyl muramic acid. This linking is done by five glycine residues. This reaction is called transpeptidation, and it is catalyzed by penicillin-binding proteins. When penicillin is administered to the patient, it binds to these penicillin-binding proteins; hence, these proteins will not be available for transpeptidation reaction, cross-linking will not be possible, and this is how a deficient cell wall is produced. Because of the deficient cell wall, the bacterium absorbs water from outside, swells, and bursts. This is how bactericidal effect comes into effect.

PBPs are transmembrane proteins. There are three important PBPs identified. PBP1 is related to transpeptidation reaction, that is, attachment of L-lysine to D-alanine. PBP 2 is responsible for the hydrolysis of D-alanine, which is important to continue cross-linking. PBP3 is related to the separation of cells after division. Its inhibition leads to filamentation, which means the newly formed bacterial cells cannot separate from one another and form a long filament-like structure.

When penicillin is administered to the patient, it binds to these PBPs. Hence, PBP1 will not be available for transpeptidation reaction. Thus, cross-linking is not possible, leading to deficient cell wall production. Because of the deficient cell wall, the bacteria absorb water from outside, swell, and burst.

Another mechanism is the activation of autolysins. The autolysins are the enzymes which are involved in degradation of worn-out cell wall components. In normal bacteria, the action of autolysins is inhibited by autolysin inhibitors. Autolysin inhibitors are naturally occurring proteins. Penicillins are known to bind to autolysin inhibitors

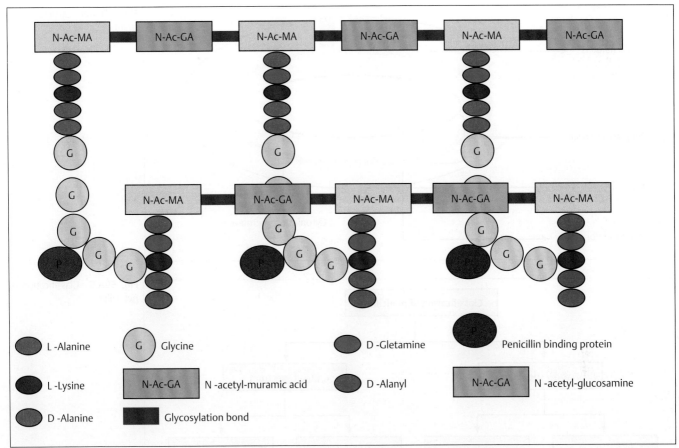

Fig. 59A.2 Note the D-alanine of one N-acetyl-muramic acid is attached to L- Lysine of the subsequent N-acetyl-muramic acid by 5 gycine residues. This is transpeptidation. This reaction is catalyzed by penicillin-binding proteins. Penicillin binds to PBP and interferes with transpeptidation reaction leading to development of deficient cell wall.

and ultimately activate autolysins, which degrade cell wall components. A deficient cell wall will allow the bacterium to absorb water, swell and burst.

Cell wall synthesis occurs in actively dividing bacteria; hence, penicillins are more active in actively dividing bacteria and are least effective in dormant bacteria. Peptidoglycan molecule is unique to the bacteria; hence, penicillins are least toxic to human beings.

In Gram-positive bacteria, this cell wall is very thick (**Fig. 59A.3**). There is easy access to PBPs and hence penicillin penetrates easily and can stop the transpeptidation reaction. This is why penicillins are more effective in Gram-positive bacteria.

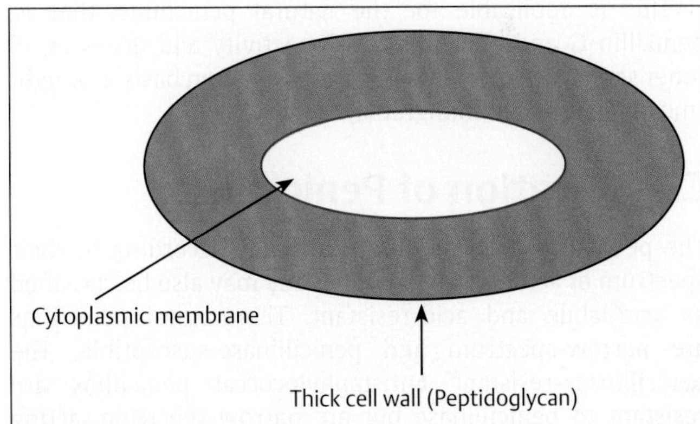

Fig. 59A.3 Structure of gram-positive bacterium

In Gram-negative bacteria, the cell wall is thin. The Gram-negative bacteria have cytoplasmic membrane surrounded by thin cell wall (**Fig. 59A.4**). There is an outermost membrane of lipids mainly made up of lipopolysaccharides. The space between the cytoplasmic membrane and lipid outer membrane is known as periplasmic space. In Gram-negative bacteria, outer lipid membrane restricts the entry of many substances, including penicillin G. There are some channels for transport of material to the bacterial cytoplasm. These channels are known as porin channels, but they are narrow; hence, penicillins are least effective in Gram-negative bacteria. Some semisynthetic penicillins, which are hydrophilic like ampicillin or amoxicillin, can be transported through porin channels; hence, they are effective in some Gram-negative bacteria. However, they are still not effective in *Pseudomonas aeruginosa*, as this organism lacks classical porin channels.

Unitage of Penicillin

1 unit of penicillin is the activity expressed by 0.6 mcg of crystalline Na or K salt of penicillin G or 600 mg equals 1 MU of crystalline Na or K salt of penicillin G

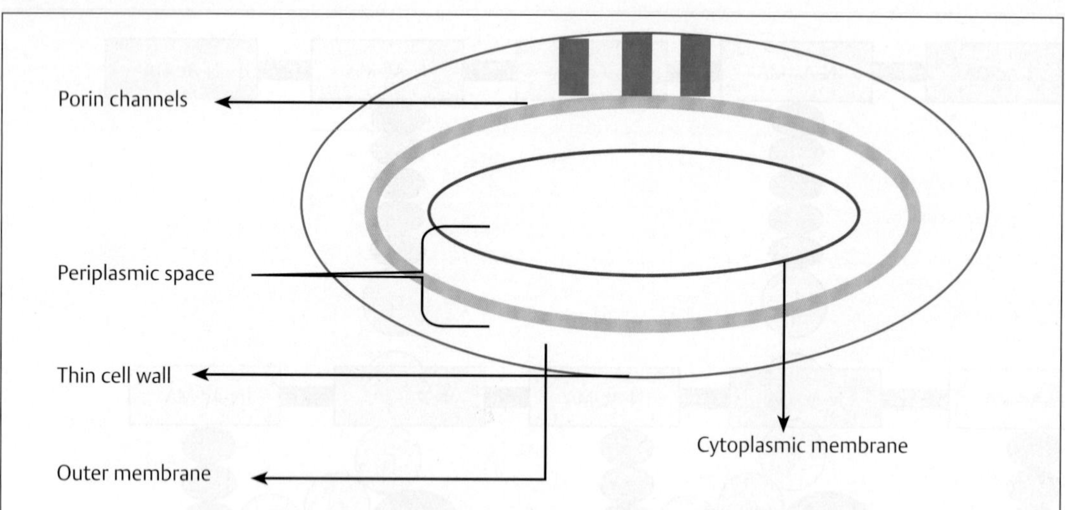

Fig. 59A.4 Structure of gram-negative bacterium.

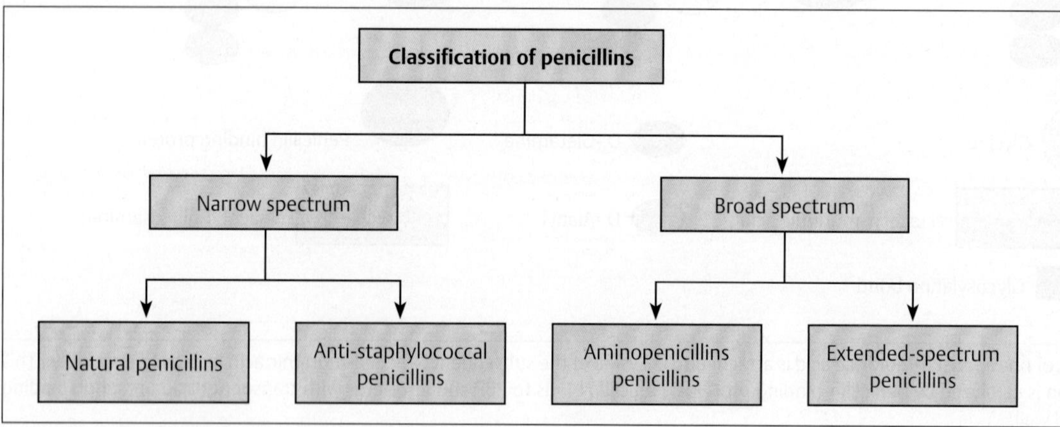

Fig. 59A.5 Classification of penicillins.

This is applicable for the natural penicillins, that is, penicillin G and penicillin V. The activity and doses of all other semisynthetic penicillin is measured on basis of weight (mostly in terms of milligrams).

Classification of Penicillins

The penicillins are classified principally according to their spectrum of activity (**Fig. 59A.5**). They may also be classified as acid-labile and acid-resistant. The natural penicillins are narrow-spectrum and penicillinase-susceptible. The penicillinase-resistant antistaphylococcal penicillins are resistant to penicillinase but are narrow-spectrum, acting against staphylococci and streptococci. The broad-spectrum penicillins are classified as aminopenicillins, which are more water-soluble and can cross the porin channels of some Gram-negative bacteria; hence, they are useful in some Gram-negative bacterial infections but not *P. aeruginosa*, because it lacks the classical porin channels. The most important group in the broad-spectrum penicillins is extended-spectrum penicillins. These are most active in seriously ill patients and cover excellent Gram-negative spectrum.

Narrow-Spectrum Penicillins

Natural penicillins and anti-Staphylococcal penicillins.

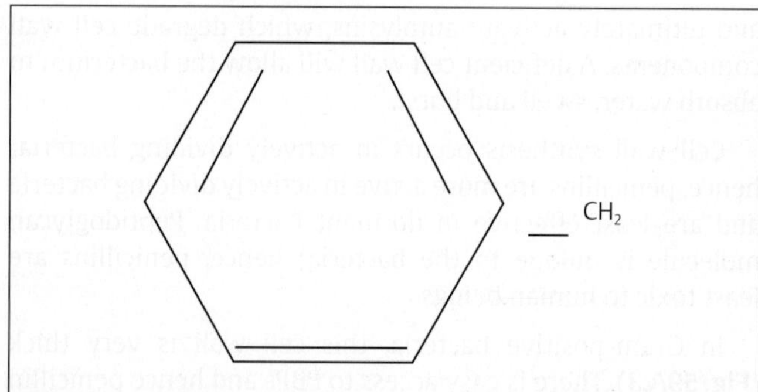

Fig. 59A.6 *R*-side chain of Penicillin G.

Natural Penicillins

Penicillin G and penicillin V are referred as natural penicillins. Penicillin G is produced by the substitution of R side chain as shown in **Fig. 59A.6**.

Penicillin V is acid-stable and hence can be given by oral route, but penicillin G is acid-labile; hence, it is given by intramuscular (IM) or intravenous (IV) route. Benzathine penicillin and procaine penicillin are depot penicillin G, as they release penicillin at extremely slow rate and hence are long-acting. Procaine penicillin acts for 12 hours to 24 hours and benzathine penicillin acts for 3 to 4 weeks.

Generally, the concentration of penicillin G in tissue is approximately equal to plasma except in central nervous system (CNS). Penetration of penicillin to CNS is poor (<1%) but in inflammation (5%), it is sufficient to control infection in meningitis. The concentration of penicillin in phagocytic cells, prostate, and ocular tissue is not significant.

Plasma half-life ranges from 30 to 90 minutes. Penicillin G is very little metabolized to penicilloic acid in liver. The excretion of the natural penicillin is by renal pathway. Tubular secretion is the major pathway (90%) and glomerular filtration (10%) is the minor pathway. Probenecid can block the tubular secretion of natural penicillin and prolongs the plasma half-life. Probenecid also reduces the active secretion of penicillin from cerebrospinal fluid (CSF) to blood, allowing more concentration of penicillin in CSF. In renal failure, the dose of penicillin should be adjusted as per the creatinine clearance.

Antibacterial Spectrum

Natural penicillins are highly active against Gram-positive cocci and bacilli and moderately active against Gram-negative cocci and *actinomyces.* They are, however, almost not active against Gram-negative bacilli and Bacteroides. Most of the *Streptococci* were sensitive but have now acquired significant resistance. This is especially important in case of *Streptococcus pneumoniae* (pneumonia) and *Streptococcus viridans* (subacute bacterial endocarditis). Notable exceptions are *meningiococci, Clostridium tetani,* and *Corynebacterium diphtheriae,* which are sensitive to penicillin G. Most species of leptospira are sensitive. *Treponema pallidum* of syphilis and *Borrlia burgdorferi* of Lyme disease are also sensitive to penicillin G.

Penicillin Testing

Penicillin must be tested intradermally before injecting. All penicillin preparations are to be prepared as and when required.

Caution

Test dose of penicillin itself can produce anaphylaxis. So, it is important to ensure all lifesaving drugs are in places like adrenalin, hydrocortisone, and pheniramine maleate. All basic life support instruments need to be at hand.

Procedure

Prepare the solution with distilled water, with 5 mL of it being poured and properly shacked. Only benzyl penicillin gives clear solution, as all other forms of penicillin solutions are turbid. Take 0.1 to 0.2 mL of the solution and inject it intradermally on extended forearm. Wait for 5 to 10 minutes, in order to observe any form of redness, itching or rash on the site of injection. Any form of hypersensitivity contraindicates use of penicillin.

Market Preparations of Penicillins

1. **Sodium penicillin G (crystalline penicillin)**—0.5–5 MU IM/IV.

   Brand—BENZYL PEN 0.5, 1 MU inj. every 6 to 12 hours for 5 days or as per the need.

2. **Procaine penicillin G**—0.5-MU IM only.

   Brand—PROCAINE PENICILLIN G 0.5/1 MU dry powder per vial once a day (OD) for 5 days.

3. **Fortified procaine penicillin**

   Brand—FORTIFIED PP OR PPF (crystalline penicillin 1 lac U and procaine penicillin 3 lac U) for 5 days OD IM only.

4. **Benzathine penicillin G**—0.6 to 2.4 MU I/M every 2 to 4 weeks as aqueous suspension and as deep IM in buttock.

   Brand—PENIDURE LA 0.6/1.2/2.4 MU as dry powder per vial every 2 to 4 weeks.

5. **Penicillin V**—Tab. 125/250 mg, 125 mg/5 mL dry syp. orally.

Penicillinase-Resistant Penicillins (PRP)

These types of penicillins are also known as antistaphylococcal penicillins.

Cloxacillin, flucloxacillin, oxacillin, dicloxacillin, methicillin, and nafcillin are the important members of this group. These types of penicillins have bulky side chain of R that protects the beta-lactam ring from hydrolysis by penicillinase. These penicillins are useful for treating the infections by penicillinase-producing *Staphylococcus aureus* and *Staphylococcus epidermidis* which are not methicillin-resistant. These types of penicillins are less effective than penicillin G in treating the infections Streptococcus pneumoniae and Streptococcus pyogenes do not produce penicillinase. Due to bulky nature of these drugs, the entry through porin channel is restricted; hence, they are not useful in treating Gram-negative infections. The only indication is staphylococcal infection caused by staphylococci-producing penicillinase. There are methicillin-resistant staphylococci known as MRSA. Penicillinase-resistant penicillins (PRP) are not resistant to beta-lactamase produced by Gram-negative bacteria.

Cloxacillin

Cloxacillin, dicloxacillin, and oxacillin are known as isoxazolyl penicillins. They are similar in pharmacological action. Only cloxacillin is available in the market. It is acid-resistant and hence is given by oral route. It has isoxazolyl side chain. It is highly penicillinase-resistant. It is inferior to penicillin G for other infection caused by other bacteria and those not producing penicillinase. It should be taken empty stomach; absorption is less but adequate. It is largely protein bound (90%). The route of elimination is liver and kidney. Plasma half-life is 1 hour. Cloxacillin can be given by parenteral routes like IM or IV in severe infections. Dose—250/500 mg four times a day (QID) orally and in severe infections 250 mg to 1 gm by IM or IV route.

Nafcillin

It is produced by the substitution of R side chain as shown in **Fig. 59A.7**.

It is a penicillinase-resistant antistaphylococcus penicillin. Its oral absorption is erratic and hence given by IV route. It is metabolized by liver and excreted in bile. The concentrations in CSF are sufficient to treat Staphylococcal meningitis; however, this type of meningitis is rare. The most important

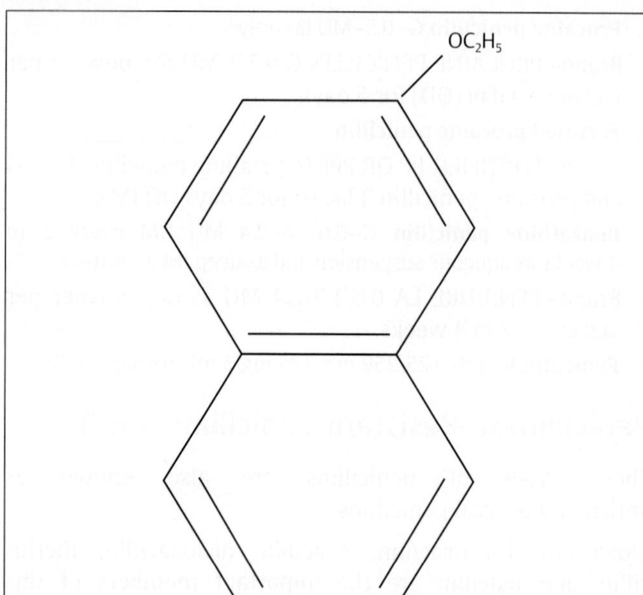

Fig. 59A.7 R side chain of nafcillin.

advantage of this drug is its usefulness in renal failure patients. It is not available in India.

Methicillin

It is acid-labile and hence can be given by IV route. Methicillin is the most active PRP from this group. Methicillin is withdrawn from market because it causes serious interstitial nephritis.

Broad-spectrum Penicillins

Semisynthetic Penicillins– Aminopenicillins

The changes in the side chain which alters the pharmacological properties as well as antimicrobial spectrum can be produced by the action of amidase on side chain (**Fig. 59A.8**).

Commercially, Penicillium chrysogenum is the right species to produce 6-aminopenicillanic acid during the fermentation process, as it contains good amount of amidase naturally. Addition of different groups to 6-aminopenicillanic acid produces different types of penicillins (**Fig. 59A.9**).

These are extended spectrum, acid-resistant, but are susceptible to penicillinase both by Gram-positive and Gram-negative organisms. The amino group added to these penicillins increases their hydrophilicity and also increases the movement through porin channels; hence they are effective in some Gram-negative bacteria which include *E. coli, H. influenza, Proteus, Salmonella, Shigella*, and *H. pylori.* With the continued use, these drugs in clinical practice developed resistance to above said organisms. Most of the *Pseudomonas, Klebsiella, Acinetobactor* and indole positive *Proteus* also are now resistant. Addition of beta-lactamase inhibitors re-establishes the activity of these drugs to originally sensitive bacteria.

Ampicillin

It is produced by the substitution of R side chain as shown in **Fig. 59A.8**. It is acid-stable and hence can be given by oral route. Food decreases the absorption; hence, it should be given 1 hour before or 1 hour after food. It can be given by parenteral routes to achieve higher plasma levels. Plasma half live is 1 to 1.5 hours. The route of elimination is hepatic as well as renal. While ampicillin is being eliminated by liver in gastrointestinal tract (GIT), some reabsorption takes place in the form of enterohepatic circulation. In renal failure, drug accumulates in blood and hence needs dose adjustment in renal failure. As it is also excreted in feces, it is more active in treating diarrhea due to *Shigella* than amoxicillin.

Dose—Cap. 250/500 mg, Syp—125/250 mg/5 mL, 100 mg/mL pediatric drops, Inj. 250 mg/500 mg/1 gm/vial.

Amoxicillin

It is close congener of ampicillin. It is acid-stable and hence is used by oral route. The oral absorption of the drug is complete. Food does not affect the absorption of amoxicillin; hence, it can be taken with food. It is fully absorbed from GIT, not excreted through bile, and hence, it is less effective than ampicillin in diarrhea due to Shigella. It also reduces the possibility of diarrhea due to irritant property. The spectrum of activity is very similar to ampicillin. The drug is almost excreted in unchanged form in urine. Probenecid competes for the tubular secretion of drug and makes it long-acting.

Doses—cap. 250/500 mg, syp. 125 mg/5 mL (dry syp), inj. 250/500 mg (dry powder).

Extended-Spectrum Penicillins

These are most active and currently the most preferred penicillins in life-threatening Gram-negative infections, especially hospital-acquired. The R side chain of natural penicillin is replaced by the group, as shown in **Fig. 59A.10**, to produce piperacillin. Piperacillin is the most commonly prescribed.

Carboxy–penicillins

Carbenicillin and ticarcillin and some other related drugs which are active against some strains of *P. aeruginosa* and certain indole-positive *Proteus* species that are resistant to ampicillin and its congeners. They are ineffective against most strains of *Staphylococcus aureus, Enterococcus faecalis, Klebsiella*, and *Listeria monocytogenes. B. fragilis* is susceptible at high concentrations of these drugs but penicillin G is more active.

Carbenicillin

Carbenicillin is sensitive to penicillinase. It is administrated by IV route in the dose of 1 to 5 g every 4 to 6 hours. It is a sodium salt; hence, at higher doses, sodium load increases, leading to sodium retention, which may complicate the patients of congestive cardiac failure (CCF) and renal failure. In higher doses, it interferes with platelet function and bleeding

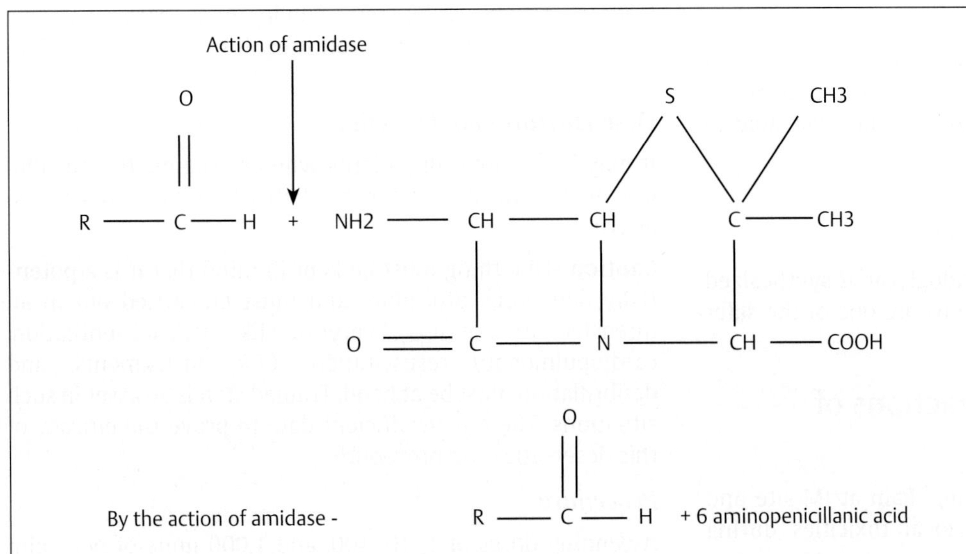

Fig. 59A.8 Action of amidase and formation of aminopenicillanic acid.

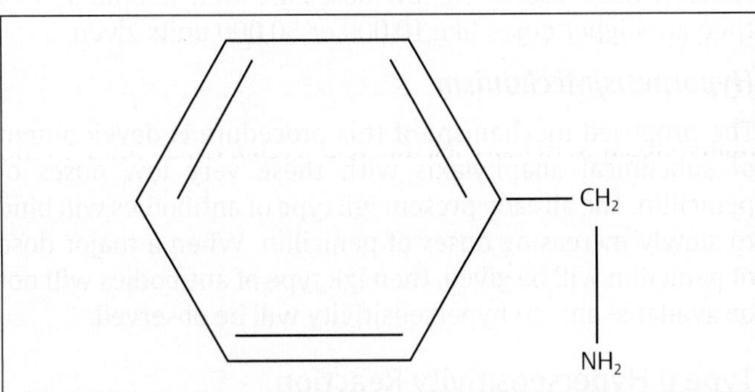

Fig. 59A.9 R side chain of ampicillin.

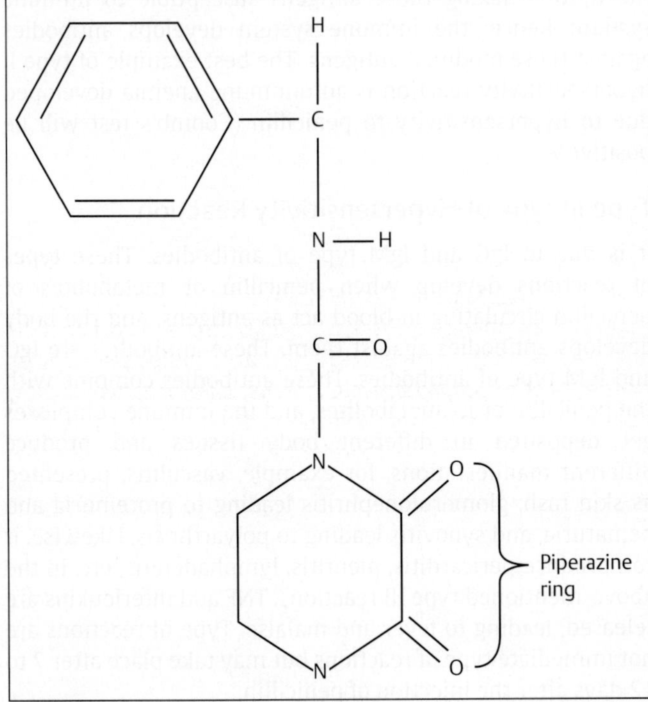

Fig. 59A.10 R side chain of piperacillin.

episodes have been observed. In place of carbenicillin, today, we prefer to use ticarcillin and piperacillin.

Dose–1-5 gm/every 6 hours

Carbenicillin Indanyl Sodium

6. It is the ester of carbenicillin which is acid resistant and hence this preparation is used orally. After absorption, the hydrolysis of the ester yields carbenicillin. The total drug absorbed is not sufficient to treat systemic infections but is excreted in urine and hence is effective in urinary tract infection (UTI) caused by proteus and pseudomonas type of Gram-negative organisms. It is not available in India.

Ticarcillin

It is 2-4 times more active with fewer side effects as compared to carbenicillin; hence, it is preferred to treat *pseudomonas* and *proteus*. It is sensitive to penicillinase and hence is combined with clavulanic acid. For serious Gram-negative septicemia, it can be combined with one of the newer aminoglycosides.

Dose–available with clavulanic acid 3.1 g/vial every 6 hours.

Ureidopenicillins

Piperacillin

This is extended-spectrum antipseudomonal penicillin covering *P. aeruginosa*, *Klebsiella*, indole-positive *proteus*, nonbeta-lactamase-producing *Enterobacteriaceae* and many *Bacteroides*, which are not inhibited by penicillin G or aminopenicillins. It is frequently used to treat serious Gram-negative infections like septicemia, UTI, burns, lower respiratory tract infection (LRTI) and infections in immunocompromised patients. Usually, it is combined with aminoglycosides to cover best Gram-negative spectrum.

Dose–1 g, 2 g, and 4 g vial every 6 to 12 hours, with maximum dose of 16 g/day.

Mezlocillin

Mezlocillin belongs to the ureidopenicillins group and is more active for Klebsiella than carbenicillin. It is more active than ticarcillin in treating *E. faecalis*. It is not available in India.

Adverse Drug Reactions

It must be remembered that no peptidoglycan is synthesized by human beings and hence penicillins are one of the safer antibiotics used clinically.

Common Adverse Drug Reactions of Penicillins

Oral doses cause nausea and vomiting. Pain at IM site and thrombophlebitis of the vein are local toxicities during administration of penicillins.

Hypersensitivity Reactions

Intradermal skin testing is must before injecting penicillin to the patient.

1. Skin testing itself may show hypersensitivity, and even anaphylaxis has been reported.
2. A negative skin test does not completely exclude hypersensitivity reaction.
3. A person taking penicillin regularly may show hypersensitivity with future dose.
4. There is cross-sensitivity between different penicillin and even cephalosporins.
5. The allergy may be to penicillin or may be to the added substances like procaine.

Type I Hypersensitivity Reaction

Hypersensitivity reactions are most commonly associated with penicillin and is the most important cause of decline in use of penicillins. The incidence is about 0.7 to 10%. It is generally manifested as maculopapular rash, urticarial rash, fever, bronchospasms, vasculitis, serum sickness, exfoliative dermatitis, Stevens–Johnson syndrome, and anaphylaxis in decreasing order.

This is IgE-mediated reaction. With the prior exposure directly or indirectly, our body develops IgE type of antibodies which are attached to mast cells and basophils. When penicillin is administered to these patients, there is activation of mast cells and basophils, leading to their degranulation and releasing so many different chemical mediators in the blood such as prostaglandins, interleukins, TNF, histamines, leukotrienes, and different proteolytic enzymes.

The most serious form of type I hypersensitivity reactions are angioedema and anaphylaxis/anaphylactoid reactions. The incidence estimated to be between 0.004 and 0.04%. Fatal outcome is seen in 0.001% reactions. Angioedema is presented as swelling of lips, tongue and face, and periorbital tissue. In anaphylaxis or anaphylactoid reaction, there is sudden drop in blood pressure (BP), bronchoconstriction leading to breathlessness, abdominal pain, extreme weakness, and nausea and vomiting. It may lead to death in severe cases.

Desensitization of Penicillin

It may be required in patients who are allergic to penicillin but need penicillin as a part of this treatment, having no alternative.

Caution—One thing must be kept in mind that it is a potentially dangerous procedure and must be carried out in an intensive care unit (ICU). Everything like artificial ventilation, cardiopulmonary resuscitation (CPR) instruments, and defibrillation must be at hand. Trained staff is an asset in such situations. There is insufficient data to prove the efficacy of this desensitization procedure.

Procedure

Ascending doses of 1, 10, 100, and 1,000 units of penicillin should be given with an interval of 60 minutes by intradermal route. If these ascending low doses are well-tolerated, only then are higher doses like 10,000 or 50,000 units given.

Hypothesis/Mechanism

The proposed mechanism of this procedure is development of subclinical anaphylaxis with these very low doses of penicillin. The already present IgE type of antibodies will bind to slowly increasing doses of penicillin. When a major dose of penicillin will be given, then IgE type of antibodies will not be available and no hypersensitivity will be observed.

Type II Hypersensitivity Reaction

It is IgG type of reaction. The breakdown products of penicillin react with the inherently present antigens in the tissue, making those antigens susceptible to immune system; hence, the immune system develops antibodies against these modified antigens. The best example of type II hypersensitivity reaction is autoimmune anemia developed due to hypersensitivity to penicillin (Coomb's test will be positive).

Type III type of Hypersensitivity Reaction

It is due to IgG and IgM type of antibodies. These types of reactions develop when penicillin or metabolites of penicillin circulating in blood act as antigens, and the body develops antibodies against them. These antibodies are IgG and IgM type of antibodies. These antibodies combine with the penicillin or its metabolites, and the immune complexes get deposited in different body tissues and produce different manifestations, for example, vasculitis, presented as skin rash, glomerulonephritis leading to proteinuria and hematuria, and synovitis leading to polyarthritis. Likewise, it can produce pericarditis, pleuritis, lymphadenitis, etc. In the above-mentioned type III reactions, TNF and interleukins are released, leading to fever and malaise. Type III reactions are not immediate type of reactions but may take place after 7 to 12 days after the injection of penicillin.

1. The extended-spectrum penicillins when given for longer duration can alter the microflora of the GIT and can lead to diarrhea or even pseudomembranous colitis.

2. Jarisch–Herxheimer reaction is a reaction when penicillin is injected in a patient of secondary syphilis, which leads to shivering, fever, myalgia, and sometimes vascular collapse. It is due to sudden release of lytic enzymes by spirochetes. It does not recur. Treatment is symptomatic.
3. Penicillins at high doses or accumulated penicillins in blood irritate CNS and can lead to CNS toxicity which, in turn, leads to seizures. It may be seen in renal failure.
4. Methicillin is a known nephrotoxic drug leading to interstitial nephritis and hence has been withdrawn from the market. Nafcillin is known to be hepatotoxic, as it is metabolized and excreted by liver.
5. Ampicillin-related maculopapular rash is due to the direct toxic effect of ampicillin and not the hypersensitivity reaction. It is seen in Epstein–Barr virus infection (infectious mononucleosis). The same maculopapular rash is seen when ampicillin and allopurinol are given concurrently.
6. Oxacillin and nafcillin are known to produce hepatitis as adverse drug effect.
7. Carbenicillin and ticarcillin may bind to surface proteins of platelets and alter their function, leading to nonaggregation of platelet and bleeding.
8. Neutropenia is seen sometimes. It is due to alteration in surface proteins and development of antibodies against neutrophils.
9. Electrolyte disorders, that is, hypernatremia and hyperkalemia can occur with higher doses or in renal failure of crystalline Na salt and K salt of penicillin G, respectively

Uses of Penicillins

Upper Respiratory Tract Infections (URTIs)

Streptococci, Staphylococci, Haemophilus influenzae are common pathogens of URTI. It causes pharyngitis, tonsillitis, sinusitis, and otitis media. These infections respond well to penicillin. Procaine penicillin or fortified procaine penicillin is used for this purpose. Procaine penicillin is used for 5 days. Fortified procaine penicillin is more preferred, especially in the pediatric age group. Use of penicillin G for the above purpose has declined now. Ampicillin and amoxicillin are more effective in URTIs, because both of them are active against Gram-positive as well as Gram-negative organisms. Amoxicillin with clavulanic acid is more active in this regard. It is frequently prescribed in tonsillitis, pharyngitis, sinusitis, otitis media, and other oropharyngeal infections.

Lower Respiratory Tract Infections (LRTI)

In bronchitis, the infection is of mixed type, especially in elderly patients, and hence ampicillin or amoxicillin with clavulanic acid is a better choice. In *Pneumococcal* pneumonia, penicillin G can be used, provided the strain is susceptible. Now significant resistance has been developed to penicillin G and hence the better choice is amoxicillin with clavulanic acid or piperacillin with tazobactam (pneumonia)

Rheumatic Fever

Rheumatic fever is poststreptococcal manifestation. Benzathine penicillin is used for this purpose. 1.2 MU every 3 to 4 weeks maintains minimum inhibitory concentrations and hence colonization is prevented. These doses of benzathine penicillin are used for 5 years or up to the age of 18, whichever is longer.

Skin and Soft-tissue Infections

Staphylococcus aureus and *Staphylococcus epidermidis* are common organisms and are best covered by cloxacillin.

Syphilis

Treponema pallidum has not shown resistance to penicillin G; hence, it can be used to treat syphilis. 1.2 MU of procaine penicillin daily for 10 days. For advance cases, 2.4 MU weekly for 4 weeks is administered.

Gonorrhea

Neisseria gonorrhoeae was susceptible but now has got significant resistance. Fluoroquinolones are a better choice.

Urinary Tract Infections (UTIs)

Most of the uncomplicated UTIs can be treated with ampicillin because the most common pathogen is *E. coli* or other organisms from *Enterobacteriaceae* family, but they have now acquired significant resistant because of production of beta-lactamase. Addition of beta-lactamase inhibitor can re-establish the sensitivity. Fluoroquinolone are preferred for this purpose now.

Salmonella Infection

Administration of high dose of ampicillin or trimithoprim-sulfamethoxazole was in use, but due to resistance over time, ceftriaxone remains the best choice. Fluoroquinolone were also effective but now significant resistance to it has been developed.

Meningitis (IM17.13)

The most common organism in the pediatric age group is *Streptococcus pneumoniae* or *Neisseria meningitis*. As much as 20 to 30% of cases show resistance to ampicillin. Listeria monocytogenes causes meningitis in immunocompromised patients. Today, empirical treatment of meningitis should be vancomycin and/or one of the third-generation cephalosporins.

Serious Gram-Negative Infections

Most hospital-acquired, serious Gram-negative infections are *Pseudomonal* infections. In septicemia, pneumonia, complicated UTIs, burns, and immunocompromised patients, there is dominance of *Pseudomonas*. Today, the best choice is piperacillin with tazobactam. This combination covers best spectrum as compared to all other penicillins.

Bacterial Endocarditis

In bacterial endocarditis, benzyl-penicillin in doses of 0.5 to 1 MU every 6 hours should be given for 2 to 4 weeks.

It is observed that 25% of cases having valve deformity are followed by endocarditis after tooth extraction. In such situations, penicillin G can be used as prophylactic antibiotic, but nowadays, amoxicillin with clavulanic acid is preferred.

Leptospirosis

Penicillin G in doses of 1.5 MU injected every 6 hours for 7 days is curative. Benzyl-penicillin is used for this purpose.

Diphtheria

Antitoxin forms a major part of treatment, but procaine penicillin in doses of 1 to 2 MU can be used to prevent carrier stage.

Tetanus and Gas Gangrene

Clostridial infections are treated with penicillin G. Antitoxin forms the main part of the treatment but penicillin G is used as an adjuvant.

Some Rare Diseases

Penicillin G is used to treat anthrax, actinomycosis, and rat bite fever.

Posteurella Multocida

This organism is the cause of infection after a dog or cat bite. It is uniformly susceptible to penicillin G and ampicillin.

Resistance to Penicillins

Natural Resistance

Natural resistance means the bacteria were never susceptible to penicillin.

Intracellular Organism

The organisms that are present inside the human-cell-like *Rickettsia* and *Legionella* are naturally protected from the action of penicillin, as penicillin does not penetrate the human cells.

Lack of Peptidoglycan

Some bacteria do not produce peptidoglycan and hence penicillin will not be an effective antibiotic in organisms such as *Chlamydia* and *Mycoplasma*.

Acquired Resistance

Organisms which were originally sensitive to penicillin but have now acquired a resistance because of repeated use of the same antibiotic, in the same individual, for a similar type of infection.

Inactivation of Beta Lactam Ring by Beta-lactamase

This is not a single enzyme but the group of enzymes produced by bacteria against beta-lactam antibiotics to hydrolyze the beta lactam ring and convert penicillin into penicilloic acid (**Fig. 59A.11**). In Gram-positive bacteria, beta-lactamase is secreted in surrounding tissue and penicillin (beta-lactam antibiotics is inactivated before it comes in contact with the bacteria), but in Gram-negative bacteria, it is accumulated in periplasmic space and hence the antibiotic will be inactivated when it enters the bacteria.

They are classically divided into four classes. Continuous research is going on, and new information is coming out. This molecular classification was initially done by AMBLER.

Class A—extended-spectrum beta-lactamase (ESBL). These are plasmid-mediated beta-lactamases (TEM, SHV, CTX-M). They hydrolyze penicillin, oxyimino cephalosporins (e.g., cefotaxime, ceftriaxone, ceftazidime) and oxyimino monobactams (aztreonam) but not 7-alpha methoxy cephalosporins (e.g., cefoxitin, cefotetan) and carbapenems.

Class D—OXA (oxacillinase) ESBL. These are plasmid-mediated beta-lactamase which hydrolyze oxacillin and related antistaphylococcal penicillin. It differs from other beta-lactamases in its molecular structure. The beta-lactamase inhibitors have minimum effect on their activity.

Class C—ampC beta-lactamase is chromosome-mediated beta-lactamase and is inducible (upregulation or downregulation is possible). ampC hydrolyzes extended-spectrum cephalosporins– oxyimino cephalosporins (e.g., cefotaxime, ceftriaxone ceftazidime) and 7-alpha methoxy-cephalosporins (e.g., cefoxitin, cefotetan), and it cannot be blocked by common beta-lactamase inhibitors like clavulanic acid/sulbactam/tazobactam.

Class B—IMP-VIM beta-lactamases. These are metallobeta-lactamases as Zn^{2+} is required for their activity. These are also called as carbepenemeses. They hydrolyze penicillins, cephalosporins, and carbapenems but not monobactams (aztreonam). They cannot be blocked by beta-lactamase inhibitors.

NDM-1—*E. coli* and *K. pneumoniae* exhibit mutation in gene, resulting in resistance to all beta-lactams by production of beta-lactamase. This was first demonstrated in New Delhi; hence, the name is NMD-1. These mutant organisms exhibit efflux pumps as well as some other mechanisms, which make them resistant to fluoroquinolone, macrolides,

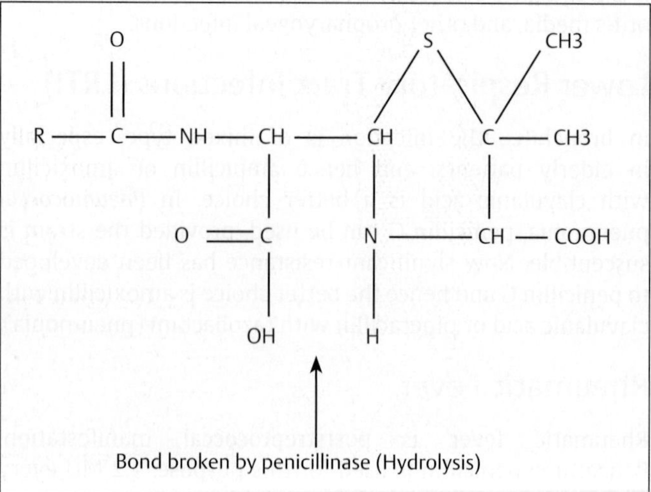

Fig. 59A.11 By the action of penicillinase the penicillin converts intopenicilloic acid.

and chloramphenicol. These organisms can be treated by tigecycline and colistin. This beta-lactamase is class-B beta-lactamase.

Permeability

The bacteria may interfere with the size of the porin channels, reducing the permeability of the penicillin and developing resistance. This typically happens in Gram-negative bacteria like *P. aeruginosa.*

Activation of Efflux Mechanism

There may be activation of efflux pump like P-glycoprotein pump, which pumps out the antibiotic from periplasmic space in Gram-negative bacteria. This actually prevents the accumulation of penicillin and ultimately its action in bacteria, for example, development of resistance to nafcillin by *Salmonella typhi.*

Change in Affinity of PBPs

To have action of penicillins they must bind to PBPs, should interfere with transpeptidation reaction, and produce deficient cell wall. With the repeated use of antibiotics, the bacteria make some changes in the structure of PBPs, so that the penicillin cannot bind to PBPs. This typically happens with MRSA. It must be noted that once the bacteria make changes in PBPs, then none of the penicillins will be effective.

Beta-Lactamase Inhibitors

These are the chemicals which bind to beta-lactamase and inhibit their action. The hydrolysis of the beta-lactam ring is prevented, and it reestablishes the activity of penicillin against organisms to which it was effective.

The beta-lactamases are as follows:

1. Clavulanic acid.
2. Sulbactum.
3. Tazobactum.
4. Avibactam
5. Vaborbactam.

Clavulanic Acid

It has beta-lactam ring but does not carry out antimicrobial activities. It is active against a variety of beta-lactamases produced by both Gram-positive and Gram-negative bacteria. Clavulanic acid can penetrate outer membrane of Gram-negative bacteria and inactivate the periplasmic accumulated beta-lactamase. It is mostly used orally, as absorption is good, and bioavailability is 60%. It pharmacokinetically matches with amoxicillin, having plasma half-life of 1 to 1.5 hours. It is important to note that excretion is not affected by probenecid. The major route of excretion is glomerular filtration. Generally, combined with amoxicillin, it restores the activity of amoxicillin to those organisms where it was effective, for example, *H. influenzae, S. aureus* (not MRSA), *N. gonorrhoeae, E. coli, Proteus, Klebsiella, Salmonella, Shigella.*

Dose

Tab. amoxicillin 500/875 mg + clavulanic acid 125 mg.

Dry syp. amoxicillin 200/400 mg + clavulanic acid 28.5/57 mg.

Sulbactam

It is a semisynthetic beta-lactamase inhibitor generally combined with ampicillin, which is given administered through parenteral route. It inhibits many beta-lactamases both by Gram-positive as well as Gram-negative bacteria. It can be used in gonorrhea, mixed infections like burns, gynecological infections, and surgical, especially hospital-acquired, infections.

Dose

Inj. ampicillin 1 gm + sulbactam 0.5 gm every 6 to 8 hours.

Tazobactam

It is structurally similar to sulbactam. Its pharmacokinetics is similar to piperacillin; hence, it is combined with piperacillin. This combination covers largest spectrum in all penicillins and is superior to all other penicillins in treating life-threatening infections. It does not inhibit chromosome-mediated beta-lactamase; hence, it is ineffective in piperacillin-resistant *Pseudomonas.* It cannot be used in resistant cases of *Pseudomonas*, where the resistance is developed by change in porin channels.

Dose

Piperacillin 2 g/4 g + tazobactum 0.25/0.5 g vial every 8 hours.

Avibactam

It is a comparatively new beta-lactamase inhibitor approved for use with ceftazidime in 2015. It blocks the beta-lactamases produced by different Gram-negative organisms. Avibactam inhibits class A, including KPC, class D and Class C beta-lactamases but shows poor activity for class B beta-lactamases.

P/K

Avibactam is not metabolized in body and is excreted by kidney. Plasma half-life is 2.7 to 3 hours.

Side Effects

Common side effects include nausea, vomiting, fever, hepatotoxicity, headache, and insomnia. Severe side effects include anaphylaxis, seizures, and pseudomembranous colitis. Doses need to be adjusted in renal insufficiency. Safety in pregnancy is not well-established.

Uses

The combination of avibactam with ceftazidime is preferred for serious Gram-infections like UTI, intra-abdominal infections, hospital-acquired infections, and pneumonia. This combination is indicated only when no other option is available. It is not available in India.

Vaborbactam

It is a beta-lactamase inhibitor approved in 2017 by US Food and drugs Administration (FDA) for use with meropenem. It inhibits the beta-lactamases of class A (KPC) and class C. but not effective against class B and Class D beta-lactamases.

P/K

Plasma half-life is 3 hours. Drug is eliminated almost completely by kidney.

Side Effects

Diarrhea, nausea, vomiting, and hypokalemia are common side effects. Liver toxicity is also noted. Severe side effects include anaphylaxis, seizures, and pseudomembranous colitis.

Uses

The combination of vaborbactam and meropenem is used to treat complicated infections, especially by Gram-negative bacteria. The indications include UTI, pneumonia, intra-abdominal infections, and hospital-acquired infections. It is not available in India.

Carbapenems

General Structure

Carbapenems are also beta-lactam antibiotics but having some differences with the penicillin molecule. Sulfur molecule is replaced by carbon molecule in the thiazoline ring of penicillin, and one double bond is there in this ring, making the structure unsaturated. Two side chains of R1 and R2 determine the pharmacokinetic and pharmacodynamic properties of carbapenems (**Fig. 59A.12**). These drugs have the broadest spectrum of all beta-lactam antibiotics.

Three important properties make them broad spectrum and they are as follows:

1. They can easily pass through porin channels because of their chemical structure.
2. They have affinity for wide range of PBPs from a variety of bacteria.
3. They are resistant to most of the beta-lactamases from most of the bacteria.

Imipenem

It is derived from Streptomyces cattleya. The mechanism of action is same as that of other beta-lactam antibiotics, that is, inhibition of cell of synthesis and bacterial lysis. Imipenem is resistant to most of the beta-lactamases.

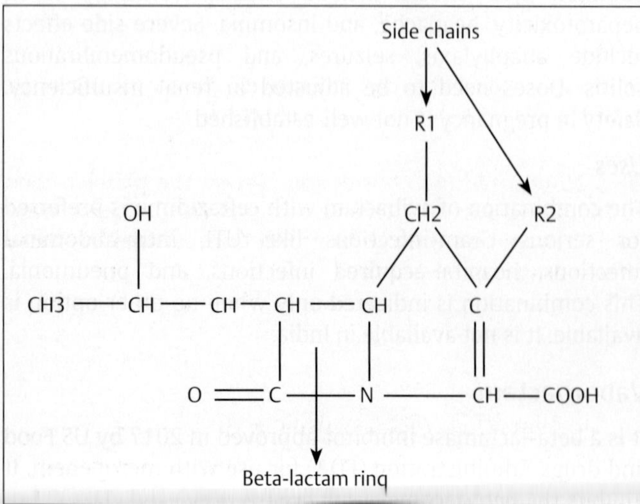

Fig. 59A.12 General structure of carbapenems.

Spectrum of Activity

It is very effective in large number of aerobic and anaerobic microorganisms. Streptococcus pneumoniae, enterococci, staphylococci, and Listeria, which are resistant to all other penicillins are susceptible to imipenem, but many of the MRSA are resistant. Most strains of Pseudomonas and Acinetobacter are inhibited. Anaerobes including B. fragilis are highly susceptible. C. difficile is resistant to imipenem. Now carbapenemase-producing strains are also evolving.

Pharmacokinetic Properties

Imipenem does not have R1 side chain, which makes the drug susceptible to dihydropeptidase I, an enzyme which is responsible for hydrolysis of imipenem in proximal part of nephron of kidney, making it less effective. Cilastatin, a synthetic inhibitor of dihydropeptidase I, is always combined with imipenem to overcome this problem of hydrolysis. The plasma half-life of both the drugs is 1 hour, which makes them compactable for coadministration. Imipenem is given only by parenteral route, mostly IV. Dose adjustment is needed in renal insufficiency.

Dose

Imipenem + cilastatin (250 mg/500 mg/1 g +250 mg/500 mg /1g) every 6 hours; maximum dose 4 g per day.

Meropenem

It is very similar to imipenem so far as the properties are concerned. Its R1 side chain is of methyl group, which make it resistant to dihydropeptidase l; hence, there is no need to combine with cilastatin. As compared to imipenem, it is less active against Gram-positive cocci but covers some of the Pseudomonas species which are resistant to imipenem. Clinically, it seems to be very similar to imipenem.

Dose

500 mg to 2 g by slow IV infusion over 1 hour three times a day (TDS).

Doripenem

Pseudomonas species is more susceptible to doripenem than other carbapenems. Other properties are similar to imipenem and meropenem.

Dose

500 mg by slow IV infusion over 1 hour TDS.

Ertapenem

It is the longest-acting carbapenem and once daily administration is sufficient. This is the most important advantage of this drug. It is less effective so far as Pseudomonas and Acinetobacter infections are concerned but is very effective in Gram-positive and Gram-negative especially organisms from Enterobacteriaceae family. It also covers anaerobes.

Dose

1 g powder for injection. After reconstitution and dilution in normal saline (NS), infused over 1 hour OD.

Faropenem

It is an orally active carbapenem. It is very effective for Gram-positive, Gram-negative, and anaerobes. The important organisms are Streptococcus pneumoniae, *H. influenzae*, and Moraxella catarrhalis.

Dose

Oral tab/cap 150 to 300 mg TDS.

Adverse Drug Reactions

Nausea and vomiting are the most common side effects. Seizures are seen especially when the patient is having some disease related to CNS. Patient is more prone to have seizures, especially in renal insufficiency. Seizures are comparatively more with imipenem (1.5%) and less with meropenem (0.5%). Patients showing hypersensitivity to penicillin should not be given carbapenems.

Uses

They are useful in variety of infections like UTIs, RTIs, intra-abdominal infections, gynecological infections, and skin and soft-tissue infections. The main indication is resistant cases of cephalosporins and extended penicillins, especially hospital-acquired infections. Ertapenem is more preferred in resistant intra-abdominal and resistant gynecological infections. Aminoglycosides are always added to broaden the spectrum and reduce the chances of development of resistance to carbapenems.

Multiple choice questions

1. A 65-years-old woman had met a road accident. She developed wounds on the body surface. She is diabetic and blood sugar level (BSL) is 340 mg/dL. She is in diabetic nephropathy, her urea is 125 mg/dL, and creatinine is 3.4 mg/dL. What would be the best choice of antibiotic for her?

A. Nafcillin.
B. Amoxicillin.
C. Piperacillin.
D. Benzyl-penicillin.

Answer: A

Nafcillin is a drug from anti-staphylococcal penicillins. These drugs are penicillinase-resistant. The most important property of nafcillin is that it is mainly metabolized and excreted by liver. In the given case, patient is suffering from renal failure due to diabetes mellitus (DM), so the drugs which are excreted by kidneys can accumulate and can lead to toxicity. All other drugs given as options are excreted by kidneys.

Note: Nafcillin is not available in India today.

2. A 12-year-old girl is having recurrent attacks of tonsillitis and pharyngitis every 2 to 4 weeks. Now, she developed joint pain and inflammation accompanied by fever. What would be the best step to prevent its recurrence?

A. Amoxicillin + clavulanic acid for 5 days.
B. Ampicillin + sulbactam for 7 days.
C. Ampicillin + cloxacillin for 5 days.
D. Benzathine penicillin 0.6 MU every 3 weeks till 15 years of age.

Answer: D

Benzathine penicillin is depot penicillin and is released extremely slow from the depot. It maintains very low concentration in the blood but is sufficient to prevent infections of beta hemolytic streptococci. Today, benzathine penicillin in the dose of 0.6/1.2 MU per 3 weeks is the drug of choice to prevent rheumatic arthritis and subsequent rheumatic heart disease.

3. A 43-year-old woman is tested negative in intradermal skin testing of penicillin. This negative testing means?

A. It is safe to give penicillin to her.
B. She does not have penicillin antibodies in her body.
C. She will not develop any reaction to penicillin.
D. It is unlikely that she will develop any immediate type of hypersensitivity reaction to penicillin.

Answer: D

This is important to note that negative skin test does not guarantee any reaction for use of penicillin, including hypersensitivity reaction. A negative skin test only suggests very less chances of developing immediate type of hypersensitivity reaction.

4. In a 32-years-old, benzyl-penicillin was given by intradermal route for testing. After some time, he developed urticaria, swelling of lips, and itching. What does it mean to the treating physician?

A. Benzyl-penicillin should not be administrated to this person.
B. He can be given any other oral forms of penicillin like amoxicillin.
C. He should not be treated by any other penicillin which has to be injected.
D. All natural and semisynthetic penicillins are contraindicated in this person.

Answer: D

It must be noted that hypersensitivity shown to any of the penicillins is applicable to all type of penicillins.

5. A 39-year-old man has dengue fever. The platelet count is 36000. He is in an intensive care unit (ICU). Doctor wants to give prophylactic drugs to prevent nosocomial infections. Which drug is to be avoided?

A. Ampicillin + sulbactam.
B. Carbenicillin.
C. Benzathine penicillin.
D. Amoxicillin with clavulanic acid.

Answer: B

Carbenicillin is known to interfere with platelet function and can lead to bleeding episodes, especially in susceptible patients;

hence, carbenicillin must be avoided in the patient having thrombocytopenia. It is important to note that studies in healthy volunteers show the similar effect of piperacillin on platelet function but is less than carbenicillin.

6. A 34-years-old-man was suffering from gout. He is on regular treatment with allopurinol. He had diarrhea and he had been treated with ampicillin. He developed rash on his back. What should be done in such case?

A. It is a hypersensitivity to ampicillin.

B. It is a toxic effect of ampicillin.

C. All types of penicillins must be not be used.

D. All beta-lactam type of antibiotics must not be used.

Answer: B

Ampicillin shows maculopapular rash as a toxic effect and is more commonly observed if allopurinol is given concurrently. It is generally not the hypersensitivity shown to ampicillin.

7. Amoxicillin + clavulanic acid combination is effective against the following except?

A. Methicillin-resistant *S. aureus* (MRSA).

B. Penicillinase-producing *S. aureus.*

C. Penicillinase-producing *N. gonorrhea.*

D. Beta-lactamase-producing *E. coli.*

Answer: A

In case of MRSA, there is change in PBP structure. If this is the mechanism of resistance, then no penicillin will work. Addition of clavulanic acid can reestablish the activity of penicillins where the resistance is developed due to production of penicillinase or beta-lactamase. Clavulanic acid cannot work for resistance developed due to change in PBP structure.

8. A bedridden 67-years-old woman developed urinary tract infection (UTI) by beta-lactamase-producing E coli. What should be the drug of choice?

A. Cloxacillin.

B. Ampicillin.

C. Amoxicillin + clavulanic acid.

D. Second-generation cephalosporin.

Answer: C

Amoxicillin and clavulanic acid can be used as the combination to treat beta-lactamase-producing microorganisms.

9. A 58-year-old man had road traffic accident. He had severe head injury. Glasgow coma scale (GCS) score is 9. He is semiconscious. Surgeon wants to give prophylactic antibiotics. Which one should be better avoided in such situation?

A. Piperacillin.

B. Carbenicillin.

C. Meropenem.

D. Nafcillin.

Answer: C

Meropenem is from the carbapenem group. Carbapenems are known to have seizure as side effect. It is more pronounced when the patient is suffering from central nervous system (CNS) disorders. With a Glasgow coma scale (GCS0 score of 9, he seems to have sustained a major injury to brain. Patient is already prone to develop seizures, so it is better to avoid any of the carbapenems.

10. A 21-year-old man clinic with an erythematous, swollen, painful left elbow. History was significant for untreated impetigo on his left forearm. A joint aspirate reveals Gram-positive cocci in clusters. In culture results, it was found to be methicillin susceptible. Which of the following would be the best drug of choice?

A. Amoxicillin.

B. Ampicillin.

C. Cloxacillin.

D. Penicillin G.

Answer: C

Methicillin and cloxacillin are from group of antistaphylococcal penicillin. They are penicillinase-resistant. Most of the time, the skin infection is due to staphylococci; hence, cloxacillin will be a better choice.

Chapter 59B Cephalosporins

Sonali Karekar

Learning Objectives

- First-generation cephalosporins.
- Second-generation cephalosporins.
- Third-generation cephalosporins.
- Fourth-generation cephalosporins.
- Fifth-generation cephalosporins.

Origin and Structure

Cephalosporins belong to the β-lactam group of antibiotics. Following the isolation of a fungus *Cephalosporium* in Sardinia in 1945, cephalosporin C, a compound with antibacterial activity, was discovered in 1953 at Oxford. Most of the cephalosporins available today are semisynthetic derivatives of cephalosporin C generated by addition of different side chains at position 7 of the β-lactam ring (governing spectrum of action) and at position 3 of the dihydrothiazine ring (governing pharmacokinetic profile) (**Fig. 59B.1**).

Mechanism of Action

Stability of the bacterial cell wall is attributed to the peptidoglycan component. Cephalosporins, being a part of β-lactam group of antibiotics, act by interfering with the bacterial cell wall synthesis. They inhibit the last step in peptidoglycan synthesis. The targets for the actions of β-lactam antibiotics are collectively termed penicillin-binding proteins (PBPs). The transpeptidase, which is a part of the peptidoglycan synthesis, is one of these PBPs. Transpeptidation governs the cross-linking of peptidoglycan, which is composed of two alternating amino sugars (*N*-acetylglucosamine and *N*-acetylmuramic acid). Cephalosporins bind to different sets of PBPs than penicillins, but eventually result in a bactericidal effect due to interference with the cell wall synthesis (**Fig. 59B.2**).

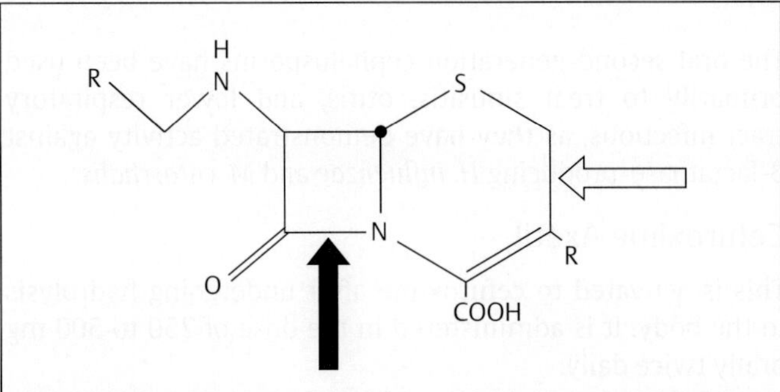

Fig. 59B.1 Structure of cephalosporins. The *solid arrow* indicates the core β-lactam ring. The *open arrow* indicates six-membered side ring for cephalosporins. "R" indicates additional side chains at which various chemical groups are substituted to vary antimicrobial spectra, pharmacokinetic properties, or stability to β-lactamases.

Classification

There are five generations of cephalosporins (**Fig. 59B.3**). The various generations differ with respect to the following:

1. Antibacterial spectrum and relative potency against specific organisms.
2. Susceptibility to β-lactamases.
3. Pharmacokinetic properties—route of administration, metabolism by liver/kidney, half-lives, tubular secretion (probenecid inhibits their tubular secretion).

First-Generation Cephalosporins

Spectrum

First-generation cephalosporins have high activity against Gram-positive bacteria but weaker activity against Gram-negative bacteria. All drugs have nearly identical spectra, with no activity against enterococci, methicillin-resistant *Staphylococcus aureus* (MRSA), or *Listeria*.

Oral

Cephalexin

It is the most commonly used orally effective first-generation cephalosporin. It is less active against penicillinase-producing staphylococci. Oral therapy with cephalexin (usually 0.5 g

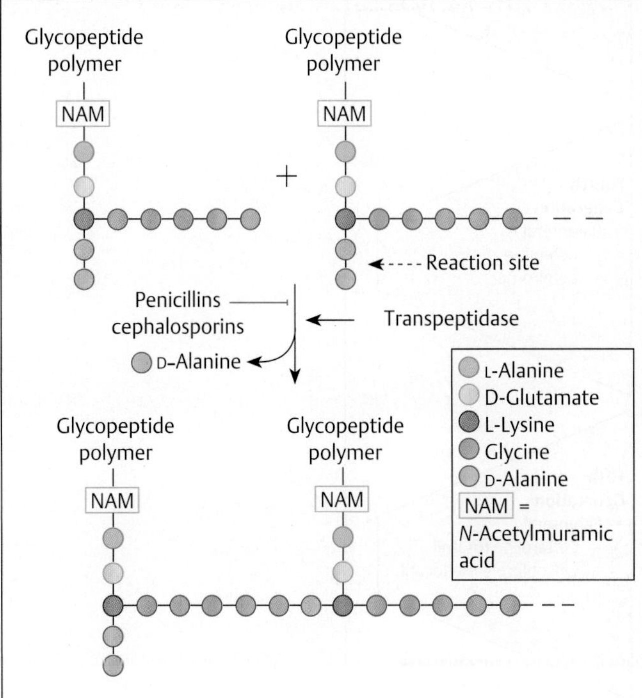

Fig. 59B.2 Mechanism of action of cephalosporins.

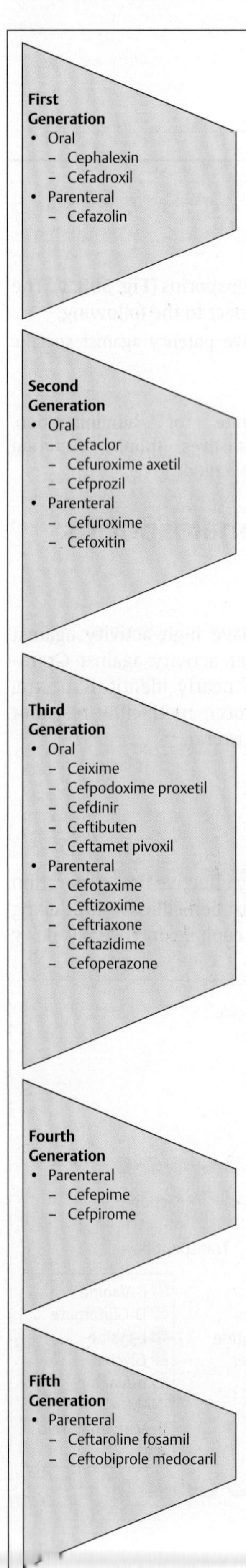

Fig. 59B.3 Five generations of cephalosporins.

twice to four times daily) results in peak concentrations in plasma, adequate for the inhibition of many Gram-positive and Gram-negative pathogens. It attains high concentration in the bile, and excretion occurs by renal route.

Cephradine and cefadroxil are oral agents with a similar pharmacokinetic and activity profile to cephalexin. Cefadroxil is administered every 12 hours, in contrast to cephalexin, which is administered every 6 to 8 hours.

Parenteral

Cefazolin

It is the prototype of first-generation cephalosporins. It is given intramuscularly or intravenously; it exhibits renal excretion and is about 85% bound to plasma proteins. It is the preferred drug for surgical prophylaxis and for many streptococcal and staphylococcal infections requiring treatment by intravenous route.

Adverse Drug Reactions

Gastrointestinal symptoms include nausea, vomiting, or diarrhea, usually mild in nature. Sometimes, pseudomembranous colitis also occurs. Nephrotoxicity is of mild grade. Elevation in liver enzyme has also been reported. Less frequent reactions include thrombocytopenia, leukopenia, and eosinophilia.

Second-Generation Cephalosporins

Spectrum

This class demonstrates enhanced activity against many Enterobacteriaceae, *Haemophilus influenzae*, and *Moraxella catarrhalis*, due to greater stability against β-lactamases, but they have less activity against Gram-negative organisms in comparison with third-generation cephalosporins. They show weak activity against Gram-positive organisms.

Some agents have activity against anaerobic organisms, but none of the agents show activity against *Pseudomonas* species. Their use has been superseded by third-generation cephalosporins.

Oral

The oral second-generation cephalosporins have been used primarily to treat sinusitis, otitis, and lower respiratory tract infections, as they have demonstrated activity against β-lactamase-producing *H. influenzae* and *M. catarrhalis*.

Cefuroxime Axetil

This is activated to cefuroxime after undergoing hydrolysis in the body. It is administered in the dose of 250 to 500 mg orally twice daily.

Cefaclor

This drug is dosed every 8 hours and is effective against *H. influenzae*, *Escherichia coli*, *Proteus mirabilis* and some anaerobes. Its use is limited due to high susceptibility to β-lactamases.

Cephamycins

Some second-generation cephalosporins are termed "cephamycins." They are derived from *Streptomyces* spp. and are regarded as members of the cephalosporin class. They demonstrate a higher level of anaerobic activity, especially against *Bacteroides fragilis*. They include cefoxitin and cefotetan.

Used parenterally, it has demonstrated activity against rapidly growing nontuberculous mycobacteria and is often included in multiple-drug combination regimens to treat serious infections caused by them.

Cefotetan

It could be considered as an alternative agent for prophylaxis in patients undergoing elective bowel surgery. It can also be employed in the treatment of patients with acute pelvic inflammatory disease and endometritis. It is given at a dose of 1 to 2 g every 12 hours.

Parenteral

All second-generation parenteral cephalosporins are cleared by renal route and need dosage adjustment in renal dysfunction.

Cefuroxime

It is administered by intramuscular route. Now, the third-generation drugs are preferred over cefuroxime. However, a single dose of 1.5 g intramuscularly has been used for the treatment of gonorrhea, due to penicillinase-producing *Neisseria gonorrhoeae*. It is administered intramuscularly or intravenously every 8 hours at a dose of 0.75 to 1.5 g.

Adverse Drug Reactions

Cefaclor and cefprozil are most commonly associated with serum sickness–like reactions along with rash, fever, and arthritis. Pseudomembranous colitis is observed more commonly with cefoxitin.

Third-Generation Cephalosporins

Spectrum

They are less active than first-generation agents against Gram-positive cocci; however, ceftriaxone and cefotaxime are exceptions, as these two have excellent antistreptococcal activity. They are also much more active than prior generations against Enterobacteriaceae, although resistance is dramatically increasing to this class as well. Some drugs have good blood–brain membrane permeability, making them useful for meningitis.

Parenteral

Cefotaxime

It is the prototype of this class. A unique pharmacokinetic feature is that it undergoes deacetylation, which forms an active metabolite (weaker) that serves to prolong its action, allowing for 12-hourly dosing. It attains high levels in cerebrospinal fluid (CSF) and is used in meningitis caused by Gram-negative bacilli. It is also used for resistant hospital-acquired infections, septicemias, and infections in immunocompromised patients. In typhoid fever, it can be used as an alternative to ceftriaxone.

Ceftriaxone

It is highly protein-bound, unlike other cephalosporins. This results in prolongation of its half-life, allowing once- or twice-daily dosing. It has good penetration into CSF and is eliminated equally in the urine and bile. It has shown high efficacy in a number of serious infections including bacterial meningitis, multidrug-resistant typhoid fever, abdominal sepsis, complicated urinary tract infections (UTIs), and septicemias. It can be given in doses ranging between 1 and 4 g daily. While for most serious infections a dose of 1 g daily is enough, doses of 2 g every 12 hours are recommended for meningitis, and 2 g daily dose is recommended for endocarditis.

Ceftazidime

It is known for its excellent activity against *Pseudomonas aeruginosa*. It is also used for patients with hematological malignancies developing febrile neutropenia, burn patients, etc. It is less active against *S. aureus*, other Gram-positive cocci, and anaerobes such as *B. fragilis*, but shows good activity against Enterobacteriaceae. The plasma $t_{½}$ of ceftazidime is 1.5 to 1.8 hours and its dose is 0.5 to 2 g every 8 hours intravenously or intramuscularly.

Cefoperazone

It has a strong activity against *Pseudomonas* and weaker activity on other organisms. It has also shown activity against *Salmonella typhi* and *B. fragilis* but is susceptible to β-lactamases. It is indicated in severe urinary, biliary, respiratory, and skin and soft-tissue infections (SSTIs), as well as in typhoid and septicemias. It is administered in doses of 1 to 3 g every 8 to 12 hours intravenously or intramuscularly. Primarily, it is excreted in the bile.

Adverse Drug Reactions

Adverse drug reactions have been observed at a rate of 1 to 12% across this generation of cephalosporins. Hypersensitivity reactions, both immediate and delayed, have been observed. There can be pain at injection sites. Nephrotoxicity, hepatotoxicity, and gastrointestinal disturbances can also occur. An adverse effect that has been observed with a higher frequency than with first-generation agents is decreased vitamin K synthesis due to suppression of endogenous bacterial flora, occasionally leading to clinically significant bleeding. Hypoprothrombinemia and bleeding occur specifically with ceftriaxone. Pseudomembranous colitis also occurs.

Acute ethanol intolerance occurs due to inhibition of acetaldehyde dehydrogenase. This is restricted to compounds that contain a methyltetrazolethiol group. This has been specifically observed with cefoperazone.

Fourth-Generation Cephalosporins

Spectrum

This class of cephalosporins is more effective against Gram-positive microbes and *P. aeruginosa* and exhibits sufficient stability against class 1 chromosomal cephalosporinases (type of β-lactamases).

Cefepime

It is a semisynthetic, broad-spectrum cephalosporin to be administered parenterally. It is highly resistant to hydrolysis by most β-lactamases and exhibits rapid penetration into Gram-negative bacteria. It is administered at doses of 0.5 to 2 g every 12 hours. Cefepime is primarily eliminated by the renal route in unchanged form. Reduction of dose is warranted in patients with renal failure. It has been approved for the treatment of moderate-to-severe infections, including pneumonia, uncomplicated and complicated UTIs, SSTIs, intra-abdominal infections, and febrile neutropenia.

Adverse Drug Reactions

It has been associated with local reactions such as phlebitis, pain, inflammation, and rash. Colitis (including pseudomembranous colitis), diarrhea, headache, nausea, vomiting, fever, oral moniliasis, pruritus, urticaria, and vaginitis have been observed in less than 1% of patients. Higher doses have been associated with an increase in frequency of adverse events. Cases of neurotoxicity have been reported.

Cefpirome

It demonstrates activity against most of the pathogens involved in hospital-acquired infections such as Enterobacteriaceae, methicillin-susceptible *S. aureus*, coagulase-negative staphylococci, and viridans group streptococci. The adverse event profile appears similar to other third-generation cephalosporins, with the most commonly observed adverse event being diarrhea.

Fifth-Generation Cephalosporins

Spectrum

They are active against multidrug-resistant Gram-positive bacteria, including MRSA, vancomycin intermediate *S. aureus* (VISA), hetero-VISA, and vancomycin-resistant *S. aureus*. It demonstrates broad-spectrum activity against many of the important community-acquired Gram-positive and Gram-negative pathogens, which is an added advantage in contrast to most of the other anti-MRSA drugs.

It also has efficacy against respiratory bacterial pathogens such as *Streptococcus pneumoniae* (including multidrug-resistant strains), *H. influenzae*, and *M. catarrhalis*. It is inactive against extensively resistant Gram-negative bacteria and exhibits limited activity against *P. aeruginosa* and many anaerobic species.

Ceftaroline

Ceftaroline fosamil is a novel fifth-generation parental cephalosporin with bactericidal activity against multi-drug resistant Gram-positive bacteria, including methicillin resistant S. aureus (MRSA), vancomycin intermediate S. aureus (VISA), hVISA, and VRSA. It has the advantage of exhibiting broad-spectrum activity against many of the important community-acquired Gram-positive and Gram-negative pathogens in contrast to most of the other anti-MRSA drugs. It also has efficacy against respiratory bacterial pathogens such as Streptococcus pneumoniae (including multidrug-resistant strains), Haemophilus influenzae, and Moraxella catarrhalis. It is inactive against extensively-resistant Gram-negative bacteria and exhibits limited activity against Pseudomonas aeruginosa and many anaerobic species.

It has been approved specifically for the treatment of complicated SSTIs and community-acquired pneumonia (CAP).

Mechanism to Overcome Resistance

Ceftaroline possesses an ethoxyimino side chain mimicking a portion of a cell wall structure, which acts as a "Trojan horse," allosterically opening and facilitating access to the active site of the PBP2a (mutated penicillin-binding protein) (**Fig. 59B.4**).

The anti-MRSA efficacy of ceftaroline results from its high affinity for the MRSA-associated PBP2a (almost ≥256 times over other β-lactams).

Pharmacokinetics

Ceftaroline is the active metabolite of its water-soluble prodrug, ceftaroline fosamil, and is formed as a result of hydrolysis by plasma phosphatases. Its chemical stability and water solubility are partly related to its improved crystallization and hygroscopicity imparted by modification of its chemical structure. This requires it to be administrated in the form of its prodrug, via intravenous or intramuscular routes.

Adverse Drug Reactions

The most common adverse drug reactions include diarrhea, nausea, and rash.

Uses

It has been approved to be used in acute bacterial skin and skin structure infections and community-acquired bacterial pneumonia by susceptible bacteria.

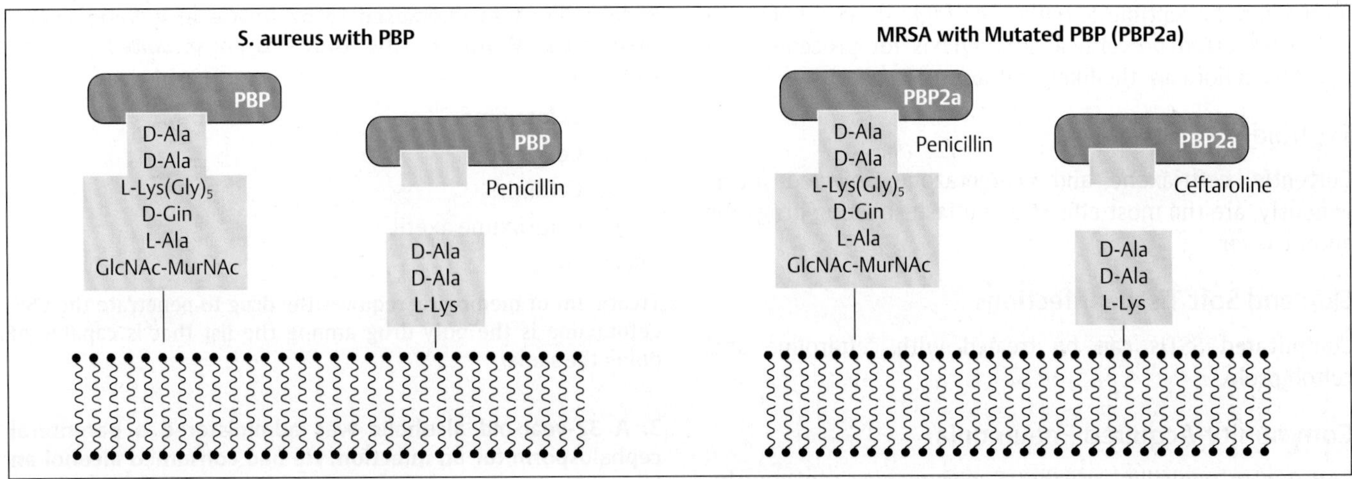

Fig. 59B.4 Mechanism to overcome resistance.

Ceftobiprole

Ceftobiprole is an extended-spectrum cephalosporin, which exhibits tight binding to several different PBPs of Gram-positive and Gram-negative organisms. Its key characteristic is the ability to also inhibit PBPs that are either resistant or weakly susceptible to conventional β-lactam antibiotics, including PBP2a of MRSA and PBP2x of penicillin-resistant pneumococci (PRP).

Spectrum

It is a broad-spectrum cephalosporin that covers MRSA and coagulase-negative staphylococci, streptococci (including PRP strains), *H. influenzae*, *M. catarrhalis*, *P. aeruginosa*, and *Enterococcus faecalis*. It has little or no activity against *Enterococcus faecium*, *Acinetobacter*, *Burkholderia*, *Proteus vulgaris*, and most Gram-negative anaerobes.

Pharmacokinetics

Ceftobiprole is the active moiety formed as a result of rapid activation of its water-soluble prodrug ceftobiprole medocaril by plasma esterases. It is administered at the dosage of 500 mg every 8 hours infused over 2 hours, by intravenous route. It has a very short $t_{1/2}$ of around 3 hours and is excreted by the renal route. Modification of dosage is required in patients with renal impairment.

Adverse Drug Reactions

Overall, the most common adverse events observed include gastrointestinal (such as nausea, vomiting, diarrhea), infusion site reactions, dysgeusia, and hypersensitivity reactions (urticaria, rash, and pruritus).

Indication

It has been approved for use in CAP and in patients with SSTIs, infective endocarditis, bloodstream infections, mediastinitis, and osteomyelitis.

Advantages

The exceptional activity against methicillin resistant staphylococci and PRP, in comparison with that of conventional β-lactams, is the key highlight of the fifth-generation of cephalosporins.

Resistance to Cephalosporins

Resistance to cephalosporins can arise broadly due to either of the following mechanisms:

1. Modification of the PBP, particularly the transpeptidases.
2. Production of β-lactamases or "permeability barriers."

Hence, target-mediated resistance can occur as a result of either reduced affinity of an existing PBP component or the acquisition of additional β-lactam-insensitive PBP. The production of β-lactamases by bacteria is determined by chromosomal or plasmid DNA. The degree of β-lactamase-mediated resistance is dependent on several factors such as the amount of enzyme produced as well as the location of the enzyme (extracellular for Gram-positive organisms and periplasmic in Gram-negative ones).

Combinations of Cephalosporins

In order to combat resistance, several novel cephalosporin–β-lactamase inhibitor combinations have been developed. Ceftolozane–tazobactam and ceftazidime–avibactam have been approved for complicated abdominal infections and UTIs. They have demonstrated potent in vitro activity against Gram-negative organisms, including *P. aeruginosa* and extended-spectrum β-lactamase-producing Enterobacteriaceae. They should be combined with metronidazole when treating complicated intra-abdominal infections, as neither of them is active against anaerobes. Both agents have short half-lives and are administered intravenously every 8 hours. Excretion occurs primarily by the kidneys, and dose adjustment is needed in patients with impaired renal clearance.

Indications

Surgical Prophylaxis

First-generation cephalosporins are highly effective against SSTIs due to their activity against *Streptococcus pyogenes* and methicillin-susceptible *S. aureus*. A single dose of cefazolin is the preferred presurgical prophylaxis for procedures in which skin flora are the likely pathogens.

Typhoid

Currently, ceftriaxone and cefoperazone, injected intravenously, are the most effective and fastest acting drugs for enteric fever.

Skin and Soft Tissue Infections

Complicated SSTIs can be treated with ceftaroline and ceftobiprole.

Community-Acquired Pneumonia

CAP due to penicillin-resistant *S. pneumoniae* can now be treated by ceftaroline fosamil.

Gonorrhea

Ceftriaxone is used for the single-dose therapy of gonorrhea with status of penicillinase production being unknown. Higher doses are recommended due to resistance. It is also advised to be combined with azithromycin.

Meningitis

Third-generation cephalosporins such as cefotaxime and ceftriaxone having good blood–brain barrier permeability are used for meningitis.

Abdominal Infections

Ceftriaxone and cefepime are used for abdominal sepsis.

Urinary Tract Infections

Ceftriaxone is effective parenterally and cefixime is effective orally in UTIs.

Acute Otitis Media and Sinusitis

Second-generation drugs have been used for these conditions.

Multiple Choice Questions

1. A 58-year-old man was being treated with an antimicrobial agent for an infection. His biochemical analysis after2 weeks showed elevated levels of serum creatinine and he was found to have developed renal failure. Which of these drugs is unlikely to have caused this effect?

A. Cefadroxil.

B. Amphotericin B.

C. Cefoperazone.

D. Cephaloridine.

Answer: C

Although most cephalosporins are excreted by the renal route, cefoperazone and ceftriaxone are secreted in the bile. Hence, cefoperazone is unlikely to have caused the renal dysfunction.

2. A 43-year-old female patient presented to the emergency OPD with headache, neck stiffness, and fever for the past 3 days. She was diagnosed to be a case of meningococcal meningitis. Which of the drugs is most suited for her condition?

A. Cefotaxime.

B. Cefazolin.

C. Cefdinir.

D. Cefuroxime axetil.

Answer: A

Treatment of meningitis requires the drug to penetrate the CSF. Cefotaxime is the only drug among the list that is capable of doing the same.

3. A 32-year-old alcoholic was administered a parenteral cephalosporin for an infection. He had consumed alcohol an hour prior to reporting to the OPD. He reported experiences similar to a disulfiram-like reaction. Which of the drug could be a possible cause?

A. Cefuroxime.

B. Cefazolin.

C. Cefoperazone.

D. Cefoxitin.

Answer: C

Cefoperazone has been known to cause alcohol intolerance attributed to the presence of a methyltetrazolethiol group.

4. Which of the following is also known as the "Trojan horse" antibiotic?

A. Cefepime.

B. Ceftaroline.

C. Ceftobiprole.

D. Cefoperazone.

Answer: B

Ceftaroline is also known as "Trojan horse" antibiotic due to allosterically opening and facilitating access to the active site of the PBP2a, conferring activity against MRSA.

5. Which cephalosporin has been associated with a "caramel-like" dysgeusia?

A. Ceftaroline.

B. Ceftobiprole.

C. Ceftibuten.

D. Ceftazidime.

Answer: B

A caramel-like dysgeusia has been observed with ceftobiprole attributed to a diacetyl product of conversion.

6. A 32-year-old sexually active man presents to OPD with penile discharge, dysuria, and a right knee joint swelling. His joint aspirate revealed many neutrophils as well as some Gram-negative diplococci. Which is the best drug to treat him?

A. Cefazolin.

B. Cephalexin.

C. Ceftriaxone.

D. Ciprofloxacin.

Answer: C

This patient's presentation is suggestive of infection with *Neisseria gonorrhoeae*. Ceftriaxone is usually the drug of choice for gonorrhea because most strains are now resistant to other classes such as penicillins and fluroquinolones.

7. Which of the following drugs belongs to the "cephamycin" group?

A. Cefazolin.
B. Ceftriaxone.
C. Cefoxitin.
D. Cefepime.

Answer: C

Some second-generation cephalosporins demonstrating higher level of anaerobic activity are designated a term known as "cephamycins." They include cefoxitin and cefotetan.

8. Which of the following cephalosporins is combined with tazobactam?

A. Cefixime.
B. Ceftaroline.
C. Ceftazidime.
D. Ceftolozane.

Answer: D

This is used in combination with β-lactamase inhibitor. The combination ceftolozane–tazobactam has been approved for complicated abdominal and urinary tract infections.

Chapter 60 Broad-Spectrum Antibiotics

Prasan R. Bhandari

Learning Objectives

- Tetracyclines.
- Chloramphenicol.

Tetracyclines

They have four cyclic rings in the structure; hence, they are known as tetracyclines. These agents are obtained from soil actinomycetes, for example, *Streptomyces aureofaciens*. They inhibit gram-positive bacteria, rickettsiae, chlamydiae, mycoplasma, and some protozoa; hence, they are also known as broad-spectrum antimicrobial agents (AMAs).

Classification

1. Short-acting ($t_{½}$–6 hours): tetracycline, oxytetracycline.
2. Intermediate-acting ($t_{½}$–12 hours): demeclocycline.
3. Long-acting ($t_{½}$–18 hours): doxycycline, minocycline.

Intermediate- and long-acting preparations are semisynthetic.

Mechanism of Action

They enter in susceptible microorganisms by active transport. Mammalian cells lack active transport and have different ribosomes. Bacterial ribosomes have 50S and 30S subunits. Tetracyclines bind to 30S ribosomal subunit. Ribosomes have three binding sites, that is, A, P, and E sites. Tetracyclines bind to "A" site and prevent binding of tRNA to this site. tRNA carries amino acid for protein synthesis. Amino acids cannot be added and hence they inhibit protein synthesis. Thus, they are bacteriostatic (**Fig. 60.1**).

Spectrum of Activity

Tetracyclines have a broad spectrum of activity against a wide range of microorganisms including gram-positive bacteria, gram-negative bacteria, rickettsiae, chlamydiae, actinomyces, plasmodia, *Entamoeba histolytica*, and mycoplasma. Additionally, streptococci, staphylococci, gonococci, meningococci, clostridia, *Bacillus anthracis*, *Listeria*, corynebacteria, *Propionibacterium acnes*, *Haemophilus influenzae*, *Vibrio cholerae*, *Yersinia pestis*, *Haemophilus ducreyi*, *Campylobacter*, *Brucella*, *Bordetella*, *Pasteurella*, and spirochetes are also inhibited.

Resistance

Many organisms have now developed resistance. Hence, this has decreased their utility. Resistance develops due to decreased uptake or increased efflux, displacing tetracyclines from target ribosomes, or due to production of inactivating

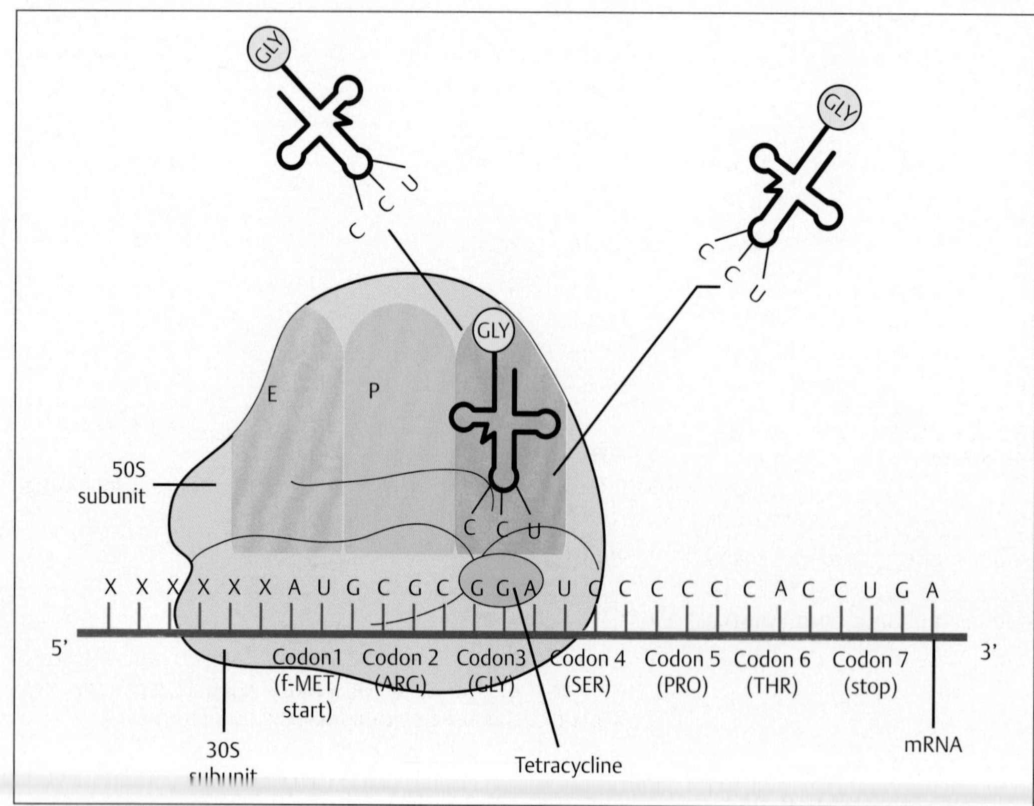

Fig. 60.1 Mechanism of action of tetracyclines.

enzymes. Cross-resistance among different tetracyclines is seen.

Pharmacokinetics

The older tetracyclines are incompletely absorbed. Food interferes with absorption (except doxycycline and minocycline). Calcium and other metals chelate tetracyclines; hence, they should not be given with milk, milk products, antacids, iron preparations, or zinc supplements. These agents are widely distributed, and they accumulate in the liver, spleen, bone, teeth, cerebrospinal fluid (CSF), synovial fluid, urine, and prostrate. They are secreted in milk, and they cross the placenta. Tetracyclines are excreted in the kidneys (except doxycycline and minocycline); hence, doxycycline and minocycline are safe in renal dysfunction.

Administration

They can be administered via oral, parenteral, or topical routes. Tetracyclines may be administered with food to reduce gastrointestinal (GI) irritation. Milk, dairy products, antacids, iron, and aluminum decrease GI absorption, therefore, avoid their coadministration. Cholestyramine and colestipol reduce absorption. Intramuscular (IM) absorption is poor and unreliable and causes irritation. Intravenous (IV) administration can lead to thrombophlebitis (except doxycycline and minocycline).

Adverse Effects

Teeth and Bone

Since tetracyclines chelate calcium, calcium–tetracycline orthophosphate complex gets deposited in developing teeth and bone. Hence, this leads to their deformities. Onycholysis and nail pigmentation also occur. Therefore, tetracyclines are teratogenic.

Superinfections

This occurs due to the suppression of GI flora. Tetracyclines are the most common AMAs to cause superinfection.

GI Irritation

Epigastric burning, esophageal ulcers, nausea, and vomiting are seen. Hence, these agents are given with food.

Hepatotoxicity

Hepatotoxicity occurs with large doses. Acute hepatic necrosis can develop in pregnant women.

Nephrotoxicity

This occurs due to the antianabolic effects and increased nitrogen. Fanconi's syndrome occurs because of outdated tetracyclines. This is manifested as polyuria, proteinuria, glycosuria, and acidosis.

Phototoxicity

It is common with doxycycline and minocycline.

Pseudotumor Cerebri

This is a condition with increase in intracranial pressure in infants, manifested as bulging of anterior fontanelle.

Antianabolic Effects

This occurs with large doses administered for prolonged duration.

Nephrogenic Diabetes Insipidus

Demeclocycline inhibits action of antidiuretic hormone (ADH) on the kidneys; hence, it used in syndrome of inappropriate antidiuretic hormone (SIADH).

Local

IM administration causes pain and irritation, while IV administration leads to thrombophlebitis (except doxycycline and minocycline).

Uses

Its use has decreased due to emergence of resistance and availability of safer AMAs.

Drug of Choice

1. Tick typhus, Q fever, Rocky Mountain spotted fever.
2. Chlamydial infections:
   a. Lymphogranuloma venereum.
   b. Trachoma.
   c. Inclusion conjunctivitis.
   d. Urethritis/cervicitis.
   e. Pneumonia.
   f. Psittacosis.
3. Mycoplasma pneumonia.
4. Granuloma inguinale, caused by *Calymmatobacterium granulomatis*.
5. Cholera—Treatment of dehydration is life-saving.
6. Brucellosis—along with rifampicin.
7. Plague—combined with aminoglycoside.

Other Infections

1. Traveler's diarrhea.
2. Sexually transmitted diseases—syphilis, gonorrhea, chancroid.
3. Acne—low dose for long time.
4. Tularemia—along with aminoglycoside.
5. Miscellaneous—Lyme disease, relapsing fever, leptospirosis, postexposure prophylaxis of anthrax.
6. Protozoal infections—chronic intestinal amebiasis, multidrug-resistant malaria (doxycycline + quinine).
7. SIADH - demeclocycline.

Contraindications

1. Pregnancy, lactation, and children younger than 8 years, since it can lead to deformities of teeth and bone, acute hepatic necrosis in pregnant, and pseudotumor cerebri in infants.
2. Renal/hepatic impairment.

Advantages/Features of Doxycycline and Minocycline

1. Bioavailability is 95 to 100%.
2. Food does not interfere with absorption.
3. Highly lipid soluble.
4. Long $t_{1/2}$; hence, once-daily administration.
5. Excreted in gastrointestinal tract (GIT) and hence safe in renal dysfunction.
6. Given both orally and parenterally.
7. Minocycline used as an alternative to rifampicin in eradicating meningococcal carrier state, that is, from nasopharynx.
8. Doxycycline preferred for postexposure prophylaxis of anthrax.

Comparison of Tetracycline and Doxycycline

A comparison of tetracycline and doxycycline is presented in **Table 60.1**.

Tigecycline

It is a glycylcycline, a derivative of minocycline, and has a wide antibacterial spectrum. It is effective against methicillin- and vancomycin-resistant staphylococci, streptococci, multidrug-resistant enterococci, *Streptococcus pneumoniae*, anaerobes, enterobacter, mycobacteria, rickettsiae, chlamydiae, and legionella. Tigecycline has a long $t_{1/2}$ (36 hours) and good tissue penetration. It is excreted from GIT; hence, no dosage reduction is required in renal impairment. Generally, it is well-tolerated, with only nausea and vomiting reported as its side effects. It is used for life-threatening infections due to resistant organisms, nosocomial infection, or intra-abdominal infections.

Chloramphenicol

It is a broad-spectrum antibiotic obtained from *Streptomyces venezuelae*.

Mechanism of Action

It is bacteriostatic in nature. It binds to 50S ribosomal subunit and inhibits transpeptidation reaction. Hence, it inhibits protein synthesis (**Fig. 60.2**).

Spectrum of Activity

It is effective against gram-negative, some gram-positive, anaerobes, rickettsiae, mycoplasma, *H. influenzae*, *Salmonella*, *Shigella*, *Bordetella*, *Brucella*, gonococci, meningococci, streptococci, staphylococci, clostridium, *Escherichia coli*, and *Klebsiella*. It is bactericidal to *Neisseria meningitidis* and *H. influenzae*.

Mechanism of Resistance

It occurs by drug-inactivating enzymes, reduced permeability to drug, or decreased sensitivity of target ribosome.

Pharmacokinetics

Chloramphenicol has good oral absorption and excellent tissue penetration. It achieves a high CSF concentration. Additionally, it is a microsomal enzyme inhibitor.

Adverse Effects

Bone Marrow Depression

This is a dose-dependent adverse reaction caused due to inhibition of mammalian cell protein synthesis. It is manifested as anemia, leukopenia, and thrombocytopenia. However, these are reversible in nature. Idiosyncratic reaction can be caused due to a toxic metabolite, for example, aplastic anemia, which could be fatal. This has reduced its use in clinical scenarios.

Gray Baby Syndrome

This is observed in newborn babies given high doses of chloramphenicol. Signs and symptoms comprise vomiting,

Table 60.1 Comparison of tetracycline and doxycycline

	Tetracycline	Doxycycline
Source	Semisynthetic	Semisynthetic
GI absorption	Incomplete	Complete
Bioavailability	75%	95%
$t_{1/2}$	8–10 h	18–24 h
Lipid solubility	Low	High
Dosing	Four times a day	Once a day
Excretion	Kidney	GIT
Safety in renal impairment	Not safe	Safe
GI flora	High suppression	Low suppression
Phototoxicity	Low	High

Abbreviations: GI, gastrointestinal; GIT, gastrointestinal tract.

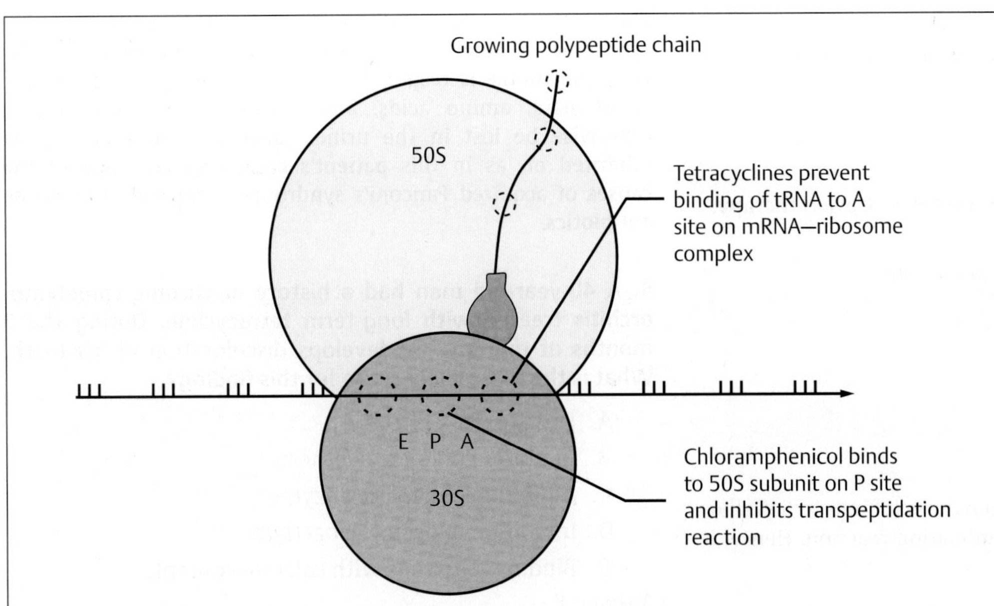
Growing polypeptide chain
50S
Tetracyclines prevent binding of tRNA to A site on mRNA–ribosome complex
E P A
30S
Chloramphenicol binds to 50S subunit on P site and inhibits transpeptidation reaction

Fig. 60.2 Mechanism of action of chloramphenicol.

refusal to feed, hypotonia, hypothermia, abdominal distention, metabolic acidosis, and ashen gray cyanosis. This complication can be fatal. It occurs due to inability to metabolize or due to inadequate hepatic glucuronidation.

Superinfection

This occurs as it is broad-spectrum antibiotic.

GI Toxicity

This is manifested as nausea, vomiting, and diarrhea.

Hypersensitivity

It is uncommon.

Drug Interactions

This occurs due to enzyme inhibition, which is manifested as toxicity of phenytoin, warfarin, or tolbutamide.

Uses

Its uses have decreased due to the risk of bone marrow depression. However, specific uses include the following:

1. Typhoid fever–earlier it was a drug of choice.
2. Bacterial meningitis–as an alternative to penicillin and cephalosporins.
3. Anaerobic infections–as an alternative to metronidazole and clindamycin, combined with aminoglycoside and penicillin.
4. Rickettsial infections–as alternative to tetracyclines.
5. Eye/ear infection–since it has good aqueous humor concentration.

Multiple Choice Questions

1. Tetracycline is used for the prophylaxis of:

A. Cholera.

B. Brucellosis.

C. Leptospirosis.

D. Meningitis.

Answer: A

Tetracyclines are used for prophylaxis of both cholera and leptospirosis.

2. Which of the following is not true regarding tetracycline?

A. It is not teratogenic.

B. It can cause tooth discoloration.

C. It can result in superinfection.

D. It can lead to pseudomembranous colitis.

Answer: A

Since tetracyclines chelate calcium, calcium–tetracycline orthophosphate complex gets deposited in developing teeth and bone. Hence, this leads to their deformities. Onycholysis and nail pigmentation also occur. Therefore, tetracyclines are teratogenic.

3. Tetracyclines inhibit protein synthesis by:

A. Inhibition of initiation and misreading of mRNA.

B. Binding to 30S subunit and inhibiting the binding of aminoacyl-tRNA to A site.

C. Inhibiting peptidyl transferase activity.

D. Inhibiting translocation.

Answer: B

Bacterial ribosomes have 50S and 30S subunits. Tetracyclines bind to 30S ribosomal subunit. Ribosomes have three binding sites, that is, A, P, and E sites. Tetracyclines bind to "A" site and prevent binding of tRNA to this site. tRNA carries amino acid for protein synthesis. Amino acids cannot be added and hence they inhibit protein synthesis. Thus, they are bacteriostatic.

4. Which one of the following statements about doxycycline is false?

A. It is bacteriostatic.

B. It is excreted mainly in the feces.

C. It is more active than tetracycline against *Helicobacter pylori*.

D. It is used in Lyme disease.

Answer: C

Tetracycline (and not doxycycline) is useful in *H. pylori* therapy.

5. Chloramphenicol acts through action on:

A. 50S ribosome.

B. 30S ribosome.

C. Nucleus.

D. Mitochondria.

Answer: A

Chloramphenicol is bacteriostatic in nature. It binds to 50S ribosomal subunit and inhibits transpeptidation reaction. Hence, it inhibits protein synthesis

6. A 15-year-old boy complains of rash on the palms and soles of his feet along with fever and headache. He was camping the previous weekend and admits to being bitten by a tick. His Weil–Felix test result is positive, suggesting Rocky Mountain spotted fever. What antibiotic should be given?

A. Ciprofloxacin.

B. Doxycycline.

C. Erythromycin.

D. Streptomycin.

E. Bacitracin.

Answer: B

Doxycycline, a tetracycline (30S ribosome inhibitor), is the antibiotic of choice to treat Rocky Mountain spotted fever, a rickettsial disease.

7. A 21-year-old woman complains of polydipsia and polyuria. She is found to have high levels of amino acids, phosphates, bicarbonate, and glucose in her urine. She reports that her friend gave her some old acne medication that she had in her medicine cabinet. Which medication did she likely use?

A. Erythromycin.

B. Isotretinoin.

C. Tetracycline.

D. Benzoyl peroxide.

E. Clindamycin.

Answer: C

This patient's manifestations are consistent with Fanconi's syndrome, a defect in proximal renal tubule function. The proximal tubule is responsible for reabsorbing the phosphate, bicarbonate, amino acids, and glucose filtered that would otherwise be lost in the urine. Fanconi's syndrome can be inherited or, as in this patient's case, acquired. One of the causes of acquired Fanconi's syndrome is expired tetracycline antibiotics.

8. A 40-year-old man had a history of chronic epididymo-orchitis treated with long-term tetracycline. During the 3 months of therapy, he develops discoloration of his teeth. What is the most likely cause for this finding?

A. Drug toxicity effect.

B. Inhibition of folate synthesis.

C. Inhibition of hepatic enzymes.

D. Inhibition of osteoclast activity.

E. Binding to tissues with calcium content.

Answer: E

Tetracyclines concentrate in the liver, kidney, spleen, and skin; and they bind to tissues undergoing calcification (e.g., teeth and bones). Deposition in the bone and primary dentition occurs during calcification in growing children. This causes discoloration and hypoplasia of the teeth and a temporary stunting of growth.

9. An 8-month-old female infant is brought to the emergency department by her parents. She is febrile, tachycardic, and hypotensive. Sepsis is suspected and the physician wants to give chloramphenicol but is worried about gray baby syndrome. Why does chloramphenicol sometimes cause gray baby syndrome in infants?

A. Chloramphenicol's narrow spectrum means empiric therapy is often ineffective.

B. Clindamycin, not chloramphenicol, causes gray baby syndrome.

C. Decreased absorption from the intestines.

D. Decreased conjugation in infant liver.

E. Decreased excretion by infant kidneys.

Answer: D

Chloramphenicol is a broad-spectrum antibiotic often used as empiric treatment in cases of sepsis. It is metabolized and inactivated via conjugation in the liver by glucuronyl transferase. The glucuronyl conjugate is easily excreted by the kidneys. Neonates and infants have decreased glucuronyl transferase activity, allowing chloramphenicol to build up to toxic levels. This is the supposed mechanism behind gray baby syndrome.

Chapter 61 Aminoglycosides

D. Thamizh Vani

Learning Objectives

- Mechanism of action.
- Antibacterial spectrum.
- Drug reactions.

Introduction

Aminoglycosides are antibiotics that are bactericidal, as they inhibit protein synthesis of bacteria and disturb the ribosomal functions. They may be natural or semisynthetic and are products of deliberate research, unlike penicillin. The term "aminoglycosides" is derived from the structure. Two amino sugars are joined to a nonsugar (aminocyclitol) by a glycosidic bond (–O–). The aminocyclitol moiety is 2-deoxystreptamine placed centrally in the majority of drugs in this group: amino sugar–O–2-deoxystreptaminen–O–amino sugar. In streptomycin, the nonsugar is streptidine placed laterally. Streptomycin was the first drug to be discovered by Waksman in 1944. There are two types of aminoglycosides

1. Systemic aminoglycosides—streptomycin, gentamicin, kanamycin, tobramycin, amikacin, sisomicin, netilmicin, paromomycin. New drug plazomicin has been approved by the FDA recently.
2. Topical aminoglycosides—neomycin, framycetin.

The salient features of aminoglycosides are given in **Box 61.1.**

Box 61.1 Salient features of aminoglycosides

- They are sulfate salts; all are highly soluble in water and are stable for months.
- They are not absorbed orally, as they ionize in solution. Distribution is only extracellular, they do not enter brain or cerebrospinal fluid (CSF).
- Excretion is via glomerular filtration, and it is excreted unchanged in the urine.
- They are active at alkaline pH and are bactericidal.
- They act by disrupting bacterial protein synthesis.
- They do not inhibit anaerobes, as their penetration involves oxygen-dependent active process. They are primarily active against aerobic gram-negative bacilli.
- Among them, there is only partial cross-resistance.
- Safety margin of this group is relatively narrow.
- All drugs exhibit ototoxicity and nephrotoxicity.

Mechanism of Action

Aminoglycosides enter bacterial cell walls through porin channels by passive diffusion. In periplasmic space, the transport is carrier mediated and is linked to electron transport chain by oxygen-dependent active process and high pH. After entry into bacterial cell, they bind to 30S ribosome and the formation of "initiation complex" freezes. Polysome formation is prevented and it is disintegrated into monosomes. This results in misreading of code and entry of wrong amino acid. Due to cell membrane disintegration, permeability is increased, and proteins and amino acids leak out, causing cell death. Their action is concentration dependent, and they also exert postantibiotic effect.

Antibacterial Spectrum

Gram-negative aerobic bacilli such as *Escherichia coli*, *Klebsiella*, *Shigella*, *Proteus*, *Enterobacter*, and *Pseudomonas aeruginosa* are inhibited. Only a few gram-positive cocci such as *Staphylococcus aureus*, *Streptococcus viridans*, and *Enterococcus faecalis* are inhibited. They are not effective against gram-positive bacilli, gram-negative cocci, and anaerobes.

Mechanism of Resistance

- Cell membrane-bound inactivating enzymes are acquired by conjugation and transfer of plasmids, which phosphorylate and adenylate/acetylate the antibiotic. This is the most important mechanism of resistance.
- Mutation decreases affinity to bind to ribosomal proteins. This is specific for a particular aminoglycoside.
- Efficiency of transporting mechanism is decreased. Pores may be less permeable or active transport is disrupted.

Drug Reactions

Ototoxicity

They are concentrated in the labyrinthine and affect vestibular or cochlear region. Degeneration of auditory nerves leads to permanent deafness.

Nephrotoxicity

Tubular damage occurs. Urine concentrating ability is lost. Low glomerular filtration rate, nitrogen retention, and albuminuria can occur.

Neuromuscular Blockade

They reduce acetylcholine release from nerve endings and also prevent fusion of synaptic vesicles and terminal membrane. This can be reversed by calcium and neostigmine. Neomycin and streptomycin have higher propensity.

Uses

Gentamicin has higher potency and broad spectrum of activity. It is used empirically in respiratory tract infections, postoperatively after tracheostomy or while on respirators, postoperative pneumonias, and peritonitis. It is used in infections caused by *Klebsiella*, *Proteus*, and *Pseudomonas* such as in burns, urinary tract infections, septicemia, osteomyelitis, and middle ear infections. It is combined with third-generation cephalosporin for meningitis and with penicillin/vancomycin/ampicillin for subacute bacterial endocarditis (SABE).

Streptomycin is used mainly in tuberculosis. It is also used in SABE (in conjunction with penicillin), plague, and tularemia. Kanamycin is more cochleotoxic, and therefore, it used occasionally as second-line drug in resistant tuberculosis. Tobramycin is used in *Pseudomonas* and *Proteus* infections.

Amikacin is resistant to inactivating enzymes and has widest spectrum of activity. Its uses are similar to those of gentamicin, and it is mainly used as a reserve drug in hospital-acquired infections. Sisomicin is used against *Pseudomonas*, *Streptococci*, and SABE. Netilmicin is used in conditions where gentamicin is resistant.

Neomycin and framycetin are used topically for infected wound, ulcers, burn, external ear infections, and conjunctivitis. They are used orally in preparation of bowel before surgery and in hepatic coma, where it kills bacteria and diminishes production of ammonia.

Precautions

Single daily dosing rather than three times a day shows lesser nephrotoxicity. Avoid concurrent use of other nephrotoxic drugs such as nonsteroidal anti-inflammatory drugs (NSAIDs), amphotericin B, vancomycin, and cyclosporine.

Caution should be exercised while using in elderly (age >60 years) and in those with kidney damage. Aminoglycosides should be avoided during pregnancy, due to risk of fetal ototoxicity. Avoid other ototoxic drugs such as minocycline and furosemide. Cautious use of muscle relaxants is required in patients receiving aminoglycoside.

Multiple Choice Questions

1. A 72-kg patient with gram-negative infection is administered amikacin intramuscularly at a dose of 5 mg/kg every 8 hours. The patient's creatinine clearance is 80 mL/min, which decreases to 40 mL/min. What is the most reasonable management?

A. Increase time interval of dose administration.
B. Decrease dosage to 200 mg daily.
C. Switch to gentamicin and discontinue amikacin.
D. Decrease dosage to 180 mg every 8 hours.

Answer: D

Monitoring plasma drug levels is important when aminoglycosides are used. In this case, the patient seems to be improving; hence, a decrease of the amikacin dose in proportion to decreased creatinine clearance is most appropriate. Because creatinine clearance is only one-half of the starting value, a dose reduction should be made to one-half of that given initially.

2. A 76-year-old diabetic man complains of pain behind the ear. Physical examination reveals edema of external canal with pus. Gram stain of exudate shows polymorphs and gram-negative rods. Which treatment is most appropriate?

A. The patient should be hospitalized and started with gentamicin plus ticarcillin.
B. Analgesics should be given, and the patient should be sent home.
C. The patient should be hospitalized and treated with imipenem.
D. Amikacin should be injected intramuscularly and the patient should be sent home.

Answer: A

The diabetic patient with otitis externa is at risk of spread of infection to middle ear; thus, hospitalization is advisable. Antibiotic coverage must include *E. coli*, *Pseudomonas*, and other gram-negative rods. Combination of aminoglycoside and wide-spectrum penicillin is synergistic and most suitable.

3. Which statement about "once daily dosing" with aminoglycosides is not accurate?

A. Dose adjustment is less important in renal dysfunction.
B. Convenient for outpatient treatment.
C. Less time required for drug administration.
D. Underdoing is less of a problem.

Answer: A

In "once daily dosing" with aminoglycosides, selection of an appropriate dose is particularly critical in patients with renal insufficiency. Aminoglycosides are eliminated in kidney in proportion to creatinine clearance. Knowledge of the degree of insufficiency based on plasma creatinine is essential for the estimation of appropriate single daily dose of an aminoglycoside.

4. A patient experiences aminoglycoside toxicity. Which problem will he/she encounter?

A. Pain.
B. Rash.
C. Tinnitus.
D. Difficulty in breathing.

Answer: C

As aminoglycosides are ototoxic, the first symptom to occur is tinnitus.

5. Which aminoglycoside is most commonly used in patients with cystic fibrosis affected with Pseudomonas aeruginosa?

A. Streptomycin.
B. Tobramycin.

C. Gentamicin.

D. Amikacin.

Answer: B

Tobramycin may be delivered via inhalational route and is frequently used in cystic fibrosis patients.

6. With regard to the toxicity of aminoglycosides, which statement is accurate?

A. Gentamicin and tobramycin are least likely to cause renal damage.

B. Ototoxicity due to amikacin and gentamicin includes vestibular dysfunction, which is irreversible.

C. Ototoxicity of aminoglycosides is reduced if used along with loop diuretics.

D. Reduced blood creatinine is an early sign of aminoglycoside toxicity.

Answer: B

The first indication of toxicity is increased through serum levels of aminoglycosides, followed by increase in blood creatinine.

Chapter 62

Macrolides and Miscellaneous Antimicrobials and Pharmacotherapy of STD and UTI

Asha B.

PH1.48: Describe the mechanisms of action, types, doses, side effects, indications, and contraindications of the drugs used in urinary tract infection/sexually transmitted diseases and viral diseases including HIV.

Learning Objectives

- Macrolide.
- Ketolides.
- Lincosamides.
- Glycopeptides.
- Lipoglycopeptides.
- Lipopeptides.
- Oxazolidinones.
- Streptogramins.
- Polypeptides.
- Drug treatment of urinary tract infections.
- Drug treatment of sexually transmitted diseases.

Macrolide

The name "macrolide" is given due to the large (macro) lactone ring of 12 or more elements, which are attached to multiple deoxy sugars. The macrolides that are 14-, 15-, and 16-membered rings are widely used as antimicrobial agents. The first macrolide, erythromycin (14-membered macrolide), isolated from *Streptomyces erythreus*, was discovered in 1952 and is used in clinical practice. The other macrolides added to this category are roxithromycin, clarithromycin, azithromycin, and fidaxomicin. Macrolides have been widely used as alternatives to penicillin.

Mechanism of Action

Macrolides inhibit protein synthesis, act as bacteriostatic agents, and can have cidal action only in higher doses. They bind to the 23S rRNA part of 50s ribosomal subunit and inhibit the translocation of nascent peptide from A (acceptor) site to the P (peptidyl) site, thereby blocking the attachment of the new amino acyl tRNA to the A site. As a result of its action on elongation stage of protein synthesis, short nascent peptides are synthesized by bacterial RNA polymerase, which ultimately stops the translation.

Development of Drug Resistance

Chromosomal mutations (mainly in gram-positive organisms) can alter 50S ribosomal protein, thereby preventing the binding of macrolide. Drug efflux by an active pump mechanism is mainly seen in gram-negative organisms. Ribosomal protection by production of methylase enzymes decreases drug binding by modifying ribosomal target, and esterases cause hydrolysis.

Erythromycin

Erythromycin is one of the earliest macrolide antibiotics used clinically. It has a narrow spectrum. It gets destroyed in acidic pH (acid labile), whereas alkaline medium enhances its activity due to increased proportion of the unionized form of the drug. It is available as enteric-coated tablet and its absorption is affected by food. The distribution of erythromycin is wide and it achieves good concentration in cavity (abscess, serous cavity) and crosses the placental barrier. It is metabolized in the liver and excreted in the bile. It is safe to use in patients with renal failure. The plasma $t_{1/2}$ is 1 to 2 hours, but the action lasts up to 4 to 6 hours.

The spectrum includes majority of gram-positive and a few gram-negative organisms, such as *Streptococcus pyogenes*, *Streptococcus pneumoniae*, *Neisseria gonorrhoeae*, *Clostridium*, *Corynebacterium diphtheriae*, *Haemophilus influenzae*, and *Bordetella pertussis*. It is effective on atypical organisms such as *Legionella*, *Chlamydia*, *Mycoplasma*, *Branhamella catarrhalis*, *Gardnerella vaginalis*, and *Rickettsia*.

Nonantimicrobial Effects

Erythromycin acts as mucolytic agent by altering the consistency of secretions; in addition, it increases the transport of mucous. It is known to reduce inflammation in bronchus and bronchioles. The anti-inflammatory action is due to inhibition of adhesion particles that assist in white blood cell (WBC) infiltration. Macrolides have membrane-stabilizing action and inhibit oxidative stress. Macrolides also inhibit cytokine production and macrophage proliferation.

Uses

Respiratory Tract Infections

Erythromycin is preferred in acute exacerbations of chronic bronchitis, tonsillitis, laryngitis, acute otitis media, acute streptococcal pharyngitis, and acute bacterial sinusitis.

Skin and Soft-tissue Infections

Erythromycin is used in the treatment of erysipelas and cellulitis due to *Staphylococcus aureus*. Recently, erythromycin was found to be ineffective against *S. aureus*.

Whooping Cough

Erythromycin can be used for 2 weeks for treating pertussis. The treatment is more effective when started in the early stages of infection.

Diphtheria

Erythromycin for 1 week is very effective in treating diphtheria.

Tetanus

Erythromycin along with tetanus toxoid is effective.

Sexually Transmitted Diseases

Erythromycin is used as a second-line drug to treat syphilis, gonorrhea, and chancroid.

Miscellaneous Uses

Erythromycin's immunomodulatory action is used in asthma, bronchiectasis, and chronic bronchitis. It also stimulates gastrointestinal (GI) motility by action on motilin receptors; hence, it is used in diabetic gastroparesis.

Adverse Effects

GI Toxicity

Erythromycin causes moderate-to-severe epigastric distress. Erythromycin stimulates GI motility by acting on motilin receptors and increases the gastric motility in intensive care setups and diabetic gastroparesis.

Hepatotoxicity

When used for long duration (more than 10 days), it is associated with manifestations of cholestatic hepatitis. It presents as nausea, abdominal discomfort, and occasional vomiting. Few people may further develop jaundice with elevated liver enzymes, which will subside on stopping the drug.

Cardiac Toxicity

Erythromycin intake has been reported to cause QT prolongation and related cardiac arrhythmias such as ventricular tachycardia. The risk increases with addition of drugs that increase QT interval. Caution is advised to avoid such combinations.

Hypersensitivity Reactions

Few people may have allergic reactions such as flulike symptoms, fever, eosinophilia, and skin eruptions, which disappear immediately after stopping the drug.

Ototoxicity

Rarely, auditory impairment with or without tinnitus has been reported with erythromycin.

Clarithromycin

Clarithromycin differs from erythromycin only by methylation of the hydroxyl group at the 6th position, due to which there is improved acid stability and tissue penetration and broad spectrum of activity.

Clarithromycin has better sensitivity for the strains of streptococci and staphylococci, *Moraxella catarrhalis*, *Chlamydia*, *Legionella pneumophila*, *Borrelia burgdorferi*, *Mycoplasma pneumoniae*, *Mycobacterium leprae*, *Mycobacterium avium* complex, and *Helicobacter pylori*. It is active against *Toxoplasma gondii*, *Cryptosporidium*, and *Plasmodium* species.

Clarithromycin has less food–drug interaction when compared to erythromycin. The extended-release preparation can be given with food to improve bioavailability. Clarithromycin achieves higher concentration throughout the body, more so in the middle ear. It inhibits CYP3A4 and has a $t_{1/2}$ of 4 to 7 hours; it is metabolized in the liver and follows zero-order kinetics in elimination; hence, increasing its dose will increase its half-life (lower-dose $t_{1/2}$: 4–7 hours; higher-dose $t_{1/2}$: 6–10 hours). Dose adjustment is not needed in hepatic failure and mild-to-moderate renal impairment.

Uses

Clarithromycin is mainly used in *H. pylori* treatment as one of the components in the triple-drug regimen. It is effective in eradicating *H. pylori* in 1 to 2 weeks. It is the first-line drug in the combination regimens for *M. avium* complex infection, especially in immunocompromised individuals such as AIDS patients. It is also used in combination to treat leprosy. Other indications are similar to erythromycin, such as pharyngitis, tonsillitis, otitis media, diphtheria, whooping cough, and skin with soft-tissue infection.

Adverse Effects

Apart from the common side effects similar to erythromycin, it causes pseudomembranous enterocolitis, myalgia, and myopathy due to rhabdomyolysis. The gastric irritation is less compared to erythromycin.

Roxithromycin

Roxithromycin is similar to erythromycin with regard to spectrum; however, it has more potency against *G. vaginalis*, *Legionella*, and *B. catarrhalis*. It has better gastric tolerance with a longer duration of action compared to erythromycin. The oral bioavailability is good, with plasma $t_{1/2}$ being 12 hours. The drug interaction with regard to cytochrome P450 is less.

Uses

Its uses are similar to those of erythromycin, such as in acute precipitation of chronic bronchitis, tonsillitis, laryngitis, acute otitis media, acute streptococcal pharyngitis, and acute bacterial sinusitis. It can be used in *Legionella* pneumonia, skin with soft-tissue infections, and bacterial vaginitis.

Adverse Effects

Roxithromycin has minimum adverse effects, as it is well-tolerated. The compliance is better due to less gastric irritation and decreased frequency of intake compared to erythromycin; therefore, roxithromycin is commonly used in children to treat upper respiratory tract infections.

Azithromycin

Azithromycin is a 15-membered lactone ring, which is an azalide derivative of erythromycin. It differs from erythromycin by the addition of a methyl-substituted nitrogen atom into the lactone ring due to which there is improved acid stability and tissue penetration and broader spectrum of activity. Azithromycin has similar activity as erythromycin against sensitive strains of streptococci and staphylococci. Azithromycin is more effective against *H. influenzae, M. catarrhalis, Chlamydia* species, *L. pneumophila, B. burgdorferi, M. pneumoniae, H. pylori, M. avium* complex, *T. gondii, Cryptosporidium*, and *Plasmodium* species.

Azithromycin has a good oral bioavailability; when administered orally, it is absorbed rapidly and distributed widely, and it achieves higher concentration within the cells and tissues, except to the brain and cerebrospinal fluid (CSF). Azithromycin should not be given just before or after food when administered orally. Azithromycin is metabolized in the liver into inactive metabolites and is excreted in the bile. The plasma $t_{1/2}$ is 50 to 68 hours; hence, there is prolonged duration of action. It does not affect the hepatic CYP3A4 and therefore drug interactions are minimum.

Uses

It is used in community-acquired pneumonia, Legionnaires' pneumonia, pharyngitis, or sinusitis. A dose of 500 mg is given once daily for 3 to 5 days, depending on the severity.

The treatment or prophylaxis of *M. avium* complex infection in HIV-infected patients requires higher doses: 500 to 600 mg daily in combination with one or more other agents for treatment or 1,200 mg once weekly for primary prevention.

Azithromycin is useful in the treatment of sexually transmitted diseases (STDs) such as nonspecific urethritis and vaginitis, especially during pregnancy when tetracyclines are contraindicated. The treatment of uncomplicated nongonococcal urethritis and chancroid requires a single 1-g dose of azithromycin. If the infection is of severe type, then three weekly doses are required. In donovanosis, caused due to *Klebsiella granulomatis*, the dose used is 500 mg once a day for 7 days.

In children, azithromycin oral suspension is preferred for acute otitis media and pneumonia, and the dose is 10 mg/kg on the first day and 5 mg/kg for 4 days. A single 30-mg/kg dose is approved as an alternative for otitis media.

Rarely, azithromycin is used in typhoid fever and toxoplasmosis.

Adverse Effects

GI Toxicity

Oral or intravenous (IV) administration of azithromycin is very rarely associated with gastric upset, accompanied by moderate-to-severe epigastric distress.

Hepatotoxicity

On prolonged use, elevated liver enzymes have been reported with azithromycin, which subsides on stopping the drug.

Cardiac Toxicity

Azithromycin intake has been reported to cause QT prolongation and cardiac arrhythmias. A long-term cohort study reports sudden cardiac arrest due to azithromycin compared to placebo.

Hypersensitivity Reactions

Allergic reactions such as rashes, fever, and eosinophilia have been reported, but the incidence is less compared to erythromycin.

Fidaxomicin

Fidaxomicin is the first narrow-spectrum macrolide antibiotic obtained from actinomycete *Dactylosporangium aurantiacum*. It does not get absorbed systemically when given orally. It is currently used to treat diarrhea induced by *Clostridium difficile*, where a dose of 200 mg twice daily for 10 days is advised. It is a well-tolerated drug with few side effects such as nausea, abdominal pain, tenderness, and, rarely, fever.

Spiramycin

Spiramycin is a 16-membered ring macrolide, which was isolated in 1954 from *Streptomyces ambofaciens*. It is effective against gram-positive cocci and rods, gram-negative cocci, and certain atypical organisms such as legionellae, mycoplasmas, and chlamydiae; it is more effective on *T. gondii* and *Cryptosporidium* species. Spiramycin achieves higher concentration in tissues compared to plasma and specifically concentrates in placental tissue. It is mainly indicated for the treatment of acquired toxoplasmosis in early pregnancy to prevent transmission to the fetus. Spiramycin is available through the investigational new drug process at the U.S. FDA. It is a well-tolerated drug with rare occurrence of mild gastritis and nausea.

Ketolides

Telithromycin

Telithromycin belongs to ketolide group and differs from erythromycin in that 3-keto group replaces the α-L-cladinose of the 14-member macrolide ring. This modification makes it less susceptible to the efflux-mediated drug resistance mechanism. Ketolides are active against macrolide-resistant gram-positive strains such as *S. pneumoniae*, *Bacteroides fragilis*, and *M. avium* complex. Telithromycin is the only ketolide currently available.

It is well absorbed orally, with about 60% bioavailability. Telithromycin penetrates well into the cells (phagocytes and WBCs) and tissue, and achieves higher concentrations compared to plasma. The plasma $t_{1/2}$ is of 10 hours, and it is given once daily. The drug is eliminated by hepatic metabolism, 50% by CYP3A4 and 50% by other metabolism. The recommended dose in adults is 800 mg orally once daily. It is not available for parenteral use.

Telithromycin is effective in the treatment of community-acquired pneumonia, acute exacerbations of chronic bronchitis, and acute bacterial sinusitis resistant to other macrolides. The major drawback is its potential to cause severe hepatotoxicity due to which FDA approval is limited to community-acquired pneumonia.

Lincosamides

The drugs under lincosamides are lincomycin and its derivative clindamycin, which were introduced for medical use in 1964. It is isolated from the actinomycete *Streptomyces lincolnensis*. The mechanism of action and spectrum is similar to that described for erythromycin with spectrum extending to *Mycoplasma* and *Plasmodium* species. The oral bioavailability is poor; hence, parental preparations (intramuscular [IM], IV) are preferred. It was mainly used for severe and resistant gram-positive infections associated with allergy to penicillin.

Clindamycin

Clindamycin is a chlorinated lincosamide antibiotic, which has largely replaced lincomycin. It binds to 50S ribosome exclusively and inhibits protein synthesis. Concomitant administration of other drugs, such as chloramphenicol and other macrolides, along with clindamycin may reduce their binding to ribosome. The bacterial strains susceptible to clindamycin are pneumococci and penicillinase-producing strains of *S. aureus* but not methicillin-resistant *S. aureus* (MRSA) and coagulase-negative *S. aureus*. Clindamycin has increased activity against *B. fragilis*, a few *Clostridium* species, *Actinomyces israelii*, and *Nocardia asteroides*. Along with primaquine and pyrimethamine, clindamycin is sensitive against *Pneumocystis jirovecii* and *T. Gondii*, respectively.

Clindamycin is not a substrate for macrolide efflux pumps due to which the strains that are resistant to macrolides by this mechanism are susceptible to clindamycin. The chances of developing resistance are less compared to other macrolides.

Clindamycin is well absorbed orally and has a good bioavailability and minimal food–drug interaction. The plasma $t_{1/2}$ is 3 to 4 hours. Clindamycin is widely distributed in fluid pockets and tissues and crosses placental barrier but not CSF barrier when meninges are normal. In inflamed meninges, the drug levels are sufficient to treat cerebral toxoplasmosis. The drug readily crosses the placental barrier. Clindamycin is primarily metabolized in the liver and dose adjustment is required in patients with severe hepatic failure.

Uses

Clindamycin is a second-line agent for the treatment of mixed infections such as pelvic and lung abscess. It is also used in other skin and soft-tissue infections such as abdominal-penetrating injuries and septic abortion, especially in patients with allergy to β-lactam antibiotics. Topical clindamycin is used for acne. Clindamycin is also administered vaginally for bacterial vaginosis.

It is used orally to treat MRSA-induced osteomyelitis (due to good penetration into the bone) and other infections involving the bone and joint. It is also effective in *Clostridium perfringens*–induced necrotizing fasciitis or gas gangrene.

It is used as an alternative agent for treatment of sinusitis, pharyngitis, and otitis media. Clindamycin along with primaquine is useful for the treatment of mild-to-moderate cases of *P. jirovecii* pneumonia in AIDS patients. Clindamycin in combination with pyrimethamine is used in encephalitis caused by *T. gondii* in patients with AIDS. Clindamycin plus quinine is used as an unconventional regimen for malaria.

Adverse Effects

Superinfection with *C. difficile* is common, which manifests as watery diarrhea, fever, and elevated peripheral WBC counts. Adequate hydration along with the administration of metronidazole or vancomycin can treat the superinfection and prevent fatality.

Skin rashes, urticaria, and, rarely, Stevens–Johnson syndrome and anaphylactic reaction can occur. The liver enzymes can temporarily increase along with decrease in WBC and platelet counts. Local thrombophlebitis may occur during IV administration of the drug. It may cause mild neuromuscular blockade, and thus it should be avoided in myasthenia gravis patients.

Glycopeptides

Vancomycin

Vancomycin was the first tricyclic glycopeptide antibiotic derived from *Streptococcus orientalis* in 1956 to treat MRSA infections resistant to penicillins. Vancomycin is active against gram-positive bacteria including MRSA, penicillin-resistant streptococci, ampicillin-resistant enterococci, *C. difficile*, *Neisseria*, and diphtheria. All species of gram-negative bacilli and mycobacteria are resistant to vancomycin.

Mechanism of Action

Vancomycin inhibits the synthesis of the cell wall in gram-positive bacteria by binding with high affinity to the D-alanyl-D-alanine terminus of cell wall units. Due to its large molecular size, it cannot penetrate the outer membrane of gram-negative bacteria. After binding to the terminal sequence of peptidoglycan units, vancomycin prevents release from lipid carrier in order to prevent assembly and cross-linking of precursor units. Thus, the formation of firm, rigid cell wall is inhibited.

Vancomycin resistance is transferred through transposon in enterococci and streptococci and *S. aureus*. Alteration of the D-alanyl-D-alanine target to D-alanyl-D-lactate or D-alanyl-D-serine prevents binding of vancomycin.

Vancomycin is poorly absorbed orally; hence, for systemic indications, it is administrated as IV infusion. It is widely distributed when given in IV to the various tissues, cavities, and meninges when inflamed. The elimination half-life is about 5 to 6 hours. Dose adjustment is needed during renal impairment.

Uses

In serious MRSA infections such as osteomyelitis, endocarditis, meningitis, and pneumonia, IV infusion of vancomycin 500 mg every 6 hours is used. It is also used in enterococcal endocarditis along with amikacin or gentamicin. In pseudomembranous colitis due to *C. difficile* in patients not responding to metronidazole and in staphylococcal enteritis, oral vancomycin 125 to 500 mg every 6 hours is advised, depending on the severity of the infection.

Vancomycin is used for surgical prophylaxis in MRSA-predominant areas. In serious skin and soft-tissue infections, either suspected MRSA or mixed infection, vancomycin alone or with ceftriaxone is used. Also, it is empirically used in community-acquired bacterial meningitis in areas where streptococcal pneumonia is prevalent; in addition, it is preferred in nosocomial meningitis.

It is prophylactically used in dialysis patients on immunosuppressive therapy and in patients with prolonged fever and neutropenia.

Adverse Effects

Oral Formulation

Vancomycin when given orally is well tolerated with few side effects such as abdominal discomfort and diarrhea due to alteration in intestinal microbiota.

Intravenous Preparation

On administering IV infusion, vancomycin can cause infusion-related reactions such as hypotension, dizziness, tachycardia, flushing, and rashes. It is known to release histamine; hence, it can lead to diffuse rash and redness, called red man or red neck syndrome. It is known to cause nephrotoxicity due to impurities in the formulation. Adequate hydration and switching over to formulation with less or no impurities can reduce nephrotoxicity. Rarely, it can lead to maculopapular eruptions and anaphylactic reactions. Ototoxicity is reported when there is higher concentration achieved in plasma.

Teicoplanin

Teicoplanin is a semisynthetic glycopeptide antibiotic isolated from *Actinoplanes teichomyceticus*, with the mechanism of action similar to vancomycin. The oral bioavailability is poor; hence, it is administered as IV or IM injection. The plasma half-life is 2 to 3 days; hence, once a day administration is sufficient. Systemically, teicoplanin 400 mg is given on the first day, followed by 200 mg daily for treating severe infection. It is mainly eliminated through the renal system; hence, dose adjustment is required in patients with renal impairment.

Teicoplanin is more effective against enterococci, MRSA, and vancomycin-resistant enterococci (VRE; but not effective in vancomycin-resistant *S. aureus* [VRSA]); hence, it is used in serious enterococcal endocarditis, penicillin-resistant streptococcal infections, and MRSA osteomyelitis.

Spectrum and Uses

As an alternative drug, it can be used in surgical prophylaxis and febrile neutropenia. Teicoplanin is used to prevent vascular catheter–related infections and mixed soft-tissue infections due to gram-positive organisms.

Adverse Effects

Hypersensitivity reactions such as rashes and urticaria anaphylaxis can occur, albeit rarely. Red man syndrome due to histamine release during IV injection is not reported. Rarely, auditory impairment can occur. Nephrotoxicity is less with teicoplanin.

Lipoglycopeptides

Lipoglycopeptides are a recently introduced group of antibiotics that have lipophilic side chain linked to glycopeptides. This class includes telavancin, dalbavancin, and oritavancin. The lipophilic chain confers a longer half-life and converts these agents into concentration-dependent bactericidal antibiotics.

Mechanism of Action

The mechanism of action of lipoglycopeptides is similar to vancomycin, but they are more robust compared to it. They bind to peptidoglycan precursor and inhibit transglycosylation along with transpeptidation, which is 10-fold higher than vancomycin. In addition to this, lipoglycopeptides also alter the membrane function associated with adenosine triphosphate, potassium leakage due to which there is increased cell permeability, and decreased cell viability. Due to this additional mechanism, there is rapid bactericidal activity compared to vancomycin.

Telavancin is administered intravenously at a dose of 10 mg/kg daily, with dosage adjustment required for patients with renal dysfunction. The approved dosage of IV dalbavancin for treatment of skin and soft-tissue infection is 1,000 mg at the initiation of treatment, followed by a 500-mg dose 7 days later. Oritavancin has been studied for skin and soft-tissue infections as a single 1,200-mg IV dose.

Uses

Telavancin, dalbavancin, and oritavancin are used as alternatives in serious MRSA infections such as osteomyelitis, endocarditis, meningitis and pneumonia. Enterococcal endocarditis, including vancomycin-resistant infections, is treated along with amikacin or gentamicin. Lipoglycopeptides are used for surgical prophylaxis in MRSA- and VRSA-predominant areas. They are used as alternatives in community-acquired bacterial meningitis in areas with streptococcal pneumonia and nosocomial meningitis.

Adverse Effects

Oritavancin is to be used cautiously with warfarin due to its effect on CYP-mediated metabolism. It should not be combined with nephrotoxic drugs as there is risk of additional toxicity. It can cause hypersensitivity reactions such as rashes, urticarial, and anaphylaxis, which will be difficult to treat due to its long half-life. Telavancin can cause QT interval prolongation, so one should be careful not to combine with other drugs with similar action. It is contraindicated in pregnancy due to teratogenic effects observed in animal studies.

Lipopeptides

Daptomycin

Daptomycin is a cyclic lipopeptide antibiotic derived from *Streptomyces roseosporus*. Daptomycin is effective against most gram-positive organisms including MRSA, vancomycin-resistant strains, e.g., VRSA, and VRE. It binds to bacterial cell membrane and inhibits membrane potential, and has bactericidal activity against aerobic and anaerobic gram-positive bacteria. It has concentration-dependent killing of bacteria. There is evidence for development of resistance to daptomycin, but the mechanism is not clear, and it could be due to alteration in the cell membrane binding site. Surprisingly, the combination of daptomycin and β-lactam antibiotics could reverse the resistance; hence, daptomycin and β-lactam antibiotics can be combined for better efficiency.

Daptomycin has a poor oral bioavailability; hence, it is administered only through the parental route. Due to direct toxicity to muscle on IM injection, currently only IV route preparations are available. The plasma $t_{1/2}$ is 8 to 10 hours, and the drug is mainly eliminated through the renal system. It is used in complicated skin and soft-tissue infections such as pelvis infection, deep-seated abscess, septicemia, bacteremia, and right-sided endocarditis. Daptomycin is ineffective in pulmonary diseases, as it gets inactivated by lung surfactant. It should be used cautiously in patients with renal impairment (once in 2 days). It is a relatively well-tolerated drug with rare occurrence of rhabdomyolysis, myopathy, arthralgia, insomnia, hypersensitivity reaction, and elevation of creatine kinase; hence, care is to be taken while combining with aminoglycosides.

Oxazolidinones

Linezolid

Linezolid belongs to a novel class of the synthetic group oxazolidinones. The second agent in this group is tedizolid, which was approved in 2014. The latest drug is sutezolid designed for drug-resistant tuberculosis. Drugs in this class are specifically active against gram-positive organisms such as staphylococci, streptococci, and enterococci, gram-positive anaerobic cocci, and gram-positive rods such as *Corynebacterium*, *Nocardia*, and *Listeria monocytogenes* including MRSA, VRSA, VRE, *Mycobacterium tuberculosis*, and *B. fragilis*. It is not effective against gram-negative aerobic and anaerobic organisms. It inhibits protein synthesis, hence bacteriostatic action against all susceptible organisms except streptococci, where it exhibits bactericidal action.

Mechanism of Action

Linezolid inhibits bacterial protein synthesis by binding to the specific site 23S fraction of the 50S ribosomal subunit at P site and prevents formation of the larger ribosomal ternary *N*-formylmethionine–tRNA complex that initiates protein synthesis. It does not exhibit cross-resistance with any group, and due to its distinctive mechanism of action, it is effective in most resistant strains of gram-positive organisms (MRSA, VRSA, VRE). Resistance may occur due to point mutation of 23S rRNA and transferable methyltransferase that causes ribosomal modification.

Linezolid has an exceptionally good oral bioavailability, nearing 100%, due to which the dose in oral and parenteral route are similar (600 mg). Food does not affect bioavailability; hence, no specific instructions are needed with regard to intake of drug. It gets metabolized without enzymes through oxidation into aminoethoxyacetic acid and glycerin derivatives. The plasma half-life is 5 to 6 hours. Linezolid gets distributed to fairly perfused organs and is eliminated mainly in the urine; however, dose adjustment is not required in renal impairment.

Uses

Linezolid is most commonly administered at a dose of 600 mg twice daily orally or intravenously for uncomplicated skin and soft-tissue infection due to streptococci and *S. aureus* (MRSA, VRSA). In respiratory tract infections such as community-acquired pneumonia, including nosocomial infection, it is also used. Linezolid can be used in urinary tract infection (UTI), prostatitis, intra-abdominal infections due to *Enterococcus faecalis* and *Enterococcus faecium*. It can also be used in extensively drug-resistant tuberculosis.

Adverse Effects

Suppression of bone marrow leading to anemia, leukopenia, pancytopenia, and thrombocytopenia has been reported in patients taking linezolid for more than 10 days, which is reversible on discontinuation of the drug. Complete hemogram should be advised if prolonged therapy is planned and patients are warned about the risk of bleeding. Peripheral neuropathy, optic neuritis, and, rarely, lactic acidosis can develop due to mitochondrial toxicity only on treatment for more than 6 weeks.

Concomitant intake of tyramine-rich food or selective serotonin reuptake inhibitors (SSRIs) and serotonin and norepinephrine reuptake inhibitors (SNRIs) along with linezolid may lead to sudden increase in serotonin levels, leading to hypertensive crisis, restlessness, uneasy sensation, palpitations, and headache. Consequently, serotonin syndrome occurs due to weak nonspecific MOA inhibition by linezolid.

Mild GI disturbances such as nausea, vomiting, and abdominal pain, taste alteration, and rashes can occur.

Tedizolid

Tedizolid was approved in 2014 and has similar spectrum to linezolid; in addition, it is active against linezolid-resistant isolates.

It is available as prodrug tedizolid phosphate, which gets hydrolyzed to tedizolid. It has a good oral bioavailability of more than 85%. It has longer plasma half-life of 12 hours compared to linezolid. The metabolism primarily occurs in the liver, and the drug gets eliminated in feces. The mechanism of action is similar to linezolid. Tedizolid is given as a 200 mg IV or oral daily dose for skin and soft-tissue infections caused by gram-positive organism resistant to other antimicrobial agents, community-acquired pneumonia, and nosocomial infections. Tedizolid's 6-day regimen is as effective as linezolid given for 10 days. It is a well-tolerated drug, as the myelosuppression and mitochondrial toxicity is less compared to linezolid.

Streptogramins (Quinupristin and Dalfopristin)

Streptogramins are semisynthetic derivatives obtained from *Streptomyces pristinaespiralis*. Fixed combination of quinupristin (a streptogramin B) with dalfopristin (a streptogramin A) in a 30:70 ratio is approved for clinical use. Quinupristin and dalfopristin inhibit protein synthesis by binding to two adjacent sites on 50S ribosomal subunit. Quinupristin binds at 23S rRNA part of 50s ribosomal subunit and inhibits translocation, and dalfopristin binds to another site nearby and causes conformational changes and increases binding of quinupristin. Both components synergistically inhibit protein synthesis and exhibit bactericidal action. Drug resistance occurs due to gene encoding a ribosomal methylase, leading to its protection from binding by streptogramins. Another gene encoding lactonases inactivates quinupristin.

Streptogramins are active against gram-positive cocci including MRSA, VRSA, *M. pneumoniae*, *Legionella*, and *Chlamydia*, but are inactive against gram-negative organisms and *E. faecalis*. Quinupristin/dalfopristin is not absorbed orally; hence, it is administered by IV infusion for over 60 to 90 minutes. It is primarily metabolized in the liver and eliminated by the bile. Dosage alteration is required in hepatic impairment as the plasma concentration may increase.

Uses

Streptogramins are used in complicated skin and soft-tissue infection due to MRSA, VRSA, and other resistant strains of *S. aureus*. They are also used in nosocomial infections such as nosocomial pneumonia and infections caused by MRSA. Vancomycin-resistant *E. faecium* infections such as endocarditis and surgical prophylaxis are also treated with streptogramins.

Adverse Effects

Infusion-related reactions such as flushing, phlebitis, and rashes are noted. They are known to cause arthralgia and myalgia. These adversities can be minimized by slow infusion over longer time. Rarely, they can cause QT prolongation; hence, caution is to be taken when they are administered along with other drugs with similar effect.

Mupirocin

Mupirocin is a complex combination of many pseudomonic acids isolated from *Pseudomonas fluorescens*. It is available only for topical use against gram-positive bacteria and few gram-negative organisms. The mechanism of action is unique—by inhibiting isoleucyl–tRNA synthetase, thereby inhibiting bacterial protein synthesis. Due to this distinctive action, it does not exhibit cross-resistance with other classes of antibiotics. Resistance can be mediated through plasmid that codes for another enzyme alternative to isoleucine synthase, which has poor binding to mupirocin.

Uses

Mupirocin 2% cream and 2% ointment are used for skin lesion to prevent secondary infection. Intranasal mupirocin ointment is used to eradicate intranasal *S. aureus* colonization. It is also used in impetigo, furunculosis, folliculitis, eruptions, and boils.

Adverse Effects

This is a well-tolerated, safe drug, which, on topical use, can cause irritation, burning sensation, and rash. Avoid applying on large damaged surface in renal impairment, as it may precipitate failure due to polyethylene glycol component in the ointment.

Fusidic Acid

Fusidic acid is a steroidal antibiotic derived from the fungus *Fusidium coccineum* and used topically to treat skin infections caused by gram-positive organisms. It inhibits bacterial protein synthesis by preventing the turnover of elongation factor G from the ribosome. It is used topically for furunculosis, carbuncle, cellulitis, impetigo, and skin infections. On topical application, it can cause burning and stinging sensation in the skin soreness and dryness when applied to the eye.

Polypeptides

Polymyxins (Polymyxin B and Polymyxin E)

They are polypeptide antibiotics that have low molecular weight and are used only topically due to their systemic toxicity. Polymyxin E is also known as colistin and is obtained from *Bacillus colistinus*. They are used due to their activity against resistant gram-negative organisms such as *Pseudomonas*, *Acinetobacter*, *Salmonella*, and *Shigella*. Their absorption is poor via oral route as well as the intact skin. Elimination is mainly through the renal system; hence, when applied on large abraded skin or mucous membrane, caution is to be taken in patients with renal impairment.

Mechanism of Action

They are smaller peptides with amphipathic ends, which act as cationic detergents, bind to phospholipids, form multiple pores, and disrupt the bacterial cell membrane. They are bactericidal in action.

Uses

It is topically used in burns and skin injury to prevent secondary infection. It is also used as eye/ear drops in bacterial conjunctivitis, corneal ulcer, and otitis externa due to gram-negative organisms. It is used orally for local action in *Shigella*- or *Salmonella*-infected diarrhea and enteritis. It is very rarely used systemically for serious resistant infections such as cystic fibrosis, bacteremia, septicemia, endocarditis, meningitis, and pelvic inflammatory disease.

Adverse Effects

Locally, it causes minor irritation, rashes, and redness. When given orally, it can cause nausea, abdominal discomfort, and bloating sensation. Systemically, it can cause dose-related nephrotoxicity, neuropathy, dizziness, and slurred speech.

Bacitracin

Bacitracin belongs to polypeptide antibiotic obtained from *Bacillus subtilis*. It is active against gram-positive organisms such as gram-positive cocci and bacilli, *Neisseria*, *H. influenzae*, *Treponema pallidum*, and certain atypical organisms such as *Actinomyces* and *Fusobacterium*. The mechanism of action is not well defined; it may inhibit bacterial cell wall and is thus bactericidal. Topically, bacitracin is used in conjunctivitis, blepharitis, infected skin abrasions, eczema, and other superficial bacterial infections. On topical application, rarely it can cause hypersensitivity reactions, and on systemic administration, nephrotoxicity occurs; hence, it is not preferred systemically.

Chemotherapy of Urinary Tract Infections (PH1.48)

Uncomplicated UTI is a bacterial infection of the bladder and associated structures. Uncomplicated UTI is also termed as cystitis or lower UTI. Several cases of uncomplicated UTI will resolve spontaneously without treatment; however, numerous patients take treatment for symptoms. Treatment is intended at averting spread to the kidneys or evolving into upper tract disease/pyelonephritis, which could lead to damage of the delicate constituents in the nephrons, causing hypertension.

Escherichia coli is one of the prime causes in the majority of UTI; however, other organisms of importance comprise *Proteus*, *Klebsiella*, and *Enterococcus*. The diagnosis of UTI is made from the clinical history and urinalysis, but the proper collection of the urine sample is important.

Urinary antiseptics have only local antibacterial activity but no systemic activity, for example, nitrofurantoin and methenamine mandelate. Other agents for UTI include cotrimoxazole, nalidixic acid, fluroquinolones, tetracyclines, and cephalosporins.

Nitrofurantoin

It is bacteriostatic in nature, but bactericidal at high concentration. It is effective against gram-positive and gram-negative bacteria. It is rapidly reduced by bacteria to highly reactive derivatives. These derivatives damage DNA and RNA synthesis. This agent attains high concentration in urine.

Side effects include hemolysis in G6PD-deficiency patients; the urine turns dark brown (due to metabolites). Pneumonitis and interstitial pulmonary fibrosis are seen with long-term therapy.

Use

It is used in acute UTI, since alkaline urine reduces efficacy, acidify urine with ascorbic acid. It is also used in long-term suppression of chronic UTI and prophylaxis of UTI.

Methenamine Mandelate

It is a salt of mandelic acid and methenamine, which releases formaldehyde in acidic urine (pH 5.5). Formaldehyde is bactericidal to the organisms. Urea-splitting organisms such as *Proteus* increase urinary pH; hence, acidified urine with ascorbic acid, mandelic acid, or hippuric acid improves the efficacy.

Use

It is used in chronic UTI that is resistant to other drugs.

Adverse Reactions

Adverse reactions include nausea and epigastric distress (due to release of formaldehyde in stomach). Hence, it is given as enteric-coated tablets to reduce these side effects. Hematuria, chemical cystitis, and painful micturition are seen with long-term use. It is avoided in renal failure (since mandelic acid adds to acidosis).

Drug Interactions

It neutralizes the action of sulfonamides and precipitates sulfonamides in acidic urine.

Urinary Analgesic

Phenazopyridine

It is an azo dye, which has an analgesic action on urinary tract. However, it has no antibacterial action. It reduces dysuria, urgency of cystitis, and UTI. However, as a side effect, it colors urine orange-red.

Treatment/Management

The treatment can range from 3 days to 6 weeks. There are outstanding rates with "mini-dose therapy" that includes 3 days of treatment. *E. coli* resistance to common antimicrobials differs in diverse areas of the country, and if the resistance rate is higher than 50%, select an alternative drug.

Trimethoprim/sulfamethoxazole for 3 days is a decent mini-dose therapy; however, resistance rates are high in several areas. First-generation cephalosporins are useful choices for mini-dose therapy. Nitrofurantoin, too, is a reliable alternative for uncomplicated UTI; however, it is bacteriostatic, rather than bactericidal, and should be administered for 5 to 7 days. Fluoroquinolones have demonstrated high levels of resistance; nonetheless, they are the favorite of urologists for a certain purpose.

In recent times, the FDA permitted fosfomycin as a single-dose therapy for uncomplicated UTI caused by *E. coli*. Adjunctive treatment with phenazopyridine for some days could offer symptom relief.

Even without management, the UTI will naturally resolve in around 20% of women. The probability that a female will advance to acute pyelonephritis is very insignificant.

Asymptomatic bacteriuria is fairly common and necessitates no treatment, except in pregnant women or persons who are immunosuppressed, have undertaken a transplant, or have undergone a urological procedure.

Chemotherapy of Sexually Transmitted Diseases (DR10.8)

1. Gonorrhea—ceftriaxone 250 mg IM single dose

   Or

   Cefixime 400 mg oral, single dose

   Or

   Ciprofloxacin 500 mg oral, single dose.
2. Syphilis—benzathine penicillin G 2.4 MU IM single dose

   Or

   Doxycycline 100 mg twice daily orally × 2 weeks.
3. Chancroid—ceftriaxone 250 mg IM single dose

   Or

   Cotrimoxazole DS two times a day orally × 1 week.
4. Granuloma inguinale—doxycycline 100 mg two times a day orally × 3 weeks

   Or

   Cotrimoxazole DS twice daily orally × 2 weeks.
5. Lymphogranuloma venereum—doxycycline 100 mg twice daily orally × 3 weeks.
6. Trichomoniasis—metronidazole/secnidazole 2 g orally, single dose.

Chemoprophylaxis

Postexposure prophylaxis of syphilis/gonorrhea can be implemented with either of the following:

1. Penicillin 4 to 8 MU IM.
2. Doxycycline 100 mg twice daily × 15 days (for postexposure prophylaxis of syphilis/gonorrhea/lymphogranuloma venereum/chancroid/granuloma inguinale).

Multiple Choice Questions

1. A male patient suffering from high-grade fever was admitted to the hospital. The patient was not responding to empirical antimicrobial agents. After culture sensitivity report, he was started on clindamycin. After 5 days, the patient developed severe diarrhea, abdominal pain, and bloating sensation. The consultant suspected drug-induced infection and started on a new drug after which the patient started recovering. Which antimicrobial agent could have been started in this patient?

A. Streptogramins.
B. Linezolid.
C. Azithromycin.
D. Vancomycin.

Answer: D

Clindamycin is lincosamide antibiotic with similar mechanism of action as erythromycin. The patient has developed pseudomembranous enterocolitis due to *Clostridium difficile*–induced superinfection caused due to clindamycin. The drugs used to treat superinfection are metronidazole and vancomycin.

2. The macrolide predominantly used to treat lung infections is:

A. Erythromycin.
B. Azithromycin.
C. Spiramycin.
D. Telithromycin.

Answer: D

Telithromycin is a ketolide with similar spectrum like erythromycin but with better tissue penetrability. Telithromycin is effective in the treatment of community-acquired pneumonia, acute exacerbations of chronic bronchitis, and acute bacterial sinusitis resistant to other macrolides.

3. The site of action for erythromycin is:

A. 30s ribosome.
B. 50s ribosome.
C. tRNA.
D. mRNA.

Answer: B

Erythromycin inhibits protein synthesis by binding to 23S rRNA part of 50s ribosomal subunit and inhibit the translocation of nascent peptide from A (acceptor) site to the P (peptidyl) site, thereby blocking the attachment of the new aminoacyl tRNA to the A site. As a result of its action on elongation stage of protein synthesis, short nascent peptides are synthesized by bacterial RNA polymerase, which ultimately stops the translation

4. A 45-year-old woman came to the medicine outpatient department with complaints of repeated pain in the nose. On examination, her vitals were normal and pustular lesions were found in the nasal passage. She was referred to the ENT department for further evaluation. On probing, she revealed that for the past 2 years, she has been suffering from these lesions recurrently, which are painful, and she was prescribed antimicrobial agents after which the lesions would subside and later reoccur. On culture, *S. aureus* were isolated. She was prescribed systemic antimicrobial agent and nasal antibiotic ointment. Which of the following drug could be prescribed as nasal ointment?

A. Mupirocin.
B. Fusidic acid.
C. Bacitracin.
D. Colistin.

Answer: A

Mupirocin is a complex combination of many pseudomonic acids isolated from *Pseudomonas fluorescens*. It is available only for topical use against gram-positive bacteria and a few gram-negative organisms. Mupirocin 2% cream and 2% ointment are used for skin lesion to prevent secondary infection. Intranasal mupirocin ointment is used to eradicate intranasal *S. aureus* colonization.

5. From the following list, choose an appropriate drug used to treat vancomycin-resistant *S. aureus*–induced infection:

A. Lincomycin.
B. Azithromycin.
C. Spectinomycin.
D. Daptomycin.

Answer: D

Daptomycin is a cyclic lipopeptide antibiotic derived from *Streptomyces roseosporus*. It is effective against most gram-positive organisms including MRSA, vancomycin-resistant strains like VRSA, and VRE. It binds to bacterial cell membrane and inhibits membrane potential and has bactericidal activity against aerobic and anaerobic gram-positive bacteria.

6. Erythromycin can be used in:

A. Diabetic gastroparesis.
B. Bronchial asthma.
C. Tetanus.
D. All of the above.

Answer: D

Erythromycin acts as mucolytic agent by altering the consistency of secretions and in addition increases the transport of mucous. It is known to reduce inflammation in bronchus and bronchioles and hence is useful in bronchial asthma. It is used in tetanus, whooping cough, and respiratory tract infections. It also stimulates GI motility by action on motilin receptors; hence, it is used in diabetic gastroparesis.

7. A pregnant woman with a history of repeated miscarriages visited an obstetrician and wanted to be evaluated for pregnancy complications. She complained of repeated body aches, mild fever, and tiredness. On examination, the temperature was raised, vitals were normal, and lymph nodes were enlarged. On investigation, high titer for IgG antibodies for *T. gondii* was present. Which of the following drug can be used in this patient?

A. Spiramycin.
B. Telithromycin.
C. Vancomycin.
D. Clindamycin.

Answer: A

Spiramycin achieves higher concentration in tissues compared to plasma and specifically concentrates in placental tissue, and is mainly indicated for the treatment of acquired toxoplasmosis in early pregnancy to prevent transmission to the fetus. Spiramycin is available through the investigational new drug process at the U.S. FDA. It is a well-tolerated drug with rare occurrence of mild gastritis and nausea.

8. Linezolid can cause all adverse effects except:

A. Taste alteration.
B. Nephrotoxicity.
C. Thrombocytopenia.
D. Optic neuropathy.

Answer: B

Leukopenia, pancytopenia, thrombocytopenia, and anemia due to suppression of bone marrow have been reported in patients taking linezolid for more than 10 days, which are reversible on discontinuation of the drug. Peripheral neuropathy, optic neuritis, and rarely lactic acidosis can develop due to mitochondrial toxicity only on treatment for more than 6 weeks. Concomitant intake of tyramine-rich food or SSRIs and SNRIs along with linezolid may lead to sudden increase in serotonin levels leading to hypertensive crisis, restlessness, uneasy sensation, palpitations, and headache, leading to serotonin syndrome due to weak nonspecific MOA inhibition by linezolid.

9. Colistin is also known as:

A. Polymyxin B.
B. Polymyxin E.
C. Polymyxin N.
D. Polymyxin G.

Answer: B

Polymyxins (polymyxin B and polymyxin E) are polypeptide antibiotics that have low molecular weight and are used only topically due to their systemic toxicity. Polymyxin E is also known as colistin and is obtained from *Bacillus colistinus*.

10. The following statements regarding tedizolid are true except:

A. It is a new oxazolidinone approved by FDA.
B. Effective against linezolid-resistant strains.
C. Dose adjustment required in hepatic disease.
D. It is a weak MAO inhibitor.

Answer: C.

It gets metabolized without enzymes through oxidation into aminoethoxyacetic acid and glycerin derivatives. It mainly gets eliminated in the urine. Therefore, dose adjustment is not required in hepatic impairment.

Chapter 63 Antituberculosis Drugs

Jitendra H. Vaghela

PH1.44: Describe the first-line antitubercular drugs, their mechanisms of action, side effects, and doses.

PH1.45: Describe the drugs used in multidrug-resistant (MDR) and extensively drug-resistant (XDR) tuberculosis.

Learning Objectives

- Tuberculosis.
- Antituberculosis drugs.
- Treatment of tuberculosis.

Tuberculosis

Tuberculosis (TB) is a chronic granulomatous disease caused by *Mycobacterium tuberculosis*. It is the leading cause of death from an infectious disease.

Type of Bacilli

M. tuberculosis is a highly aerobic, gram-positive, slowly dividing, rod-shaped bacillus, which spreads by inhalation of air from infected people. Among mycobacteria, *Mycobacterium avium* can also cause infection in immunocompromised persons. Bacilli can be extracellular or intracellular, i.e., inside macrophage. Also, they can be rapidly growing or slowly growing. Different types of drugs are used according to the type of bacilli.

Peculiar features of *M. tuberculosis* are as follows:

1. Rapid growers: in the wall of cavitary lesion, i.e., extracellular.
2. Slow growers: intracellular, within macrophages at inflamed sites.
3. Spurters: intermittent growth spurts.
4. Dormant: do not grow for long time; become active at times of low-host resistance.
5. Atypical: *M. avium, Mycobacterium kansasii.*
6. Lipoarabinomannan: helps survival in macrophages.
7. Bacilli continuously shift from one subpopulation to another.

Pathophysiology

Tuberculous bacilli, via inhalation route, enter the human body and get lodged in the lungs primarily and then spread throughout the body over time. They predominantly affect the lungs, causing pulmonary TB. Common extrapulmonary TB sites are the lymph nodes, bones, intestine, genitourinary tract, eye, and meninges. After entry into the lungs, bacilli get engulfed by macrophages and reach the hilar lymph node. This stage is called the primary stage. In the second stage, macrophages and cell-mediated immunity cells (T lymphocytes) attempt to contain the infection by forming granulomas. In the third stage, bacilli escape from the primary focus and infect other organs in individuals with weaker immune systems and at areas with low-oxygen tension. The most severe form is miliary TB, which affects the whole-body organs including the liver and spleen.

Symptoms and Diagnosis

TB is characterized by purulent cough, evening rise of fever, loss of weight, muscle weakness, and loss of appetite for more than 2 weeks. TB is diagnosed by chest radiogram and sputum smear microscopy. For testing, 2-day sputum testing is the most widely used method. Liquid probe assay and liquid culture media are the other methods.

Management (PE34.3)

In developing countries, TB is a major health care burden. The Revised National Tuberculosis Control Programme (RNTCP) has been carrying out activities for control of TB in India since 1997. Recently, anti-TB drug treatment has shifted from weekly basis to daily basis through RNTCP across India.

Antituberculosis Drugs (CT1.14, CT1.15)

Drugs are classified as first-line drugs and second-line drugs. First-line drugs are highly efficacious and less toxic. Second-line drugs have either low efficacy or high toxicity, or both.

First-line drugs are isoniazid, rifampin, pyrazinamide, ethambutol, and streptomycin. Second-line drugs include fluoroquinolones (FQs)—ciprofloxacin, ofloxacin, levofloxacin, and moxifloxacin; injectable drugs—capreomycin, amikacin, and kanamycin; and other oral drugs—cycloserine, rifabutin, rifapentine, ethionamide, para-amino salicylic acid (PAS), and terizidone.

All first-line drugs are bactericidal except ethambutol. Individual drug usage is not recommended because of chances of resistance. All drugs are used in combination. According to a recent guideline, RNTCP has started using fixed-dose combinations (FDCs) for four first-line drugs. Streptomycin is given only intramuscularly or intravenously.

The World Health Organization (WHO) has given another classification, dividing drugs into groups (**Table 63.1**). This classification helps delineate multidrug-resistant (MDR) TB treatment formulation to be made easily.

First-Line Drugs

Isoniazid (Isonicotinic Acid Hydrazide)

It is one of the most important first-line drugs. It is bacteriostatic for slowly growing or resting bacilli and

Table 63.1 WHO classification of antitubercular drugs

First-line drugs	Group 1 (oral)	Isoniazid Rifampin Pyrazinamide Ethambutol
Second-line drugs	Group 2 (injectables)	Streptomycin Capreomycin Amikacin Kanamycin
	Group 3 (fluoro-quinolones—oral and injectable)	Ciprofloxacin Ofloxacin Levofloxacin Moxifloxacin
	Group 4 (oral)	Cycloserine Rifabutin, rifapentine Ethionamide PAS Terizidone
	Group 5 (reserve drugs)	Bedaquiline Clarithromycin Clofazimine Amoxycillin + clavulanic acid Linezolid Imipenem/cilastatin

Abbreviation: PAS, para-aminosalicylic acid.

bactericidal for rapidly growing bacilli. It can act on both intra- and extracellular bacilli.

Mechanism of Action

It inhibits mycolic acid synthesis. Mycolic acid, arabinogalactan, and peptidoglycan are integral parts of mycobacterial bacilli cell wall. Isoniazid is a prodrug, and it gets converted to activated isoniazid in the presence of catalase-peroxidase enzyme, which is encoded by *katG*. Then, this active metabolite of isoniazid combines with NAD and inhibits two genes, namely, *inhA* and *kasA*. These genes are important for mycolic acid synthesis. By inhibiting these, isoniazid inhibits mycolic acid synthesis. The most common mechanism of resistance to isoniazid is due to mutation in *katG* gene. Other causes of isonicotinic acid hydrazide (INH) resistance are mutation of other genes.

Pharmacokinetics

Isoniazid is well absorbed orally. It gets distributed all over the body. It is metabolized in the liver by acetylation. Acetylation differs among the Indian population because of genetic variation. Around 30 to 40% Indians are fast acetylators (half-life of 1 hour) who need increased dose of isoniazid. Approximately, 60 to 70% Indians are slow acetylators (half-life of 3 hours) with chances of isoniazid toxicity.

Drug–Drug Interactions

Aluminum-containing antacids decrease isoniazid absorption. Isoniazid is a microsomal enzyme inhibitor. It decreases metabolism of some anticonvulsants, warfarin, and theophylline. It also inhibits pyridoxine conversion from pyridoxal phosphate, thus causing pyridoxine deficiency. Alcoholics tend to develop hepatitis.

Adverse Effects

Peripheral neuritis, a dose-dependent toxicity, is an adverse effect of isoniazid. This can be managed by administering pyridoxine 10 mg daily as prophylaxis or 100 mg daily as treatment. Hepatotoxicity is one of the serious side effects. Hypersensitivity reactions can also occur. Systematic lupus erythematosus, allergic reaction, abdominal discomfort, and neurotoxicity are also seen with isoniazid.

Dosage

The recommended dose is 300 mg/day or 10 mg/kg/day. FDC of isoniazid with rifampicin, pyrazinamide, and ethambutol is also available. In FDC, dose of isoniazid is 75 mg per tablet. According to a new guideline, drug dosage is decided according to weight band, which is described later in the chapter. Isoniazid is safe during pregnancy. It is used in combination with other drugs and also as single drug for prophylactic purposes.

Rifampin

It is a semisynthetic derivative of rifamycin B derived from *Amycolatopsis rifamycinica*, formerly named *Streptomyces mediterranei*. Rifabutin and rifapentine are other derivatives of this family. Rifampin is a bactericidal drug mainly acting against slow-growing bacilli. It acts both intra- and extracellularly. In combination with isoniazid, it prevents chances of resistance and also helps in complete eradication of bacilli. It also functions as a sterilizing agent.

Mechanism of Action

Rifampin inhibits bacterial RNA synthesis. Rifampin inhibits bacterial DNA-dependent RNA polymerase by binding with it and inhibiting further polymerization. It selectively binds to bacterial RNA polymerase only. Rifampin resistance develops due to mutation in gene encoding β subunit of RNA polymerase (rpoβ).

Pharmacokinetics

Rifampin is well absorbed orally. Food decreases its absorption, so it is taken before meal. It gets distributed all over the body. It also attains high levels in cerebrospinal fluid (CSF) in the case of meningeal infection. It is metabolized and excreted through the liver. It is excreted in the bile also. It causes harmless red-orange discoloration of body fluids such as urine and also of contact lenses. It is a potent microsomal cytochrome P450 (CYP) enzyme inducer. All major CYP isoenzymes such as CYP3A4, CYP2C, and CYP1A2 are induced by rifampin.

Drug–Drug Interactions

It increases metabolism of own as well as many other drugs such as warfarin, oral contraceptive pills (OCPs), anticoagulants, antiretroviral drugs, and antifungal drugs. An alternate method of contraception is advised for patients taking rifampin. Rifampin is replaced by rifabutin, a less potent enzyme inducer, in patients taking antiretroviral drugs.

Adverse Effects

Dose-dependent hepatotoxicity is a major adverse effect of rifampin. Flulike syndrome, abdominal cramps, red-orange discoloration of urine, and thrombocytopenia are also seen.

Dosage

The approved dose of rifampin is 600 mg/day. In FDC, the dose of rifampin is 150 mg.

Rifampin is also useful in leprosy, meningococcal meningitis, *Haemophilus influenzae* meningitis, and *Legionella* infection as treatment or for prophylactic purpose. It is also drug of choice for brucellosis in combination with doxycycline.

Pyrazinamide (Pyrazinoic Acid)

It is an important chemical drug used especially for intracellular bacilli. It is active at acidic pH as well as in macrophages. It is one of the important first-line drugs due to good sterilizing activity.

Mechanism of Action

Pyrazinamide inhibits cell wall synthesis. After getting entry into *Mycobacterium*, it gets converted to pyrazinoic acid, an active metabolite, by pyrazinamidase enzyme. This active metabolite inhibits mycobacterial fatty acid synthase-I enzyme and thus cell wall synthesis. Resistance mainly develops due to mutation in *pncA* gene encoding for pyrazinamidase enzyme.

Pharmacokinetics

It is well absorbed orally. It is widely distributed. It has good penetration in CSF, so it is useful in meningeal TB. However, isoniazid has the maximum CSF penetration. It is metabolized in the liver and excreted in the urine.

Adverse Effects

It is the most hepatotoxic drug. It can also cause gouty arthralgia and hyperuricemia. It is contraindicated in liver disease. It is safe during pregnancy.

Dosage

The recommended dose is 1,500 mg/day orally. In FDC, the dose of pyrazinamide is 400 mg per tablet.

Ethambutol (Bacteriostatic)

It is a synthetic drug developed mainly to combat mycobacteria resistant to INH and also some nontuberculous mycobacteria. It is added to the first-line drugs to decrease the chances of resistance and also to decrease the duration of treatment to a short course.

Mechanism of Action

It inhibits bacterial cell wall synthesis. It inhibits arabinosyltransferase enzyme and interrupts arabinogalactan production, an integral component of the cell wall of bacilli. It is active against rapidly growing bacilli. It has also good activity against *M. avium* complex (MAC) infection.

Pharmacokinetics

It is a less absorbed drug comparatively. Only 70% of oral dose is absorbed. Half of its dose gets excreted rapidly unchanged in the urine.

Adverse Effects

After prolonged therapy with ethambutol, dose-dependent toxicity is seen. Major adverse effects include visual loss and loss of red-green color discrimination due to retrobulbar optic neuritis. It is only allowed under strict monitoring in children, as they may not report visual problems properly. Visual disturbances are reversible on discontinuation of the drug. It is well tolerated and a comparatively safe drug. It is safe during pregnancy.

Dosage

Ethambutol is given at a dose of 800 mg/day orally. In FDC, the dose of ethambutol is 275 mg per tablet.

Streptomycin

Streptomycin is an aminoglycoside antibiotic. It was the first clinically useful drug developed. It is bactericidal. As of now, it has only supplemental use in first-line drugs due to comparatively lower efficacy, high toxicity, and increased resistance.

Mechanism of Action

As it is an aminoglycoside, it inhibits bacterial protein synthesis. It binds to 30S ribosome and interrupts protein synthesis. It acts on extracellular bacilli only, as it does not penetrate into macrophages. It is also less concentrated in CSF.

Pharmacokinetics

It is given by intramuscular route only. It is not absorbed orally. Injection is painful. It is very cautiously used in the elderly and in those with renal impairment.

Adverse Effects

Nephrotoxicity and ototoxicity are the main adverse effects associated with its use. Because of adverse effects and widespread resistance due to mutation in genes for ribosomal protein synthesis, its used has become only an add-on purpose. It is only used during the intensive phase (IP).

Dosage

Streptomycin is given at a dose of 1,000 mg/day via intramuscular injection. The dose is reduced to 500 to 750 mg/day in elderly and those with renal impairment. It is given intramuscularly, so it is not a part of FDC preparation. It is contraindicated in pregnancy.

Second-Line Drugs

These drugs are similar or less efficacious and used only as replacement or when there is resistance. They are also used when there is intolerance to one or more first-line drugs. Mostly, they are useful for drug-resistant TB and also against some nontuberculous mycobacterial infections by atypical mycobacteria. They are more toxic than first-line drugs.

Fluoroquinolones

Ciprofloxacin, ofloxacin, levofloxacin, and moxifloxacin are the mainly used FQs. They are bactericidal, well-tolerated drugs. They inhibit DNA gyrase enzyme. Moxifloxacin and levofloxacin are the most widely used drugs among them. Moxifloxacin has the highest activity among them against *M. tuberculosis*. Ciprofloxacin and levofloxacin show good activity against nontuberculous mycobacteria such as MAC. They are used as reserved drugs, despite good activity as first-line drugs, to be used for drug-resistant TB. They are given both orally and parenterally. Moxifloxacin dose is 400 mg once a day.

Kanamycin, Amikacin

They are bactericidal injectable drugs. They are also aminoglycoside drugs like streptomycin. There is less nephrotoxicity and ototoxicity compared to streptomycin. They are mainly used for drug-resistant TB. The recommended dose is 750 to 1,000 mg/day intramuscularly.

Capreomycin

It is a peptide antibiotic. Its usage and other effects are comparable to those of aminoglycoside. It is mainly used as an alternative for aminoglycoside-resistant mycobacteria.

Ethionamide

It is similar to isoniazid structurally and in terms of mechanism of action. It is more toxic than isoniazid. Allergic reactions, vomiting, neurological disturbances, and hepatotoxicity can occur. It is active against drug-resistant TB and also nontuberculous infection by mycobacteria. The approved dose is 250-mg tablet twice daily orally.

Cycloserine

It is a bacteriostatic drug. It inhibits peptidoglycan synthesis, and thus, there is cell wall synthesis inhibition. It is effective against drug-resistant TB. Its major adverse effect is neurotoxicity. Its main side effect is neuropsychotoxicity. It is reserved for drug-resistant and nontuberculous mycobacterial infection such as MAC infection. The approved dose is 250 mg twice daily orally.

Para-Amino Salicylic Acid

It is a bacteriostatic drug. It inhibits folate synthase. It is one of the least active drugs. It is reserved for use only in drug-resistant TB. It is given with other bactericidal drugs to prevent resistance. Hypothyroidism, hypersensitivity reactions, and gastrointestinal disturbances are the main adverse effects. It is given in granular form and taken whole with liquids. The recommended dose is 2 to 3 g/day four times a day orally.

Terizidone

It is a combination of two molecules of cycloserine. It inhibits cell wall synthesis by peptidoglycan synthesis inhibition. It is similar to cycloserine and is used as its replacement. It is used for pulmonary and extrapulmonary TB. It is given at a dose of 250 to 750 mg/day orally.

Rifabutin

It is similar to rifampin. It only differs from rifampin in that it has less microsomal enzyme–inducing property, less *M. tuberculosis* activity, more MAC activity, and longer half-life. Its main use is in TB coinfection with HIV infection. Rifampin, being a microsomal enzyme inducer, decreases antiretroviral drug effect. Rifabutin can replace rifampin for this purpose.

Rifapentine

It is a bacterial RNA polymerase inhibitor. Microsomal enzyme induction and toxicity are similar to those of rifampin. Its half-life (13–15 hours) is longer compared to that of rifampin. It can be used in place of rifampin in the continuation phase (CP) and also for latent TB.

Clarithromycin/Azithromycin

These macrolide drugs are mainly indicated for MAC infection.

Bedaquiline

Bedaquiline fumarate (Sirturo 100 mg tablet) is approved by the U.S. Food and Drug Administration (FDA) for use as part of a combination therapy for MDR TB. It targets the proton pump of adenosine triphosphate (ATP) synthesis, leading to inadequate ATP synthesis, which is necessary for bacterial metabolism. Bedaquiline kills both rapidly dividing and slowly dividing bacilli. Resistance develops mainly due to mutation of ATP synthase enzyme or efflux pump. The half-life of bedaquiline is very long (160 hours). It is given at a dose of 400 mg daily for 2 weeks, and then 200 mg three times a week for 22 weeks. Hepatotoxicity, cardiac conduction defects, and QTc prolongation are the main adverse effects.

Linezolid

This is the drug of last choice for drug-resistant TB. Adverse effects such as bone marrow depression overweigh the benefits against *Mycobacterium*.

Treatment of Tuberculosis

In the present era, a newer short-course regimen of 6 to 9 months is preferred over older 18- to 24-month regimen. In India, anti-TB drugs are given under RNTCP. They are given under the direct supervision of the medical professional (i.e., DOTS [directly observed treatment] using short course). To increase the success rate of treatment, a combination of two or more drugs is used. An FDC of four drugs is aimed to eliminate poor patient compliance and rate of resistance. Commonly, isoniazid, rifampin, pyrazinamide, and ethambutol are given together for various reasons. Isoniazid kills rapidly multiplying organisms, rifampin kills both extra- and intracellular organisms, pyrazinamide predominantly acts against intracellular organisms, and ethambutol delays resistance to other anti-TB drugs and shortens the treatment duration.

Understanding the Biology of TB Infection

There is continuous shifting of bacilli between the following subpopulations:

- Rapidly growing: High bacterial load is present in areas where oxygen tension is high and pH is neutral, so susceptible drugs are in this order: isoniazid > rifampin > ethambutol > streptomycin.
- Slow growing: They are present in low pH sites (intracellularly and at inflamed sites), so susceptible drugs are in this order: pyrazinamide > isoniazid > rifampin > ethambutol.
- Spurters: They are present at sites where oxygen tension is low and pH is neutral, so the only susceptible drug is rifampin.
- Dormant: They are inactive for prolonged period. No first-line drug is susceptible. Bedaquiline can be useful against them.

Short-Course Treatment Regimen (PE34.3)

According to the new guidelines by RNTCP, anti-TB drugs are to be given in FDC as daily doses (**Table 63.2**); drug doses for adult TB are given in **Table 63.3**. The numbers of FDC tablets required are shown in **Table 63.4**.

In patients older than 50 years, the maximum dose of streptomycin should be 0.75 g.

Drug-sensitive TB for new cases is treated with a 6-month duration regimen: 2 months of IP with isoniazid, rifampin, pyrazinamide, and ethambutol for complete sterilizing activity, and 4 months of CP with isoniazid, rifampin, and ethambutol. For previously treated cases, an 8-month duration regimen is used: 2 months of isoniazid, rifampin, pyrazinamide, and ethambutol with streptomycin injection, followed by 1 month of isoniazid, rifampin, pyrazinamide, and ethambutol in IP, a total of 3 months. It is then followed

Table 63.2 Treatment regimen for new and previously treated patients

Treatment group	Type of patient	Regimen		Total duration
		IP	CP	
New	Microbiologically confirmed TB case Clinically diagnosed TB case	2 HRZE	4 HRE	6 mo
Previously treated	Recurrent TB Treatment after failure Treatment after lost to follow-up Other previously treated patients	2 HRZES + 1 HRZE	5 HRE	8 mo

Abbreviations: CP, continuous phase; HRE, isoniazid, rifampin, ethambutol; HRZE, isoniazid, rifampin, pyrazinamide, ethambutol; HRZES, isoniazid, rifampin, pyrazinamide, ethambutol, streptomycin; IP, intensive phase; TB, tuberculosis.

Table 63.3 Daily doses of first-line antituberculosis drugs as per body weight

Name of drug	Daily dose (mg/kg)	
	Adult	Children
Isoniazid	5 (4–6)	5 (4–6)
Rifampin	10 (8–12)	15 (10–20)
Pyrazinamide	25 (20–30)	35 (30–40)
Streptomycin	15 (12–18)	15 (12–18)
Ethambutol	15 (15–20)	20 (15–25)

Table 63.4 Numbers of FDCs of first-line drugs according to weight

Weight category (kg)	Number of tablets (FDCs)		Injection of streptomycin (g)
	IP	CP	
	HRZE	HRE	
	75/150/400/275 mg	75/150/275mg	
25–39	2	2	0.5
40–54	3	3	0.75
55–69	4	4	1
≥70 kg	5	5	1

Abbreviations: CP, continuous phase; FDC, fixed-dose combination; HRE, isoniazid, rifampin, ethambutol; HRZE, isoniazid, rifampin, pyrazinamide, ethambutol; IP, intensive phase.

by CP for 5 months with isoniazid, rifampin, and ethambutol. These are standard regimens for pulmonary TB. For extrapulmonary TB, the same regimen is advocated with 3- to 6-month increase in CP, as per severity.

Drug-Resistant Tuberculosis

Because of the increasing cases of drug resistance to various first-line drugs, MDR cases of TB are increasing. Different forms of drug-resistant TB are defined, according to their resistance status.

- Monoresistant TB: Resistance to a single drug of first-line drugs. In this case, apart from the resistant drug, two sensitive first-line drugs, one injectable second-line drug, and one FQ, making up a five-drug combination, is used in the IP for 3 to 6 months.
- Polyresistant TB: Resistance to more than one drug, but not the combination of isoniazid and rifampicin. In this case, rifampin, one injectable, one FQ, and two oral second-line drugs are used in the IP. For mono- and polyresistant TB, CP of 9 to 12 months with omission of the injectable drug is given.
- MDR or rifampicin-resistant TB: Resistance to at least isoniazid and rifampicin.
- Extensively drug-resistant (XDR) TB: MDR plus resistance to FQs and at least one of the three injectable drugs (amikacin, kanamycin, capreomycin).

Treatment regimens for rifampin-resistant TB, MDR TB, and XDR TB are given in **Table 63.5**. The regimen for drug-resistant TB should have at least four drugs that are known to be effective. Normally, six drugs are included for better efficacy. Drugs according to the WHO classification are used from groups 1 to 4. Two drugs from group 1 (pyrazinamide, ethambutol), one injectable from group 2, one FQ from group 3, and two second-line oral drugs from group 4 are included in the regimen to make it effective.

Tuberculosis in Special Conditions

Tuberculous Meningitis (IM17.13)

In tuberculous meningitis, streptomycin replaces ethambutol in IP. CP should be extended by 3 months. Steroids should be given initially and gradually tapered over 6 to 8 weeks.

TB during Pregnancy and Postnatal Period

In pregnancy, streptomycin is absolutely contraindicated. Isoniazid, rifampin, and ethambutol are found safe during pregnancy. Breastfeeding can be continued. Mothers should continue to practice cough hygiene. Children should be administered preventive chemoprophylaxis of isoniazid.

TB with Renal Failure

Rifampicin, isoniazid, and pyrazinamide can be safely given. Dosage of streptomycin and ethambutol should be adjusted according to the creatinine clearance.

TB with Women on OCPs

Rifampin decreases the efficiency of OCPs by increasing their metabolism. Increase in dosage of the OCP or switching over to alternate methods of contraception is advisable.

TB in HIV-Positive Patients

Significant drug interactions can occur with protease inhibitors (PIs) and rifampicin; hence, PIs should not be used with rifampicin-containing regimens. Another rifamycin, rifabutin, is a less potent inducer of CYP 3A4 liver enzyme and is equally safe and effective. Boosting drugs such as ritonavir alters the metabolism of rifabutin and hence the dose of rifabutin should be reduced. Cotrimoxazole preventive therapy has shown reduced mortality among TB with HIV patients. Efavirenz should be replaced with nevirapine, as efavirenz is less affected by rifampin. After anti-TB drug therapy for at least 2 weeks, antiretroviral therapy is instituted.

Patient on Treatment Developing Hepatitis (IM5.16)

In this condition, first stop all anti-TB drugs. Rule out other causes of hepatitis. Do not restart treatment till symptoms resolve and liver enzymes return to baseline levels. Restart treatment with one drug at a time, starting with rifampicin, followed by INH and then pyrazinamide. In patients with severe disease in whom treatment cannot be stopped, use a nonhepatotoxic regimen consisting of streptomycin and ethambutol.

Table 63.5 Treatment regimen for different drug-resistant TB

Type of TB case treatment	Treatment regimen in IP	Treatment regimen in CP
Rifampin resistant + isoniazid sensitive or unknown	(6–9) Km, Lfx, Eto, Cs, Z, E, H	(18) Lfx, Eto, Cs, E, H
MDR TB	(6–9) Km, Lfx, Eto, Cs, Z, E (modify treatment based on the level of INH resistance)[a]	(18) Lfx, Eto, Cs, E
XDR TB	(6–12) Cm, PAS, Mfx, high-dose H, Cfx, Lzd, Amx/Clv	(18) PAS, Mfx, high-dose H, Cfx, Lzd, Amx/Clv

Abbreviations: Amx/Clv, amoxicilin/clavulanic acid; Cfx, ciprofloxacin; Cm, capreomycin; CP, continuous phase; Cs, cycloserine; E, ethambutol; Eto, ethionamide; H, isoniazid; INH, isonicotinic acid hydrazide; IP, intensive phase; Km, kanamycin; Lfx, levofloxacin; Lzd, linezolid; Mfx, moxifloxacin; MDR TB, multidrug-resistant tuberculosis; PAS, para-amino salicylic acid; XDR TB, extensively drug-resistant tuberculosis; Z, pyrazinamide.

[a]All MDR TB cases would be subjected to liquid culture (LC) and drug sensitivity test (DST) at baseline for kanamycin and levofloxacin. Appropriate modification of the treatment regimen can be done in case of additional resistance

Chemoprophylaxis

It is indicated for contacts of open cases who show recent Mantoux conversion; children with positive Mantoux and a TB patient in the family; neonate of tubercular mother; patients with leukemia, diabetes, silicosis, or those who are HIV positive or are on corticosteroid therapy who show a positive Mantoux; and patients with old inactive disease who are assessed to have received inadequate therapy. INH 300 mg (10 mg/kg in children) once a day for 6 to 12 months is recommended.

Due to increased INH resistance, a combination of INH (5 mg/kg) and rifampin (10 mg/kg) is given daily for 6 months.

Immunoprophylaxis

It is achieved by intradermal injection of live attenuated vaccine Bacillus Calmette–Guérin. The strain causes self-limited lesion and induces hypersensitivity and immunity. It converts a tuberculin-negative person to positive reactor. Immunity lasts for 10 to 15 years. Immunity is 60 to 80%.

Role of Steroids in TB Management

Steroid is not commonly used in TB patients. It is contra-indicated in intestinal TB, as perforation may occur. However, steroid is indicated in some serious cases, for example, hypersensitivity reaction management, in AIDS patients, and in meningeal TB. It should be gradually tapered over time.

Mycobacterium Avium Complex Infection

Clarithromycin 500 mg twice a day and azithromycin 500 mg once a day are very effective newer macrolide drugs for MAC and other nontuberculous bacterial infection. Clarithromycin 500 mg twice daily or azithromycin 500 mg once daily, ethambutol 15 mg/kg and rifabutin 300 mg once a day for IP of 2 to 6 months, and clarithromycin/azithromycin same dose with ethambutol or one FQ for CP of 9 to 12 months are given for treatment.

Multiple Choice Questions

1. A 35-year-old Canadian man presents to his family physician because his mother, who is on a visit from India, was found to have tuberculosis (TB). The family physician recommends prophylaxis against TB. Which of the following is indicated for TB prophylaxis in exposed adult patients?

A. Rifampin.

B. Ethambutol.

C. Isoniazid.

D. Streptomycin.

Answer: C

Isoniazid can be used alone for the prophylaxis of tuberculosis (TB) in the case of such exposure.

2. A 28-year-old pregnant woman develops tuberculosis. Which of the following drug should not be used?

A. Rifampin.

B. Ethambutol.

C. Isoniazid.

D. Streptomycin.

Answer: D

As streptomycin has been shown to have fetotoxicity, it is contraindicated in pregnancy.

3. A patient presents with a 10-day history of high fever, cough, and purulent sputum. A chest X-ray (CXR) shows a dense consolidation in the right upper lobe. The next step is:

A. Obtain sputum specimens for acid-fast bacilli (AFB) and start tuberculosis (TB) treatment.

B. Start a course of moxifloxacin.

C. Obtain sputum specimens for AFB and culture/sensitivity examination and start azithromycin.

D. Refer the patient to a TB hospital.

Answer: C

An acute presentation suggests acute bacterial infection. There is a history of less than 14 days. Sputum specimens should be obtained before starting conventional antibiotics. Fluoroquinolones should be avoided if TB is at all suspected as they will result in temporary improvement because TB is sensitive to this class of drugs, leading to delay in diagnosis.

4. A 30-year-old laborer complained of fever, cough, and loss of weight for 15 days. On sputum examination, he was found to be positive for pulmonary tuberculosis. He was put on category 1 regimen of treatment as new case. After some days, the patient complained of vomiting, malaise, lethargy and joint pain, and his laboratory investigation showed high levels of AST and ALT. The consulting physician diagnosed him to have hepatotoxicity. Which of the following drug would be the culprit drug for causing hepatotoxicity?

A. Rifampin.

B. Pyrazinamide.

C. Isoniazid.

D. Ethambutol.

Answer: B

Pyrazinamide is the most hepatotoxic drug. There is also a history of joint pain, which mostly occurs due to pyrazinamide. Thus, the culprit drug here is pyrazinamide.

5. A 35-year-old patient complained of fever, cough, and loss of weight for 15 days on consultation. On sputum examination, he was found to be positive for pulmonary tuberculosis. He was put on category 1 regimen of treatment as new case. After some months, the patient complained of visual disturbances, line blurring of vision, difficulty in color discrimination with some haziness, nausea, and anorexia. Which of the following drug would be the culprit drug for this side effect?

A. Rifampin.

B. Pyrazinamide.

C. Ethambutol.

D. Isoniazid.

Answer: C

Ethambutol is known to cause visual disturbances. On prolonged therapy with ethambutol, such scenario develops in some cases.

6. A 35-year-old AIDS patient on antiretroviral drugs develops tuberculosis. As there are chances of drug–drug interactions with rifampin, which NNRTI is not affected from these drug–drug interactions?

A. Stavudine.
B. Nevirapine.
C. Efavirenz.
D. Lamivudine.

Answer: C

There are less interactions noted with rifampin and efavirenz than any other NNRTI.

7. Which antituberculosis drug acts by inhibiting folate synthesis?

A. Clofazimine.
B. Para-amino salicylic acid.
C. Cycloserine.
D. Ethionamide.

Answer: B

Para-amino salicylic acid is a folate synthase inhibitor.

8. Which antituberculosis drug dose needs to be adjusted in patient having renal impairment?

A. Rifampin.
B. Pyrazinamide.
C. Ethambutol.
D. Isoniazid.

Answer: C

Ethambutol dose needs to be adjusted in renal impairment since nearly 80% of it is excreted unchanged by the kidneys.

9. A 28-year-old patient was diagnosed to have *Mycobacterium avium* complex (MAC) infection caused by *Mycobacterium avium* and *Mycobacterium intracellulare*. As it is atypical mycobacterial infection, which antibiotic drugs are preferred for treatment with ethambutol or rifampin?

A. Streptomycin/azithromycin.
B. Capreomycin/clarithromycin.
C. Clarithromycin/azithromycin.
D. Linezolid/amikacin.

Answer: C

These two macrolides are preferred over other mentioned drugs for MAC infection since these two macrolides are indispensable for the treatment of MAC.

10. A 30-year-old woman was diagnosed to have multidrug resistant tuberculosis (MDR TB). She was put on short-course regimen for MDR TB. After initial 2 months' treatment, the patient developed slurred speech, hallucinations, and psychotic reactions. Which second-line drug from MDR TB regimen is most likely to have caused the condition?

A. Para-amino salicylic acid.
B. Cycloserine.
C. Ethionamide.
D. Clofazimine.

Answer: B

Cycloserine is known to cause neuropsychotic adverse reactions.

11. A 24-year-old patient was newly diagnosed with pulmonary tuberculosis and was put on category 1 regimen as per RNTCP. The regimen contains fixed-dose combination (FDC) of four first-line drugs, namely, isoniazid (H), rifampin (R), pyrazinamide (Z), and ethambutol (E). Choose the right dose combination per single tablet for H/R/Z/E from the given doses.

A. 75/150/275/400 mg.
B. 150/75/275/400 mg.
C. 75/400/150/275 mg.
D. 75/150/400/275 mg.

Answer: D

Each tablet contains the right dose as per RNTCP.

12. A 45-year-old patient diagnosed with multidrug-resistant tuberculosis (MDR TB) has been put on short-course regimen for MDR TB as per RNTCP. The patient was eligible to be put on newer drug bedaquiline in MDR TB with other three drugs. What would be the dosage schedule for bedaquiline?

A. 400 mg daily for 2 weeks, then 400 mg three times a week for 22 weeks.
B. 400 mg daily for 2 weeks, then 200 mg three times a week for 22 weeks.
C. 200 mg daily for 2 weeks, then 400 mg three times a week for 22 weeks.
D. 200 mg daily for 2 weeks, then 200 mg three times a week for 22 weeks.

Answer: B

As per the RNTCP guideline, bedaquiline 400 mg should be given daily for 2 weeks, followed by 200 mg three times a week for 22 weeks.

13. Which fluoroquinolones has the highest activity against mycobacterial tuberculosis?

A. Ciprofloxacin.
B. Moxifloxacin.
C. Ofloxacin.
D. Levofloxacin.

Answer: B

Moxifloxacin has highest activity against *Mycobacterium tuberculosis*.

14. Isoniazid-induced peripheral neuropathy can be treated with pyridoxine. In which dose pyridoxine is used per day to treat peripheral neuropathy?

5. 10 mg/day.
6. B 100 mg/day.
7. C 1000 mg/day.
8. D 100 g/day.

Answer: B

It is given in a dose of 10 mg/day as preventive dose and 100 mg/day for treatment purpose.

15. How is extensively drug-resistant tuberculosis (XDR TB) defined?

A. Multidrug-resistant (MDR) TB + resistant to one FQ.

B. MDR TB + resistant to one second-line oral drug.

C. MDR TB + resistant to one FQ + one injectable drug.

D. MDR TB + resistant to one FQ + one second-line oral drug + one injectable drug.

Answer: C

This is as per RNTCP.

Chapter 64 Chemotherapy of Leprosy

Sachin Parab and Prasan R. Bhandar

PH1.46: Describe the mechanisms of action, types, doses, side effects, indications, and contraindications of antileprotic drugs.

Learning Objectives

- Drugs used in leprosy.
- Treatment of leprosy.

Introduction

Leprosy is also known as Hansen's disease. It is a chronic granulomatous infection commonly caused by *Mycobacterium leprae* and *Mycobacterium lepromatosis*, both of which predominantly affect the skin and peripheral nerves.

Types (DR9.4)

The histopathological manifestations of leprosy are diverse and depend on the cellular immune response to the *M. leprae* complex.

Tuberculoid Leprosy and Borderline Tuberculoid

This type is characterized by infiltration of dermis and subcutaneous fat with well-defined epithelioid noncaseating granulomas and few or absent acid-fast bacilli (AFB). In this type, there is intact cell-mediated immunity (CMI) with a predominant peripheral nerve involvement. Patients have a single or few lesions. Bacilli are rarely seen in the lesion.

Lepromatous Leprosy and Borderline Lepromatous Leprosy

This type consists of macrophages with a vacuolar cytoplasm, plasma cells, lymphocytes, and numerous AFB. In this type, there is impaired CMI, with a rapid progression of disease and extensive bilateral skin lesions, and the lesions contain numerous bacilli.

Depending on clinical features, leprosy is classified as:

1. Indeterminate leprosy.
2. Paucibacillary leprosy.
3. Borderline tuberculoid leprosy.
4. Borderline borderline leprosy.
5. Borderline lepromatous leprosy.
6. Multibacillary leprosy.

WHO Classification of Leprosy

Paucibacillary

The number of *M. leprae* in the body is small (less than 1 million), and a skin smear test is negative. Patients with this type of leprosy have five or fewer skin lesions. Most cases of leprosy are paucibacillary.

Multibacillary

M. leprae can multiply in the body almost without any check and is thus present in high numbers. In this type, the bacillus has likely spread to almost all areas of skin and peripheral nerves. A skin smear test is positive, and patients present with more than five skin lesions.

Drugs Used in Leprosy (DR9.5)

Diaminodiphenyl sulfone or dapsone, rifampicin, clofazimine, ethionamide, ofloxacin, minocycline, and clarithromycin are some of the drugs used in the treatment of leprosy.

Dapsone (Diaminodiphenyl Sulfone)

It is a sulfone. It is one of the oldest and cheapest agents; hence, it is widely used. Being chemically related to sulfonamides, it has the same mechanism of action as sulfonamides (**Fig. 64.1**). Lepra bacilli utilize para-aminobenzoic acid (PABA) for synthesis of folic acid. Folic acid is necessary for its growth and multiplication. Dapsone is structurally similar to PABA; thus, it competitively inhibits folate synthetase. Hence, it prevents formation of tetrahydrofolic acid. Therefore, dapsone is leprostatic in nature. It has a complete oral absorption and is widely distributed, especially in the infected skin, muscle, liver, and kidney. It undergoes enterohepatic circulation and is metabolized by acetylation, the degree of which is genetically determined. Adverse effects are dose-related hemolytic anemia and methemoglobinemia in patients with glucose-6-phosphate dehydrogenase (G6DP) deficiency. Sulfone syndrome can occur, that is, exacerbations of lesions/symptoms such as fever, dermatitis, pruritus, lymphadenopathy, hepatitis, anemia, and methemoglobinemia. Other adverse effects include allergic dermatitis, itching, and peripheral neuropathy. In general, these symptoms will occur within the first 6 weeks of therapy, or not at all, and may be treated by corticosteroid therapy.

Acedapsone is a repository form of dapsone whose single intramuscular injection maintains inhibitory levels of dapsone in tissues for up to 3 months. Dapsone is also

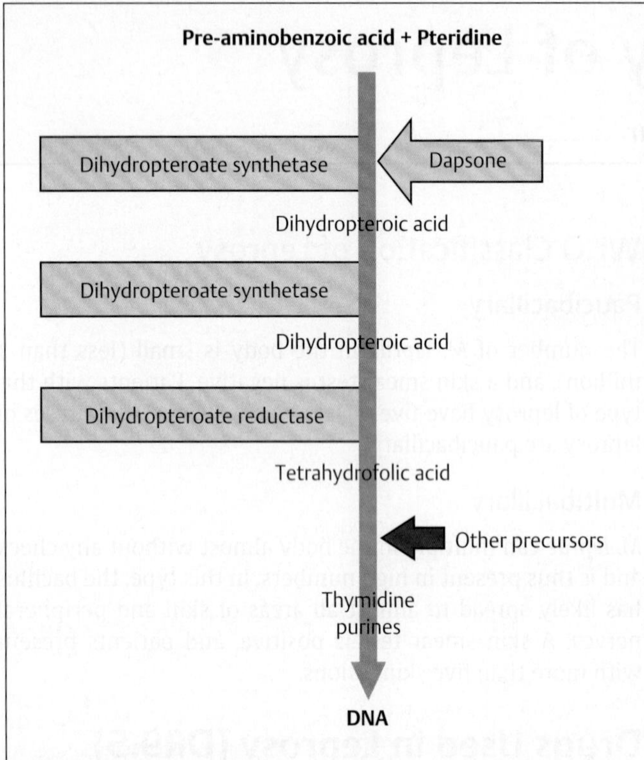

Fig. 64.1 Mechanism of action of dapsone.

an alternative drug for the treatment of *Pneumocystis jirovecii* infection in AIDS patients. It is the drug of choice for treatment of dermatitis herpetiformis.

Rifampicin

It is the most effective, bactericidal antileprotic agent, which acts on rapidly multiplying lepra bacilli. It prevents development of resistance to dapsone. The WHO recommends it for all types of multidrug regimens.

Clofazimine

It is a phenazine dye with weak bactericidal effect. It has additional anti-inflammatory effect and hence is useful for type 2 lepra reaction. This agent binds to mycobacterial DNA to inhibit its template function. The beneficial effect is that it acts against dapsone-resistant bacilli. Clofazimine is given orally, and food increases its absorption. It is not metabolized and is excreted in the feces via the bile. Adverse drug reactions (ADRs) include: red-brown discoloration of exposed skin; conjunctival and corneal pigmentation; discoloration of hairs, tears, sweat, urine, etc. Other side effects comprise nausea, vomiting, diarrhea, and abdominal pain.

Ethionamide

It is a second-line antituberculosis agent, which is effective against lepra bacilli. It is reserved as an alternative to clofazimine. Its major ADR is its hepatotoxic potential.

Newer Agents

These include clarithromycin administered 500 mg daily for 28 days. Minocycline is the only tetracycline effective against lepra bacilli, which is used in combination regimens. Ofloxacin is a bactericidal agent used in multidrug regimen in combination with rifampicin, in a regimen of ofloxacin 400 mg and rifampicin 600 mg for 28 days.

Treatment of Leprosy

The WHO recommends multidrug therapy (MDT) for all leprosy cases. The objectives of MDT are to render patients noncontagious at the earliest (by killing rapidly multiplying bacilli), prevent resistance, prevent relapse (by destroying persisters), and shorten the duration of treatment.

Treatment Schedule

All drugs are given orally.

For Multibacillary Leprosy (Lepromatous Leprosy, Borderline Lepromatous Leprosy, and Borderline Borderline)

Rifampicin is administered 600 mg once monthly, supervised; clofazimine 300 mg once monthly, supervised; dapsone 100 mg daily, unsupervised (self-administered); and clofazimine 50 mg daily, unsupervised (self-administered). The treatment duration is approximately 2 years. Follow-up should be for at least 5 years. If clofazimine is ineffective use ethionamide 250 mg daily, unsupervised.

For Paucibacillary Leprosy (Tuberculoid Leprosy, Borderline Tuberculoid, and Indeterminate Leprosy)

Rifampicin 600 mg is given once monthly, supervised; dapsone 100 mg is administered daily, unsupervised, for 6 months.

Alternative Regimens

These include clofazimine 50 mg plus any two newer drugs (clarithromycin/minocycline/ofloxacin) daily for 6 months, followed by clofazimine 50 mg and any one newer drug for another 18 months. For single-lesion paucibacillary leprosy, the following regimen is recommended:

1. Rifampicin 600 mg.
2. Ofloxacin 400 mg as a single dose.
3. Minocycline 100 mg.

Lepra Reactions

These are immunologically mediated reactions that occur during the course of disease. The cause is not known; however, it is precipitated by infection, trauma, stress, etc. They are of two types, as discussed in the following.

Type 1 (Reversal Reaction)

It is a delayed-type hypersensitivity seen in borderline leprosy cases. It is characterized by neuropathy, painful tender lesions, and cutaneous ulcerations. When it occurs after initiation of treatment, it is known as reversal reaction. This is treated by oral prednisolone.

Type 2 (Erythema Nodosum Leprosum)

It is a type III hypersensitivity commonly seen in lepromatous leprosy. This reaction is more severe than type 1 and is characterized by tender, inflamed subcutaneous nodules. It is associated with fever, lymphadenopathy, arthritis, nerve pain, orchitis, iridocyclitis, etc. It occurs due to the release of antigen from dying lepra bacilli. Treatment includes thalidomide (contraindicated in pregnancy) and other drugs such as clofazimine, chloroquine, corticosteroids (prednisolone), and aspirin.

Multiple Choice Questions

1. The most common side effect of dapsone is:

A. Hemolytic anemia.
B. Thrombocytopenia.
C. Cyanosis.
D. Bone marrow depression.

Answer: A

Hemolysis develops in almost every individual treated with 200 to 300 mg dapsone per day. Doses of less than 100 mg in healthy persons and less than 50 mg per day in persons with G6PD deficiency do not cause hemolysis. Methemoglobinemia is also very common.

2. In leprosy, the best bactericidal agent is:

A. Clofazimine.
B. Dapsone.
C. Rifampicin.
D. Ethionamide.

Answer: C

The best and fastest acting drug for leprosy is rifampicin.

3. In lepra reaction, the useful drug is:

A. Penicillins.
B. Clofazimine.
C. Dapsone.
D. Rifampicin.

Answer: B

Anti-inflammatory drugs are used in lepra reaction. Steroids, clofazimine, and thalidomide can be used.

4. Which of the following drugs can produce dramatic improvement in patients with type 2 lepra reaction?

A. Thalidomide.
B. Steroids.
C. Dapsone.
D. Clofazimine.

Answer: A.

Steroids are drug of choice for both type 1 and type 2 lepra reactions. Thalidomide is used in steroid-resistant type 2 lepra reaction.

Chapter 65 Antifungal Agents

Amrita Sil

Learning Objectives

- Types of fungal infections.
- Classification of antifungal agents.
- Individual antifungal agents.

Introduction

Fungal infections affect over a billion people, with global mortality rates estimated at 1.5 million per year. This mortality rate is similar to tuberculosis and threefolds more than malaria. Modern medicine advancements in the form of solid organ and bone marrow transplants and antineoplastic chemotherapy and also the AIDS pandemic cause immunosuppression. They are associated with a dramatic increase in opportunistic fungal infections.

The fungi are also showing some ominous shifts in terms of virulence and pathogenicity in recent times. This rising trend of fungal infection is persistently continuing, even in the presence of advanced antifungal agents.

Factors responsible for emerging infections

Human fungal infections are on a steady rise. Their causes are multifactorial.

1. Emergence of intrinsically resistant fungal species affecting humans.
2. Use of immunosuppressive agents (like corticosteroids) and immunomodulatory agents in transplant patients, treatment of cancers, autoimmune diseases, rheumatoid arthritis, etc. lowers host defense.
3. The AIDS pandemic has led to an increased number of immunocompromised hosts who have fungal infections like mucocutaneous candidiasis, Pneumocystis carinii pneumonia, cryptococcal meningitis, coccidioidomycosis, and histoplasmosis.
4. Indwelling catheters, stents, dentures, and implants breaks down host barriers and defense mechanisms and saprophytic fungi can invade easily.
5. Indiscriminate use of topical corticosteroids alone or in combination with other molecules, including topical antifungal agents.
6. Use of broad-spectrum antibiotics.
7. Inadvertent and uncontrolled use of antifungal agents in hospital settings and over-the-counter use in the community.

Types of Fungal Infections

Depending on cell morphology, fungi fall into four classes (**Table 65.1**):

Yeasts

They are unicellular fungi and reproduce by budding. The only pathological yeast-causing disease in humans is *Cryptococcus neoformans*. Cryptococcus causes opportunistic infection in AIDS patients, causing meningitis.

Yeast-Like Fungi

They grow partly as yeast and partly as elongated cells resembling hyphae and form pseudomycelium. Such fungi are Candida and *Malassezia furfur*. Candida causes oral (thrush), vulvovaginal, and systemic candidiasis. *Malassezia furfur* is responsible for pityriasis versicolor infection, which presents as hyper or hypopigmented macules with fine scaling on skin.

Molds or Filamentous Fungi

They form true mycelia and reproduce by forming spores, for example, dermatophytes, *Aspergillus fumigatus*, and Mucor.

Table 65.1 Types of fungal infections

Fungi causing superficial infections	Fungi causing deep infections	
	Subcutaneous	**Systemic**
▪ Candida ▪ Malassezia furfur ▪ Dermatophytes/ringworm/Tinea (Trichophyton, Epidermophyton, Microsporum)	▪ Sporothrix sp ▪ Chromoblastomycoses ▪ Blastomyces	▪ Aspergillus ▪ Candida ▪ Mucor ▪ Histoplasma capsulatum ▪ Coccidioides immitis ▪ Blastomyces dermatides ▪ Cryptococcus neoformans

Dermatophytes cause skin or nail infections and are termed as Tinea infections, according to the body site they affect: Tinea capitis (scalp), Tinea facii (face), Tinea barbae (beard), Tinea corporis (body), Tinea cruris (groin), Tinea manuum (hand), Tinea pedis (feet/ athlete's foot), and Tinea unguium (nails). Aspergillus cause aspergillosis.

Dimorphic Fungi

They can grow both as yeast in host tissues at 37°C or as filaments in soil and cultures at 22°C. Most fungi causing systemic infections are dimorphic fungi, for example, *Blastomyces dermatitidis* causing blastomycosis, *Histoplasma capsulatum* causing histoplasmosis, *Coccidiodes immitis* causing coccidioidomycosis, and Paracoccidiodes causing paracoccidiodomycosis. All of the above dimorphic fungi cause pulmonary infections followed by dissemination. *Sporothrix schenckii* cause sporotrichosis, a subcutaneous mycoses which can spread by lymphatic route.

Classification of Antifungal Agents (DR7.3)

Fungi are eukaryotes with distinctive cell walls containing glucans and chitin, and their eradication requires different strategies than those for treatment of bacterial infections. Antifungal agents can be classified according to their sites of action as mentioned below and demonstrated in **Tables 65.2** and **65.3** and **Figure 65.1.**

Individual Antifungal Agents

Echinocandins

They are large cyclic peptides linked to a long-chain fatty acid. Three echinocandins are currently licensed for use: Caspofungin, Micafungin, and Anidulafungin

Pharmacokinetics

These agents are available only for intravenous (IV) use as they are not absorbed orally. Loading dose is required during administration. They are water-soluble and highly protein bound (>97%). Metabolites are excreted by kidney and gastrointestinal tract (GIT). However, dose adjustments are required only during severe hepatic compromise.

Mechanism of Action

Echinocandins inhibits the synthesis of 1, 3-β-glucan, an essential component of fungal cell wall. This causes disruption of the fungal cell wall, cell lysis, and death of the fungus. Mammalian cells do not require 1, 3-β-glucan and thus contribute to the selective toxicity of these agents.

Antifungal Spectrum

- Invasive Aspergillus infections.
- Invasive Candidiasis (esophageal, intra-abdominal peritonitis).
- Febrile neutropenic patients with suspected fungal infections.

Table 65.2 Classification of antifungal agents according to sites of action

Target site	Mechanism of action	Class	Examples
Cell wall	Inhibition of cell wall synthesis	Echinocandins	Caspofungin Micafungin Anidulafungin
Cell membrane	Binds to fungal cell membrane ergosterol and increase membrane permeability which disrupts membrane function	Polyene	AmB Nystatin
Cell membrane	Inhibition of ergosterol + lanosterol synthesis	Allylamine	Terbinafine
Cell membrane	Inhibition of ergosterol synthesis	Azole	Ketoconazole Fluconazole Itraconazole Voriconazole Posaconazole Topical: Clotrimazole, Miconazole, Oxiconazole, Econazole, Sertaconazole
Nucleic acids	Inhibition of synthesis of nucleic acids		5-FC
Mitotic spindle	Inhibition of fungal mitosis by disruption of mitotic spindle		Griseofulvin
Miscellaneous	Miscellaneous		Ciclopirox Tolnaftate Amorolfine Butenafine

Abbreviations: 5-FC, flucytosine; AmB, Amphotericin B.

Table 65.3 Antifungal agents used for superficial and invasive fungal infections

Antifungal agents used for superficial fungal infections	Antifungal agents used for invasive fungal infections
Azoles	Echinocandins
Terbinafine	AmB
Griseofulvin	5-FC
Topical antifungal agents	Azoles

Abbreviations: 5-FC, flucytosine; AmB, Amphotericin B.

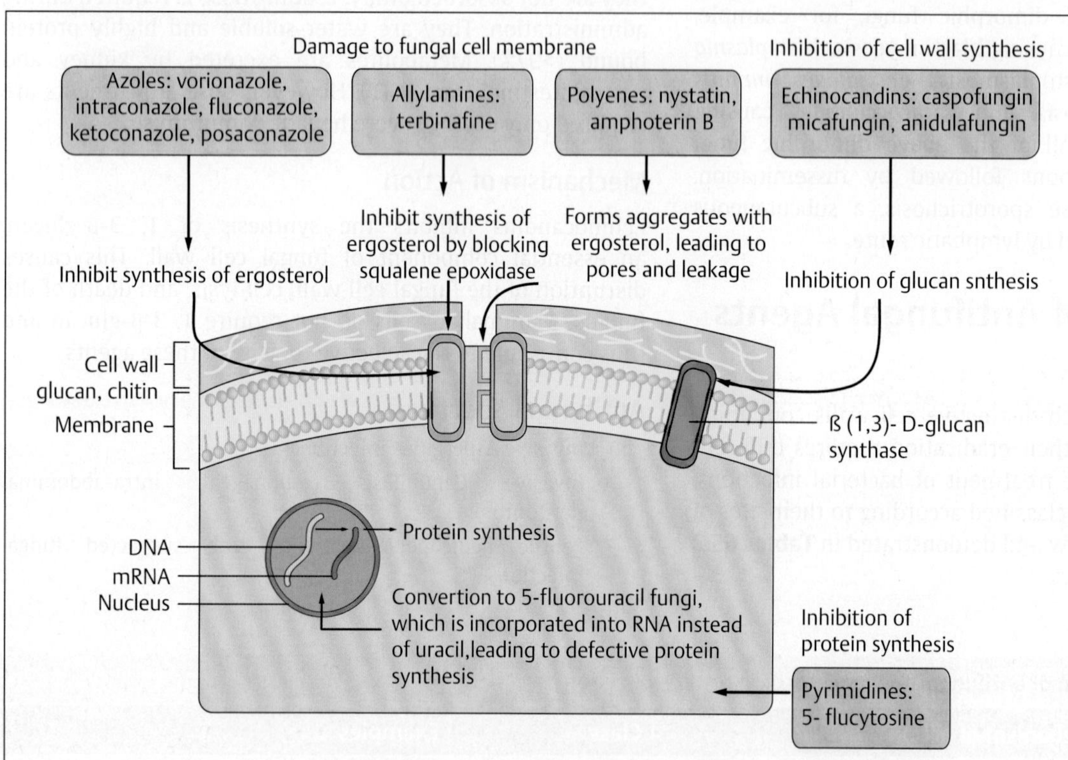

Fig. 65.1 Classification of antifungal agents.

Adverse Effects

These agents are remarkably well-tolerated. Phlebitis of the infusion site has been reported. Histamine-like effects have been reported with rapid infusions.

Polyenes/Polyene Antibiotics

This group of polyene antibiotics is so named because they have several conjugated double bonds attached to a large lactone ring. This portion is highly lipophilic. The other end with many -OH bonds is hydrophilic. Amphotericin-B (AmB) and nystatin are drugs in this group. Polyenes will be discussed with AmB as prototype.

Pharmacokinetics

AmB is poorly absorbed from GIT. Therefore, it is IV administered as a suspension made with deoxycholate (DOC). Oral AmB can be given for intestinal candidiasis without systemic toxicity. The drug is widely distributed in most tissues except cerebrospinal fluid (CSF). It binds to sterols in tissues and lipoproteins in plasma and stays in the body for long periods. AmB is metabolized in liver. Excretion occurs slowly both in urine and bile. Since plasma concentrations are not affected much, dose adjustments are not needed in renal and hepatic compromise.

Mechanism of Action

The polyene molecules have high affinity for ergosterol present in fungal cell membrane. They combine with it, get inserted into the membrane, and several polyene molecules together orient themselves to form pores. The hydrophilic side of the polyene molecule forms the interior of the pore through which ions, amino acids, and other water-soluble substances move out. The micropore is stabilized by membrane sterols, which fill up the spaces between the AmB molecules on the lipophilic side which, in turn, constitute the outer surface of the pores. Therefore, permeability of the membrane is increased and leakage of small molecules occurs.

Cholesterol, present in human cell membranes, closely resembles ergosterol. Polyenes bind with cholesterol but with low affinity. Therefore, the selectivity of action of polyenes is low.

Antifungal Spectrum

- Invasive Aspergillosis.
- Invasive Candidiasis.
- Mucormycosis.
- Histoplasmosis.
- Coccidioidomycosis, Paracoccidioidomycosis.
- Blastomycosis.
- Cryptococcal meningitis (used with fluconazole or with flucytosine [5-FC]).
- Topical as 3% cream, lotion, ointment in oropharyngeal candidiasis, cutaneous candidiasis, mycotic corneal ulcers, otomycosis.
- Reserve drug for kala-azar and mucocutaneous leishmaniasis.

Adverse Effects

Acute Reactions

Chills, fever, aches, pain, nausea, vomiting, and dyspnea occur with each infusion of AmB. This is probably due to release of cytokines (IL, TNFα). When these are severe, the dose is increased gradually. This infusion-related reactions are least with liposomal AmB (L-AmB). The intensity of reaction decreases with continued medication, pretreatment with paracetamol, or use of hydrocortisone hemisuccinate 0.7 mg/kg.

Long-Term Toxicity

1. Nephrotoxicity: Azotemia, reduced glomerular filtration rate (GFR), acidosis, hypokalemia, hypomagnesemia, renal tubular acidosis, and inability to concentrate urine occur fairly uniformly and are dose related. It reverses slowly and incompletely after stoppage of therapy. Keeping the patient well-hydrated by prior infusion of 1 Liter of normal saline reduces risk of renal toxicity.
2. Anemia: Hypochromic, normocytic anemia occurs commonly during treatment with AmB. This anemia occurs due to decreased production of erythropoietin and reverses slowly following stoppage of AmB.
3. Central nervous system (CNS) toxicity: Arachnoiditis, headache, vomiting, and nerve palsies have been observed following intrathecal injection.

Drug Interactions

- 5-FC has synergistic action with AmB. AmB facilitates permeation of 5-FC through fungal cell membrane.
- Since AmB is nephrotoxic, concomitant nephrotoxic drugs such as aminoglycosides, vancomycin, and cyclosporine enhance impairment caused by AmB.

New AmB Formulations

To improve tolerability, decrease the nephrotoxicity of AmB and achieve targeted delivery, the following three formulations have been made:

AmB Colloidal Dispersion (ABCD)

It contains AmB and cholesteryl sulfate formulated for injection (**Fig. 65.2**). ABCD is less nephrotoxic than conventional AmB but causes more fever and chills.

Liposomal AmB (L-AmB)

AmB is incorporated in liposomes (small unilamellar vesicles made up of lecithin and biodegradable phospholipids). L-AmB produces milder acute reaction. L-AmB delivers AmB particularly to reticuloendothelial cells of liver and spleen (targeted delivery) and is especially useful for kala-azar and immunocompromised patients (**Fig. 65.3**).

AmB Lipid Complex (ABLC)

AmB is incorporated in ribbon-like particles of dimyristoyl phospholipids. ABLC is more nephrotoxic than L-AmB.

The cost of lipid formulations of AmB is greater than conventional AmB.

Azole Antifungals

Azoles are synthetic antifungals with a broad-spectrum antifungal activity and are extensively used. They may be fungistatic or fungicidal, depending on concentration. Azoles are subdivided into two groups:

Imidazole Group

Two nitrogens in azole group—Clotrimazole, Econazole, Miconazole, Oxiconazole, Sertaconazole, Eberconazole, Luliconazole, and Ketoconazole. The only imidazole that can be used both systemically and topically is Ketoconazole. The rest are used topically.

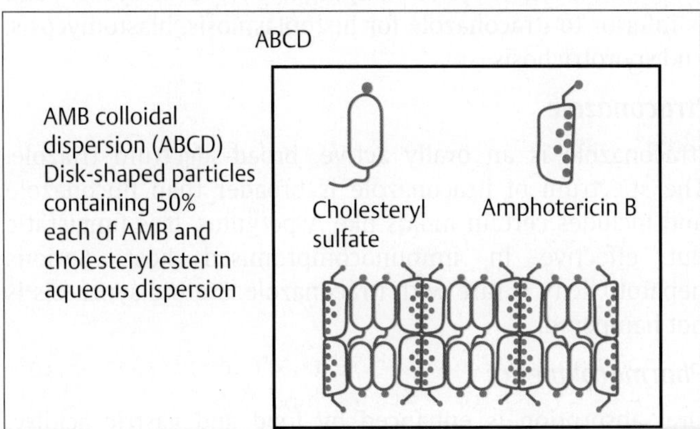

Fig. 65.2 AmB colloidal dispersion (ABCD).

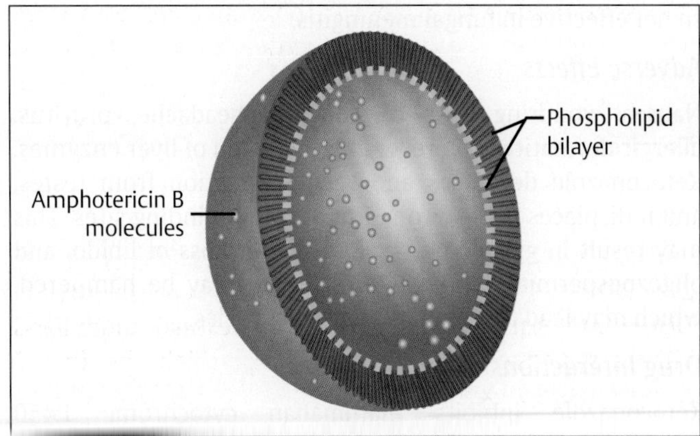

Fig. 65.3 Liposomal amphotericin (L-AmB).

Triazole Group

Three nitrogens in azole ring—Fluconazole, Itraconazole, Voriconazole, and Posaconazole. Triazoles are used systemically.

Mechanism of Action

Azoles bind to fungal cytochrome P-450-dependent 14-α-demethylase enzyme. Demethylation of lanosterol to ergosterol is hampered, which results in damaged and leaky fungal cell membrane.

Azoles also inhibit fungal respiration under aerobic conditions; hence, blockade of respiratory chain electron transport may also be another mechanism of action.

Antifungal Spectrum

Dermatophytes, Candida, and other fungi are involved in deep mycosis (except mucor).

Bacteria such as Nocardia, *Staph aureus, Streptococcus faecalis, Bacteroides fragilis*, and parasites like Leishmania.

Topical Imidazoles

Clotrimazole, Econazole, Miconazole, Oxiconazole, Sertaconazole, Eberconazole, Luliconazole, and Ketoconazole. They are effective against superficial mycoses such as tinea cruris, tinea corporis, tinea pedis, pityriasis versicolor, cutaneous, and oropharyngeal candidiasis. Since systemic absorption is negligible, adverse effects are rare. Various forms of topical application such as cream, ointment, lotion, vaginal cream, and vaginal tablets are available. Ketoconazole is available as shampoo for treating seborrheic dermatitis of scalp.

Ketoconazole

This was the first orally effective antifungal. At present, its systemic use is limited due to its toxicity and availability of newer triazoles like fluconazole and itraconazole.

Therapeutic Uses

- Mucocutaneous candidiasis, dermatophytosis.
- Cushing's syndrome (since it inhibits steroid synthesis).
- Deep mycoses (but not preferred due to toxicity).

Pharmacokinetics

Oral absorption of ketoconazole is facilitated by gastric acidity. It is metabolized in liver. Penetration to CSF is poor, so not effective in fungal meningitis.

Adverse Effects

Nausea, vomiting, loss of appetite, headache, pruritus, allergic dermatitis, and reversible elevation of liver enzymes. Ketoconazole decreases androgen production from testes, and it displaces testosterone from protein-binding sites. This may result in gynecomastia, loss of hair, loss of libido, and oligozoospermia. Synthesis of estradiol may be hampered, which may lead to irregular menstrual cycles.

Drug Interactions

Ketoconazole inhibits mammalian cytochrome P450 (CYP3A4). Therefore, plasma level of drugs metabolized by CYP3A4 is raised.

1. Dangerous interaction with terfenadine, astemizole, and cisapride (all metabolized by CYP3A4), resulting in polymorphic ventricular tachycardia.
2. Rifampicin and phenytoin accelerate ketoconazole metabolism and reduce its efficacy.
3. H_2 receptor blockers, proton-pump inhibitors, and antacids decrease ketoconazole absorption by decreasing acidity.

Fluconazole

It is a water-soluble, broad-spectrum triazole. Fluconazole has least effect on mammalian cytochrome P450.

Pharmacokinetics

Orally, 94% is absorbed; absorption of drug is not affected by gastric acidity or food. Half-life is long (25–30 hours), needing administration once daily. Fungicidal concentrations reached in nails, vagina, and saliva. Fluconazole penetrates well into brain, CSF, and saliva. Fluconazole is eliminated by renal route in unchanged form; therefore, it can be used in hepatic impairment. Dose reduction is needed in renal impairment.

Adverse Effects

Very few side effects like GI disturbance, headaches, and rashes may occur but are well tolerated. Increase in hepatic transaminases and alopecia has been reported after prolonged therapy. Since it has minimum effect on mammalian cytochrome P450, drug interactions are not clinically significant. Contraindicated in pregnancy and lactation. Total fluconazole dose >300 mg is contraindicated throughout pregnancy (FDA category D) and lactation. However, recent FDA guidelines state that a single low dose (≤300 mg total dose) of fluconazole does not increase the risk of congenital disorders and may be considered in the absence of a topical alternative after the first trimester.

Therapeutic Uses

1. Cryptococcal meningitis—after amphotericin B.
2. Coccidioidal meningitis in AIDS—drug of choice also for prophylaxis.
3. Candidiasis—oropharyngeal, esophageal candidiasis, mucocutaneous candidiasis, candidemia in ICU patients (given IV), vaginal candidiasis (single 150 mg dose is curative).
4. Dermatophytes/Tinea infections.
5. Histoplasmosis—itraconazole preferred as it has better efficacy.

Fluconazole is ineffective in aspergillosis, mucormycosis, and is inferior to itraconazole for histoplasmosis, blastomycosis, and sporotrichosis.

Itraconazole

Itraconazole is an orally active, broad-spectrum triazole. The spectrum of itraconazole is broader than fluconazole and includes certain molds like Aspergillus. It is fungistatic but effective in immunocompromised host. Serious hepatotoxicity is rare with itraconazole. Steroid synthesis is not hampered.

Pharmacokinetics

Oral absorption is enhanced by food and gastric acidity. It is highly protein bound (99%) and has a large volume of distribution. It accumulates in vaginal mucosa, nails, and skin. CSF penetration is poor. It is metabolized by CYP3A4 and excreted via feces.

Adverse Effects

Although well-tolerated, headache, nausea, and epigastric distress may occur. Some cases of congestive cardiac failure and transient rise in plasma transaminases have been reported.

Drug Interactions

Since itraconazole inhibits CYP3A4, drug interactions are similar to ketoconazole.

1. Ventricular arrhythmias are reported with terfenadine, astemizole, cisapride, and class III antiarrhythmics.
2. Rifampicin and phenytoin accelerate itraconazole metabolism and reduce its efficacy. Clarithromycin and protease inhibitors inhibit metabolism and increase itraconazole blood levels.
3. H_2 receptor blockers, proton-pump inhibitors, and antacids decrease itraconazole absorption by decreasing acidity.

Therapeutic Uses

1. Systemic mycoses not associated with meningitis.
2. Vaginal candidiasis, dermatophytosis, onychomycosis.
3. Drug of choice for paracoccidioidomycosis and chromomycosis.
4. Aspergillosis.

Newer Triazoles

Voriconazole

It is a second generation triazole with high-oral bioavailability and good CSF penetration. It undergoes extensive hepatic metabolism. Plasma half-life is short (6 hours). It is a drug of choice for invasive aspergillosis, esophageal candidiasis, molds like Fusarium and *Pseudallescheria boydii*, and candida isolates resistant to fluconazole.

Posaconazole

This newer triazole is orally well-absorbed better with fatty meals. It is therapeutically used for mucormycosis, zygomycosis (for which only AmB was available), fluconazole-resistant oropharyngeal candidiasis, and aspergillus infection in immunocompromised. It inhibits CYP3A4 and causes drug interaction akin to ketoconazole.

Flucytosine (5-FC)

5-FC is closely related to the anticancer agent 5-fluorouracil (5-FU). It is devoid of anticancer activity but has antifungal properties.

Mechanism of Action

5-FC is transported into fungal cells with the help of cytosine permease enzyme. It is converted to 5-FU by fungal cytokine deaminase enzyme. 5-FU is further converted to 5-fluorodeoxyuridine monophosphate (5-FdUMP), which then acts as a competitive inhibitor of thymidylate synthetase. Thus, inhibition of thymidylate synthetase inhibits fungal DNA synthesis. Thymidylate synthetase is responsible for the conversion of deoxyuridine monophosphate to thymidine monophosphate and for DNA synthesis. Human cells are devoid of cytokine deaminase, which prevents conversion of 5-FC to 5-FU; thus, selective toxicity to fungal cells occurs.

Therapeutic Use

5-FC has limited antifungal spectrum. It is not preferred as a monotherapy due to therapeutic failure and development of resistance. 5-FC is currently used as a part of combination therapy for cryptococcal meningitis (along with AmB).

Adverse Effects

Major toxicity is bone marrow depression.

Griseofulvin

It is a fungistatic agent extracted from *Penicillium griseofulvum.*

Pharmacokinetics

Griseofulvin is administered orally. Micronization and fatty meal improve the bioavailability. It gets deposited in keratin, forming cells of hair, nails, and skin. Since it is fungistatic, the fungus persists in already infected keratin till it is shed off. The duration of treatment depends on the site of infection, thickness of the infected keratin and its turnover rate.

Mechanism of Action

Griseofulvin causes disruption of mitotic spindles, as a result of which multinucleated cells are formed and mitosis is inhibited. It also binds to newly synthesized keratin of skin, hair, and nails, and makes them resistant to fungal infection (**Fig. 65.4**).

Therapeutic Uses

It is used orally for dermatophytosis only and ineffective topically. The duration of treatment for the following areas are mentioned in **Table 65.4.**

Adverse Effects

Headache, GIT disturbances, peripheral neuritis, and photosensitivity. It induces CYP P-450 and can reduce effectiveness of warfarin and oral contraceptives. Hepatotoxicity has been observed.

Terbinafine

Terbinafine is an orally and topically effective allylamine. It is effective against Dermatophytes and Candida. It is fungicidal. It inhibits "squalene epoxidase," which is an early step in ergosterol synthesis.

Bioavailability is decreased to 40% due to first-pass metabolism in the liver. Terbinafine does not inhibit CYP450. It is effective for dermatophytosis and onychomycosis but less effective in candidiasis. Side effects are gastric upset,

Table 65.4 Duration of treatment at various sites

Site	Duration of treatment
Skin	4 weeks
Fingernails	3 months
Toenails	6 months

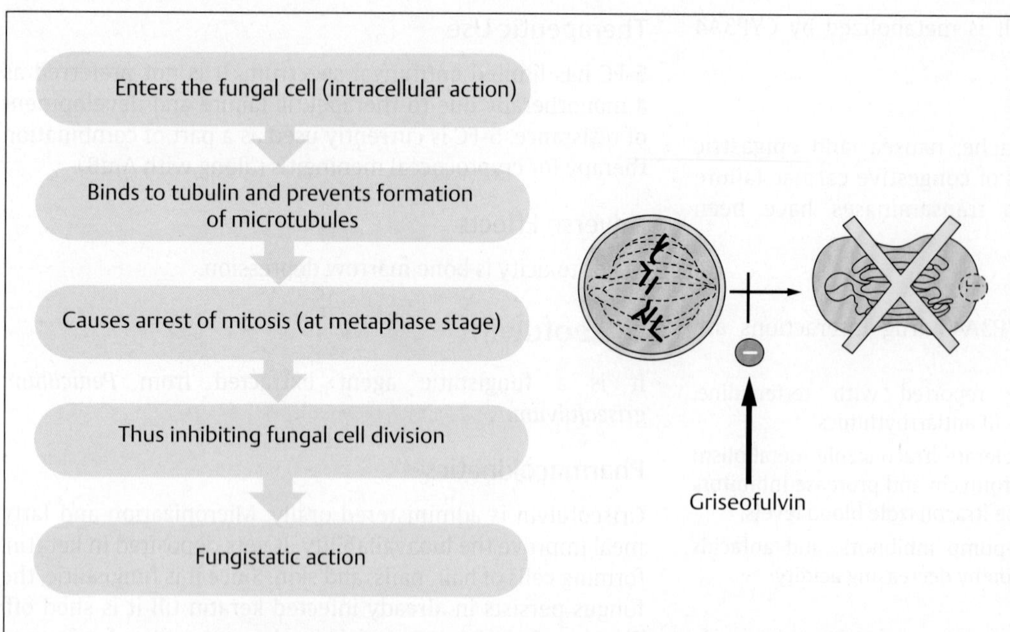
Enters the fungal cell (intracellular action)
Binds to tubulin and prevents formation of microtubules
Causes arrest of mitosis (at metaphase stage)
Thus inhibiting fungal cell division
Fungistatic action
Griseofulvin

Fig. 65.4 Mechanism of action of griseofulvin.

rashes, and liver enzyme elevation. Some cases of severe cutaneous reaction have been reported.

Topically Used Antifungals

Nystatin

It is a topical polyene antifungal agent with structure and mechanism of action similar to AmB. It is mainly used to treat candidal infections of skin, GIT, mucosa, and vagina.

Topical Allylamines

Terbinafine, butenafine, and naftifine are available as cream for topical use. They are used for dermatophytosis and candida infections.

Amorolfine

It is used as nail lacquer for treatment of onychomycosis and as cream for dermatophytosis. Amorolfine inhibits squalene epoxidase and disrupts ergosterol biosynthesis.

Topical Azoles

Clotrimazole, Econazole, Miconazole, Oxiconazole, Sertaconazole, Eberconazole, Luliconazole, and Ketoconazole are topical imidazoles. They are effective against superficial mycoses like tinea cruris, tinea corporis, tinea pedis, pityriasis versicolor, and cutaneous and oropharyngeal candidiasis. Since systemic absorption is negligible, adverse effects are rare. Various forms of topical application like cream, ointment, lotion, vaginal cream, and vaginal tablets are available. Ketoconazole is available as shampoo for treating seborrheic dermatitis of scalp.

Ciclopirox Olamine

It is available as cream and lotion for treatment of dermatophytosis, cutaneous candidiasis, tinea versicolor, seborrheic dermatitis of scalp, and onychomycosis (higher concentration required).

Tolnaftate, Clioquinol, Sodium thiosulfate, and Benzoic Acid

These are less commonly used agents.

Drugs Used in Superficial and Deep Mycoses

Drugs Used in Superficial Mycoses

1. Dermatophytoses (ringworm).
   a. Topical: azole/terbinafine.
   b. Oral: terbinafine/itraconazole/griseofulvin

For limited tinea involving single site, use of topical agents only is recommended. For generalized tinea involving more than one site, use of both oral and topical agents is recommended. Due to the resurgence of tinea infections in India, "rule of 2" is followed where the topical antifungal should be applied 2 cm beyond the margin of the lesion for at least twice daily for 2 weeks beyond clinical resolution.

2. Cutaneous candidiasis.
   a. Topical: AmB/azole/nystatin/ciclopirox.
   b. Oral: fluconazole.
3. Oropharyngeal candidiasis.
   a. Topical: azole/nystatin/AmB.
   b. Oral: itraconazole.
4. Vaginal candidiasis.
   a. Topical: azole/nystatin.
   b. Oral: fluconazole.

Drugs for Systemic Fungal Infections

- Aspergillosis (invasive)—voriconazole.
- Blastomycosis—AmB/itraconazole.

- Candidiasis–fluconazole/voriconazole.
- Coccidioidomycosis–AmB ± 5-FC.
- Histoplasmosis–itraconazole/AmB.
- Mucormycosis–AmB/5-FC, posaconzole.
- Paracoccidioidomycosis–itraconazole.
- Sporotrichosis–itraconazole.

Multiple Choice Questions

1. Which of the following antifungal drug is available for both topical and systemic dosing?

A. Ketoconazole.
B. Terbinafine.
C. Amphotericin B (AmB).
D. All of the above

Answer: D

Ketoconazole is available as cream, shampoo (for seborrheic dermatitis), and tablets.

2. A patient with hepatic compromise has presented with extensive Tinea cruris. Which oral antifungal drug would you prefer for him?

A. Itraconazole.
B. Fluconazole.
C. Griseofulvin.
D. Terbinafine.

Answer: B

Fluconazole is eliminated unchanged by renal route. It is not metabolized in liver.

3. A HIV patient on highly active antiretroviral therapy (HAART) is diagnosed to be suffering from aspergillosis. Which antifungal agent is preferred in him?

A. Voriconazole.
B. Itraconazole.
C. Posaconazole.
D. Fluconazole.

Answer: C

Nevirapine and efavirenz decrease the plasma level of voriconazole and itraconazole when coadministered, leading to therapeutic failure. Fluconazole is not effective in Aspergillosis.

4. Nephrotoxicity of Amphotericin B (AmB) can be decreased by the following modality except:

A. Saline loading of the patient prior to start of therapy.
B. Coadministration of aminoglycosides.
C. Decreasing the dose of administered AmB.
D. Using a lipid formulation of AmB.

Answer: B

Aminoglycosides are nephrotoxic and increase the nephrotoxicity of AmB.

5. Echinocandins are preferred antifungal agents for the following except:

A. Dermatophytosis.
B. Esophageal candidiasis.
C. Aspergillosis.
D. Febrile neutropenia.

Answer: A

Caspofungin is approved for initial therapy of deeply invasive candidiasis and as salvage therapy for patients with invasive aspergillosis failing on voriconazole or Amphotericin B (AmB). Caspofungin is also approved for treatment of persistently febrile neutropenic patients with suspected fungal infections. Micafungin and anidulafungin are given for deeply invasive candidiasis. Dermatophytosis does not respond to echinocandins.

Chapter 66 Antiviral Drugs

Niti Mittal and Jitendra H. Vaghela

PH 1.48: Describe the mechanisms of action, types, doses, side effects, indications, and contraindications of the drugs used in urinary tract infections (UTIs)/sexually transmitted diseases (STDs) and viral diseases including human immunodeficiency virus (HIV).

Learning Objectives

- Antiherpetic drugs.
- Anti–hepatitis B virus drugs.
- Anti–hepatitis C virus drugs.
- Anti-influenza drugs.
- Nucleoside reverse transcriptase inhibitors.
- Nonnucleoside reverse transcriptase inhibitors.
- Protease inhibitors.
- Integrase inhibitors.
- HIV treatment guideline.

Viral Infections

Viruses are generally labeled as obligate intracellular parasites, acellular infectious agents that need the existence of a host cell for them to reproduce. Viruses infect all types of cells—humans, animals, plants, bacteria, yeast, archaea, and protozoa. Some scientists have even claimed that they have found a virus that infects other viruses! However, this is not possible without some cellular assistance. Viruses comprise a nucleic acid (either deoxyribonucleic acid [DNA] or ribonucleic acid [RNA]) linked with proteins programmed by the nucleic acid. A virus could also possess a lipid bilayer membrane (or envelope); however, this is attained from the host cell, generally by budding through a host cell membrane. If a membrane exists, it should comprise one or more viral proteins to act as ligands for receptors on the host cell.

1. Antiviral drugs need to have a high degree of specificity to discriminate viral and host targets. In contrast to antibacterials, there is limited information regarding pharmacodynamics of antiviral agents, as well as lack of established guidelines to adjust their dosages. Hence, the clinical use of antivirals demands more stringent monitoring to maximize benefits and minimize toxicity.
2. An important determinant of the outcome of viral infections, like any other infections, is the state of host defense mechanisms, for example, preexisting immunity, ability to mount the desired immune responses, and innate immunity, which need to be considered while treating them.
3. Determining a specific and timely diagnosis is required for optimal use of antiviral drugs. Diagnosis can be made on various grounds such as characteristic clinical manifestations (e.g., herpes zoster), epidemiologic information (e.g., influenza outbreak), or rapid viral diagnostic techniques.
4. All the existing antiviral drugs are virustatic, that is, active only against replicating viruses, with no effect on latent viruses.

Reproductive Cycle of Viruses and Various Targets of Antiviral Drugs

Fig. 66.1 represents various stages of the life cycle of a virus and targets of action of existing different antiviral drugs.

Table 66.1 enlists various clinically important DNA and RNA viruses and diseases caused by them (excluding HIV).

On the basis of its metabolic and replication profile, institution of viral chemotherapy was considered difficult and toxic. However, since the past 50 odd years, understanding of these steps has made treatment with the antiviral drugs relatively easier and tolerable. Additionally, antiviral agents that target virus-specific steps, such as cell penetration, uncoating, reverse transcription, and virus assembly or maturation, have been developed. Furthermore,

Table 66.1 Clinically important DNA and RNA viruses and diseases caused by them

Viruses	Diseases caused in humans
DNA viruses	
Herpes viruses	
▪ HSV-1	Oral/orolabial herpes
▪ HSV-2	Genital herpes
▪ VZV	Chicken pox
▪ EBV	Infectious mononucleosis
▪ CMV	Retinitis
▪ HBV	Hepatitis, hepatocellular carcinoma, cirrhosis, liver failure
RNA viruses	
▪ Rhinovirus	Common cold
▪ HCV	Hepatitis, hepatocellular carcinoma, cirrhosis, liver failure
▪ CoV	Common cold, SARS-CoV
▪ Parainfluenza virus	Croup, pneumonia, bronchiolitis
▪ Respiratory syncytial virus	Common cold, pneumonia, bronchiolitis
▪ Influenza A, B, and C viruses	Respiratory tract infection—influenza/flu

Abbreviations: CoV, coronaviruses; CMV, Cytomegalovirus; EBV, Epstein–Barr virus; HBV, hepatitis B virus; HCV, hepatitis C virus; HSV, herpes simplex virus; SARS, severe acute respiratory syndrome; VZV, varicella zoster virus.

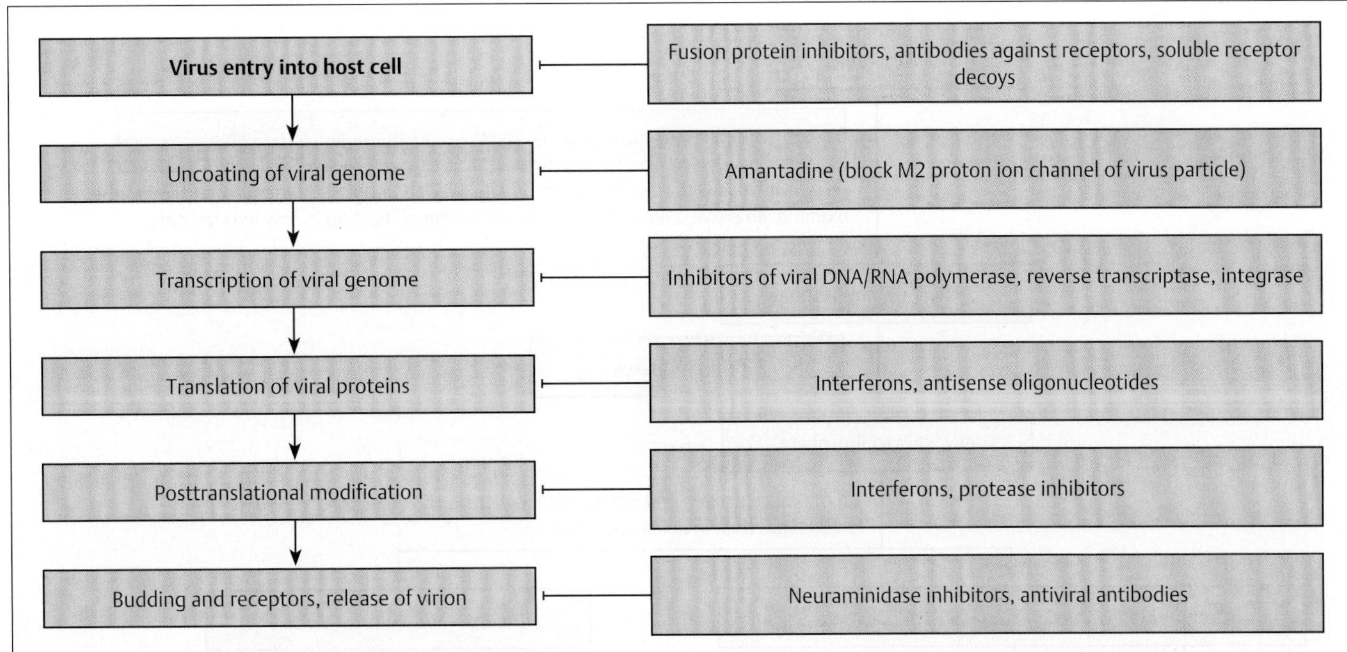

Fig. 66.1 Stages of viral replication and various drug targets.

another drawback of such therapy is that in most acute infections, viral reproduction is already at its highest when symptoms manifest. Hence, for better efficacy, the therapy should usually be initiated during the incubation period, that is, it has to be prophylactic or preemptive.

Antiherpetic Drugs

These are drugs that have activity against the herpes group of viruses.

Acyclovir and Valacyclovir

Acyclovir is the prototype of nucleoside analogs, a class of antiviral drugs that act by inhibiting viral DNA synthesis. Acyclovir is an acyclic guanosine derivative, which requires three phosphorylation steps to be activated (**Fig. 66.2**). In 1988, Gertrude Elion and George Hitchings were awarded the Nobel Prize for their discovery of acyclovir.

Resistance to acyclovir can develop due to mutation in viral thymidine kinase (TK; more commonly) or DNA polymerase. Acyclovir is active against herpes simplex viruses (HSVs) types 1 and 2, varicella zoster virus (VZV), and Epstein–Barr virus, and has relatively less activity against *Cytomegalovirus* (CMV) infections.

Pharmacokinetics

Acyclovir has oral bioavailability ranging from 10 to 30%, which decreases with increase in dose. The bioavailability of orally administered drugs is not altered in the presence of food. It is widely distributed in body fluids including cerebrospinal fluid (CSF), vesicular fluid, aqueous humor, amniotic fluid, breast milk, and placenta. The concentration in saliva is low compared to plasma and vaginal concentrations, demonstrating wide interindividual variability. With topical formulations, the intralesional concentration of the drug is quite good but poor percutaneous absorption leads to low systemic levels.

The principal route of elimination of unmetabolized acyclovir is renal (both glomerular filtration and tubular secretion). The elimination half-life of acyclovir is 1 to 6 hours in adults with normal renal function. Dosage needs to be reduced in patients having creatinine clearance less than 50 mL/min.

Valacyclovir is the L-valyl ester of acyclovir, which, after oral administration, undergoes rapid and almost complete conversion to acyclovir by hepatic and intestinal hydrolysis. Valacyclovir offers a better pharmacokinetic profile than acyclovir in terms of greater oral bioavailability (55–70%), higher blood levels, and need of less frequent administration (twice or thrice daily as compared to five times daily for acyclovir).

Adverse Effects

Acyclovir is generally well tolerated. Few side effects include nausea, diarrhea, and rash. Rarely, it is associated with renal toxicity due to drug crystallization, especially when the drug is administered rapidly intravenously or in the presence of inadequate hydration. Central nervous system (CNS) side effects such as lethargy and tremors are mainly reported in immunocompromised recipients. In neonates, the drug is associated with neutropenia. No fetal abnormalities have been reported with its use in pregnant women.

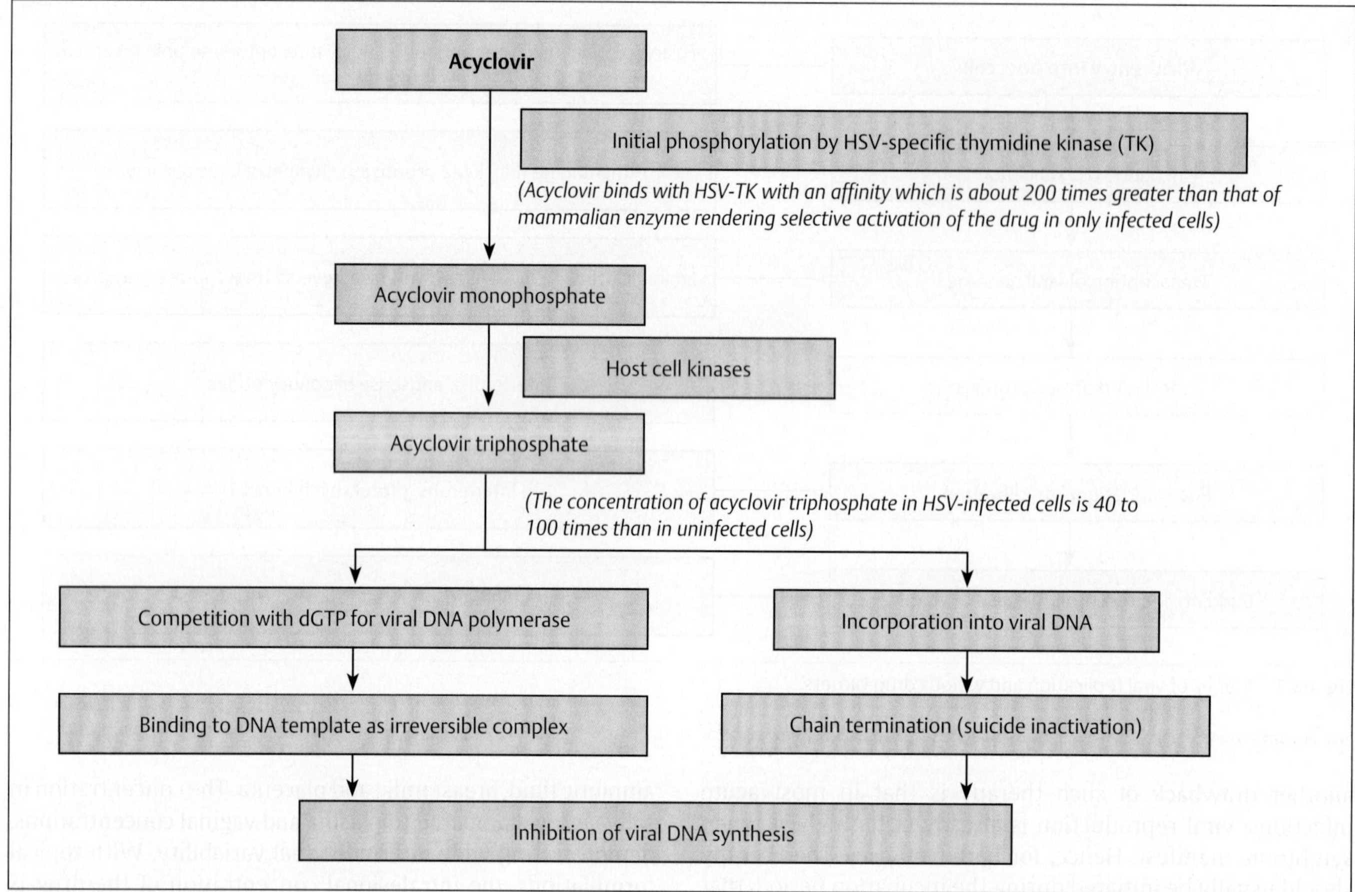

Fig. 66.2 Mechanism of action of acyclovir.

The safety profile of valacyclovir is similar to acyclovir; high dose of valacyclovir is associated with thrombotic thrombocytopenic purpura/hemolytic uremic syndrome in immunocompromised patients.

Most acyclovir-resistant strains respond to foscarnet, cidofovir, and trifluridine, as these drugs are not dependent on viral TK for activation.

Clinical Uses

Table 66.2 provides a list of clinical uses of acyclovir in various infections caused by the herpes group of viruses.

Famciclovir and Penciclovir

Famciclovir is the diacetyl 6-deoxyester of the guanosine analog penciclovir. It undergoes rapid deacetylation and oxidation in the liver and intestine to get converted to penciclovir. The mechanism of action and spectrum of activity of penciclovir are similar to those of acyclovir; penciclovir, however, does not cause chain termination. Acyclovir-resistant strains (due to mutated TK) exhibit cross-resistance to penciclovir and famciclovir. Famciclovir is also active against hepatitis B virus (HBV).

Famciclovir is well absorbed orally, having 75 to 77% bioavailability. Oral penciclovir has low bioavailability (~5%). The serum half-life of penciclovir is 2 hours; however, the drug is retained intracellularly at high concentrations with prolonged half-life (7–20 hours). Hence, famciclovir has a less frequent dosing schedule (twice daily) as compared to acyclovir. Penciclovir primarily undergoes renal elimination, requiring dose adjustment in renal insufficiency.

Oral famciclovir is clinically used in the treatment of primary and recurrent genital herpes, herpes zoster, and chronic HBV infection (less effective than lamivudine). Topical penciclovir (1% cream) is used in orolabial herpes. Intravenous (IV) penciclovir can be used in mucocutaneous HSV infections in immunocompromised hosts, with efficacy comparable to IV acyclovir.

Oral famciclovir is generally well tolerated, although it may cause nausea, headache, and diarrhea. There are reports of urticaria, rash, hallucinations, or confusional states in the elderly. Penciclovir is mutagenic at high doses, and its safety during pregnancy is not well documented. Long-term administration of penciclovir is not reported to affect spermatogenesis in males.

Ganciclovir and Valganciclovir

Ganciclovir is structurally and mechanistically similar to acyclovir. Valganciclovir is the L-valyl ester prodrug of ganciclovir.

Ganciclovir shows higher activity against CMV infections where the initial phosphorylation of the drug is mediated by a viral phosphotransferase encoded by the *UL97* gene. Ganciclovir is not active against acyclovir-resistant strains of HSV.

Table 66.2 Clinical uses of acyclovir

Acyclovir, oral	Primary genital/orolabial herpes 200 mg five times daily/400 mg thrice daily for 7–10 days
	Recurrent genital herpes 800 mg thrice daily for 2 days or 800 mg twice daily/400 mg thrice daily for 5 days
	Recurrent orolabial herpes 200–400 mg five times daily for 5 days
	Suppression of genital/orolabial herpes 400–800 mg two to three times daily
	Herpes proctitis 400 mg five times daily until healed
	Varicella infection 20 mg/kg (maximum 800 mg) four times a day for 5 days
	Zoster infection 800 mg five times daily for 7–10 days
Acyclovir, topical (5% cream)	Orolabial herpes Five times daily for 4 days
Acyclovir, IV	Severe HSV infection or HSV infection in immunocompromised host 5–10 mg/kg every 8 hours for 7–14 days
	Severe VZV infection or VZV infection in immunocompromised host 10–15 mg/kg every 8 hours for 7 days
	Herpes encephalitis 10–15 mg/kg every 8 hours for 21 days
	Neonatal HSV infection 10–20 mg/kg every 8 hours for 14–21 days

Abbreviations: HSV, herpes simplex virus; IV, intravenous; VZV, varicella zoster virus.

The oral bioavailability of ganciclovir is very low (5–9%). On the other hand, valganciclovir possesses good oral bioavailability (~60%), which is further increased in the presence of food. Ganciclovir primarily (more than 90%) undergoes renal elimination in unchanged form, necessitating dose adjustment in renal failure.

Ganciclovir triphosphate gets concentrated intracellularly at much higher concentrations (10-fold) than acyclovir triphosphate. Hence, it shows greater activity against CMV. Also, a longer intracellular elimination half-life (more than 24 hours) of ganciclovir allows for less frequent dosing schedule (single daily doses) than acyclovir.

Ganciclovir is used in the treatment of CMV retinitis (IV, intravitreal injection, intraocular sustained release implant). For oral use in this indication, valganciclovir is preferred to ganciclovir due to favorable pharmacokinetics. It is also used for prophylactic and preemptive therapy of CMV infections in acquired immunodeficiency syndrome (AIDS) patients and transplant recipients (IV followed by oral ganciclovir or high-dose oral acyclovir).

The most common adverse effect of ganciclovir is myelo-suppression (neutropenia in 15–40% of patients), which is reversible and dose-limiting. In persistent cases of neutropenia, recombinant granulocyte colony-stimulating factor (filgrastim, lenograstim) may be useful. CNS side effects (5–15%) reported include headache, behavioral disturbances, convulsions, and coma. Other rare side effects may be hepatotoxicity, vitreous hemorrhage and retinal detachment (with intravitreal ganciclovir), infusion-related phlebitis, azotemia, anemia, rash, and eosinophilia.

Cidofovir

Cidofovir is a cytidine nucleotide analog. Like other antiherpes drugs, it inhibits viral DNA polymerase and causes chain termination; however, the conversion of cidofovir to its active diphosphate form takes place with the help of cellular kinases and is independent of viral enzymes; hence, the drug attains similar concentrations in infected and uninfected cells. Also, because of its nonidentical mechanism of action, the drug shows activity against acyclovir-resistant TK-deficient or TK-altered HSV or VZV strains, ganciclovir-resistant CMV strains with *UL97* mutations (but not those with DNA polymerase mutations), and some foscarnet-resistant CMV strains. Cidofovir resistance in CMV is due to mutations in viral DNA polymerase. Cidofovir-resistant isolates show cross-resistance to ganciclovir and respond to foscarnet.

Cidofovir has very poor oral bioavailability and CSF penetration. The drug undergoes renal elimination mainly by active renal tubular secretion. The terminal half-life is approximately 2.6 hours. Apart from the active metabolite cidofovir phosphate, which has a prolonged intracellular half-life (17–65 hours), there is another separate metabolite, cidofovir phosphocholine, which serves as an intracellular reservoir of active drugs. Cidofovir phosphocholine has a half-life of at least 87 hours, thus allowing infrequent dosage regimen (weekly or biweekly).

IV cidofovir is indicated in the treatment of CMV retinitis, acyclovir-resistant mucocutaneous HSV infection, adenovirus disease in transplant recipients, extensive molluscum contagiosum in HIV patients, and BK virus nephropathy in patients with renal transplant. Topical cidofovir gel is used in acyclovir-resistant mucocutaneous HSV infections, anogenital warts and molluscum contagiosum in immunocompromised patients, and cervical intraepithelial neoplasia in women. Intralesional cidofovir is used to induce remissions in respiratory papillomatosis.

The major dose-limiting toxicity of cidofovir is nephro-toxicity; saline prehydration and concomitant administration of probenecid decrease the risk of nephrotoxicity. The risk of renal toxicity is increased with concurrent intake of other nephrotoxic drugs such as aminoglycosides, IV pentamidine, amphotericin B, foscarnet, nonsteroidal anti-inflammatory drugs, or contrast dye. Other reported side effects include neutropenia, dose-related application site reactions such as burning and itching (topical cidofovir), and anterior uveitis and low intraocular pressure (IV formulation). Cidofovir is a potential human carcinogen and gonadotoxic.

Foscarnet

Foscarnet is an inorganic pyrophosphate analog that does not require activation by phosphorylation to inhibit viral DNA polymerase in herpes viruses; hence, the drug is active against acyclovir- and ganciclovir-resistant HSV, CMV, and VZV viruses. The drug also shows inhibitory activity against HIV reverse transcriptase enzyme. Resistance to foscarnet in herpes viruses occurs due to mutations in viral DNA polymerase.

The drug has very poor oral bioavailability; IV, intravitreal, and topical formulations are used to treat various infections such as mucocutaneous HSV infections, CMV retinitis, and genital herpes. More than 80% of the dose administered undergoes renal elimination in unchanged form, thus requiring dose adjustment in renal failure. Around 10 to 20% of the dose is sequestered in bone with gradual release.

Nephrotoxicity and symptomatic hypocalcemia are the major dose-limiting toxicities with foscarnet. Among other adverse effects are generalized rash, fever, nausea, anemia, leukopenia, deranged liver function tests, electrocardiographic changes, infusion-related thrombophlebitis, and painful genital ulcerations.

Trifluridine

Trifluridine is a fluorinated pyrimidine nucleoside that is phosphorylated intracellularly by host cell enzymes and inhibits viral DNA polymerase. It is active against HSV-1, HSV-2, CMV, vaccinia, and some adenoviruses. The drug gets incorporated in both viral and host DNA due to which systemic use is limited. Topical formulation is used in the treatment of primary keratoconjunctivitis and recurrent epithelial keratitis owing to HSV types 1 and 2 and acyclovir-resistant HSV cutaneous infections. Discomfort on instillation and palpebral edema are few reported side effects of the drug when applied locally.

Idoxuridine

Idoxuridine is an iodinated thymidine analog having activity against herpes viruses and poxviruses. The mechanism of action is similar to other antiherpes drugs. Lack of selectivity (due to incorporation into both viral and cellular DNA) limits its systemic use; topical formulation is used to treat HSV keratitis, herpes labialis, herpes genitalis, and zoster.

Docosanol

Docosanol is a long-chain saturated alcohol that prevents fusion of the HSV envelope with host cell plasma membrane, which, in turn, prevents the entry of virus into cells and its replication. Topical (10% cream) is available for the treatment of recurrent orolabial herpes.

Fomivirsen

Fomivirsen, a 21-base phosphorothioate oligonucleotide, provides antisense oligonucleotide (ASO) therapy for CMV retinitis.

Fomivirsen is complementary to messenger transcripts of the immediate-early transcriptional region of CMV, which codes for proteins regulating viral gene expression. In addition to its antisense mechanism of action (**Fig. 66.3**), it causes inhibition of viral binding to cells as well as directly inhibits viral replication. The drug shows activity against CMV strains resistant to ganciclovir, foscarnet, and cidofovir. Intravitreal administration of fomivirsen is approved for treatment of CMV retinitis unresponsive to other treatments. Major ocular side effects are vitritis, iritis, cataracts, and rise in intraocular pressure.

Antihepatitis B Drugs

Interferons

Interferons (IFNs) are potent cytokines produced by host cells in response to various stimuli. They possess antiviral (**Fig. 66.4**), immunomodulatory, and antiproliferative properties.

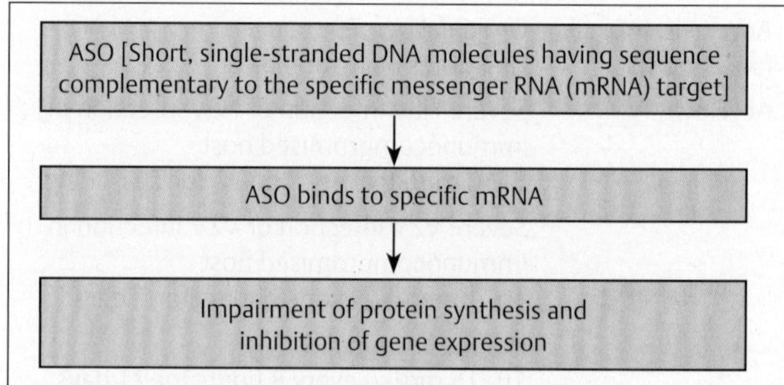

Fig. 66.3 Mechanism of action of antisense therapy.

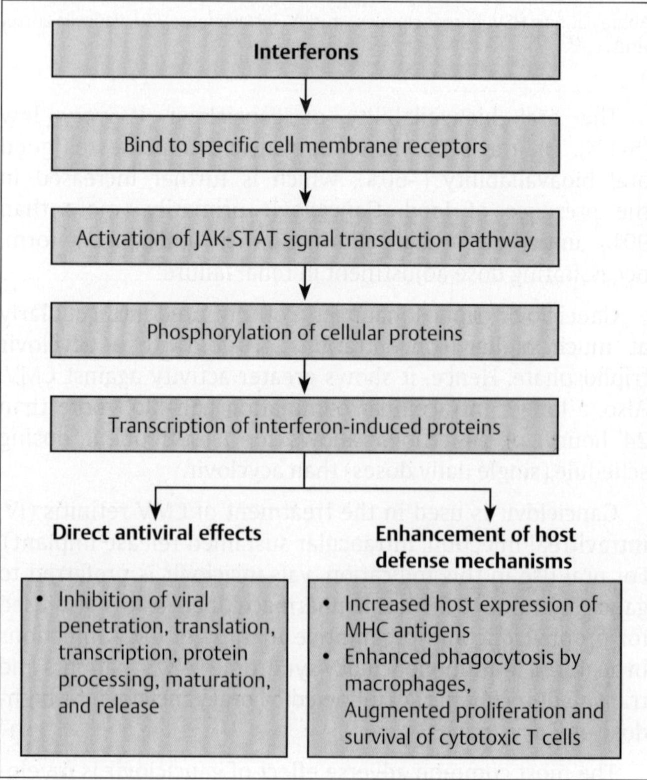

Fig. 66.4 Mechanism of antiviral actions of interferons.

The disadvantages of IFNs are that they are expensive, have a less than 50% response rate, need parenteral injections, and show unfavorable safety profile. Side effects of IFNs include flulike syndrome, transient hepatic enzyme elevations, neurotoxicities (mood disorders, somnolence, seizures), myelosuppression, alopecia, tinnitus, reversible hearing loss, retinopathy, pneumonitis, and, possibly, cardiotoxicity. Induction of autoantibodies may occur, leading to exacerbation or unmasking of autoimmune disorder (especially thyroiditis). Use of IFNs in pregnancy is not recommended due to their demonstrated abortifacient potential in primates. Serum-neutralizing antibodies may develop during IFN therapy, which may lead to loss of clinical responsiveness.

Pegylated IFNs (Peg IFN; with attached polyethylene glycol) have slower absorption, decreased clearance, better tolerability, and more sustained serum concentrations, thereby permitting a more convenient, once-weekly dosing schedule.

IFN-a2b and Peg IFN-a2a are approved for the treatment of hepatitis B. The advantages of IFN over nucleoside/nucleotide analogs for treatment of HBV are finite duration of treatment (nucleoside/nucleotide analogs may require lifelong treatment), absence of resistance, and achievement of higher rates of viral agglutinin reduction. For HCV, IFN-a2a, IFN-a2b, Peg IFN-a2a, Peg IFN-a2b, and IFN alfacon-1 are approved—however, with the advent of newer and highly effective antiviral drugs for HCV, their use has considerably diminished for this indication.

Nucleoside/Nucleotide Analogs

The mechanism of action of the nucleoside/nucleotide analogs used in the treatment of HBV infections is depicted in **Fig. 66.5**.

All the nucleoside/nucleotide analogs may be associated with lactic acidosis and hepatomegaly with steatosis as well as exacerbations of hepatitis upon drug withdrawal; hence, close monitoring for liver function is routinely recommended, and some cases may even demand resumption of antiviral therapy. All the nucleoside/nucleotide analogs undergo renal excretion as the primary route of elimination; hence, dose adjustment should be made in the presence of renal dysfunction.

Lamivudine

Lamivudine also inhibits HIV reverse transcriptase. The intracellular half-life of the drug is greater in HBV-infected cells (17–19 hours) as compared to HIV-infected cells (10–15 hours); hence, the drug is recommended at relatively lower doses and less frequency of administration for the treatment of HBV infection.

Lamivudine causes rapid and potent suppression of HBV load but emergence of resistance with chronic use is a major drawback (up to 70% of patients develop resistance after 5 years of use). Lamivudine-resistant strains show cross-resistance to emtricitabine and entecavir and may respond to adefovir and tenofovir. The safety profile of the drug is quite favorable with rarely reported side effects such as headache, nausea, diarrhea, dizziness, myalgia, malaise, and aminotransferase elevations.

Telbivudine

About 22% of patients develop resistance to telbivudine after 2 years of use. The oral bioavailability of the drug is about 68%, with no effect of food. The primary route of elimination of the unchanged drug is renal. Telbivudine has greater efficacy than lamivudine and adefovir with respect to virologic response. The drug does not show activity in

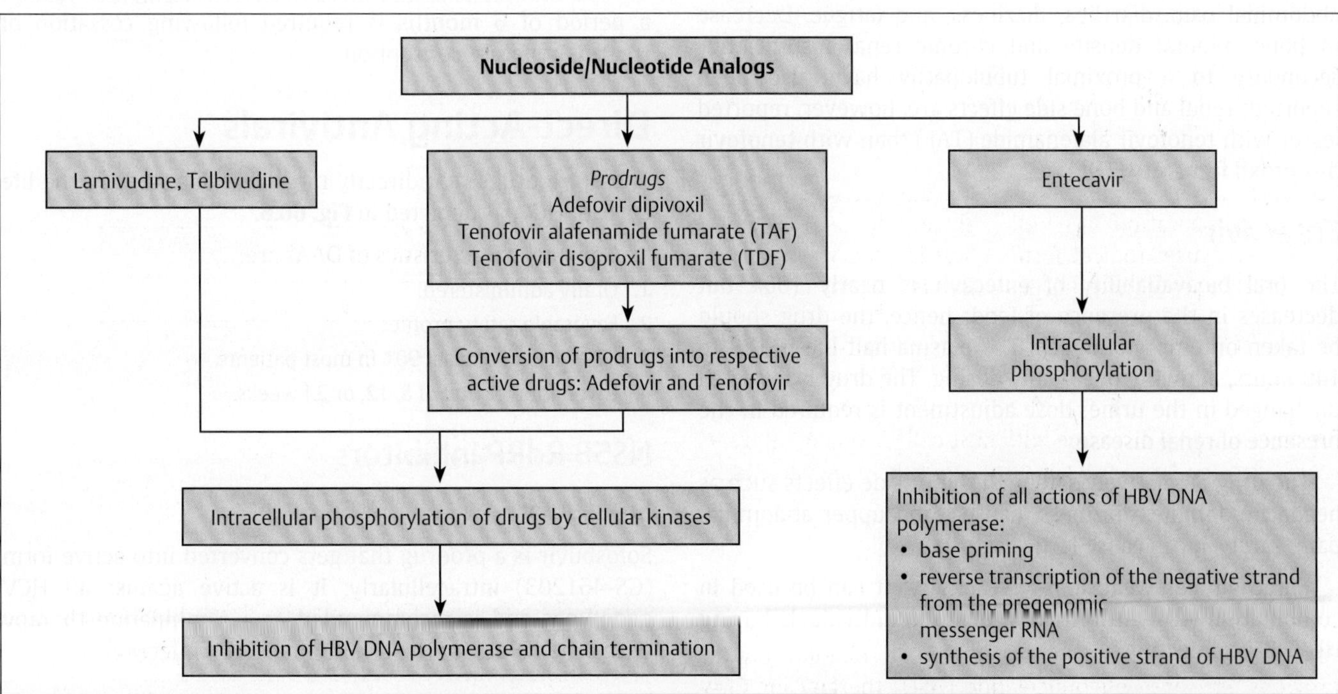

Fig. 66.5 Mechanism of action of various nucleoside/nucleotide analogs used in the treatment of HBV infection.

lamivudine-resistant strains. Few reported adverse effects include uncomplicated myalgia, myopathy with elevated creatinine kinase, and peripheral neuropathy.

Adefovir

The incidence of development of resistance with adefovir is 29% after 5 years of use. There is no cross-resistance with lamivudine or entecavir. The drug is administered as prodrug due to poor oral bioavailability (<12%) of the parent compound. The major pathway of elimination from the body is renal excretion of the unchanged drug. Dose-related nephrotoxicity and tubular dysfunction are the major side effects of adefovir.

Of the available oral anti-HBV drugs, development of virologic response to adefovir is slower. Adefovir has demonstrated mutagenic and genotoxic potential in preclinical studies and therefore should be used with caution in pregnancy.

Due to high rates of emergence of resistance and subsequent increased risk of hepatic decompensation associated with chronic use of lamivudine, adefovir, and telbivudine, the use of these three drugs is not currently recommended for the treatment of HBV infection.

Tenofovir

When used as monotherapy, no cases of resistance have been reported with tenofovir. The oral bioavailability is 25%, which increases with high-fat meal. Excretion of the unchanged drug occurs through the renal route. Tenofovir is active against lamivudine- and entecavir-resistant HBV strains; however, the drug does not show activity against strains resistant to adefovir and having double mutations (A181T/V and N236T).

The side effects reported with tenofovir include nausea, abdominal pain, diarrhea, dizziness, and fatigue. Decrease in bone mineral density and chronic renal insufficiency secondary to a proximal tubulopathy have also been reported; renal and bone side effects are, however, reported lesser with tenofovir alafenamide (TAF) than with tenofovir disoproxil fumarate (TDF).

Entecavir

The oral bioavailability of entecavir is nearly 100% but decreases in the presence of food; hence, the drug should be taken on empty stomach. The plasma half-life is 128 to 149 hours, allowing once-daily dosing. The drug is excreted unchanged in the urine; dose adjustment is required in the presence of renal disease.

The drug is relatively safe with minor side effects such as headache, fatigue, dizziness, nausea, and upper abdominal pain; rarely, it can cause lactic acidosis.

Entecavir has weak anti-HIV activity; it can be used in combination with antiretroviral drugs in individuals having HIV/HBV coinfection.

Hepatitis C

The hallmark of HCV is remarkable within and between subject genetic heterogeneity, which serves as a hindrance to the development of a universal treatment or vaccine for this virus. There are six genotypes (with subtypes) of HCV, which exhibit wide variability with respect to disease progression and response to existing treatments. The most common genotype worldwide is genotype 1 followed by genotype 3. Genotype 1 subtype a is reported to have higher relapse rates with certain anti-HCV drugs as compared to subtype 1b.

The goal of treatment in HCV infection is viral eradication and achievement of sustained viral response (SVR), which is defined as absence of detectable HCV RNA in the blood following cessation of treatment.

Anti-HCV Drugs

Interferons

(Kindly see the discussion under HBV infection.)

Ribavirin

Ribavirin is a purine nucleoside analog having activity against various DNA and RNA viruses such as orthomyxo-, paramyxo-, arena-, bunya-, and flaviviruses in vitro. The drug undergoes phosphorylation by host cell enzymes and exerts antiviral actions such as inhibition of HCV RNA-dependent RNA polymerase (RdRP) and nucleic acid synthesis. It can be administered through oral, IV, and inhalation routes. For the treatment of chronic HCV infection, ribavirin is administered in combination with various direct-acting antivirals (DAAs).

Adverse effects of ribavirin include anemia, fatigue, cough, rash, and pruritus. The drug is teratogenic and hence contraindicated in men and women attempting conception; a period of 6 months is required following cessation of treatment before conception.

Direct-Acting Antivirals

These are drugs that directly target various steps in the life cycle of HCV, as depicted in **Fig. 66.6**.

General characteristics of DAAs are:

1. Orally administered.
2. Favorable safety profile.
3. SVR rates of at least 90% in most patients.
4. Given for a period of 8, 12, or 24 weeks.

NS5B RdRP Inhibitors

Sofosbuvir

Sofosbuvir is a prodrug that gets converted into active form (GS-461203) intracellularly. It is active against all HCV genotypes and is recommended as a combination therapy with other DAAs for the treatment of HCV infection.

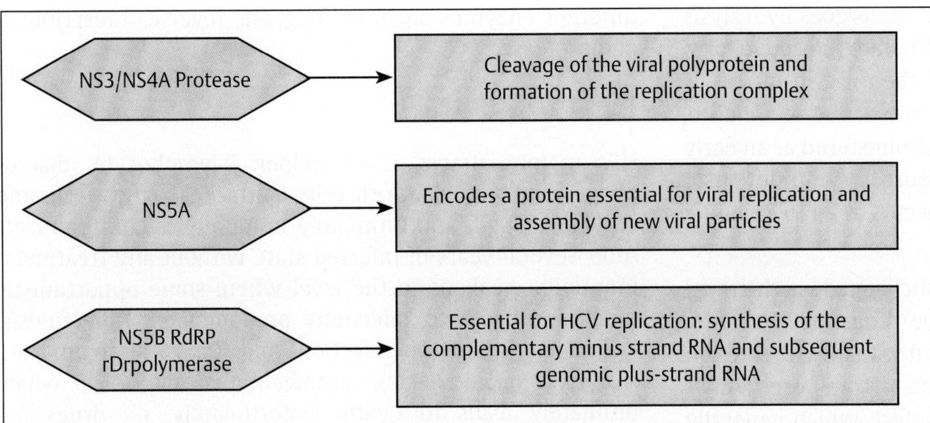

Fig. 66.6 Major structural proteins in HCV serving as targets of direct-acting antivirals (DAAs).

The oral bioavailability of the drug is approximately 80%, which is further increased by high-fat meals. The drug primarily undergoes renal elimination, demanding dose adjustment in renal impairment, and is contraindicated in patients with estimated glomerular filtration rate of less than 30 mL/min/1.73 m^2 or those with end-stage renal disease. The use of sofosbuvir in pediatric population is not currently approved.

NS5A Inhibitors

Ledipasvir

It is available only as fixed-dose combination (FDC) with sofosbuvir (LDV/SOF). LDV/SOF is approved for the treatment of HCV infection with genotypes 1, 4, 5, and 6, coinfection with HIV, and in patients having decompensated cirrhosis. In decompensated cirrhosis, addition of ribavirin is advised to achieve high SVR rates.

Daclatasvir

Daclatasvir is approved for use in combination with sofosbuvir to treat HCV infection due to genotype 3, HIV coinfection regardless of HCV genotype, and in patients having advanced liver disease.

Velpatasvir

This drug is available as part of a FDC product with sofosbuvir (SOF/VEL). SOF/VEL is the only currently available DAA combination therapy that is approved for the treatment of all HCV genotypes (1–6).

NS3 Protease Inhibitors

Simeprevir

Simeprevir is indicated for the treatment of HCV-infected individuals with genotype 1 or 4 in combination with sofosbuvir (SIM/SOF) or with ribavirin + Peg INFa.

Simeprevir contains a sulfonamide moiety and can cause photosensitivity, rash, and itching, more commonly encountered in cirrhotic patients receiving SIM/SOF.

Anti-influenza Drugs

Amantadine and Rimantadine

These drugs act by inhibiting the viral M2 protein (an ion channel), thereby preventing uncoating of the viral genome inside the infected cell. Mutation in M2 protein leads to the development of resistance to these drugs.

Amantadine and rimantadine are active against influenza A virus, but not against influenza B and H1N1 (swine flu) or H5N1 (bird flu) strains of influenza A.

Both the drugs are available in oral formulations (tablet, syrup) and have >90% oral bioavailability. Amantadine is largely excreted unchanged in the urine (>90%), necessitating dose adjustment in renal impairment and elderly patients. Rimantadine, in contrast, undergoes mainly hepatic metabolism (~75%) prior to renal excretion. Minor dose-related side effects with amantadine include nausea, loss of appetite, nervousness, insomnia, difficulty concentration, etc. Both the drugs are pregnancy category C drugs.

The advantages of rimantadine over amantadine are as follows:

1. Rimantadine, as compared to amantadine, is longer acting ($t_{1/2}$: 24–36 hours vs. 12–18 hours).
2. Rimantadine has better tolerability and less frequent CNS side effects (e.g., delirium, hallucinosis, seizures, coma) as compared to amantadine.

Due to the emergence of resistance to adamantine in influenza strains and the availability of broad-spectrum and more efficacious drugs (e.g., neuraminidase inhibitors), the use of this group of drugs has declined in the recent past.

Neuraminidase Inhibitors: Oseltamivir, Zanamivir, Peramivir

These drugs act by inhibiting the influenza virus neuraminidase enzyme and hence prevent the release of progeny virions from the infected cell. They exhibit broad spectrum of action and are effective in the treatment and prophylaxis of influenza A and B, including adamantine-resistant H5N1 and H1N1 strains.

Oseltamivir is an ester prodrug that undergoes hydrolysis by intestinal and hepatic esterases to liberate the active form "oseltamivir carboxylate." Efficacy of the drug in infants is doubtful due to inability to generate the active metabolite. Neuraminidase inhibitors should be administered at an early stage of infection, that is, within 48 hours of symptom onset because the peak of viral replication occurs at 24 to 72 hours of onset of illness.

All the drugs are mainly excreted unchanged via the renal route. IV formulations of all the three drugs are available; oseltamivir can be given orally and zanamivir through inhalation route as well. Side effects of oral oseltamivir include nausea and abdominal discomfort, which generally resolve within 2 to 3 days and can be prevented by taking the medicine with food. Inhaled zanamivir is associated with side effects such as wheezing, bronchospasm, and acute deterioration in lung function; hence, it is not recommended in patients having underlying disease of the airways. Adverse effects reported with peramivir include diarrhea, hypersensitivity reactions, and neuropsychiatric events, for example, behavioral abnormalities, delirium, hallucinations, etc.

Antiretroviral Drugs (IM6.17, IM6.18)

Introduction

Antiretroviral drugs are mainly used against HIV. HIV is a retrovirus, in which DNA is made from RNA. Normally, RNA is made from DNA. HIV is comparatively a new and resistance-prone virus. It is a single-stranded RNA virus. It has viral cell envelope, viral nucleocapsid, viral RNA, and different enzymes such as integrase, reverse transcriptase, and protease.

HIV Cycle

HIV mainly attacks CD4+ helper T-lymphocyte, macrophages, and brain dendritic cells. It attaches to these cells and replicates itself, and ultimately immunity is compromised. After several years of infected state without any treatment, immunity weakens to the level where some opportunistic fungal or bacterial infections predominate. Tuberculosis, *Pneumocystis jirovecii* infection, and Kaposi's sarcoma are mainly seen. Severe stage of infection is called AIDS, which ultimately leads to death. Unfortunately, no drugs are available to cure the disease completely. Antiretroviral drugs mainly delay viral load to the level that immunity is not compromised and CD4+ cell level in blood remains in normal level (>500 cells/mm^3).

- The most noteworthy development in the medical management of HIV-1 infection has been the treatment of patients with antiviral drugs, which inhibits HIV-1 replication to undetectable levels. The finding of HIV-1 as the causal agent of AIDS, together with an ever-increasing understanding of the virus multiplication cycle, has been helpful in this work by providing scientists with the information and tools vital to drug discovery struggles, dedicated to directed inhibition with specific pharmacological agents. These drugs are classified into six distinct classes, based on their molecular mechanism and resistance profiles: (1) nucleoside reverse transcriptase inhibitors (NRTIs), (2) nonnucleoside reverse transcriptase inhibitors (NNRTIs), (3) integrase inhibitors, (4) protease inhibitors (PIs), (5) fusion inhibitors, and (6) coreceptor antagonists. In this chapter, we will review the basic principles of antiretroviral drug therapy, the mode of drug action, and the factors leading to treatment failure (i.e., drug resistance) (**Fig. 66.7** and **Box 66.1**).

Box 66.1 Types of antiretroviral drugs

NRTIs				
Zidovudine	Didanosine	Stavudine		
Lamivudine	Abacavir	Emtricitabine		
Tenofovir				
NNRTIs				
Nevirapine	Efavirenz	Delavirdine	Etravirine	Rilpivirine
PIs				
Ritonavir	Atazanavir	Indinavir	Nelfinavir	
Saquinavir	Fosamprenavir	Lopinavir	Darunavir	
Integrase inhibitors				
Raltegravir	Dolutegravir			
Entry inhibitors				
Enfuvirtide				
CCR5 receptor inhibitors				
Maraviroc				

Abbreviations: NRTIs, nucleoside reverse transcriptase inhibitors; NNRTIs, nonnucleoside reverse transcriptase inhibitors; PIs, protease inhibitors.

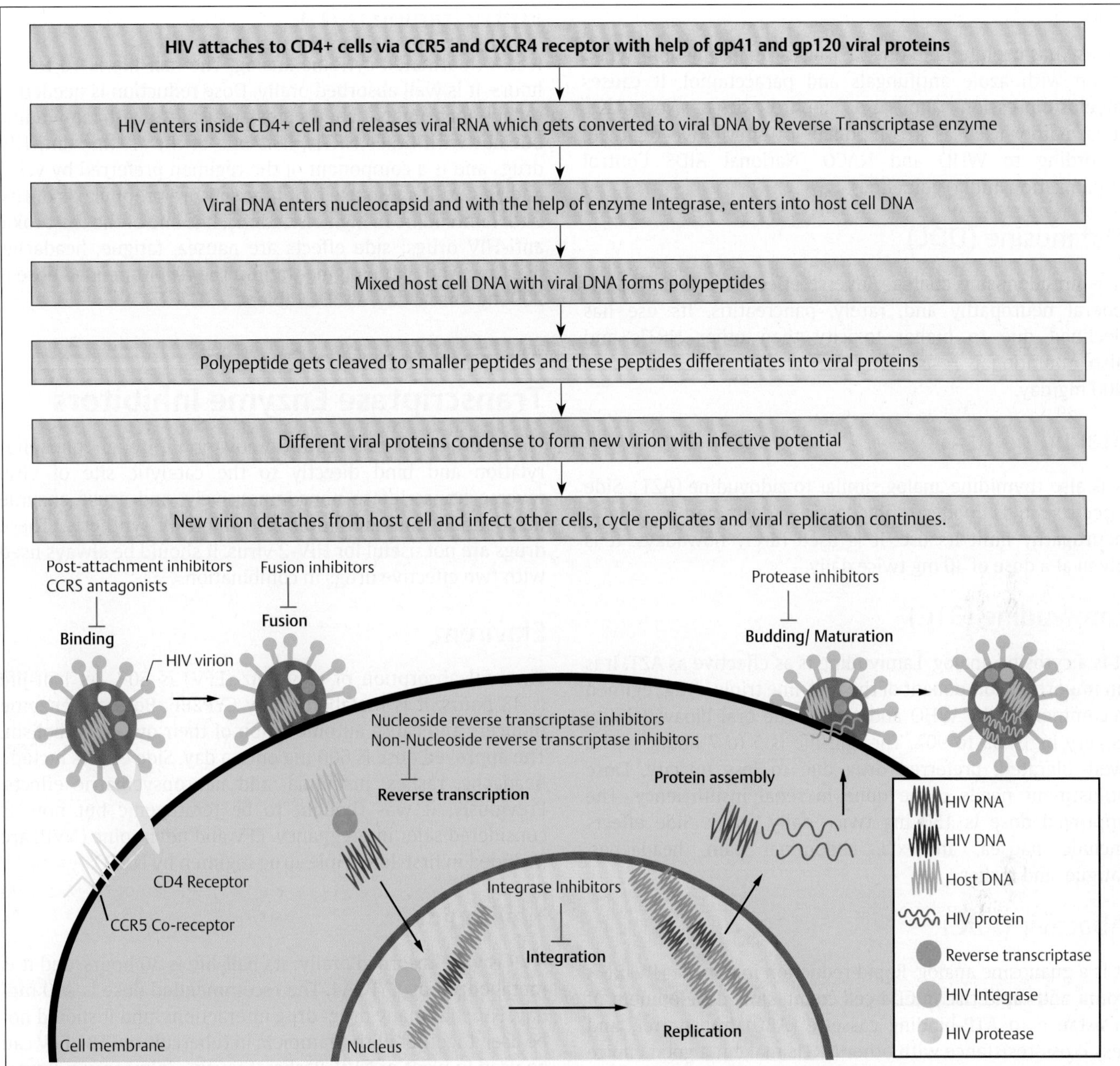

Fig. 66.7 Mode of drug action.

Nucleoside Reverse Transcriptase Inhibitors

NRTIs get activated inside the cell via phosphorylation by cellular enzymes to triphosphate form; then, they inhibit reverse transcriptase enzyme and restrict further processes. NRTIs also get incorporated into viral DNA and cause chain termination, ultimately stopping viral replication. These drugs are useful for both HIV-1 and HIV-2.

Zidovudine

It is a thymidine analog. It was the successful drug for HIV. It was first employed as anticancer drug and later got established as antiviral drug. It is given at a dose of 300 mg twice daily.

Pharmacokinetics

The oral absorption is rapid; bioavailability is 65%. It is metabolized by hepatic glucuronidation. The half-life is 1 hour. It gets excreted unchanged in the urine.

Side Effects

Anemia and neutropenia are mostly seen. Nausea, anorexia, abdominal pain, headache, insomnia, and myalgia are some initial side effects of the drug. Myopathy, pigmentation of nails, lactic acidosis, and hepatomegaly are infrequent. The reason for all these side effects is inhibition of cellular mitochondrial DNA polymerase γ.

Use

Its use has been limited due to drug–drug interactions when given with azole antifungals and paracetamol. It causes myelosuppression and also nephrotoxicity. Nowadays, it is mainly used as a component of alternative regimen, according to WHO and NACO (National AIDS Control Organization, India) guidelines.

Didanosine (DDL)

It is an adenosine analog. Adverse effects are mainly peripheral neuropathy and, rarely, pancreatitis. Its use has declined due to higher toxicity than other NRTIs and also mutational resistance. The recommended dose is 400 mg/day.

Stavudine (d4T)

It is also thymidine analog similar to zidovudine (AZT). Side effects such as lipodystrophy, lactic acidosis, and peripheral neuropathy limit its use. It is used rarely nowadays. It is given at a dose of 30 mg twice daily.

Lamivudine (3TC)

It is a cytosine analog. Lamivudine is as effective as AZT. It is an important component of the first-line triple-drug regimen recommended by WHO and NACO. The oral bioavailability is very high—85 to 90%. The half-life is 5 to 7 hours. It is a well-tolerated, preferred drug due to less toxicity. Dose adjustment needs to be done in renal insufficiency. The approved dose is 150 mg twice daily orally. Side effects include nausea, anorexia, abdominal pain, headaches, fatigue, and rashes.

Abacavir (ABC)

It is a guanosine analog. Rapid reduction in plasma HIV-RNA count and rapid rise in CD4 cell count, slow development of resistance to ATP-binding cassette (ABC) transporter, and less cross-resistance with other NRTIs make it a good choice drug for AIDS.

The oral bioavailability is 80%. The half-life is 1 to 1.5 hours. Hypersensitivity reactions are the main problem with its use. Combination regimens including abacavir are frequently used, and it is a component of the preferred "I" line WHO regimen for children. It is not advised in alcoholics and in patients with cardiovascular problems. The recommended dose is 300 mg twice a day.

Tenofovir (TDF)

Tenofovir (TDF) is a nucleotide (not nucleoside) analog. It is the preferred and the only nucleotide analog being used by WHO and NACO as first-line drug for HIV. Tenofovir-containing regimens are effective and less toxic compared to other first-line regimens. The oral bioavailability is 25 to 40%. The half-life is 17 hours. Nausea, vomiting, and diarrhea are the common side effects. It is given at a dose of 300 mg twice daily.

Emtricitabine (FTC)

It is a fluorinated cytidine analog. The half-life is 10 to -40 hours. It is well absorbed orally. Dose reduction is needed in renal impairment. It shows cross-resistance with lamivudine but not with other NRTIs. It is one of the "I" line anti-HIV drugs and is a component of the regimen preferred by WHO and NACO. It is also used for preexposure prophylaxis of HIV with lamivudine in high-risk adults. It is one of the least toxic anti-HIV drugs; side effects are nausea, fatigue, headache, diarrhea, and photo pigmentation. The recommended dose is 200 mg once a day, as FDC tablets.

Nonnucleoside Reverse Transcriptase Enzyme Inhibitors

These drugs do not require activation through phosphorylation and bind directly to the catalytic site of viral reverse transcriptase noncompetitively, and cause enzyme inactivation and inhibition of viral DNA synthesis. These drugs are not useful for HIV-2 virus. It should be always used with two effective drugs in combination.

Efavirenz

The oral absorption of efavirenz (EFV) is 50%. Its half-life is 48 hours. It is metabolized by CYP2B6. Both are enzyme inducers and cause autoinduction of their own metabolism. The approved dose is 600 mg once a day. Side effects include headache, rashes, insomnia, and neuropsychiatric effects. Previously, it was thought to be teratogenic but now is considered safer in pregnancy. EFV and nevirapine (NVP) are included in first-line triple-drug regimen by NACO.

Nevirapine

NVP is well absorbed orally; its half-life is 30 hours, and it is metabolized by CYP3A4. The recommended dose is 200 mg/day. NVP has many drug–drug interactions, and it should not be used together with rifampicin in tuberculosis (TB). EFV can be used in place of NVP. Rashes, Stevens–Johnson syndrome, vomiting, headache, fever, and hepatotoxicity are adverse effects usually seen. Prevention of mother to newborn transmission is an important indication of this drug.

Etravirine

This is a newer drug in this class, specifically indicated for those that have already been treated and resistant cases. It is a well-absorbed drug with a half-life of around 40%. It is metabolized by CYP3A4. It is approved for use only in combination. Nausea and skin rashes are main side effects. It is given at a dose of 200 mg twice daily. Delavirdine and rilpivirine are the other drugs in this class, which are not used usually.

Protease Inhibitors

These drugs are not activated by intracellular phosphorylation. This class of drugs is effective on both newly and already infected cells. These drugs competitively inhibit the viral protease enzyme and form immature, noninfectious virions. They are less effective with other enzyme-inducer drugs. When combined with NRTIs, these drugs are more effective than when used alone, and chances of resistance are also reduced. Low-dose ritonavir (RTV) is added to increase the efficacy of other PIs, which are known as booster PI. RTV, in 100-mg dose, reduces first-pass metabolism, increases bioavailability, slows systemic metabolism, and decreases clearance of other PIs. Only nelfinavir does not need to be given with RTV. Frequent doses and complex schedules affect patient compliance. Gastrointestinal tract intolerance, headache, dizziness, rashes, asthenia, tingling, numbness, lipodystrophy (central obesity), raised cholesterol, and insulin resistance are the common side effects with PI. Significant drug–drug interactions are found with antifungals, antimycobacterial drugs, hormonal contraceptives, and statins. They are avoided as first-line regimen and reserved for failure cases. They are recommended in combination only.

Atazanavir

Atazanavir (ATV) is better absorbed when given with food. It should not be given with antacids. It is metabolized by CYP3A4. When combined with RTV as booster PI, efficacy and bioavailability are better. Its half-life is 6 to 8 hours. Gastric discomfort is a major side effect. There are less lipid abnormalities and insulin resistance compared to other PIs. The approved dose is 300 mg once a day.

Ritonavir

RTV is given at a dose of 600 mg twice a day. It can be used as an antiretroviral drug, but it is more commonly used in a low dose of 100 mg orally as booster PI with other PIs except nelfinavir. It is a potent CYP3A4 inhibitor. Nausea, vomiting, diarrhea, and lipid abnormalities are major side effects but are less seen with low dose.

Lopinavir

Lopinavir (LPV) is a potent PI employed commonly nowadays. It has similar properties as RTV. It is better absorbed and efficacious with booster RTV. The recommended dose is 400 mg twice daily. FDC with RTV is available. Nausea, vomiting, diarrhea, and lipid abnormalities are major side effects.

Darunavir

It is a potent newer PI, especially useful in resistant cases. It is also approved for use in combination only with booster RTV or cobicistat, a new booster drug. The recommended dose is 600 mg twice daily. It is better tolerated compared to other PIs, with mild side effects such as nausea and diarrhea.

Indinavir, nelfinavir, fosamprenavir, and saquinavir are other PIs, which are less used nowadays due to toxicity and efficacy issues.

Integrase Inhibitors

These drugs inhibit the viral enzyme integrase, preventing the insertion of HIV viral DNA into host cell's DNA and restricting viral replication.

Raltegravir

It is well absorbed orally. The half-life is 12 hours. It should not be given with supplements containing big ions such as Ca^{2+} and Mg^{2+}. Headache, diarrhea, weakness, and myopathy are some of the side effects. It has good activity against both types of DNA virus, acts rapidly to clear viral load, and is also efficacious in both new and already on treatment cases with NRTIs. The recommended dose is 400 mg twice daily.

Dolutegravir

It is similar in profile to raltegravir but is also active against raltegravir-resistant viruses. It has shown better efficacy than raltegravir. It is absorbed slowly and the half-life is of 12 hours. Skin rash and hypersensitivity reactions are the side effects. It is given at a dose of 50 mg once daily. It is a costly drug and therefore is not used routinely in developed countries.

Entry Inhibitor

Enfuvirtide

It inhibits attachment of gp41 and gp120 viral proteins to the cell and restricts further processes. It is one of the newer drugs. It is given subcutaneously twice daily and is used in multidrug-resistant cases of HIV. Pain at the site of injection and cost are the limiting factors for its use.

CCR5 Receptor Inhibitors

Maraviroc

It blocks attachment of HIV RNA to CCR5 receptors on CD4+ cells. It has no activity for HIV RNA attachment to CXCR4 receptors. It is useful in resistant cases. Cough, fever, rashes, and abdominal pain are the common side effects.

HIV Treatment Guideline

The treatment of HIV infection should be started as soon as possible after the diagnosis. As none of the currently available drugs can completely cure infection, increased life expectancy and disease-free state are the primary objectives. Triple-drug regimen, containing two NRTIs and one NNRTI or integrase inhibitor, is the first-line regimen. Due to cost problems, in developing countries, PIs are still being used in place of integrase inhibitors. Emergence of resistance to monotherapy has restricted single-drug usage. Newer highly effective drugs such as integrase inhibitors and entry inhibitors have also changed the treatment protocol.

In the case of TB, anti-TB drugs are first instituted and within 4 to 6 weeks of initiating anti-TB treatment, antiretroviral drugs are started.

The goal of therapy is to decrease the viral load below 50 copies/μL and maintain CD4+ cell level to optimum level so that immune system remains intact enough to counter opportunistic infections. To decrease high-viral load, abacavir + lamivudine + dolutegravir is the preferred regimen. Tenofovir + emtricitabine + EFV can also be used as an alternative regimen.

Booster PI–containing regimens are reserved for resistant cases. Immune reconstitution inflammatory syndrome can occur due to long-time usage of these drugs, as treatment is needed lifelong. At present, FDCs of mentioned drugs are available and can be used as first- or second-line drugs.

In pregnancy, zidovudine, lamivudine, tenofovir, emtricitabine, EFV, NVP, and nelfinavir are considered safer and can be used as needed, as per triple-drug regimen.

The whole drug regimen should be changed in case of resistance or failure of first-line drugs.

Prophylaxis of HIV Infection (IM6.18)

Prophylaxis of HIV infection is also an important consideration for preexposure prophylaxis, postexposure prophylaxis (PEP), or mother-to-child transmission prophylaxis. Homosexual partners, multiple sexual partners, injecting drug users, health care workers working with HIV patients, and sex workers are prone to develop HIV infection. Hence, prophylactic measures are important among these groups of people.

Preexposure Prophylaxis

Tenofovir 300 mg daily ± emtricitabine 200 mg daily.

Postexposure Prophylaxis

For adults and adolescents, preferred two NRTIs: tenofovir (300 mg) + emtricitabine (200 mg) daily ± preferred PI: LPV/r (400 + 100 mg) or ATV/r (300 + 100 mg) daily.

Alternative third drug: darunavir/r (600 + 100 mg twice daily) or raltegravir (400 mg twice daily) or EFV (600 mg daily).

For children younger than 10 years, preferred two NRTIs: AZT + lamivudine.

Alternative two NRTIs: abacavir + lamivudine or tenofovir + lamivudine.

Preferred PI: emtricitabine, LPV/r.

Alternative third drug: ATV/r or darunavir/r or EFV or raltegravir.

Duration of regimen: 4 weeks.

Prophylaxis after Sexual Exposure

The same PEP regimen as for needle-stick may be employed after sexual exposure to HIV. In the United States, a 28-day regimen of tenofovir + emtricitabine (as FDC once daily) + raltegravir (400 mg twice daily) is the most popular.

Perinatal HIV Prophylaxis HIV

All HIV-positive women who are not on antiretroviral therapy should be put on the standard three-drug antiretroviral therapy. This should be continued through delivery and into the postnatal period. It has been shown to prevent vertical transmission of HIV to the neonate as well as benefit mother's own health. The first-line regimen for pregnant women includes:

Tenofovir 300 mg + lamivudine 300 mg + EFV 600 mg (as FDC tablet) once daily.

(WHO guidelines, 2016); r = RTV as booster dose of 100 mg.

Multiple Choice Questions

1. MS is a 57-year-old man who developed vesicles unilaterally around his waist associated with stabbing irritation in the area. He is diagnosed with herpes zoster. The treatment of choice for this patient is:

A. Acyclovir 200 mg five times daily for 7 days.
B. Ganciclovir.
C. Acyclovir 800 mg thrice daily for 5 days.
D. Acyclovir 800 mg five times daily for 7 to 10 days.

Answer: D

2. A 32-year-old nursing woman presented with genital herpes. There is a previous history of similar episodes, which responded to some topical treatment. Which is the best antiviral drug to be prescribed now?

A. Foscarnet.
B. Trifluridine.
C. Valacyclovir.
D. Lamivudine.

Answer: C

This is a case of recurrent genital herpes. Valacyclovir, a prodrug of acyclovir, is the drug of choice in this case.

3. Which of the following drugs is not dependent on viral thymidine kinase for activation?

A. Acyclovir.
B. Valacyclovir.
C. Famciclovir.
D. Foscarnet.

Answer: D

4. A 65-year-old woman with chronic obstructive pulmonary disease reports to the physician with flulike symptoms since day 1. She is diagnosed with influenza. Which is the most appropriate drug to be prescribed to her?

A. Amantadine.
B. Oseltamivir.
C. Zanamivir.
D. Rimantadine.

Answer: B

Oseltamivir is the most preferred agent due to low level of resistance and oral administration.

5. A 50-year-old woman with renal failure undergoes renal transplant surgery. Which of the following antiviral drugs should be prescribed for prophylaxis of CMV infections?

A. Acyclovir.

B. Ganciclovir.

C. Trifluridine.

D. None of the above.

Answer: B

For prophylaxis and treatment of CMV infections, antiviral drugs of choice include ganciclovir, cidofovir, and foscarnet.

6. Which of the following is an antisense therapy approved for treatment of CMV retinitis?

A. Foscarnet.

B. Fomivirsen.

C. Mipomersen.

D. Cidofovir.

Answer: B

Intravitreal fomivirsen is the antisense oligonucleotide therapy approved for the treatment of CMV retinitis resistant to ganciclovir, foscarnet, and cidofovir.

7. A 58-year-old man with chronic hepatitis B is on treatment with tenofovir alafenamide (TAF). Which of the following statements is true?

A. TAF has better renal and bone safety profile as compared to tenofovir disoproxil fumarate (TDF).

B. TAF and TDF are both prodrugs of tenofovir.

C. Both TAF and TDF should be taken with food to increase oral bioavailability.

D. All are true.

Answer: D

8. A 45-year-old woman on treatment for chronic HBV infection develops nephrotoxicity. Which is the most likely drug being taken by patient?

A. Adefovir.

B. Lamivudine.

C. Ribavirin.

D. Entecavir.

Answer: A

Most common anti-HBV drug implicated in the causation of nephrotoxicity is adefovir.

9. A 41-year-old woman is having chronic hepatitis C genotype 1a infection. The treating physician prescribes her a fixed-dose combination of ledipasvir/sofosbuvir. One month later, the patient presents with symptoms of gastroesophageal reflux disease. Which of the following statements is true in the context of her management?

A. A proton pump inhibitor (PPI) can be safely administered with ledipasvir/sofosbuvir.

B. PPI should be taken during fasting state to avoid any drug interactions.

C. Absorption of sofosbuvir is affected by gastric pH.

D. Absorption of ledipasvir is increased with increasing pH.

Answer: B

The absorption of ledipasvir is pH dependent: there is reduced absorption with increase in gastric pH; hence, concurrent administration of antacids, H2 receptor antagonists, and PPIs should be avoided. In cases when absolutely indicated, PPIs and other antacids should be given in fasting conditions to ensure that gastric pH is sufficiently lowered at the time of intake of ledipasvir/sofosbuvir.

10. Which class of direct-acting antivirals (DAAs) used in hepatitis C acts by inhibiting replication of HCV?

A. NS3/NS4A protease inhibitors.

B. NS5A inhibitors.

C. NS5B polymerase inhibitors.

D. Interferons.

Answer: C

NS5B polymerase inhibitors act by inhibiting RNA polymerase responsible for HCV replication.

11. A 45-year-old person is being treated for human immunodeficiency virus (HIV)-1 infection and is stable on treatment. He developed hypertriglyceridemia and hypercholesterolemia after some time. The most likely drug implicated for these adverse effects is:

A. Ritonavir.

B. Raltegravir.

C. Didanosine.

D. Efavirenz.

Answer: A

Ritonavir is a protease inhibitor and can cause hypertriglyceridemia and hypercholesterolemia.

12. A dental surgeon consults you with the following problem: during a dental procedure, he got exposed to a 26-year-old female patient's blood and saliva through a piercing injury on the finger. A needle had penetrated across his gloves and skin to a depth of 2 to 3 mm, but was withdrawn immediately and the area washed under running water. On inquiry, the patient revealed that 1 year back, she had tested HIV-positive but was asymptomatic and not taking any anti-HIV medication. (I) Should the dental surgeon be advised to take post-exposure prophylactic medication for HIV? (II) If medication is advised, which drug/drugs, doses, and duration of use would be appropriate? Answer I and II.

A. I: Yes. II: Only lopinavir–ritonavir (400 mg + 100 mg) for 4 weeks.

B. I: Yes. II: Tenofovir 300 mg + emtricitabine 200 mg + lopinavir–ritonavir (400 mg + 100 mg) or atazanavir–ritonavir (300 mg + 100 mg) each once daily for 4 weeks.

C. I: No. II: Take any anti-HIV drug regimen for 4 weeks.

D. I: No. II: No need to worry, no drug needed.

Answer: B

Considering the facts of injury and exposure in this case, the risk of contracting HIV infection by the dental surgeon is low. However, HIV disease can only be prevented, but not cured, and has serious life-long implications. Moreover, even a few virions entering the body can set up an infection. Therefore, it would be prudent to give prophylactic medication to further cut down chances of acquiring the infection. According to current WHO guidelines, a three-antiretroviral drug regimen, namely, two nucleoside reverse transcriptase inhibitors (NRTIs) + one boosted protease inhibitor (PI) postexposure prophylactic (PEP) regimen is considered superior to the two NRTIs regimen. As such, the dental surgeon should be advised to immediately start taking: tenofovir 300 mg + emtricitabine 200 mg + lopinavir–ritonavir (400 mg + 100 mg) or atazanavir–ritonavir (300 mg + 100 mg) each once daily for 4 weeks.

13. A 32-year-old pregnant woman was previously found HIV-positive and better with anti-HIV drug. Which of the following drugs is used to prevent HIV transmission from an HIV-positive pregnant mother to child?

A. Lamivudine.

B. Stavudine.

C. Nevirapine.

D. Didanosine.

Answer: C

Nevirapine and zidovudine are used to prevent vertical transmission of HIV from pregnant females to the baby.

14. A 40-year-old man was started on antiretroviral therapy after being found positive for HIV. The patient was put on tenofovir, lamivudine, and abacavir. After some months of treatment, the patient was not responsive to the therapy, a resistant case. The consulting physician decided to start a new drug of NNRTI class to overcome the resistance. Which drug from the following options can be started?

A. Zidovudine.

B. Efavirenz.

C. Etravirine.

D. Oseltamivir.

Answer: C

Etravirine, a newer NNRTI, can be used for resistant cases specially.

15. A 46-year-old man was started on antiretroviral therapy after being found positive for HIV. The patient was put on zidovudine, lamivudine, and abacavir. After 4 to 8 weeks of treatment, the patient developed some type of hypersensitivity reaction syndrome. This syndrome was characterized by fever, abdominal pain and other gastrointestinal (GI) complaints, rash, malaise, and fatigue. Identify the potential drug/cause responsible for this reaction:

A. Zidovudine.

B. Lamivudine.

C. No drug involved.

D. Abacavir.

Answer: D

The presence of fever, abdominal pain, and rash within 6 weeks of starting abacavir is diagnostic and necessitates the discontinuation of the drug. Abacavir is associated with a unique and potentially fatal hypersensitivity syndrome.

Chapter 67 Chemotherapy of Malaria

Prasan R. Bhandari

PH1.47: Describe the mechanisms of action, types, doses, side effects, indications, and contraindications of the drugs used in malaria, kala-azar, amebiasis, and intestinal helminthiasis.

Learning Objectives

- Classification of antimalarials.
- Regimens for malaria chemoprophylaxis.
- Regimens for malaria treatment.

Introduction

Malaria was thought to be due to bad air ("mala"–bad, "aria"– air) on account of the protozoa of genus plasmodia. It is transmitted by the bite of the female anopheles mosquito, blood transfusion, or vertical transmission (mother to fetus). There are four species of malaria, namely, *P. falciparum* which causes most severe form of malaria, malignant tertian malaria, associated with high mortality. The parasite in red blood cells (RBCs) complete their life cycle in 48 hours and ruptures every third day (hence called tertian), which results in fever. There is no exoerythrocytic stage; hence, there is no relapse. *P. vivax* which is a less severe malaria, that is, benign tertian associated with low mortality. It has exoerythrocytic stage (hypnozoites), hence has relapses. *P. ovale*, which is seen more in Africa, is similar to P. vivax. P. malariae is of a mild type. A total of 72 hours is required for its maturation; fever is present every fourth day, hence termed as benign quartan malaria. An additional species, which is known as P. knowlese and is seen mostly in South-East Asian countries, has a 24-hour erythrocytic cycle and fever is there every day.

Life Cycle of Malaria Parasite

The bite of infected female anopheles mosquito introduces sporozoites into the human blood, which then enter hepatocytes. Sporozoites multiply there; subsequently, the cells rupture, releasing merozoites (preerythrocytic stage). These merozoites enter RBCs and develop and mature in 48 hours (72 hours in P. malaria; erythrocytic stage). The rupture of RBCs releases the merozoites, which invade fresh RBCs and multiply. The merozoites from ruptured RBCs release cytokines and other inflammatory mediators, which are responsible for fever and other symptoms. In P. vivax and P. ovale, the sporozoites in hepatocytes enter the hypnozoite stage (dormant stage). Hypnozoites multiply later, causing relapse (exoerythrocytic stage). Most merozoites continue this replicative cycle. However, some merozoites, upon infecting red blood cells, differentiate into male or female sexual forms called gametocytes. These gametocytes circulate in the blood until they are taken up when a mosquito feeds on the infected vertebrate host, taking up blood which includes the gametocytes (**Fig. 67.1**).

Clinical Features

These generally include fever with chills, myalgia, arthralgia, headache, and fatigue. Diarrhea, abdominal pain, dizziness, hypotension, and, rarely, convulsions are seen. Mild anemia, hepatomegaly, and splenomegaly too are manifested.

Classification of Antimalarials (IM4.22, IM4.23, IM4.26)

The aims of using drugs in relation to malarial infection are to prevent clinical attack of malaria (prophylactic), to treat clinical attack of malaria (clinical curative), completely eradicate the parasite from the patient's body (radical curative), and cutdown human-to-mosquito transmission (gametocidal) (**Fig. 67.2**).

Therapeutic classification

1. Causal prophylactics–primaquine, pyrimethamine.
2. (primary tissue schizontocides destroy parasites in liver cells and prevent RBC invasion).
3. Blood schizontocides–chloroquine, quinine, mefloquine, halofantrine, atovaquone, pyrimethamine, artemisinin derivatives (clinical suppressives destroy RBC parasites and terminate clinical attack).
4. Tissue schizontocides–primaquine (hypnozoitocidals prevent relapse).
5. Radical curatives–blood schizontocides + hypnozoitocidals (2 + 3) (eradicate all forms of P. vivax and P. ovale from body).
6. Gametocidals–primaquine, chloroquine, quinine (destroys gametes and prevent transmission).

Chemical Classification

1. 4-aminoquinolines–chloroquine.
2. 8-aminoquinoline: primaquine.
3. Quinolone methanols–quinine, quinidine, mefloquine.
4. Sesquiterpene lactones–artemisinin, artesunate, artemether, arteether.
5. Folate antagonists–sulfadoxine, pyrimethamine, proguanil.
6. Phenanthrene methanol–halofantrine, lumefantrine.
7. Napthaquinone–atovaquone.

Chloroquine

It is one of the highly effective blood schizontocides, with activity against all five species. It is rapidly acting, and

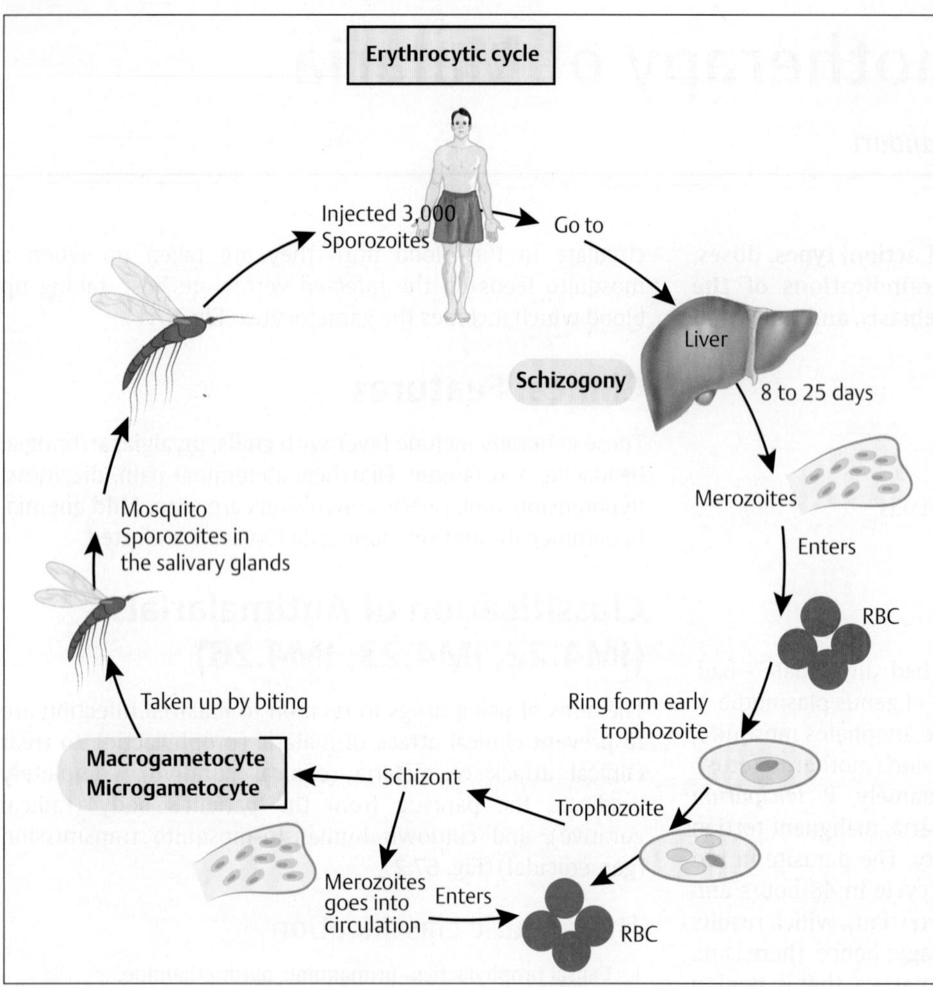

Fig. 67.1 Life cycle of malarial parasite.

patients become afebrile in 24 to 48 hours. Chloroquine is gametocidal for P. vivax, P. ovale, and P. malaria, however, there is no effect on hypnozoites in liver. It is safe during pregnancy.

Mechanism of Action

It acts by (**Fig. 67.3**) entering the parasite-infected RBC and subsequently the acidic food vacuoles (since chloroquine is base). Parasites digest host hemoglobin (source of its amino acid) and transport it to acidic food vacuole. Toxic heme is formed in the process, which is detoxified to hemozoin by heme polymerase. Chloroquine, quinine, and mefloquine inhibit heme polymerase; thus, there is accumulation of toxic heme in the parasite, resulting in the death of parasite. Chloroquine also prevents digestion of hemoglobin by parasite, which disrupts the parasites' amino acid supply.

Mechanism of Resistance

Chloroquine-resistant P. falciparum is very common. It occurs due to the mutant gene that encodes for chloroquine transporter; hence, chloroquine is transported out of food vacuoles. In P. vivax, resistance is modulated by P-glycoprotein and other transporters. Resistance may be prevented by verapamil, desipramine, and chlorpheniramine (however, the benefits need to be confirmed). These drugs prevent chloroquine efflux from parasite.

Other Actions

Chloroquine is also effective against Giardia lamblia and entamoeba histolytica. It is concentrated in liver, hence useful in hepatic amoebiasis. Additionally, it has anti-inflammatory properties, hence also useful in rheumatoid arthritis and lepra reactions.

Pharmacokinetics

Chloroquine can be given both orally and parenterally. Toxic concentration is reached following its rapid parenteral administration; hence, it is administered as slow infusion in divided doses. It is rapidly absorbed orally and has wide tissue distribution. The volume of distribution (Vd) is large, approximately > 100 L/kg. It has high affinity for melanin-rich tissues and nuclear chromatin; hence, chloroquine accumulates in retina (this leads to retinopathy on long-term use).

Adverse Effects

It is a reasonably safe drug. However, it can lead to nausea and vomiting, which is very severe, hence give antiemetic 30 minutes before its administration. Pruritus, dizziness, visual disturbances, and insomnia are also seen. Intravenous (IV) chloroquine can lead to hypotension, widening of QRS complex, and arrhythmias, therefore avoid parenteral use.

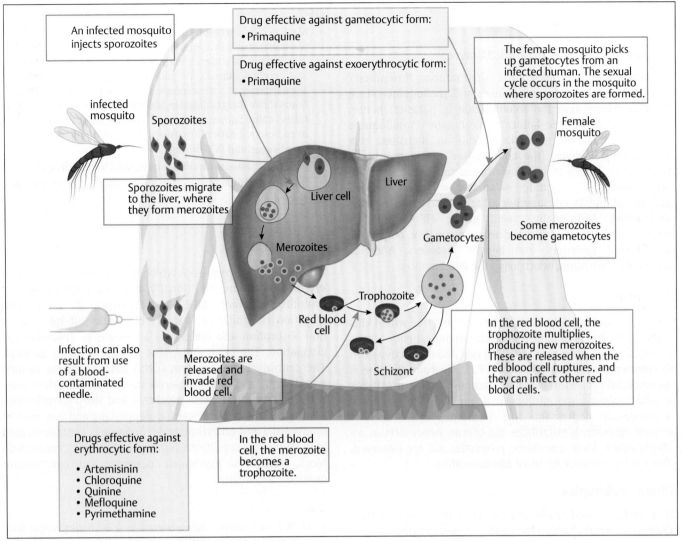

Fig. 67.2 Sites of action of antimalarial drugs.

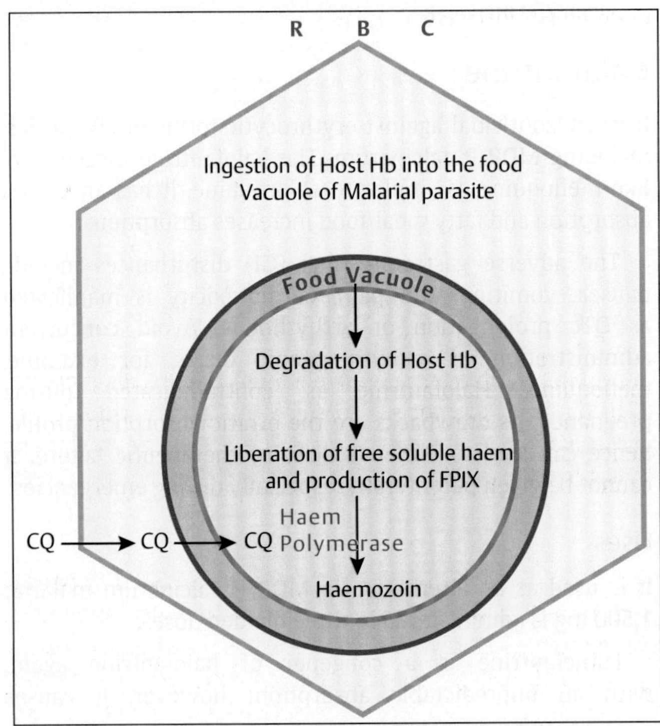

Fig. 67.3 Mechanism of action of chloroquine.

High dose can lead to cardiomyopathy, peripheral neuropathy, ototoxicity, and convulsions. Long-term use causes blurring of vision, bleaching of hair, myopathy, irreversible retinopathy, and reversible corneal deposits.

Uses

1. Malaria

   Chloroquine is highly effective in the treatment of sensitive strains of all four species. Chloroquine phosphate 250 mg (150 mg base) is administered in the following dosage: 1 gm (600 mg), that is, four tablets at 0 hour, 0.5 gm (300 mg), that is, two tablets at 6 hours, 0.5 gm (300 mg), that is, two tablets at 24 hours, and 0.5 gm (300 mg), that is, two tablets at 48 hours. The World Health Organization (WHO) regimen is 1 gm (600 mg), that is, four tablets at 0 hour, 1 gm (600 mg), that is, four tablets at 24 hours, and 0.5 gm (300 mg), that is, two tablets at 48 hours. The prophylaxis dose is 300 mg base—two tablets/week.

   Because of its anti-inflammatory actions, chloroquine is used in the following:

2. Extraintestinal (hepatic) amoebiasis (as it is completely absorbed from small intestine and concentrated in liver).
3. Rheumatoid arthritis.
4. Lepra reactions.
5. Photogenic reactions.

6. Infectious mononucleosis.
7. Discoid lupus erythematosus.

Precautions and Contraindications

Avoid parenteral administration (slow infusion if required), and also avoid concurrent quinine and mefloquine (since there is competition for accumulation in parasite; hence, it leads to therapeutic failure). Chloroquine + mefloquine combination should be avoided (due to increased risk of seizures). Likewise, the combination of chloroquine + halofantrine is also to be avoided (due to increased risk of arrhythmias). Chloroquine + gold/penicillamine should not be administered together (due to increased risk of dermatitis). Additionally, avoid giving chloroquine in patients afflicted with retinal disease, myopathy, porphyria, neurological disorders, and hepatic disorders. Antacids reduce its absorption, hence avoid the combination.

Quinine

It is an alkaloid from the bark of the cinchona tree which kills erythrocytic forms of parasite like chloroquine, hence acts as a clinical suppressive. It is rapidly acting and is effective even in chloroquine-resistant strains of P. falciparum. Quinine is gametocidal for all three species except P. falciparum. It has a mild analgesic and antipyretic action. Quinine possesses a myocardial depressant (like quinidine) and a skeletal muscle relaxant. It stimulates the uterus, hence acts as an abortifacient. Local anesthetic properties too are observed. There is hypotension on its IV administration.

Pharmacokinetics

It is well-absorbed orally and has wide tissue distribution. Quinine is metabolized in liver and excreted in urine.

Adverse Effects

Being an alkaloid in nature, it is highly bitter; as a gastric irritant, it causes nausea, vomiting, and epigastric distress and is thus poorly tolerated. Hypoglycemia can occur due to the stimulation of pancreatic beta cells; additionally, the parasite utilizes host glucose. Cinchonism is manifested as tinnitus, high-tone deafness, visual impairment, and vertigo, which are important manifestations. The cardiovascular system (CVS) adverse effects include hypotension (on rapid IV injection), widening of QRS complex, atrioventricular (AV) block, and arrhythmias. Hence, frequent monitoring of CV functions is a must. The neurological adverse effects comprise neurotoxicity; hence, it can lead to convulsions. Allergic reactions include blackwater fever, that is, acute hemolytic anemia, hemoglobinuria, and fever with renal failure.

Precautions and Contraindications

Quinine is administered orally preferably; if IV injection is given, then give as a slow infusion. Hypoglycemia can occur, thus caution is recommended. Avoid concurrent use of mefloquine due to risk of cardiotoxicity (even if mefloquine is given 20–30 days before).

Uses

1. Malaria: For uncomplicated falciparum malaria (chloroquine-resistant), it is administered at a dose of 600 mg orally TDS × 3 to 7 days. In patients with complicated falciparum malaria and cerebral malaria, IV quinine 20 mg/kg over 4 hours is administered as a slow infusion, followed by 15 mg/kg over 4 hours thrice daily (diluted in 500 mL of 5% dextrose) till patient takes orally. Subsequently, oral quinine 600 mg TDS is given to complete 7 days of treatment. Monitor blood pressure (BP), blood sugar, and ECG during its administration.
2. Babesiosis: along with clindamycin, which is the drug of choice.
3. Nocturnal muscle cramps: low dose i, that is, 200 to 300 mg is given at night.
4. Myotonia congenita.

Mefloquine

It is a quinolone methanol which is highly effective against erythrocytic forms. Additionally, it is also effective against multidrug-resistant (MDR) P. falciparum. Its mechanism of action is similar to that of chloroquine. It has a good oral absorption and undergoes an extensive enterohepatic circulation. The t½ is long, that is, nearly 20 to 30 days. The central nervous system (CNS) adverse effects include visual and auditory impairment, ataxia, disorientation, seizures, encephalopathy, psychosis, and sleep disturbances. On the CVS, it is a myocardial depressant and can lead to bradycardia and arrhythmias. Mefloquine is contraindicated in the following conditions, namely, arrhythmias, conduction block, epileptics, psychiatric patients, and concomitant quinine/halofantrine.

Uses

1. MDR P. falciparum: administered as a 20 mg/kg single dose combined with artesunate.
2. Prophylaxis in travelers (areas with chloroquine resistance): given 250 mg/week.

Halofantrine

It is schizonticidal against erythrocytic forms of all species, including MDR P. falciparum. The halofantrine mechanism, like mefloquine, is similar to chloroquine. It has an erratic absorption and fatty meal/food increases absorption.

The adverse gastrointestinal (GI) disturbances include nausea, vomiting, and pain. Cardiotoxicity is manifested as QTc prolongation or arrhythmias. Avoid concurrent administration of arrhythmogenic drugs, for example, mefloquine. Halofantrine is contraindicated during pregnancy. Its drawbacks are the erratic absorption profile, hence can lead to either toxicity or therapeutic failure. It cannot be given parenterally, especially during emergencies.

Uses

It is used as an alternative in MDR P. falciparum malaria; 1,500 mg is administered in three divided doses.

Lumefantrine is a congener of halofantrine again, with an unpredictable absorption; however, it causes less cardiotoxicity. It is administered with artemisinin/mefloquine for MDR P. falciparum. It has a 99% plasma protein binding and is generally well-tolerated. Adverse drug reactions (ADRs) include minimal GI disturbances, headache, and dizziness.

Primaquine

This is an agent which is effective against all forms of malaria parasites; however, it is not effective against erythrocytic forms. It kills hepatic parasites and prevents RBC invasion. Although it acts a casual prophylactic, it is not used for this. Primaquine kills hepatic hypnozoites (exoerythrocytic forms), hence prevents relapse of P. vivax and P. ovale. It is gametocidal for all four species. However, its mechanism is not known. The pharmacokinetics profile includes good oral absorption and wide tissue distribution. Generally, it is well-tolerated. The metabolite of primaquine causes hemolysis in G6PD-deficient patients, since the enzyme G6PD protects RBCs from oxidative damage.

Uses

1. Radical cure of P. vivax and P. ovale malaria: along with blood schizonticide, it kills gametocytes of vivax and ovale. It is administered at a dose of 15 mg/day × 14 days (30 mg in areas of resistance).
2. Gametocidal: as 45 mg single dose for P. falciparum.
3. Chemoprophylaxis: Generally, it is not routinely recommended, as it has to be given daily in a dose of 30 mg. However, it is used as alternative to mefloquine/doxycycline.
4. Terminal prophylaxis: After visiting endemic area, it is used with regular chloroquine prophylaxis at a dose of 15 to 30 mg × 14 days.
5. Pneumocystis jirovecii: For these patients, it is administered with clindamycin as an alternative to cotrimoxazole.

Folate Antagonist—Pyrimethamine

It is related to trimethoprim and is effective against erythrocytic forms of all four species. It is slow acting if given alone; hence, when it is combined with sulfadoxine, it acts faster. Since it has a long t½ of nearly 3 to 4 days, it is administered once a week.

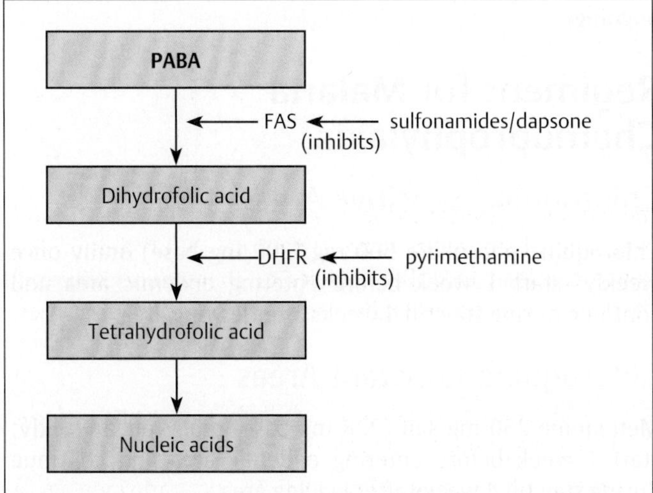

Fig. 67.4 Synergistic sequential blockade of folate synthesis by sulfonamides and pyrimethamine.

Mechanism of Action

It is a dihydrofolate reductase (DHFR) inhibitor, which is 2,000 times more selective for plasmodial DHFR than mammalian DHFR. Sulfadoxine inhibits folic acid synthetase (FAS), hence prevents conversion of para-aminobenzoic acid (PABA) to dihydrofolic acid. Therefore, there is a sequential blockade of nucleic acid synthesis. As there is a synergistic combination between these two drugs, there is slow development of resistance. Additionally, it can also be combined with dapsone (**Fig. 67.4**).

Resistance is widespread, due to the mutation of DHFR/FAS. It is generally well-tolerated. ADRs include megaloblastic anemia (high dose) and Stevens–Johnson syndrome (with sulfadoxine).

Uses

1. Malaria
   a. Treatment: as an alternative in uncomplicated chloroquine-resistant falciparum malaria and as an adjunct to quinine. Three tablets single dose (pyrimethamine 25 mg + sulfadoxine 500 mg—one tablet) is administered.
   b. Prophylaxis: MDR falciparum malaria at a dose of one to two tablets/week. However, it is usually not preferred.
2. Toxoplasmosis: It is the drug of choice, being administered at 200 mg pyrimethamine bolus, followed by 50 mg daily for 4 to 6 weeks + sulfadoxine 4 g/day. Leucovorin (folinic acid) 10 mg daily is given to prevent severe folate deficiency.
3. Pneumocystosis: as an alternative to cotrimoxazole.

Proguanil (Chloroguanide)

It belongs to the biguanide class and is a prodrug. Proguanil is an erythrocytic schizontocide and also a causal prophylactic, that is, it acts against preerythrocytic forms. However, it has a slow onset of action. It is generally combined with atovaquone, as there is resistance to monotherapy. Proguanil, which is a prodrug, is converted to active cycloguanil, which inhibits plasmodial DHFR. It is used with atovaquone for MDR falciparum malaria treatment and as a causal prophylaxis of falciparum malaria, as an alternative to pyrimethamine + sulfadoxine.

Atovaquone

It is a naphthoquinone derivative which is effective against erythrocytic forms and also effective against *T. gondii* and *P. jirovecii*. Resistance develops with monotherapy, hence it is synergistically combined with proguanil. It inhibits mitochondrial electron transport, thus causing the collapse of mitochondrial membrane potential in parasite. This action is potentiated by proguanil. It also inhibits pyrimidine and adenosine triphosphate (ATP) synthesis in parasite (dependent on electron transport). Atovaquone has a low oral absorption, which is increased by fatty food. It has a high-plasma protein binding and a long $t_{1/2}$ of 2 to 3 days. ADRs include vomiting, headache, diarrhea, abdominal pain, rashes and insomnia. It is contraindicated in pregnancy.

Use

1. Atovaquone + proguanil: MDR falciparum malaria. Atovaquone 250 mg + proguanil 100 mg four tablets are administered daily for 3 days. However, it is not used in India. For chemoprophylaxis of falciparum malaria, one tablet daily is given.
2. Atovaquone alone: As an alternative to cotrimoxazole at a dose of 750 mg BD with food × 3 weeks for *P. jirovecii* infections.

Artemisinin and Derivatives

Artemisinin is a sesquiterpene lactone derived from Artemisia annua plant, which was used in China as "Quinghaosu" for 2,000 years. Its semisynthetic derivatives, which have better efficacy and pharmacokinetics, include artesunate, artemether, arteether, and dihydroartemisinin. These agents interact with heme, and there is generation of free radicals. The free radicals damage macromolecules and parasite membrane; in addition, they also inhibit calcium ATPase. Resistance to artemisinin derivatives develops less readily. However, reports of resistance are emerging, hence avoid monotherapy.

They are potent, rapid-acting erythrocytic schizonticide effective against all four species. These drugs are also effective against MDR P. falciparum and gametocytes (not liver stage). They are also effective against cerebral malaria. Since their $t_{1/2}$ is short, recrudesce (resumption of symptoms after period of remission) is common. This is avoided by combing with mefloquine. Artemisinin derivatives are also effective against *T. gondii*, leishmania, and schistosomes.

Pharmacokinetics

Artemisinin has poor water and oil solubility. Artesunate is water-soluble; hence, it is given orally, rectal, intramuscularly (IM), and IV. Artemether is lipid-soluble, hence given orally, rectally, and IM. Artemether is long-acting, hence given IM, whereas dihydroartemisinin is water-soluble, hence given orally. Oral bioavailability of artemisinin is poor. Artemisinin and artemether are prodrugs, which are converted to active dihydroartemisinin. In addition, they are microsomal enzyme inducers.

Adverse Effect

Generally, they are well-tolerated. Mild GI symptoms, itching, and bradycardia are seen with its administration. Raised liver enzymes can occur. It can lead to bone marrow toxicity, hence anemia, neutropenia, and decreased reticulocyte count are seen. It is used with caution during pregnancy (as it is embryotoxic in animals).

Uses

1. MDR falciparum malaria: complicated and severe infections and cerebral malaria.
2. Severe malaria during pregnancy.
3. Artemisinin-based combination therapy (ACT): It is a WHO-recommended therapy for the treatment of chloroquine-resistant/MDR falciparum malaria. ACT increases efficacy, decreases resistance, decreases side effects, and decreases the duration of treatment. For uncomplicated MDR falciparum malaria, oral treatment is recommended, whereas for complicated, severe MDR falciparum malaria, parenteral treatment is given. The short t½ of artemisinin is compensated by giving a second drug. The common regimens include the following:
   a. Artesunate + mefloquine.
   b. Artesunate + sulfadoxine + pyrimethamine.
   c. Artesunate + lumefantrine.
   d. Artesunate + amodiaquine.
   e. Artesunate + pyronaridine.
   f. Dihydroartemisinin + piperaquine.

Antibiotics in Malaria

These include the following: tetracycline shows weak activity against erythrocytic forms, whereas doxycycline is combined with quinine for the treatment of falciparum malaria and chemoprophylaxis of falciparum malaria. Sulfadoxine along with pyrimethamine can also be used. Clindamycin is active against erythrocytic forms. It is used as an alternative to doxycycline, following quinine/artemisinin therapy. Fluoroquinolones as well as azithromycin demonstrate some antimalarial activity.

Immunity in Malaria

People residing in endemic areas develop antibodies both humoral and cell-mediated. These are species- and strain-specific forms of immunity; hence, many people living in endemic areas do not develop malaria. Passive immunity with IgG Ab is effective in children. Maternal Ab is transferred to infants which protects them for few months after birth. There is loss of immunity if person resides away from endemic area for 6 to 12 months.

Malaria Vaccine

It is developed against different parasite stages, for example, sporozoite vaccine, merozoite vaccine, gametocyte vaccine. Development of effective vaccine poses a major problem due to the presence of multiple strains. However, studies are ongoing.

Regimens for Malaria Chemoprophylaxis

Chloroquine-Sensitive Areas

Chloroquine phosphate 500 mg (300 mg base) orally once weekly; start 1 week before entering endemic area and continue during stay till 4 weeks after leaving area.

Chloroquine-Resistant Areas

Mefloquine 250 mg salt (228 mg base) orally once weekly; start 1 week before entering endemic area and continue during stay till 4 weeks after leaving area

or

Doxycycline hyclate 100 mg orally daily; start 1 day before entering endemic area and continue during stay till 4 weeks after leaving area (contraindicated in pregnancy and children)

or

Atovaquone 250 mg + proguanil 100mg fixed-dose combination (FDC) tablet; start 1 day before entering endemic area and continue during stay till 1 week after leaving area

Regimens for Malaria Treatment

Treatment of Uncomplicated Malaria

1. For acute attack of P. vivax, P. ovale, P. malariae, and chloroquine-sensitive P. falciparum, oral chloroquine is the drug of choice. The dosage regimen includes the following: chloroquine 600 mg base (10 mg/kg) stat at 0 hour, followed by 300 mg base (5 mg/kg) at 6 hours on the first day; thereafter, 300 mg base on second day and 300 mg base on third day.
2. For radical cure of P. vivax and P. ovale: chloroquine (as above) + primaquine 15 mg base orally × from day 4 daily for 14 days. Primaquine kills hepatic hypnozoites and prevents relapse of P. vivax and P. ovale. Chloroquine alone can produce radical cure in chloroquine-sensitive P. falciparum, as there are no hypnozoites.
3. For chloroquine-resistant P. falciparum: quinine sulfate 600 mg orally TDS × 3 to 7 days + doxycycline 100 mg BD × 7 days or clindamycin 600 mg BD × 7 days or pyrimethamine 25 mg + sulfadoxine 500 mg FDC three tablets as single oral dose
4. MDR P. falciparum: mefloquine HCl 750 mg orally stat, followed 12 hours later by second dose of 500 mg. Alternatives include artemisinin and atovaquone + proguanil.

Severe or Complicated P. Falciparum Malaria (Cerebral Malaria)

1. Quinine is the drug of choice at a dose of 20 mg/kg. Quinine dihydrochloride is diluted in 500 mL of 5% dextrose and infused slowly over 3 to 4 hours. Subsequently, 10 mg/kg is repeated every 8 hours till patient takes orally. Then, oral quinine sulfate 600 mg TDS should be substituted to complete 1 week of therapy. Frequently monitor the BP, blood sugar, and ECG. Along with quinine orally, use either doxycycline/clindamycin/sulfadoxine + pyrimethamine (see above for doses). Supportive treatment should be given, that is, tepid sponging for fever, NaHCO3 for acidosis correction, IV diazepam if convulsions occur, and 10 % dextrose to control hypoglycemia. Blood transfusion is given to correct anemia.
2. For quinine-resistant P. falciparum, artesunate 2 mg/kg IM/IV stat is administered, followed by 1 mg/kg, then 1 mg/kg for next 4 days.
3. Mixed infection (P. vivax + P. falciparum).
4. Full course of ACT + primaquine 15 mg/day × 14 days is administered.

Multiple Choice Questions

1. A person who traveled to a location where chloroquine-resistant P. falciparum is endemic used a drug for prophylaxis; however, he developed a severe attack of P. vivax malaria. The drug taken for chemoprophylaxis was possibly:

A. Atovaquone.
B. Quinine.
C. Mefloquine.
D. Artemisinin.
E. Quinine.

Answer: C

Mefloquine is used for prophylaxis in places where chloroquine-resistant P falciparum is endemic. One dose of mefloquine weekly prior to the visit and till 4 weeks after leaving the region is recommended.

2. The oral treatment of the acute attack of P. vivax malaria which does not eradicate exoerythrocytic forms of the parasite could be which of the following?

A. Chloroquine.
B. Atovaquone.
C. Pyrimethamine-sulfadoxine.
D. Primaquine.
E. Mefloquine.

Answer: A

Chloroquine is the drug of choice for the oral treatment of an acute attack of malaria due to P. vivax, however it will not eradicate exoerythrocytic forms of the parasite.

3. Which drug eradicates schizonts and latent hypnozoites in the patient's liver?

A. Primaquine.
B. Mefloquine.
C. Halofantrine.
D. Quinine.
E. Chloroquine.

Answer: A

Primaquine is the only antimalarial drug which acts on tissue schizonts in liver cells.

4. The antimalarial agent which can lead to a dose-dependent toxic state, manifested as blurred vision, dizziness, flushed and sweaty skin, nausea, diarrhea, and tinnitus, could be which of the following?

A. Halofantrine.
B. Atovaquone.
C. Proguanil.

D. Primaquine.
E. Quinine.

Answer: E

These dose-related symptoms are due to cinchonism. These are specific to alkaloids like quinine and quinidine. These agents are obtained from the bark of the cinchona tree.

5. A 45-year-old man has been diagnosed with malaria. He is prescribed chloroquine. For subsequent evaluation, which of the following investigations be advised?

A. Echocardiogram.
B. Electrocardiogram.
C. Serum sodium.
D. Serum potassium.
E. Serum creatinine.

Answer: B

Chloroquine therapy can lead to electrocardiographic (ECG) changes due to its quinidine-like activity. Hence, electrocardiogram is recommended for this patient.

6. A 25-year-old foreigner returns from a trip to India with symptoms of fever and malaise. A peripheral blood smear verifies that he has malaria. The clinician gives him only chloroquine as treatment. What is incorrect with the treatment of this patient?

A. Chloroquine is not recommended since malaria infection is self-limiting.
B. He should have been prescribed mefloquine.
C. He should have been prescribed artemisinin derivative.
D. He should have been prescribed primaquine in addition to chloroquine.
E. There is nothing wrong with this prescription.

Answer: D

He should have been prescribed primaquine in addition to chloroquine. This is necessary, since chloroquine will only kill organisms infecting erythrocytes. Due to travel history, this patient could have been infected with P. vivax or P. ovale and thus presumed to have infected hepatocytes as well as erythrocytes. Primaquine is the drug of choice for killing the organisms in hepatocytes and must be administered along with chloroquine when infection by P. vivax or P. ovale is expected.

7. A 23-year-old woman prepares to visit a malaria-laden area for a fortnight. Her doctor prescribes mefloquine prior to her visit for malaria prophylaxis instead of the conventional chloroquine due to frequent resistance to chloroquine. Which one of the following is responsible to cause chloroquine resistance?

A. Increased activity of efflux pumps.
B. Antigenic variation.
C. Chloroquine inactivation.
D. Enhanced protozoal metabolism.
E. Altered target proteins.

Answer: A

Chloroquine acts by inhibiting conversion of heme to hemozoin, leading to the accumulation of heme, which poisons the malarial parasites. For efficacy, chloroquine should be present in the parasite's food vacuole. Resistance develops when efflux pumps remove chloroquine from the food vacuoles, consequently chloroquine is not able to achieve the therapeutic concentrations.

8. A 27-year-old man decides to visit Africa. The physician prescribes a drug for malaria prophylaxis starting 2 weeks prior to his visit. Following the administration of the antimalarial prophylactic drug, the patient develops scleral icterus. Which drug is implicated for the condition?

A. Ampicillin.
B. Atovaquone.
C. Sulfadoxine.
D. Mefloquine.
E. Chloroquine.

Answer: E

G6PD deficiency is a frequent occurrence in patients of South Asian, African, or Middle Eastern origin. This enzyme is especially significant in red blood cells (RBCs) to preserve levels of glutathione. G6PD deficiency by itself is not responsible for any problems; however, it makes RBCs highly vulnerable to oxidative stress. Numerous oxidating drugs can lead to hemolysis and jaundice in patients who have G6PD deficiency, including chloroquine.

9. A 35-year-old man visited his physician for a regular foreign trip preparation. He is visiting a malaria-endemic area in 1 month. Medications for the prevention of diarrhea and malaria are recommended to him. The patient has a history of epilepsy and dormant tuberculosis (TB), which had developed on his previous visit. Which drug is contraindicated for this patient?

A. Chloroquine.
B. Mefloquine.
C. Diphenoxylate.
D. Minocycline.
E. Loperamide.

Answer: B

Mefloquine is contraindicated for patients with a history of epilepsy, psychiatric illness, arrhythmia, cardiac conduction defects, or hypersensitivity to similar drugs. More serious adverse effects comprise depression, confusion, acute psychosis, and seizures. It is an efficacious antimalarial for several strains of chloroquine-resistant P. falciparum and is used commonly in malaria-endemic regions where resistance to chloroquine is frequent.

Chapter 68

Antiamebics and Drugs for Leishmaniasis, Trypanosomiasis, and Pneumocystosis

Anuja Jha and Prasan R. Bhandari

Learning Objectives

- Antiamebic drugs.
- Treatment of pneumocystosis.
- Treatment of leishmaniasis.
- Treatment of trypanosomiasis.

Antiamebic Drugs

Amebiasis is caused by *Entamoeba histolytica.* It spreads by fecal contamination of food and water. The primary site of infection is the colon, whereas the secondary site of infection includes the liver, lungs, and brain. Acute amebiasis is manifested as bloody mucoid stools and abdominal pain, whereas chronic amebiasis symptoms include anorexia, abdominal pain, intermittent diarrhea, and constipation. Cyst passers/carriers are generally asymptomatic.

Classification of Antiamebic Drugs (Fig. 68.1)

1. Tissue amebicides—attain high-tissue concentration following oral/parenteral administration:
   a. Nitroimidazoles—metronidazole (MTZ), tinidazole, secnidazole, ornidazole.
   b. Emetine group—emetine, dehydroemetine (DHE).
   c. 4-aminoquinoline—chloroquine (only extraintestinal amebiasis).
2. Luminal amebicides—poorly absorbed after oral administration, they attain high concentration in bowel and act on mucosal cysts and trophozoites:
   a. Amide—diloxanide furoate (DF).
   b. Halogenated hydroxyquinolines—iodoquinol, iodochlorhydroxyquin.
   c. Antibiotics—tetracyclines, paromomycin, erythromycin.

Metronidazole

It belongs to the nitroimidazole class of drugs. It is highly effective against most anaerobic bacteria, such as *E. histolytica*, *Giardia lamblia*, *Trichomonas vaginalis*, and *Balantidium coli.* It is also effective against *Dracunculus medinensis.*

Mechanism of Action

MTZ is a prodrug, which enters susceptible microorganisms. Its nitro group is reduced by nitroreductase and an active cytotoxic metabolite is formed, which breaks and damages microbial DNA and kills organism (bactericidal) (**Fig. 68.2**). Aerobic bacteria lack nitroreductase and hence they are not sensitive.

Pharmacokinetics

It is available for oral, parenteral, and topical administration. It has good oral absorption but poor protein binding. It attains therapeutic concentration in various body fluids such as saliva, semen, vaginal secretions, bile, breast, milk, and cerebrospinal fluid. It is metabolized by glucuronide conjugation and excreted in urine.

Adverse Drug Reactions

Adverse drug reactions (ADRs) are rarely severe and include the following:

1. Gastrointestinal: anorexia, nausea, metallic taste, epigastric distress, abdominal cramps.
2. Allergic: rashes, urticarial, itching, flushing.
3. Central nervous system (CNS): dizziness, vertigo, confusion, irritability, headache; rarely, convulsion and polyneuropathy on long-term use.

Drug Interactions

1. Disulfiram-like reaction (nausea, vomiting, abdominal cramps, headache, flushing) is seen with alcohol (hence, avoid alcohol during treatment).
2. It increases effect of warfarin, as it inhibits metabolism and hence increases prothrombin time.
3. It increases lithium toxicity, as it reduces renal clearance.

Uses

1. Amebiasis—drug of choice:
   a. 400 to 800 mg thrice daily for 7 to 10 days.
   b. Does not eradicate cysts.
2. Giardiasis—drug of choice:
   a. 200 mg thrice daily for 7 days.
3. *T. vaginalis*—drug of choice:
   a. 200 mg thrice daily for 7 days or
   b. 2 g single dose
4. Anaerobic infections:
   a. Intra-abdominal infections.
   b. Pelvic inflammatory disease.
   c. Lung abscess.
   d. With third-generation cephalosporins.

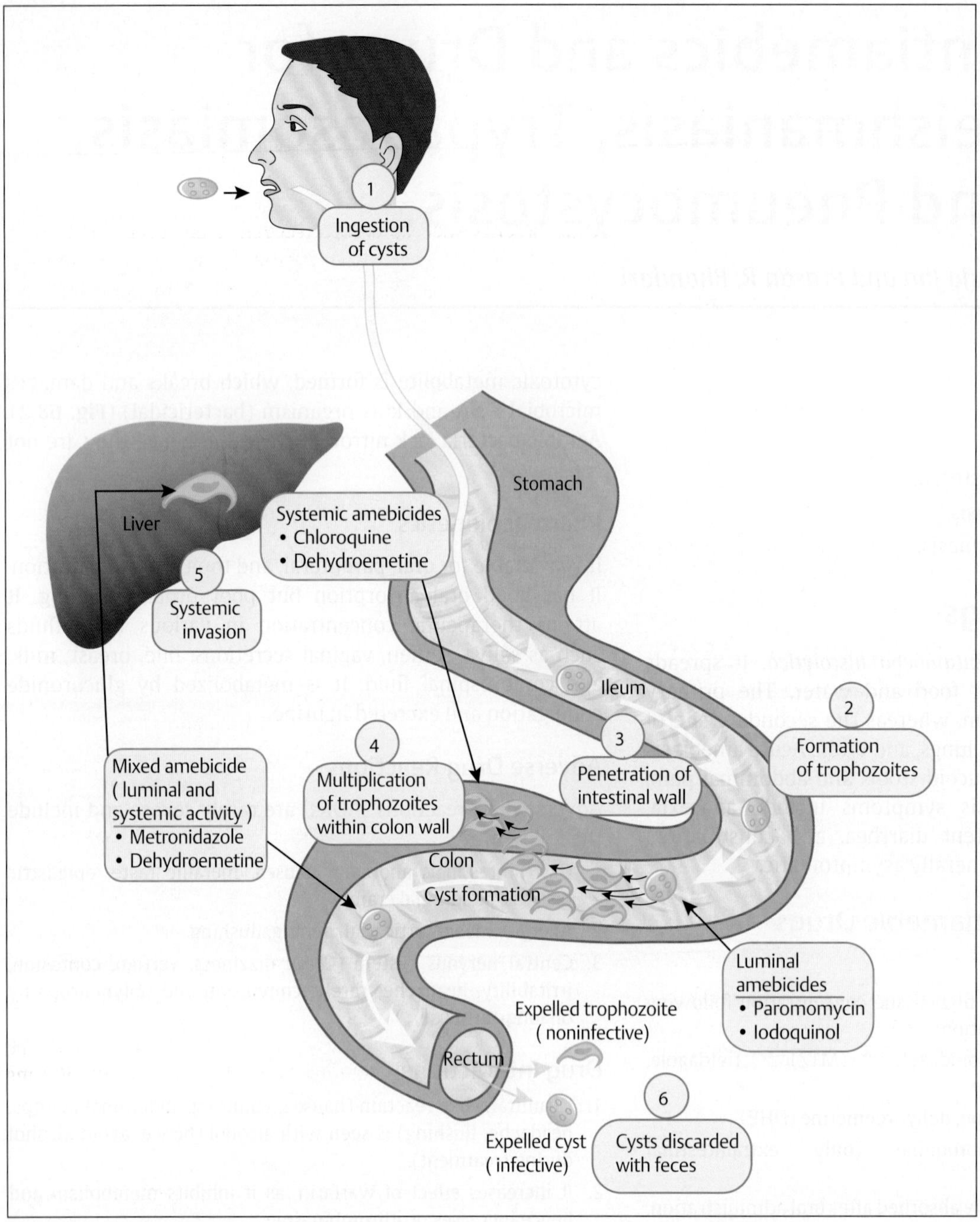

1
Ingestion of cysts
Stomach
Liver
Systemic amebicides
• Chloroquine
• Dehydroemetine
5
Systemic invasion
Ileum
2
Formation of trophozoites
3
Penetration of intestinal wall
4
Multiplication of trophozoites within colon wall
Mixed amebicide (luminal and systemic activity)
• Metronidazole
• Dehydroemetine
Colon
Cyst formation
Luminal amebicides
• Paromomycin
• Iodoquinol
Expelled trophozoite (noninfective)
Rectum
6
Expelled cyst (infective)
Cysts discarded with feces

Fig. 68.1 Antiamebic drugs.

CH₂CH₂OH
O₂N
CH₃
Metronidazole
Freedoxin (reduced)
Metronidazole
Inside microorganism
Ferredoxin (oxidized)
Metabolite with reduction at 5' nitro group
Act on DNA
DNA fragmentation

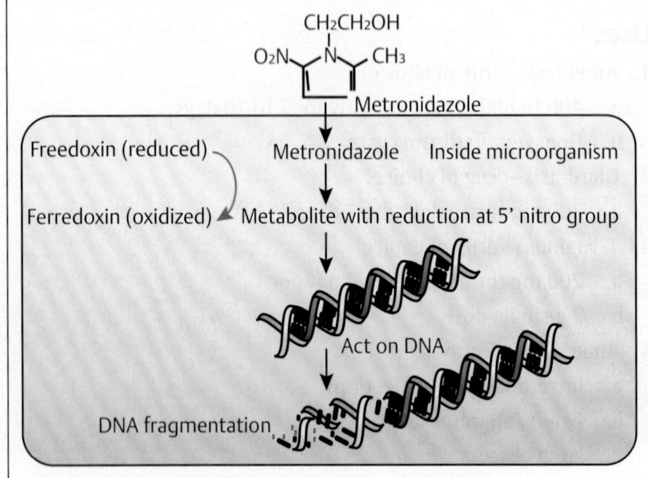

Fig. 68.2 Mechanism of action.

5. *Helicobacter pylori* infection—with clarithromycin + proton-pump inhibitor.
6. Pseudomembranous colitis—caused by *Clostridium difficile*.
7. Acute ulcerative gingivitis (Vincent's angina) as an alternative to penicillin G.
8. Dracunculosis—facilitates extraction of guinea worm.
9. Acne/skin infections—topical 1% gel.

Tinidazole

It is a long-acting and better-tolerated analog of MTZ. It is administered as 2 g once a day for 3 days for amebiasis and as single dose for other indications.

Secnidazole and Ornidazole

These are long-acting; 2 g single dose is adequate.

Emetine and Dehydroemetine

Emetine is derived from an alkaloid from ipecac (Brazil root), whereas DHE is semisynthetic in nature. They directly affect the trophozoites but not cysts. They have improper oral absorption and hence are administered subcutaneously/ intramuscularly (IM) but not intravenously (IV).

Adverse Drug Reactions

1. Pain at the site of injection.
2. Thrombophlebitis.
3. Nausea, vomiting, diarrhea.
4. Cardiotoxicity, arrhythmia, hypotension, cardiac failure.

These ADRs are observed lesser with DHE.

Uses

It is used in cases of severe amebiasis, where MTZ cannot be used.

Diloxanide Furoate

It is a direct luminal amebicidal, which is split in the intestine to diloxanide and furoic acid. ADRs include flatulence, nausea, and abdominal cramps. It is used alone in asymptomatic cyst passers and mild intestinal amebiasis. It is used with MTZ to cure amebiasis in a dose of 500 mg orally thrice daily for a duration of 10 days.

Nitazoxanide

It is a congener of niclosamide (anthelminthic), which is effective against *E. histolytica*, *T. vaginalis*, and *G. lamblia*. It is also effective against intestinal helminths such as *Ascaris* and *Hymenolepis nana*.

Nitazoxanide and its active metabolite interfere with pyruvate ferredoxin oxidoreductase (PFOR) enzyme-dependent electron transfer in anaerobic metabolism. It has good oral absorption. It is highly plasma protein bound (99%) and is converted to tizoxanide. ADRs are rare and include greenish tinge to urine. It is used in the treatment of giardiasis and diarrhea due to *Cryptospora*, *Cryptosporidium parvum*, *H. nana*, *Ascaris*, *Trichuris trichiura*, and *Enterobius vermicularis*.

Iodoquinol and Quiniodochlor

Both belong to 8-hydroxyquinoline class and are directly acting luminal amebicides. Their mechanism is not known. ADRs include the following:

1. Iodine present in these agents results in thyroid enlargement, pruritus, and skin rashes.
2. Long-term use can cause neurotoxicity such as subacute myelo-optico-neuropathy, causing irreversible loss of vision.

It is used in treating asymptomatic amebiasis, which requires 20-day treatment; hence DF, which is given for 10 days, is safe and preferred.

Paromomycin

It is an aminoglycoside, which is given orally. Since it is poorly absorbed from the gut, it acts as intestinal amebicide/ luminal amebicide.

Tetracycline

Older agents such as chlortetracycline are used. Since they are not absorbed well, they inhibit the intestinal flora. This breaks symbiosis between intestinal flora and amebae. Hence, these are used as adjuvants in chronic cases.

Chloroquine

Since it is completely absorbed from the small intestine, it is highly concentrated in the liver. It has direct toxicity to trophozoites. It is used in hepatic amebiasis but is not effective against colonic amebae. It is used as an alternative to MTZ at a dose of 300 mg for a duration of 21 days. It has to be combined with a luminal amebicide (DF).

Treatment of Amebiasis

1. Asymptomatic carriers (luminal amebicide is used):
   a. DF 50 mg thrice daily for 10 days.
      Or tetracycline or iodoquinol or paromomycin.
2. Intestinal amebiasis:
   a. MTZ/tinidazole + luminal agent.
   b. MTZ 400 to 800 mg thrice daily for 7 to 10 days.
      Or tinidazole 2 g once daily for 3 days.
      Or secnidazole 2 g single dose + DF 500 mg thrice daily for 7 to 10 days.
3. Severe intestinal amebiasis and extraintestinal amebiasis:
   a. Similar to intestinal amebiasis + DHE if the patient is not responding to MTZ.
4. Hepatic amebiasis:
   a. Similar to severe intestinal amebiasis + chloroquine phosphate orally 500 mg twice daily for 2 days, 500 mg once daily for 3 weeks.

Treatment of Pneumocystosis

Pneumocystis jirovecii demonstrates features of both protozoa and fungi. Pneumocystosis in humans is caused by *P. jirovecii*. Pneumocystosis in animals is caused by *Pneumocystis carinii*. *P. jirovecii* causes opportunistic infections such as pneumonia in patients with AIDS.

Treatment includes:

1. Cotrimoxazole is given in high oral dose: trimethoprim 20 mg/ kg + sulfamethoxazole 100 mg/kg daily.
2. Pentamidine–4 mg/kg daily for 14 days parenterally.
3. Atovaquone–as an alternative to cotrimoxazole.

Treatment of Leishmaniasis

Kala-azar/visceral leishmaniasis is caused by *Leishmania donovani*. Oriental sore is caused by *Leishmania tropica*, and mucocutaneous leishmaniasis is due to *Leishmania braziliensis*. Leishmaniasis is an infection transmitted by bite of female sandfly *Phlebotomus*.

Treatment includes:

1. Antimony compounds–sodium stibogluconate, meglumine antimonite.
2. Diamidines–pentamidine.
3. Miscellaneous–amphotericin B, ketoconazole, miltefosine, allopurinol, paromomycin.

Antimony Compounds–Sodium Stibogluconate

It is a pentavalent antimonial, which is most effective in kala-azar. It is also effective in mucocutaneous and cutaneous leishmaniasis. Its mechanism is unknown. It is administered at a dose of 4% solution 10 to 20 mg/kg IM/IV for 20 days.

Adverse Drug Reactions

1. Metallic taste, nausea, vomiting, diarrhea.
2. Myalgia, arthralgia, headache.
3. Pain at the site of injection.
4. Hematuria, jaundice.
5. Sudden death due to shock.
6. Arrhythmias, hence requires ECG monitoring.

Pentamidine

It is an aromatic diamidine, which is effective against *L. donovani*, trypanosomes, *P. jirovecii*, and some fungi. It is IM administered.

Adverse Drug Reactions

1. It liberates histamine and hence leads to flushing, pruritus, rashes, hypotension, tachycardia, vomiting, and diarrhea.
2. Hepatotoxicity.
3. Renal impairment.
4. ECG changes.
5. Diabetes mellitus.

Uses

1. Visceral leishmaniasis–alternative to sodium stibogluconate.
2. Trypanosomiasis (sleeping sickness).
   a. Alternative to suramin.
   b. (Or) combined with suramin.
   c. Chemoprophylaxis.
3. Pneumocystosis–as alternative to cotrimoxazole.

Miltefosine

It is the first oral drug for leishmaniasis. It is highly effective against visceral and cutaneous leishmaniasis. It is also effective against leishmaniasis resistant to stibogluconate.

Adverse Drug Reactions

Vomiting, diarrhea, and raised liver enzymes and creatinine. It is contraindicated in pregnancy.

Miscellaneous

1. Amphotericin B–attempted where antimonials are ineffective.
2. Ketoconazole–effective in cutaneous leishmaniasis, since it inhibits ergosterol synthesis in Leishmania.
3. Allopurinol–its metabolite inhibits leishmania protein synthesis; used with antimonials.
4. Paromomycin–aminoglycoside for all forms of leishmaniasis; used alone or with antimonials.

Drugs for Dermal Leishmaniasis (Oriental Sore)

1. Sodium stibogluconate injected around the sore: 2-mL solution containing 200 mg infiltrated.
2. Alternative is paromomycin ointment topically,

Treatment of Trypanosomiasis

Trypanosomiasis is caused by protozoa of genus *Trypanosoma*. *T. brucei gambiense* and *T. brucei rhodesiense* cause African trypanosomiasis (sleeping sickness). *Trypanosoma cruzi* causes South American trypanosomiasis. Drugs used include suramin, pentamidine, melarsoprol, eflornithine, nifurtimox, and benznidazole.

Suramin Sodium

It is the drug of choice for early stages. Since it does not cross the blood–brain barrier, it is not used in later stages. It is IV administered. It has high plasma protein binding; hence, it is present in plasma for nearly 3 months. It is also effective in eradicating adult forms of *Onchocerca volvulus*.

Adverse Drug Reactions

ADRs include high incidence of vomiting, shock, loss of consciousness, neuropathy, hemolytic anemia, and agranulocytosis.

Eflornithine

It is used as an alternative in CNS trypanosomiasis.

Melarsoprol

This is preferred in later stages of trypanosomiasis associated with meningitis and encephalitis.

Nifurtimox and Benznidazole

These are useful in Chagas' disease (American trypanosomiasis).

Multiple Choice Questions

1. A 14-year-old boy returns from a trip with foul-smelling watery diarrhea. On further questioning, he admits to drinking water from a mountain stream without first boiling it. His stool is sent for ova and parasites, confirming the

diagnosis of Giardia lamblia infection. Which of the following drugs is appropriate for treatment?

A. Metronidazole.

B. Nifurtimox.

C. Suramin.

D. Mebendazole.

Answer: A

Metronidazole is used to treat protozoal infections caused due to *Giardia*, *Entamoeba*, and *Trichomonas* spp.

2. A 54-year-old diabetic woman complains of swelling, warmth, and pain in her foot. She is diagnosed with cellulitis and is administered a 10-day course of an oral first-generation cephalosporin. She comes back with severe diarrhea, and Clostridium difficile is the causative organism. What is the primary treatment for this condition?

A. Clindamycin.

B. Metronidazole.

C. Ciprofloxacin.

D. Neomycin.

Answer: B

Metronidazole is the ideal treatment for *Clostridium difficile* colitis, which is possibly caused due to the patient's use of a broad-spectrum antibiotic for her initial infection.

3. In a patient suffering from pseudomembranous colitis, caused due to C. difficile, with proven hypersensitivity to metronidazole, the best drug to be of clinical importance is:

A. Chloramphenicol.

B. Clindamycin.

C. Doxycycline.

D. Vancomycin.

Answer: D

Vancomycin is beneficial in the treatment of pseudomembranous colitis in patients with proven hypersensitivity to metronidazole.

4. A male patient complains of lower abdominal discomfort, flatulence, and infrequent diarrhea. A diagnosis of intestinal amebiasis is done, and E. histolytica is detected in his diarrheal stools. An oral drug is administered, which decreases his intestinal complaints. Subsequently, he develops severe dysentery, right upper quadrant pain, weight loss, fever, and an enlarged liver. Amebic liver abscess is established, and the patient is hospitalized. He has a current history of drug treatment for tachyarrhythmia. The ideal treatment that he should have got for the initial symptoms (which were indicative of mild to moderate disease) is:

A. Diloxanide furoate.

B. Iodoquinol.

C. Metronidazole.

D. Metronidazole plus diloxanide furoate.

Answer: D

Metronidazole plus a luminal amebicide is the treatment of choice in mild-to-moderate amebic colitis. Diloxanide furoate (or iodoquinol, or paromomycin) can be administered as the singular agent in asymptomatic intestinal infection.

5. The drug best expected to be efficacious in treating severe extraintestinal disease in this patient is:

A. Chloroquine.

B. Diloxanide furoate plus iodoquinol.

C. Emetine plus diloxanide furoate plus chloroquine.

D. Tinidazole plus diloxanide furoate.

Answer: D

Metronidazole administered for 10 days, or tinidazole for 5 days, along with a luminal agent is efficacious in most circumstances of hepatic abscess, and these treatments have the double benefit of being equally amebicidal and active against anaerobic bacteria.

6. Metronidazole is ineffective in the treatment of:

A. Amebiasis.

B. Infections due to *Bacteroides fragilis*.

C. Infections due to *Pneumocystis jirovecii*.

D. Pseudomembranous colitis.

Answer: C

Metronidazole is the drug of first choice for all of the conditions listed except pneumocystosis.

7. A 39-year-old woman with repeated sinusitis has been treated with several antibiotics on numerous occurrences. In the course of one such treatment, she had an episode of severe diarrhea and was hospitalized. Sigmoidoscopy showed colitis, and pseudomembranes were established histologically. Which of the following drugs, given orally, is in all probability effective in the treatment of colitis caused due to Clostridium difficile?

A. Ampicillin.

B. Cefazolin.

C. Metronidazole.

D. Trimethoprim-sulfamethoxazole.

Answer: C

The anaerobic bacterium *Clostridium difficile* results *in* life-threatening pseudomembranous colitis. The main drugs used in the management of such infections are vancomycin (not listed) or metronidazole.

Chapter 69 Anthelmintic Drugs

Alka Bansal

PH1.47: Describe the mechanisms of action, types, doses, side effects, indications, and contraindications of the drugs used in helminthiasis.

Learning Objectives

- Mebendazole.
- Albendazole and thiabendazole.
- Narrow-spectrum anthelmintic drugs: pyrantel pamoate and piperazine citrate.
- Antifilarial drugs DEC, ivermectin.
- Diethylcarbamazine (DEC) and ivermectin.
- Niclosamide and praziquantel.

Helminths

Anthelmintics (Ant = against, helminths = parasitic worm).

Helminths are macroscopic pathogenic organisms which cause disease of intestine and/or tissues in humans. They are categorized into three main classes, namely, nematodes (collectively called roundworms), trematodes (flukes), and cestodes (tapeworms). Trematodes and cestodes together are called flatworms or platyhelminths. Common names of individual helminths along with treatment are summarized in **Table 69.1** and **Fig. 69.1**.

Helminthic Infection

Most nematode and cestode infections enter through the fecal-oral route except in filariasis, hookworm, and schistosomes (blood flukes). Helminths are not fatal but harm the host by depriving him of food, causing blood loss, damaging organs like liver, lung, and brain, causing intestinal and lymphatic obstruction, and producing hypersensitivity reactions due to endotoxins released. Mostly, adult helminths cannot multiply in humans except Strongyloides and echinococcus.

General Principles of Anthelmintic Therapy (IM16.13)

Anthelmintic drugs are taken by oral route, act locally in intestine, or are absorbed to act systemically in tissues. They either expel (purge) or kill the worms. These drugs more or less either affect the central nervous system (CNS) of helminths, causing flaccid/tonic muscle paralysis, affecting the uptake of glucose and energy stores, or interfering with polymerization of β tubulin (**Box 69.1**). No anthelmintic, however, is equally active against all worms. They are selectively toxic to helminths and do not affect the host cells. The effect of therapy is sustained till reinfection occurs. Resistance is not a problem with anthelmintics.

Classification of the Drugs (Box 69.2)

On the basis of their spectrum of activity anthelmintic drugs are classified into

1. **A-Broad spectrum-**
   a. Effective against all three categories of helminths—benzimidazoles, mebendazole, and albendazole.
   b. Against trematodes and cestodes—praziquantel.
   c. Against many nematodes—pyrantel pamoate.
2. **B-Narrow spectrum**– They are further subdivided into
   a. For certain nematodes only—levamisole, piperazine, DEC, ivermectin, triclabendazole, and thiabendazole.

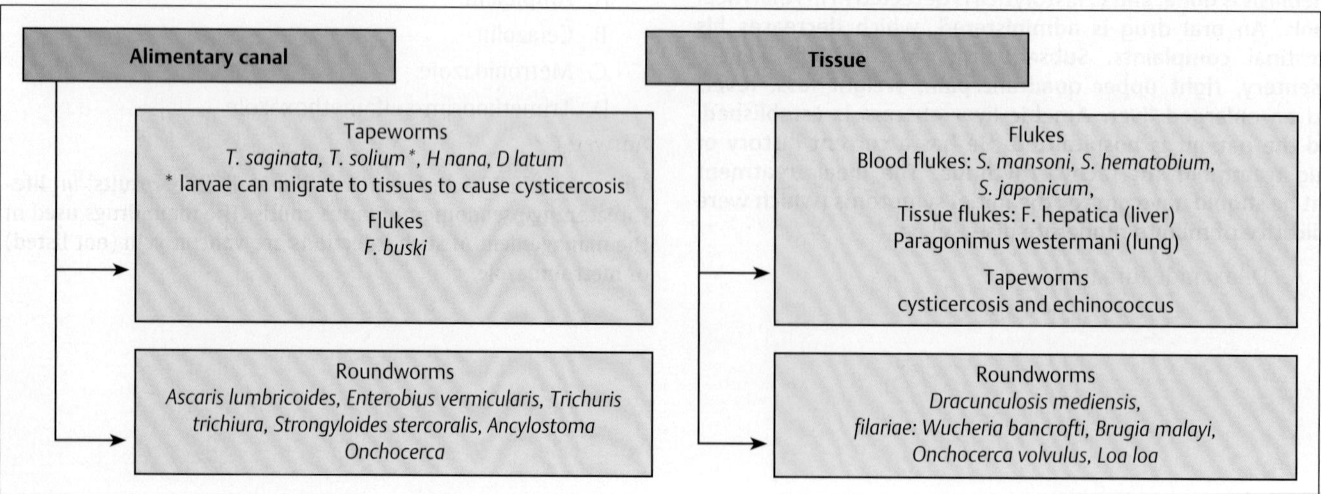

Fig. 69.1 Common helminths causing infestations.

Table 69.1 Different helminths infesting humans with their common names, mode of transmission, important signs, symptoms, diseases caused by them, and treatment

Class	Common name	Organism	DOC	Alternative drugs
Nematodes	Giant roundworm	*Ascaris lumbricoides*	Albendazole/mebendazole	Pyrantel pamoate/ piperazine/ levamisole
	Threadworm	*Strongyloides stercoralis*	Ivermectin	Albendazole
	Pinworm/oxyuris	*Enterobius vermicularis*	Albendazole/mebendazole During pregnancy: Pyrantel pamoate is the DOC	Pyrantel pamoate/ piperazine
	Hookworms	*Necator americanus* *and Ancylostoma duodenale*	Albendazole/mebendazole For cutaneous larva migrans: albendazole	Pyrantel pamoate/ levamisole Ivermectin
	Trichinella/pork roundworm	*Trichinella spiralis*	Albendazole	Mebendazole
	Whipworm	*Trichuris trichura*	Mebendazole	Albendazole
	Filarial	*Wucheria bancrofti,* *Brugia malayi,* *Onchocerca volvulus,* *Loa*	DEC Ivermectin: used in areas where onchocerciasis is prevalent, as DEC can worsen onchocercal eye disease	Albendazole
	Guinea worm	*Dracunculus medinensis*	Metronidazole	Mebendazole/niridazole
	Dog roundworm Cat roundworm	*Toxocara canis (mystax)* *Toxocara cati*	Albendazole	DEC/ivermectin
Cestodes/ tapeworms	Pork tapeworm	*Taenia solium*	Praziquantel Albendazole	Niclosamide, albendazole, nitazoxanide Praziquantel
	Beef tapeworm	*Taenia saginata*	Praziquantel	Niclosamide
	Fish tapeworm	*Diphyllobothrium latum*	Praziquantel	Niclosamide
	Dog tapeworm/ hydatid larva	*Echinococcus granulosis* *E. multilocularis,* *E. vogeli (alveolar)*	Surgery/albendazole For cysts in tissues like liver and lung, albendazole is DOC. It may be required lifelong	Praziquantel/mebendazole
	Dwarf tapeworm	*Hymenolepis nana*	Praziquantel	Nitazoxanide and niclosamide
Trematodes / flukes	Liver fluke	*Faschiola hepatica*	Triclabendazole	Bithionol
	Lung fluke	*Paragonimus westermani*	Praziquantel	Triclabendazole
	Blood flukes/ schistosomes	*S. haematobium (bilharzia, genitourinary)* *S. mansoni, S. japonicum (intestine/liver/spleen)*	Praziquantel	Different for each, given in text.
	Intestinal fluke	*Fasciola buski*	Praziquantel	Niclosamide
	Chinese liver fluke/ oriental liver fluke	*Clonorchis sinensis*	Praziquantel	Albendazole

Abbreviations: DEC, diethylcarbamazine; DOC, drug of choice.

Box 69.1 History/timeline of development of anthelmintics

- 1948–DEC.
- 1950–Piperazine.
- 1953–Niclosamide.
- 1960–Levamisole.
- 1969–Pyrantel pamoate.
- 1972–Mebendazole.
- 1975–Ivermectin.
- 1970s–Praziquantel.

Box 69.2 Classification on the basis of mechanism of action

- Inhibit polymerization of beta tubulins: benzimidazoles like mebendazole, albendazole.
- NN receptor agonist (cause spastic paralysis): pyrantel pamoate, levamisole.
- GABAA agonist (cause flaccid paralysis): piperazine
- Glutamate-gated Cl^- channel (tonic paralysis): ivermectin.
- Increase phagocytosis by altering microfilarial membrane: DEC.
- Increase calcium influx (tonic paralysis): praziquantel.
- Uncoupling of oxidative phosphorylation: bithionol, niclosamide.

b. For cestodes only—niclosamide.

c. For trematodes only—metrifonate, oxamniquine, and bithionol.

Mebendazole

Benzimidazoles with modifications at 2 and/or 5 positions of ring are therapeutically useful as anthelmintics. They include mebendazole, albendazole, thiabendazole, and triclabendazole.

We will discuss mebendazole as the prototype drug.

Mechanism of Action

Mebendazole is a synthetic drug which primarily acts by binding to β tubulin and inhibiting the microtubule polymerization. Other supported mechanisms of action are inhibition of mitochondrial fumarate reductase, uncoupling of oxidative phosphorylation, reduced glucose transport and glycogen synthesis.

Pharmacokinetics

Benzimidazoles are poorly absorbed but absorption is increased by fatty meals. However, mebendazole is minimally absorbed. It is highly protein-bound and excreted by fecal route after glucuronide conjugation. Half-life of mebendazole is 3 to 6 hours.

Pharmacological Effects

Mebendazole is more active than albendazole against trichuris and guinea worm but less effective than albendazole against Strongyloides, hookworm, and tissue-dwelling forms of helminths cutaneous larva migrans/creeping eruption (by ancylostoma), visceral larva migrans (by toxocara), neurocysticercosis (by *T. solium* larva) and hydatid disease (by echinococcus). Mebendazole and albendazole are equally effective against ascariasis and Enterobius. In case of trichinella spiralis, mebendazole acts in intestine only and not against larva migrated to muscles. It has no action against *H. nana*. Benzimidazoles are active against both adults and larva forms in above-mentioned infections and have additional ovicidal actions in Ascaris and trichuris. Hatching of eggs is inhibited in Strongyloides.

Mebendazole is a less toxic alternative to albendazole and is effective even in the presence of anemia and malnutrition. However, multiple doses are required, so albendazole is drug of choice for most of the above-mentioned indications (except trichuriasis and multiple infestations where mebendazole is drug of choice).

Resistance is not seen with benzimidazoles except rarely in *W. bancrofti* and *T. trichiura* due to β tubulin gene mutations.

Indications and Doses

Mebendazole is given orally in the dose of 100 mg single dose to 400 mg BD (twice a day)/TD (thrice a day) for 3 to 4 weeks, depending on the organism. No fasting and purging is required with all benzimidazoles. For children less than 2 years of age, dose is half.

Uses

1. Drug of choice in trichuriasis and multiple infestations by roundworm—100 mg BD for 3 consecutive days.

Alternative to albendazole in-

2. Pinworm—100 mg single dose for 2 years and above, which is repeated after 2 to 3 weeks if required. Maintain proper hygiene and treat all contacts simultaneously.
3. Ascaris/hookworm—100 mg BD for 3 days or 500 mg single dose (less effective).
4. Trichinella spiralis—200 mg BD for 4 days.
5. Hydatid—200 to 400 mg BD or TD for 3 to 4 weeks.

Alternative to metronidazole in guinea worm infection.

Adverse Effects

They are mild and well-tolerated even by patients with poor health. They include nausea, vomiting, abdominal pain, and diarrhea. At higher doses, alopecia, rash, urticaria, and granulocytopenia are seen. Certain incidences of starvation of Ascaris and its migration, leading expulsion from mouth and nose have been reported.

Contraindications

Pregnancy; however, WHO recommends it can be preventively used in second and third trimester for soil-transmitted helminths (Strongyloides, ancylostoma, necator) in endemic areas.

Drug Interactions

Cimetidine increases plasma levels of mebendazole by inhibiting CYP 450 chromosomes.

Albendazole

Albendazole has the same spectrum as mebendazole but is more effective because it produces active sulfoxide metabolite and has better tissue penetration. It requires less number of doses than mebendazole in many infections. Albendazole is less effective than mebendazole against trichuriasis but more effective against Strongyloides, hydatid, and cutaneous larva migrans, hookworm. However, it is still not a dependable treatment for Strongyloides and tapeworm (except in neurocysticercosis) where ivermectin and praziquantel are preferred, respectively.

Albendazole shows erratic absorption. Fatty meal increases absorption. It is taken on an empty stomach for local action in intestine and with fatty meals for action in tissues. After absorption, it is metabolized into an active sulfoxide metabolite, which is widely distributed to different tissues, bile, and cerebrospinal fluid (CSF), making albendazole more effective in tissue infections. Hence, it is the drug of choice in neurocysticercosis, hydatid cysts, and visceral/cutaneous larva migrans. $T_{1/2}$ is 8 to 12 hours. It is different from mebendazole as mebendazole has no relation to meals and no active metabolite is formed in it.

Dose and Indications of Albendazole

1. Drugs of choice in Ascaris, necator, Enterobius, ancylostoma is single dose of 400 mg. It is taken for 3 days for heavy infestation. Dose is reduced to 200 mg in children less than 2 years of age. In Enterobius, second dose is given 2 weeks apart.
2. For tapeworms and Strongyloides—400 mg once a day (OD) for 3 days.
3. For trichinella, 400 mg BD for 3 days but not effective on larva migrated to muscles.
4. For cutaneous larva migrans caused by Ancylostoma braziliense and Ancylostoma caninum—400 mg OD for 3 to 5 days.
5. In visceral larva migrans by Toxocara canis and catti—400 mg BD for 28 days.
6. Neurocysticercosis caused by T. solium cercariae reaching the brain—400 mg BD for 3 to 28 days, depending on number, size and activity of cysts. Steroids and anticonvulsants are added to suppress the inflammation and check the convulsions. Despite being a tapeworm infection, albendazole is preferred over praziquantel for its better penetration, high cure rate, shorter duration of action, and cost effectiveness.
7. Hydatid disease by Echinococcus granulosis and alveolar Echinococcosis by *E. multilocularis*—400 mg BD for 28 days.
8. Alternative and equally effective drug for trichuriasis and enterobius infection in 400 mg single dose.
9. Clonorchis sinensis (liver fluke)—400 mg BD for 7 days.
10. Filariasis—400 mg albendazole annually added to DEC/ivermectin as adjuvant for mass prophylaxis as recommended by WHO.
11. Other uses of albendazole are *T. vaginalis, G. lamblia,* and microsporidial species (Enterocytozoon bieneusi, Encephalitozoon intestinalis) which cause intestinal infection in AIDS.

Adverse Effects

Albendazole is more toxic than mebendazole and causes gastrointestinal tract (GIT) distress, nausea, fatigue, headache, dizziness, alopecia, and jaundice.

Contraindicated in pregnancy and used with caution in renal and hepatic disease.

Triclabendazole

It is used in dose of 10 mg/kg body weight to treat liver flukes, specifically Fasciola hepatica and Paragonimus westermani. Side effects include abdominal pain and headaches. Biliary colic may occur due to dying worms.

Thiabendazole

It is a water-soluble drug having additional anti-inflammatory, analgesic, and antipyretic properties. It can be applied locally for cutaneous larva migrans and trichinella two to three times daily for 5 days.

Uses

Same as albendazole. Oral dose is 25 mg/kg/day in two divided doses.

Adverse Effects

Besides fever, rash, and GIT-related adverse effects, it shows erythema multiforme, hallucination, Steven–Johnsons syndrome, angioneurotic edema, shock, tinnitus, convulsions, cholestatic jaundice, crystalluria, and visual side effects.

Caution is advised against activity requiring mental alertness. It is not used now because of frequent side effects.

Benzimidazoles are also frequently used in veterinary medicine.

Narrow-Spectrum Anthelmintic Drugs

Pyrantel Pamoate

It acts by increasing the acetylcholine concentration at N_n junction by inhibiting acetylcholinesterase enzyme (AChE) and is also a direct N_n agonist. Excess of AChE causes persistent depolarization. Helminths are unable to maintain their intestinal attachment and are expelled out. Spectrum of infection is similar to albendazole on nematodes. In Aascaris, it does not provoke abnormal migration of worms. Pyrantel pamoate is used in the dose of 10 mg/kg of base. *E. vermicularis* may require single dose and may be repeated after 2 weeks. Necator americana/Strongyloides require treatment for 3 consecutive days.

Pyrantel pamoate does not act against trichuris but its analog oxantel is effective in single dose; hence, in many countries, they are available in combination to cover it.

Adverse Effects

They cause mild nausea, vomiting, diarrhea, and abdominal pain. Contraindicated in pregnancy and in children less than 2 years.

Drug Interaction

Not given with piperazine as they have opposite mechanism of action. While pyrantel causes spastic paralysis, piperazine causes flaccid paralysis.

Piperazine

Piperazine is a narrow-spectrum GABA agonist used as an alternative drug for ascariasis and pinworm only. It activates GABA-mediated chloride channel and causes hyperpolarization, which leads to flaccid paralysis. Worms are expelled alive and purgatives should be given with it. Dose is 2 g OD consecutively for 2 days in ascariasis and 7 days for pinworm.

Adverse Effects

They are nausea, vomiting, diarrhea, headache and, rarely, neurotoxicity, respiratory failure, and allergic reaction. It is safe in pregnancy but contraindicated in epilepsy and compromised hepatic and renal function.

Drug Interaction

Pyrantel pamoate.

Antifilarial Drugs (DEC, Ivermectin)

Diethylcarbamazine (DEC)

DEC is drug of choice for lymphatic filariasis caused by *W. bancrofti*, *B. malayi*, Loa loa, and Onchocerca volvulus. Chemically, it is related to piperazine, but it has additional mechanisms of action besides GABA chloride-mediated hyperpolarization of worm. DEC also increases the phagocytosis of both adult worm and microfilaria (mf) form by tissue phagocytes. Moreover, release of prostaglandins causes vasoconstriction and makes it difficult for microfilaria to travel through the vessels. Both adults and mf are killed in wucheria, brugiya but only mf in onchocerciasis and Loa infection.

It is available as citrate salt, well-absorbed orally, widely distributed, and excreted in urine. Its half-life depends on pH of urine. In acidic urine, more of DEC is excreted, so half-life is less (2–3 hours) and alkalization of urine increase half-life to 8 to 12 hours. Dose needs to be reduced in renal impairment.

Indications

1. Filariasis—DEC kills both adults and mf in filarial infection whereas albendazole kills only adults. Recommended dose is 2 mg/kg thrice a day for 12 to 21 days (total dose 72–126 mg/kg). After 7 days of treatment, mf in lymphatics/blood become undetectable but mf in nodules and hydrocoele are not killed. Elephantiasis once developed is not reversed.
2. Tropical pulmonary eosinophilia (TPE).
3. For prophylaxis of filariasis, DEC 6 mg/kg with 400 mg albendazole single dose is given annually. In case of ocular filariasis by Onchocerciasis and oculodermal filariasis by Loa, ivermectin is used in place of DEC, because of risk of severe hypersensitivity reaction, leading to risk of river blindness due to dying microfilariae.
4. Other uses of DEC—mf and adult in dipetalonema streptocara and toxocariasis.

Adverse Effects

They are mainly due to destruction of mf and adult worms—fever, rash, pruritus, enlarged lymph nodes, broncho-spasm, enlarged lymph nodes, arthralgia, and tachycardia (Mazzotti reaction). These adverse effects are minimized by administering nonsteroidal anti-inflammatory drugs (NSAIDs), antihistamines, and steroids.

Ivermectin

It is a semisynthetic macrocyclic lactone derived from Streptomyces avermitilis. It acts by activating glutamate-gated Cl^- channels found specifically in nematodes. It is taken on an empty stomach, is well-absorbed orally, has a wide distribution, and excreted in feces. Plasma half-life is 12 hours. Ivermectin acts only on larval (mf) stages and decreases transmission to its vector Simulium black fly.

Uses

1. It is drug of choice (DOC) for onchocerciasis and strongyloidiasis in single dose of 20 mg/kg and is also very effective in disseminated strongyloidiasis where it is given for 2 consecutive days in same dose of 20 mg/kg. Ivermectin does not kill the adult onchocerca but keeps in check the infection. Hence, it is repeated every 6 to 12 months as prophylaxis to prevent blindness. Corticosteroids are given with it for their anti-inflammatory action.
2. Brugian and bancroftian filariasis—40 mg/kg per year single dose.
3. Oculodermal filariasis caused by Loa is also treated by ivermectin.
4. **Other uses**—given orally for cutaneous larva migrans, pediculosis, and scabies.

Adverse Effects

Mazzotti-like reaction (milder) due to killed mf. Give aspirin, antihistamines, steroids for it.

Ivermectin is contraindicated in pregnancy and children less than 5 years of age,

Drug Interaction

Shows no significant drug interaction, although it is metabolized by CYP3A4.

Levamisole

Levisamole is used as an immunostimulant in vitiligo and as adjunct in colorectal cancer and mucositis due to chemotherapy. For anthelmintic purpose, it is used in Ascaris, ancylostoma, and Strongyloides infestation. The mechanism of action is similar to pyrantel pamoate (N_n agonist). It is used as single-dose treatment for ascariasis. The dose is weight-dependent; 50 mg OD for 10 to 20 kg, 100 mg for 21 to 40 kg, and above 150 mg for 40 kg. In ancylostoma infection, double dose, that is, 300 mg for 2 consecutive days is given.

It is generally well-tolerated as only one or two doses are used in helminthiasis.

Role of Doxycycline in the Treatment of Filariasis

Doxycycline is a broad-spectrum antibacterial and anti-protozoal drug useful in filariasis. The logic of using it is that Onchocerca volvulus and W. bancrofti have a symbiotic organism called Wolbachia. Doxycycline slowly eliminates Wolbachia, and it also results in long-term embryogenesis block of the adult worms. In addition, doxycycline is potentially microfilaricidal as well. It is used at dose of 100 mg per day for 6 weeks. *Loa loa* is the only filarial nematode that does not possess Wolbachia endosymbionts and hence doxycycline is not useful in it.

Comparison between DEC and Ivermectin

Table 69.2 provides comparison and contrast between DEC and ivermectin

Treatment Regimens for Acute Treatment for Filarial Fever and Mass Prophylaxis of Filariasis

Acute Treatment for Filarial Fever

DEC in dose of 6 mg/kg every day in three divided doses for 2 weeks in case of W. bancrofti (total dose 84 mg/kg) and 3 weeks in case of Brugia malayi (total dose 126 mg/kg).

Mass Prophylaxis of Filariasis

The aim of mass prophylaxis against filariasis is to reduce the microfilarial concentration in blood to subinfective level for mosquitoes. DEC in dose of 6 mg/kg every 6 to 12 months is given with 400 mg of albendazole. The regions where oncocerciasis or *Loa* is more common, ivermectin 40 mg/kg is used in place of DEC along with albendazole to prevent river blindness.

Niclosamide and Praziquantel

Praziquantel

It is another broad-spectrum drug very effective against cestodes (except neurocysticercosis and echinococcus where DOC is albendazole) and trematodes (except F. hepatica where DOC is triclabendazole). However, it is not useful in nematodes. Praziquantel works by increasing the influx of calcium from endogenous stores. In cestodes, praziquantel produces tetanus-like contractions of the musculature of the worm and finally expulsion of the worm. In trematodes, the contractions cause appearance of vacuoles in the tegument. This exposes the antigen, and antibodies present in the host bind to them, causing their phagocytosis. Unlike albendazole, praziquantel is readily absorbed from the intestinal tract.

Indications

1. Praziquantel is drug of choice. In most tapeworm infections *T. solium, T. saginata, T., H. nana, D. latum* 10 mg/kg single dose is given as it kills encysted larva also (niclosamide does not kill encysted)
2. Schistosomes and other flukes (except *F. hepatica*) 40–75 mg/kg single dose
3. Used as alternate drug in *F. hepatica* next to triclabendazole and bithionol. Contraindicated in pregnancy.

Neurocysticercosis and hydatid disease—50 mg/kg in three divided doses for 15–30 days.

Drug Interactions

Carbamazepine, phenytoin, and steroids induce praziquantel metabolism and decrease its bioavailability.

Niclosamide

Niclosamide is cheaper alternative of praziquantel for similar uses and is safe in pregnancy and poor health. Niclosamide definitely requires purgation after the drug in case of T. solium infection (in contrast to benzaimidazoles and

Table 69.2 Compare and contrast between DEC and ivermectin

Parameters	DEC	Ivermectin
Action on	mf as well as adult worm	mf only
Mechanism of action	increase phagocytosis by altering microfilarial membrane	Cause paralysis by glutamate-gated Cl^- channel
Additional action	Nil	Anti-inflammatory action also
First choice	DOC in *W. bancrofti, Brugia malayi, Loa loa* and tropical eosinophilia	DOC in *O. volvulus* (river blindness, also known as Robles disease)
Other uses	Dipetalonema streptocara and toxocariasis.	Also used in rosacea, scabies, pediculosis
Adverse effects	Mazotti reaction risk is high	Less severe and low risk
Special condition	Safe in pregnancy	Avoided in pregnancy, children below 5 years

Abbreviation: mf, microfilaria.

Table 69.3 Comparison and contrast between niclosamide and praziquantel

Characteristics	Praziquantel	Niclosamide
Mechanism of action	Increase calcium influx, tonic paralysis.	Uncoupling of oxidative phosphorylation
Spectrum	Tapeworms and flukes.	Tapeworms and pinworm (nematode)
Pharmacokinetics	Well-absorbed, extensive first-pass metabolism, excreted in urine.	Poorly absorbed
Effective against	Adult and larval stages, kills encysted larva also.	No effect on encysted larva.
Serious adverse event	Useful in neurocysticercosis (DOC is albendazole) but not in ocular cysticercosis where ivermectin is used.	Rather can cause cysticercosis by partly digesting T. solium segments and releasing eggs/larvae into intestine which penetrate intestine and migrate into tissue.
DI	Phenytoin, carbamazepine, dexamethasone induce metabolism of praziquantel.	Absent
Side effects	More—fever, arthralgia, myalgia, rash, CNS-related headache, dizziness, sedation	Less and mild
Use in special population	Safe in pregnancy, children more than 4 years.	safe in pregnancy and poor health
DOC	All cestodes except cysticercus cellulosae by T. solium and echinococcus (albendazole) and trematodes except F. hepatica (triclabendazole)	Alternative to praziquantel for similar cestodic indications. Amongst trematodes used as alternate to praziquantel only in *F. busci*.
Cost	Expensive	Cheaper

Abbreviations: CNS, central nervous system; DI, drug interactions; DOC, drug of choice.

praziquantel) to prevent the development of cysticercosis, and scolex should be searched in stools to ensure complete removal. Saline purgation is done 2 hours after breakfast.

Indications and Dose

1. *T. solium*—1 gm and again 1 gm after 1 hour.
2. *H. nana*—2 gm for 5 days (praziquantel is single dose alternative 15–25 mg/kg)

Comparison between Niclosamide and Praziquantel

Table 69.3 compares and contrasts between niclosamide and praziquantel.

Miscellaneous Limited Spectrum Drugs

1. Nitazoxanide is a drug approved for treating human protozoan infections. It was serendipitously shown to have therapeutic activity against soil-transmitted helminths. It is comparable to albendazole for treatment of *Ascaris* infections and is approved for use in children ≥ 12 months of age.
2. Artemisinin-based therapy– Artether shows promise as an antischistosomal 6 mg/kg once every 2 to 3 weeks. Concern is raised for increased risk of resistant malaria.
3. Against flukes.
   a. Bithionol—It is useful against liver and lung flukes. It is suggested that bithionol is an uncoupler of oxidative phosphorylation. It is given orally at a dose of 30 to 50 mg per kg of body weight on alternate days for 10 to 15 doses for the treatment of fascioliasis and paragonimiasis. WHO recommends 30 mg/kg daily for 5 days in liver fluke infection. Adverse effects are mostly related to GIT and CNS, namely, nausea, vomiting, diarrhea, headache, dizziness, and skin rashes. It is not used below 8 years of age.
   b. Metrifonate—It is an alternative drug effective against Schistosoma hematobium (blood fluke causing bilharziasis). It is a long-acting cholinesterase inhibitor, which is well-tolerated but still not a first-line treatment, as it is not effective against eggs, and these eggs continue to pass in urine for months. Recommended dose is a single oral dose of 7.5 to 10 mg/kg repeated 2 weeks apart. Important adverse effects are due to excess of acetylcholine such as diarrhea, nausea, vomiting, bronchospasm, sweating, and tremors. It is contraindicated in pregnancy. Metrifonate shows drug interactions with insecticide exposure, leading to neuromuscular blockade as adverse effects increase due to cholinergic toxicity.
   c. Oxamniquine—It is a tetrahydroquinoline derivative which is esterified in liver to produce reactive metabolite. This metabolite alkylates DNA of Schistosoma mansoni, resulting in contraction, paralysis of the worms, eventual detachment from terminal venules in the mesentery, and death. Pharmacokinetic and well-absorbed orally, but with unpredictable effects, as it shows high-interindividual variability in response. Adverse effects are CNS-related, nausea, colic, pruritus, and urticaria. Common effects are drowsiness, dullness, headache and, rarely, seizures. Contraindicated are pregnancy and history of seizures.

Questions and Answers

1. A 5-year-old child presented with complaints of abdominal pain and perianal pruritus. Microscopic examination of an adhesive tape stuck to perianal area revealed small, white, roundworms and translucent eggs. Which is the best treatment for this child?

A. Fluconazole.
B. Mebendazole.
C. Metronidazole.
D. Praziquantel.

Answer: B

This child has an *Enterobius vermicularis*, or "pinworm," infection. A simple way to ascertain infection is by the adhesive tape test described in the question stem. This test ideally should be done at night to maximize the chance of collecting worms for identification. A single dose of mebendazole is best choice to treat this type of infection.

2. An adult gave history of eating pork, and he was found to be infested with both tapeworm and schistosomes. Drug which is effective against both is?

A. Praziquantel.
B. Albendazole.
C. Niclosamide.
D. Ivermectin.

Answer: A

Praziquantel is the drug of choice for both tapeworms and flukes.

3. A person presented with complaints of headache, vomiting, and seizures. On CT scan, some active and some calcified cysts were found. What is the most appropriate treatment for this patient?

A. Albendazole.
B. Niclosamide.
C. Tetracycline.
D. Watchful waiting.

Answer: A

Neurocysticercosis is caused by *Taenia solium* larvae called cysticerci in the brain. Cysticercosis is diagnosed by CT scan or biopsy. Therapy is albendazole and/or surgery. Corticosteroids are beneficial in reducing inflammation and swelling and are used as an adjunct to albendazole therapy.

4. A rural woman presents with complaint of cyst on the foot. On examination, dracunculosis was suspected. We have to give which drug?

A. Albendazole.
B. Metronidazole.
C. Mebendazole.
D. Piperazine.

Answer: B

The larvae of guinea worm (*naaru rog*) enter the body through the fecal-oral route and mature in tissues. After maturation, it migrates to subcutaneous tissue usually at leg and forms a cyst. Metronidazole is the drug of choice. At times, they try to remove worm by slowly rotating it on a stick.

5. It was decided to give mass prophylaxis for filariasis in areas where coinfection with onchocerciasis is common. Combination preferred is?

A. Diethylcarbamazine (DEC) with albendazole.
B. Pyrantel with ivermectin.
C. Ivermectin with albendazole.
D. Niclosamide with albendazole.

Answer: C

Filariasis is common in certain areas. There mass prophylaxis programs are run where 6 monthly or annual dose is given.

6. A woman who recently immigrated to the United States from Africa presents with diffuse abdominal pain and an unusual rash. The erythematous linear rash spreads from her right upper quadrant to the umbilicus. Laboratory testing confirms the diagnosis of *Toxocara canis* infection. What is the most appropriate treatment?

A. Diethylcarbamazine (DEC).
B. Ivermectin.
C. Praziquantel.
D. Albendazole.

Answer: D

The patient is most likely suffering from visceral larva migrans caused by *Toxocara canis*. Albendazole is treatment of choice in visceral larva migrans by Toxocara canis and cati.

7. Which of the following drug causes flaccid paralysis of Ascaris?

A. Praziquantel.
B. Piperazine.
C. Pyrantel pamoate.
D. Niclosamide.

Answer: B

Piperazine is the drug which causes flaccid paralysis (see Table 69.3).

8. Uses of ivermectin include all except?

A. Scabies.
B. Onchocerciasis.
C. Visceral larva migrans.
D. Strongyloides.

Answer: C

It is drug of choice for onchocerciasis and strongyloidiasis. It is also used in Brugian and bancroftian filariasis, Oculodermal filariasis. It is also given orally for cutaneous larva migrans, pediculosis, and scabies.

9. Which drug shows acetylcholine-like side effects and can cause bronchospasm?

A. Metrifonate.
B. Niridazole.

C. Oxamniquine.

D. Albendazole.

Answer: A

It is effective against S. hematobium, and because of cholinergic side effects, it is not used with neuromuscular blockers.

10. A 35-year-old woman with a history of world travel is found to have a hookworm infection. She has begun therapy with mebendazole therapy orally and now returns home for follow-up. Which of the following statements regarding the pharmacodynamics of this agent is correct?

A. Best results are obtained with intravenous (IV) doses.

B. Hepatic first-pass metabolism is achieved.

C. Low-fat meals enhance absorption.

D. Side effect profile is unfavorable.

Answer: B

Mebendazole is nearly insoluble in aqueous solution. Little of an oral dose (that is chewed) is absorbed, unless it is taken with a high-fat meal.

It undergoes first-pass metabolism to inactive compounds. Mebendazole is relatively free of toxic effects, although patients may complain of abdominal pain and diarrhea. It is, however, contraindicated in pregnant women, because it has been shown to be embryotoxic and teratogenic in experimental animals.

11. Why piperazine and pyrantel pamoate are not given together? Choose the most appropriate answer.

A. Adverse effects are added.

B. Both have similar spectrum.

C. Oppose each other's mechanism of action.

D. Both are costly.

Answer: C

Not given with piperazine as they have opposite mechanism of action. While pyrantel causes spastic paralysis, piperazine causes flaccid paralysis.

12. Purgation is required with which of the following drugs?

A. Albendazole.

B. Niclosamide.

C. Piperazine.

D. Ivermectin.

Answer: B

Niclosamide to avoid risk of cysticercosis.

Chapter 70 Cancer Chemotherapy

C. S. Suthakaran and Prasan R. Bhandari

PH1.49: Describe mechanism of action, classes, side effects, indications, and contraindications of anticancer drugs.

Learning Objectives

- Phases of cell cycle.
- Common adverse effects of anticancer agents.
- Anticancer agents.

Introduction (IM13.6, IM13.13, IM13.14, IM13.17)

Cancer is one of the major causes of death worldwide. In developed countries, one in three patients is diagnosed as a cancer patient. An increase in life expectancy has increased its incidence. Cancer is characterized by progressive, persistent, perverted (abnormal), purposeless, and uncontrolled proliferation of tissues. Special characteristics of cancer cells include uncontrolled proliferation, invasiveness, metastasis, and dedifferentiation. Generally, cancer cells multiply faster than host cells and cancer cells are own cells, unlike microbes; hence, anticancer drugs which destroy cancer cells also kill host cells. Host defense does not attack cancer cells, as they are also host cells. Additionally, cancer cells enter a resting phase, only to multiply and recur later. Anticancer agents do not act during resting phase, hence making its treatment difficult.

Phases of Cell Cycle

There are four phases of cell cycle: G1, S, G2, and M. G1 is the presynthetic phase and is of variable duration. S is the synthesis phase during which DNA synthesis occurs. Replicating enzymes like polymerases, topoisomerases, thymidine kinases, and dihydrofolate reductases are active for a maximum duration of 12 to 18 hours. G2 is the postsynthetic phase with a duration ranging from 1 to 8 hours. M, the mitosis phase, has a duration of 1-2 hours. The daughter cells divide or remain dormant in the G0 phase. Knowledge of cell cycle is used for staging and treatment schedule. Different drugs act on different phases (cell-cycle- specific) and some drugs are cell-cycle-nonspecific (**Fig. 70.1**).

Cell-cycle-specific drugs (mainly acts on dividing cells)

- S phase: antimetabolites, doxorubicin, epipodophyllotoxins.
- G2 and M phase: bleomycin.
- M phase: taxanes, vinca alkaloids.

Cell-cycle-nonspecific drugs (mainly acts on dividing & resting cells)

- Alkylating agents.
- Anticancer antibiotics.

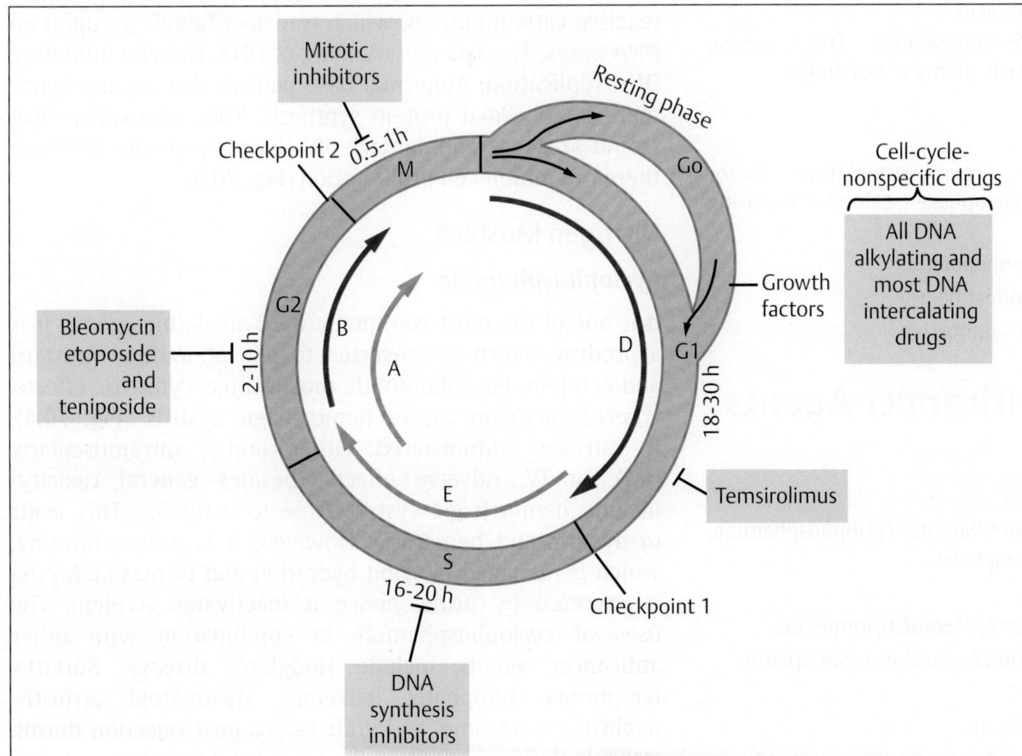

Fig. 70.1 Phases of cell-cycle and drugs acting on it.

- Cisplatin.
- Procarbazine.
- Camptothecins.

Common Adverse Effects of Anticancer Agents

Most anticancer agents act on rapidly multiplying cells (both cancer cells and normal cells); hence, normal multiplying cells of bone marrow, gonads, and epithelial cells of skin and mucous membrane are affected. The common side effects of anticancer medications include:

Bone marrow depression is manifested as leukopenia, anemia, thrombocytopenia, infections, and bleeding. Gastrointestinal tract (GIT) side effects are manifested as stomatitis, glossitis, esophagitis, proctitis, diarrhea, and ulcers. Alopecia could be partial/total but is reversible. There is reduced spermatogenesis in men and amenorrhea in women. Immediate side effects include nausea and vomiting, which is very common due to chemoreceptor trigger zone (CTZ) stimulation. It starts after 4 to 6 hours and lasts 1 to 2 days. Hence, prophylactic antiemetic is a must. Hyperuricemia occurs due to rapid tumor cell lysis. There is increase in plasma uric acid, hence there is tumor lysis syndrome and renal failure. Teratogenicity is common, hence these drugs are contraindicated in pregnancy. Carcinogenicity, that is, secondary cancers (e.g., leukemia following treatment of Hodgkin's lymphoma) can occur. Some unique adverse effects are discussed individually.

Measures to Prevent Adverse Effects

- Nausea, vomiting–antiemetics, for example, ondansetron, metoclopramide.
- Hyperuricemia–allopurinol.
- Methotrexate toxicity–folinic acid.
- Cyclophosphamide cystitis–intravenous (IV) mesna, N-acetyl cysteine bladder wash, plenty of oral fluids.
- Myelosuppression.
  - Anemia–erythropoietin.
  - Leukopenia–granulocyte colony-stimulating factor (G-CSF), granulocyte/macrophage colony-stimulating factor (GM-CSF).
  - Thrombocytopenia–thrombopoietin.
- Cisplatin nephrotoxicity–amifostine.
- Xerostomia due to radiation–amifostine.

Classification of Anticancer Agents (Fig. 70.2)

1. **Alkylating agents**
   a. Nitrogen mustards–mechlorethamine, cyclophosphamide, ifosfamide, chlorambucil, melphalan.
   b. Alkyl sulfonate–busulfan.
   c. Nitrosoureas–carmustine, streptozotocin, lomustine.
   d. Platinum-containing compounds–cisplatin, carboplatin.
2. **Antimetabolites**
   a. Folate antagonist–methotrexate.
   b. Purine antagonist–6 mercaptopurine, 6-thioguanine.
   c. Pyrimidine antagonist–5-fluorouracil, cytarabine.
3. **Natural products**
   a. Plant products.
      i. Vinca alkaloids–vincristine, vinblastine.
      ii. Taxanes–paclitaxel, docetaxel.
      iii. Epipodophyllotoxins–etoposide.
      iv. Camptothecins–topotecan, irinotecan.
   b. Antibiotics–actinomycin D, bleomycin, mitomycin C, mithramycin, doxorubicin, daunorubicin.
   c. Enzymes–L-asparaginase.
4. **Hormones and antagonists**
   a. Estrogens–ethinyl estradiol, fosfestrol.
   b. Antiestrogens–tamoxifen.
   c. Progestins–hydroxyprogesterone caproate, medroxy-progesterone acetate.
   d. Androgens–testosterone propionate.
   e. Antiandrogens–flutamide.
   f. 5-α reductase inhibitors–finasteride.
   g. Gonadotropin-releasing hormone (GnRH) analogs–buserelin, goserelin, naferelin.
   h. Corticosteroids–prednisolone and others.
5. **Biological response modifiers**
   a. Interferon α, interleukin 2, amifostine, hematopoietic growth factors.
6. **Miscellaneous**–hydroxyurea, imatinib, thalidomide, monoclonal antibodies.

Anticancer Agents

Alkylating Agents

All alkyl group (s) are capable of introducing "alkyl" groups into nucleophilic sites of DNA bases with covalent bonds. These are cell-cycle-nonspecific drugs. These agents also have radiomimetic actions. They act by forming highly reactive carbonium ion, which transfers "alkyl" group(s) on DNA bases. There is cross-linking of DNA, thereby inhibiting DNA replication. Abnormal base pairing also occurs, hence there is abnormal protein synthesis. They also cause DNA strand breakage and damage of RNA and proteins. All these therefore inhibit cell proliferation (**Fig. 70.3**).

Nitrogen Mustard

Cyclophosphamide

It is one of the most commonly used alkylating agents. It is a prodrug which is converted to phosphoramide mustard and acrolein. Phosphoramide mustard has cytotoxic effects, whereas acrolein causes hemorrhagic cystitis (**Fig. 70.4**). It can be administered either orally, intramuscularly (IM), or IV. Adverse effects (besides general toxicity) include hemorrhagic cystitis (due to acrolein). This leads to dysuria and hematuria. However, it is a dose-limiting, which is managed by good hydration and IV mesna. Mesna is excreted by urine, hence it inactivates acrolein. The uses of cyclophosphamide in combination with other anticancer agents include Hodgkin's disease, Burkitt's lymphoma, lymphatic leukemia, rheumatoid arthritis, nephrotic syndrome, and graft versus host rejection during transplantation due to immunosuppressant action.

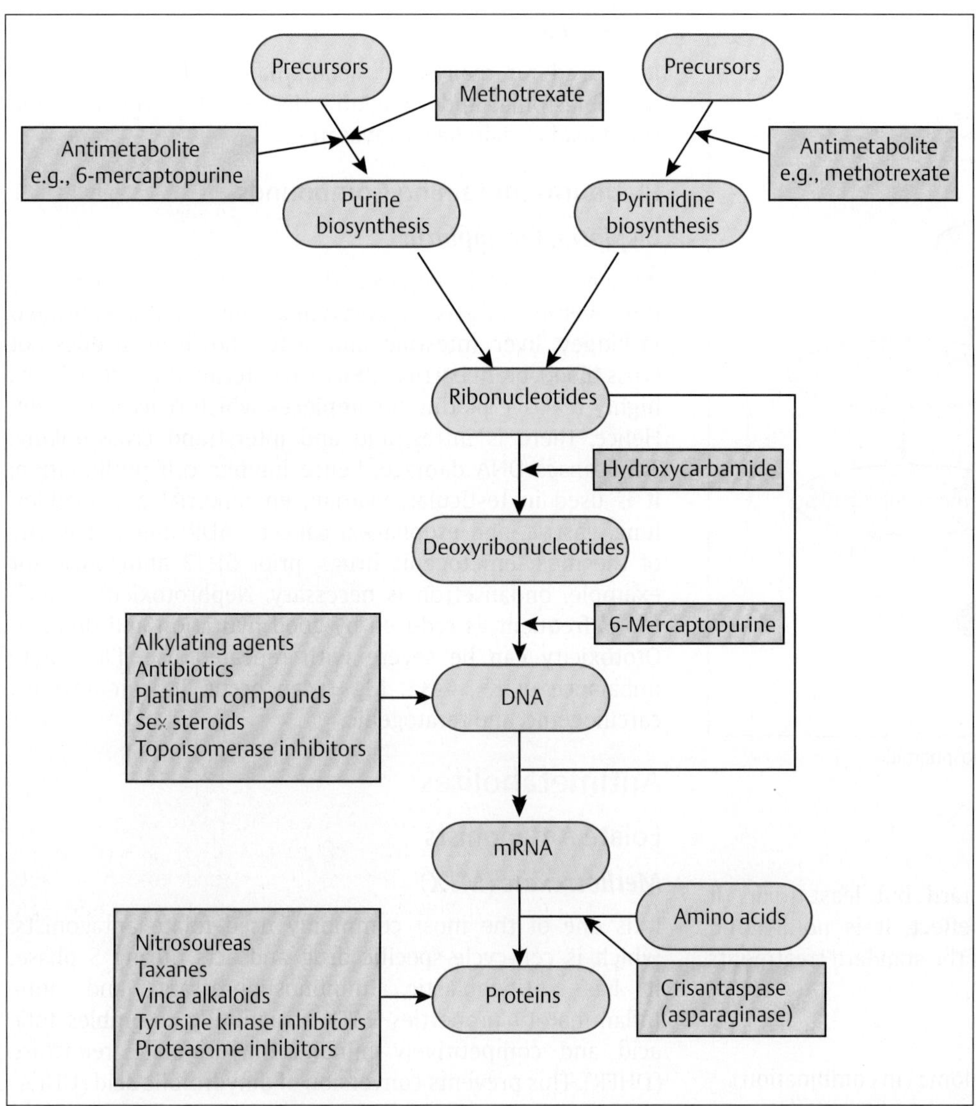

Fig. 70.2 Sites of action of anticancer agents.

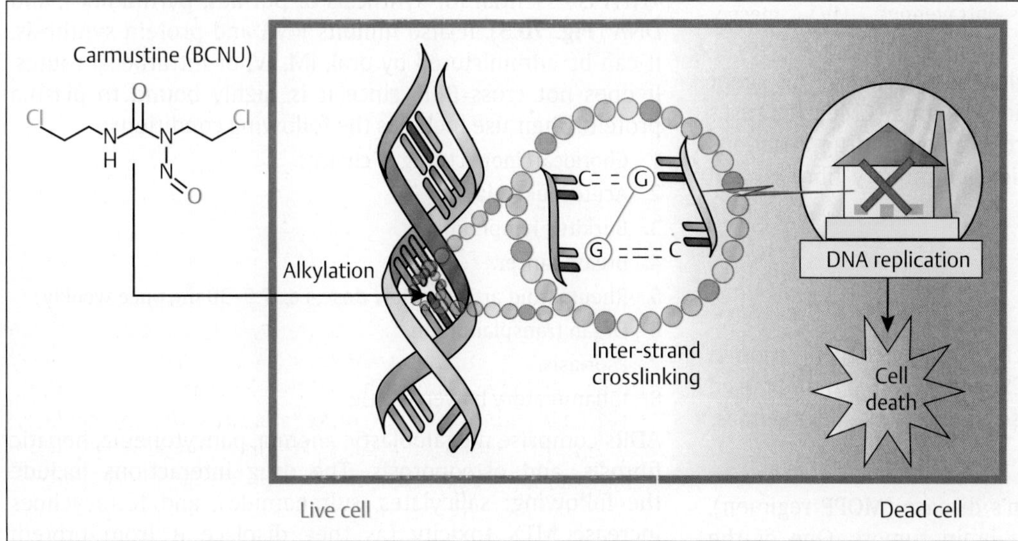

Fig. 70.3 Mechanism of alkylating agents.

Mechlorethamine

It is a prodrug at physiological pH, which is spontaneously converted to a highly reactive cytotoxic product. It is one of the components of mechlorethamine, vincristine procarbazine, and prednisone (MOPP) regimen for Hodgkin's disease (nitrogen mustard, oncovin, prednisone, and procarbazine). It is an extreme irritant, hence care should be taken during IV administration (avoid extravasation).

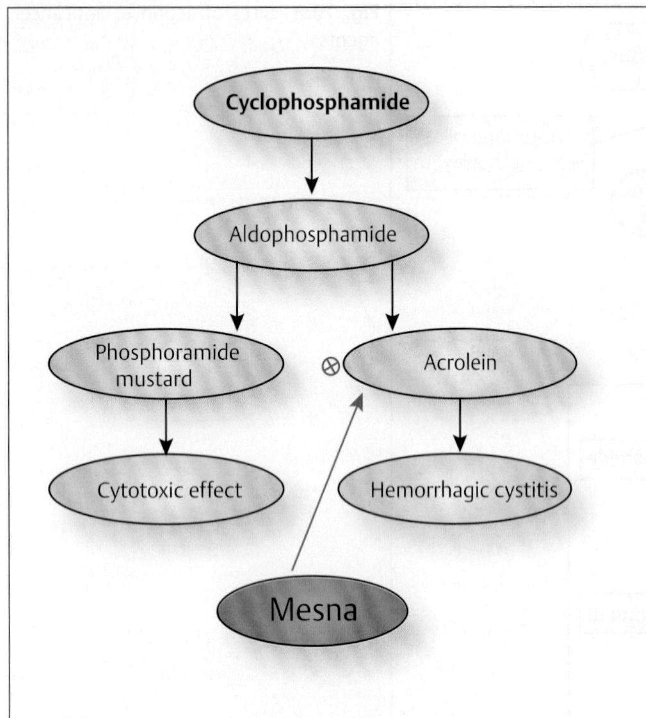

Fig. 70.4 Mechanism of action of cyclophosphamide.

Chlorambucil (Leukeran)

It is a slow-acting, nitrogen mustard but least toxic. It possesses a marked lymphocytic effect. It is nonirritant, hence can be given orally. It is one of the standard treatments of chronic lymphatic leukemia (CLL).

Melphalan

It is highly effective in multiple myeloma (in combination).

Alkyl Sulfonates

Busulfan (Myleran)

It has a selective action on myeloid series. Hence, this agent is preferred for chronic myeloid leukemia (CML). It causes bone marrow suppression. Other adverse drug reactions (ADRs) include skin pigmentation, pulmonary fibrosis, and hyperuricemia.

Nitrosoureas

Carmustine, Lomustine

It is highly lipid soluble, thus achieves high concentration in brain and cerebrospinal fluid (CSF). Hence. it is mainly used in brain tumor, Hodgkin's disease, and meningeal leukemias.

Procarbazine

It is effective orally in Hodgkin's disease (MOPP regimen), non-Hodgkin's lymphoma, and brain tumors. One of the metabolites is a monoamine oxidase (MAO) inhibitor, hence it can lead to food/drug interactions.

Streptozocin

It is an antibiotic used in pancreatic islet cell tumors. Its most important ADR is nephrotoxicity.

Dacarbazine

It is used for malignant melanoma, soft-tissue sarcomas, neuroblastoma, and Hodgkin's disease. It is given IV and could lead to pain on extravasation.

Platinum-Containing Compounds

Cisplatin, Carboplatin

It is a heavy metal complex and a cell-cycle-nonspecific drug. It is given IV and has high protein binding. It is concentrated in kidney, liver, intestine, and testes; however, it does not cross blood-brain barrier (BBB). On entering the cell, it forms highly reactive platinum complexes which react with DNA. Hence, there is intrastrand and interstrand cross-linking. This causes DNA damage, hence inhibits cell proliferation. It is used in testicular, ovarian, endometrial and bladder, lung, gastric, and esophageal cancers. ADR: Since it is one of the most emetogenic drugs, prior 5HT3 antagonist, for example, ondansetron is necessary. Nephrotoxicity, which too is frequent, is reduced by good hydration and diuresis. Ototoxicity can be severe with repeated use. Electrolyte imbalance of K^+, Ca^{++}, Mg^{++} can occur. It is mutagenic, carcinogenic, and teratogenic.

Antimetabolites

Folate Antagonists

Methotrexate (MTX)

It is one of the most commonly used folate antagonists, which is cell-cycle-specific drug and acts during S phase. It has antineoplastic, immunosuppressant, and anti-inflammatory properties. MTX structurally resembles folic acid and competitively inhibits dihydrofolate reductase (DHFR). This prevents conversion of dihydrofolic acid (DHFA) to tetrahydrofolic acid (THFA), thus decreasing the latter. THFA is essential for synthesis of purines, pyrimidines, and DNA (**Fig. 70.5**). It also inhibits RNA and protein synthesis. It can be administered by oral, IM, IV, or intrathecal routes. It does not cross BBB, since it is highly bound to plasma protein. Their use includes the following conditions:

1. Choriocarcinoma (drug of choice).
2. Acute leukemia.
3. Burkitt's lymphoma.
4. Breast cancer.
5. Rheumatoid arthritis (low dose, i.e., 7.5–30 mg once weekly).
6. Organ transplantation.
7. Psoriasis.
8. Inflammatory bowel disease.

ADRs comprise megaloblastic anemia, pancytopenia, hepatic fibrosis, and osteoporosis. The drug interactions include the following: salicylates, sulfonamides, and tetracyclines increase MTX toxicity (as they displace it from protein binding sites). Nonsteroidal anti-inflammatory drugs (NSAIDs) and sulfonamides increase MTX toxicity (since they reduce its excretion). This can be managed by folinic acid rescue/leucovorin rescue. This agent decreases toxic effects on normal cells, hence permitting use of very high doses (mega pulse therapy) of MTX. Folinic acid is an active

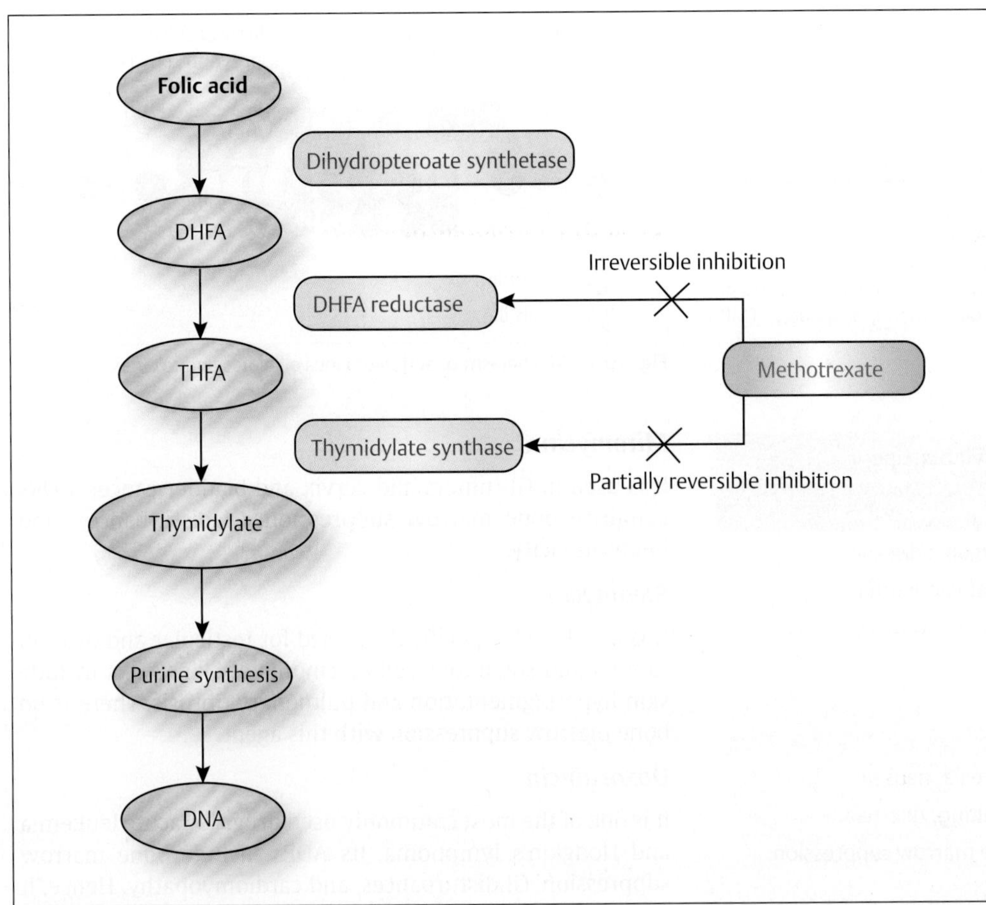

Fig. 70.5 Mechanism of action of methotrexate. DHFA, dihydrofolic acid; THFA, tetrahydrofolic acid.

coenzyme form, which bypasses block produced by MTX toxicity.

Purine Antagonists

6-Mercaptopurine (6-MP)

6-MP is activated to its ribonucleotide, which inhibits purine ring biosynthesis and nucleotide interconversion. It is a cell-cycle-specific drug that acts on S phase. It also has immunosuppressant effects. 6-MP is given orally. It does not cross BBB. It is metabolized by xanthine oxidase and excreted in urine. Allopurinol inhibits xanthine oxidase, hence it not only interferes with metabolism of 6-MP but also increases the effects of 6-MP. Therefore, allopurinol is combined to reduce the dose of 6-MP and prevent hyperuricemia. It is used for acute lymphoblastic leukemia and choriocarcinoma.

Fludarabine

It is an analog of vidarabine, an antiviral agent. It is converted to an active triphosphate derivative, which inhibits DNA polymerase and causes DNA chain breakage and termination. It is used for CLL and non-Hodgkin's lymphoma.

Pyrimidine Antagonist

Fluorouracil (FU)

It is a prodrug activated to deoxyuridine monophosphate. This interferes with DNA synthesis by inhibiting thymidylate synthetase enzyme. It is used mainly in GI, breast, ovary, and skin carcinomas and premalignant keratosis (topically) (**Fig. 70.6**).

Gemcitabine

It is a recently developed analog of cytarabine, which is used in pancreatic, lung, cervical, bladder, ovarian, and breast cancers.

Natural Products

Plant Products

Vinca Alkaloids

Vincristine and vinblastine are derived from the periwinkle plant. These are cell-cycle-specific drugs and act during M phase. The mechanism of action is identical for both these agents, that is, they bind to β-bulin and form drug-tubulin complex. Thus, there is disruption of mitotic spindle. Hence, chromosomes fail to move apart during mitosis, leading to a metaphase arrest and inhibition of cell division (**Fig. 70.7**). The uses of vincristine and vinblastine are mentioned in **Table 70.1**.

Taxanes

Paclitaxel is derived from the bark of the Western yew tree, while docetaxel is a newer taxane. These agent binds to β-tubulin and stabilizes polymerized tubulin. There is formation of abnormal microtubules (spindle poison), thus leading to inhibition of mitosis. It is administered by IV infusion for advanced breast and ovarian cancers, lung, esophageal, and bladder cancers. The ADRs include bone marrow suppression, peripheral neuritis, arthralgia, myalgia, and hypersensitivity reactions.

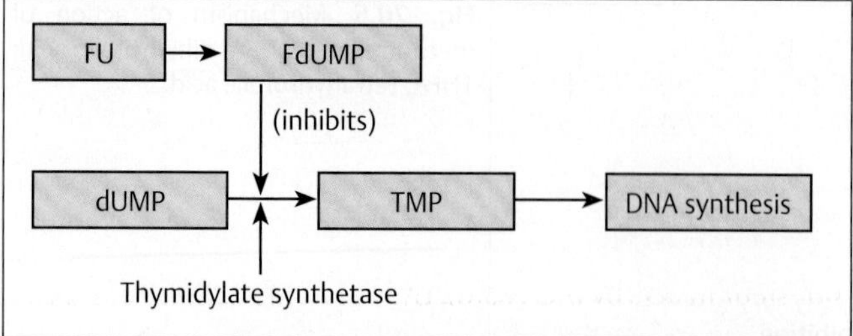

Fig. 70.6 Mechanism of action of fluorouracil. dUMP, deoxyuridine monophosphate; FdUMP, fluorodeoxyuridine monophosphate; TMP, Thymidine monophosphate

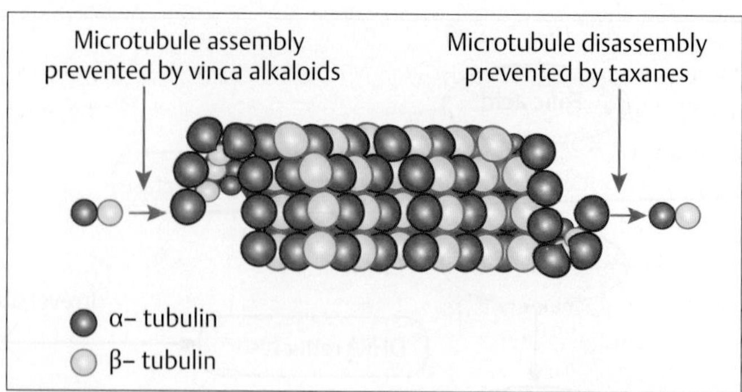

Fig. 70.7 Mechanism of action of vinca alkaloids and taxanes.

Table 70.1 Uses of vincristine and vinblastine

Vincristine	Vinblastine
Childhood leukemias	Hodgkin's disease
Childhood tumors	Breast carcinoma
Wilm's tumor	Testicular tumors
Neuroblastoma	
Hodgkin's disease	
ADR	
Peripheral neuritis	Anorexia, nausea
Constipation	Vomiting, diarrhea
Bone marrow sparing	Bone marrow suppression

Camptothecins

These agents bind and stabilize the DNA-topoisomerase 1 complex, hence inhibiting resealing function. However, the strand-breaking action is not affected. Hence, there is cell death. It is used for advanced ovarian, lung, colon, and cervical cancers. ADRs comprise bone marrow suppression and GI disturbances.

Epipodophyllotoxins

These include etoposide and teniposide which act in the S-G2 phase. It forms complex with DNA-topoisomerase II. This leads to DNA damage and strand breakage, hence there is cell death. Uses include testicular and lung cancer, non-Hodgkin's lymphoma, breast cancer, and AIDS-related Kaposi's sarcoma. The important ADRs are bone marrow suppression, GI side effects, and hepatotoxicity in high doses.

Anticancer Antibiotics

All are cell-cycle-nonspecific agents except bleomycin. They all have a direct action by causing an intercalation between adjoining nucleotide pairs on the same strand of DNA. This interferes with cell division.

Actinomycin D

It is used in Wilm's tumor, Ewing's sarcoma, and methotrexate-resistant choriocarcinoma. ADRs include bone marrow suppression and GI disturbances.

Mitomycin C

It is used in GI tumors and cervix and bladder cancer. ADRs comprise bone marrow suppression, GI disturbances, and nephrotoxicity.

Bleomycin

It is a cell-cycle-specific drug used for testicular and ovarian tumors and squamous cell carcinoma of skin. ADRs include skin hyperpigmentation and pulmonary fibrosis. There is no bone marrow suppression with this agent.

Doxorubicin

It is one of the most commonly used drugs for acute leukemia and Hodgkin's lymphoma. Its ADRs include bone marrow suppression, GI disturbances, and cardiomyopathy. Hence, it can cause congestive cardiac failure (CCF), hypotension, and arrhythmias.

Mithramcin

This drug decreases blood calcium by inhibiting the osteoclasts, hence it is used in hypercalcemia with bone metastasis.

Enzymes

L-Asparaginase

This agent is isolated from bacteria. Asparagine is an amino acid essential for protein synthesis. Normal cells can synthesize asparagine, since they contain enzyme asparagine synthetase. Cancer cells lack this enzyme, hence depend on external source, that is, extracellular fluid. L-asparaginase converts asparagine to aspartic acid. Its inhibition reduces the source of aspargine, hence inhibits protein synthesis. It is used in acute lymphocytic leukemia. The ADRs include:

- **H**ypersensitivity reactions, since it is an enzyme; it is allergic.
- **H**emorrhage due to inhibition of synthesis of clotting factors.
- **H**yperglycemia, due to insulin deficiency.
- **H**eadache.
- **H**allucinations and coma.

Hormonal Agents

They have only palliative effects.

Glucocorticoids

They have a marked lympholytic effect, hence it is used in acute leukemia and lymphomas. The other beneficial actions include the following:

- Anti-inflammatory action.
- Increases effect of antiemetics.
- Nonspecific antipyretic effect.
- Reduces hypersensitivity reactions due to certain anticancer agents.
- Controls bleeding.
- Controls hypercalcemia.
- Improves appetite.
- Produces euphoria.

Oestrogens

They are physiologic antagonists of androgens, hence used in androgen-dependent prostatic tumors. Fosfeterol, a prodrug, is activated to stilbesterol. Since it achieves a high concentration in prostate, it is used in prostate carcinoma.

Tamoxifen

It is an antiestrogen used in palliative treatment of hormone-dependent breast carcinoma.

Progestins

They are used in endometrial carcinoma.

Antiandrogens

Flutamide is a nonsteroidal agent which blocks androgen at receptor level, hence used for palliative treatment of advanced prostate carcinoma.

Finasteride

It blocks conversion of testosterone to dihydrotestosterone by blocking enzyme 5-α-reductase. Both flutamide and finasteride are used for palliative treatment of advanced prostate carcinoma. Finasteride is also useful for benign prostatic hyperplasia (BPH).

GnRH Agonists

Pulsatile and continuous administration of buserelin, goserelin, leuprolide, follicle-stimulating hormone (FSH), and luteinizing hormone (LH) suppresses pituitary gonadotropins (FSH and LH) by downregulating GnRH receptors. They are used in palliative treatment of advanced prostate and breast cancer.

Biological Response Modifiers

Hematopoietic Growth Factors

These include erythropoietin, myeloid growth factors like G-CSF, M-CSF, GM-CSF, and thrombopoietin, which are used to treat bone marrow suppression.

Interferons

The commonly used interferon is interferon α. It is used in hairy cell leukemia, Kaposi's sarcoma, and condylomata acuminate.

Interleukin 2

Aldesleukin acts by increasing the cytotoxic activity of T-cells. It induces effects of natural killer cells and also induces interferon production. It is used to induce remission of renal cell carcinoma. Its most important ADR is hypotension.

Tretinoin (All Transretinoic Acids)

This agent induces differentiation in leukemic cells. Hence, the leukemic promyelocytes lose their ability to proliferate. Therefore, it is used to induce remission in acute promyelocytic leukemia.

Amifostine

It provides selective cytoprotection to normal tissues. It activates an enzyme in normal tissues, which can inactivate the active form of cisplatin and radiation. This agent may stimulate bone marrow.

Miscellaneous

Hydroxyurea

It is an analog of urea which inhibits enzyme ribonucleotide reductase. Hence, it inhibits DNA synthesis. It acts on S phase and is orally effective. The most common ADR is skin pigmentation. It is used in patients with CML.

Protein Tyrosine Kinase Inhibitors

Imatinib

It is a selective inhibitor of tyrosine kinase. These enzymes take part in signal transduction and are also involved in pathogenesis of CML. Hence, it is a drug of choice in CML. It is also used in GI tumors that express tyrosine kinase. Dasatinib and nilotinib are used in imatinib-resistant cases.

Gefitinib inhibits epidermal growth factor receptor (EGFR) tyrosine kinase. EGFR is overexpressed in several malignancies. Hence, it is used in nonsmall cell lung cancers (NSCLCs) not responding to first-line drugs.

Sunitinib is used in renal cell carcinoma.

Thalidomide

This drug had been banned since many years and is now used again in patients of multiple myeloma. Its exact mechanism is unknown. It may act by stimulating T-cells and NK cells. Thalidomide inhibits angiogenesis, tumor cell proliferation, and modulation of hematopoietic stem cell differentiation. Its ADRs include sedation, constipation, peripheral neuropathy, and carpal tunnel syndrome.

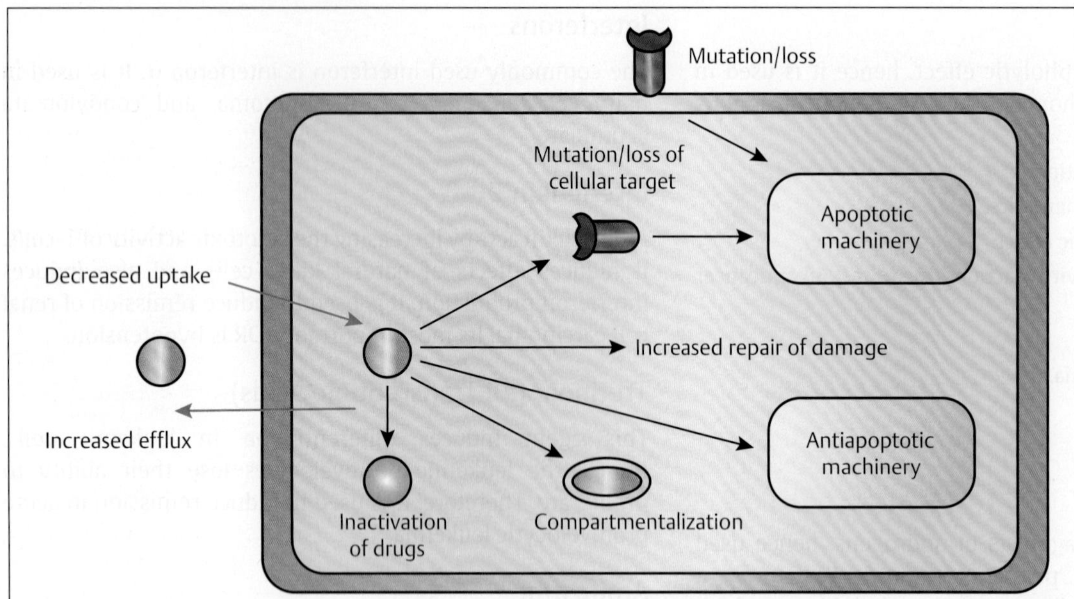

Fig. 70.8 Mechanism of anticancer drug resistance.

Monoclonal Antibodies

Since cancer cells express several antigens, these antigens are targeted by monoclonal antibodies. These agents are used for lymphomas and solid tumors. Rituximab targets CD20 antigen on B-cell and is used in B-cell lymphoma and CLL. It is also used as maintenance therapy to delay progression. It has a synergistic effect with chemotherapy. Rituximab sensitizes lymphoma cells susceptible to apoptotic effects of chemotherapy. Alemtuzumab binds to CD52 antigen on B- and T-cells and is used in lymphomas and CLL. Trastuzumab is a humanized antibody against human epidermal receptor 2 (HER2). HER2 receptor belongs to the family of EGFR. HER2 receptors are overexpressed in breast cancer cells and are also involved in resistance to chemotherapy. Hence, it is used along with or following chemotherapy in breast cancers (HER2 +ve).

Radioactive Isotopes

Radiophosphorus P32 is used in polycythemia vera. Its t½ is 14 days and is taken up by bone. They emit beta rays from bones. Strontium chloride also emits beta rays from bones. It has a longer $t_{1/2}$. It decreases pain in painful bony metastases. Radioactive iodine I131 is used in thyroid cancers.

Resistance to Anticancer Drugs

It could be primary, that is, nonresponsiveness from first exposure or secondary, that is, acquired during treatment (**Fig. 70.8**). The mechanisms include the following:

1. Reduced drug uptake.
2. Drugs are expelled from cells by transport proteins like P-glycoprotein.
3. Decreased activation of prodrug (MP, FU).
4. Increased inactivation (cytarabine).
5. Production of target enzymes.
6. Use of alternate metabolic pathway.
7. Altered target protein (e.g., modified topoisomerase II).

Hence, appropriate treatment of cancers is important for success

General Principles of Cancer Treatment

Chemotherapy is generally palliative and suppressive (except curable ones). Since cancers recur, avoid this by killing all the cells or as many cells as possible during treatment. This is known as "total cell kill." Besides chemotherapy, other modalities are surgery and radiotherapy. A combination of drugs is used for synergism to reduce adverse effects, and to prevent resistance. Avoid drugs with overlapping adverse effects. Maintain good nutrition, treat anemia, protect against infection, and adequately control pain and anxiety. Provide good emotional support, which helps in the management of this dreaded disease successfully.

Multiple Choice Questions

1. Cyclophosphamide is one of the most widely used alkylating agents because of its:

A. High-oral bioavailability.
B. Availability in both enteral and parenteral formulations.
C. Does not cause systemic toxicity.
D. Wide spectrum of action.

Answer: A

Cyclophosphamide is one of the most widely used alkylating agents because of its high-oral bioavailability.

2. Hemorrhagic cystitis is associated with:

A. Cisplatin.
B. Carboplatin.
C. Methotrexate.
D. Ifosfamide.

Answer: D

Hemorrhagic cystitis is a common manifestation of urothelial toxicity, which is caused by the metabolite acrolein. Mesna reacts specifically with this metabolite in the urinary tract, preventing toxicity. The agents implicated are cyclophosphamide and ifosfamide.

3. Ifosfamide skin pigmentation is associated with:

A. Busulfan.

B. Melphalan.

C. Cyclophosphamide.

D. Mechlorethamine.

Answer: A

Skin pigmentation is associated with busulfan.

4. Ototoxicity is seen with:

A. Methotrexate.

B. Cisplatin.

C. Carboplatin.

D. Oxaliplatin.

Answer: B

Ototoxicity is seen with cisplatin.

5. The drug that forms a complex with topoisomerase II to have antitumor activity is:

A. Etoposide.

B. Paclitaxel.

C. Vincristine.

D. Vinorelbine.

Answer: A

Epipodophyllotoxins such as etoposide form a complex with topoisomerase II to have antitumor activity.

6. The drug that acts by inhibiting the activity of topoisomerase I, the key enzyme responsible for cutting and relegating single DNA strand is:

A. Etoposide.

B. Irinotecan.

C. Paclitaxel.

D. Vincristine.

Answer: B

The drug that acts by inhibiting the activity of topoisomerase I, the key enzyme responsible for cutting and relegating single DNA strand, is irinotecan.

7. The drug that reduces renal toxicity associated with repeated administration of cisplatin is:

A. Leucovorin.

B. Mesna.

C. Amifostine.

D. Penicillamine.

Answer: C

The drug that reduces renal toxicity associated with repeated administration of cisplatin is amifostine.

Chapter 71 Antimicrobial Stewardship

Vasudeva Murthy, T. Smitha, and Asha B.

PH1.43: Rational use of antimicrobials including antimicrobial stewardship program.

Learning Objectives

- The emergence of antibiotic resistance.
- Antimicrobial stewardship program.
- Antibiotic stewardship program activities in India.
- Hospital antibiotic stewardship programs.

Background

Modern medicine uses antibiotic treatment as one of the approaches to combat infections. A number of antibiotics were developed between 1930 and 1960, and hence this period is considered the "golden era" of antibiotics. The advent of antibiotics made lethal infections treatable. The prompt initiation of antimicrobials reduced the morbidity and mortality.

The Emergence of Antibiotic Resistance

The misuse and overuse of antibiotics have resulted in the emergence of antibiotic resistance. The emergence of antibiotic resistance reduces the effectiveness of the antibacterial agent due to mutant strain.

The broader term antimicrobial resistance encompasses resistance to drugs to treat infections due to various types of pathogens, including bacteria, viruses such as influenza and HIV, malaria-causing parasites, and fungi such as *Candida* spp. The failure to treat infections due to bacteria is a serious threat to public health. Antibiotic resistance is imperiling the value of antibiotics, leading to the global crisis of therapeutic management. This is ascribed to the "exploitation" of antibiotics, unavailability of newer antibiotics, and demanding regulatory requirements. Factors such as subtherapeutic utilization of antibiotics also led to drug resistance, adverse effects, and the economic burden associated with extended hospital stay. Nonjudicious clinical uses of antibiotics are predisposing factors for antibiotic resistance. It is essential to optimize the use of antibiotics in treating infections, preventing adverse effects caused by unnecessary use of antibiotics, and combating resistance. The antimicrobial stewardship program promotes regularization of antibiotic utilization which helps to prevent the emergence of microbial mutant strains. This program is promoted by Infectious Diseases Society of America (IDSA), the Society for Healthcare Epidemiology of America (SHEA), and the American Society of Health-System Pharmacists (ASHP).

Antimicrobial Stewardship Program

The concept of stewardship involves the management of something, such as property, which is assigned to care. Antimicrobial stewardship program (AMSP) can be defined "as an organizational systemic health care strategy promoting appropriate use of antimicrobials through implementation of evidence-based interventions." According to the IDSA, antimicrobial stewardship covers "optimizing the indication, selection, dosing, route of administration and duration of antimicrobial therapy to maximize the clinical cure or prevention of infection, whilst limiting the collateral damage of antimicrobial use, including toxicity, the selection of pathogenic organisms and the emergence of resistance." This encourages an effective antibiotic prescription to improve the clinical outcomes. The main purpose of the antimicrobial stewardship includes making use of the antimicrobial agent in appropriate patient, appropriate indication, proper drug(s), proper administration of the dose, route, duration of treatment, use of antibiotics in appropriate combination, and its cost. The important constituents of antimicrobial stewardship include dedicated leadership, responsibility, pharmacy practice, diagnosis testing, and interventions for the better use of antibiotics. This part of the chapter deals with strategies for antibiotic preauthorization, formulary restriction, facility and infrastructure for antibiotic treatment along with tracking and reporting mechanism, conversion of intravenous (IV) antibiotics to oral dose, and consideration of pharmacokinetics and pharmacodynamic for drug dosage optimization.

Antimicrobial resistance (AMR) results in complicated illness, with prescription intervention for antibiotic replacement. The severity sometimes demands physician consultations, and it may result in death caused by the infections. The most common types of AMR are observed in skin infections, urinary tract infection (UTI), sexually transmitted disease (STD), and respiratory tract infection (RTI). Preponderance of antibiotic resistance is majorly due to the unwarranted use of antibiotics. AMR is seen more commonly in hospital-acquired infections than community-acquired infections. Colonization of microorganisms is seen in patients who have longer duration of exposure to the antibiotics. Approximately 30% of mortality correlates with multidrug-resistant (organisms, for example, *Staphylococcus aureus* and Enterococcus species. The meta-analysis data suggested a heightened risk of mortality among patients with methicillin-resistant *S. aureus* (MRSA) bacteremia compared to those with methicillin-susceptible *S. aureus*.

The antimicrobial stewardship team usually comprises a certified infectious disease (ID) physician, a clinical pharmacist, and a highly qualified director of clinical microbiology laboratory (**Fig. 71.1**). The microbiology laboratory works in tandem with infection control professionals, epidemiologists, clinical microbiologists, and information technology specialists. With the appropriate utilization of the antimicrobial agents, clinical pharmacologists and pharmacists play a major role in achieving goals and administering the antimicrobial stewardship program.

Antibiotic Stewardship Program Activities in India

In India, the giant responsibility of dealing with infectious diseases and related health issues are due to the unwarranted use of antibiotics. The uncontrolled abuse and overuse of the antibiotics in many conditions are baseless and are ungrounded, and result in AMR both in hospitals and in communities. The burden to reduce AMR and set up effective infection control in hospital settings is now on the health care system.

In a survey conducted by Indian Council of Medical Research (ICMR), infection control and antibiotics stewardship program at various government and private hospitals ascertained their clinical setup. This survey reviewed the approach of the hospitals to infection control guidelines, their AMS guidelines, and strategies engaged for AMSP. It recorded AMR data of the pathogens and the standard guidelines for treatment. The survey also noted the method of monitoring and auditing pattern practiced in the hospitals. It observed the deficiency of the infrastructure, in spite of the availability of the guidance document in the hospitals. Additionally, the inquiry revealed the lack of standard treatment guidelines in hospitals; even if the guidelines exist, they are not followed strictly. The survey

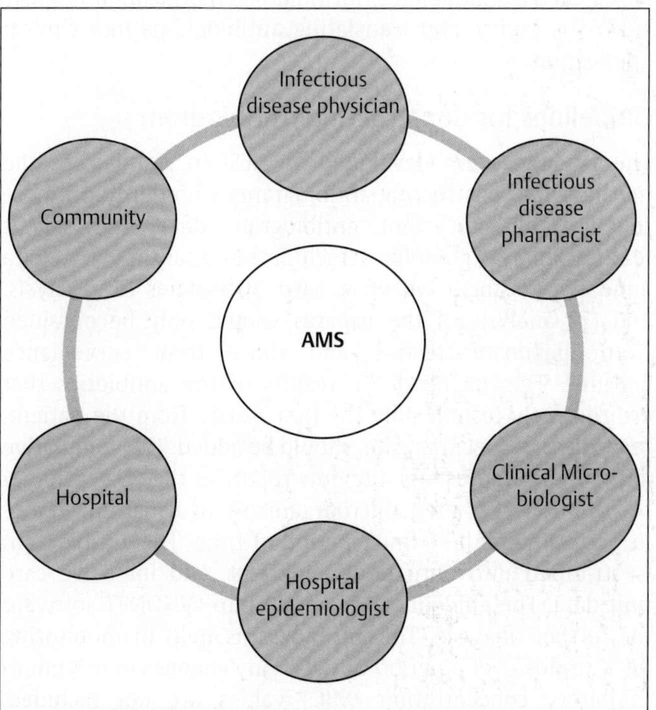

Fig. 71.1 Team of antimicrobial stewardship program (AMSP)

revealed that infection management practices in the country need to be strengthened and recommended customization of the guidelines based on hospital requirements. The ICMR survey stressed upon the need for coordination between microbiologists and physicians and called for monitoring and auditing mechanisms in all hospitals.

A survey, consisting of a detailed questionnaire, involving health care institutions is being carried out since 2013 in order to ascertain the practice of AMSP in India. Based on existing AMSP practices in India, a steering committee was set up by ICMR in 2013. On their recommendations, treatment guidelines are prepared for the clinical infection and hospital infections control (HIC). The survey was conducted based on the recommendation of the AMSP steering committee to gauge ground realities, plug loopholes, and strengthen AMSP. The questionnaire contained information such as bed strength, superspecialty services, audit of compliance, and antimicrobial agents (AMA) usage data analysis. Frequency, AMA prescription guidelines, AMA usage audit and feedback, and AMSP implementation outcome studies are included in the questionnaire.

Antimicrobial Stewardship Program in India

In February 2016, a recognized AMSP was established in India by adopting its contents from IDSA, SHEA, and the Centers for Disease Control and Prevention, centered around intervention and improvement of the institutional guidelines and postprescriptive audit with feedback. This AMSP encompasses physicians, intensivists, microbiologists, and clinical pharmacists.

Antimicrobial Resistance Surveillance and Research Network in India

The Antimicrobial Resistance Surveillance and Research Network (AMRSN) was initiated in India to collect data on six pathogenic groups mainly responsible for the AMR. This network's main aim is to identify the degree and prototype of AMR, in order to guide and plan for various approaches to control the expansion of AMR. This section describes the conception and implementation of AMR in India, focusing on the challenges, limitations, and benefits of the program. The combined resistance of the third-generation cephalosporins and fluoroquinolones, as well as the resistance of carbapenem, is a matter of concern, as it has effects on patients' outcome.

The data generated through AMRSN are used for preparing treatment guidelines and harmonizing treatment practices. The data demonstrated the process of resistance, prototype applicable to the community, and supporting efforts for the expansion of the AMR activities, which are helpful initiatives of the surveillance system. The test before health care settings is the expansion of present activities to the next levels. The ICMR, New Delhi, initiated the AMRSN in 2013 to gather data to understand the molecular mechanisms of bacterial resistance. The onus is with ICMR-AMRSN to institute the network of hospitals to observe the antimicrobial susceptibility profiles and identify clonality of the resistant antimicrobials. Data on resistant pathogens and AMR are disseminated to the concerned health care professionals for alternatives in disease prevention in addition to other treatment options for the emerging resistant strains. The network also promotes data management for collection and analysis.

Some of the key findings of ICMR-AMRSN targeted majorly clinically important bacterial and fungal pathogens. The data showed the dominance of gram-negative pathogens responsible for 90% of respiratory, 86% of urine, 73% of cerebrospinal fluid, 76% of sterile body fluids, and 55% of blood isolates in severe hospital-acquired infections. This information is based on the data and choice of antibiotics (ICMR-AMRSN 2016–2018). This surveillance network has been burdened with many challenges, from streamlining the quality data collection to data entries in each laboratory, apart from dedicated human resources to sustain the network. Periodic training sessions are also essential for sustaining the quality data collection. The ICMR network initiated the holistic approach toward AMR by engaging the relevant stakeholders, including the veterinary and environmental sectors in India. This step and understanding the epidemiological linkages help in identifying the opportunities for intervention, in order to control AMR in India.

Tertiary-care hospitals in India received the evidence for the trends of AMR found by the ICMR-AMRSN. Still certain tools are essential to draw meaningful outcomes from the data collected. The challenge is to scale up the data which truly represent the country and then permeate to the next levels of the health care system in both government and private hospitals while maintaining the quality. The latest scientific initiative also helps us to understand each component of AMR and devise suitable interventions.

The survey divulged various details based on its outcome, including standardization of health care system in India, accreditation of all hospitals including their diagnostic laboratories, provision of infection disease physicians in all secondary and tertiary care hospitals, appointment of clinical pharmacists in tertiary and secondary health care institutes for better medicines audit and proper therapeutic use, and frequent audit to assess how well guidelines are being followed.

Regularly reviewing the comprehensive record of health care-associated infections, analyzing the data of antimicrobial agents to specific infections, and promoting continuous research in all aspects of AMSP along with regular education and availability of guidelines are essential.

Limitations of Implementation of the AMSP

There are several barriers to the successful implementation of the AMSP in India: lack of (1) funding for the developing clinical protocol, (2) development of indigenously diagnostic tools, (3) antibiotic cycling, (4) training programs and surveillance studies, and (5) human resources in the area of infectious disease education programs and active involvement of the clinical pharmacists and microbiologists. The information technology (IT) tools must be made available to use computer-assisted programs and there also should be development of mobile phone applications. Lack of awareness among administrators can be stemmed by providing suitable platforms for discussion and making AMSP a part of the accreditation process. Prescriber education, refresher training, evidence-based guidelines, and frequent reminders on guidelines through electronic circulation are needed. Prescription audit and use of mobile applications for disseminating information on therapy would also go a long way in overcoming the above-mentioned limitations.

Antibiogram

The hospital antibiogram particularly helps in guiding empiric therapy and tracking the emergence of the bacterial resistance. This review of susceptibilities of the bacterial isolates is helpful to the clinicians, and they routinely use it in their clinical microbiology laboratory. Antibiograms track the resistance trends and facilitate the pattern of susceptibility of the organisms across various medical hospitals.

The free software WHONET, available for analysis, supports the extraction of data to report. The strategies developed by the Clinical and Laboratory Standards Institute (CLSI) help in standardizing and constructing antibiograms.

The WHONET software for data analysis enters only the first isolate from the patient. The patient's location and specimen type are included for the analysis. The most frequently isolated bacteria are presented in the antibiogram in a tabular format. The intranet facilities are adopted for an easy access for all clinicians. For the accreditation requirements, antibiotic policy is mandatory, and making an antibiogram foundation is essential prior to framing the antibiotic policy. To make the reliable information about antibiograms available, patients' details are incorporated for predicting the outbreaks. The role of a clinical microbiologist involves reporting of bacterial culture of susceptibility, based on CLSI guidelines, formulating the hospital empiric antibiotic policy, and translating antibiograms into clinical applications.

Guidelines for Constructing Antibiogram

The guidelines are developed by CLSI to standardize the methods for constructing antibiograms, in order to promote reliable and consistent antibiogram data. The salient features of the guidelines include (1) analyzing the data annually, (2) inclusion of at least 30 isolates for analysis, and (3) analysis of the isolates should only be obtained from diagnostic testing and those from surveillance cultures. This included the results of the antibiotics that are routinely tested. Only the first isolate from the patient, regardless of specimen site, should be added. The cumulative antibiogram represents a review report of the susceptibility of commonly isolated microorganisms to usual antibiotics in percentage in a definite period of time. The antibiogram is stratified into outpatient, inpatient, and intensive care unit data. The guidelines are added into WHONET software for further analysis. The antibiograms help in monitoring AMR trends over a period of time. Any changes in minimum inhibitory concentration (MIC) values are not included, and subtle changes below the resistance threshold (known as "MIC creep") are not included. The data do not pick up the patient's past antimicrobial history or infection, as the resistance pattern significantly changes with age. The data of antibiogram cannot be generalized to a specific population or location based on the hospital data.

Syndromic Surveillance

Syndromic surveillance is adopted where treatment is likely empirical and syndromic and where laboratory facilities are limited. Instituting an AMSP is demanding, particularly in community hospitals where resources are often limited. Nonavailability of clinical pharmacists and microbiologists who are trained in infectious diseases is the main concern for the management of community hospitals. The training must be provided to the clinical pharmacist and microbiologist in the area of syndrome-based action plans, together with definitions, severity, empiric regimens, and de-escalation and length of the treatment. The pharmacist must be involved in the prospective audit, and this must be established in the community hospitals. When the program is implemented in a hospital, it must be supervised by the ID physician. Antimicrobial therapy in certain sample size must be assessed for a minimum period of time, and assessment is carried out prior and subsequent to AMSP. Periodically, prospective audit and feedback are reviewed in a hospital.

Syndromic surveillance results in utilization of antimicrobial agents and expenditure incurred on the purchase of antimicrobials. This surveillance study reveals various types of infections occurring as a common syndrome. Such measures also help in intervention and de-escalation from broad-spectrum antibiotics, and this particularly helps in noncritical settings. Syndromic surveillance decreases the antibiotic use, helps to choose alternative antibiotics, and lessens antibiotic expenditure. Still AMSP remains a challenge in critically challenged ill patients. Access to ID physicians and guidelines are necessary to provide adequate support to the clinical pharmacist and microbiologist, in order to curb unnecessary antibiotic use. Expanding the list of syndromes may further force the physicians to choose antibiotics rationally.

Access, Watch, and Reserve

The World Health Organization (WHO), in the year 2019, developed a database on the recommendations of the expert committee on the selection and use of essential medicines.

The WHO initiated the global action plan to fight against antibiotic resistance, in order to improve the quality of antibiotic use in the hospitals. The Access, Watch, and Reserve (AWaRe) classification of the list of medicines speed up the stewardship interventions which are relevant to the inclusiveness of the overall hospitals. The data provided by the AWaRe antibiotic therapeutic applications could be used for their respective countries' stewardship intervention program. Various details of 180 antibiotics are categorized as access, watch, or reserve, together with their pharmacological classes and anatomical therapeutic chemical (ATC) codes.

Goals of AMSP in Reducing the Emergence of Antimicrobial Resistance

Awareness and understanding helps clinicians to prescribe the right drugs for the right disease at right doses. Optimal use of antimicrobials extends the lifetime of the effective antibiotics through their judicial use. Minimization of the adverse effects results in improved clinical outcomes. Integrated data surveillance improves the detection and control of the drug-resistant organisms. Implementation of the public health programs, reporting antibiotic resistance, and fostering antibiotic stewardship in health care setup and in the community are critical steps towards containing and mitigating AMR. Innovative diagnostic tests help in identification and characterization of resistant bacteria and aid in favorable treatment. Identification of the new drug target and nature of the microbes and accelerating the development of the new antibiotics reduce the development of resistant strains. Antibiotic resistance is a big issue worldwide. Hence, research and development and improving the international collaboration in antibiotic-resistance prevention program, surveillance, and control are needed.

Hospital Antibiotic Stewardship Programs

Many advances in the medical practices transformed the treatment of infections. Efficient initiation of antibiotics to treat infections lowers the morbidity and saves lives. To make AMSPs an effective tool, it needs appropriate drug selection, dosing interval, route of administration, and length of therapy. The clinicians improve patient care and safety, thereby lessening treatment failure, reducing the duration of the treatment by using appropriate therapy and prophylaxis, and decreasing AMR.

For a successful AMSP, evidence-based education is a must, as it not only favors de-escalation and optimal use of antibiotics but also promotes awareness on AMR to the public. This includes selection of an appropriate drug, dose, and dose interval. The main aim of AMSP includes the optimization and safe use of antibiotics to enhance clinical outcomes, appropriate therapy, reducing health care expenditure, and framing antibiotic policies and antimicrobial prescription.

The main components of the AMSP include active strategy, monitoring outcome, leadership commitment, accountability, drug expertise, action, tracking, reporting, and education. The success of AMSP leadership support is critical for the successful implementation and monitoring of the program. This consists of a regular schedule to report stewardship activity, resources, and outcomes to the clinicians, executives, and hospital management; monitoring of current resources, prioritizing resources and intervention plans, and implementing business plans; and regular meetings with stakeholders of the hospital and integration of the stewardship activities for quality improvement and safety of the patients.

Physicians, along with pharmacists, play an important role in leading an accountable program. A formal training in stewardship management helps program leaders with continued presence of full-time physicians improving the inpatient care with their supportive efforts. Epidemiologists and infection control professional skills help in auditing, analyzing, and reporting the data. The antibiogram report is generated and interpreted by the laboratory staff, which guides empiric therapy. The staff involved in the quality improvement team is concerned with medical quality and patient safety issues. By reviewing the medications, nurses too contribute and participate in the discussion of antibiotic treatment, indication, and duration.

With the help of pharmacodynamic dose optimization and review of doses, keeping in mind their therapeutic bioavailability, the pharmacist ideally acts as a coleader of the stewardship program to improve the effective use of the antibiotics. He/she also audits the antibiotics, resulting in significant cost savings. His/her expertise in the pharmacokinetics of antimicrobial agents is essential in proper utilization of the antimicrobial agents in patients with any organ failure or dysfunction. The policies of stewardship program promote the optimal use of antibiotics and interventions of three types: broad, pharmacy-driven, and infection syndrome–specific, prioritized on the needs of the hospital. Documenting the dose, duration, and indication is also essential to choose the interventions, based on the needs of the facilities and empirical management of antibiotics, while diagnostic information is pending. This part also involves dose adjustments and optimization of the therapy.

Action includes implementation of interventions, which is categorized based on infection, provider, pharmacy, microbiology, and nursing-based interventions. It is critically focused on indications such as lower RTI, UTI, and skin and soft-tissue infection for antibiotic use. The stewardship program should select the interventions that address the gaps between antibiotic prescriptions and to prioritize rational prescribing strategies such as prospective audit and feedback, preauthorization, and facility-specific treatment guidelines. Such approaches recommend evidence-based or foundational interventions for stewardship program, and this approach optimizes the therapy. Evaluation of tracking, reporting, and antibiotic use and outcomes demands the periodic assessment of the use of antibiotics or management of infections. This resolves the quality and quantity of use of antibiotics for therapeutic purposes in the clinical setup. Separate antibiotic audit forms assist in reviewing the drug use. To keep an eye on the emergence of resistance patterns, antibiotic prescription is evaluated along with their impact on interventions and other outcomes. Outcome measures consist of impact of interventions to improve antibiotic use and reduce antibiotic resistance. The antibiotic stewardship program minimizes drug cost, and a part of this program regularly updates on antibiotic use and its resistance to the prescribers, pharmacists, and nursing staff members. The prospective audit and feedback and preauthorization offer an effective and affordable method of antibiotic use. Several options are available that provide education on antibiotic use: by employing various methods such as developing algorithms, didactic presentation, flyer, posters, and newsletters among hospital staff members. Also, hospital staff members, physicians, pharmacists, and nurses can be educated on side effects, adverse reactions, antibiotic resistance, and optimal prescribing dose of antibiotics. All these are part of the stewardship program, along with patient education on antimicrobial agents.

Antimicrobial Stewardship Program Detailed in Intensive Care Units

Transmission of drug-resistant strains is highly prominent in patients admitted to intensive care unit (ICU) with acute illness, comorbidities, and aligned complications. These patients with reduced immunity are considered vulnerable to various infections and colonization by the resistant bacilli. Furthermore, the use of invasive medical devices or surgical procedures or insertion of catheters exposes them to the higher risk of nosocomial transmission of infections along with massive consumption of antibiotics, leading to the development and dissemination of drug-resistant strains. Generally, patients with critical clinical conditions are subjected to high-potent antibiotics and often for a longer duration.

In 2003, the Centers for Disease Control and Prevention reported that 60% of *S. aureus* isolates are resistant to methicillin in ICUs in the United States. It also mentions the select microorganisms developing resistance over time (**Table 71.1**). Likewise, **Table 71.2** from IDSA depicts the emergence of resistant strains in ICUs (ESKAPE).

The nosocomial transmission of infections is estimated to be 20 to 30%, resulting in prolonged hospital stay, development of complications, morbidity, mortality, and allied economic burden. Hence, the trained stewardship pharmacist in infectious diseases needs to apply stringent policy to observe carefully dispensing of antimicrobials. The nonjudicial prescribing practices of antimicrobials result in less improved outcomes, increased morbidity and mortality from adverse reactions and toxicity, superinfection, and colonization with drug-resistant bacilli and development of altered gut flora, for example, development of *Clostridium difficile*.

The strategies of the stewardship team in the ICU include:

1. Providing evidence-based interventions.
2. Setting definite goals, indicators, and targets for improved outcome.
3. Proper data handling system with feedback provided to prescribers.
4. Identifying and solving the knowledge gaps.

The optimized and appropriate antibiotic use is obtained by following the framework of antibiotic care bundle (ACB) in the ICU. This includes:

1. Documenting the purpose of indication of the antibiotic, which helps in understanding the pathology and institutional antibiogram.

Table 71.1 Select germs showing resistance over time

Antibiotic approved or released	Year released	Resistant germ identified	Year identified
Penicillin	1941	Penicillin-resistant *Staphylococcus aureus*	1942
		Penicillin-resistant *Streptococcus pneumoniae*	1967
		Penicillinase-producing *Neisseria gonorrhoeae*	1976
Vancomycin	1958	Plasmid-mediated vancomycin-resistant *Enterococcus faecium*	1988
		Vancomycin-resistant *Staphylococcus aureus*	2002
Amphotericin B	1959	Amphotericin B-resistant *Candida auris*	2016
Methicillin	1960	Methicillin-resistant *Staphylococcus aureus*	1960
Extended-spectrum cephalosporins	1980 (Cefotaxime)	Extended-spectrum β-lactamase-producing *Escherichia coli*	1983
Azithromycin	1980	Azithromycin-resistant *Neisseria gonorrhoeae*	2011
Imipenem	1985	KPC-producing *Klebsiella pneumoniae*	1996
Ciprofloxacin	1987	Ciprofloxacin-resistant *Neisseria gonorrhoeae*	2007
Fluconazole	1990 (FDA approved)	Fluconazole-resistant *Candida*	1988
Caspofungin	2001	Caspofungin-resistant *Candida*	2004
Daptomycin	2003	Daptomycin-resistant methicillin-resistant *Staphylococcus aureus*	2004
Ceftazidime-avibactam	2015	Ceftazidime-avibactam-resistant KPC-producing *Klebsiella pneumoniae*	2015

Abbreviation: KPC, *Klebsiella pneumoniae* carbapenemase.
Source: Reproduced with permission from the website of the Centers for Disease Control and Prevention,.

Table 71.2 IDSA depicting the emergence of resistant strains in ICUs (ESKAPE)

Microorganism	Resistant to the antibiotic
Enterococcus faecium	Vancomycin-resistant *Enterococci*
Staphylococcus aureus	Methicillin-resistant *Staphylococcus aureus*
Klebsiella pneumoniae	Carbapenem-resistant *Klebsiella pneumoniae*
Acinetobacter baumannii	Carbapenemase-producing *Acinetobacter baumannii*
Pseudomonas aeruginosa	Imipenem-resistant *Pseudomonas aeruginosa*
Enterobacteriaceae	Extended-spectrum, β-Lactamase-producing *Enterobacteriaceae*

2. Performing the culture in sterile.
3. Prescribing empiric antibiotics, considering susceptible organisms in the ICU and institutional guidelines.
4. Recording the initiation and anticipated hold dates of antibiotics to help reduce misuse.
5. De-escalation of therapy, based on the active pathogen, from broad-spectrum antibiotics to the pathogen-specific, narrow-spectrum antibiotic.
6. Mentioning the antibiotic "time-out" strategy. This is preferred 48 to 72 hours after the initiation of antimicrobial agents to determine the need to continue the antimicrobial therapy. This helps in shorter course of therapy with health benefits and cost effectiveness.
7. Medical devices acting as nidus for infection must be removed when not in need, for example, catheters.

Therapeutic Drug Monitoring

Therapeutic drug monitoring (TDM) is an approach measuring the drug concentrations in patients to determine the pharmacodynamics of the dose. The key aspect of TDM is to attain the accurate plasma concentration of narrow therapeutic index drugs, based on clinical practice of drug–effect relationship. The dosage should be purposed based on the individual patients' clinical condition. TDM is preferred for those drugs with narrow therapeutic index or therapeutic window and those with pharmacokinetic differences. The narrow therapeutic index of the drugs lies between the maximum and minimum therapeutic dosages (**Fig. 71.2**). These drugs may cause therapeutic failure due to subtherapeutic dosages or may cause adverse drug reactions,

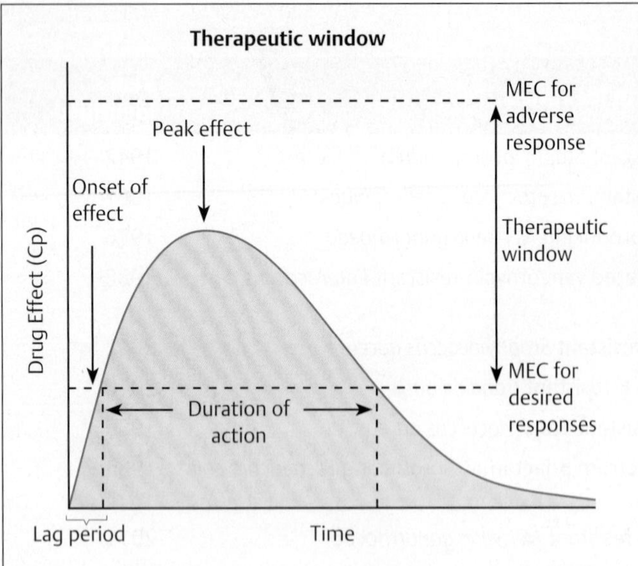

Fig. 71.2 Graph representing narrow therapeutic index.

life-threatening events requiring hospitalization, or morbidity or mortality. The following are the few antibiotics with narrow therapeutic index: β-lactams, quinolones, linezolid, aminoglycosides (gentamicin, tobramycin, amikacin), and glycopeptides (vancomycin, teicoplanin). It helps in avoiding overdose and toxicity in acute and critical conditions of the patients, improving the drug efficacy. In general, the recommended dosing of the antimicrobials is based on the derivations from noncritical clinical conditions or from healthy volunteers. Using TDM, the recommended maximum daily dose of a drug can be calculated for attaining adequate serum level and trough concentration in altered pharmacokinetics, drug–drug interactions, liver and renal dysfunctions, aged individuals, newborn, pregnancy, and obesity.

Vancomycin is used to treat serious and life-threatening infections of MRSA. The trough serum concentrations of vancomycin should be maintained at 10 mg/L for all infections to reduce the emergence of resistance and at 15 to 20 mg/L for complicated infections. According to the 2020 vancomycin monitoring guidelines of DoseMeRx pharmacokinetics model, it requires a loading dose of 25 to 35mg/L in critically infected patients with MRSA with normal renal function.

The high doses of vancomycin result in serious events such as ototoxicity and nephrotoxicity. The steady-state concentration is maintained by dosing the patient at regular intervals. The drug distributes throughout the body and is removed through renal system, which depends on the age, body mass index, renal function, comorbidities, and medications. Nephrotoxicity, a life-threatening side effect of vancomycin, usually occurs in few patients in the first 10 days of dosing. Baseline investigations are much required to monitor such side effects, and pharmaceutical care monitoring is mandatory in patients receiving concomitant medications that have an influence on renal function, for example, aminoglycosides and amphotericin B.

The maximum dose should not exceed beyond 3,000 mg per day. Sometimes, it is preferential to measure area under the curve (AUC) to reduce the toxicities of the drug. Although TDM is a burden to the patient, it is a cost-effective approach, and implementing TDM in regular clinical practice among antimicrobial stewardship may reduce the risk of emergence of resistance and bring therapeutic benefit.

The software tools that help adjust the doses according to altered pharmacokinetic conditions are Kinetidex, WinNonlin, PK Solver, PharmPK, Kinetica, etc.

Surgical Site Infection

The Surgical Care Improvement Project (SCIP) suggests measures to focus on antibiotic use to prevent surgical site infections (SSIs). These include:

1. The initiation of prophylactic antibiotics.
2. Appropriate antibiotic selection and dosing.
3. Discontinuation of antibiotics within 24 hours of surgery (48 hours for patients with cardiac surgery).
4. Appropriate redosing for patients undergoing prolonged procedures.

Antibiotics in Neonatal ICU

Infections are the main causes of hospitalization in newborns. The common organisms include group *B. streptococcus*, *Listeria monocytogenes*, and *Escherichia coli*, which cause a variety of infections such as sepsis, pneumonia, meningitis, and UTIs. The rational medication of antibiotics should consider anticipated pathogens, indications of the drugs, age, and proportional drug formulations with efficacy and safety. The major categories of drugs in neonates include drugs belonging to β-lactam antibiotics, aminoglycosides, vancomycin, which requires adjustment in duration, route, dosage, and its duration of administration. The antimicrobial therapy should be discontinued by 36 hours after the initiation of therapy and on recovery of patient's clinical condition, negative blood culture, and clinical diagnosis suspected for infection lessening. Procalcitonin (PCT), a 116-amino acid precursor of calcitonin and a biomarker of inflammation, can be used to evaluate and direct the duration of antibiotic therapy. Its level in the blood elevates within 2 to 4 hours in conditions such as bacterial infections, sepsis, malaria, and pancreatitis, and peaks on the second day. The level falls off rapidly during the recovery period. Although PCT is considered for shortening antibiotic courses, it is to be weighed for its impact on clinical decisions and economic burden on the patient.

Antimicrobial Stewardship Metrics on Consumption and Costs

Antimicrobial stewardship is an effectual process that brings changes in economic realities in health care. In the late 1980s, the inventory of antimicrobials emerged with 40% of the hospital expenditure, which surmounts those for all other drugs in hospitals in the current scenario. A simple approach for reducing the cost is by switching from IV to oral antibiotic. At the same dosage, oral antimicrobials cost less compared to their IV formulations. Moreover, IV forms involve cost of administration, IV tubing, injections, and, sometimes with phlebitis, requirement of dressing, as well as antiseptics in any complication. The same antibiotics given in oral formulation would not bear all the cost implied in IV administration nor have any complications.

The measure of economical and clinical outcomes can be assessed with the rate of antimicrobial use, as per a standardized number of patients. This is performed by considering the metrics of the defined daily dose (DDD), day of therapy (DOT), or length of therapy (LOT).

Rate of antimicrobial use, as per a standardized number of patients = DDD/ DOT.

The WHO promotes the use of DDD, which is based on the "assumed average maintenance dose per day for a drug used for its main indication in adults. To estimate the antibiotic use, the total numbers of grams of antibiotic used over the period of interest are divided by the WHO-assigned DDD. Comparisons with antibiotic use by other hospitals can then be done, usually by expressing DDDs per 1,000 patient days (PD). DDD defines the average daily dose in a patient, which ignores the patient-specific health-related factors and considers similar health profiles in all patients treated. Hence, it is replaced by DOT, which represents the administration of a single agent on a given day, regardless of the number of doses administered or the dose strength.

Rational Prescribing Strategies in Terms of Minimizing Resistance

The active stewardship program in hospital generally reduces antimicrobial prescribing for nonbacterial infections, preserves the efficacy, reduces the development of resistant strains, and prevents the occurrence of adverse effects of the drugs. It ensures the algorithmic approach for antimicrobial prescribing for patient's safety and efficacy, and helps in attaining quality-adjusted life year.

The mission of the antibacterial stewardship team in reducing the AMR is to initiate and execute research that detects and reduces the emergence of antibacterial resistance. Economically beneficial, novel, and rapid molecular diagnostic tests that allow the detection of pathogens and drug resistance help in optimizing the antimicrobial therapy, for example, monoplex polymerase chain reaction (PCR) testing and multiplex PCR panels, microarray panels, peptide nucleic acid fluorescent *in situ* hybridization (FISH) technologies, magnetic resonance–based testing, and matrix-assisted laser desorption ionization-time of flight mass spectrometry (MALDI-TOF MS). The IDSA/SHEA recommend two fundamental strategies: preauthorization and formulary restrictions, and prospective audit and feedback strategies for rationale prescribing for the effective antibiotic stewardship. The following are the strategies that enhance rational prescribing of antimicrobials.

Preauthorization and Formulary Restriction

Prior approval from the stewardship team is essential to the front-line prescriber for the use of certain antibiotics. It helps optimize the initiation of empiric therapy, as it allows the decision of expert input on antibiotic selection and dosing, which prevents adverse effects, for example, sepsis. The preauthorized restrictions for antimicrobial formulary may be absolute or conditional and are based on specific patient health-related factors, such as specific disease states, allergies, and antimicrobial history, or on drug-specific criteria, such as maximum LOT and limitation to combination therapy. The formulary restrictions on the antimicrobial order form placed prospectively allows the hospital stewardship evaluating to evaluate the quantity and the quality of prescribing practice. The antimicrobial stewardship team plays a crucial role in validating the antimicrobial agent for a clinical condition and hence enhances safety of the patient by the restricted use approach of antimicrobial agents.

Outcomes

Restricting the utilization and proper usage of antimicrobials reduces the emergence of resistant strain and horizontal transmission from one individual to another.

Advantages

Outcome of patients can be predicted with the help of prior and proper screening of suitable active antibacterial agent. The prior screening of an antimicrobial agent enhances the right therapy and builds the education process. The stewardship team involved in discussions with the prescribers ensures optimal therapy to the patient.

Limitations

Generally, the interventions are exempted only in few cases and have a limitation in implementing the same for all the patients with similar health profile. In few instances, patient health may be affected due to delay in the approvals in the antimicrobial therapy.

Prospective Audit and Feedback Strategies or Postprescription Review or Handshake Stewardship

Antimicrobial stewardship provides prescribing recommendations after an antibiotic has been used for approximately 72 hours. It is an oversight process in which there is prescription audit and feedback (verbal or written communication–medical notes) to the prescriber for any improper use of the antimicrobial agent. The priority is to identify the clinical conditions and correct the order for optimal antimicrobial medication. These strategies are employed after the dispensing of the drug to the patient. It authorizes a specialist to audit the disproportionate agents, provide feedback to the prescriber, and enhance the antimicrobial care among the patients. Prospective audit and feedback in hospitals employ antimicrobial specialist or a pharmacist trained in infectious diseases. The antimicrobial use is evaluated against a set of approved guidelines to ensure the optimal use of drug therapy. The computerized clinical decision support system (CDSS) identifies patients' antibiograms, tracks antimicrobial consumption, identifies patients to target by disease state, hospital location, or infecting organism, and interacts with clinicians to provide feedback for the required therapy in any resistance. The implementation of CDSS in hospital improves health outcomes and minimizes the cost.

Outcomes

It reduces inappropriate antimicrobial use, drug resistance, and economic burden.

Advantage

Discussions among the specialist, stewardship personnel, and the prescriber output the best antimicrobial therapeutic approach. The review by the pharmacist, ideally trained in infectious diseases, or physician directs the appropriateness of the antimicrobial agent targeted at a pathogen, points toward alternative agents, and offers cost-effective alternatives and rationalized therapy. It facilitates an individualized patient care and improves the global hospital-based outcomes. It is one of the sources for any interventional approach in need. It also allows minimizing the prescription of broad-spectrum antimicrobial agents, preventing mutant strains.

Facility-Specific Treatment Guidelines

It enhances the effectiveness of the prospective audit and feedback and preauthorization. It establishes clear recommendations for optimal antibiotic use at the hospital. These guidelines optimize antibiotic selection and duration, particularly for common indications, for example, community-acquired pneumonia, UTI, intra-abdominal infection, skin and soft-tissue infection, and surgical prophylaxis.

Strategies of Rational Drug Use in ICU

These include de-escalation of empiric antibiotics to narrow spectrum, based on culture sensitivity results and regular clinical assessments. In few instances, the longer antibiotic courses of 7 to 14 days with broad-spectrum antimicrobials may not necessarily improve the patient outcomes and may increase the risk of multidrug-resistant organisms, adverse events, and higher health care costs.

The strategies to reduce the duplication of antimicrobials include:

1. A thorough review for any medication errors, essential to investigate similarities of the agents prescribed or being utilized by the patient.
2. Maximization of the efforts of stewardship by regulating stringent operations for formulary tracking antimicrobial usage, maintaining an adequate inventory, and reordering.
3. Fortifying the prescription with the specific active antimicrobial agent against the involved microorganism, with appropriate economic benefit approach.
4. A thorough analysis of medical literature review that supports a clinical indication, providing equivalent therapeutic effect.
5. Limiting the time duration while utilizing the broad-spectrum antibiotics for empiric treatment with antimicrobials to 48 or 72 hours.
6. Streamlining or de-escalation reduces antibiotic use and saves costs. Additional clinical documentation reviewed for continuation of the empiric treatment or for considering alternative agent.

Recommendations of ABS Program

Antimicrobial agents are known for their efficacy and low risk of toxicity. This tendency of low toxicity led to exploitation and inappropriate utilization of these drugs, which led to the establishment of antimicrobial stewardship. New molecules have been invented with proven potent efficacy than the earlier existing ones. The guidelines framed by the IDSA in collaboration with the SHEA serve to configure various stewardship programs. California has made it compulsory to assess the antimicrobial utilization in acute illness. The antimicrobial stewardship must be involved in quality improvement programs for the judicious usage of antimicrobials. It requires the documentation of the clinical and economic burden of the activities involved with AMSP for the continual conductance of the program.

The antimicrobial agent should be characterized for its use in empiric therapy, culture sensitivity, resistance, or prophylactic use in surgery. The empiric treatment of broad-spectrum antimicrobials should be specified for 48 or 72 hours and the need should be reviewed. The interventions essential in treating specific infectious diseases and syndromes with improved antibiotic use should be implemented, along with regular evaluations. This adaptation improves prescribing and reinforces clinical guidelines and algorithms, with sustained improvement in the outcome. Regular review of antimicrobial medication order enforces a prompt regulation of the antibiotic time-outs and stop orders. Tracking the retrospective records provides feedback and educates the proper prospective utilization of the antimicrobial agent. For precise clinical outcomes, it depends on the goals and size of the interventions, and this will have an impact on the improved antibiotics usage. Inappropriate antibiotics use can be minimized in neonatal ICUs by suitably employing the antibiotic stewardship interventions, which also prevent antibiotic resistance. The team of stewardship must offer its help to the clinical practitioners, in order to minimize the antibiotics usage in terminally ill patients.

The timely conversion of IV to oral antibiotics reduces the economic burden on the patient, and the appropriate choice of antibiotics reduces length of hospital stay. To enhance the clinical outcomes in immunocompromised patients, properly employing the antifungal antibiotics is helpful in hospitals and to the clinicians who work closely for the interventions with primary teams of hematology-oncology and solid organ transplant providers.

Allergy assessments, penicillin skin testing, and treatment strategies should be developed and promoted, for example, β-lactam antibiotics. Antibiotic use in the hospitals should be measured using DOT in preference to DDD. Antibiotic costs should be measured based on antimicrobial prescription order or administrations instead of assessing expenditures on antibiotic use. Implementation of computerized CDSS into the electronic medical record (EMR) at the time of prescribing helps in streamlining the work of antimicrobial stewardship team by identifying opportunities for interventions.

Pharmacokinetic monitoring and dosage adjustment programs for aminoglycosides and vancomycin should be implemented to reduce costs and decrease adverse effects. Stratified antibiograms (by location, age) should be developed and compared with nonstratified antibiograms in association with microbiology department for improved empiric therapy. This stratification identifies the differences in susceptibility and helps establish optimized treatment recommendations and guidelines. Rapid diagnostic tests along with the conventional culture sensitivities on blood specimens should be encouraged to optimize antibiotic therapy with improved clinical outcomes. Clinical guidelines for management of fever and neutropenia in hematology and oncology patients should be developed to reduce unnecessary antibiotic use and improve outcomes.

The AMSP should help in execution and provide integrated pharmacy training to the hospital staff members. Pedagogic guidance among health professionals in the form of lectures and informational pamphlets should be implemented to reduce the inappropriate antibiotic use. Development of necessary facilities is essential for a specific clinical practice guidelines and algorithms to standardize the pattern and implementation of the antimicrobial medical practices to a specific region. A structured program collaborating various departments of the hospital, facility-based treatment, competent staffing, and stringent vigilance on the open formularies at community level helps reduce the emergence of the mutant and resistant strains in the patients and environment.

Part XI

Endocrine Pharmacology

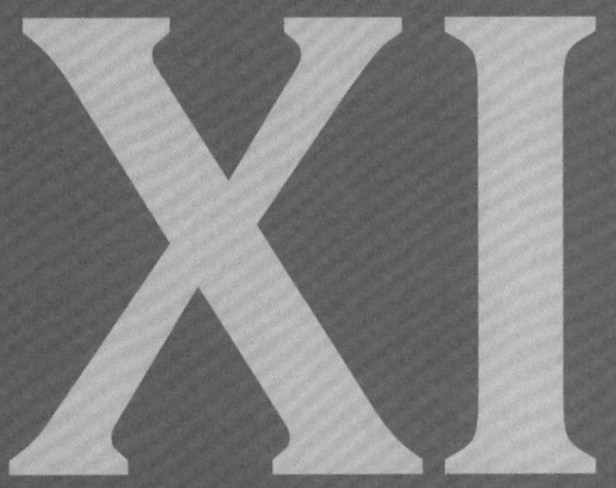

Chapter 72

Hypothalamic and Anterior Pituitary Hormones

Arunachalam Muthuraman, Aswinprakash Subramanian, and Jagadeesh Dhamodharan

PH1.37: Describe the mechanisms of actions, types, doses, side effects, indications, and contraindications of hypothalamic and anterior pituitary hormones and their drugs.

Learning Objectives

- Anterior pituitary gland hormones.
- Growth hormone.
- Octreotide.
- Prolactin inhibitors.
- Gonadotropin preparations.
- Gonadorelin agonists.
- Diagnostic uses of thyroid-stimulating hormone (TSH) and adrenocorticotropic hormone (ACTH).
- Vasopressin and its analogs.

Hormones Secreted by Anterior Pituitary Gland

The hypothalamus region lies in the center of the brain and the inferior and anterior side of the thalamus. Further, it is a master of all glands and controls the body functions. The gland of the hypothalamus is located in the middle part of the basal brain. It is encapsulated within the central portion of the third ventricle of the brain. It has an interconnection to the pituitary gland via a stalk-like infundibulum (a funnel-shaped cavity or structure).

Functional Anatomy of Hypothalamus and Pituitary Gland

This hypothalamus-pituitary complex acts as the "commanding center" of all active endocrine systems. Because the hypothalamus-pituitary complex has a strongly correlated function to secrete several hormones and produce the response of various target tissues, it especially regulates the synthesis and secretion of other gland hormones. Further, it also coordinates functions between endocrine and nervous systems. Sometimes, the nervous system stimulates the hypothalamus-pituitary complex to secrete hormones and initiate responses. The pituitary gland is a bean-sized organ which lies beneath the hypothalamus and rests at the base of the skull. It consists of two lobes, that is, anterior and posterior lobes. Both lobes secrete different hormones in response to the arrival of signals from the hypothalamus regions. Commonly, the pituitary gland is called the *hypophysis* (roundish) organ. The anterior pituitary gland is known as the *adenohypophysis* (mainly covered with glandular tissue and developed from the primitive digestive tract) organ, while the posterior pituitary gland is known as the *neurohypophysis* (mainly covered with neural tissue) organ. Various hormones are secreted from anterior and posterior pituitary glands. Further, the intermediate zone (tissue located between the lobes) is also able to secrete a specialized hormone, that is, melanocyte-stimulating hormone (MSH). The details of pituitary gland hormones and their functions are summarized in **Table 72.1**.

The connection between the hypothalamic and anterior pituitary glands is involved in the neurovascular system. Moreover, some of the neuron connections also contribute to the regulation of pituitary gland hormone secretion either directly or indirectly. Based on vascular connections, anterior pituitary hormones' secretion is strictly controlled by hypothalamic hormones. The supply of hypothalamic hormones to the anterior pituitary gland occurs via the following routes: (1) branches of hypophyseal arteries ramify as a capillary bed in lower hypothalamus regions via capillary blood flow; (2) hormones drain from those blood capillaries into *hypothalamic-hypophyseal portal veins*. The branch of hypothalamic-hypophyseal portal veins allows the blood flow toward the adjuvant branch of capillaries in the anterior pituitary gland; (3) anterior pituitary gland capillaries carry the hormones and drain into the systemic blood vessels (vein). The same veins also collect posterior pituitary gland hormone via capillary blood flow mechanism (**Fig. 72.1**).

Moreover, the secretion of the hypothalamic hormone is controlled by complex autonomic neuronal connections. This autonomic neuronal connection has two kinds of neurons, that is, afferent and efferent neurons toward hypothalamic tissue. Both afferent and efferent neuron pathways are involved in the regulation of hypothalamic hormone secretion. These neurons are mostly unmyelinated, and they are well-connected to limbic, midbrain tegmentum, pons, and hindbrain areas of the brain. This autonomic neuron can release norepinephrine (also called noradrenaline) in cell bodies and nerve terminal sites, that is, hindbrain end and different parts of the hypothalamus area of the brain. Furthermore, hypothalamic neuronal control mechanisms are mainly dominated by the posterior pituitary gland (**Fig. 72.2**).

In the posterior pituitary gland, the paraventricular neurons are connected to the hindbrain and spinal cord neurons. It plays a role in the regulation of oxytocin and vasopressin secretions of the posterior pituitary gland via the

Table 72.1 Pituitary gland hormones and their functions

Pituitary regions	Associated hormones	Chemical nature	Target organs	Functions
Anterior lobe	GH	Protein	Liver, adipose tissue	Promotes body tissue growth by direct as well as indirect actions. Controls the protein, lipid, and carbohydrate metabolism.
Anterior lobe	PRL	Peptide	Mammary glands	Promotes milk production and milk secretion.
Anterior lobe	TSH	Glycoprotein	Thyroid gland	Stimulates the synthesis, secretion, and release of thyroid hormone.
Anterior lobe	ACTH	Peptide	Adrenal gland (cortex)	Stimulates the secretion of corticosteroids.
Anterior lobe	FSH	Glycoprotein	Ovary and testis	Regulates reproductive organs via reproductive hormones.
Anterior lobe	LH	Glycoprotein	Ovary and testis	Control of reproductive function.
Posterior lobe	ADH	Peptide	Kidney	Stimulates water reabsorption (conservation) of body water.
Posterior lobe	Oxytocin	Peptide	Mammary glands and uterus	Induces the milk ejection from breastfeeding women (after the birth of the baby) and uterine contractions (during childbirth).
Intermediate zone	MSH	Peptide	Hypothalamus, skin and fat cells	Stimulates melanin formation in melanocytes. Suppresses appetite.

Abbreviations: ACTH, adrenocorticotropic hormone ADH, antidiuretic hormone; FSH, follicle-stimulating hormone GH, growth hormone; LH, luteinizing hormone; MSH, melanocyte-stimulating hormone; PRL, prolactin; TSH, thyroid-stimulating hormone.

release of epinephrine in the hindbrain and the end of the ventral hypothalamus. Moreover, intrahypothalamic system, composed of dopaminergic neurons which release dopamine in the arcuate nucleus, end hypothalamic-hypophyseal portal artery and capillaries. Further, the serotonin-secreting neurons also project to hypothalamus regions of the brain from the raphe nuclei area. Therefore, hypothalamic nuclei function and secretion of the hormone are under the control of certain specialized cells of the midbrain. The specialized neuron cells secrete and release dopamine, noradrenaline, and serotonin at their nerve terminals. These biomolecules also known as neurotransmitters are responsible for excitation of hypothalamic nuclei. This system is called "monoaminergic neurotransmitter neurons." Furthermore, it is highly sensitized with visceral (deep inward feelings rather than to the intellectual) responses like environmental and emotional factors (stress). The release of nanogram quantities of hypothalamic hormones is sufficient to influence the release of a microgram level of trophic hormones, and target glands release milligram levels of hormones. Thus, this amplifier cascade system regulates the original hypothalamic signals via the multiply and remultiply processes of interlinked endocrine functions. Endocrine gland secretion molecules are known as "hormone." The hormone is defined as the presence of known chemical structures, which is synthesized by specialist cells of the endocrine gland. It is released in the bloodstream and passes the message to various parts of the body and vital organs. Hence, they are known as "chemical messengers." Moreover, hypothalamic hormones are categorized as hypothalamic regulatory hormones. Based on function, there are two varieties of hypothalamic regulatory hormones, the hypothalamic releasing hormones and hypothalamic inhibitory hormones. The details of hypothalamic regulatory hormones are listed in **Box 72.1** and **Fig. 72.3**.

Box 72.1 Hypothalamic regulatory hormones

I. Hypothalamic releasing hormones

- Gonadotropin-releasing hormone (GnRH)
- Thyrotropin-releasing hormone (TRH)
- Somatotropin-releasing hormone (SRH)/growth hormone-releasing hormone (GHRH)
- Corticotropin-releasing hormone (CRH)
- Melanocyte stimulating hormone (MSH)
- Prolactin-releasing hormone (PRH)

II. Hypothalamic inhibiting hormones

- Somatotropin release inhibiting hormone (SRIH)/growth hormone release inhibiting hormone (GHRIH)
- Melanocyte release inhibiting hormone (MRIH)
- Prolactin release inhibiting hormone (PRIH)

These hypothalamic regulatory hormones play a vital role in the regulation of the pituitary gland. Besides, anterior pituitary lobe has vascular connections from the hypothalamus region of the brain, while posterior pituitary lobe undertakes major neural communication arriving from the central part of the hypothalamic region. In the embryo, the neuronal evagination process starts from the floor of the

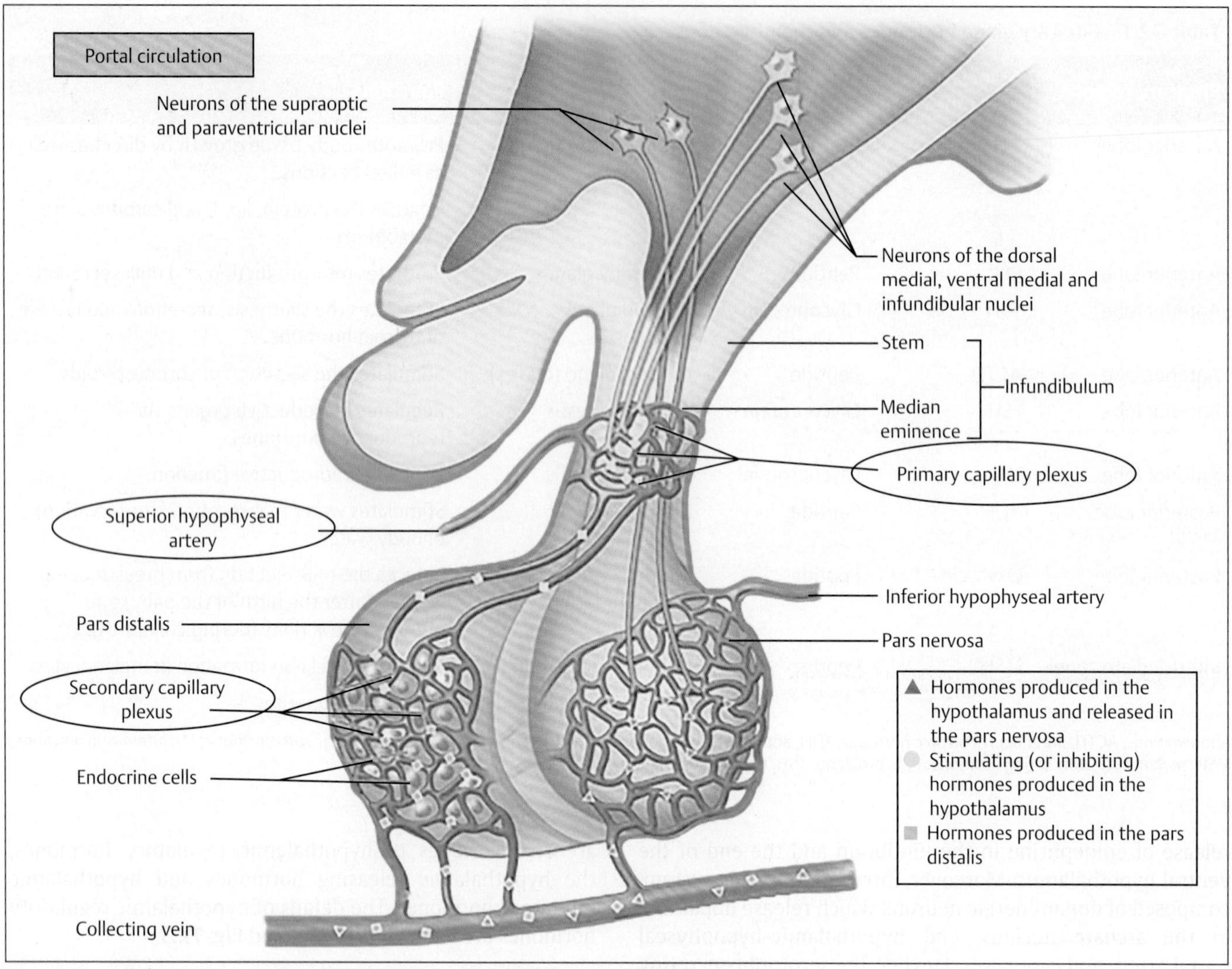

Portal circulation
Neurons of the supraoptic and paraventricular nuclei
Neurons of the dorsal medial, ventral medial and infundibular nuclei
Stem
Infundibulum
Median eminence
Primary capillary plexus
Superior hypophyseal artery
Inferior hypophyseal artery
Pars distalis
Pars nervosa
Secondary capillary plexus
Endocrine cells
Collecting vein
▲ Hormones produced in the hypothalamus and released in the pars nervosa
● Stimulating (or inhibiting) hormones produced in the hypothalamus
■ Hormones produced in the pars distalis

Fig. 72.1 The pattern of hypothalamic-hypophyseal portal circulation on the pituitary gland.

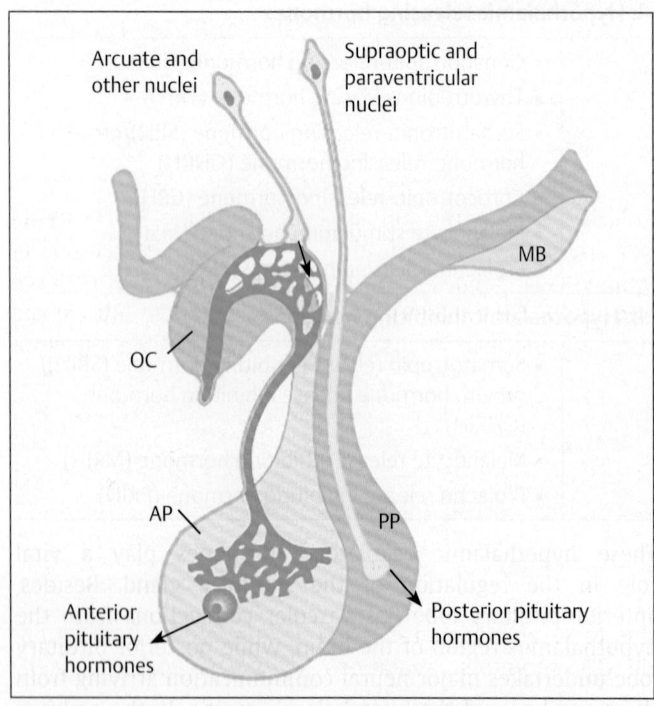

Fig. 72.2 Pituitary hormones and their control. AP, Anterior pituitary; MB, mammillary body; OC, optic chiasma; PP, Posterior pituitary.

third ventricle. In the adult, a large part of nerve endings is arranged from cell bodies of supraoptic and paraventricular nuclei. Further, it spread over to the posterior pituitary gland (known as a hypothalamohypophysial tract). The supraoptic fibers ended in the posterior lobe of the pituitary gland, whereas the paraventricular fibers partially ended in the median eminence of the pituitary gland. This autonomic (sympathetic) unmyelinated nerve fiber has a wide area of connection with the brain, that is, limbic, pons, and hindbrain areas. Hence, it is rapidly sensitized with multiple visceral stimuli (factors), that is, temperature, neuroendocrine hormone, appetitive, defensive reactions, and body rhythms (circadian rhythms: physical, mental, and behavioral changes). The list of primary hypothalamic regulatory mechanisms is summarized in **Table 72.2**.

Anterior pituitary hormones are considered as drugs for various hormone-associated ailments, as they regulate the body homeostasis condition via control of other endocrine glands. Besides the condition of hormonal imbalance and deficiency, pituitary (endogenous and/or exogenous) hormones contribute to maintaining the health status. They have agonistic and antagonistic effects on various tissues, depending upon the condition of the biological environment. Hence, they are used in replacement therapy, as a diagnostic

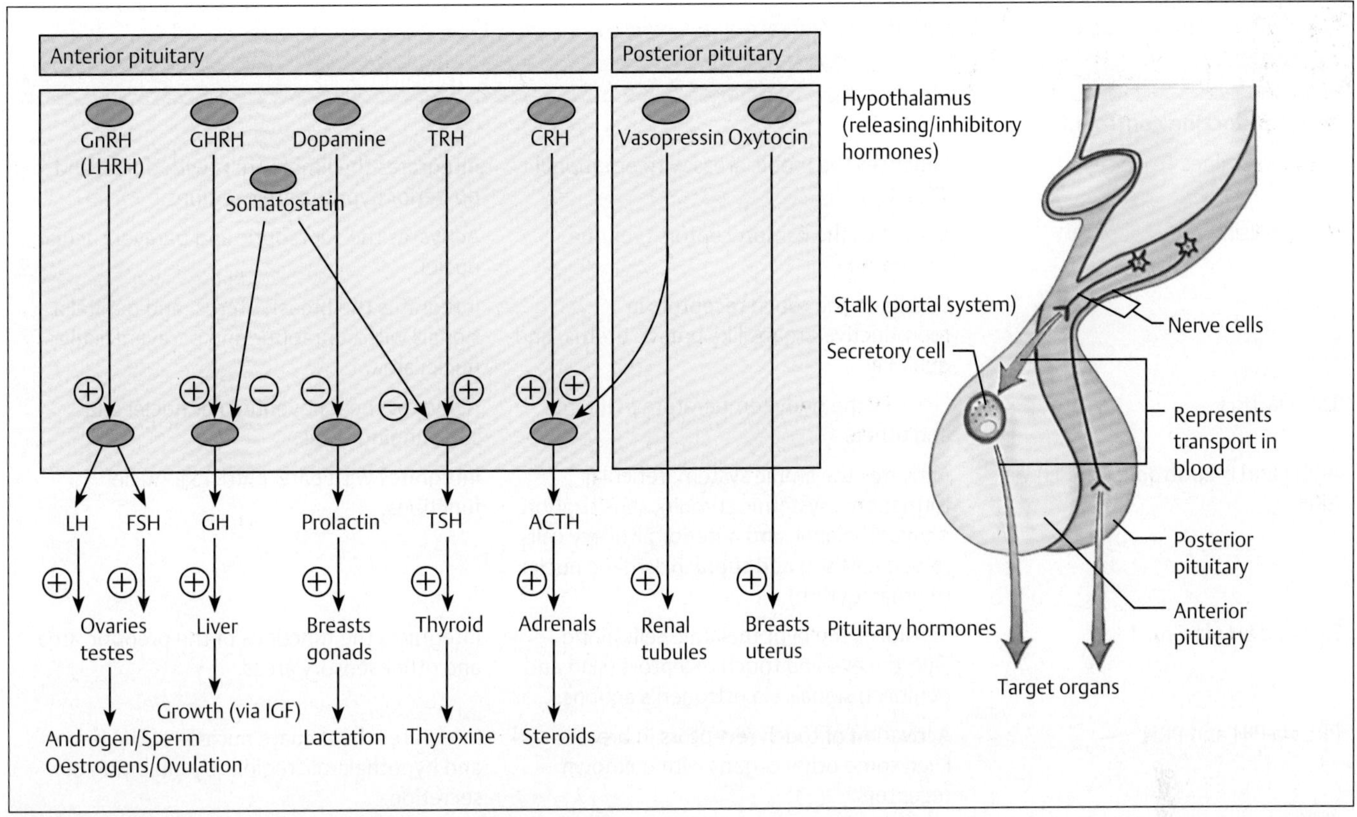

Fig. 72.3 Hypothalamic releasing and pituitary trophic hormones

agent, and as a blocking agent of anterior pituitary hormones. Some of the features of anterior pituitary hormones are cited in **Table 72.3**.

Growth Hormone

The growth hormone is an anterior pituitary hormone. It is an essential hormone promoting body growth in childhood and adolescence. It produces lipid and carbohydrate metabolism and regulates body mass and bone density. The major mechanism of GH promotes body mass growth via insulin-like growth factor-1 (IGF-I). IGF-I is also known as somatomedin-C (somatotropin). In congenital or acquired deficiency of GH in childhood or adolescent stage, the patient fails to reach the normal adult height and body mass while there is disproportional body fat and decrease the muscle mass.

Chemically, GH has 191-amino-acid peptide with two sulfhydryl bridges. The structure of the GH closely resembles prolactin. Earlier, GH was isolated from the pituitaries of human cadaver tissue for the treatment of GH disorders. However, it was found to have various complications such as Creutzfeldt–Jakob disease due to contaminated peptides with prions; hence, this approach was discontinued. Currently, the recombinant technology-based GH is produced and known as somatropin from GH. It has an identical GH peptide chain (191-amino-acid sequence) which mimics the native form of human GH actions.

Mechanism (Pharmacodynamics)

GH binds to cell surface receptors and activates the Janus kinase (JAK)/ signal transducer and activator of transcription (STAT) signaling pathway. The JAK/STAT pathway is a cytokine receptor superfamily. Briefly, it has two distinct GH receptor-binding sites. Further, it enhances the dimerization of two GH receptors and activates the JAK/STAT signaling process. In this condition, cells undergo complex effects, that is, cell growth, increase in body composition, and carbohydrate, protein and lipid metabolism raising the production of IGF-I in liver tissue. Further, it acts on bone, cartilage, muscle, kidney, and other tissues, which leads to enhancement of the autocrine or paracrine functions. In bone, it stimulates longitudinal growth until the closing of epiphyses (it happens near the end of puberty). In children and adults, GH enhances the anabolic effects in muscle and catabolic effects in adipose cells, which leads to maintenance of the balance of body mass via an increase in muscle mass and reduces the adiposity signals. These (direct and indirect) effects of GH are mixed due (**Fig. 72.4**) to opposite actions of GH and IGF-I on the insulin sensitivity process in tissue compartments. GH reduces insulin sensitivity, leading to mild hyperinsulinemia, and raises blood glucose levels. In contrast, IGF-I has insulin-like effects on glucose transport. In the clinical setup, GH is unable to respond to patients due to severe resistance to GH. It occurs due to mutations of GH receptors, mutations of postreceptor signaling

Table 72.2 Primary factors of the hypothalamic regulatory mechanism

Hormone/Factors	Mechanisms	Integrating areas
Neuroendocrine control of		
Catecholamines	Enhances the limbic areas with emotional stimuli.	Integrates the limbic areas with dorsal and posterior hypothalamic regions.
Vasopressin	Sensitizes the osmoreceptors (volume receptors).	Activates the supraoptic and paraventricular nuclei.
Oxytocin	Sensitizes the touch receptors in reproductive organs like breast, uterus, and genitalia.	Integrates the breast, uterus, and genitalia signals with supraoptic and paraventricular nuclei area.
TSH via TRH	Elevates the body temperature in infants and others.	Activates the paraventricular nuclei and surrounding areas.
ACTH and b-lipotropin (b-LPH) via CRH	Activates the limbic system; reticular formations (systemic stimuli); sensitization of hypothalamic and anterior pituitary cells (blood cortisol) and suprachiasmatic nuclei (diurnal rhythm).	Integrates with paraventricular nuclei functions.
FSH and LH via GnRH	Sensitizes the hypothalamic cells along with the eye and touch receptors (skin and genitalia) signals via estrogen's actions.	Integrates the functions of the preoptic area and other sensory areas.
PRL via PIH and PRH	Activation of touch receptors in breasts. Even some other organs with unknown receptors.	Integrates the arcuate nucleus of the brain and hypothalamic regions by inhibition of secretion.
Growth hormone via somatostatin and GHRH	Unknown receptors	Integrates the functions of the periventricular nucleus and arcuate nucleus.
Appetitive behaviors		
Thirst	Activation of osmoreceptors in organum vasculum; and uptake of angiotensin II in the subfornical organ.	Integrates the communication of lateral superior hypothalamus to thirst sensory areas.
Hunger	Sensitization of glucostat cells for glucose utilization; and leptin receptors for polypeptides action.	Integrates the function of ventromedial, arcuate and paraventricular nuclei, and lateral hypothalamic regions.
Sexual behavior	Anterior ventral hypothalamus plus and piriform cortex cells sensitized with circulating estrogen, androgen, and other local hormones.	Integrates the anterior ventral hypothalamus and piriform cortex information.
Body temperature		
Temperature	Sensitizes the thermoreceptors of skin, deep tissues, spinal cord, hypothalamus, and various parts of the brain.	Integrates with anterior hypothalamus for heat; and posterior hypothalamus for cold stimuli.
Defensive reactions		
Fear and rage (violent uncontrollable anger)	Sensitizes the sense organs and neocortex area of the brain.	Integrates with deep limbic system and hypothalamus.
Circadian rhythms		
Body rhythmicity	Activation of the retina via retinohypothalamic fibers.	Integrates with suprachiasmatic nuclei.

Abbreviations: CRH, corticotropin-releasing hormone; ACTH, adrenocorticotropic hormone ADH, antidiuretic hormone; FSH, follicle-stimulating hormone; GHRH, growth hormone releasing hormone; GnRH, gonadotropin-releasing hormone; GH, growth hormone; LH, luteinizing hormone; LPH, lipotropic hormone; PIH, prolactin-inhibiting hormone; PRH, prolactin-releasing hormone; PRL, prolactin; TRH, thyrotropin-releasing hormone; TSH, thyroid-stimulating hormone.

Table 72.3 Analogs of anterior pituitary hormones

Drugs	Drug descriptions
Sermorelin	Recommended for the treatment of dwarfism and prevention of HIV-induced weight loss.
Somatotropin (rhGH)	Recommended for the treatment of dwarfism, deficiency of GH, acromegaly, and prevent weight loss in HIV patients.
Pegvisomant	It acts as a GH receptor antagonist. Recommended for the treatment of acromegaly.
Mecasermin	It is recombinant IGF-1. Recommended for the treatment of growth failure in pediatric patients with primary IGF-1 deficiency.
Tetracosactide	Acts as a diagnostic agent for the screening of adrenocortical insufficiency patients.
Corticotropin	
Tesamorelin	GHRF analog. Recommended for the treatment of excess loss of abdominal fat in HIV patients (lipodystrophy condition).
Somatrem (rhGH)	Recommended for the treatment of adult growth hormone deficiency, Turner's syndrome, chronic renal failure, and SGA.
Thyrotropin alfa	It is a recombinant TSH. As a diagnostic agent for thyroid cancer.
Mecasermin rinfabate	Used for the treatment of severe primary IGF deficiency.

Abbreviations: GH, growth hormone; GHRF, growth hormone-releasing factor; IGF, insulin-like growth factor; rhGH; recombinant human growth hormone; SGA, small for gestation age; TSH, thyroid-stimulating hormone.

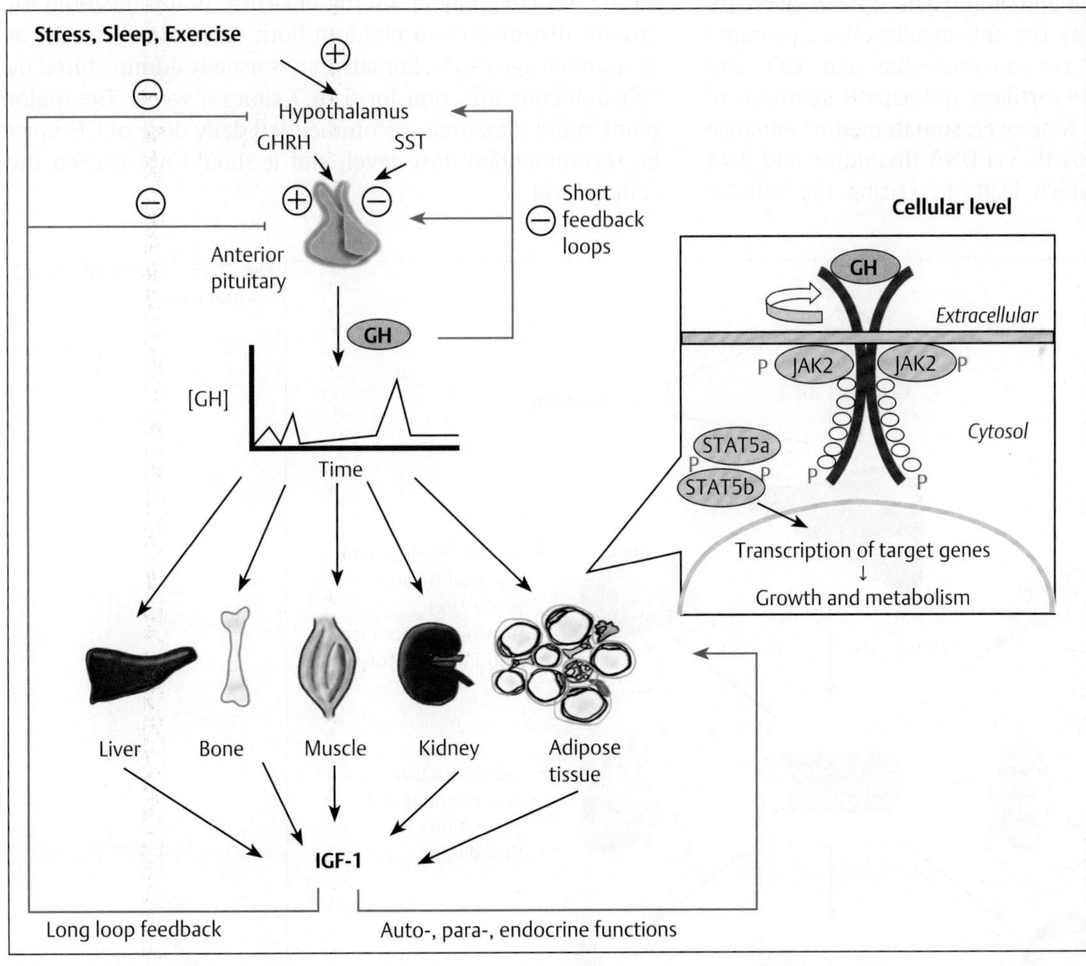

Fig. 72.4 Mechanism of action of growth hormone (GH).

proteins, and/or development of GH antibodies. Moreover, the administration of recombinant human IGF-I may cause hypoglycemia due to its insulin-like effects.

Pharmacological Effects

Pharmacologically, GH acts as a regulator of metabolism of carbohydrate and lipids along with controlling the body mass and bone density. The pharmacokinetics of GH is variable, based on the preparations. The naturally circulating endogenous GH has 20 minutes of half-life duration, and it is metabolized by the liver. The recombinant human GH (rhGH) is administered via a subcutaneous (SC) route 6 to 7 times per week. The peak plasma levels of GH are reached within 2 to 4 hours and these levels persist for 36 hours in circulation (**Fig. 72.5**).

There are two different types of GH, that is, somatropin and somatotropin, which are employed in the regulation of the growth process via the metabolism process of carbohydrate and lipids. Somatotropin is a naturally biosynthesized form of the pituitary hormone, whereas somatropin is synthesized with the help of recombinant DNA technology. GH has various pharmacological actions like insulin-like effects that lead to raising the glucose and amino acid uptake, decrease the lipolysis process, delay the anti-insulin effect, promote the longitudinal growth via somatomedins and IGFs, and stimulate the growth plate cartilage and hepatic synthesis of IGF-I and IGF-II peptides. Moreover, somatomedins enhance the processes of bone growth, via DNA thymidine and RNA uridine incorporation, which leads to raising the cellular proliferation and conversion of proline to hydroxyproline for cartilage synthesis. The GH deficiency conditions are because the reduction of somatomedin levels lead to short stature. Short stature occurs with various conditions like IGF-I deficiency due to a higher level of GH secretion. The development of dwarfism is due to the absence of IGF-I during the pubertal surge (pygmies).

Dosage and Administration

The normal dose of GH is 0.375 mg/kg/week. The maintenance of the GH phase is less dose-dependent on GH. The response with GH treatment is variable, based on age, child height standard deviation score (SDS), midparental height, and a dose of GH. The normal catch-up phase (at 2 to 3 years of age) of GH treatment produces the height gain from 1.2 to 2.0 SDS. The dosage of somatropin preparation is administered with the variable dose, based on individual child growth patterns and variability of child condition. For GH deficiency condition, 23 to 39 mg of GH/kg/day or 0.7 to 1.0 mg of GH/m^2 is recommended. For Turner syndrome and chronic renal insufficiency (CRI), about 45 to 50 mg of GH/kg/day or 1.4 mg of GH/m^2 is administered. Moreover, 35 mg of GH/kg/day or 1.0 mg of GH/m^2 is administered for growth disturbance in children born (premature) small for gestational age (SGA). Somatropin is usually administered by subcutaneous injection for 6 to 7 times a week. The major point is the maximum recommended daily dose of GH must be recommended dose level, and it should not exceed the ceiling level.

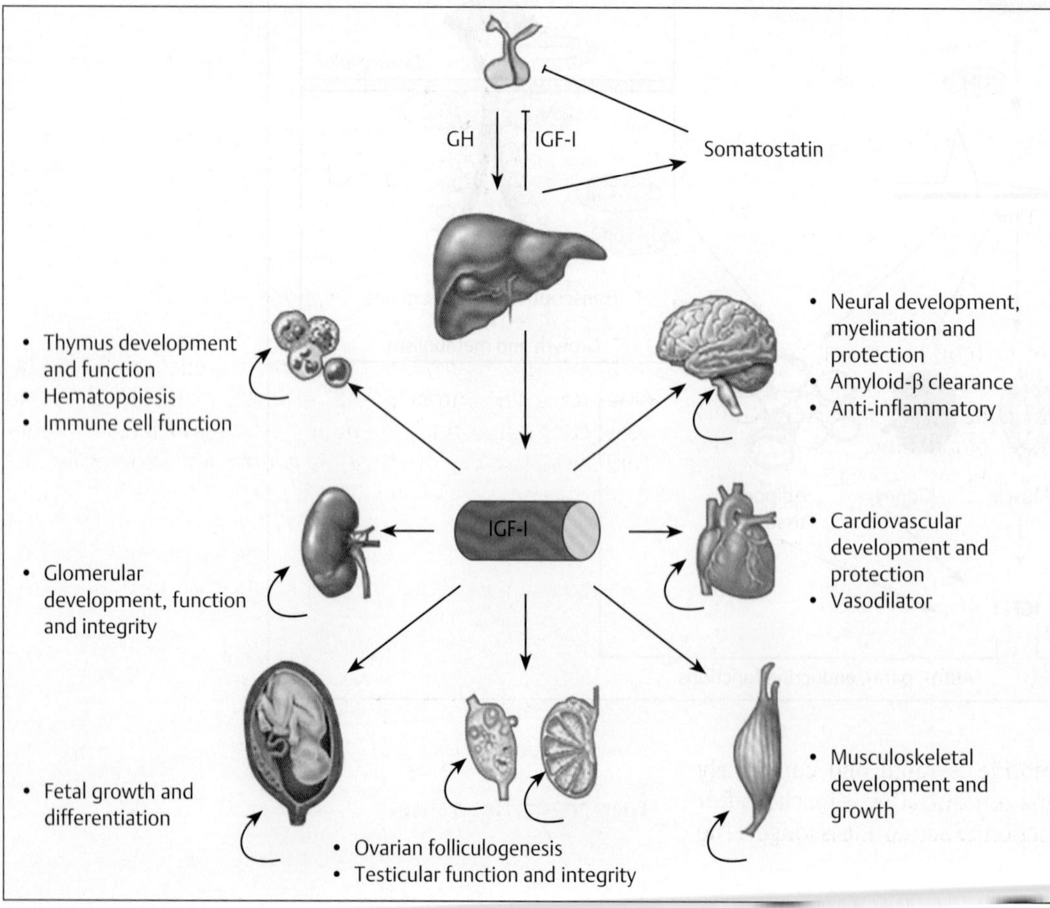

Fig. 72.5 Effects of growth hormone (GH).

Side Effects

Headache, edema, growth failure, acromegaly, arthralgia, myalgia, and carpal and tarsal tunnel syndromes are very common. Rarely, it produces tinnitus, atrial fibrillation, hypertension, acute intracranial hypertension, Reynaud's syndrome, and gynecomastia. The major adverse effects of hypersecretion of GH are rapid growth due to slipped capital femoral epiphysis in limps, especially in the lower extremity, and development of slow progression of leukemia incidence. The impairment of GH occurs due to untreated hypothyroidism, diabetes mellitus, and diabetes insipidus.

Indications

Generally, GH is used for GH deficiency, Turner syndrome, CRI (mainly with pretransplantation), and SGA.

Contraindications

Acute malignancy, other endocrinological disorders, benign intracranial hypertension, proliferative diabetic retinopathy, pregnancy, and lactation.

Octreotide

Octreotide is a synthetic analog of somatostatin. The acetate salt of a cyclic octapeptide is mimicked the natural somatostatin. It has 40 times more potent inhibitory action on GH, glucagon, and insulin than its natural hormone. First, octreotide was synthesized by Wilfried Bauer in 1979.

Mechanism

Octreotide is readily bound to the somatostatin receptor, and it belongs to G-protein coupled receptor superfamily (GPCR). Octreotide inhibits the pertussis toxin, which is sensitive to the GPCR receptor, followed by adenylate cyclase activity and calcium influx. Further, it also enhances the phosphotyrosine phosphatase enzyme activity and activation of sodium-hydrogen (Na^+/H^+) exchanger functions.

Pharmacological Action

The pharmacologic actions of octreotide are similar to that of natural somatostatin. It inhibits GH, glucagon, and insulin. It reduces the luteinizing hormone (LH) response to GnRH stimuli, reduces the splanchnic blood flow, and decreases serotonin, gastrin, cholecystokinin secretin, motilin, pancreatic polypeptide, vasoactive intestinal peptide, and TSH release. Moreover, it also reduces the secretion of intestinal and pancreatic fluids, reduces the motility of gastrointestinal (GI) content, inhibits gallbladder contraction, decreases certain anterior pituitary hormones, induces the vasoconstriction, and reduces portal blood vessel pressures. Besides, it has potential analgesic effects via partial agonistic action on the mu-opioid receptor.

The SC injection of octreotide is rapid and completely absorbed. The maximal plasma concentration is reached after 30 minutes. The duration of action of octreotide is longer. The half-life ($t_{1/2}$) of octreotide is 90 minutes. Octreotide is mainly eliminated via biliary excretion. The average elimination $t_{1/2}$ of octreotide is 100 minutes (1.7 hours) by SC injection, whereas the elimination rate of octreotide by intravenous (IV) injection is faster than SC injection ($t_{1/2}$ 10–90 minutes).

Dosage

The starting dose of octreotide is 20 mg every 4 weeks, and in subsequent weeks, the dose of octreotide is increased 30 mg/every week. Rarely, the dose needs to increase up to 40 mg/every week when octreotide resistance is developed. The SC administration of octreotide can start with an initial dose of 50 µg for three to four times per day. The maximal permitted dose of octreotide is 1.5 mg per day.

Side Effects

Generally, octreotide is well-tolerated by most patients. The discontinuation of octreotide treatment causes transient GI symptoms. The common side effects of octreotide are nausea, abdominal pain, intestinal discomfort, flatulence, and diarrhea due to the inhibition of pancreatic exocrine secretions. Rarely, it develops the malabsorption and steatorrhea via alteration of pancreatic enzymes. Octreotide also produces the lithogenic effect and gallbladder sludge and gallstones due to inhibition of cholecystokinin secretion. Some patients also showed erythema and burning sensations at the injection site. The repeated administration also showed the formation of painful subcutaneous nodules. The direct effect of octreotide on the reduction of gastrin secretion alters the intrinsic factor of the coagulation cascade, and it can raise the risk of chronic gastritis and pernicious anemia. Other side effects of octreotide are loss of hair, bradycardia, and diffuse alopecia.

Indications

Octreotide is commonly used for the treatment of acromegaly due to negative feedback regulation of GH (which inhibits the GH release) from the pituitary gland. Further, it is also recommended for the treatment of GI fistula via the reduction of GI secretions and inhibition of gastrointestinal motility. It is also used for refractory hypoglycemia in neonates and sulphonylurea drug-induced hypoglycemia in adults.

Moreover, it provides symptomatic relief of the metastatic carcinoid tumors, that is, flushing and diarrhea and vasoactive intestinal peptide (VIP)-associated adenocarcinoma (watery diarrhea). It is used for acromegaly due to normalizing action on GH and/or IGF-I levels. It is also used as a treatment choice for adenoma of thyrotrope due to the inhibitory action of TSH secretion. Octreotide treats the acute hemorrhage of esophageal varices associated with liver cirrhosis. It is also used as a diagnostic agent for noninvasive imaging of neuroendocrine tumors. It is labeled with carbon-11, yttrium-90, indium-111, gallium-68, and lutetium-177 in nuclear medicine imaging and positron emission tomography (PET) techniques.

Contraindications

The adequate study of octreotide contraindications has not been made in the treatment of children and pregnant and lactating women. However, it is contraindicated in some conditions such as untreated level of thyroid hormones (decreased), diabetes, low-blood sugar, inadequate vitamin B_{12}, slow heartbeat (abnormal cardiac rhythm), hardening of the liver, gallstones, disorder of gallbladder, and stage 5 chronic kidney disease. Very commonly, octreotide shows the hypersensitivity (allergy) reactions.

Prolactin Inhibitors

Prolactin is a potential bioactive hormone which is released from the anterior pituitary gland. It is also known as luteotropic hormone or luteotropin. It affects different hormones of the body and presents in both men and women. Prolactin promotes the production of breast milk in lactating women via proliferation of breast alveolar epithelium and ductal and acinar cells of breast tissue. It is synthesized from anterior pituitary gland as well as the uterus, breasts, prostate, adipose tissue, skin, and immune cells. A minimal amount of prolactin is present in the blood circulation. The administration of oxytocin causes the milk ejection process (**Fig. 72.6**).

Mechanism

Prolactin has a diverse mechanism of action in target tissues via prolactin receptors (PrlR). PrlR may be "internalized" into target cells and amplify the intracellular signals. Further, these receptors are members of cytokine receptors. They lack the major intrinsic kinase domain activity in this receptor; however, they have a JAK_2-associating region. Hence, they transduce the plasma membrane signals via activation of JAK_2 activity which, in turn, enhances the phosphorylation process of various JAK_2 signal pathways. The net effects of prolactin include stimulation by RNA synthesis. Subsequently, it has the following cellular actions:

1. Increase the intracellular concentration of potassium and a reduce the level of sodium;
2. Raise the level of cGMP and reduce the level of cyclic adenosine monophosphate (cAMP);
3. Enhance the rate of prostaglandin biosynthesis via stimulation of phospholipase-A_2 activity; and iv) activate the polyamine synthesis process.

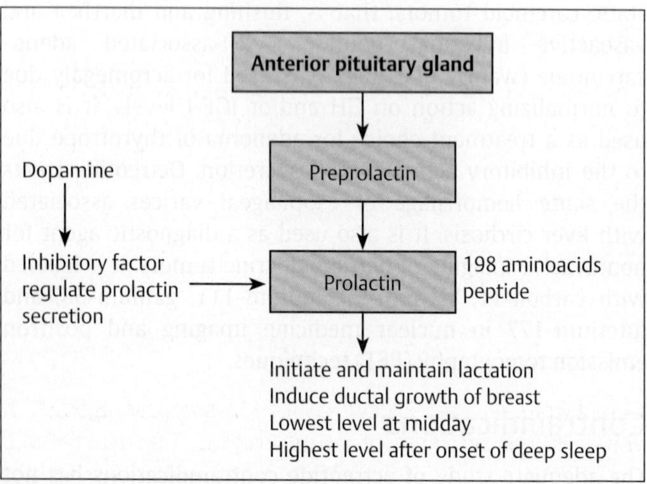

Fig. 72.6 Control of prolactin (PRL) secretion.

Pharmacological Effects

Prolactin has two main functions, stimulating the milk production from breast tissues and enhancing the development of breasts via stimulating actions of estrogen and progesterone. Prolactin is involved in the biosynthesis of milk constituents via activation of cell membrane PrlR and cellular transcription cascade. After parturition, estrogen and progesterone levels fall, and during suckling, the prolactin level is maintained very stable (elevated level in pregnancy; with each episode of feeding producing peak prolactin levels). If the mother is not nourishing the baby, prolactin levels become normal (as nonpregnant levels) after 1 or 2 weeks.

The secretion of prolactin is very low in childhood and increases in girls at puberty. The higher level is reached in adult females. It is progressively raised in pregnancy. Besides, prolactin suppresses the hypothalamic-pituitary-gonadal axis by inhibiting the GnRH, causes lactational amenorrhea and infertility, loss of libido, and impotence in male. Furthermore, the regulation of prolactin secretion occurs under constant release of PRIH (dopamine, DA) via dopamine-2 (D_2) receptors. DA receptor agonists bromocriptine and cabergoline inhibit the release of prolactin secretion, while DA antagonists such as chlorpromazine, domperidone, metoclopramide, haloperidol, risperidone, sulpiride, TRH, and VIP increase the levels of prolactin.

Clinical Applications

Natural prolactin does not have any clinical use. However, DA agonists and antagonists play a role in the modification of prolactin levels and their actions. DA modulators, on the other hand, are employed in the clinical setup and act on prolactin.

Bromocriptine

Bromocriptine is a natural medicine, and it is obtained from ergot derivatives such as2-bromo-α-ergocryptine. It has potent dopamine agonists which weakly act on alpha-adrenergic receptors in the neuronal tissue. The affinity is greater on the D_2 receptor, and there is partial agonist/antagonist action on the D_1 receptor.

Pharmacological Actions

Bromocriptine reduces the release of prolactin via antigalactopoietic action, while it raises the GH level in a normal person and decreases it in pituitary tumor (acromegaly) patients. Further, it has antiParkinsonian effects similar to that of like levodopa. It stimulates the chemoreceptor trigger zone (CTZ) center, leading to nausea and vomiting. It causes the hypotensive effects via alteration of postural reflex and alpha-blockade. It also decreases GI motility.

Pharmacokinetics

Bromocriptine is partially absorbed (1/3rd) and has high first-pass metabolism. The peak plasma concentration of bromocriptine is reached in 1 to 2 hours. The half-life ($t_{1/2}$) of bromocriptine is 3 to 6 hours. It readily crosses the membrane of the blood–brain barrier (BBB). The metabolites of bromocriptine are excreted via the bile excretion method.

Mechanism of Action

Prolactin is constantly inhibited with PRIH (dopamine) on pituitary lactotrophs via D_2 receptors agonistic actions by dopamine, bromocriptine, and cabergoline.

Therapeutic

(I) It is used for hyperprolactinemia-associated galactorrhea, amenorrhea and, female infertility, and impotence and sterility in males. A lower dose of bromocriptine, that is, 2.5 to 10 mg/day produces responses within weeks. (II) Acromegaly: 5 to 20 mg of bromocriptine per day is used for nonoperable cases of pituitary tumors. (III) Parkinsonism disease. (IV) It reduces breast engorgement and neonatal death. (V) It treats diabetes mellitus via D_2 receptor action in the hypothalamus. (VI) It also reduces the severity of hepatic coma. However, it should be stopped during pregnancy.

Side Effects

It has a potential role in CTZ; hence it shows levodopa like side effects, that is, nausea, vomiting, and constipation. It also produces postural hypotension, behavioral alterations, hallucinations, psychosis, mental confusions, and abnormal movements.

Cabergoline

Its is newer D_2 receptor agonist. It is more selective and a potential D_2 receptor agonist. It has a long half-life, that is, 60 days. Cabergoline is administered twice per week. It is mainly used for hyperprolactinemia and acromegaly, although it produces nausea and vomiting via activation of the CTZ center. The details of dopamine receptor antagonists have been discussed in drugs acting on the central nervous system (CNS).

Gonadotropin Preparations

The preparations of gonadotropin mimic the endogenous effects of gonadotropin hormones. They are therapeutically recommended for the treatment of fertility-related disorders via ovarian hyperstimulation and induction of ovulation. They are also known as menotropins. Consisting of LH and follicle-stimulating hormone (FSH) and extracted from human urine from menopausal women, currently, recombinant variants are also available.

Mechanism

Gonadotropin preparations act on plasma membrane GPCR receptors and induce the release of gonadotropin. They regulate multiple varieties of their own gonadotropin receptors which lead to targeted cell responses. Gonadotropin preparations act on the GPCR family of FSH and LH receptors. Further, they activate cAMP and produce gametogenesis via the influence of cholesterol-pregnenolone pathways.

Pharmacological Effects

Gonadotropin preparations stimulate the gonads and promote gametogenesis and secretion of gonadal hormones, that is FSH and LH. FSH enhances the follicular growth, development of the ovum, and secretion of estrogen. In the male, FSH induces spermatogenesis and is trophic to seminiferous tubules. In the absence of FSH, atrophy of ovary and testes are observed. LH aids in ripening of Graafian follicles, triggers ovulation, rupture follicles, and sustains corpus luteum. In the male, it stimulates testosterone secretion. The regulation of gonadotropin occurs with the influence of the following factors: (i) high and low frequency; high and low amplitude variability associated secretion of gonadotropin pulses; (ii) estrogen and progesterone producing the feedback inhibition of GnRH; (iii) weak inhibition of FSH and LH secretion via testosterone; (iv) release of inhibin leads to blocking the FSH action; and (v) dopamine-mediated inhibition of LH secretion.

Dosage

A typical dose of FSH is 75 to 300 IU/day. Rarely, FSH is administered at a high dose of 600 IU/day. The dose of LH is 75 to 150 IU/day.

Side Effects

The most common side effects of LH preparations are pain, swelling of the GI system, irritation at the injection site, skin rashes, and stomach and/or pelvic pain. Feeling of stomach fullness, bloating and tenderness of the lower abdomen, mood swings, fatigue, and hypertrophy of the ovaries are common side effects of FSH preparations. Besides, hyperstimulation of gonadal tissue also produces ovarian bleeding and polycystic ovary disorder. Further, it causes precocious puberty, allergic reactions, edema, headache, and mood swings.

Indications

Generally, gonadotropins are identified as fertility drugs. They consist of FSH, LH, or both. The primary uses of gonadotropin preparations involve stimulating ovulation and enhancing fertilization *in vitro* and *in vivo*. Moreover, they are also used for amenorrhea patients, controlled ovarian hyperstimulation, oligospermia effect in male (hypogonadism effect), male sterility, sexual maturation via stimulation of androgens, and cryptorchism (undescended testes).

Contraindications

Gonadotropin preparations are contraindicated in the following conditions: prostatic and testicular cancers, tumors of the pituitary gland, premature puberty, obstructed blood vessel with blood clot, hyperstimulated ovary, abnormal hypertrophy of ovaries, condition of water retention, and pregnancy. Some allergic conditions with biopeptides, especially chorionic gonadotropins, are contraindicated.

Gonadorelin Agonists

Gonadorelin is also known as GnRH receptor agonist. It enhances the secretion of gonadotropins, that is, FSH and LH from anterior pituitary gland, followed by sex hormone production by gonadal tissue.

Mechanism

The natural gonadorelin is physiologically released by the FSH and LH in a pulsatile manner. The synthetic gonadorelin acts on the pituitary gland and continuously downregulates GPCR. The activation of the GPCR family of the GnRH receptor enhances the calcium (Ca^{2+}) ions from the endoplasmic reticulum (ER) and activation of extracellular signal-regulated kinase (ERK) via activation of phospholipase C (PLC) and phospholipase A2 (PLA_2) pathways. After 1 to 2 weeks of gonadorelin administration, there is desensitization of GnRH receptors which, in turn, inhibits the FSH and LH release, followed by suppressing the gonadal functions, ovulation, and spermatogenesis. In this condition, testosterone and estrogen levels fall to the castration level.

Pharmacological

Gonadorelin is rapidly absorbed from the injected site. The plasma half-life of gonadorelin is shorter, that is, 4 to 8 minutes. It is rapidly degraded by an enzymatic reaction. It is rapidly hydrolyzed to inactive peptide components by hepatic enzymes. Further, the gonadorelin effect is terminated within 10 to 40 minutes and excreted via urine. The major gonadorelin is responsible for releasing the FSH and LH from the anterior pituitary. It can control the complex process of follicular growth, ovulation, corpus luteum of the ovary, and spermatogenesis from the testis. The pulsatile exposure to GnRH releases FSH/LH which desensitizes the pituitary gonadotropes. The lack of gonadorelin release is not used in the treatment of hypogonadism.

Dose

The IV administration of 100 mg of synthetic GnRH induces the release of FSH and LH. The preparation of synthetic gonadorelin acetate is available with various doses, 0.5 mg, 0.8 mg, 100 mcg, and 500 mcg per vial for IV and SC administration.

Indications

It is commonly used as a diagnostic tool for testing of the pituitary-gonadal axis in male and female hypogonadism. Besides, it is also used for the induction of follicular growth, ovulation, corpus luteum of the ovary, and spermatogenesis from testis via increasing the secretion of FSH and LH from the anterior pituitary. Moreover, it is used for the evaluation of the residual gonadotropic function of the pituitary after removal of a pituitary tumor.

Side Effects

The common side effects of gonadorelin are headache, flushing, nausea, abdominal discomfort, dizziness, light-headedness, skin rash, itching, and pain and swelling at the injection site.

Contraindications

The contraindications of gonadorelin are hypersensitivity, ovarian cysts, hormonal-dependent tumors, and pregnancy. Also, it is cautioned to multiple gestations, treatment with reproductive medicine and pulsatile LHRH/GnRH delivery.

Gonadorelin Analogs

The superactive/long-acting GnRH agonists such as leuprolide, goserelin, histrelin, triptorelin, and nafarelin are used as an alternative for natural gonadorelin. It is 15 to 150 times more potent than natural gonadorelin. The duration of action is observed in 2 to 6 hours. Further, it has a high affinity to GnRH receptors and a lack of enzymatic hydrolysis.

Nafarelin

It produces the long-acting action on the GnRH receptor, and it is 150 times more potent than natural gonadorelin. The plasma half-life is 2 to 3 hours. Moreover, the peak downregulation of pituitary GnRH receptors occurs within 1 month. It is very commonly used for reproduction with intranasal administration of 400 mcg BD, followed by 200 mcg BD when menstrual bleeding starts. Further, suppression of endogenous LH surge is altered with nafarelin, and it is used for uterine fibroid damage (with 200 mcg BD), endometriosis (200 mcg for 6 months), precocious puberty (800 mcg BD nasal spray formulation). Besides, it arrests the breast and genital developments with goserelin (long-acting gonadorelin), and prostate and endometriosis damage with the administration of goserelin before 1 to 3 weeks of ovulation.

Triptorelin

This long-acting agent is administered by SC injection once a month for regular release for female infertility. It is also administered by intramuscular (IM) injection for long-term use. Similarly, the long-acting *leuprolide* is administered via IM/SC injection.

GnRH Antagonists

The administration of GnRH antagonists, that is, cetrorelix and ganirelix block the GnRH membrane receptors in the pituitary gland and suppress the release of FSH and LH. The SC injection of GnRH antagonist is used for the inhibition of gonadotropin hormone without initial stimulation of histamine release. Further, it is used for *in vitro* fertilization to suppress the LH surge. The advantages of GnRH antagonists are rapid competitive antagonistic action, lower risk of ovarian hyperstimulation, and complete suppression of gonadotropin hormone.

Diagnostic Uses of TSH and ACTH

TSH

The abnormalities of the thyroid gland either produce hyperthyroidism (too high) or hypothyroidism (too low). The symptoms of hyperthyroidism are anxiety, weight loss, hand tremors, tachycardia, eye-bulging, and insomnia, whereas those of hypothyroidism are body weight gain, hair loss, lack of tolerance to cold temperature, abnormal menstruation, tiredness, and constipation. Generally, thyroid hormone changes occur during pregnancy (usually not significant).

Sometimes, it can develop as thyroid disease in pregnancy. The prevalence rate of hyperthyroidism is one case in 500 pregnancies, and hypothyroidism cases is one in 250 pregnancies.

The inference of the TSH test indicates that the thyroid gland is to lose its ability of thyroid hormone synthesis and secretion (hypothyroidism). If the thyroid gland releases too large amounts of hormone, it is called hyperthyroidism. Furthermore, the TSH test does not explain directly the level of TSH secretion (too high or too low). This test includes the testing of the following hormones: triiodothyronine (T_3) and thyroxine (T_4) hormones. Usually, the TSH test is carried out in less than 5 minutes in blood samples. The samples must be taken in fasting condition (fasting condition including liquid drink for several hours). TSH test is used for testing of Addison's disease. In Addison's disease, the TSH test shows the excess level of TSH with or without low thyroxine, thyroid autoantibodies, and symptoms of hypothyroidism. Moreover, the TSH test is also used for the diagnosis of Graves' disease with the detection of antibodies based on autoimmune reaction with hyperthyroidism. Similarly, the TSH test is used for the diagnosis of "Hashimoto's thyroiditis," with an autoimmune reaction of hypothyroidism.

ACTH

ACTH test is used for the quantification of ACTH level in blood. It is secreted from the anterior pituitary gland and controls the biosynthesis of cortisol by adrenal glands (present above the kidneys). Normally, cortisol is a response to various pathophysiological events like stress, infections, to regulate the glucose in the blood, blood pressure, and metabolism process. The abundant/little production of cortisol leads to provoking serious health care problems. ACTH test is used for testing of secondary adrenocortical insufficiency and isolated ACTH deficiency. ACTH test shows the low level of cortisol. Moreover, the administration of cortisol is slowly reversible to the level of cortisol content. It is also used as a diagnostic aid for "Cushing's syndrome." The indication is to release a large amount of stress hormone cortisol by adrenal glands. Further, the chronic condition of "Cushing's syndrome" can be caused by a tumor of the pituitary gland/chronic administration of steroidal drugs. Moreover, the ACTH test is also used for the diagnosis of "Addison's disease," with low production of cortisol from the adrenal gland. Similarly, the "hypopituitarism" condition is characterized by low production of ACTH from the pituitary gland. The symptoms of hypercortisol are body-weight gain, fat deposition in shoulders, pink/purple stretch marks in abdomen, thighs, and breasts, skin bruises, lack of muscle strength, fatigue, and acne. Hypocortisol is referred to as a lack of body weight, dizziness, fatigue, GI disturbance (nausea, vomiting, diarrhea, and abdominal pain), skin color darkening, and salt craving behavior.

The symptoms of hypopituitarism vary depending upon the severity of the disease; such symptoms are lack of appetite, abnormal menstruation, female infertility, lack of hair growth in body and facial regions in men, lack of sexual desire in both men and women, more sensation to a cold environment, unusual frequent urination, and fatigue.

Usually, the ACTH test is carried out in less than 5 minutes in blood samples. The samples must be taken in overnight fasting (not eat or drink) conditions. It is tested in the early morning due to the variability of cortisol levels throughout the day. The inference of cortisol levels before and after injection of ACTH indicates various complications. High levels of ACTH and cortisol indicate the "Cushing's disease." The identification "Cushing's syndrome" and/or "tumor of adrenal gland" is based on the level of ACTH; low level of ACTH and high-cortisol levels indicate the "Cushing's syndrome" and/or "tumor of adrenal gland." Paradoxically, high ACTH and low-cortisol levels are indicated as "Addison disease." In "hypopituitarism" conditions, the levels of ACTH and cortisol are lower than normal.

Vasopressin and Its Analogs (PH1.24)

Vasopressin is also known as antidiuretic hormone (ADH), arginine vasopressin (AVP), and argipressin. This hormone is biosynthesized from neurons of the hypothalamus and converted to AVP. These neuron terminals traveled down toward the axon of the posterior pituitary. AVP is highly stored in posterior pituitary gland cells. Further, vasopressin plays a role in maintaining the process of osmolality and water volume in extracellular fluid. Besides, it acts on collecting ducts of renal nephron tubules via activation vasopressin-2 (V_2) receptor. Further, it raises the level of water permeability from collecting duct by active cAMP-dependent mechanism. This reaction is to enhance the reduction of urine formation which is called antidiuretic action. Hence, it is also known as ADH. The rising of water retention leads to a rise in blood volume, cardiac output, and arterial pressure (vasoconstrictor action). The secretion of vasopressin is controlled by osmoreceptors of the hypothalamus neuron. The activation of this osmoreceptor enhances the release of vasopressin release and stimulation of thirst.

Mechanism

Vasopressin acts on a specialized cell surface receptor known as vasopressin (V) receptor, and it regulates the isotonicity of body biofluids. In hypertonicity conditions, it is secreted by the posterior pituitary gland, reabsorbing the solute-free water from the kidney. Further, water returns to circulation, thereby restoring the normal tonicity of the body fluids. This action occurs via activation of V_2 receptors via the generation of water channel, that is, aquaporin-2. In vasodilatory shock condition, vasopressin enhances the systemic vascular resistance and mean arterial pressure (MAP) and reduces the heart rate and cardiac output level (**Fig. 72.7 a, b, c**)

Pharmacological Effects

The pharmacological action of vasopressin involves reducing the portal collateral blood flow and variceal pressure via activation of V_1 receptors. In the kidney, vasopressin has three major effects, (i) enhancing the water permeability from renal proximal and cortical collecting tubules of

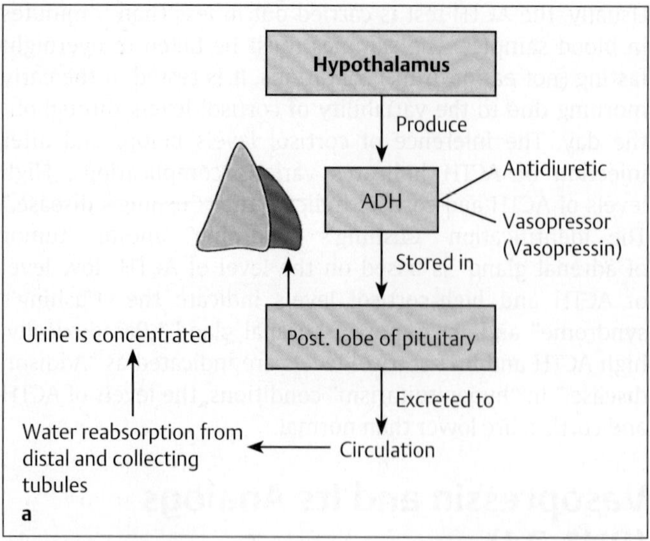

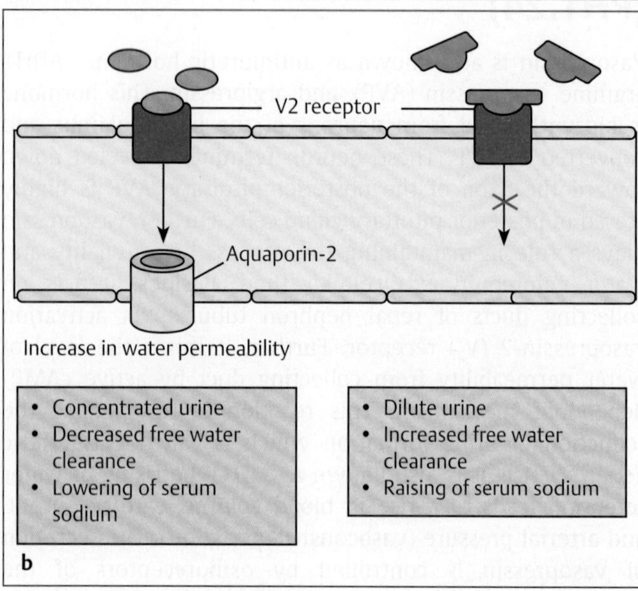

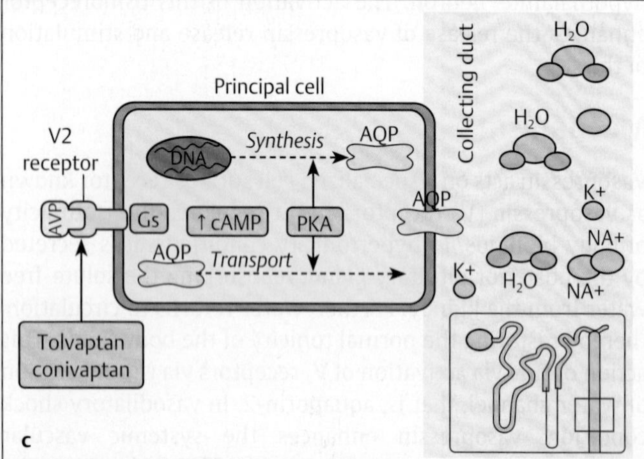

Fig. 72.7 **(a, b)** Mechanisms of vasopressin. **(c)** Mechanism of action of vasopressin and its antagonists.

nephron and inner an outer medullary collecting duct, (ii) increasing the permeability of urea in the inner medullary portion of the collecting duct via urea transporters, (iii) increasing the sodium absorption across the ascending loop of Henle. The net effect of vasopressin is reabsorption of water and excretion of concentrated urine. In the CNS, vasopressin is synthesized by the hypothalamus and secreted in the pituitary gland. In the brain, it has several actions, that is, enhancing the vasopressin release with alteration of circadian rhythmic signal in the suprachiasmatic nucleus. It is also released from central projecting hypothalamic neurons with stimuli of aggression and alteration of blood pressure and temperature. Currently, it is evidenced to have analgesic effects, depending on stress and sex. Pharmacologically, it increases the systemic vascular resistance (SVR) and MAP and decreases cardiac index; pulmonary artery pressure is usually unchanged or decreased, whereas urine output is either unchanged or increased.

Pharmacokinetics

Vasopressin is administered via IV, IM, and SC routes. The duration of action of vasopressin is variable (30–60 minutes) based on the mode of administration. The half-life of vasopressin is 10 to 20 minutes, and it is distributed in entire body via circulation of blood. Furthermore, vasopressin is rapidly metabolized by the liver and excreted via kidneys.

Dose

AVP is administered with a dose of 20 U (1 ampoule). Generally, it is administered via IV route. Rarely, it is also administered via the endotracheal and intraosseous route.

Side Effects

The common side effects of vasopressin are nausea, dizziness, trembling, fever, angina, heartburn, abdominal pain, and water intoxication. The most serious adverse reactions of vasopressin are angina pectoris and skin hypersensitivity. Rarely, it causes peripheral vascular edema, a decrease of cardiac output and coronary regional blood flow, bowel ischemia, raising of liver enzymes, and reduced platelet count. At higher doses, it shows myocardial ischemia, hyponatremia, cutaneous necrosis, extravasation, and allergy.

Indications

AVP is used for the management of hypovolemic and refractory shocks (with 1–10 U dose of AVP). Septic shock is managed with an infusion of 0.04 U/min of AVP. At higher doses, it may cause side effects. Hypovolemic cardiac arrest is managed with IV bolus administration of 40 U of AVP. For postcardiopulmonary bypass surgery, associated vasodilation condition is managed with an infusion of 0.1 U/min of AVP, and it starts with downward titrated dose as tolerated; following which, catecholamine is recommended for the reduction of 0.02 U/min of AVP before ceasing tolerance. Vasopressin is also used as an off-label treatment for circulatory shock, bleeding in the GI system, and tachycardia and fibrillation of ventricular tissue. It is recommended for the treatment of diabetes insipidus-associated decrease of ADH.

Contraindications

The preparation of lysine vasopressin is contraindicated with hypersensitivity patients due to the presence of beef or pork proteins. It is also contraindicated to elevated blood urea nitrogen and chronic kidney failure due to interaction with the urea molecule. Further, it is sensitive to seizures, migraines, bronchial asthma, and heart failure with polyuria conditions.

Vasopressin Analogs

Vasopressin analogs are produced in a similar function, but it is not structurally similar to vasopressin. Such vasopressin analogs are desmopressin and terlipressin. Desmopressin acts on vasopressin's receptors. It is used for childhood bedwetting and abnormal circadian rhythmicity behavior of children. It is recommended 30 to 45 minutes before sleeping time, and it makes the concentration of urine production and experience fill the urination reflex in the urinary bladder. The mechanism of desmopressin is similar to vasopressin in renal collecting duct via V_2 receptors and aquaporin channels. This medication is also recommended for the treatment of hemophilia-A, diabetes insipidus, von Willebrand disease, and polyurea conditions. Moreover, it produces headaches, diarrhea, and low-blood sodium (cause seizure). It is contraindicated to kidney problems or low-blood sodium. Moreover, it is safer for pregnancy. The synthetic analog of vasopressin agonist, that is, desmopressin is therapeutically used in low-vasopressin secretion, control of bedwetting in children, and internal bleeding. Terlipressin produces a similar action of naturally occurring vasopressin hormone. It is used for certain vasoconstrictor conditions like esophageal bleeding and portal hypertension. Further, it is also treats the hepatorenal syndrome via reversal of renal failure and liver disease. Terlipressin increases the blood flow in the kidneys tissue via constricting blood vessels, and it is relatively used for decompensated cirrhosis. It is administered via an IV route with 1 mg (over a minute) every 4 to 6 hours for 72 hours as a starting dose, followed by 1.5 and 2 mg (over a minute) for every 4 to 6 hours for 72 hours, which is administered for hepatorenal syndrome. The detailed summary of pituitary hormones and their drugs properties has been indicated in **Fig. 72.8** and **Tables 72.4 and 72.5**.

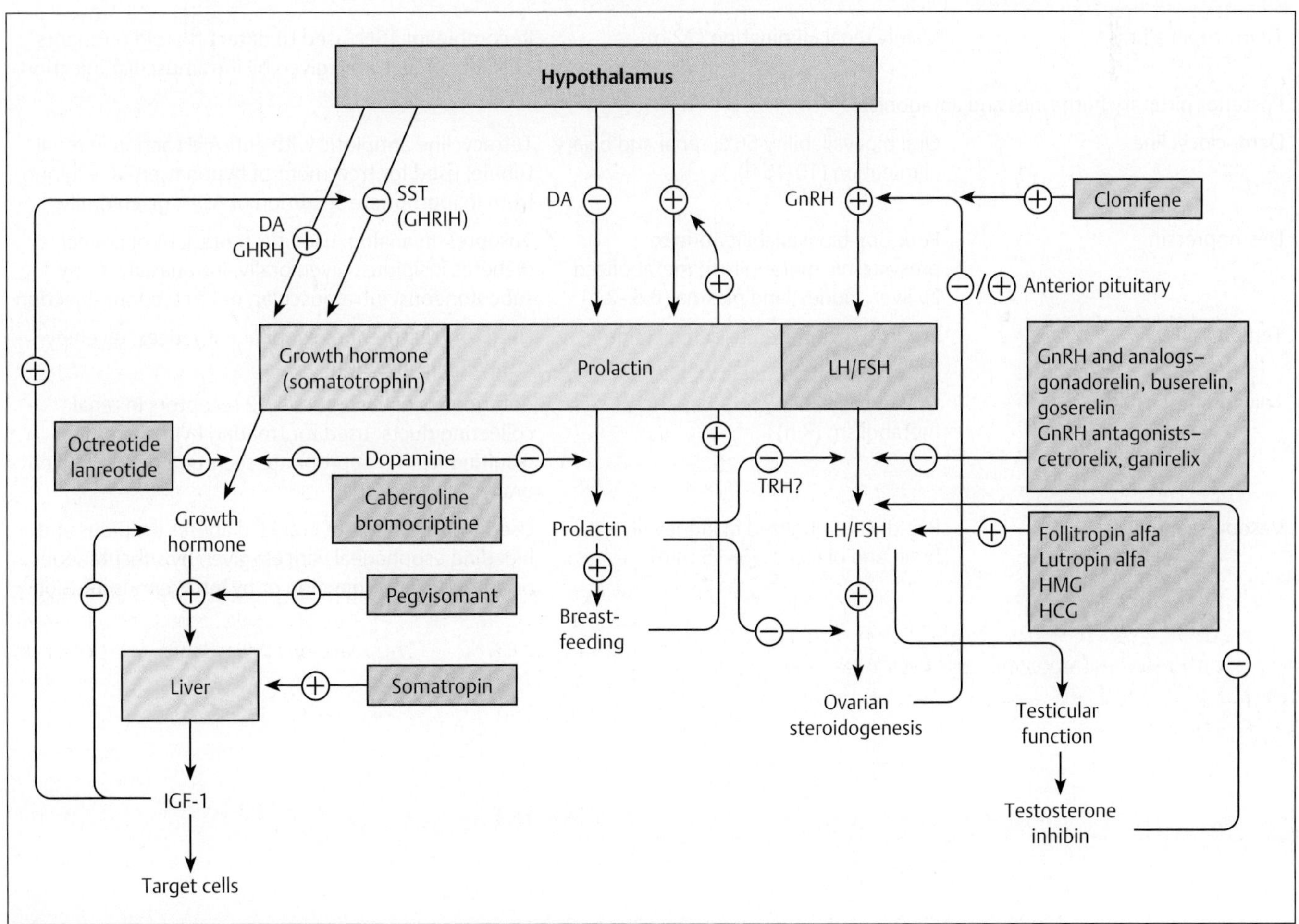

Fig. 72.8 Summary of control mechanisms for the release of growth hormone (GH), gonadotropins, and prolactin (PRL) from the anterior pituitary.

Table 72.4 Summary of pituitary hormones and antagonists

Hormone/Factors	Mechanisms	Integrating areas
Choriogonadotropin alfa	Metabolic routes not defined; about 100% is excreted in urine (29 h)	Recombinant HCG; given by subcutaneous injection
Corifollitropin alfa	Slow release from injection site; renal elimination (59–79 h)	Synthetic FSH (modified); given by subcutaneous injection
Growth hormone		
Somatropin	Slow release from injection site; proteolytic degradation (4 h)	Synthetic form of growth hormone (somatotropin); given by subcutaneous or intramuscular injection
Growth hormone receptor antagonists		
Pegvisomant	Route of elimination not defined (6 days)	Pegylated synthetic antagonist of growth hormone receptors: given by subcutaneous injection
Prolactin antagonists		
Used to suppress lactation.		
Bromocriptine	See Ch. 24	D_2 receptor agonist; given orally (Ch. 24)
Cabergoline	See Ch. 24	D_2 receptor agonist; better tolerated than bromocriptine: given orally (Ch. 24)
Ouinagolide	Well absorbed; hepatic metabolism; renal and fecal excretion (17 h)	Non-ergot D_2 receptor agonist; better tolerated than bromocriptine; given orally
TSH		
Thyrotropin alfa	Mainly renal elimination (22 h)	Recombinant TSH; used to detect thyroid remnants post-thyroidectomy: given by intramuscular injection
Posterior pituitary hormones and antagonists		
Demeclocycline	Oı al bioavailability 66%: renal and biliary elimination (10-15 h)	Tetracycline antibiotic with anti-ADH action in renal tubule; used for treatment of hyponatremia resulting from inappropriate secretion of ADH: given orally
Desmopressin	Poor oral bioavailability due to presystemic metabolism; metabolized by liver, kidney, and plasma (0.5–2 h)	Vasopressin analog: used for treatment of cranial diabetes insipidus; given orally, intranasally, or by subcutaneous, intramuscular, or intravenous injection
Terlipressin	Prodrug hydrolyzed to activeLysine vasopressin (which has half-life of 0.5 h)	Used for treatment of esophageal varices; given by intravenous injection
Tolvaptan	Oral bioavailability 56% hepatic metabolism (8 h)	Antagonists of vasopressin V2 receptors in renal collecting ducts; used for treating hyponatremia resulting from inappropriate secretion of ADH: given orally
Vasopressin (ADH)	Rapidly metabolized in kidney, liver. brain and placenta (5–15 min)	Used for treatment of cranial diabetes insipidus and bleeding esophageal varices; given by subcutaneous or intramuscular injection or by intravenous infusion

Table 72.5 Anterior and posterior pituitary hormones

Generic (brand)	Route and dosage	Uses and considerations
Anterior lobe		
GH		
Somatropin (nutropin, genotropin)	C: SC/IM: Nutropin: 0.006 mg/kg/d; Genotropin: 0.04 mg/kg in 6–7 equal daily doses; *max*: 0.08 mg/kg/wk	For GH deficiency. Promotes bone growth at epiphyseal plates of long bones. Pregnancy category: Nutropin: C; Genotropin: B; PB: 20%; half-life: 15–60 min
GH suppressant drugs		
Bromocriptine mesylate (parlodel)	A: PO: 1.25–2.5 mg/d for 3 d; range: 10–30 mg/d; max: 100 mg/d	For acromegaly. Also used with pituitary radiation or surgery to decrease GH levels. Decreases lactation and prolactinoma. Pregnancy category: B; PB: 93%; half-life: 3-6 h
Octreotide acetate (sandostatin)	A: SC: 50–100 mcg t.i.d.	For acromegaly. To treat severe diarrhea associated with metastatic carcinoid and other tumors. Pregnancy category: B; PB: 65%; half-life: 1.5 h
Lanreotide acetate (Somatuline Depot)	A: SC: Initially, 90 mg q4wk for 3 mo; then 60–120 mg q4wk for 4 mo	To suppress GH. Monitor glucose levels. Pregnancy category: C; PB: 69–78%; half-life: 23–30 d
TSH		
Thyrotropin (thyrogen)	Thyroid cancer: A: IM: 0.9 mg into gluteus maximus, repeat in 24 h for 2 doses; *max*: 0.9 mg/d	For thyroid cancer. Radioiodine study follows last injection. Pregnancy category: C; PB: UK; half-life: 15–35 h
ACTH		
Corticotropin (H.P. acthar gel)	In the treatment of infantile spasms, the recommended dose is 150 U/m2 divided into twice daily intramuscular injections of 75 U/m2.	In the treatment of acute exacerbations of multiple sclerosis, daily intramuscular or subcutaneous doses of 80–120 units for 2–3 weeks may be administered.
Cosyntropin (cortrosyn)	A/C: > 2 y: IM/IV: 0.25 mg over 2 min or slow infusion over 6 hC: < 2 y: IM/IV: 0.125 mg slow infusion over 6 h	For diagnostic testing to differentiate between pituitary and adrenal cause of adrenal insufficiency. Obtain plasma cortisol levels before and 30 min after administration. Pregnancy category: C; PB: UK; half-life: 15 min
Posterior lobe		
ADH		
Desmopressin acetate (DDAVP, Stimate)	DDAVP: A: Intranasal: 0.1–0.4 mL/d in divided doses. Stimate: A: SC/IV: 0.2–0.4 mcgA/C: > 11 mo: intranasal: 150 mcg/kg	For DI, hemophilia A, and von Willebrand disease. Can have a long duration of action (5–21 h). Pregnancy category: B; PB: UK; half-life: 1.5-2.5 h
Vasopressin (aqueous) (pitressin)	Diabetes insipidus: A: SC/IM: 5–10 units, b.i.d./q.i.d. C: SC/IM: 2.5–10 units, b.i.d./q.i.d.	For DI. For relief of intestinal distention. Decreases GI bleeding from esophageal varices. Can also be given intranasally. Promotes reabsorption of water from renal tubules. Duration of action is 2–8 h. Pregnancy category: C; PB: UK; half-life: 15 min
Demeclocycline (declomycin)	A: PO: 600 mg/d in 3–4 divided doses	For treatment of SIADH. Inhibits ADH-induced water reabsorption in renal distal tubules. Closely monitor sodium levels. Pregnancy category: C; PB: 99%; half-life: 12 h
Conivaptan (vaprisol)	A: IV: Loading dose 20 mg over 30 min; maintenance dose 20 mg continuous IV over 24 h; then 20 mg/d for 1–3 d; max: 4 days therapy	For hypervolemic hyponatremia associated with SIADH. Closely monitor sodium levels. Pregnancy category: C; PB: 99%; half-life: 5 h
Tolvaptan (samsca)	A: PO: Initially 15 mg/d; then 15–30 mg/d; *max*: 60 mg/d	For hyponatremia associated with SIADH. Closely monitor sodium levels. Pregnancy category: C; PB: 99%; half-life: 12 h

Abbreviations: ACTH, adrenocorticotropic hormone; A, adult; ADH, antidiuretic hormone; b.i.d., twice a day; C, child; d, day; DI, diabetes insipidus; GH, growth hormone; GI, gastrointestinal; h, hour; IM, intramuscular; IV, intravenous; LD, loading dose; min, minute; NSS, normal saline solution; PB, protein-binding; PO, by mouth; q.i.d., four times a day; SC, subcutaneous; SIADH, syndrome of inappropriate antidiuretic hormone secretion; t.i.d., three times a day; TSH, thyroid-stimulating hormone; UK, unknown; wk, week; y, year; >, greater than; <, less than.

Multiple Choice Questions

Case History: 1

A 62-year-old man was inspected for the condition of severe chronic back pain. The man was constituted to osteosclerotic bone metastases by prostate carcinoma. An analgesic agent with sufficient doses of nonsteroidal anti-inflammatory drugs (NSAIDs) successfully controlled his osteosclerotic pain. Thereafter, he was administered with gonadotropin-releasing hormone (GnRH) analog agent with goserelin (3.6 mg subcutaneously/month). After 1 week, his pain worsened at night and observed no evidence for spinal compression.

1. What one of the following points is NOT correct in this deterioration effect of his symptoms?

A. Tumor flare reaction.
B. Acute secretion of follicle-stimulating hormone (FSH)/luteinizing hormone (LH).
C. Initial increase the testosterone.
D. Increase spinal disc herniation.

Answer: D

His symptoms worsen in the first week of treatment with GnRH analog for "tumor flare reaction." Normally, GnRH analog agents enhance the secretion of FSH/LH level within 1/2 weeks, and it can cause acute elevation of testosterone levels. Later, it causes the downregulation of the receptor and reduces the level of FSH/LH and testosterone hormone.

2. Which one of the statements is NOT appropriate for treatment for chronic back pain with gonadotropin-releasing hormone (GnRH) analog therapy?

A. Initiate GnRH analog therapy after several weeks.
B. Goserelin can be recommended for the initial management of back pain.
C. Androgen receptor antagonist administered with GnRH analog therapy.
D. It starts with an analgesic agent along with an androgen receptor antagonist.

Answer: B

Metastatic prostate cancer patients are treated with the initial administration of GnRH analog therapy for several weeks, followed by androgen receptor antagonists like flutamide, cyproterone acetate, and bicalutamide. The antiandrogens are recommended for the treatment of "tumor flare" conditions. Generally, adequate analgesic agent and androgen receptor antagonist (i.e., oral flutamide) is started at once, and goserelin is restarted after several weeks.

Case History: 2

A 55-year-old pale skin-colored woman was admitted with complications of hematemesis. She was also identified in a case of alcohol-induced cirrhosis. Her medical history was documented as the presence of recurrent upper gastrointestinal (GI) bleeding and esophageal varices. Further, she had not taken any medicines and had no known allergies to drugs. The examination reports revealed that her blood pressure (BP) was 77/42 mm Hg, pulse rate was 112 beats per minute, and respiratory rate was 21 breaths per minute. She felt cold in the skin. Cardiac examinations were observed as normal level. Abdominal examinations were observed as ascites and palpable spleen. The sounds of the bowel were normal. Serum electrolytes were normal levels. An electrocardiogram (ECG) graph expressed her condition as sinus tachycardia.

3. Which one of the following approaches is the immediate and highest priority to manage her hematemesis conditions?

A. Initiate with volume resuscitation.
B. Acute/rapid treatment of bleeding.
C. Immediately starts the portal decompressive shunt surgery.
D. Prevention of recurrence of bleeding of variceal region.

Answer: C

The observation of the acute effect of variceal bleeding provokes medical emergency conditions and is treated immediately. The major treatment goals are volume resuscitation, reduction of bleeding, and prevention of reappearance of variceal bleeding. Generally, 10% of patients undergo endoscopic and medical intervention for life-saving portal-decompressive shunt surgery and/or transjugular intrahepatic portosystemic shunt (TIPS).

Case History: 3

A 55-year-old pale skin-colored woman was admitted with complications of hematemesis. She was also identified in a case of alcohol-induced cirrhosis. Her medical history was documented as the presence of recurrent upper gastrointestinal (GI) bleeding and esophageal varices. Further, she had not taken any medicines and had no known allergies to drugs. The examination reports revealed that her blood pressure (BP) was 77/42 mm Hg, pulse rate was 112 beats per minute, and respiratory rate was 21 breaths per minute. She felt cold in the skin. Cardiac examinations were observed as normal level. Abdominal examinations were observed as ascites and palpable spleen. The sounds of the bowel were normal. Serum electrolytes were at normal levels. An electrocardiogram (ECG) graph expressed her condition as sinus tachycardia.

The treatment was initiated with three units of whole blood transfusion and two units of fresh frozen plasma transfusion. Her gastric tissue was lavaged with saline, followed by gastric aspirated via nasogastric (NG) tube. It continued to bring a strong positive response for blood homeostasis. The 4 hours later observation of her conditions was expressed as the bleeding persisted.

4. Which one of the pharmacological interventions is most suitable for controlling her esophageal bleeding?

A. Highly preferred the octreotide administration.
B. Prefer the short-acting vasoconstricting agents.
C. Highly preferred the vasopressin administration.
D. Prefer the ultrashort-acting vasoconstricting agents.

Answer: A

Variceal bleeding is controlled by various vasoconstricting drugs. The initial gold standard drug was vasopressin. It is an

endogenous hormone, and it is called 8-arginine vasopressin and antidiuretic hormone (ADH). Originally, it is developed for the treatment of diabetes insipidus in pituitary insufficiency patients. Clinically, its recommended for the prevention of variceal bleeding, and it produces advantages in the form of reduction of intense smooth muscle and vasoconstriction associated bleeding. The efficacy of vasopressin in the prevention of esophageal bleeding is limited. Moreover, the adverse effects like arrhythmias, abdominal cramping, and gangrenes are very common. Therefore, it is replaced with a newer agent, that is, octreotide. However, clinicians are still prescribing vasopressin for variceal bleeding.

Case History: 4

An 18-year-old man was admitted to hospital with a 2-month medical history of irritability of mood, uncontrolled sweating, and enlargement of breast. His past medical history was unremarkable. He smoked 5 cigarettes/day, occasional drinking of alcohol, and did not take any drugs. His clinical examination revealed mild thyrotoxic condition, small size of goiter in the thyroid gland, and gynecomastia. Besides, he was unable to do eye response with examiner finger upward movements. The clinical report revealed that blood cell count, electrolytes, and liver function tests were normal. His luteinizing hormone (LH) level was 25 U/L (normal value is 3–8 U/L), follicle-stimulating hormone (FSH) level was 5.0 U/L (normal value is 0.5 to 5.0 U/L); free T4 level was 36 pmol/L (normal value is 9 to 25 pmol/L), thyroid-stimulating hormone (TSH) level was 0.1 mU/L (normal level is 0.5 to 5 mU/L), testosterone level was 60 nmol/L (normal value is 9 to 42 nmol/L), and 17-β-estradiol level was 638 pmol/L (normal value is 220 pmol/L).

5. Which one of the following is the most appropriate option for the diagnosis of this condition?

A. LH-secreting pituitary adenoma.
B. Testosterone self-administration.
C. Leydig cell tumor of the testis.
D. Pinealoma.

Answer: D

The beta subunit of human chorionic gonadotropin (HCG) mimics the LH. It stimulates the Leydig cells which, in turn, leads to enhancement of the production of testosterone. Further, it cross-reacts with the diagnostic assay of LH. The development of seminiferous tubule is completely dependent upon FSH, leading to the precocious puberty and small testicles, due to the development of human chorionic gonadotropin (HCG)-secreting tumors. On the other hand, TSH-like actions of HCG lead to acceleration of the goiter, and hyperthyroidism (without alteration of ophthalmic vision changes). The most common causes of HCGs are teratoma, choriocarcinoma, and pinealoma. Furthermore, it frequently secretes the estrogen, leading to gynecomastia and/or dysmenorrhea. Besides, it makes the loss of upgaze striking of the pineal region which leads to Parinaud's syndrome.

Case History: 5

A 45-year-old spinster showed heavy body weight, lethargy, and depression. She smoked 10 cigarettes/day and drank 30 units of alcohol/weekly. Her examination showed a Cushingoid condition without stigmata of chronic liver abnormalities. Her clinical examination report revealed that the level of cortisol at 9 a.m. was 800 nmol/L and at midnight cortisol level was 780 nmol/L. Her adrenocorticotropic hormone (ACTH) level at 9 a.m. was 60 ng/L and at midnight ACTH level was 45 ng/L. The physician was administered dexamethasone dose 0.5 mg every 6 hours for 48 hours, and at 9 a.m., cortisol level was 90 nmol/L.

6. Which one of the following conditions is appropriate with this case study report?

A. Pseudo-Cushing's syndrome.
B. Adrenal adenoma.
C. Adrenal carcinoma.
D. Micronodular adrenal hyperplasia.

Answer: A

The primary protocols for the identification of Cushing's syndrome vary between institutions. The general protocol's principles are as follows:

1. **Screening of hypercortisolism, that is, the level of free cortisol in urine after 24 hours duration.**
2. **Confirmation of hypercortisolism, that is, dexamethasone suppression test with low-dose level.**
3. **Identify the pseudo-Cushing's syndrome by assessment of ACTH levels. Further, establish the ACTH-dependent or/and ACTH-independent pseudo Cushing's syndrome, with an assessment of circadian rhythmic actions of ACTH, cortisol, and corticotropin-releasing hormone (CRH).**
4. **Further, the ACTH-dependent ectopic form of pituitary actions confirmed CRH test, bilateral inferior petrosal sinus sampling (BIPSS) test, and dexamethasone suppression test with high-dose level.**
5. **The identification of possible sites of hormone hyper-secretion via high-resolution images.**

The administration of dexamethasone at a low-dose level has more sensitive action with 98% of hypercorticism functions. Nowadays, CRH stimulation with ACTH has revealed that the various centers of the pituitary gland are activated. In pseudo-Cushing's syndrome conditions, there are no changes in ACTH level; however, brisk administration of ACTH causes the adenoma of corticotroph region of the pituitary gland.

7. Which one of the following diagnostic test is more appropriate to take a decision for further treatment of this patient?

A. Glucagon stimulation test (GST).
B. Corticotropin-releasing hormone (CRH) stimulation test (CST).
C. Chest CT imaging test.
D. Dexamethasone suppression test for overnight changes.

Answer: B

The major discrepancy of ectopic adrenocorticotropic hormone (ACTH) levels is observed in Cushing's syndrome, and it is a primary demanding factor for this diagnostic procedure. Furthermore, there is no successful test with 100% sensitivity and specificity. Moreover, the inducers of hepatic

enzymes like phenytoin and/or rifampicin can accelerate the metabolism of dexamethasone, leading to false-positive result in dexamethasone suppression test with low-dose level. Pseudo-Cushing's syndrome also shows severe type of depression, alcoholism, and lack of circadian rhythmic support in dexamethasone suppression tests with low-dose level. Whereas, in real-life situations, this suppressive action occurs with a high dose of dexamethasone. The additional diagnostic test is an insulin tolerance test (ITT) with cortisol response. The ITT test results lead to mimicking the depression without Cushing's syndrome. *Men are more prone to Cushing's disease than women.* **Moreover, the rare case of Carney's syndrome, that is, due to autosomal dominant gene leads to causes the tumor of endocrine and peripheral nerves, myxoma, color spots in the skin, McCune–Albright syndrome, and hyperfunctions of adrenal, thyroid, gonads, and pituitary glands.**

The details of ACTH-dependent factor of Cushing's syndromes are as follows:

- **80% with pituitary adenoma.**
- **20% of cases with ectopic ACTH along with small-cell lung carcinoma, phaeochromocytoma, carcinoid, and medullary thyroid carcinoma.**
- **Very rarely, ectopic CRH.**

The details of non-ACTH-dependent factor of Cushing's syndromes are as follows:

- **Mainly, exogenous glucocorticoid.**
- **40 to 50% with adrenal adenoma and adrenal carcinoma.**
- **50% with complex pigmented adrenal nodular tissue damage.**
- **Rare case with McCune–Albright syndrome, and idiopathic macronodular adrenal disease (MAD) via ectopic and elevated receptors in adrenal cells.**

Case History: 6

A 22-year-old woman has higher medical attention due to severe irregularity of menstrual periods and problems with the conceiving process. She was admitted to the hospital for fatigue and pulsatile headaches; she expressed reasons which were part of a stressful job. Further, she was not taking any medicines. The clinical examination revealed that she had bitemporal lower quadrantanopia. Moreover, her blood cell count, electrolyte levels, and liver function tests were normal. Her luteinizing hormone (LH) level was 2.2 U/L, follicle-stimulating hormone (FSH) level was 1.1 U/L, prolactin level was 3000 U/L, thyroid-stimulating hormone (TSH) level was 1.9 mU/L, and free thyroxine (T3 and T4) levels were pmol/L. Her insulin stress test results were expressed to minimize the level of blood glucose at 1.6 mmol/L.

8. Which of the following conditions exactly correlates to these conditions?

A. Prolactin-dependent macroadenoma.
B. Hypothyroidism.
C. Craniopharyngioma.
D. Anterior pituitary-associated sarcoidosis.

Answer: C

The elevated prolactin at a moderate level is caused by a tumor of nonprolactin-secreting pituitary stalk tissue. It reduces the dopamine levels in the pituitary. In these conditions, all pituitary axis underwent the sizeable tumors, compression of the chiasma, and progression of craniopharyngioma. In addition to that, nonfunctional pituitary adenoma and tumors have undergone the eccentric growth which leads to produce the meningioma.

9. Which of the following method is most likely to be used in these conditions?

A. Cabergoline then surgical method.
B. Surgical method.
C. Stereotactic radiotherapy method.
D. Thyroxine treatment method.

Answer: B

The replacement therapy of hydrocortisone is necessary during the application of the surgical process. Generally, prolactinoma is treated with dopamine agonists like cabergoline. The effective remission of the tumor is achieved. The surgical intervention of these kinds of tumors is high. Mostly, large tumors cause the compression of surrounding structures, and sometimes, patients are intolerant to the medical treatment.

Case History: 7

A 26-year-old-woman delivered a nonviable fetus at 24 weeks gestation. She informs her obstetrician about wanting to avoid her lactation process.

10. Which one of the following approaches is suitable for the suppression of lactation?

A. Bromocriptine.
B. Mild analgesic.
C. Ice pack application on breasts.
D. Stimulation of anterior pituitary gland.

Answer: D

Women with stillborn infants and abortion are expected to stop breastfeeding. The drugs and nonpharmacologic methods were used in 1988. The recommendation of the Food and Drugs Administration (FDA) is analgesics to relieve breast pain. Further, bromocriptine was also approved for postpartum suppression of lactation. Moreover, FDA is concerned about the fact that it can cause cardiovascular complications, followed by stroke and myocardial infarctions. Moreover, the stimulation of breast is restricted (with and/or without breast binder), production of breast milk leads to engorgement, distension of breast alveoli were increased. Then, there is termination of lactation vessels for several days. About 40% of women are using this method to avoid breast discomfort conditions and breast pain, while 30% of women are experiencing forceful milk leakage. Besides, ice packs are also recommended for the same purpose to apply to the breast tissues.

Chapter 73

Thyroid Hormones and Antithyroid Drugs

Kiran Rajendra Giri, Kamlesh M. Palandurkar, and Reena Rajendra Giri

PH1.36: Describe the mechanism of action, types, doses, side effects, indications, and contraindications of drugs used in endocrine disorders (diabetes mellitus, thyroid disorders, and osteoporosis).

Learning Objectives

- Thyroid hormone.
- Hypothyroidism.
- Hyperthyroidism.
- Antithyroid drugs.

Introduction

Antithyroid drugs have been in use for the management of hyperthyroidism for more than half a century. The drugs play a principal role in the management of hyperthyroidism, and Graves' disease. Before 1940, surgery was the only treatment for hyperthyroidism. In 1942, scientist Prof. Edwin B. Astwood successfully treated patients of hyperthyroidism with thiourea.

Regulation of Thyroid Axis (Fig. 73.1) (IM12.13, IM12.14, IM12.15)

Thyroid-Stimulating Hormone

The release of thyroid-stimulating hormone (TSH) is pulsatile and has a diurnal rhythm. Its levels increase at night. It is composed of α and β subunits. The α subunit of TSH is common to luteinizing hormone, follicle-stimulating hormone, and human chorionic gonadotropin, while the β subunit is unique to TSH. The normal TSH level excludes primary abnormality of thyroid function. Immunochemiluminometric assay is used for measurement of TSH level. The binding of TSH to its receptor stimulates the Gs adenylyl cyclase–cyclic AMP pathway. A higher concentration also activates the Gq–PLC pathway. TSH attaches to TSH receptor at the basolateral surface of the follicular cell. The normal TSH level is 0.4 to 4.0 mIU/L. It stimulates T3 and T4 secretion, whereas somatostatin and dopamine inhibit TSH release.

The details of the important sources, levels of daily intake of Iodine, and their daily production of thyroid hormones are given in **Table 73.1**, **Table 73.2**, and **Table 73.3**.

Steps of Biosynthesis of Thyroid Hormone

1. Uptake of iodide.
2. Oxidation and iodination.
3. Formation of thyroxine and triiodothyronine from iodotyrosine.

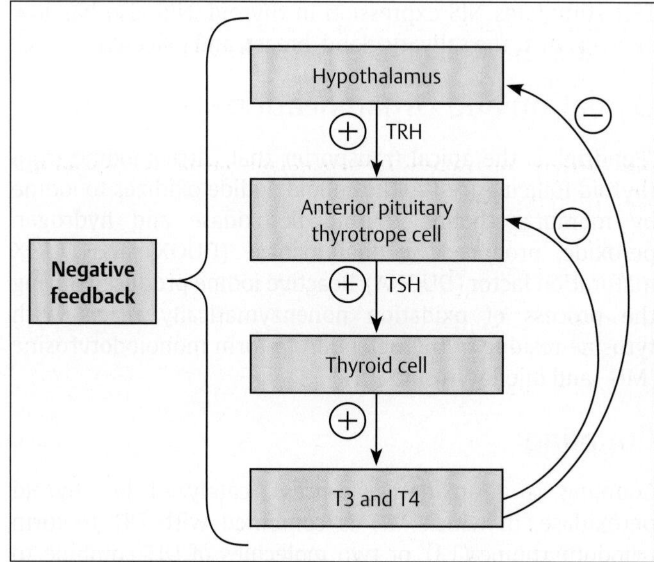

Fig. 73.1 Regulation of thyroid axis.

Table 73.1 Daily intake of iodine	
Adult	150 µg/d
Pregnant women	220 µg/d
Breastfeeding	290 µg/d

Table 73.2 Daily production of thyroid hormones	
T4	80–100 µg
T3	30–40 µg

Table 73.3 Source of iodine	
High source of iodine	Dairy product, fish
Minimal source of iodine	Vegetables, meat

Note: 75-µg iodine is daily utilized for hormone synthesis.

4. Synthesis and secretion of thyroid hormone.
5. Conversion of T4 to T3 in peripheral tissue.

Iodide Uptake or Pump

Iodine is reduced to iodide in the intestine and reaches the systemic circulation in the form of iodide ion (I^-). The thyroid gland has an active transport mechanism, sodium/iodide symporter (NIS; specific membrane-bound protein), located at the basolateral membrane of thyroid follicular cell.

Iodide Uptake Enhancer

1. TSH.
2. Iodine deficiency.

Iodine Uptake Inhibitor

1. Iodide ion.
2. Drugs: digoxin, thiocyanate, perchlorate.

TSH stimulates NIS expression in thyroid. NIS also has low expression at the salivary gland, breast, and placenta.

Oxidation and Organification

"Pendrin" is the apical transporter that carries iodine from thyroid follicular cell to the colloid. Iodide oxidizes to iodine by membrane-bound thyroid peroxidase and hydrogen peroxide, produced by dual oxidase (DUOX) and DUOX maturation factor (DUOXA). Reactive iodine produced during the process of oxidation nonenzymatically reacts with tyrosine residue of thyroglobulin to form monoiodotyrosine (MIT) and diiodotyrosine (DIT).

Coupling

Coupling is an oxidative process, catalyzed by thyroid peroxidase, in which MIT is combined with DIT to form triiodothyronine (T3), or two molecules of DIT combine to form thyroxine (T4). In the case of hormone deficiency, more amount of T3 is formed to produce high amount of active hormone. This process of coupling is stimulated by TSH.

Synthesis and Secretion of Thyroid Hormone

T4 and T3 are still within thyroglobulin, which is then taken up by the follicular cell by the process of endocytosis and broken down by lysosomal proteases. Simultaneously, MIT and DIT are deiodinated by enzyme dehalogenase, and then recycled and metabolized within the cell. TSH enhances the activity of lysosomal thiol endopeptidases. T3 is five times more potent than T4 but has shorter half-life of 1 to 2 days. T4 has half-life of 6 to 7 days. T4 and T3 enter circulation from follicular cells.

Peripheral Conversion

The liver and kidney are the main sites for peripheral conversion. T4 is converted to T3 by iodothyronine deiodinase enzymes.

Types of Deiodinase Enzymes

1. D1: thyroid, liver, kidney; lower affinity for T4. D1 is inhibited by propylthiouracil but D2 remains unaffected.
2. D2: pituitary gland, brain, brown fat, thyroid gland. D2 deiodinase enzyme has higher affinity for T4 and is regulated by thyroid hormone.
3. D3: human placenta; convert T4 to rT3 (Reverse T3).

Transport, Metabolism, and Excretion

Thyroid hormones bind to plasma proteins such as thyroxine-binding globulin (TBG), transthyretin, and albumin reversibly.

T4 secretion is 20 times more than T3 secretion. As much as 99.98% of T4 and 99.7% of T3 is protein bound.

Out of all protein bound hormones, 80% is bound to TBG. TBG has low concentration and higher affinity for the hormone. Only free T3 and T4 is responsible for all the metabolic processes and action. The metabolic products of this hormone are excreted in the bile by enterohepatic circulation and excreted in urine.

Receptor Mechanism of Thyroid Hormones

Thyroid hormones bind to nuclear receptor. TRα is mainly present in the brain, kidney, gonads, muscles, and heart, and TRβ is mainly present in the pituitary and liver. TRβ2 isoform has a unique amino terminal that selectively expresses at hypothalamus, playing an important role in the negative feedback mechanism.

There are two binding domains, DNA-binding domain and C-terminal ligand-binding domain. Thyroid hormone binds to central specific DNA sequence, which is also known as thyroid response element. T3 has 10 to 15 times greater than T4 affinity for binding to the receptor. After binding, the receptor either homodimerizes or heterodimerizes with retinoid X (RXR) receptor. This brings conformational change in the receptor, depending upon the nature of regulator, which either stimulates or inhibits gene transcription and protein synthesis. Conformational change releases the corepressor and binds the coactivator.

Indication for Uses of Thyroid Hormones

1. Hypothyroidism.
2. Hypothyroidism during pregnancy.
3. Myxedema coma.
4. Congenital hypothyroidism.
5. Thyroid cancer.
6. Thyroid nodule.

Adverse Effects/Precautions While Taking Thyroid Hormone

1. Overtreatment leads to hyperthyroidism.
2. Increased risk of atrial fibrillation, especially in the elderly population.
3. Increased risk of osteoporosis in postmenopausal women.

Drug Interaction

1. Antacids, bile acid sequestrants, and food impair thyroxine absorption.
2. Rifampicin and phenytoin increase thyroxine metabolism.
3. Amiodarone impairs T4 to T3 conversion.
4. Metformin decreases TSH without changing free T4 in levothyroxine-treated patient.

Preparation Available

1. Levothyroxine sodium: tablets or liquid-filled capsules for oral administration and lyophilized powder for injection.
2. Liothyronine: salt of T3 in tablet or in an injectable form, liothyronine absorption is nearly 100%.

Thyroxine (T4) is the hormone of choice for thyroid hormone replacement therapy. Lower doses are recommended for older individuals. In cases of cardiovascular disorders, replacement dose is 12.5 to 50 µg/ day. Levothyroxine is used off-label in infertility, refractory anemia, and chronic constipation.

Hypothyroidism

Neonatal hypothyroidism is due to thyroid gland dysgenesis in 82 to 85% of newborns. Inborn errors of thyroid hormone synthesis affect 18% of the neonatal population. Congenital hypothyroidism is due to TSH-blocking antibodies in mother or due to intake of antithyroid drugs. Autoimmune hypothyroidism may be associated with goiter, for example, Hashimoto's disease due to immune reaction against thyroglobulin.

Clinical Features

Clinical features of hypothyroidism are mentioned in **Box 73.1**.

Diagnosis

Mainly elevation of TSH level; in some patients, unbound T4 level is required to confirm clinical hypothyroidism.

Treatment

For congenital hypothyroidism, the average dosage for an infant between 1 and 6 months of age is 10 to 15 µg/kg/day. For hypothyroidism in adults, levothyroxine 1.7 µg/kg body weight is given daily 30 minutes before breakfast.

Subclinical Hypothyroidism

Subclinical hypothyroidism is thyroid hormone deficiency with no clinical feature of hypothyroidism. Raised low-density lipoprotein and lower high-density lipoprotein levels are also important features in some patients. Generally, no treatment is required, but if TSH level is severely increased (>10 mU/L), levothyroxine 25 to 50 µg/day is given.

Myxedema Coma

Myxedema coma is an emergency condition due to long-standing hypothyroidism precipitated by infection, congestive heart failure, or stress. Cardinal features are hypothermia, seizures, hallucination respiratory depression, edema, bradycardia, muscle weakness, tendency to gain weight, pleural effusion, and pericardial effusion. Elderly population is mostly affected.

Treatment

1. Intravenous (IV) thyroid hormone: levothyroxine 200 to 400 µg, followed by a daily full replacement dose (adding levothyroxine 10 µg IV, followed by 2.5–10 µg every 8 hours, is also advised in some patients).
2. Ventilator support.
3. Rewarming.
4. IV glucocorticoid (hydrocortisone 100 mg IV, followed by 25–50 mg every 8 hours) is recommended until coexisting adrenal insufficiency is excluded.

Hypothyroidism in Pregnancy

Hypothyroidism during pregnancy is due to estrogen-induced high serum concentration of TBG and small amount of placental transfer of levothyroxine from mother to fetus. Hypothyroidism increases the risk of miscarriage and premature delivery. Assessment of T4 level is important. In pregnant women, levothyroxine should be adjusted for maintenance of TSH at lower reference range. In some pregnant patients, however, increased dose of levothyroxine is required for stringent control of TSH. Thyroxine should be

Box 73.1 Clinical features of hypothyroidism
Neonates
Jaundice
Photophobia
Enlarged tongue
Feeding problem
Delayed bone maturation
Adult
Dry skin
Feeling of cold
Hair loss
Weight gain
Paresthesia
Puffy face
Bradycardia
Peripheral edema
Carpal tunnel syndrome
Hypoglycemia
Hypercholesterolemia
Hypertriglyceridemia

administered after at least a 4-hour gap from vitamins and calcium doses.

Thyroid Cancer

Thyroid papillary or follicular carcinoma requires surgical thyroidectomy or radioiodine therapy and then levothyroxine treatment lifelong to maintain TSH at lower level.

Thyroid Nodule

Thyroid nodule, which causes discomfort in the neck region, is common in females. Ionizing radiation increases the chances of nodule formation. If TSH is elevated, it requires levothyroxine treatment.

Hyperthyroidism

Overfunction of thyroid gland is known as hyperthyroidism. Thyrotoxicosis means excess level of thyroid hormone in blood circulation. Major etiologies of thyrotoxicosis are Graves' disease and toxic nodular goiter.

Different Types of Thyrotoxicosis

Primary:

- Graves' disease.
- Toxic nodular goiter.
- Toxic adenoma.
- Drugs such as iodine access (Jod-Basedow phenomenon).

Thyrotoxicosis without hyperthyroidism:

- Subacute thyroiditis.
- Thyroid hormone ingestion.

Secondary hyperthyroidism:

- TSH-secreting pituitary adenoma.
- Gestational thyrotoxicosis.

Symptoms and Signs

- Hyperactivity.
- Diarrhea.
- Weight loss with increased appetite.
- Palpitation.
- Heat intolerance.
- Tachycardia.
- Atrial fibrillation in the elderly.
- Skin retraction.
- Warm moist skin.
- Exophthalmos.
- Hyperglycemia.
- Decreased triglycerides and cholesterol.

Antithyroid Drugs

Antithyroid drugs disrupt thyroid hormone synthesis, metabolism, and release process.

Classification

1. *Iodide uptake inhibitor*: perchlorate, thiocyanate, nitrate.
2. *Drugs interfering with organification of iodine*: thionamides, thiocyanate, sulfonamides.
3. *Interfering with coupling reaction*: sulfonamide, thionamides.
4. *Hormone release inhibitor*: lithium salt, iodide.
5. *Drugs interfering with peripheral iodothyronine deiodination*: propylthiouracil, amiodarone.
6. *Thioamide derivative*: propylthiouracil, methimazole, carbimazole.

Thioamide Derivatives Mechanism of Action

1. Interference with incorporation of iodine into tyrosyl residue of thyroglobulin.
2. Inhibition of the coupling of iodotyrosyl residues to form iodothyronines by inhibiting peroxidase enzyme.
3. Propylthiouracil partially inhibits peripheral deiodination of T4 to T3.

Pharmacokinetics

Metabolism of methimazole decreases during liver disease. Propylthiouracil dosing frequency is one to four times daily. Methimazole dosing frequency is once or twice daily.

Carbimazole is converted to methimazole after absorption. Comparison between propylthiouracil and methimazole can be seen in **Table 73.4.**

Therapeutic Indication

1. Graves' disease.
2. In conjugation with radioactive iodine treatment.
3. Pretreatment before thyroid surgery to make the patient euthyroid.

Adverse Effect

Reversible agranulocytosis (< 1%) is a rare side effect, which occurs mostly in the first few weeks or months. Symptoms include sore throat, mouth ulcer, and fever.

Periodic prospective monitoring of granulocyte count is essential for early identification of agranulocytosis. Mild urticaria and rashes should be managed by antihistaminic drugs and corticosteroids.

Table 73.4 Comparison between propylthiouracil and methimazole

Characteristics	Propylthiouracil	Methimazole
Plasma protein binding	75%	Nil
Volume of distribution	0.4 L/kg	0.7 L/kg
Plasma half-life	75 min	4–6 h
Transplacental passage and level in breast milk	Low	Low

Other adverse effects include hepatitis and nephritis. Overtreatment leads to hypothyroidism. Thyroid function test should be done every 2 to 4 months. Due to hepatotoxicity of propylthiouracil, its indication is limited in the first trimester of pregnancy. Cholestasis is a major adverse effect due to carbimazole and methimazole.

Ionic Inhibitors

Ionic inhibitors interfere with the concentration of iodide within the thyroid gland. Thiocyanate and perchlorate resemble iodide ion. Higher concentration of thiocyanate inhibits organification of iodine. Perchlorate inhibits NIS actively and competitively, thus inhibiting iodide trapping. A major adverse effect of perchlorate is fatal aplastic anemia.

Iodine

It is the oldest remedy. Iodine inhibits its own transport and interferes with expression of NIS. This effect is acute and temporary, with beneficial effects remaining only for 10 to 15 days. Iodine inhibits synthesis of iodotyrosines and iodothyronines (Wolff–Chaikoff effect). It inhibits thyroid hormone release. Patients get rapid response in hyperthyroidism. Vascularity of the gland reduces, gland becomes firm, and colloid reaccumulates. Iodine is used for the treatment of the following:

1. Thyrotoxic crisis with antithyroid drug and propranolol.
2. Pretreatment before thyroidectomy.

Other preparations of iodine are Lugol's solution (5% iodine and 10% potassium iodide) and tincture iodine (antiseptic). Adverse effects are acute hypersensitivity reactions (type III) such as angioedema, laryngeal edema, multiple cutaneous hemorrhages, and thrombocytopenic purpura. Chronic intoxication (iodism) is related to dose and leads to sore throat, increased salivation, coryza, sneezing, irritation of the eyes, pulmonary edema, and fatal eruption (ioderma).

Radioactive Iodine

Radioactive I^{123} and I^{131} isotopes of iodine are used for diagnosis and treatment of thyroid diseases.

I^{123} emits gamma rays having half-life of 13 hours and is mainly used for diagnosis purpose. I^{131} emits gamma rays and beta particles; half-life is 8 days and is used therapeutically for thyroid destruction in thyroid carcinoma and for treatment of metastatic diseases. It causes progressive destruction of thyroid cells. Pretreatment with antithyroid drug reduces or eliminates the complications. Carbimazole should be stopped 2 to 3 days before radioiodine use to increase uptake, and it should start 3 to 7 days after treatment of radioactive iodine, till effect of radioiodine arrives.

Indication

1. Hyperthyroidism in the elderly with cardiovascular diseases.
2. Graves' disease persistent or recurring after subtotal thyroidectomy.
3. Toxic nodular goiter.

Available Preparation

Sodium iodide solution for oral administration is available at a dose 4 to15 mCi, with recommended target of delivering 8 mCi to the thyroid gland, based on the 24-hour radioiodine uptake.

Gradual decrease in hyperthyroidism takes over 2 to 3 months.

Radioactive iodine dose = (thyroid mass [g] × 80–200 mCi/g)% uptake.

Persistent hyperthyroidism can be treated with a second dose of radioiodine, usually 6 months after the first dose.

Advantage

1. Decreases risk of surgery.
2. Less expensive.
3. Patients do not require hospitalization.

Disadvantage

1. Delayed hypothyroidism.
2. Some studies state increased risk of stomach, kidney, and breast carcinoma linked with the presence of NIS transporter.

Radioiodine is contraindicated in pregnancy, young children, and breastfeeding women.

Graves' Disease

Graves' disease is an autoimmune disorder due to defect in suppressor T-lymphocyte, which stimulates B-lymphocyte to synthesize antibodies to thyroidal antigens that are directed against TSH receptor. In laboratory diagnosis, T3, T4, fT3, and T4 are elevated and TSH is suppressed. Cytokines appear to play an important role in thyroid-associated ophthalmopathy. The first-line treatment is antithyroid drug therapy controlling hyperthyroidism. Destruction of the thyroid gland with radioactive iodine and surgical thyroidectomy also play important roles in management. Antithyroid drug therapy is preferred in young patients. In mild-to-moderate disease, methimazole 20 to 40 mg is given as early morning dose for 4 to 8 weeks, and the maintenance dose required is 5 to 15 mg once daily.

Principles of Management of Hyperthyroidism

The **Fig. 73.2** gives the management for hyper hyperthyroidism

Thyroid Storm

Thyroid storm is an extreme manifestation of thyrotoxicosis present in association with Graves' disease, toxic multinodular goiter, and acute thyroiditis. Immunological involvement and cytokines' release are precipitated by trauma, surgery, sepsis, diabetic ketoacidosis, and toxemia of pregnancy. Induction of anesthesia may lead to precipitation of thyrotoxicosis.

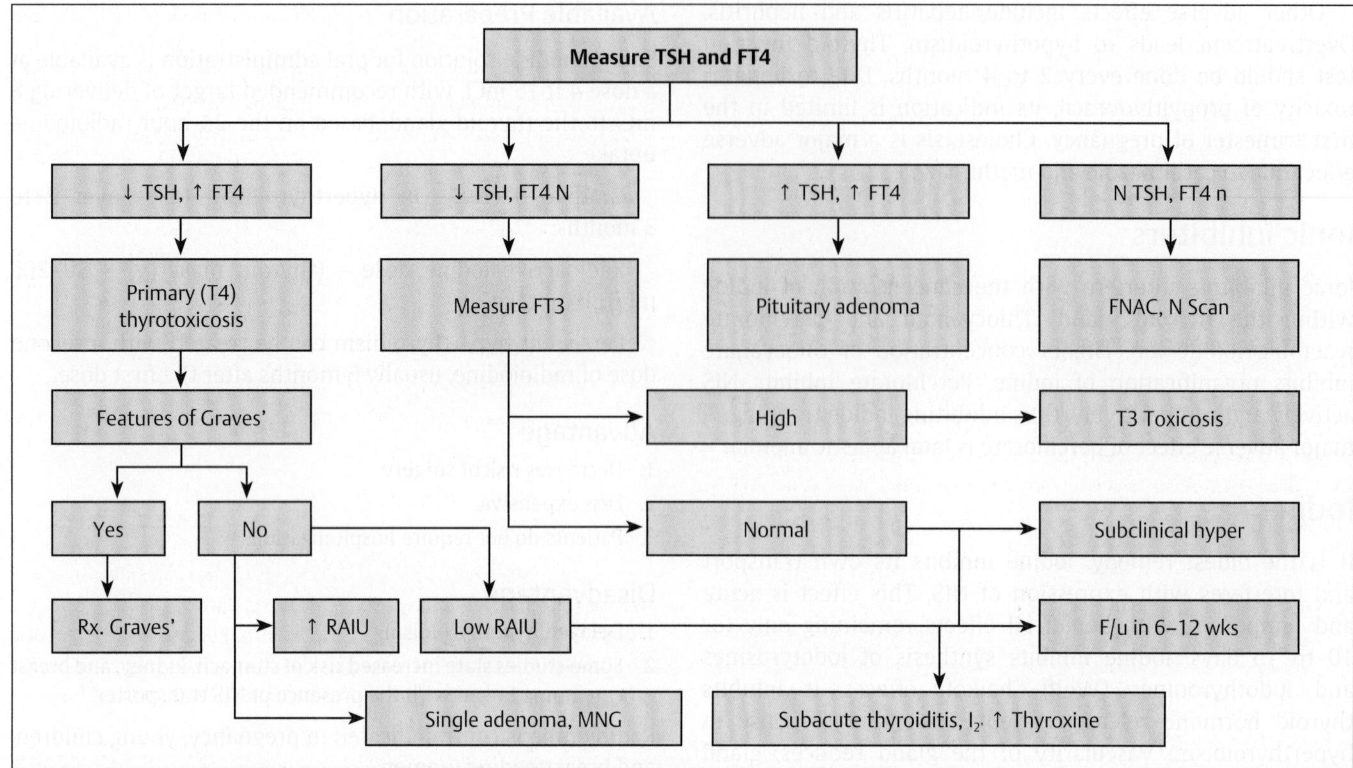

Fig. 73.2 Algorithm for hyperthyroidism. RAIU, radioiodine uptake.

Clinical manifestations include fever, profuse sweating, tachycardia, arrhythmia, pulmonary edema, congestive heart failure, weight loss, and respiratory distress.

Management

Emergency situation requires rapid management:

1. Ventilator support.
2. IV fluid: dextrose preferred to cope with high-metabolic demand.
3. Propylthiouracil: 500 to 1,000 mg loading dose, then 250 mg four times a day.
4. Saturated KI solution 6 mg daily orally.
5. Propranolol 60 to 80 mg oral four times a day to minimize sympathetic symptoms.
6. IV radiocontrast such as ipodate and iopanoic acid can be used to suppress T4 and T3 release from thyroid.
7. Hydrocortisone 300 mg IV bolus, 100 mg IV every 8 hours.
8. Plasmapheresis to remove large amount of protein-bound thyroid hormone, which plays life-saving role.
9. Iodine preparation should be stopped once acute phase is resolved.
10. Diltiazem for complications such as heart failure.

Pharmacological Basis of Propranolol

Role of β-Blocker

Propranolol and atenolol help to control adrenergic symptoms and cardiovascular symptoms (β1 blockade). Propranolol prevents peripheral conversion of T4 to T3 by inhibition of monodeiodinase. Propranolol 20 to 40 mg every 6 hours is used in the treatment of thyroid storm. β-Blockers are useful in patients with thyrotoxicosis, till the response to carbimazole or radioactive iodine is achieved.

Contraindications: asthma, airway diseases.

Toxic Nodular Goiter

Toxic nodular goiter is common in elderly women, in whom free thyroxine level is moderately elevated. Cardiac symptoms are tachycardia, palpitation, atrial fibrillation, nervousness, tremors, and weight loss. Toxic multinodular goiter is treated with antithyroid drugs, followed by subtotal thyroidectomy.

Subacute Thyroiditis

Subacute thyroiditis may be due to acute viral infection and transient release of thyroid hormone due to destruction of thyroid parenchyma. Supportive treatments such as β-blocking drugs without intrinsic sympathomimetic activity, corticosteroids, and nonsteroidal anti-inflammatory drugs are used to reduce pain and inflammation.

Management of Thyrotoxicosis during Pregnancy and Lactation

1. Use of lowest dosage of thionamides (normal range of total T4 during pregnancy is estimated to be 1.5 times of nonpregnant state).
2. Monitoring of maternal T4 concentration, dose titration of drug, and risk–benefit ratio, and keeping T4 just above reference range.
3. Thyroidectomy; if persistently high dose of thionamide is required, β-blocker and low dose of iodine may be given before surgery.

Treatment Modality/Drug for Following Conditions

1. Hyperthyroidism in the elderly: high risk of cardiac morbidity; radioactive iodine is safe as primary treatment option.
2. No remission to prolonged treatment with antithyroid drugs: total or near-total thyroidectomy or radioactive iodine.

Multiple Choice Questions

1. A patient was hospitalized in the emergency department with symptoms of racing heart rate, exceeding 140 beats per minute, high fever, persistent sweating, shaking, agitation, restlessness, and confusion. The patient was stabilized. The patient had excess sweating, excessive hunger, fatigue, and heat intolerance for several weeks. What is the diagnosis?

A. Hyperthyroidism.
B. Hypothyroidism.
C. Hashimoto's thyroiditis.
D. Thyroid storm.

Answer: D

Clinical manifestations of thyroid storm include fever, profuse sweating, tachycardia, arrhythmia, pulmonary edema, congestive heart failure, weight loss, and respiratory distress.

2. Symptoms of menstrual changes or lack of menstruation (amenorrhea), mood swings, hot flashes, and insomnia, anxiety, and warm moist skin may be due to which thyroid disorder?

A. Hypothyroidism.
B. Hyperthyroidism.
C. Hashimoto's thyroiditis.
D. Thyroid storm.

Answer: B

Hyperactivity, diarrhea, weight loss with increased appetite, palpitation, heat intolerance, tachycardia, atrial fibrillation in the elderly, skin retraction, warm moist skin, exophthalmos, hyperglycemia, decreased triglycerides and cholesterol, and anemia due to increased RBC turnover are the clinical manifestations of hyperthyroidism.

3. A 50-year-old housewife complains of progressive weight gain of 20 pounds in 1 year, fatigue, postural dizziness, loss of memory, slow speech, deepening of her voice, dry skin, constipation, and cold intolerance. What is the diagnosis?

A. Hypothyroidism.
B. Hyperthyroidism.
C. Hashimoto's thyroiditis.
D. Thyroid storm.

Answer: A

Dry skin, feeling cold, hair loss, weight gain, paresthesia, puffy face, bradycardia, peripheral edema, carpal tunnel syndrome, hypoglycemia, hypercholesterolemia, hypertriglyceridemia, anemia due to decreased RBC production, and mental retardation are the symptoms of hypothyroidism.

4. A 55-year-old nurse complained of nervousness, weakness, and palpitations with exertion for the past 6 months. Recently, she noticed excessive sweating and wanted to sleep with fewer blankets than her husband. She had maintained a normal weight of 120 pounds but was eating twice as much as she did 1 year ago. Menstrual periods have been regular but there was less bleeding. Her thyroid contained three nodules, two on the right and one on the left, with a total gland size of 60 g (three times the normal size), all nodules being of firm consistency, and there was no lymphadenopathy. In laboratory diagnosis, TSH level is low, T4 normal, and T3 level elevated. What is the diagnosis?

A. Hypothyroidism.
B. Hyperthyroidism.
C. Hashimoto's thyroiditis.
D. Toxic nodular goiter.

Answer: D

Toxic nodular goiter is common in elderly women, in whom free thyroxine level is moderately elevated. Cardiac symptoms are tachycardia, palpitation, atrial fibrillation, nervousness, tremors, and weight loss. Toxic multinodular goiter is treated with antithyroid drugs followed by subtotal thyroidectomy.

5. Which hormone should be followed for treatment compliance of hypothyroidism?

A. T3.
B. T4.
C. fT3.
D. Thyroid-stimulating hormone (TSH).

Answer: D

High and low thyroid-stimulating hormone (TSH) levels are important for thyroid disease; high TSH level indicates underactive thyroid gland, leading to hypothyroidism, while low TSH level indicates overactive thyroid gland, leading to hyperthyroidism.

6. What is the normal level of thyroid-stimulating hormone (TSH) for a normal adult?

A. 0.4 to 4 mIU/L.
B. 2 to 8 mIU/L.
C. 0.1 to 0.8 mIU/L.
D. 6 to 12 mIU /L.

Answer: A

Normal level of TSH for a normal adult is 0.4 to 4 mIU/L.

7. Radioactive iodine is contraindicated in:

A. Elderly.
B. Adult with cardiovascular disease.
C. Pregnant women.
D. None of the above.

Answer: C

Radioactive iodine is contraindicated in pregnancy and young children. Breastfeeding leads to fetal hypothyroidism.

8. Agranulocytosis is major adverse effect of:

A. Propylthiouracil.

B. Iodine.

C. Radioactive iodine.

D. None of the above.

Answer: A

Propylthiouracil leads to reversible agranulocytosis (< 1%), which is a rare adverse effect occurring in the first few weeks or months; symptoms are sore throat, mouth ulcer, and fever. Periodic prospective monitoring of granulocyte count is essential.

9. Following is/are the advantage/s of radioactive iodine:

A. Decreases risk of surgery.

B. Less expensive.

C. Hospitalization not required.

D. All of the above.

Answer: D

Advantages of radioactive iodine are that it is less expensive, patients do not require hospitalization, and there is no surgical risk.

10. Drug (s) interfering with organification of iodine is/are:

A. Perchlorate.

B. Sulfonamides.

C. Thiocyanate.

D. Both B and C.

Answer: D

Drugs interfering with organification of iodine are thionamides, thiocyanate, and sulfonamides.

Pharmacology of Estrogens and Related Drugs

Sheshidhar Bannale

PH1.37: Describe the mechanisms of action, types, doses, side effects, indications, and contraindications of the drugs used as sex hormones, their analogs, and anterior pituitary hormones.

PH1.39: Describe mechanism of action, types, doses, side effects, indications, and contraindications of drugs used for contraception.

Learning Objectives

- Estrogen.
- Progestins.
- Contraceptive drugs.

Estrogen

Estrogens are naturally occurring endogenous hormones. They control and influence various physiological actions. In women, they affect developmental process, ovulation, cyclical changes in reproductive tract, and metabolic actions. In males, they influence bone development, spermatogenesis, and behavior. Pharmacological actions are mainly extension of physiological roles.

Classification (Fig. 74.1)

Synthesis of these endogenous compounds in the ovary is primarily influenced by gonadotropins. Luteinizing hormone (LH) stimulates theca cells of ovarian follicle to produce androgens, androstenedione, and testosterone. These are taken up by granulosa cells of ovarian follicles. In ovarian follicles, under the influence of follicle-stimulating hormone (FSH), there is expression of aromatase enzymes. Aromatase converts the androgens into estrogens, estrone, and estradiol. Adipose tissue and liver cells also contain aromatase, which converts circulating androgen into estrogen (**Fig. 74.2**).

1. Estradiol is the major naturally secreted estrogen by the ovary. Steps of production are depicted in **Fig. 74.2**. Estradiol, estrone, and estriol are circulating natural estrogens.
2. In males, small quantity (2–20 µg/day) of estradiol is produced by aromatization of testosterone in the testes. Natural estrogen, given orally, has lesser bioavailability due to high first-pass metabolism in the liver. Hence, to overcome this, synthetic estrogens have been produced.
3. Daily secretion of estrogen in menstruating women varies from 10 to 100 µg, depending on the phase of the menstrual cycle. Blood level of estrogen increases gradually under the influence of FSH during the follicular phase. Due to preovulatory surge in FSH, corresponding increase in estrogen is also seen.

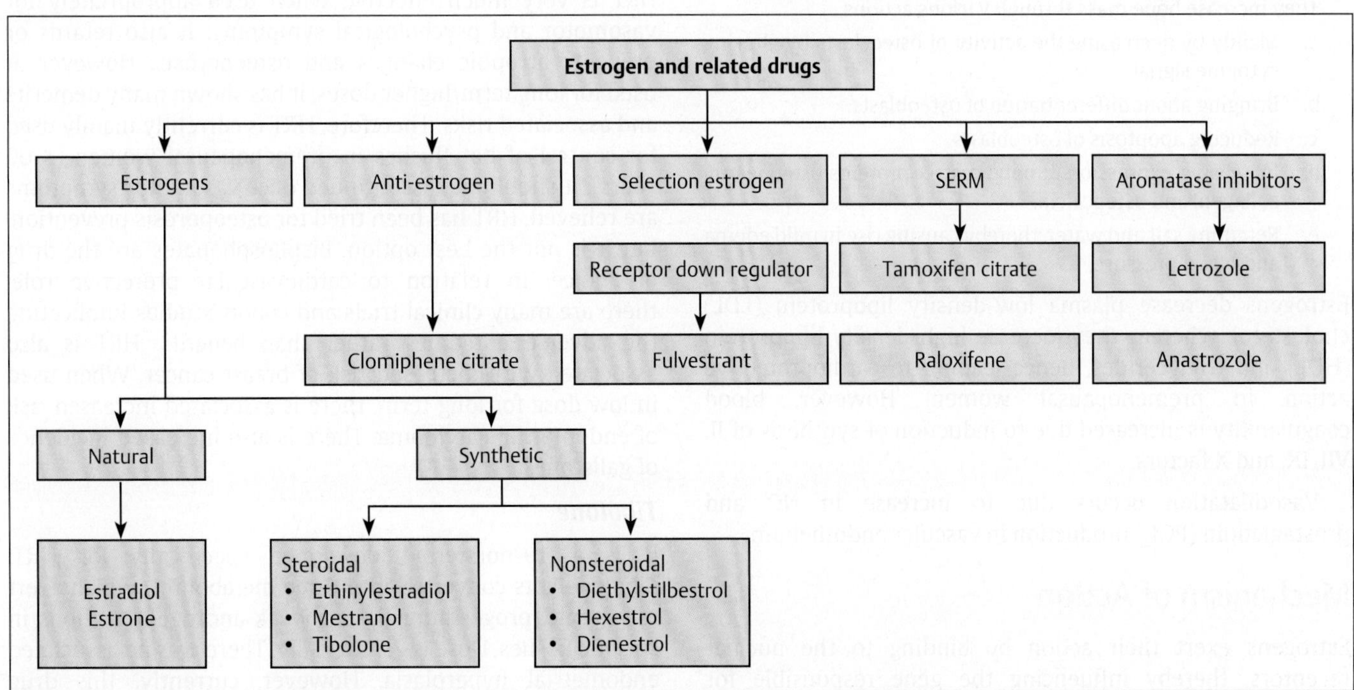

Fig. 74.1 Classification of estrogen and related drugs. SERM, selective estrogen receptor modulators.

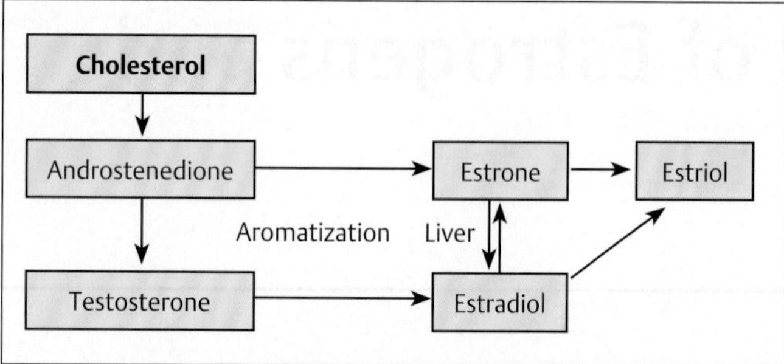

Fig. 74.2 Steps depicting conversion of cholesterol to estrogen.

Postovulation, corpus luteum continues to secrete estrogen. They exert feedback inhibition of FSH by acting on pituitary and hypothalamus. During pregnancy, placenta secretes large quantities of estrogen, which subsides after delivery (**Fig. 74.2**).

Physiological Actions

1. Reproductive tract: Estrogens bring pubertal change, that is, growth of uterus, fallopian tubes, and vagina. Vaginal epithelium gets thickened, stratified, and cornified. Endometrial proliferation occurs during the preovulatory phase.
   a. Estrogens favor sperm penetration by increasing rhythmic contractions of fallopian tubes and uterus. They also induce watery alkaline cervical secretion and sensitizes uterus to oxytocin.
2. Secondary sexual characters: Estrogens at puberty cause thelarche (growth of breast), growth of pubic and axillary hair and feminine body contours, and behavior changes. They also influence Voice changes.
3. Estrogens cause vasodilatation of capillaries in general and endometrial in particular.
4. They promote union of epiphyses influencing height.
5. Metabolic actions: Estrogens are weekly anabolic in nature and they increase bone mass through various actions.
   a. Mainly by decreasing the activity of osteoclasts by altering cytokine signal.
   b. Bringing about differentiation of osteoblasts.
   c. Reducing apoptosis of osteoblasts.
   d. Increasing expression of bone matrix proteins osteonectin, collagen, and osteocalcin.
   e. Retaining salt and water, thereby causing rise in mild edema and blood pressure.

Estrogens decrease plasma low-density lipoprotein (LDL) cholesterol, whereas they increase high-density lipoprotein (HDL) and triglycerides, hence leading to cardioprotective action in premenopausal women. However, blood coagulability is increased due to induction of synthesis of II, VII, IX, and X factors.

Vasodilatation occurs due to increase in NO and prostaglandin (PGI_2) production in vascular endothelium.

Mechanism of Action

Estrogens exert their action by binding to the nuclear receptors, thereby influencing the gene responsible for synthesis of various proteins through estrogen response elements. There are two subtypes of estrogen receptors (ER), ER_α and ER_β.

ER_α is predominantly present in the female genital tract, breasts, endometrium, hypothalamus, and vascular smooth muscles.

ER_β is mainly expressed in the brain, bone, ovary, and prostate.

Some of the rapid actions of estrogens are carried out by ER present on cell wall.

Pharmacokinetics

Estrogens are available for oral, parenteral, transdermal, and topical administrations, but natural estrogens are inactive orally, as they get extensively metabolized in the liver.

Estradiol esters injected intramuscularly (IM) are slowly absorbed and exert longer action. Transdermal application also leads to continuous absorption over a period of a week and is to be changed later. Natural estrogens bind to sex hormone–binding globulin (SHBG) as well as albumin.

Estrogens are conjugated with glucuronic acid and sulfate, which are excreted in the urine and bile. They undergo some amount of enterohepatic circulation.

Ethinylestradiol is metabolized very slowly, with a $t_{1/2}$ of 12 to 20 hours, and is administered orally and is considered potent.

Uses

Mainly, they are used as part of contraception and hormone replacement therapy (HRT).

Hormone Replacement Therapy

HRT is very much effective when used appropriately for vasomotor and psychological symptoms; it also retards or prevents atrophic changes and osteoporosis. However, if used for long term/higher doses, it has shown many demerits and associated risks. Therefore, HRT is currently mainly used for control of hot flushes in premenopausal women (≤ 60 years). It should be discontinued once vasomotor symptoms are relieved. HRT has been tried for osteoporosis prevention, but it is not the best option. Bisphosphonates are the drug of choice. In relation to cardiovascular protective role, there are many clinical trials and cohort studies implicating the adverse outcomes rather than benefits. HRT is also associated with increased risk of breast cancer. When used in low dose for long term, there is associated increased risk of endometrial carcinoma. There is also increased incidence of gallstones.

Tibolone

It is a 19-norsteroid developed specifically for HRT. Tibolone gets converted into three metabolites, which exert estrogenic, progestational, and weak androgenic actions in specific tissues. Dose is 2.5 mg daily. There was no associated endometrial hyperplasia. However, currently, this drug popularity has declined.

Primary Hypogonadism

It is associated with Turner's syndrome or hypopituitarism, leading to delayed puberty among girls. In this case, cyclic estrogen is administered and progestin can be added.

Senile Vaginitis

Estrogen, when applied topically, brings changes in vaginal tissue, reduces atrophic changes, and even relieves pruritis.

Other Uses

Estrogen is also used in treating dysmenorrhea, acne, and dysfunctional uterine bleeding, and for palliative therapy in prostate carcinoma.

Antiestrogens

Clomiphene Citrate

It is an estrogen antagonist. It blocks both α and β receptors in all tissues, thereby blocking the estrogen-induced feedback inhibition of FSH and LH. Thus, there is increased release of FSH and LH, leading to enlargement of ovaries and ovulation. This drug is used mainly as "ovulation-inducing agent." Dose is 50 mg daily for 5 days, starting from the fifth day of the cycle. Therefore, it leads to conception in women who previously had anovular cycles. It is well-absorbed orally and its half-life is around 6 days. It is metabolized in the liver and excreted in the bile. Side effects include hot flushes, gastric upset, polycystic ovaries, vertigo, and allergic dermatitis.

This drug can be used for a maximum of six cycles. Other uses involve aiding males with oligozoospermia and in in vitro fertilization.

Selective Estrogen Receptor Modulators

There are drugs that have estrogen agonistic as well as antagonistic actions, depending on the tissue/organ. Hence, these are known as selective estrogen receptor modulators (SERMs). Examples include tamoxifen citrate, toremifene, and raloxifene.

Tamoxifen Citrate

It is a SERM, chemically related to clomiphene. It interacts differently with many coactivators and subcellular signaling mechanisms, depending on the tissue.

Agonistic Actions

It acts as a partial agonist at the uterus, bone, liver, and pituitary, and reduces LDL cholesterol level. Hence, there is proliferation of the endometrium, decrease in gonadotrophin levels, and increase in bone density. It is also associated with increased risk of deep vein thrombosis.

Antagonistic Actions

It acts as a potent antagonist at the breast and blood vessels. Hence, it is effective in carcinoma of the breast.

Pharmacokinetics

It is available as 10 mg tablet; 20 mg is effective orally, with biphasic half-life of 10 hours and 7 days. Also, it is long acting with active metabolites and excreted primarily in the bile.

Uses

It is one of the common drugs used in the management of ER-positive breast carcinoma. It is approved for metastatic breast carcinoma in premenopausal women. It is also used to prevent recurrent postmastectomy and is given prophylactically to those who have high-risk potential for breast carcinoma. It can be given for up to 5 years, whereas in postmenopausal women it can be given for 2 years, followed by aromatase inhibitors.

Side Effects

Hot flushes, vomiting, rashes, vaginal bleeding, menstrual irregularities, and increased risk of venous thromboembolism are common side effects. Other side effects include anorexia, depression, and ocular changes.

Toremifene

It is similar to tamoxifen but has lesser agonistic action at ER.

Raloxifene

It is also a SERM and differs from tamoxifen in tissue-specific actions.

Partial Agonist

In cardiovascular system and bone and lipid metabolism.

Antagonist

Breast and endometrium.

Mode of Action

It acts by binding to nuclear receptors, with a specific DNA target named raloxifene response element. Its advantages are that it does not cause endometrial stimulation and related adverse effects such as risk of endometrial carcinoma and has positive effect on bone health. However, bisphosphonates are more efficacious for osteoporosis. Studies have shown that it reduces breast carcinoma by 60 to 68%.

It is available as 60-mg tablet. It is well-absorbed orally, but has low bioavailability. Its $t_{1/2}$ is 28 hours and it is excreted mainly in the feces.

Side Effects

Side effects include leg cramps, hot flushes, and serious risk of venous thromboembolism and pulmonary embolism.

Uses

1. It is approved for prevention of breast carcinoma in high-risk patients.
2. It is used as a second line of treatment for management of osteoporosis.

Aromatase Inhibitors

These are the drugs that block aromatase enzyme, which governs the final key step in the production of estrogen from androstenedione and testosterone by aromatization.

1. Reversible, nonsteroidal inhibitors: letrozole, anastrozole.
2. Irreversible, steroidal inhibitors: exemestane.

These drugs are orally active, and they block aromatization in breast tissue and cause complete deprivation of estrogen in postmenopausal women. These drugs are not effective when functioning ovaries are intact. They are devoid of SERMs-related venous thromboembolism risk.

Letrozole has 100% oral bioavailability; anastrozole 40 mg has long half-life, with peak action at 7 to 10 days. Exemestane, even though it irreversibly blocks 90% of enzymes, has weak androgenic activity.

Uses

Letrozole is the first-line drug for adjuvant therapy in carcinoma breast. It can be extended beyond 5 years of tamoxifen. It is also currently used as the first-line drug for advanced carcinoma breast.

Adverse Effects

Adverse effects include hot flushes, dyspepsia, vaginal dryness, and joint pain.

Progestins

Compounds that are similar to progesterone in their biological actions are termed as progestins. They mainly carry out secretory changes in the endometrium and maintain pregnancy.

Natural Progestin

Progesterone, a 21-carbon compound which is steroidal in nature, is derived from cholesterol. It is secreted under the influence of LH in second/latter half of the menstrual cycle. If ovum gets fertilized, blastocyst starts/takes up production of chorionic gonadotropin, which sustains the corpus luteum in early pregnancy. Later, placenta starts secreting estrogen and progesterone in large quantities from the second trimester onward.

Synthetic Progestins

Two groups of synthetic compounds with high oral bioavailability have been produced, namely, progesterone derivatives (21C) and 19-nortestosterone (18C) (**Table 74.1**).

Progesterone derivatives have weak antiovulatory actions and are mainly used for HRT, threatened abortion, and endometriosis.

19-Nortestosterone derivatives have weak estrogenic, androgenic, and anabolic actions and potent antiovulatory actions. They are primarily used as part of combination therapy for contraception.

Physiological/Pharmacological of Actions

Genital Organs

They cause secretory changes in estrogen-primed endometrium, that is, increase secretion, tortuosity of glands, and hyperemia. During pregnancy, they bring decidual changes in the endometrium and sensitivity to oxytocin. Pregnancy changes in vagina such as leukocyte infiltration occur. Watery secretions of cervix are converted to thick viscid and scanty cellular secretion.

Mammary Tissue

They cause proliferation of acini in the mammary glands. Continuous exposure during pregnancy stabilizes the mammary glands and prepares them for lactation. Postdelivery fall in progesterone level causes release of prolactin.

Body Temperature

They cause a small rise (0.5°C) in the body temperature by resetting hypothalamic thermostat.

Respiration

In higher doses, during pregnancy, they stimulate respiration.

Central Nervous System

Mild sedative action is seen.

Pituitary

They have negative feedback action at hypothalamic level which, in turn, reduces gonadotropin-releasing hormone (GnRH) secretion. They also reduce preovulatory LH surge and prevent ovulation.

Metabolism

Long-term administration (as oral contraceptive pill [OCP]) is associated with impaired glucose tolerance. 19-Nortestosterone derivatives tend to raise LDL and

Table 74.1 Synthetic progestins

Progesterone derivatives	19-Nortestosterone (18C)
Medroxyprogesterone acetate	Estrones
Megestrol acetate	▪ Norethindrone
Dydrogesterone	▪ Lynestrenol
Hydroxyprogesterone caproate	▪ Allylestrenol
Nomegestrol acetate	Gonanes (13 ethyl substitute)
	▪ Levonorgestrel
	▪ Desogestrel
	▪ Norgestimate
	▪ Gestodene

reduce HDL cholesterol. However, micronized progesterone formulation does not have this adverse action on HDL and LDL levels.

Mechanism of Action

Progestins act by binding to nuclear receptors; there are two isoforms of progesterone receptors, PR-A and PR coded by single gene.

These receptors are present in the monomeric form in the absence of any ligand/drug and are bound to heat shock protein. When progesterone binds to receptors, the heat shock protein gets dissociated, receptors are phosphorylated, and dimerization of receptors takes place. After dimerization, this "progesterone and receptor complex" binds to progesterone response element located on the target genes.

Pharmacokinetics

Oral bioavailability is less, as they undergo high first-pass metabolism. However, micronized large-dose preparations are available as oral preparations. Many injectable formulations, depot preparations, and implants are available.

In plasma, progesterone is bound to albumin and corticosteroid-binding globulin, whereas 19-nortestosterone compounds bind to SHBG. Overall, they have extensive binding to plasma protein, up to 90%.

Elimination $t_{1/2}$ of progesterone is 5 minutes, and it is metabolized primarily in the liver to hydroxylated metabolites and sulfate.

Uses

Contraception

As part of contraceptive pills, it is the most common indication, which is described later in detail.

Dysfunctional Uterine Bleeding

Patients who have dysfunctional bleeding, that is, heavy and irregular, are often associated with ovulation. There is often hyperplastic endometrium because of continuous stimulation by estrogen. Hence, administration of progesterone will check this process, and cyclic treatment along with estrogen regularizes the menstrual bleed.

Endometriosis

It is the presence of endometrial tissue at ectopic sites, leading to pelvic pain, dysmenorrhea, and infertility. Administration of progestins continuously leads to decrease in estrogen and GnRH. Hence, it causes atrophic changes in ectopic endometrial tissue. It may also lead to anovulation. Symptomatically, patients will be relieved usually in 3 to 6 months. Patient will also tolerate well.

Hormone Replacement Therapy

As part of combination therapy, micronized oral progesterone is added for 10 to 12 days of cycle, mainly in nonhysterectomized, postmenopausal women. It will counteract or decrease the risk of endometrial carcinoma.

Premenstrual Dysphoric Syndrome

Women will develop cluster of symptoms such as headache, irritability, fluid retention, and breast tenderness just few days before menstruation. It may even lead to depressive symptoms. Its treatment includes suppression of ovulation, especially in severe cases. Therefore, it is combined with estrogen, cyclically, to suppress ovulation.

Threatened Abortion

In India, for threatened abortion, a pure progestin is commonly used, although there is no deficiency of progesterone in most of the cases. However, in proven cases, it has to be used to support and prevent premature delivery.

Endometrial Carcinoma

High-dose progestins are used as palliative therapy in advanced stage of endometrial carcinoma.

Other Uses

Progesterone is also used in the treatment of fibrocystic disease of the breast, precocious puberty, and patients with short luteal phase. In addition, it is used for postponement of menstruation for short period.

Adverse Effects

Headache, rise in body temperature, edema, breast tenderness, lower esophageal reflux, mood swings, and acne are common side effects. When given continuously, amenorrhea and irregular bleeding can happen. Progestins lower HDL and promote atherogenesis (19-nortestosterone derivative).

Long-term use is associated with precipitation of diabetes mellitus and breast carcinoma. Its use in early pregnancy may cause masculinization of female fetus and congenital anomalies.

Antiprogestins

Mifepristone, onapristone, gestrinone, and ulipristal.

Mifepristone

It is a partial agonist and competitive antagonist for both A and B types of progestin receptors. Hence, it is known as progestin receptor modulator. When administered early, it can lead to decrease in midcycle gonadotrophin surge, causing delay in follicular development and failure of ovulation. Given in the later phase of cycle, it blocks progesterone support to the endometrium, PG release, and sensitization of myometrium to PG, leading to menstruation. In the case of implantation, mifepristone blocks decidualization, decreases human chorionic gonadotropin (HCG), and softens cervix, leading to abortion/miscarriage.

Pharmacokinetics

Oral bioavailability is about 25%. It is mainly metabolized in the liver by CYP3A4 enzymes and excreted in the bile, and its $t_{½}$ is 20 to 36 hours.

Uses

Medical Termination of Pregnancy

1. A single oral dose of 600 mg leads to complete abortion in 60 to 85% cases, where gestation age is 7 weeks or less. To improve efficiency, a singly 400 µg of oral misoprostol is administrated after 48 hours, which leads to a success rate of more than 90%.
2. Usually, it is safe, but have side effects such as uterine cramps, abdominal pain and discomfort, nausea, prolonged bleeding, and failed abortion.
3. Mifepristone and PG combination to be used carefully or avoided in patients with heart disease and asthma.

Postcoital Contraception

A single dose of 600-mg mifepristone administered within 72 hours of intercourse is used as emergency contraception. It is a highly effective method but may lead to disturbed subsequent menstrual cycles.

For Cervical Dilation

Given preoperatively, it leads to softening and dilation of the cervix and has lesser side effects compared to PG.

Induction of Labor

In case of intrauterine death of fetus.

Ulipristal

The recently approved selective progestin receptor modulator (SPRM) is used for emergency contraception (30 mg). Its efficacy is similar to levonorgestrel (1.5 mg) taken within 72 hours. It has weaker antiglucocorticoid activity compared to mifepristone.

Side Effects

Nausea, vomiting, headache, pain abdomen, delay in menstruation, and ovarian cyst.

Contraceptive Drugs (Hormonal)

Currently, the world population is increasing at an alarming rate; in order to control this, various methods of contraception are in practice.

Methods include: (1) coitus interruptus; (2) physical barriers such as condoms, pessaries, and intrauterine contraceptive devices; (3) chemical barriers using spermicidal chemicals, which contain surfactants such as nonoxynol; and (4) oral and injectable hormonal contraception.

Oral

The most commonly used is oral hormonal contraception in females. They include the following: (1) combined pills; (2) phased pills; (3) minipills; and (4) emergency pills.

These have remarkable efficacy, and are relatively safe, easy to administer, and cost-effective.

Combined Pills

These are conventional pills containing both estrogen and progestin fixed dose in a single tablet. These are also known as monophasic pills. These are to be taken from the 5th day of menstrual cycle to the 25th day (total 21 days). Then, on stoppage, some withdrawal bleeding occurs. If a pill is missed within 12 hours, it has to be taken and the cycle has to be continued; however, if a pill is missed for more than 36 hours, additional barrier methods of contraception are to be adopted.

Drugs used are ethinylestradiol, 30 µg daily, which can be reduced to 20 µg, along with 19-nortestosterone (as they have potent antiovulatory actions).

After 21 days of drug/pills, A 7-day gap is given during which withdrawal bleeding occurs, and it also decreases risk of endometrial carcinoma.

Combinations available are as follows:

1. Norgestrel (0.3 mg) + ethinylestradiol (30 µg).
2. Norgestrel (0.5 mg) + ethinylestradiol (50 µg).
3. Levonorgestrel (0.5 mg) + ethinylestradiol (50 µg).
4. Levonorgestrel (0.15 mg) + ethinylestradiol (30 µg).
5. Levonorgestrel (0.1 mg) + ethinylestradiol (20 µg).
6. Desogestrel (0.15 mg) + ethinylestradiol (30 µg).

Phased Pills

In this, estrogen dose is kept constant, whereas dose of progestin varies, depending on day/phase of cycle. In first/early phase, dose of progestin is kept low and progressively increases in later phase, mimicking menstrual cycle. Overall, it reduces the dose of steroids.

However, these are costly and commonly used in patients older than 35 years and those with no withdrawal bleeding. Evidence of superiority over conventional combined pills is lacking.

1. Levonorgestrel 50 + 75 + 125 µg + ethinylestradiol 30 or 40 µg.
2. Norethindrone 0.5 + 0.75 + 1.0 mg + ethinylestradiol 30 or 35 µg.

Minipills (Progestin-Only Pills)

These pills are aimed at eliminating estrogen content and associated adverse effects. Hence, these pills contain only progestin. These are helpful for women in whom estrogen is contraindicated. These pills are to be taken continuously throughout the cycle. Its efficacy is poor, and they are not very popular.

Emergency (Postcoital) Pills

These are used within 72 hours of sexual intercourse with failed contraception or unprotected act. Commonly used regimens are:

1. Levonorgestrel: 0.75 mg two tablets 12 hours apart or 1.5 mg single dose as soon as possible within 72 hours of unprotected intercourse. This regime is more efficacious than emergency contraception; associated adverse effects include nausea, headache, and delayed and disturbed cycles.

2. Ulipristal: It has been approved recently. A single tablet contains 30 mg of ulipristal and is to be used within 120 hours. It is also an equally effective method.
3. Mifepristone: 600 mg single dose within 12 hours is used in European countries.

In general, discontinuation of OCP leads to return of fertility within 2 to 3 months. If a woman misses a pill, she should be advised to take two tablets the next day. If there is failure of contraception, that is, occurrence of pregnancy when a woman is on pills, it should be terminated, as there is risk of fetal malformations.

Injectable Hormonal Contraceptives

In order to avoid daily consumption of tablets and improve compliance, injectable preparations have been developed.

These include the following:

1. Depot medroxyprogesterone acetate (DMPA): 150 mg IM at 3-month interval; usually, given in initial 5 days of menstrual cycle.
2. Norethindrone enanthate (NEE): 200 mg IM at 2-month interval.
3. Implants: These are special drug delivery systems implanted subcutaneously and include biodegradable and non-biodegradable implants, for example, a set of six capsules each containing 36 mg of levonorgestrel, which acts up to 5 years.

However, these injectables have certain constraints.

1. Animal studies have shown carcinogenic potential, but it has not been proven in human usage; also, a slight increase in breast carcinoma risk, especially in women younger than 35 years.
2. Menstrual irregularities, amenorrhea, and excessive bleeding have been noted.
3. Return of fertility may take 1 to 3 years.

Mechanism of Action: Hormonal Contraception

Hormonal contraceptives act by different methods:

1. By blocking feedback mechanism involved in gonadotropin release from pituitary. Block midcycle LH surge; as a result, follicles fail to develop and rupture, thus leading to suppression of ovulation.
2. Low-dose progestin and injectable also disrupt LH surge but are less efficacious.
3. Progestin-induced thick cervical secretion creates hostile environment for penetration of sperm.
4. Changes in the endometrium, making it hyperproliferative or atrophic and thus not suitable for nidation of blastocyst.
5. Modification in uterine and tubal contractions.
6. Postcoital pills dislodge blastocyst and interfere with fertilization.

Adverse Effects

Mild Adverse Effects

1. Nausea, vomiting, and headache.
2. Breakthrough bleeding, especially when progestin only pills are used.
3. Discomfort in breast.

Delayed Side Effects

1. After continuous administration, patients will have weight gain, acne, pruritis vulvae, and increase in body hair.
2. Chloasma: pigmentation of cheeks, nose, and forehead as seen in pregnancy.
3. Mood swings and depression can occur.
4. Some patients may have impaired carbohydrate metabolism, hyperglycemia, and precipitation of diabetes.

Serious Adverse Effects

1. Pulmonary embolism and leg vein thrombosis. This was more common in older preparation; however, lesser incidence is seen with newer pills having low quantity of steroids. But these low-dose pills pose greater risk in presence of certain risk factors such as age more than 35 years, diabetes, and hypertension, and in smokers.
2. Cerebral and coronary thrombosis leads to myocardial infarction. A small increase in risk with low-dose pills. Underlying mechanisms include increased coagulability, reduced antithrombin III, reduced plasminogen activators, and increased platelet aggregation.
3. Hypertension: seen in 10% of patients; again, less frequently seen with newer low-dose preparations.
4. Benign hepatoma can get converted to malignant lesions, which are seen rarely.
5. Increase in incidence of gallstones.
6. Estrogens have beneficial effect on cholesterol metabolism by increasing HDL/LDL ratio; however, progestin component counteracts and nullifies this benefit.
7. Animal study data have shown increased risk of genital, cervical, and breast carcinoma, but human data do not support this.

Contraindications

Absolute Contraindications

1. History of coronary, cerebrovascular, and thromboembolic disease.
2. Active liver disease, existing hepatoma.
3. Uncontrolled hypertension.
4. Suspected malignancy of genital tissue.
5. Porphyria.
6. Impending major surgery.

Relative Contraindications

Diabetes, obesity, smoking, mild hypertension, mentally ill, age more than 35 years, gallbladder disease, uterine leiomyoma, and undiagnosed vaginal bleeding.

Drug Interactions

Drugs that are enzyme inducers will increase the metabolism of OCPs, leading to faster metabolism and failure of OCPs, for example, phenytoin, phenobarbitone, rifampicin, carbamazepine, and ritonavir.

Noncontraceptive Uses/Benefits of OCP

1. Reduced risk of endometrial carcinoma and colorectal carcinoma
2. Regular menstrual cycles, and reduced blood loss and improved anemia.

3. Reduced endometriosis and other pelvic inflammatory diseases.
4. Symptomatic relief of fibrocystic breast disease.

Ormeloxifene (Centchroman)

It is a SERM developed in India. It has estrogen antagonist action at the uterus and breast, with little action at the vagina and cervical mucus. Endometrial proliferation is blocked. There is utero embryonic asynchrony, leading to failure of implantation. Plasma $t_{½}$ is 1 week; it is associated with weight gain and rise in blood pressure. Even though it has acceptable efficacy, it has still failed to gain popularity.

Male Contraception

Considerable efforts have been made in male contraception, mainly by suppressing spermatogenesis. If we suppress gonadotropin secretion, it will affect testosterone level, which, in turn, will affect many actions. Spermatogenesis is a long process that takes around 60 days and millions of sperms are produced unlike ovum. Acceptance of contraception by men is also low as they do not get pregnant! Drugs that have been tried are antiandrogens, estrogens and progestin, androgens, suppression of GnRH, and cytotoxic drugs.

Gossypol

It is a nonsteroidal compound derived from cotton seeds. It causes suppression of spermatogenesis and alters sperm motility. Fertility is restored after discontinuation. It is associated with hypokalemia, muscle weakness, and oligozoospermia.

Multiple Choice Questions

1. A 47-year-old woman complains of severe sweating almost every night. She had undergone a transvaginal hysterectomy 6 years ago; however, she has intact ovaries. On physical examination, it is observed that she has a body mass index (BMI) of 22, but all her vital signs are normal. Which of the following would best treat her condition?

A. Conjugated estrogens.
B. Levonorgestrel.
C. Raloxifene.
D. Calcitriol.
E. Calcium.

Answer: A

Vasomotor symptoms are the most frequent complaints of perimenopausal women. Estrogen is the only effective treatment of these symptoms.

2. An estrogen that is used in most combined hormonal contraceptives is:

A. Clomiphene.
B. Estrone.
C. Ethinyl estradiol.
D. Diethylstilbestrol (DES).
E. Norgestrel.

Answer: C

Ethinyl estradiol, a synthetic estrogen with good bioavailability, is the estrogenic component of most combined oral contraceptives, the transdermal contraceptive, and the vaginal ring contraceptive.

3. A 52-year-old woman with a positive mammogram had undergone lumpectomy and a small carcinoma was removed. Biochemical analysis of the cancer demonstrates the presence of estrogen and progesterone receptors. Following this procedure, she could possibly be given which of the following agents?

A. Danazol.
B. Flutamide.
C. Leuprolide.
D. Mifepristone.
E. Tamoxifen.

Answer: E

Tamoxifen has demonstrated efficacy in adjunctive therapy of breast cancer; the drug reduces the recurrence of cancer.

4. Which of the following is a specific property of selective estrogen receptor modulators (SERMs)?

A. Act as agonists in some tissues and antagonists in other tissues.
B. Activate a unique plasma membrane–bound receptor.
C. Possess both estrogenic and progestational agonist activities.
D. Inhibit the aromatase enzyme required for estrogen synthesis.
E. Produce estrogenic effects without binding to estrogen receptors.

Answer: A

SERMs such as tamoxifen and raloxifene demonstrate tissue-specific estrogenic and antiestrogenic effects.

5. A 50-year-old postmenopausal patient has reduced bone mineral density. Her treating doctor is considering therapy with raloxifene or a combination of conjugated estrogens and medroxyprogesterone acetate. Which of the following patient characteristics is most likely to lead them to select raloxifene?

A. Previous hysterectomy.
B. Recurrent vaginitis.
C. Rheumatoid arthritis.
D. Strong family history of breast cancer.
E. Troublesome hot flushes.

Answer: D

Conjugated estrogens and raloxifene both improve bone mineral density and protect against osteoporosis. The two advantages of raloxifene over full estrogen receptor agonists are that raloxifene has antagonist effects in breast tissue and lacks an agonistic effect in the endometrium. In patients with a strong family history of breast cancer, raloxifene may be a better choice than a full estrogen agonist because it will not further increase the woman's risk of breast cancer and may even lower her risk.

6. Combining a progestin to the estrogenic component of hormone replacement therapy for postmenopausal women confers which of the following effects?

A. Reduces thromboembolic events.

B. Provides improved control of problematic hot flushes.

C. Decreases the risk of endometrial cancer.

D. Regularizes vaginal bleeding.

E. Decreases bone loss.

Answer: C

Progestin acts on the endometrium, where estrogen agonists can cause proliferation and endometrial cancer. Progestin has demonstrated to decrease this risk.

7. A young woman has symptoms of abdominal pain during menstruation. Examination reveals the presence of prominent endometrial deposits on the pelvic peritoneum. Which of the following is the most suitable medical therapy for this patient?

A. Flutamide, orally.

B. Medroxyprogesterone acetate by intramuscular injection.

C. Norgestrel as an intrauterine device (IUD).

D. Oxandrolone by intramuscular injection.

E. Raloxifene orally.

Answer: B

In endometriosis, inhibition of ovarian function and production of gonadal steroids are useful. Intramuscular injection of relatively high doses of medroxyprogesterone confers 3 months of an ovarian suppressive action due to suppression of pituitary production of gonadotropins.

8. A young woman consults her gynecologist since she had unprotected sexual intercourse 12 hours earlier. Depending on her menstrual cycle, she feels that conception could be possible. Which drug should she use as a postcoital contraceptive?

A. Clomiphene.

B. Diethylstilbestrol plus raloxifene.

C. Flutamide.

D. Letrozole plus finasteride.

E. Levonorgestrel.

Answer: E

Levonorgestrel is a progestin. Progestins administered within 72 hours are efficacious as emergency contraception either singly or in combination with estrogens. "Progestin-only" emergency contraceptives have lesser side effects as compared to those containing estrogens.

9. On discharge from the hospital, the patient is told not to rely only on oral contraceptives to prevent pregnancy, since they could be less effective while she is taking anti-mycobacterial drugs. The drug most possible to interfere with the effect of oral contraceptives is:

A. Amikacin.

B. Ethambutol.

C. Isoniazid.

D. Pyrazinamide.

E. Rifampin.

Answer: E

Rifampin induces the formation of many microsomal drug-metabolizing enzymes, including cytochrome P450 isoforms. This increases the rate of elimination of several drugs, including anticoagulants, ketoconazole, methadone, and steroids, which are present in oral contraceptives. The therapeutic efficacy of these drugs can be decreased significantly in patients administered rifampin.

10. A 35-year-old premenopausal woman has been taking a combined oral contraceptive for 10 years. Because of this contraceptive use, she has a decreased risk of which of the following?

A. Deep vein thrombosis.

B. Episodes of migraine headache.

C. Ischemic stroke.

D. Ovarian cancer.

E. Pituitary adenoma.

Answer: D

Combination hormonal contraceptives have clinical uses and beneficial role in treatment of acne, hirsutism, and dysmenorrhea. Furthermore, with long-term use, they have demonstrated to decrease the risk of ovarian and endometrial cancer.

Chapter 75 Androgens and Anabolic Steroids

Upinder Kaur and Amit Singh

PH1.37: Describe the mechanisms of action, types, doses, side effects, indications, and contraindications of the drugs used as sex hormones, their analogs, and anterior pituitary hormones.

Learning Objectives

- Injectable testosterone derivatives.
- Oral testosterone derivatives.
- Therapeutic uses of anabolic steroids.
- Misuse in sports.
- Adverse effects.

Introduction

Testosterone, the principal male hormone, was first isolated in 1935 from bull testes by Ernst Laqueur. The hormone is known for its androgenic and anabolic roles in human physiology. Androgenic action of testosterone is responsible for spermatogenesis, development of internal and external genitalia, and appearance of secondary sexual characteristics. Anabolic action, on the other hand, is required for the development of muscle mass, strengthening of bones, and prevention of fractures. In an attempt to enhance the anabolic potential of testosterone, various derivatives of testosterone were synthesized, which could be utilized preferentially for conditions associated with poor bone and muscle mass. Such compounds are known as androgenic anabolic steroids (AAS) or anabolic steroids. Exploiting this performance-enhancing action of testosterone, the hormone and its derivatives were soon abused by athletes and bodybuilders, provoking their ban from the Olympics in 1976. In the section below, various derivatives of testosterone with stronger anabolic action are discussed along with their potential therapeutic roles.

Injectable Testosterone Derivatives

Esterification at 17-beta hydroxy position of testosterone makes the derivative long-acting and suitable for parenteral administration at 2 to 4 weeks interval. Such preparations include testosterone cypionate, testosterone enanthate, nandrolone (19-nortestosterone) decanoate, nandrolone phenylpropionate, methenolone enanthate, dromostanolone propionate, and testosterone undecanoate. The latter has been also available as capsules for oral use in many countries and was approved recently by the Food and Drugs Administration (FDA) under the brand name JATENZO. The derivatives are not only approved officially for their androgenic roles (mentioned below) but are also used off-label for their anabolic actions. Prone to abuse by athletes in order to improve performance in sports, these drugs are in the prohibited list of the World Anti-Doping Agency (WADA).

Oral Testosterone Derivatives

Testosterone when given by the oral route undergoes high first pass metabolism and hepatic inactivation. In order to improve oral bioavailability, certain modifications such as alkylation are made at the 17-alpha position of testosterone. Such 17-α alkylated preparations include methyl testosterone, fluoxymesterone, mesterolone, oxymetholone, oxandrolone, danazol, and stanozolol.

Androgenic-anabolic activity of any compound is generally estimated by myotropic androgenic (M/A) index. The index is calculated as increase in levator ani muscle weight divided by increase in prostate weight when the compound is administered to animals after orchidectomy. For testosterone, the ratio is 1, while it is > 1 for AAS. Nandrolone and oxandrolone, for example, have M/A ratio of 11 and 10, respectively.

Therapeutic Uses of Anabolic Steroids

Androgenic Indications

Ester derivatives of testosterone are approved officially for diseases associated with testosterone deficiency such as primary hypogonadism due to testicular failure, secondary hypogonadism due to disturbance or tumor affecting the hypothalamic-pituitary axis, and erectile dysfunction associated with hypogonadism and cryptorchidism.

Use in the Elderly

AAS are used in elderly men with low serum testosterone levels who develop symptoms such as osteoporosis, unexplained fatigability, poor sexual drive, and erectile dysfunction. Improvement is seen to occur in mood, sexual drive, erectile function, muscle mass, and bone mineral density (BMD). Although testosterone decline with age also occurs in females, the relationship between low testosterone levels and BMD in postmenopausal women is unclear. Vaginal preparations of testosterone are sometimes used in elderly women with low sexual desire, which is related to low serum testosterone levels.

Catabolic States

AAS are given in patients of burns, severe trauma, immobilization, postsurgery, renal failure, and chronic obstructive pulmonary disorder (COPD). The short-term use of these compounds helps to preserve bone and muscle mass and enhance body weight.

HIV-Associated Muscle Wasting

HIV patients often suffer from decrease in lean body mass and experience severe weight loss. Muscle wasting can occur despite antiretroviral therapy and is associated with poor quality of life and increased morbidity. Although significant heterogeneity exists between various studies, anabolic steroids are useful in AIDS-associated cachexia and are given to enhance body weight in patients afflicted with HIV. Liver function and lipid profile need to be monitored frequently as both anabolic steroids and HAART have been linked with disturbances in liver function and lipid abnormalities.

Osteoporosis

For the management of postmenopausal osteoporosis and osteoporosis in men, better treatments that inhibit bone resorption and stimulate bone formation are available now. These include bisphosphonates, calcitonin, and teriparatide. Employment of anabolic steroids as a primary treatment of osteoporosis is no longer a common practice but can be attempted as an adjuvant therapy, in some cases, for prevention of fractures. The bone-strengthening action of anabolic steroids can also be utilized for the prevention and treatment of glucocorticoid-induced osteoporosis.

Anemia of Chronic Disease, Hemolytic and Hypoplastic-Aplastic Anemia

Physiologically, androgens stimulate the release of erythropoietin (EPO) from the kidney. The expression of EPO receptors on erythrocyte progenitors is also increased, leading to increase in red blood cell (RBC) mass, reticulocyte count, and hemoglobin. AAS, by their androgenic action, stimulate erythropoiesis and are used in the management of hypoplastic anemia, aplastic anemia of moderate severity, and anemia of chronic disease. However, with the advent of better treatments such as bone marrow transplant, recombinant EPO, and immunosuppressive therapies, anabolic steroids possess a modest role overall in anemia management and are less preferred these days.

Hereditary Angioneurotic Edema

Hereditary angioneurotic edema (HAE) is a rare disorder that occurs due to deficiency or malfunction of the C1s esterase component of the complement system. The disease manifests as repeated attacks of edema involving the skin, upper respiratory tract, and gastrointestinal tract. The acute attacks of the disease are treated by intravenous C1s concentrates, ecallantide, a kallikrein inhibitor, and icatibant, a specific bradykinin receptor (B2R) antagonist. Prophylactic therapy to prevent attacks of HAE is needed by patients who suffer from severe or frequent attacks. Anabolic steroids such as stanozolol, danazol and methyltestosterone are most commonly used prophylactic therapies for HAE and act possibly by enhancing the synthesis of C1s in liver.

Breast Carcinoma

Androgen receptors (AR) inhibit tumor growth in a subset of ER+ and ER– breast cancer patients. Since androgenic therapy carries with it a multitude of adverse effects, certain compounds such as selective androgen receptor modulators (SARMs), with selective androgenic action on targeted tissue are being investigated in patients of carcinoma breast.

Misuse in Sports

The use of testosterone derivatives and SARMs in sports is banned by WADA. However, misuse and abuse of these compounds is common among athletes and body builders. Anabolic steroids increase body weight, bone mass, muscle mass and strength, and improve performance in sports. Increase in body weight of 2 to 5 kg is observed with short term (< 10 weeks) use of AAS, while chronic use (over years) can produce increment of 10 to 15 kg. Muscle strength is shown to improve by 5 to 20% from baseline. Hypertrophy of muscle fibers, increase in satellite cells in preexisting fibers, increase in myonuclei per fiber, and direct action on mesenchymal stem cells seem to be the mechanisms responsible for AAS-induced increased muscle mass. Central actions such as producing euphoria, and building up of confidence and competitive attitude, also contribute to the performance-enhancing effect of AAS. The action of AAS is synergistic with exercise and physical therapies and AAS also hasten recovery from exercise-induced fatigability.

Some derivatives of testosterone such as dehydroepiandrosterone (DHEA) and etiocholanolone are sold as dietary supplements in order to escape regulatory restrictions, and some "designer steroids" such as tetrahydrogestrinone (THG), also known as "the clear," are not amenable to detection by routine laboratory methods. The illegal use of such banned compounds in sports not only hampers the integrity of sports but can also produce lethal health consequences in players as mentioned below.

Mechanism of Action

Anabolic steroids act on the AR present in the cytoplasm, which then dissociate from heat shock protein and move to the nucleus. By modulating the activity of co-activators or co-repressors, AAS enhances the transcription of genes involved in protein synthesis. Anabolic steroids also inhibit glucocorticoid receptors (GR) and therefore antagonize the catabolic action of glucocorticoids. This results in increased collagen synthesis and nitrogen retention. Another action of these compounds is on the growth hormone (GH)-insulin-like growth factor 1 (IGF1) axis. The activation of this pathway also contributes to bone and muscle mass, increases BMD, and improves insulin sensitivity (**Fig. 75.1**).

Adverse Effects

Although AAS are believed to possess relatively stronger anabolic action, they are not free of androgenic potential. Conversion to dihydrotestosterone (DHT) is responsible for the androgenic adverse effects on the skin, hair, and prostate,

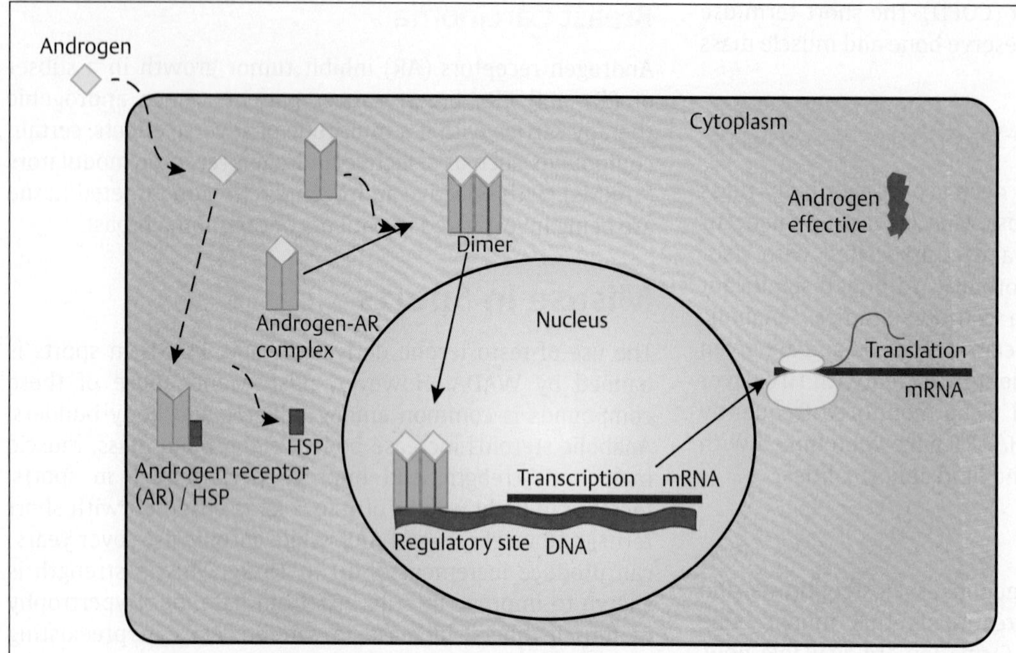

Fig. 75.1 Mechanism of action.

while conversion to estradiol by the enzyme aromatase is responsible for the estrogenic adverse effects. An important point worth mentioning here is that most of the adverse effects noticed with AAS have been from clinical studies investigating their use at normal dosage. The compounds are often abused at much higher dosage in athletes, and the exact pattern and incidence of adverse effects may be more severe than observed from the clinical studies. All anabolic steroids belong to **Schedule III** class of the U. S. Controlled Substances Act. The list of their adverse effects is as follows (**Fig. 75.2**):

Virilization and Precocious Puberty

Anabolic steroids when used in females produce androgenic features such as excessive hair growth and hoarseness of voice. Androgenic action also accounts for premature development of secondary sexual characteristics in male teenagers, leading to precocious puberty.

Acne and Alopecia

Because of androgenic action, anabolic steroids increase the sebum production from sebaceous glands and produce or precipitate acne in both males and females. Conversion to DHT is responsible for male pattern hair loss or androgenic alopecia.

Priapism

Androgenic action of AAS causes an initial increase in sexual drive. Risk of prolonged and painful penile erection also increases with AAS.

Gynecomastia and Loss of Libido

Conversion of AAS to estradiol produces enlargement of breasts in males. Males using AAS also complain of loss of libido because of hypothalamic–pituitary axis suppression.

Premature Closure of Epiphyses

The anabolic steroids produce an initial growth spurt, but this is followed by premature closure of epiphyses, leading to cessation of growth. Tendonitis and tendon rupture can also occur with the use of these compounds. Children and adolescents with short stature due to GH deficiency should be given recombinant GH supplements rather than androgenic preparations or anabolic steroids.

Behavioral Disturbances

The AAS can produce central nervous system (CNS) disturbances such as elevation of mood, aggressiveness, agitation, and hypomania/mania. Depression is also observed in chronic AAS users on withdrawal from the drug.

Edema, Salt, and Water Retention

Because of anabolic action, the drugs produce salt and water retention, leading to hypertension and worsening of heart failure in patients with poor cardiac reserve.

Erythrocytosis

Although useful in anemia management, erythrocytosis induced by anabolic steroids can lead to hyperviscosity features in patients of polycythemia vera.

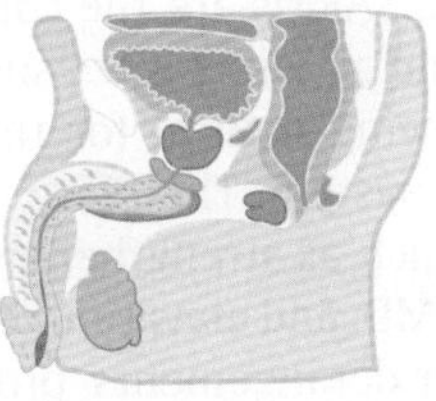

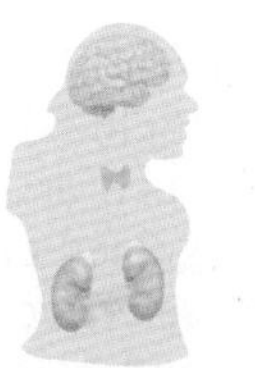

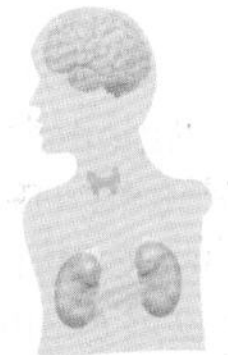

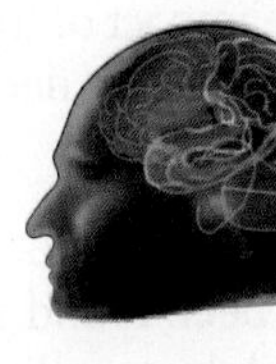

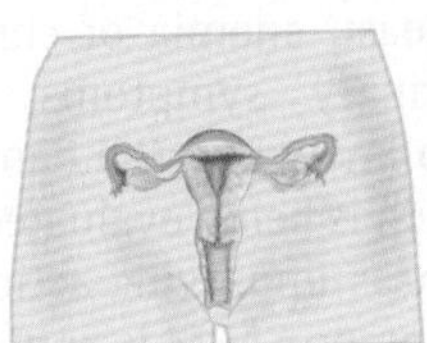

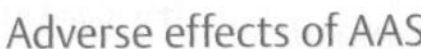

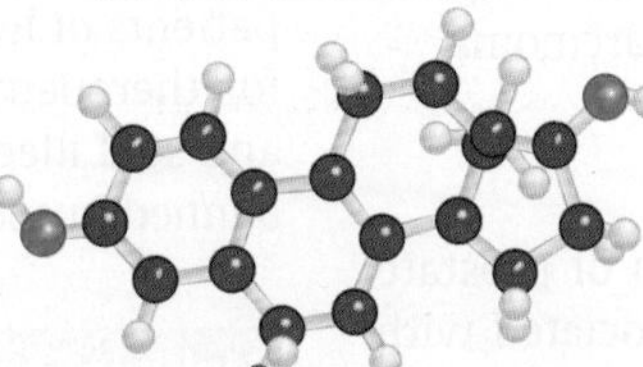

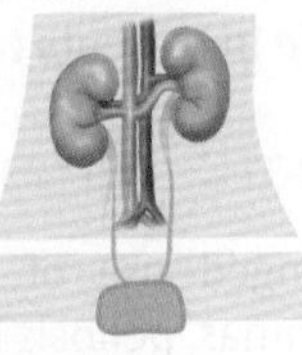

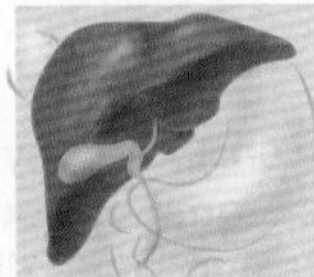

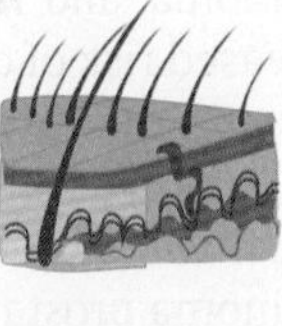

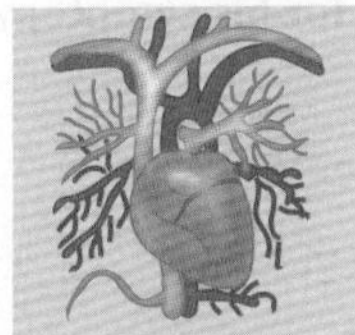

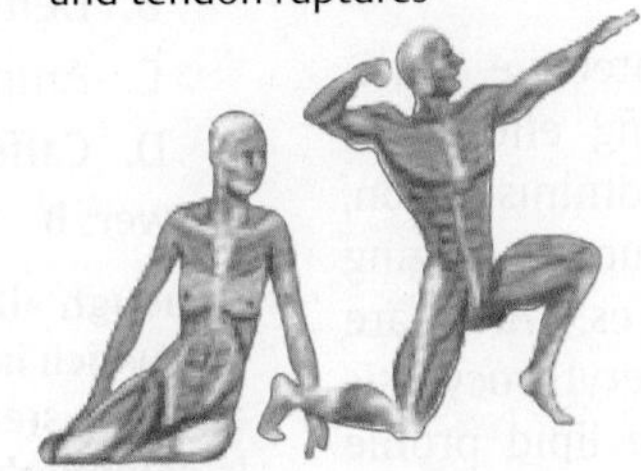

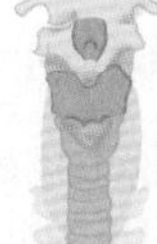

Fig. 75.2 Adverse effects of androgens and anabolic steroids.

Oligozoospermia and Infertility

AAS on long-term use suppresses the hypothalamic–pituitary axis, leading to lowering of gonadotropin-releasing hormone (GnRH), follicle-stimulating hormone (FSH), and luteinizing hormone (LH) levels. The decline in gonadotropic hormones blunts spermatogenesis, leading to oligozoospermia and poor fertility patterns.

Hepatitis and Cholestatic Jaundice

17-α alkylated AAS such as oxymetholone and stanozolol are known to produce cholestasis and obstructive jaundice. These are manifested biochemically as elevation of serum SGOT, SGPT, alkaline phosphatase, and bilirubin levels.

Lipid Derangements

Anabolic steroids such as oxymetholone and stanozolol are known to elevate serum low-density lipoprotein (LDL) levels and decrease high-density lipoprotein (HDL) levels. Lipoprotein (a) on the other hand is decreased by testosterone action. The impact of these biochemical changes on cardiovascular risk, however, needs to be determined.

Kidney Disease

Anabolic steroids have been found to produce acute decline in kidney function and hypercalcemia, particularly when given with nutritional supplements. Renal function also needs to be monitored along with liver enzymes and lipid profile in patients taking anabolic steroids.

Hepatic Tumours

Prolonged use of anabolic steroids can produce hepatic adenomas, peliosis hepatis, and hepatocellular carcinoma.

Prostate Carcinoma

Testosterone plays a pivotal role in the growth of prostate carcinoma, and high testosterone levels are associated with increased risk of carcinoma prostate over the years. Although new insights are evolving concerning androgen signaling and tumor occurrence, with many studies unable to show a positive correlation between testosterone therapy and carcinoma prostate risk, the US FDA so far has issued a black box warning of carcinoma prostate risk on all testosterone derivatives. Serum prostate-specific antigen (PSA) needs to be monitored every 3 to 6 months in patients on AAS, and the use of AAS should be stopped if serum PSA increases to > 4 ng/mL.

Cardiovascular Adverse Effects

Physiologically, androgens exert vasculoprotective, anti-inflammatory and nitric oxide (NO) releasing effects on the endothelium. Exogeneous testosterone administration, on the other hand, has been shown to produce damaging biochemical and cardiovascular disturbances. AAS are known to elevate blood pressure because of erythrocytosis and salt-water retention. They also alter the lipid profile unfavorably with most remarkable effects on LDL and HDL. Some evidence exists in relation to their potential to cause vasospasm, platelet aggregation, left ventricular hypertrophy, and direct myocardial injury. Whether these changes translate to increased cardiovascular mortality cannot be commented on at present, as clinical studies of testosterone supplementation have given inconclusive evidence so far.

Anabolic steroids should not be administered in patients of benign prostatic hyperplasia (BPH), carcinoma prostate, liver disease, kidney disease, cardiovascular diseases, and pregnancy. Caution is advised in patients with obstructive sleep apnea and migraine.

Selective Androgen Receptor Modulators

With the success of selective estrogen receptor modulators (SERMs) such as tamoxifen and raloxifene in conditions such as carcinoma breast, research in the field of SARMs gained enthusiasm. SARMs are the compounds which exert selective androgenic action at sites such as bones, muscles, and blood while being neutral for the liver, prostate, and the cardiovascular system. Therefore, the compounds exert beneficial effects such as strengthening of bone and muscle mass, increase in BMD, and elevation of hemoglobin. Adverse effects such as liver derangements, prostatic symptoms, and edema are expected to be less with these compounds. They are being explored in various areas such as osteoporosis in men and women, carcinoma breast, anemia of chronic illness, postmenopausal genitourinary symptoms, and cachexia of cancer. Enobosarm, also known by the name of ostarine, is one such compound which is being evaluated for its weight-enhancing and muscle mass-improving action in patients of lung carcinoma. At present, no SARM is approved for therapeutic use but such compounds are manufactured and sold illegally to sportspersons. The use of SARMs is also banned in sports.

Multiple Choice Questions

1. A 28-year-old man with athletic build consults a physician for anorexia, pain in abdomen, and occasional episodes of vomiting. He reports that he has been taking some dietary supplements for the past 6 months which were prescribed to him by his gym trainer to increase body weight. Biochemical tests show normal blood glucose and blood counts but elevated serum alkaline phosphatase and SGOT/SGPT levels. Which compound do you think might be present in the supplements and is responsible for his symptoms?

A. Ephedrine.
B. Dehydroepiandrosterone (DHEA).
C. Amphetamine.
D. Caffeine.

Answer: B

Although all these substances can be abused by players but the one which is used for weight-enhancing properties is androgenic anabolic steroids (AAS). DHEA is one such example of AAS that is commonly sold as herbal or nutritional supplements and on chronic use can cause liver function derangement.

2. All of these changes can be observed with androgenic anabolic steroids (AAS) supplementation in humans except:

A. Excessive hair growth.
B. Elevation in hemoglobin.
C. Elevation in sperm count.
D. Elevation in blood pressure.

Answer: C

AAS produce decrease in sperm count because of reflex inhibition of hypothalamic-pituitary axis.

3. Which of the following testosterone derivatives can be given by oral route?

A. Testosterone enanthate.

B. Testosterone undecanoate.

C. Nandrolone decanoate.

D. Nandrolone phenylpropionate.

Answer: B

Testosterone undecanoate can be given by oral route also. The remaining ester derivatives are given by intramuscular route only.

4. All of these testosterone derivatives are suitable for oral route except:

A. Oxymetholone.

B. Stanozolol.

C. Danazol.

D. Testosterone enanthate.

Answer: D

Testosterone enanthate is given by intramuscular route. The rest are all 17-α alkylated forms and suitable for oral route.

Chapter 76 Drugs for Erectile Dysfunction

Upinder Kaur and Sankha Shubhra Chakrabarti

PH1.40: Describe mechanism of action, types, doses, side effects, indications, and contraindications of:

1. Drugs used in the treatment of infertility

2. Drugs used in erectile dysfunction

Learning Objectives

- Medical treatment of erectile dysfunction.
- Precautions and contraindications for using phosphodiesterase 5 inhibitors
- Nonmedical therapy of erectile dysfunction.

Erectile Dysfunction

Normal sexual performance in males depends on four factors: sexual desire, sexual arousal (erection), ejaculation, and detumescence. Disturbance in any of these leads to sexual dysfunction. Erectile dysfunction (ED) is the most common sexual dysfunction and is seen in around one-third of men. ED is defined as the inability to attain and sustain penile erection with sufficient rigidity to allow adequate sexual performance. Some degree of ED is present in around 50% men in the age group 40 to 70 years. Incidence of ED increases with age, with three times higher prevalence in men in their 70s compared to those in their 40s.

ED can be psychogenic in nature or can be the manifestation of organic causes such as those involving vascular, neurogenic, metabolic, urogenital, and hormonal systems. Coronary atherosclerosis, hypertension, diabetes, spinal cord injury, obesity, hypogonadism, hypothyroidism, and benign prostate hypertrophy are the common etiologies responsible for ED. Depression, physical inactivity, smoking, and alcoholism are some of the other risk factors of ED. ED can also be iatrogenic, and common drugs implicated in ED are listed in **Table 76.1**.

Fig. 76.1 depicts the physiology of erection and action of phosphodiesterase inhibitors.

Medical Treatment of Erectile Dysfunction

PDE5 Inhibitors

The development of phosphodiesterase 5 (PDE5) inhibitors revolutionized the treatment of ED. PDE5 is selectively expressed in the pulmonary and penile system and is

Table 76.1 Drugs causing erectile dysfunction and their possible mechanisms

Drugs causing erectile dysfunction	Possible mechanism
Antiandrogens: flutamide, nilutamide, enzalutamide	Antiandrogenic action
Antiadrenal: ketoconazole	Decreasing testosterone levels as well as exerting antiandrogenic action
Progestin: cyproterone acetate	Antiandrogenic action
Estrogens	Blocking androgenic action
5-α reductase II inhibitors: letrozole, anastrozole	Decreasing dihydrotestosterone levels
H_2 blockers: cimetidine	Antiandrogenic action
Cardiovascular drugs	
Thiazides	By causing volume depletion (suggested)
Spironolactone	Antiandrogenic action, decreasing testosterone levels
Digoxin	Decreasing serum testosterone levels, increasing estrogens, vasoconstricting action on penile arteries (suggested)
Methyldopa, clonidine	Alpha-mediated action on penile blood vessels, decreasing central sympathetic outflow (suggested)
Beta blockers (propranolol)	By impairing penile blood flow
Antidepressants	
Mainly SSRIs	By serotonergic action in brain and blood vessels
TCAs (less common)	By anticholinergic action

Abbreviations: SSRIs, selective serotonin reuptake inhibitors; TCAs, tricyclic antidepressants.

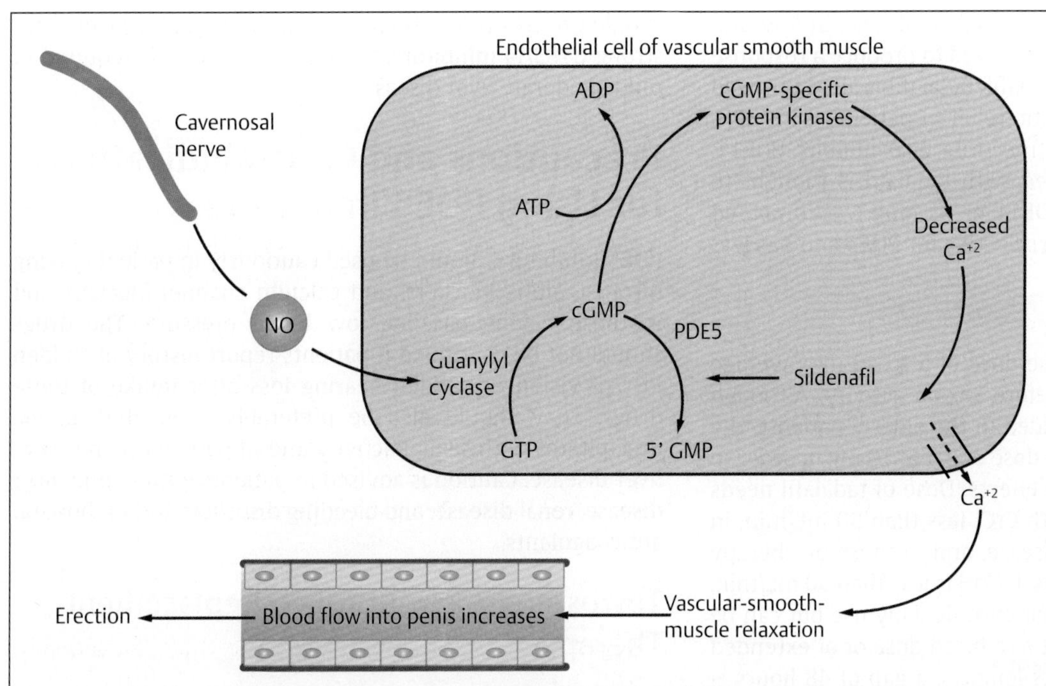

Fig. 76.1 Cellular mechanism of action of PDE5 inhibitors.

responsible for degradation of cyclic guanosine monophosphate (cGMP). These drugs, by inhibiting PDE5, increase cGMP (**Fig. 76.1**), relax the corpora cavernosal smooth muscle, and expand the lacunar spaces inside the corpora, leading to compression of tunica albuginea veins. Penile engorgement occurs and leads to erection. Sildenafil was the first agent of this class, which got approval in 1998. The remarkable success of sildenafil in improving erectile function fueled the surge of other PDE5 inhibitors in the market, such as vardenafil, tadalafil, and avanafil. The drugs are effective in ED of vascular, psychogenic, and, to a considerable extent, neurologic cause. Some difficult-to-treat patients such as those suffering from severe diabetic neuropathy and those who have undergone prostatectomy can also benefit from these drugs. However, the drugs need adequate supply of neurogenic NO in corpora cavernosa and therefore act only if preceded by adequate sexual stimulation. The drugs have no effect on sexual desire and ejaculation.

Among PDE5 inhibitors, sildenafil and tadalafil are approved for the treatment of pulmonary artery hypertension (PAH) also. Among all these drugs, tadalafil has the longest $t_{1/2}$ of 17 to 18 hours. For sildenafil, vardenafil, and avanafil, C_{max} decreases and T_{max} increases with fatty diet, and the drugs therefore should be avoided with fat-rich meal. Tadalafil has no such interactions with food. Plasma protein binding of drugs varies from 96 to 99%. Except tadalafil, all other PDE5 inhibitors have active metabolites with variable potency and activity. Common adverse effects of PDE5 inhibitors include flushing, headache, dizziness, rhinitis, epistaxis, edema, and dyspepsia. Concomitant use of PDE5 inhibitors with nitrates is contraindicated. Caution should be exercised and cardiovascular monitoring should be done when using these drugs with alpha blockers (e.g., prazosin) and calcium channel blockers (e.g., nifedipine).

Sildenafil

Sildenafil was the first PDE5 inhibitor approved for the treatment of ED. The drug inhibits PDE5 and, to some extent, PDE6. While the inhibition of the former is responsible for therapeutic benefits in ED and PAH, the inhibition of the latter can cause vision abnormalities such as blurring of vision and color blindness. The drug is also effective in relieving lower urinary tract symptoms of benign prostatic hyperplasia (BPH). CYP3A4 and CYP2C9 are involved in the metabolism of sildenafil, and the dose of sildenafil should be halved in the presence of moderate-strong CYP3A4 inhibitors such as ketoconazole, itraconazole, isoniazid, and erythromycin. A gap of 24 hours should be maintained between nitrates and sildenafil, as when taken together the drugs can result in marked lowering of blood pressure and cardiovascular collapse. Sildenafil should be avoided if there is a history of provocation of anginal attacks with sexual activity. Few cases of sudden hearing loss and sudden loss of vision related to nonarteritic anterior ischemic optic neuropathy have been reported with sildenafil.

Dose

The usual dose of sildenafil is 50 mg taken 30 minutes to 1 hour before sexual activity, to be increased to 100 mg depending upon the response. The starting dose of sildenafil should be 25 mg in men older than 65 years or in those suffering from renal disease (creatinine clearance [CrCl] < 30 mL/min) or moderate liver disease or in those consuming moderate-strong CYP3A4 inhibitors. With ritonavir, the recommended oral dose is 25 mg in 48 hours.

Tadalafil

The mechanism of action of tadalafil is similar to that of sildenafil but its action lasts longer for 36 to 48 hours.

The drug is also approved for chronic daily use in low oral dose of 2.5 to 5 mg where it is believed to produce a response close to "cure" of ED. Like sildenafil, tadalafil is also approved for PAH and gives symptomatic relief in patients with BPH. Apart from inhibiting PDE5, the drug also inhibits PDE11. Musculoskeletal pain observed with tadalafil is thought to be related to inhibition of PDE11 or its long $t_{1/2}$. Compared to sildenafil, the drug is more selective for PDE5 and has less action at PDE6.

Dose

The drug is given orally at the dose of 5 to 20 mg (average 10 mg) 60 to 90 minutes before sexual activity. Although no dose change is recommended in the elderly patients, the drug should be given at a low dose of 2.5 to 10 mg in order to avoid cardiovascular adverse effects. Dose of tadalafil needs to be reduced in patients with CrCl less than 50 mL/min, in those with moderate liver disease, and in those on therapy with potent CYP3A4 inhibitors. If CrCl is less than 30 mL/min, the drug should be avoided for chronic daily use but can be given on "as-needed" basis at a reduced dose or at extended dosing interval. Because of its long $t_{1/2}$, a gap of 48 hours is needed while administering this drug with nitrates.

Although no clinically significant difference is present between various PDE5 inhibitors, a meta-analysis of randomized controlled trials showed better psychological outcomes with tadalafil. Because of its long $t_{1/2}$ and ability to resume spontaneous sexual activity, tadalafil is preferred over sildenafil by many patients and their partners.

Vardenafil

The drug is pharmacokinetically and dynamically similar to sildenafil but carries an additional risk of prolongation of QT interval on ECG. It is usually mild, but caution should be exercised while administering the drug in patients with hypokalemia; likewise, the concomitant use of vardenafil and CYP3A4 inhibitors and other drugs known to prolong QT interval such as levofloxacin, gatifloxacin, azithromycin, and tricyclic antidepressants is not recommended. Because of its affinity for PDE6, vision-related side effects are also reported with vardenafil.

Dose

The recommended dose of vardenafil is similar to that of tadalafil—5 to 20 mg scheduled 30 minutes to 1 hour before sexual activity. A gap of 24 hours should be ensured between vardenafil and nitrates. The dose should be halved in patients with CrCl less than 30 mL/min or moderate liver disease and when used with potent CYP3A4 inhibitors and in patients older than 65 years. With ritonavir, vardenafil dose of 2.5 mg/48 hours is recommended.

Avanafil

The advantages of avanafil are that it has fast onset of action and lesser hemodynamic adverse effects.

Dose

It is given at the dose of 50 to 100 mg 20 to 40 minutes before sexual activity. A gap of 12 to 24 hours should be there between avanafil and nitrates. The drug should be avoided if CrCl is less than 30 mL/minute and if given with strong CYP3A4 inhibitors. No decrease in dose is required in mild-moderate liver disease.

Precautions and Contraindications for Using PDE5 Inhibitors

PDE5 inhibitors should be used cautiously in patients taking nitrates, alpha blockers, and calcium channel blockers and in those having baseline low blood pressure. The drugs should not be continued if patients report history of sudden loss of vision or sudden hearing loss after intake of these drugs. They should also be preferably avoided if angina precipitates with sexual activity and in patients with severe liver disease. Caution is advised in patients with peptic ulcer disease, renal disease, and bleeding disorders and in those on anticoagulants.

Testosterone or Androgen Replacement Therapy

Symptomatic hypogonadism manifesting as ED and poor sexual drive, in association with low serum testosterone levels (< 400 ng/dL), occurs in 6 to 12% of 40- to 70-year-old men. Androgen replacement therapy (ART) is given in patients with documented hypogonadism because ED in these patients often fails to respond to PDE5 inhibitors. Testosterone is given as injectable formulations such as testosterone enanthate and cypionate, given intramuscularly every 2 to 4 weeks, or as oral, sublingual, cutaneous, and transdermal forms. Response is better with transdermal forms. Common adverse effects of testosterone supplementation include fluid retention, weight gain, hypertension, erythrocytosis, and acne. Methylated derivatives such as methyltestosterone and fluoxymesterone can derange lipid levels and liver function. Serum prostate-specific antigen and hematocrit need to be monitored every 3 to 6 months if the patient is on testosterone therapy. Sexual desire, ED, muscle mass, and insulin sensitivity improve with ART. Controversy exists, however, with respect to cardiovascular risks and benefits of ART. Both worsening and improvement of cardiovascular events have been shown with ART. ART should be avoided in patients with uncontrolled heart failure, prostate carcinoma, and breast carcinoma.

Prostaglandin E1 (PGE1) Analog: Alprostadil

Given as intracavernosal or intraurethral injection, the prostaglandin E1 (PGE1) analog alprostadil has been found to be effective in many patients (50–80%) with ED. The drug stimulates Gs type of G protein–coupled receptor located on corporal smooth muscles and elevates cAMP inside the muscles. cAMP then relaxes the smooth muscles, and this leads to penile engorgement. Intracavernosal injection is given on the dorsolateral aspect of the proximal one-third of the penis. The starting dose is 1.25 to 2.5 µg and this is slowly titrated to 10 to 40 µg depending upon the response. Penile hematoma, fibrosis, hypotension, and, rarely, priapism are the risks associated with intracavernosal use of alprostadil.

Alprostadil available as MUSE (medicated urethral system for erection) is inserted into the urethra after urination. The starting dose is 125 µg, and this is increased slowly to a maximum of 1,000 µg. Compared to intracavernosal injection, this is less efficacious but is preferred by some patients because of the less invasive nature of administration. Urethral bleeding, dysuria, and hypotension can occur with MUSE. Condoms should be worn by males who use PGE1 analogs, in order to avoid the unnecessary exposure of female partners to the uterotonic effect of alprostadil.

Others

Some other drugs that can be given by intracavernosal route include the alpha blocker phentolamine and the nonselective PDE inhibitor papaverine. Because of the risk of priapism, hematoma, and permanent penile damage, the above-mentioned intracavernosal and intraurethral therapies should be avoided in patients with sickle cell anemia and multiple myeloma and in those on anticoagulants.

Nonmedical Therapy of Erectile Dysfunction

Nonmedical therapies for ED are given if patients fail to respond to the above-mentioned medical therapies. Such options include vacuum constriction device to constrict the veins of penile system, surgical implantation of inflatable prostheses, and vascular reconstructive surgeries. Stem cell therapy, gene therapy, low-intensity extracorporeal shock wave therapy (LI-ESWT), and intracavernosal administration of platelet-rich plasma are novel vascularity-improving therapeutic options, which are being explored in ED. Pharmacological and nonpharmacological therapies should always be accompanied by lifestyle modifications and treatment of underlying diseases. Such modifications include weight loss, smoking cessation, and optimal physical activity, all of which are known to improve the endothelial function and NO supply to the corpora. Psychosocial counseling involving both partners should be given concomitantly with drugs in cases of ED of psychogenic cause.

Multiple Choice Questions

1. A 45-year-old man, who is a smoker, consulted his family physician for chest pain and palpitations. His sitting and standing blood pressure values were 136/80 and 130/80 mm Hg and pulse rate was 82/minute. Upon ECG and treadmill test, the physician made an empirical diagnosis of coronary artery disease (CAD) and started the patient on oral glyceryl trinitrate 2.6 mg twice daily and sublingual Sorbitrate 5 mg (isosorbide dinitrate) on SOS basis along with oral aspirin 75 mg. Before sending the patient home, which "over-the-counter" drug history should be taken in order to avoid a potentially severe cardiovascular complication?

A. History of taking ranitidine or related drugs.
B. History of taking indomethacin or related drugs.
C. History of taking Viagra (sildenafil) or related drugs.
D. History of taking hydrocortisone or related drugs.

Answer: C

The patient, who is a smoker, was recently diagnosed with CAD. He might also be suffering from erectile dysfunction as he is having two major risk factors of erectile disorder: smoking and CAD. Before starting the patient on nitrates, history of taking sildenafil (brand name Viagra) should always be excluded. The two when given together can result in severe hypotension and cardiovascular collapse. A gap of 24 hours should be maintained between these two drugs.

2. A 40-year-old man was recently diagnosed with stage I idiopathic pulmonary artery hypertension (PAH). He reports to his doctor that he also feels problems in maintaining erection while engaging in sexual activity. The treating doctor makes a statement in jest "The drug I am recommending will be a weapon for both." Which drug do you think he must have suggested?

A. Bosentan.
B. Sildenafil.
C. Methyltestosterone.
D. Selexipag.

Answer: B

Sildenafil is approved for both idiopathic PAH and erectile dysfunction.

3. Which of the following is not an adverse effect of testosterone supplements?

A. Acne.
B. Elevations in SGOT/SGPT.
C. Fluid retention.
D. Osteoporosis.

Answer: D

Androgens are known to cause acne, liver abnormalities, hypertension, and fluid retention. They do not cause osteoporosis.

4. Which of the following statements about alprostadil use in erectile dysfunction is correct?

A. It is given by intramuscular route and is a PGI2 analog.
B. It is given by intracavernosal route and is a PGI2 analog.
C. It is given by intracavernosal route and is a PGE1 analog.
D. It is given by intramuscular route and is a PGE1 analog.

Answer: C

Alprostadil is a PGE1 analog, approved for erectile dysfunction by intracavernosal route and intraurethral route.

5. Backpain and myalgia are the characteristic adverse effects of which PDE5 inhibitor?

A. Sildenafil.

B. Tadalafil.

C. Vardenafil.

D. Avanafil.

Answer: B

Tadalafil can cause backpain and myalgia. The exact mechanism is not known but is thought to be linked with the drug's PDE11-inhibiting property.

6. PGE analogs are useful in all except:

A. Impotence.

B. Peptic ulcers.

C. Medical termination of pregnancy (MTP).

D. Glaucoma.

Answer: D

PGF2α analogs such as latanoprost are used in the management of glaucoma, not PGE analogs.

Chapter 77 Antidiabetic Drugs

Yogesh A. Kulkarni

PH1.36: Describe the mechanism of action, types, doses, side effects, indications, and contraindications of drugs used in endocrine disorders (diabetes mellitus, thyroid disorders, and osteoporosis).

Learning Objectives

- Insulin synthesis, storage, release, distribution, and degradation.
- Diabetes mellitus.
- Management of diabetes.

Introduction

The pancreas is both an endocrine gland and an exocrine gland. Pancreas can be divided into two parts: exocrine and endocrine. About 99% of pancreas consists of exocrine cells, which are arranged in clusters. These clusters are called acini. Different digestive enzymes produced by the acini flow into the gastrointestinal tract (GIT) and help in the process of digestion.

The remaining 1% of pancreas consists of tiny clusters of endocrine tissue called pancreatic islets or islets of Langerhans. Pancreas consists of about 1 to 2 million pancreatic islets scattered among the exocrine acini. Each pancreatic islet is made up of five types of cells namely α, β, δ, ε and PP. β cells secrete insulin; α cells secrete glucagon; PP cells secrete pancreatic polypeptide; δ cells secrete somatostatin; and ε cells secrete ghrelin. The core of each islet contains mainly the predominant β cells surrounded by a covering of α cells interspersed with δ cells or PP cells. The exocrine and endocrine parts of the pancreas are supplied with blood with the help of capillary network.

Regulation of Blood Glucose Level

Glucose is the essential source of energy for body tissues. In normal physiological condition, the human body maintains a blood glucose level of 120 to 140 mg/kg (4.4–5 mM) despite changing glucose consumption and metabolism. Insulin is the main hormone that controls the blood glucose level. The process of maintaining blood glucose level also involves role of many organs through systematic communication with the help of various organs, neurons, and local factors. During fasting condition, the energy requirement is fulfilled by oxidation of fatty acids. The brain cannot utilize fatty acids as effectively as other organs, so it requires glucose for normal functioning. In the fasting state, the liver plays an important role in maintaining blood glucose level in the normal range by various processes.

In normal condition, about 15 to 20 g of glucose are present in the extracellular pool of the body. Generally, 30 to 90 g of carbohydrates are consumed during each meal. The excess glucose is stored as glycogen in the liver.

When blood glucose level is decreased below normal, it is increased by the action of glucagon. In the opposite condition, that is, when blood glucose level is increased, insulin action is responsible for decreasing blood glucose level. The secretion of glucagon and insulin is controlled by blood glucose level through negative feedback mechanism (**Fig. 77.1**).

The sequence of events controlling the blood glucose level is as follows:

1. Decrease in blood glucose level below normal (hypoglycemia) is sensed by α-cells of the pancreatic islets. Thus, A cells are stimulated for secretion of glucagon.
2. Glucagon secreted by A cells enters the blood and reaches the liver. It acts on hepatocytes and increases glycogenolysis (breakdown of glycogen to glucose). Glucagon also stimulates gluconeogenesis (formation of glucose from noncarbohydrate sources such as lactic acid and certain amino acids) in the liver.
3. The glucose obtained from glycogenolysis and gluconeogenesis is released by hepatocytes into the blood. Thus, the blood glucose level is increased to normal.

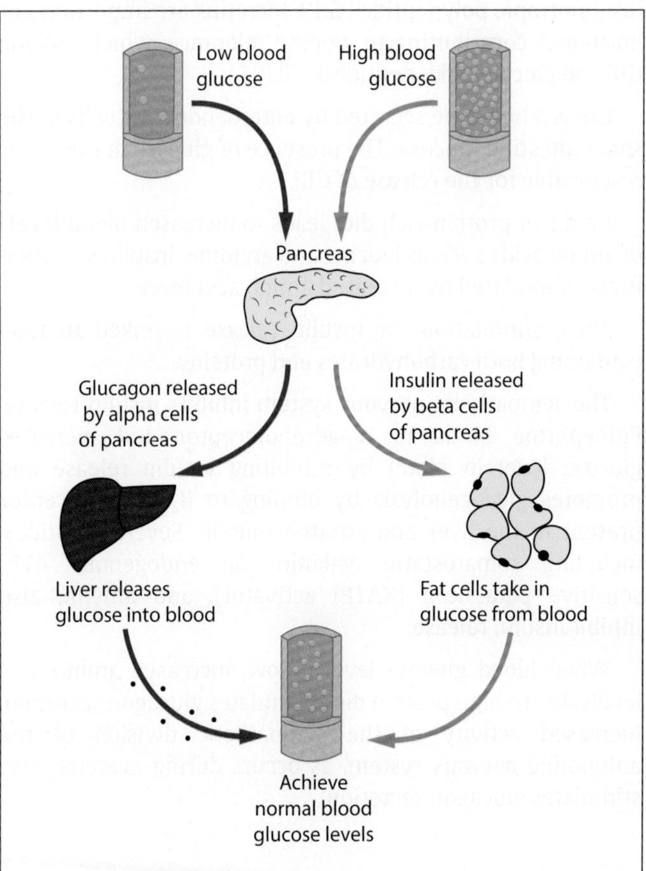

Fig. 77.1 Regulation of insulin secretion.

4. If the blood glucose level continues to increase above normal (hyperglycemia), A cells stop releasing glucagon (negative feedback).
5. Hyperglycemia stimulates secretion of insulin by B- or β-cells.
6. Insulin reaches various cells and acts to decrease blood glucose level by:
   a. Increasing facilitated diffusion of glucose into cells.
   b. Accelerating glycogenesis.
   c. Reducing glycogenolysis and gluconeogenesis.
   d. Accelerating synthesis of fatty acids (lipogenesis).
   e. Increasing uptake of amino acids by cells and increasing protein synthesis.

All these processes help in decreasing the blood glucose level to normal.

If blood glucose level falls below normal, it inhibits release of insulin by negative feedback mechanism. The lowered blood glucose level also stimulates release of glucagon.

Glucagon stimulates insulin release but insulin suppresses glucagon secretion. In the situation when blood glucose falls and less insulin is secreted from β pancreatic cell, α-cells of pancreases become activated due to inhibitory effect of insulin, which can secrete more glucagon. Various hormones such as human growth hormone and adrenocorticotropic hormone also help in insulin secretion indirectly during elevated blood glucose situation. Neural stimuli of endocrine system also stimulate insulin secretion prior to food consumption. Insulin secretion is also stimulated by acetylcholine (as pancreatic islets have innervations of parasympathetic vagus nerve fibers) and glucose-dependent insulinotropic polypeptide (GIP). Incretins are important gut hormones contributing to glucose tolerance, which include GIP and glucagonlike peptide 1 (GLP-1).

GIP is a hormone secreted by enteroendocrine cells of the small intestine mucosa. The presence of glucose in the GIT is responsible for the release of GIP.

Intake of protein-rich diet leads to increased blood levels of amino acids such as leucine and arginine. Insulin secretion is also stimulated by increased amino acid levels.

Thus, stimulation for insulin release is linked to food containing both carbohydrates and proteins.

The sympathetic nervous system inhibits insulin release. Epinephrine binds to α_2-adrenoreceptor and increases glucose level in blood by inhibiting insulin release and promotes glycogenolysis by binding to β_2-adrenoreceptor present in the liver and striated muscle. Several peptides, including somatostatin, galanin (an endogenous ATP-sensitive potassium [KATP] activator), and amylin, also inhibit insulin release.

When blood glucose level is low, increased amino acid levels due to high protein diet stimulates glucagon secretion. Increased activity of the sympathetic division of the autonomic nervous system, as occurs during exercise, also stimulates glucagon secretion.

Insulin Synthesis, Storage, Release, Distribution, and Degradation

Insulin is synthesized in β-cells of pancreatic islets. First, precursor of insulin– preproinsulin is synthesized in rough endoplasmic reticulum. Preproinsulin consists of a single polypeptide chain containing 110 amino acids. Preproinsulin is converted to proinsulin by its proteolytic cleavage in the Golgi apparatus. In the next stem, proinsulin in packed with some enzyme, which is responsible for its conversion to insulin in the secretory granule. Proinsulin undergoes cleavage to give insulin and a fragment called C-peptide. The conversion of proinsulin to insulin is carried out with the help of two endoproteases (enzymes), PC2 and PC3. These two enzymes require Ca^{2+} for their actions. These insulin and C-peptide are stored in secretory granules in B cells. Insulin and C-peptide are secreted by exocytosis in equal amounts. The physiological role and receptor of C-peptide are not yet known. Proinsulin is also secreted in smaller amounts along with insulin and C-peptide (**Fig. 77.2**).

Insulin consists of two polypeptide chains: A and B. Chain A consists of 21 amino acids and chain B consists of 30 amino acids. Chains A and B are joined with each other with the help of disulfide bonds. Chain A also consists of one intrachain disulfide bond joining amino acid residues 6 and 11.

Absolute blood glucose and rate of change of blood glucose are responsible for insulin release and synthesis from B cells of pancreas. Other stimuli for insulin release are mentioned earlier.

Insulin release is steady. Insulin is released in response to increase in blood glucose. Response to blood glucose possesses two phases–initially, a rapid phase, which reflects release of stored hormone, and then delayed phase, reflecting continued release of stored hormone and new synthesis.

The first phase is short-lived and reaches its peak after 1 to 2 minutes. The second phase has delayed onset with longer duration.

Generally, the B cell is hyperpolarized in its resting state. Depolarization of the B cell is responsible for the secretion of insulin. Increasing blood glucose levels initiate a series of events that leads to depolarization of B cells.

The resting membrane potential in B cells is determined by KATP channels.

Glucose cannot enter any cell directly; it requires transporter protein for entry inside cell. A membrane transporter called GLUT (glucose transporter) helps glucose in entering into cell. In B cell, glucose enters B cells with the help of GLUT2. After entering in the B cell, glucose metabolism starts with conversion of glucose to glucose 6-phosphate with the help of the enzyme glucokinase. Increase in concentration of glucose and glucose 6-phosphate increases adenosine triphosphate (ATP) production, thereby increasing the ATP/adenosine diphosphate ratio. This increase in ATP concentration inhibits an ATP-sensitive K^+ channel. This leads

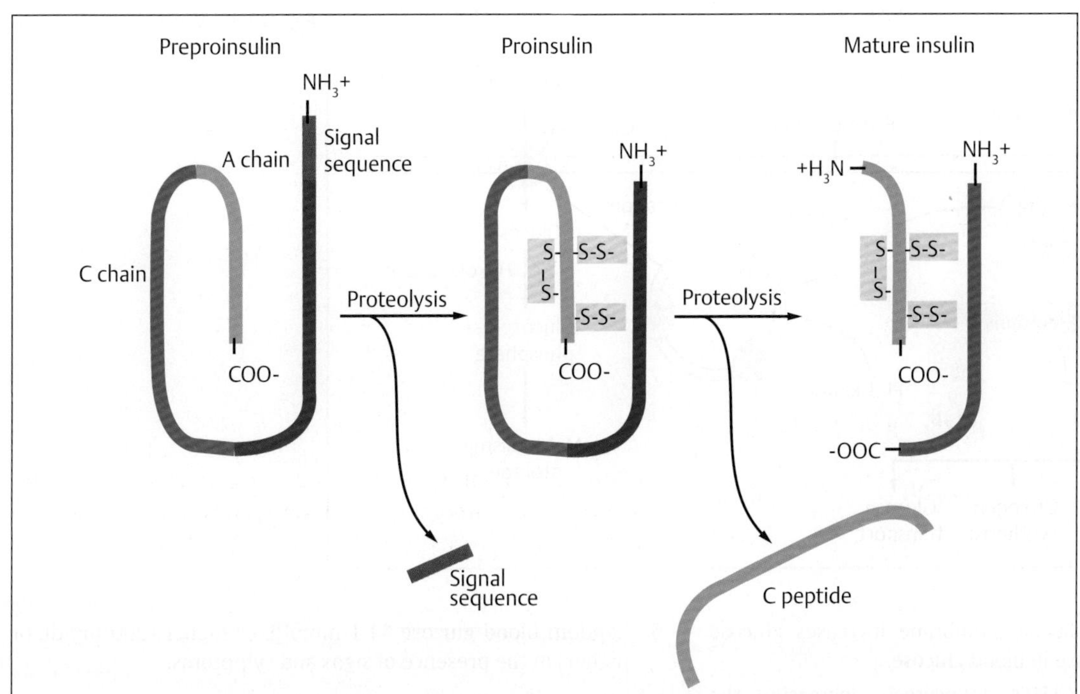

Fig. 77.2 Insulin secretion steps.

to decrease in K^+ conductance (as K^+ movement across cell is blocked) and opening of voltage-gated Ca^{2+} channels. The increase in intracellular (cytoplasmic) Ca^{2+} leads to insulin secretion.

In blood, insulin circulates as free monomer. The volume of distribution is approximately equal to the volume of extracellular fluid. The concentration of insulin is 2 to 4 ng/mL (50–100 mU/mL) in portal blood and 0.5 ng/mL (12 mU/mL) or about 0.1 nM in the peripheral circulation. During fasting, insulin secretion increases; the pancreas secretes 40 mg of insulin per hour to the portal vein, which is equal to 1 unit. After food, the concentration of food significantly increases in the portal blood, followed by a parallel but smaller increase in the peripheral circulation.

Insulin undergoes extensive hepatic clearance. In healthy individuals, $t_{1/2}$ of insulin is 5 to 6 minutes. The half-life of proinsulin is about 17 minutes. As mentioned earlier, C-peptide is released in equimolar amounts to insulin. C-peptide has lower hepatic clearance as compared to insulin; therefore, its molar concentration in plasma is higher and it has a longer half-life of about 30 minutes. Thus, C-peptide is also an important marker for acute insulin secretion.

Primarily, insulin is degraded in the liver, kidney, and muscle. The liver is the main site for degradation of insulin. About a half of the insulin concentration is degraded once it enters through the portal vein into the liver. As insulin enters the kidney, it is filtered by the glomeruli but is reabsorbed by the tubules. The tubule cells also degrade insulin. The key enzyme responsible for insulin degradation is a thiol metalloproteinase. It is mainly present in hepatocytes. However, the muscle, kidney, and brain also showed presence of immunologically related molecules. Peripheral fat also affects insulin and inactivates it.

Insulin Receptor

Insulin shows actions by binding to a cell surface receptor. The insulin receptor is a tyrosine kinase receptor. Insulin receptors are present in almost all mammalian cells. The liver, muscle, and fat are classic targets for insulin action. Some of the nonclassic targets of insulin are circulating blood cells, neurons, and gonadal cells. The maximum number of receptors are present on adipocytes and hepatocytes (about 3,00,000 per cell). The insulin receptor is composed of α/β-subunit dimers, which are linked by disulfide bonds. It consists of a transmembrane heterotetramer glycoprotein composed of two extracellular α-subunits and two membrane-spanning β-subunits.

The binding of insulin to its receptor activates a cascade of downstream signaling events (**Fig. 77.3**):

1. When insulin binds to α-subunit of receptor, the receptor is activated. This binding activates intrinsic tyrosine kinase activity. Due to tyrosine kinase activation, β-subunits of receptor are phosphorylated at tyrosine residues.
2. Binding of insulin to receptor also phosphorylates a few specific proteins such as the insulin receptor substrate (IRS) proteins, Gab-1, and Src homology 2–containing protein (Shc).
3. Each of these tyrosine-phosphorylated proteins through SH2 and SH3 domains activates different pathways, leading to specific effects on insulin.
4. Glucose transporter type 4 (GLUT4) is expressed in skeletal muscle and adipose tissue, which are important insulin-responsive tissues. After taking meal, glucose is mainly transferred to these tissues.
5. Phosphorylation of IRS activates phosphatidylinositol 3-kinase (PI3K). PI3K activates PKB/Akt. In skeletal muscle and adipocytes, Akt is responsible for the translocation of the GLUT4 glucose transporter from intracellular vesicles to the plasma membrane.

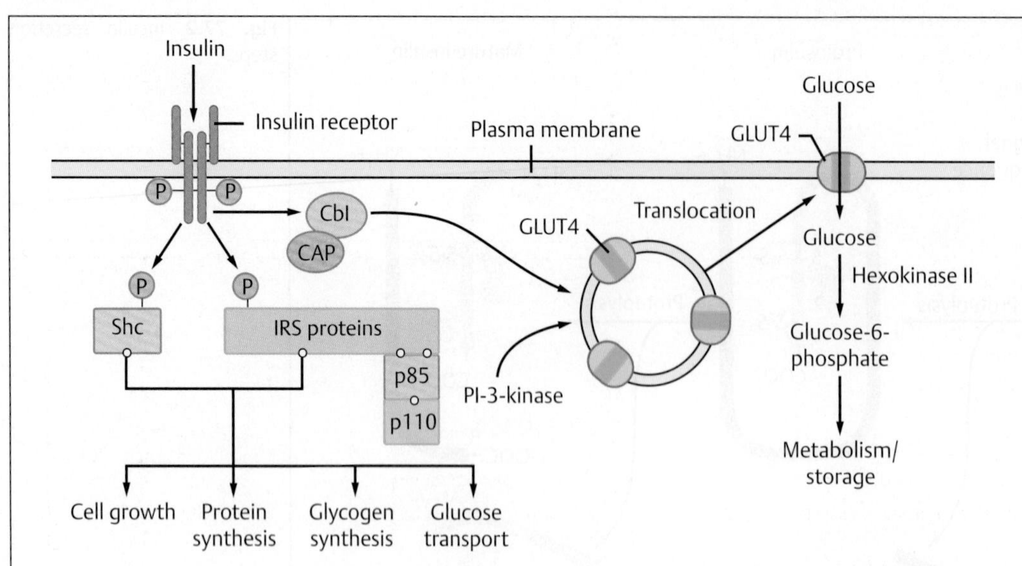

Fig. 77.3 Mechanism of action of insulin.

6. Increase in GLUT4 at plasma membrane increases glucose uptake by cell and decrease in blood glucose.
7. Insulin also decreases GLUT4 endocytosis, increasing the residence time of the protein in the plasma membrane.
8. The glucose taken inside the cell undergoes phosphorylation to form glucose 6-phosphate, which enters metabolism pathways.
9. Insulin also stimulates the plasma membrane Na^+/K^+-ATPase, which leads to accumulation of K^+ in the cell.
10. The pathways are inactivated by specific phosphoprotein phosphatases (e.g., PTB1B).

Diabetes Mellitus (IM11.16, IM11.18, IM11.19)

Diabetes mellitus (DM) is a chronic metabolic disorder characterized by high blood glucose concentration, that is, hyperglycemia. DM is characterized by defects in insulin action or insulin secretion, or both. The condition also indicates disturbance in metabolism of primary metabolites: carbohydrate, fat, and protein. The reason for the development of DM is insulin deficiency in combination with insulin resistance. Reduced glycogen synthesis with reduced uptake of glucose from skeletal muscle and uncontrolled hepatic glucose output is the key reason for the development of hyperglycemic condition.

Diagnosis

According to the World Health Organization (WHO), the diagnosis of diabetes is based on the following parameters:

1. The fasting blood glucose level (≥7.0 mmol/L or 126 mg/dL).
2. Glucose level 2 hours after an oral glucose administration (≥11.1 mmol/L or 200 mg/dL).
3. The level of hemoglobin A1c (HbA1c) (≥6.5% or 48 mmol/mol).
4. Excess glucose reacts with proteins (nonenzymatic glycation of proteins) and forms glycated end products. Glucose reacts with Hb, which is one of the proteins present in body, and forms HbA1c. Thus, the level of HbA1c represents a measure of the average glucose concentration to which the Hb has been exposed.
5. Random blood glucose 11.1 mmol/L or higher (200 mg/dL or higher) in the presence of signs and symptoms.

Classification of Diabetes

There are two main types of DM:

1. **Type 1 diabetes** (previously known as insulin-dependent diabetes mellitus [IDDM]): In type 1 diabetes, there is an absolute deficiency of insulin resulting from autoimmune destruction of pancreatic B cells.
2. **Type 2 diabetes** (previously known as non-insulin-dependent diabetes mellitus [NIDDM]).

Type 2 diabetes is accompanied both by insulin resistance (initial stage of the disease) and by impaired insulin secretion.

However, at present, diabetes cannot be classified into only two types because of increase in prevalence in young population, increase in subtype of diabetes due to developed knowledge of molecular genetics, and less distinct phenotype.

According to the WHO 2019 report, diabetes is classified as type I, type II, hybrid type, other specific type, and unclassified. Type I and type II diabetes have been differentiated based on age, severity of damage to β-cells, degree of insulin resistance, concentration of insulin needed for survival, and amount of diabetes autoantibodies required. **Table 77.1** shows a detailed classification of diabetes.

Management of Diabetes

The management of diabetes is aimed at alleviating the symptoms such as hyperglycemia and polyuria. It also focuses on preventing or reducing severity of complications of diabetes. Pharmacological and nonpharmacological management options for controlling diabetes are shown in **Fig. 77.4**.

1. Biguanides: metformin.
2. Thiazolidinediones (glitazones, insulin sensitizers): pioglitazone, rosiglitazone.
3. Sulfonylureas: glyburide, glipizide.

Table 77.1 Classification of diabetes mellitus

Class	Subclass
Type 1	
Type 2	
Hybrid forms	▪ Slowly evolving immune-mediated diabetes of adults ▪ Ketosis-prone type 2 diabetes mellitus
Other specific types	▪ Monogenic diabetes: – Monogenic defects of β-cell function – Monogenic defects in insulin action ▪ Diseases of the exocrine pancreas ▪ Endocrine disorders ▪ Drug- or chemical-induced ▪ Infection-related diabetes ▪ Uncommon specific forms of immune-mediated diabetes ▪ Other genetic syndromes associated with diabetes
Unclassified diabetes	
Hyperglycemia first detected in pregnancy	▪ Diabetes mellitus in pregnancy ▪ Gestational diabetes mellitus

Source: World Health Organization (WHO). Classification of Diabetes Mellitus. Geneva; April 2019. https://www.who.int/publications-detail/classification-of-diabetes-mellitus.

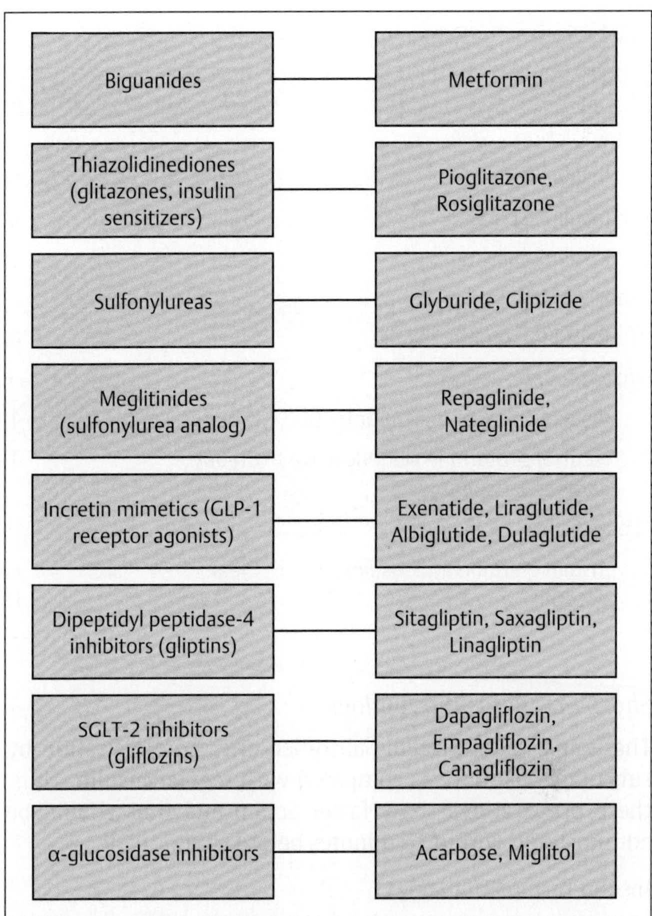

Fig. 77.4 Options for the management of diabetes mellitus.

4. Meglitinides (sulfonylurea analog): repaglinide, nateglinide.
5. Incretin mimetics (GLP-1 receptor agonists): exenatide, liraglutide, albiglutide, dulaglutide.
6. Dipeptidyl peptidase-4 inhibitors (DPP-4; gliptins): sitagliptin, saxagliptin, linagliptin.
7. Sodium-glucose cotransporter 2 (SGLT-2) inhibitors (gliflozins): dapagliflozin, empagliflozin, canagliflozin.
8. α-Glucosidase inhibitors: acarbose, miglitol.

Insulin Treatment

Insulin is the main treatment option for all types of diabetes patients. Insulin can be administered via intravenous, subcutaneous, or intramuscular route. Subcutaneous route is preferred for long-term treatment.

Insulin Preparations

Previously, porcine and bovine pancreatic extracts were used for insulin preparation.

Nowadays, human insulin is prepared from recombinant DNA technology, which is soluble in aqueous medium. Solubility of insulin can be improved when it is supplied at pH 7. International unit is the standard used clinically to express dose and concentration of insulin preparation. The amount of insulin required to reduce blood glucose concentration in fasting rabbit to 45 mg/dL (2.5 mM) is considered as one unit of insulin. Marketed preparations of insulin are available in solution or suspension at a concentration of 100 and 500 units/mL, termed U-100 and U-500. Insulin injections are generally given in subcutaneous tissues of the abdomen, the anterior thigh, dorsal arm, and buttock.

Classification of Insulin Preparations

Insulin preparations are classified based on their period of action into two classes: short-acting and long-acting (**Table 77.2**).

Pharmacokinetic profile of insulin can be altered by formulations that slow down the absorption after subcutaneous injection and by changing amino acid sequence or protein structure of human insulin.

Alteration of the amino acid sequence of insulin leads to increased or prolonged duration of action in solution or after its injection. This change in structure does not affect the ability of insulin to bind to the insulin receptor. Insulin analogs have been prepared by altering amino acid sequence.

Short-Acting Regular Insulin

This insulin preparation has neutral pH and it consists of insulin molecules associated with hexamers in aqueous solution. After subcutaneous injection, this association slows down absorption. Regular insulin should be administered 30 to 45 minutes before meal.

Table 77.2 Types of insulin preparations

Type	Appearance	Onset (h)	Peak (h)	Duration (h)
Rapid-acting				
Insulin lispro	Clear	0.2–0.3	1–1.5	3–5
Insulin aspart	Clear	0.2–0.3	1–1.5	3–5
Insulin glulisine	Clear	0.2–0.4	1–2	3–5
Short-acting				
Regular (soluble) insulin	Clear	0.5–1	2–3	6–8
Intermediate-acting				
Insulin zinc suspension or lente	Cloudy	1–2	8–10	20–24
Neutral protamine Hagedorn or isophane insulin	Cloudy	1–2	8–10	20–24
Long-acting				
Insulin glargine and insulin detemir	Clear	Glargine: 2–4 Detemir: 1–4	–	Glargine: 24 Detemir: 20–24

Short-Acting Insulin Analogs

These analogs are rapidly absorbed after administration by subcutaneous route as compared with regular insulin. Thus, these preparations show faster action and thus should be administered within 15 minutes before meal.

Insulin Lispro (Humalog)

In this preparation, the sequence of two amino acid residues at B28 and B29 is reversed. Lispro also exists as a hexamer in commercially available formulations just like regular insulin.

After administration, lispro dissociates into monomers immediately and thus leads to rapid absorption and shorter duration of action when compared with regular insulin.

Insulin Aspart (Novolog)

In this preparation, proline at B28 is replaced with aspartic acid. After administration, it dissociates rapidly into monomers. In type 1 diabetic patients, lispro and aspart have shown similar plasma insulin levels.

Insulin Glulisine (Apidra)

In this preparation, lysine is replaced by glutamic acid at B29 and asparagine is replaced by lysine at B23. Substitutions help to dissociated it into active monomers. Absorption profile of insulin glulisine is similar to that of lispro and aspart.

Long-Acting Insulins

Neutral Protamine Hagedorn (NPH; Insulin Isophane)

This preparation is a cloudy or whitish suspension of native insulin complexed with protamine and zinc in a phosphate buffer. After subcutaneous injection, insulin is dissolved more slowly (as it is in complex form), prolonging its duration of action.

NPH insulin is usually given either twice a day in combination with short-acting insulin or once a day (at bedtime). Type 2 diabetic patients are prescribed long-acting insulin at bedtime for regulating fasting blood glucose. Postprandial glucose elevation in insulin-deficient type 1 or type 2 diabetes is not controlled by long-acting basal insulin alone.

Insulin Glargine (Lantus)

This preparation of insulin is a long-acting analog of human insulin. Insulin glargine is produced after two alterations of human insulin. The C-terminus of the B-chain has been added with two arginine residues, and asparagine in position A21 is replaced with glycine. Insulin glargine has acidic pH (pH 4.0), and is available as clear solution. After administration by subcutaneous route, insulin aggregates at the site, which is responsible for prolonged release. Short-acting insulin preparations cannot be mixed with this preparation due to difference in pH.

Insulin Detemir (Levemir)

This is an insulin analog prepared by addition of a saturated fatty acid to the ε-amino group of LysB29, yielding a myristoylated insulin. After injection, fatty acid chain helps it to bind to albumin. Usually, detemir is administered twice daily. The absorption profiles of glargine and detemir insulin are similar.

Insulin Combinations

Combinations of NPH and regular insulin (70:30), lispro protamine and lispro (50:50 and 75:25), and aspart protamine and aspart (70:30) are also available in the market.

Adverse Effects

Hypoglycemia

It is a common unwanted effect of insulin. Severe hypoglycemia can cause brain damage. It can be treated by consumption of a sweet drink or snack. In the case of unconscious patient, glucose can be administered by intravenous route. In some cases, glucagon can also be used (intramuscular route). Insulin-induced hypoglycemia may be followed by the Somogyi effect or rebound hyperglycemia.

Allergy

It is a rare adverse effect of insulin but can occur. It may in the form of local or systemic reactions.

Diabetes Ketoacidosis

Diabetic ketoacidosis (DKA), also known as diabetic coma, is a serious complication of type 1 diabetes where insulin levels are insufficient to meet the body's metabolic requirement. It is less commonly observed in type 2 diabetes. Insulin deficiency can be absolute (e.g., during lapses in the administration of exogenous insulin) or relative (e.g., when usual insulin doses do not meet metabolic needs during physiologic stress). DKA happens when blood glucose level is very high and acidic substance called "ketone" builds up to dangerous level in the body. DKA is not generally observed in type 2 diabetes but may occur in the situation of unusual physiologic stress. Obese patients sometimes show ketosis-prone type 2 diabetes, which is a variant of type 2 diabetes. This is often observed in African-American or Afro-Caribbean people. People with ketosis-prone diabetes possess significant impairment of β-cell function with hyperglycemia and therefore are more prone to DAK.

Hyperosmolar (Nonketotic Hyperglycemic) Coma

Hyperosmolar (nonketotic hyperglycemia) coma (HONK) is a severe condition brought on by very high blood glucose in the elderly type 2 diabetic patients. The reason behind the development of HONK is not clear but it is found to be associated with same factor as that of ketoacidosis, especially those resulting in dehydration. Won Frerichs and Dreschfeld first described this disorder in around 1880. They described patients with DM with profound hyperglycemia and glycosuria without the classic Kussmaul breathing or acetone in the urine seen in DKA. Glycosuria of DM produces diuresis, resulting in dehydration and hemoconcentration over several days. Urine output gets reduced, which results in accumulation of glucose in the blood (> 800 mg/dL) and affects plasma osmolarity. These conditions cause coma, and death can occur if not vigorously tested. The primary symptom of hyperosmolar hyperglycemic state is altered consciousness varying from confusion or disorientation to coma, usually as a result of extreme dehydration with or without prerenal azotemia, hyperglycemia, and hyperosmolality. Patients are more prone to thrombosis and the mortality rate is high in HONK (rate of up to 20%).

Treatment is same as that of DKA, but in case of HONK faster fluid replacement is required and alkali is not usually required.

Oral Hypoglycemic Agents

Sulfonylureas

Drugs from this class are derived by substitution in arylsulfonylureas. Substitution can be done at para position on the benzene ring and at nitrogen atom in urea.

They are classified into two classes:

1. First-generation sulfonylureas: examples include chlorpropamide, tolbutamide, and tolazamide.
2. Second-generation sulfonylureas, which are more potent: examples include glimepiride, glyburide (glibenclamide), and glipizide.

Mechanism of Action

Sulfonylureas bind to a KATP channel complex known as the sulfonylurea receptor on the β-cell and inhibit its activity. Due to this action, β-cells are stimulated for release of insulin. KATP channel inhibition causes depolarization of cell membrane, leading to insulin secretion. In type 2 diabetic patients, sulfonylurea treatment promotes insulin release from the pancreas (**Fig. 77.5**). Initially, fasting plasma insulin levels and insulin responses to oral glucose challenges are increased. Long-term use decreases circulating insulin levels, but despite this reduction in insulin levels, reduced plasma glucose levels are maintained. The reason behind this effect is not yet clear.

Pharmacokinetics

All drugs from this class are absorbed from the GIT, but the rate of absorption is different for all. Hyperglycemic condition and presence of food in the GIT can decrease absorption. The detailed pharmacokinetics of sulfonylureas are shown in **Table 77.3**.

They often can be administered once daily. All drugs are metabolized by the liver and excreted in the urine. Care should be taken while giving dose of sulfonylureas to patients with either renal or hepatic insufficiency.

Adverse Effects

1. Hypoglycemia, including coma, is common in elderly patients with liver and kidney impairment function, who are taking

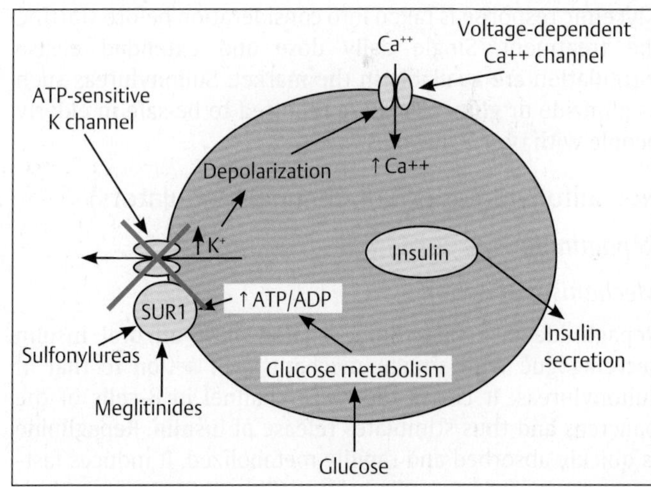

Fig. 77.5 Mechanism of action of sulfonylureas.

Table 77.3 Pharmacokinetics of sulfonylureas

Parameter	Value
Plasma protein binding	90–99%
Volumes of distribution	~0.2 L/kg
Half-lives	3–5 h
Duration of effect	12–24 h

longer-acting sulfonylureas. Due to this effect, first-generation sulfonylureas are rarely used.

2. Weight gain is a common side effect.
3. Nausea and vomiting.
4. Cholestatic jaundice.
5. Anemias.
6. Hypersensitivity and dermatological reactions.
7. Alcohol-induced flush similar to that caused by disulfiram or hyponatremia (rare).

Drug Interactions

Drugs such as sulfonamides, clofibrate, and salicylates displace sulfonylureas from binding proteins and thus increase free drug. Ethanol may enhance the action of sulfonylureas and cause hypoglycemia.

Hypoglycemia is frequently observed when sulfonylureas are taken together with other drugs such as antifungal agents, histamine H_2-antagonist, tricyclic antidepressant, and anticoagulants.

Drugs such as sympatholytics, Ca^{2+} channel blockers, cholestyramine, diazoxide, estrogens, hydantoins, isoniazid, nicotinic acid, phenothiazines, rifampin, sympathomimetics, thiazide diuretics, and urinary alkalinizers decrease effect of sulfonylureas.

Therapeutic Uses

They are used for the treatment of hyperglycemia in type 2 diabetes. These drugs should not be used in type 1 diabetes, during pregnancy, and in patient with hepatic and renal abnormalities.

Dose and Dosage Forms

Glycemic response is taken into consideration before starting the treatment. Single daily dose and extended-release formulation are available in the market. Sulfonylureas such as glipizide or glimepiride are reported to be safe in elderly people with type 2 diabetes.

Nonsulfonylureas (KATP Channel Modulators)

Repaglinide

Mechanism of Action

Repaglinide is a meglitinide analog. It is an oral insulin secretagogue with similar mechanism of action to that of sulfonylureas. It closes the KATP channel in β-cells of the pancreas and thus stimulates release of insulin. Repaglinide is quickly absorbed and rapidly metabolized. It induces fast-onset short-lasting insulin release (**Fig. 77.6**). Repaglinide is mainly metabolized by the liver. It should be used cautiously in patients with liver diseases. This drug (~10%) is also metabolized by the kidney, so it should be administered cautiously in patients with renal insufficiency. It is administered before each major meal to control postprandial hyperglycemia.

Side Effect

Hypoglycemia.

Drug Interactions

Drugs such as β-blockers, chloramphenicol, coumarins, monoamine oxidase inhibitors (MAOIs), nonsteroidal anti-inflammatory drugs (NSAIDs), probenecid, salicylates, and sulfonamide may potentiate the action of repaglinide by displacing it from plasma protein binding sites.

Drugs such as gemfibrozil, itraconazole, trimethoprim, cyclosporine, simvastatin, and clarithromycin increase the action of repaglinide by altering its metabolism.

Nateglinide

Mechanism of Action

Nateglinide is derived from D-phenylalanine. It is also an orally effective insulin secretagogue. The mechanism of action of nateglinide is same as that of repaglinide. Nateglinide is mainly used in patients with type 2 diabetes to reduce postprandial glucose level. The drug is metabolized mainly by the liver.

Treatment is risky in patients with liver diseases. This drug (~16%) is also excreted unchanged by the kidney; thus, it should be administered cautiously in patients with renal insufficiency.

Drug Interactions

Drugs such as corticosteroids, rifampicin, sympathomimetics, thiazide, diuretics, and thyroid products reduce the efficacy of nateglinide. Drugs such as alcohol, NSAIDs, salicylates, MAOIs, and nonselective β-blockers increase the risk of hypoglycemia when administered with nateglinide.

Pharmacokinetics

Pharmacokinetics of KATP channel modulators, nonsulfonylureas, are shown in **Table 77.4**.

Repaglinide and nateglinide show decrease in efficacy (secondary failure) after initially improving glycemic control.

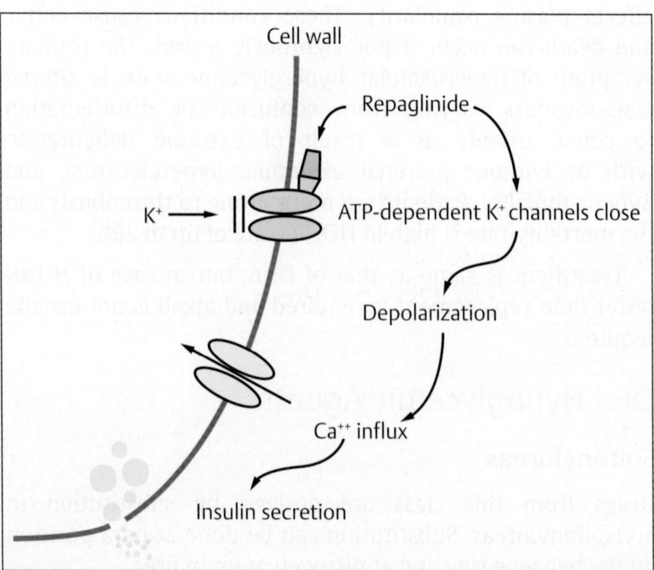

Fig. 77.6 Mechanism of action of nonsulfonylureas (KATP channel modulators).

Table 77.4 Comparative pharmacokinetics of Nateglinide and Repaglinide

Parameter	Nateglinide	Repaglinide
Time to peak concentration	≤ 1 h	≤ 1 h
Bioavailability	73%	56%
Protein binding	98%	> 98%
Cytochrome P450 isoenzymes	2C9, 3A4	3A4
Half-life	1.5 h	1 h
Fraction excreted unchanged in the urine	16%	8%
Volume of distribution	10 L	31 L

Dose and Dosage Forms

Oral administration of repaglinide, between 0.5 to 4 mg twice to thrice daily, to a maximum of 16 mg, produces glycemic control in a similar order to other antihyperglycemic agents. Repaglinide should be administered approximately 30 minutes before an intended meal, and the dose skipped if a scheduled mealtime is skipped. Dose adjustments should be reviewed a minimum of one week later. Nateglinide is available generically and under the brand name Starlix in tablets of 60 and 120 mg. The typical initial dose in adults is 120 mg three times daily before meals.

AMPK and PPARγ Activators: Biguanides

Phenformin and metformin from the class biguanides were introduced for the management of diabetes in the 1950s. Phenformin has been withdrawn due to higher risk of lactic acidosis. Thus, only metformin from this class is available in the market today.

Metformin

Mechanism of Action

Biguanides need presence of insulin for its action but it does not release insulin form pancreas. Metformin is ineffective in type 1 diabetics. Metformin enhances activity of the AMP-dependent protein kinase (AMPK). AMPK is activated by phosphorylation when concentrations of ATP and phosphocreatine, that is, cellular energy stores, are lowered (**Fig. 77.7**). Activation of AMPK leads to:

1. Stimulation of fatty acid oxidation.
2. Stimulation of glucose uptake and nonoxidative metabolism.
3. Reduction of lipogenesis.
4. Reduction of gluconeogenesis.

The net effect is increased glycogen storage in skeletal muscle, decreased hepatic glucose production, increased insulin sensitivity, and decreased blood glucose levels.

In normoglycemic state, metformin is not effective against blood glucose and has no activity on insulin release and other islet hormone release and rarely causes hypoglycemia.

Side Effects

These include nausea, indigestion, abdominal cramps or bloating, and diarrhea. Metformin affects glucose and bile salt absorption. It decreases vitamin B_{12} blood levels. Renal failure is another common comorbidity reported in patients having lactic acidosis associated with metformin use.

Uses

Metformin is accepted as the first-line treatment for type 2 diabetes. Metformin is effective as monotherapy and in combination with nearly every other therapy for type 2 diabetes. Metformin is available as fixed-dose conjugation with glipizide, glyburide, pioglitazone, repaglinide, rosiglitazone, and sitagliptin.

Dose and Dosage Forms

Metformin is an oral medication typically dosed from 500 to 2,550 mg per day and administered with a meal to decrease GI upset. The daily dose is often titrated weekly in increments of 500 or 850 mg to reduce this risk. Recommendations are to take metformin at the same time every day. Extended-release tablets are typically taken once daily with an evening meal and should be swallowed with a full glass of water.

Thiazolidinediones

Mechanism of Action

Nuclear hormone receptor peroxisome proliferation activating receptor γ (PPARγ) is involved in the regulation of genes related to glucose and lipid metabolism. Thiazolidinediones are ligands for these receptors (**Fig. 77.8**).

Rosiglitazone and pioglitazone are two thiazolidinediones currently available in the market to treat patients with type 2 diabetes. PPARγ activation increases tissue sensitivity to insulin.

Pioglitazone and rosiglitazone increase insulin-mediated glucose uptake by 30 to 50% and are considered as insulin sensitizers. Adipose tissue is the primary target for PPARγ agonists; they also act on skeletal muscle, which is the major site of glucose disposal associated with insulin. The mechanism behind improvement of insulin resistance is not clear. These drugs also reduce hepatic glucose production and uptake.

Thiazolidinediones affect lipid metabolism and reduce plasma levels of fatty acids by increasing clearance and reducing lipolysis.

They are metabolized by the liver and thus should not be used in the case of hepatic disease. These drugs can be prescribed to patients with renal defects.

Drug Interactions

The plasma level of these drugs is decreased if administered with rifampin because it induces the enzymes responsible for the metabolism of thiazolidinediones. Plasma levels of rosiglitazone and pioglitazone are increased if administered with gemfibrozil as it impedes the metabolism

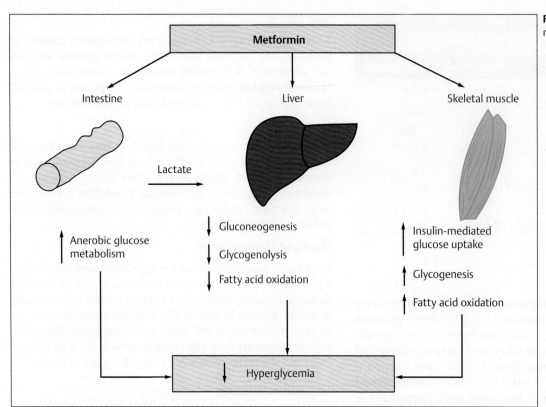

Fig. 77.7 Mechanism of metformin.

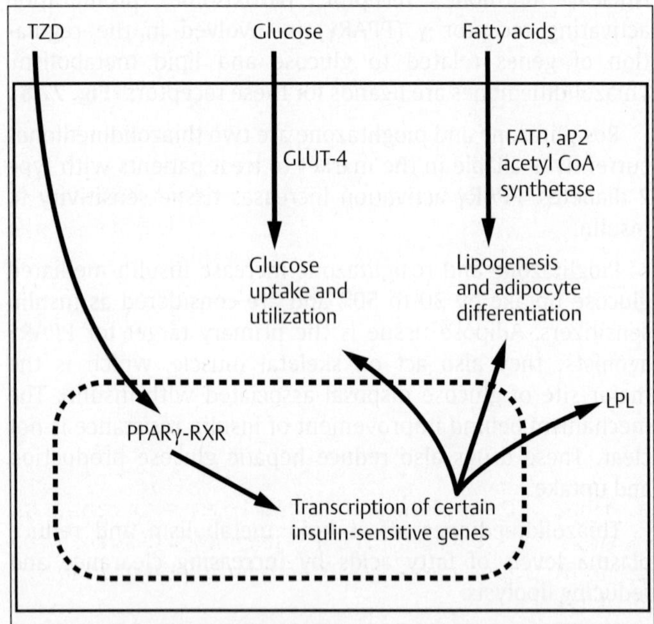

Fig. 77.8 Mechanism of action of glitazones. TZD, thiazolidinediones.

of the thiazolidinediones. Presence of insulin is required for thiazolidinediones. They are not used for type 1 diabetic patients.

Adverse Effects

Weight gain and edema, macular edema, and increased incidence of congestive heart failure are common. Rosiglitazone possesses risk of cardiovascular events. Rosiglitazone is banned in the European market.

Dose and Dosage Forms

Thiazolidinediones are administered orally once a day, with or without food. Prior to initiating treatment and regularly during treatment, liver function tests and HbA1C levels must be monitored. Maximal glucose-lowering effects of thiazolidinediones are not observed for 6 weeks to 6 months because of late onset of action via modification of gene expression. For the management of type 2 diabetes mellitus, glitazones must be used in combination with lifestyle modifications. They can be used along with biguanides, sulfonylureas, and insulin injectables.

Dosing for treatment of type 2 diabetes mellitus:

1. Pioglitazone: Initial 15 to 30 mg orally with a meal once a day; the dose may be increased by 15 mg with careful monitoring to 45 mg once a day. The maximum dose is 45 mg.
2. Rosiglitazone: Initial 4 mg orally once a day. If inadequate response after 8 to 12 weeks, the dose may be increased to 8 mg orally once a day or divided 12 hourly (4 mg twice a day).

α-Glucosidase Inhibitors

Mechanism of Action

Intestinal brush border contains an enzyme called α-glucosidase, which is responsible for the absorption of starch, dextrin, and disaccharides. α-Glucosidase inhibitors affect the enzyme activity responsible for absorption of dextrin, starch, and disaccharides (**Fig. 77.9**). These drugs also reduce the speed of absorption and digestion of polysaccharide and sucrose. They delay carbohydrate absorption and prevent postprandial rise in plasma glucose in normal and diabetic patients without increasing insulin level. The beneficial effect of α-glucosidase inhibitors is observed in

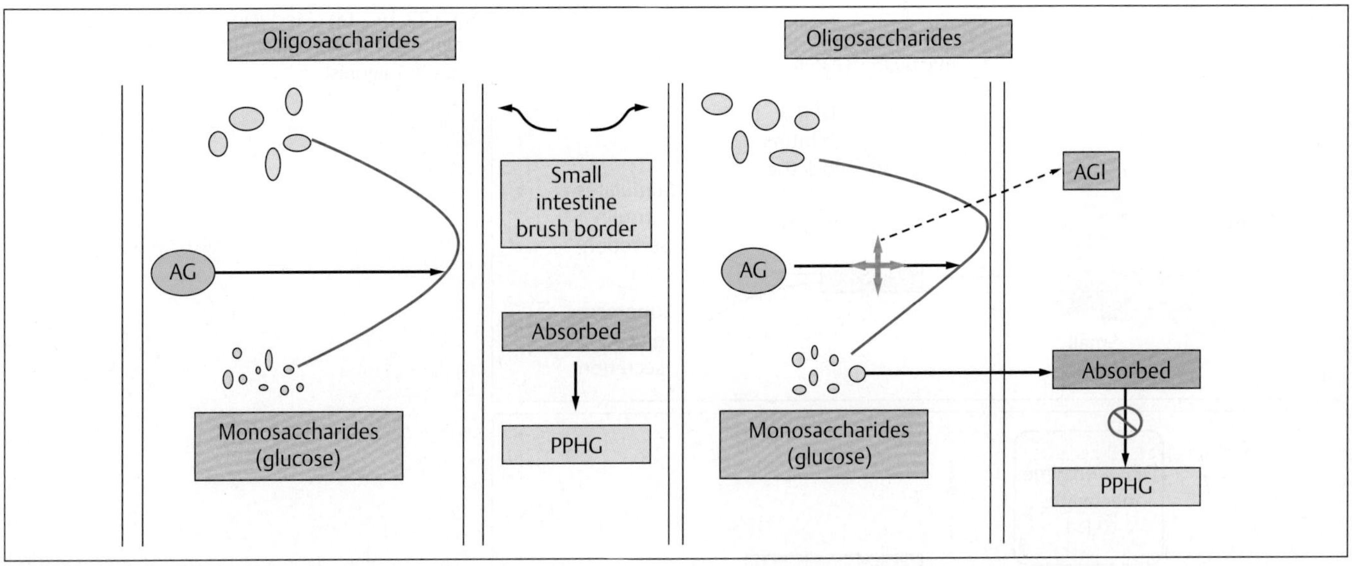

Fig. 77.9 Mechanism of action of α-glucosidase inhibitors. PPHG, postprandial hyperglycemia; AGI, α-glucosidase inhibitors.

elderly patients or patients with postprandial hyperglycemia when given as a monotherapy. Apart from this, it is also used in combination with other oral hypoglycemic agents as well as insulin. α-Glucosidase inhibitors should be taken at the start of the meal.

Acarbose and Miglitol

Acarbose is a well-known α-glucosidase inhibitor and is a complex oligosaccharide. It reversibly inhibits the enzyme activity. It has week effect on pancreatic α-amylase and competitively inhibits glucoamylase and sucrose.

Miglitol also showed the same activity but is more potent in inhibiting sucrase. Both the drugs possess HbA1c-inhibitory activity and reduce postprandial glucose in both type 1 and type 2 diabetic patients.

Pharmacokinetics

Acarbose is absorbed in a small amount and a very small amount of it that reaches the systemic circulation is excreted via the kidney. Miglitol absorption is saturable, with 50 to 100% of the drug taken into the circulation. Miglitol is completely excreted via the urine. A 50% reduction in dose is necessary for those who suffer from kidney disorder having creatinine clearance less than 30 mL/minute.

Side Effects

α-Glucosidase inhibitors do not cause hypoglycemia but are responsible for malabsorption, flatulence, diarrhea, abdominal bloating, and loose stool in about 50% of patients due to fermentation of unabsorbed carbohydrates.

Interactions

α-Glucosidase inhibitors can affect the absorption of commonly used drugs such as phenytoin, warfarin, verapamil, glyburide, L-thyroxine, and ethinyl estradiol. They may affect absorption of fat-soluble vitamins.

DPP-4 Inhibitors

Mechanism of Action

DPP-4 is a serine protease present on the endothelial cell and on the surface of T-lymphocytes and is widely distributed throughout the body in the form of ectoenzyme. DPP-4 cleaves amino acids at its N-terminal from peptide with alanine and proline in the second position. There are many substrates for this enzyme (**Fig. 77.10**). DPP-4 inhibitors prevent the degradation of incretins and endogenous GLP-1. This helps in potentiating the action of GLP-1, which ultimately inhibits postprandial hyperglycemia. DPP-4 inhibitors increase the area under curve (AUC) of GLP-1 and GIP (i.e., gastric inhibitory peptide) when their secretion is by a meal. DPP-4 inhibitor is a drug of choice and is used in combination with other hypoglycemic agents. Examples are sitagliptin, vildagliptin, saxagliptin, linagliptin, and alogliptin.

Pharmacokinetics

DPP-4 inhibitors are readily absorbed orally. Following oral ingestion, absorption occurs mainly in the small intestine, with median times to maximum (peak) plasma concentration ranging from 1 to 3 hours. The fraction of each dose absorbed ranges from approximately 30% with linagliptin to 75 to 87% for all others.

Side Effects

There are no observable adverse effects reported during clinical studies.

Dose and Dosage Forms

Among the DPP-4 inhibitors, linagliptin is available as 5 mg daily. Vildagliptin is given as 50 mg once or twice weekly, sitagliptin as 25, 50, or 100 mg once daily, and saxagliptin as 2.5 or 5 mg once daily.

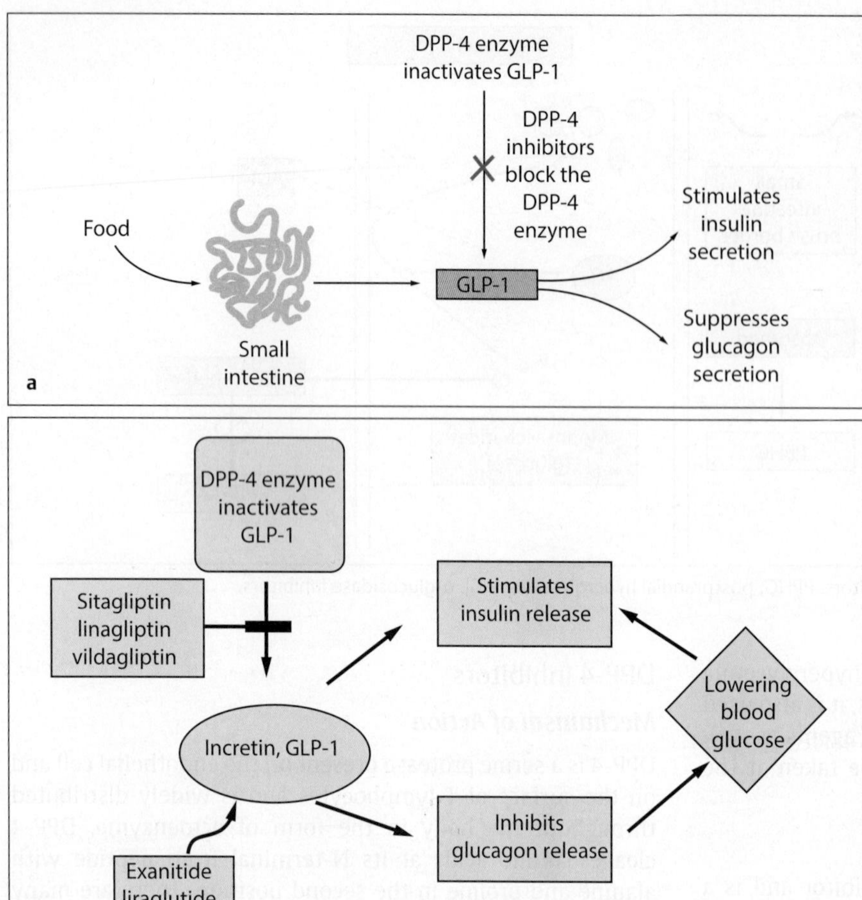

Fig. 77.10 **(a)** Mechanism of action of DPP-4 inhibitors. **(b)** Mechanism of action of glucagon-like peptide 1 agonist.

Glucagonlike Peptide 1 Agonist

Mechanism of Action

After taking a meal, GI hormone incretins are released, which help in stimulating insulin secretion. GLP-1 and GIP are the two most important incretins, which share many similarities. The difference between the two is that GLP-1 is effective in insulin release and lowering blood glucose in type 2 diabetic patients, whereas GIP is not as effective as GLP-1. GLP-1 is considered as one of the important drug targets in the diabetic population. Intravenous injection w GLP-1 agonist reduces food intake, delays gastric emptying, stimulates insulin secretion, inhibits glucagon release, and normalizes fasting and postprandial insulin secretion (**Fig. 77.11**). The insulinotropic effect of GLP-1 is glucose-dependent. Currently, there are two GLP-1 agonists, namely, exenatide and liraglutide, which are widely used for the treatment of diabetes.

Exenatide

Exendin has 39 amino acids and is a naturally occurring reptilian peptide with considerable homology to GLP-1. It is a potent GLP-1 receptor agonist that shares many of the physiological and pharmacological effects of GLP-1. Exenatide causes glucose-dependent insulin secretion. It is used as a monotherapy and as adjunctive therapy for the treatment of type 2 diabetes. In clinical trials, exenatide, alone or in combination with metformin, sulfonylurea, or thiazolidinedione, shows more specific activity in controlling glycemic levels.

Liraglutide

Liraglutide is used as adjunctive therapy in patients not achieving glycemic control with metformin, sulfonylurea, or the combination of metformin/sulfonylurea or metformin/thiazolidinedione. Liraglutide controls glycemia better and also helps in reducing weight in diabetic patients. The fatty acid side chain in the structure of liraglutide increases its $t_{1/2}$.

Pharmacokinetics

Exenatide is given via subcutaneous injection twice daily before meal. It is quickly absorbed and shows plasma peak concentration within 2 hours. It undergoes little metabolism in the circulation and has a volume of distribution of 30 L. Exenatide is excreted via the kidney. Liraglutide is also given by subcutaneous injection once daily. Peak levels are reached in 8 to 12 hours and the elimination $t_{1/2}$ is 12 to 14 hours. Liraglutide is eliminated via the intestinal and renal route.

Adverse Effects

GLP-1 receptor agonist mimics the pharmacology of native GLP-1. It causes nausea and vomiting in a dose-dependent manner. Based on data from clinical trials, up to 40 to 50% of patients given a GLP-1 receptor agonist report nausea at the initiation of therapy.

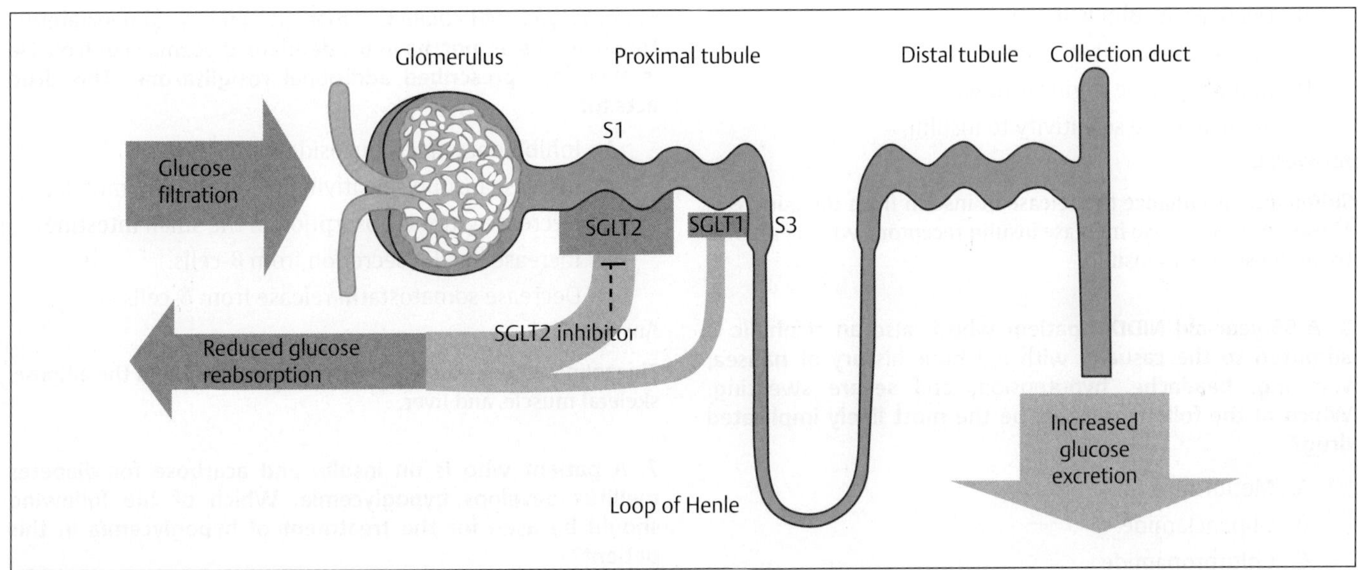

Fig. 77.11 Mechanism of action of SGLT2 inhibitors.

Dose and Dosage Forms

Many formulations of GLP-1 agonists, all of which historically were injectable and administered subcutaneously due to poor oral bioavailability can be prescribed. Lixisenatide and liraglutide are administered once daily, albiglutide, dulaglutide, and semaglutide dosing are given once weekly, and exenatide comes as either a twice-daily or a once-weekly injection. Recently, the FDA approved an oral formulation of semaglutide. Depending on the drug prescribed, the medication may come as a single- or multidose pen and may require a separate prescription for needles with various needle gauge requirements.

Newer Treatments in Diabetes

SGLT2 Inhibitors

Mechanism of Action

SGLT2 is a new class of antihyperglycemic drugs used in the treatment of type 2 diabetes. SGLT2 inhibitors have an insulin-independent mechanism of action. They inhibit the reabsorption of glucose in the kidney, which helps in increasing the level of glucose in the urine.

Canagliflozin and Dapagliflozin

Canagliflozin and dapagliflozin are well-known drugs from this class used for the improvement of glycemic control in type 2 diabetes. They are selective and reversible inhibitors of SGLT2 and possess dose-proportional pharmacokinetics. After administration, 60% of canagliflozin is absorbed orally and out of that 33% of the absorbed dose is excreted via the urine. Dapagliflozin is rapidly absorbed orally and the peak plasma concentration is reached within 2 hours. Dapagliflozin is metabolized into dapagliflozin 3-*O*-glucuronide and gets excreted in the urine.

Dose and Dosage Forms

Among the SGLT2 inhibitors, canagliflozin is initially given at a dose of 100 mg daily, which is gradually increased to 300 mg daily, and dapagliflozin is given at a dose of 5 or 10 mg daily, and empagliflozin is given at a dose of 10 or 25 mg daily.

Pramlintide

Pramlintide is an amylin analog, which is a polypeptide produced by pancreatic β-cells. It reduces glucagon secretion from α-cells and delays gastric emptying and helps in reducing postprandial hyperglycemia. It is injected subcutaneously just before meal and exerts a centrally mediated anorectic action. The duration of action is 2 to 3 hours. It is mostly used for a combination treatment with insulin, sulfonylureas, and metformin.

Multiple Choice Questions

1. A 20-year-old man with insulin-dependent diabetes mellitus is admitted in the casualty ward after collapsing during a physical cricket game. His blood sugar is 375 mg/dL. Which of the following is the best route of administration to bring the blood sugar down?

A. Intravenous.
B. Intramuscular.
C. Subcutaneous.
D. Sublingual.
E. Oral.

Answer: A

Insulin should reach the circulation for maximal effect; intravenous infusion has the fastest and highest peak blood insulin concentration.

2. The fasting blood sugar level of a 40-year-old woman is 139 mg/dL. She has type 2 diabetes mellitus. She is prescribed metformin; however, her fasting glucose levels remain higher than 100 mg/dL. Her physician decided to change the medication to a sulfonylurea. This drug acts to:

A. Reduce glucocorticoid levels.

B. Decrease insulin half-life.
C. Increase insulin secretion.
D. Inhibit enzyme α-glucosidase.
E. Reduce tissue sensitivity to insulin.

Answer: C

Sulfonylureas enhance the release of insulin from the pancreas. These agents may also increase insulin receptors, which enhance tissue sensitivity to insulin.

3. A 55-year-old NIDDM patient who is also an alcoholic is admitted to the casualty with a 1-hour history of nausea, vomiting, headache, hypotension, and severe sweating. Which of the following could be the most likely implicated drug?

A. Metformin.
B. Glibenclamide.
C. Chlorpropamide.
D. Acarbose.
E. Pioglitazone.

Answer: C

A disulfiram-like reaction could be present in NIDDM patients treated with chlorpropamide, an oral hypoglycemic, when consumed with alcohol.

4. A 50-year-old obese NIDDM patient is also an alcoholic. Metformin is relatively a contraindication or administered with extreme caution in this patient since the combination of metformin and alcohol enhances the risk of which of the following?

A. Weight gain.
B. Hypoglycemia.
C. Hepatotoxicity.
D. Lactic acidosis
E. A disulfiram-like reaction.

Answer: D

Biguanides, such as phenformin, have been documented to cause lactic acidosis. Hence, metformin, which is also a biguanide, must be avoided or given with extreme caution in patients with conditions that enhance the risk of lactic acidosis, such as alcohol consumption.

5. A 55-year-old man with NIDDM is admitted to the emergency room. He has tachycardic and tachypneic and looks disoriented. He has a history of consuming an antidiabetic medication. Which of the following agent could be responsible?

A. Metformin.
B. Glibenclamide.
C. Acarbose.
D. Glucagon.
E. Pioglitazone.

Answer: B

Any of the sulfonylureas can lead to hypoglycemia, which leads to shocklike manifestations.

6. A 55-year-old diabetic man is taking glibenclamide. However, he is not having adequate glycemic control. He is therefore prescribed additional rosiglitazone. This drug acts to:

A. Inhibit enzyme α-glucosidase.
B. Increase insulin sensitivity in adipose and muscle.
C. Decrease glucose absorption in the small intestine.
D. Increase insulin secretion from β-cells.
E. Decrease somatostatin release from δ-cells.

Answer: B

Thiazolidinediones increase sensitivity to insulin in the adipose, skeletal muscle, and liver.

7. A patient who is on insulin and acarbose for diabetes mellitus develops hypoglycemia. Which of the following should be used for the treatment of hypoglycemia in this patient?

A. Sucrose.
B. Galactose.
C. Glucose.
D. Starch.
E. Pentose.

Answer: C

Complex carbohydrates (polysaccharides and sucrose) are absorbed after conversion to simple carbohydrates by α-glucosidase. Inhibitors of this enzyme (acarbose and miglitol) decrease carbohydrate absorption from the gastrointestinal tract. Although these drugs themselves do not cause hypoglycemia, blood sugar may decrease if these are combined with insulin or other drugs releasing insulin. In such a case of hypoglycemia, simple carbohydrates such as glucose (not sucrose or other complex carbohydrates) should be used.

8. If a diabetic patient being treated with an oral hypoglycemic agent develops dilutional hyponatremia, which one of the following could be responsible for this effect?

A. Chlorpropamide.
B. Tolbutamide.
C. Glyburide.
D. Glimepiride.
E. Metformin.

Answer: A

Chlorpropamide is a first-generation sulfonylurea. It increases the risk of hypoglycemia (like other sulfonylureas and meglitinides). Other adverse effects of chlorpropamide are antidiuretic hormone (ADH)-like action leading to dilutional hyponatremia, cholestatic jaundice, and disulfiram-like reaction.

9. Insulin acts by stimulation of:

A. Ionotropic receptor.
B. Enzymatic receptor.
C. Metabotropic receptor.
D. Nuclear receptor.
E. α-receptor.

Answer: B

Insulin acts by stimulation of tyrosine kinase receptors.

10. Glibenclamide reduces blood glucose in all of the following except:

A. Nondiabetics.
B. Type 1 diabetics.
C. Type 2 diabetics.
D. Obese diabetics.
E. Thin diabetics.

Answer: B

Sulfonylureas decrease blood glucose in diabetics as well as nondiabetics. It requires at least 30% of functional β-cells for their action. Insulin is the only treatment for type 1 diabetes.

11. Metformin is *not* effective in lowering blood sugar level in which of the following patients?

A. Nondiabetics.
B. Obese diabetics.
C. Type 2 diabetics.
D. Diabetics not responding to sulfonylureas.
E. Thin diabetics.

Answer: A

Metformin is the drug of choice for the treatment of obese diabetic patients, as it causes weight loss. It does not cause release of insulin and therefore there are less chances of hypoglycemia.

12. A 15-year-old girl with type 1 diabetes is brought to the emergency department complaining of dizziness. Laboratory findings include severe hyperglycemia, ketoacidosis, and blood pH of 7.15. To achieve rapid control of severe ketoacidosis, the appropriate drug is:

A. Crystalline zinc insulin.
B. NPH insulin.
C. Tolbutamide.
D. Ultralente insulin.
E. Insulin glargine.

Answer: A

Diabetic ketoacidosis must be managed by fast-acting insulin preparations such as regular insulin (crystalline zinc insulin), insulin lispro, and insulin aspart.

13. A 54-year-old obese patient with type 2 diabetes mellitus and a history of alcoholism probably should not receive metformin because it can increase the risk of:

A. Disulfiram-like reaction.
B. Hypoglycemia.
C. Lactic acidosis.
D. Severe hepatic toxicity.
E. Nephrotoxicity.

Answer: C

Biguanides such as metformin and phenformin increase the risk of lactic acidosis particularly in patients with hepatic or renal disease. Both these drugs can cause lactic acidosis, although phenformin has more potential to cause this adverse effect than metformin. Metformin is more likely to cause megaloblastic anemia than phenformin.

14. Which of the following drug is α-glucosidase inhibitor?

A. Pioglitazone.
B. Miglitol.
C. Metformin.
D. Nateglinide.
E. Glibenclamide.

Answer: B

Complex carbohydrates (polysaccharides and sucrose) are absorbed after conversion to simple carbohydrates by α-glucosidase. Inhibitors of this enzyme (acarbose, voglibose, and miglitol) decrease carbohydrate absorption from the gastrointestinal tract.

15. A common side effect of thiazolidinediones is:

A. Dysgeusia.
B. Hypoglycemia.
C. Water retention with weight gain.
D. Anemia.
E. Lactic acidosis.

Answer: C

Glitazones have been reported to cause weight gain, edema, and plasma volume expansion. Therefore, these should be avoided in congestive heart failure patients (NYHA [New York Heart Association] class III and IV).

Chapter 78 Corticosteroids

Prasan R. Bhandari

PH 1.38: Describe the mechanism of action, types, doses, side effects, indications, and contraindications of corticosteroids.

Learning Objectives

- Pharmacological Actions.
- Mechanism of Action.
- Adverse effect.
- Synthetic corticosteroids.
- Clinical uses of corticosteroids.
- Corticosteroid withdrawal.
- Corticosteroid inhibitors.

Introduction

The Nobel Prize was credited to three searchers more than 60 years ago for their discovery of corticosteroids. This therapeutic class continues to be one of the most prescribed categories of medication in the current therapeutic armamentarium. The mechanism of action of corticosteroids has been elusive since very long and active basic research continues to be conducted in order to design new drugs capable of possessing the inhibitory properties without the agonist properties at the level of gene transcription. These novel ideas would permit better tolerability. Consequent to the documenting of the structure–activity properties of steroids, all the pharmacological aspects are studied in order to better comprehend the mechanisms of adverse drug side effects and try to recognize them best. All the advances regarding local topics, especially in the field of dermatology and asthma, have before now been a foremost step toward improved tolerance. Prescribing corticosteroids is always weighing the balance between benefits and risks primarily due to side effects and dependence.

Secretion

Corticosteroids are secreted from the adrenal cortex and the vital significance of corticosteroids has been validated. It was established that the cortical portion of adrenal gland is more essential as compared to the medullary portion. Several synthetic corticosteroids have been developed that are utilized clinically for an extensive range of nonendocrine conditions.

The adrenal (suprarenal) gland has two chief parts: the medulla and the cortex. The adrenal medulla is responsible for the control of short-term stress from moment to moment (fine adjustment) by secreting adrenaline and noradrenaline. The adrenal cortex comprises three layers: the zona glomerulosa, zona fasciculata, and zona reticularis. The adrenal cortex secretes steroidal hormones accountable for the management of long-term stress. These are together named corticosteroids, that is, steroids from the adrenal cortex. Corticosteroids are classified on the basis of source (part of the adrenal cortex) and their principal effect, as discussed in the following.

Zona Glomerulosa

The zona glomerulosa is the outermost layer, in which cells are arranged in arcuate formations. Mineralocorticoids are synthesized in the zona glomerulosa, for example, aldosterone (natural endogenous substance) deoxy-corticosterone. It possesses salt-retaining activity.

Zona Fasciculata

It is responsible for intermediary metabolism. Glucocorticoids are synthesized in the zona fasciculate, for example, hydrocortisone (natural endogenous substance). It is responsible for intermediary metabolism. Hypersecretion causes Cushing's syndrome.

Zona Reticularis

It has androgenic or estrogenic activity. Androgens are synthesized in the zona reticularis, for example, dehydroepiandrosterone (major), androstenediol, and androstenedione It has androgenic or estrogenic activity.

Hyposecretion of all these hormones leads to Addison's disease.

Synthesis

All corticosteroids have cyclopentanoperhydrophen-anthrene ring (steroid nucleus). Corticosteroids possess a 21-carbon structure, whereas sex steroids possess an 18- or 19-carbon structure and have the same steroid nucleus. All corticosteroids are synthesized in the cells of the adrenal cortex from the cholesterol under the regulation of adrenocorticotropic hormone (ACTH).

Pharmacological Actions

Natural Corticosteroids (Endogenous)

A wide-ranging diversity of physiological effects are produced by hydrocortisone (cortisol)

The control of its secretion and release in reaction to stress are shown in **Fig. 78.1**.

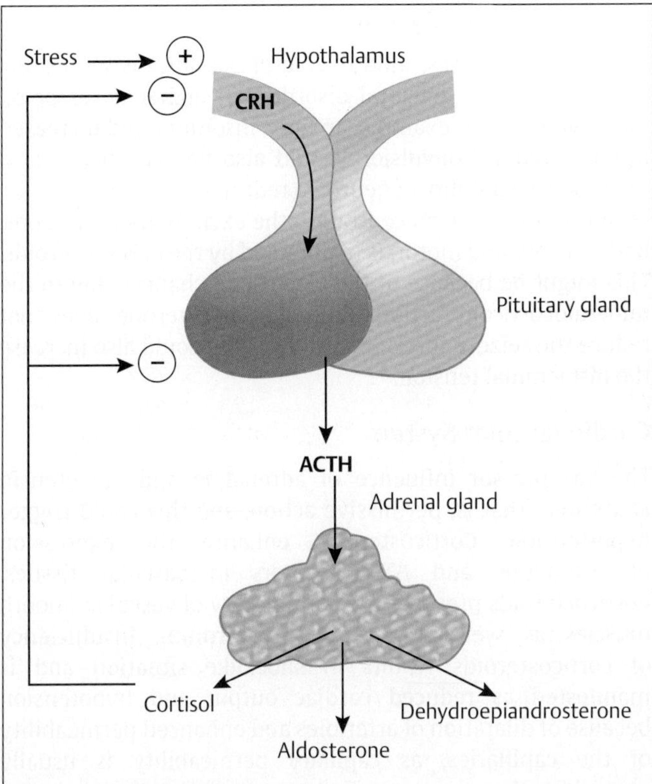

Fig. 78.1 Regulation of cortisol secretion. CRH, corticotropin-releasing hormone; ACTH, adrenocorticotropic hormone.

Physiological Effects

Effects are seen on majority of the tissues. The actions could be direct or indirect (permissive effects).

Permissive actions are those where the existence of hormone assists the action of other substances or in other words the absence of hormone causes deficient normal function.

For example, the reaction of smooth muscles such as vascular or bronchial (nonvascular) smooth muscles is decreased due to the action of catecholamines such as adrenaline and the responsiveness can be obtained again by the administration of corticosteroids in the physiological concentration.

Depending on the effect on mineral or other metabolism, the effect of corticosteroids could be classified into mineralocorticoid and glucocorticoid. Likewise, corticosteroids could be divided into glucocorticoid and mineralocorticoid on the basis of prominent action. The effects are dose-related and slight amount is secreted for the physiological action, and when corticosteroids are administered exogenously, the doses are higher and lead to toxicity.

Mineralocorticoid Effect

The main effect is sufficient sodium retention by enhancing the reabsorption of sodium (Na^+) from the distal convoluted tubule of the kidney. This is supplemented by increased excretion of potassium (K^+) and hydrogen (H^+). Consequently, deficiency of corticosteroids leads to deficiency of sodium, and if there is reduced sodium level, there is loss of circulatory volume. This causes absorption of water without associated sodium absorption and hence there is dilutional hyponatremia as well as changes associated with it. There is concomitant retention of potassium and hydrogen, which leads to hyperkalemia and acidosis result. If lack of corticosteroids is protracted, it causes circulatory failure, such as in cases of hypocorticism or adrenal insufficiency, and survival of patients could be challenging.

In overdoses, as might happen in prolonged use of exogenous corticosteroids, there is sodium and water retention and expansion in circulatory volume and hypertension. Thus, corticosteroids are avoided in hypertensive patients and extreme precaution is essential if the use of corticosteroids is compulsory in such patients. Additionally, because of this effect, deoxycorticosterone acetate (DOCA) is utilized as a pharmacological tool to induce hypertension in experimental animals for research use.

The endogenous constituent possessing mineralocorticoid effect is aldosterone. Aldosterone acts by synthesizing a protein mainly the NA^+/K^+-ATPase in the renal tubular cells.

Glucocorticoid Effect

Effect on Carbohydrate, Fat, and Protein Metabolism

Carbohydrate Metabolism

The foremost effects are glycogen synthesis by activating the enzyme hepatic glycogen synthetase and deposition of glycogen in the liver and stimulating gluconeogenesis from the amino acids released due to the breakdown of proteins. There is hyperglycemia because of suppression of uptake and utilization of glucose in the peripheral tissues (skeletal muscles), gluconeogenesis, and release of hepatic glucose. The sufficient level of glucose is preserved so that the brain gets optimum glucose throughout the starvation. Because of increased blood level of glucose, the insulin release is also activated and insulin resistance could occur. The long-term use of corticosteroids can result in precipitation of diabetes mellitus.

Fat Metabolism

They activate hormone-sensitive lipase and lipolysis. The lipolytic action of adrenaline, glucagon, growth hormone, etc., is expedited, that is, permissive action. Lipolysis in the subcutaneous tissue over the extremities releases fat that is redistributed and deposited over the face, neck, and shoulder reason. This produces the classical signs of Cushing's syndrome (hypercorticism), such as the moon face, buffalo bump, and fish mouth, if there is endogenous hypersecretion or exogenous use in the overdoses and/or prolonged use.

Protein Metabolism

The proteins are broken down and the produced amino acids are used for the synthesis of glucose, that is, gluconeogenesis. The protein breakdown (catabolic effect) produces numerous alterations based on the tissues where the protein is being broken down, for example, muscle wasting, osteoporotic modifications in the bone, thinning of skin, and catabolic changes in the lymphoid and connective tissue.

Effect on Inflammation, Immunity, and Blood Cells

Effect on Inflammation

Glucocorticoids are potent anti-inflammatory and decrease all varieties of inflammation irrespective of the cause since they act by several mechanisms. They prevent the effect of several mediators of inflammation and effect of leukocytes, cytokines, and chemokines. The inflammatory process is a complicated sequence of events comprising production of intracellular adhesion molecules such as endothelial leukocyte adhesion molecule-1 (ELAM-1) and intracellular adhesion molecule-1 (ICAM-1). These effects are vital for leukocyte localization and are suppressed by corticosteroids.

Effect on Lymphoid Tissue, Immunity, and Allergy

They primarily act on various constituents of cellular immunity but have relatively little effect on humoral immunity. The principal antibody response is reduced, and with constant use, the previously recognized antibody response is also decreased. They possess numerous mechanisms. Tissue macrophages and antigen-presenting cells react to antigens and mitogens, and this reaction is decreased by glucocorticoids. Glucocorticoids on topical application lead to vasoconstriction by suppressing the degranulation of mast cells and decreasing the capillary permeability by inhibiting histamine release from mast cells and basophils. Macrophage results in phagocytosis, kills microorganisms, and generates tumor necrosis factor α (TNF-α) and interleukin-1 (IL-1), and these functions of macrophages are suppressed by glucocorticoids. Both macrophage and lymphocyte produced fewer IL-12 and interferon gamma responsible for stimulation of cellular immunity. IL-12 is responsible for T-helper cell action and cytotoxic T-lymphocyte proliferation. In macrophages, monocyte, endothelial cells, and fibroblasts, glucocorticoids suppress the production of IL-1, IL-2, IL-4, IL-6, and TNF-α. They also inhibit the synthesis of all the mediators of inflammation (e.g., prostaglandins, leukotrienes [LTs], platelet-activating factor) due to the inhibition of phospholipase A2. They decrease expression of cyclooxygenase-2 (COX-2), an induced form of COX, in inflammation. All these effects contribute to both anti-inflammatory and immunosuppressant action.

Effect on Blood Cells

Blood cells such as the red blood cells (RBCs), neutrophils, and platelets are enhanced; however, lymphocyte (T and B), monocytes, eosinophils, and basophil decrease in the blood circulation on administration of a single dose of short-acting steroid. The increase in neutrophils in the blood circulation is due to increased migration from bone marrow and decreased migration from blood cells, leading to a decrease in the number of cells at inflammatory site. The other white cells migrate from vascular bed to lymphoid tissue; consequently, the concentration in the blood circulation is diminished. These effects are transitory and return to normal later on discontinuing the corticosteroids.

Central Nervous System

In therapeutic doses, mild degree of euphoria is witnessed. There could be behavioral disorders in higher doses or on prolonged use, for example, anxiety, insomnia, and increased motor activity. Convulsions could also be seen because of increased excitability of neurons (reduced seizure threshold), as in physiological concentration the excitability of neurons, both sensory and motor, is maintained by the corticosteroids. This might be because of the electrolyte changes due to the mineralocorticoid action, although aldosterone does not reduce the seizure threshold. Higher dose could also increase the intracranial tension.

Cardiovascular System

The vasopressor influence of adrenaline and angiotensin is assisted, that is, permissive action, and this could trigger hypertension. Corticosteroids enhance the expression of adrenergic and AT_1 receptors in vascular tissues. Corticosteroids preserve the contractility of vascular smooth muscles as well as that of myocardium. Insufficiency of corticosteroids results in shocklike situation and is manifested as reduced cardiac output and hypotension because of dilatation of arterioles and enhanced permeability of the capillaries, as capillary permeability is usually normal in the presence of corticosteroids. Administration of adrenaline produces poor response in insufficiency of corticosteroids since they possess a permissive action and hence corticosteroids reestablish the responsiveness of adrenaline and increase the blood pressure (BP). Additional contributing factor in the hypotension is loss of sodium because of reduction/absence of mineralocorticoid effect.

Bone and Skeletal Muscle

There is osteoporosis of the bone because of loss of calcium from bone (enhanced resorption) and reduced intestinal absorption of calcium. This leads to weakening of various bones. The normal muscular activity needs the physiological concentration of corticosteroids and weakness is experienced in both the hyposecretion (because of reduced circulation) and hypersecretion or excess administration of corticosteroids (because of hypokalemia, a mineralocorticoid action; due to muscle wasting, a glucocorticoid action).

Others

Water Metabolism

Generally, water absorption is associated with the absorption of sodium; however, owing to lack of corticosteroids, there is increased water retention. This glucocorticoid action is independent of sodium absorption and does not happen because of deficiency of aldosterone, a mineralocorticoid. Accordingly, glucocorticoid deficiency could lead to water intoxication if a large quantity of fluid is administered by intravenous (IV) infusion.

Gastrointestinal Tract

Corticosteroids are ulcerogenic, that is, they could worsen existing ulcer or cause ulcer. This is because of augmented release of gastric acid and pepsin. Furthermore, decrease of local immune response against *Helicobacter pylori* could also be responsible.

Fetal Lung Maturation

Fetal secretion of cortisol controls the maturation of fetal lungs and is essential for manufacture of pulmonary surfactant crucial for normal breathing. Therefore, in circumstances of premature delivery, large quantity of betamethasone is administered.

Miscellaneous

Hydrocortisone in small quantity is required for normal glomerular filtration and it also possesses a uricosuric effect. Prolonged administration of glucocorticoids results in decreased release of ACTH, growth hormone, thyroid-stimulating hormone, and luteinizing hormone from the anterior pituitary.

Intracellular Mechanism

Corticosteroids act on two categories of receptors, the glucocorticoid receptor (GR) and mineralocorticoid receptor (MR), and lead to their response (**Fig. 78.2**).

Glucocorticoid Receptor

The GR is a cytoplasmic receptor and is extensively and consistently distributed/expressed in all the tissues. It has three domains, namely, glucocorticoid-binding domain (carboxy-terminal), DNA-binding domain, and receptor regulatory domain (amino-terminal). The DNA-binding domain is located in the middle of the protein and contains nine cysteine residues. This region folds into a "two-finger" structure stabilized by zinc ions connected to cysteines to form two tetrahedrons. This is similarly termed zinc fingers and this portion of DNA-binding domain identifies specific nucleic acid sequence. The GR is inactive and retained in this state due to diverse proteins, heat shock protein 90 (HSP-90) and HSP-70, and immunophilin attached to receptor regulatory domain. These proteins possess inhibitory effect on the GR; when steroid combines with receptor, these proteins are disbanded and the steroid receptor (SR) complex is formed. The SR complex produces a homodimer, that is, SR + SR, and this homodimer is translocated to nucleus where it interacts with glucocorticoid-responsive element (GRE), a precise DNA sequence on chromatin. GRE also has a duplicate sequence, which is appropriate to combine with SR homodimer. The binding of SR dimer with GRE affects the transcription process by a group of proteins termed steroid receptor coregulators either by initiation of transcription coactivators (induction) or by inhibition of transcription corepressor (suppression).

Induction

The particular desired m-RNA generated is moved to cytoplasm for necessary protein (enzyme) synthesis to facilitate several processes. The proteins synthesized are cyclic adenosine monophosphate–dependent kinases, which mediate metabolic processes, and annexin 1 (previously known as lipocortin I). Annexin 1 stimulates enzyme phospholipase A2 besides mediating negative feedback mechanism. The negative feedback suppresses the release of ACTH probably by acting at cell membrane receptor

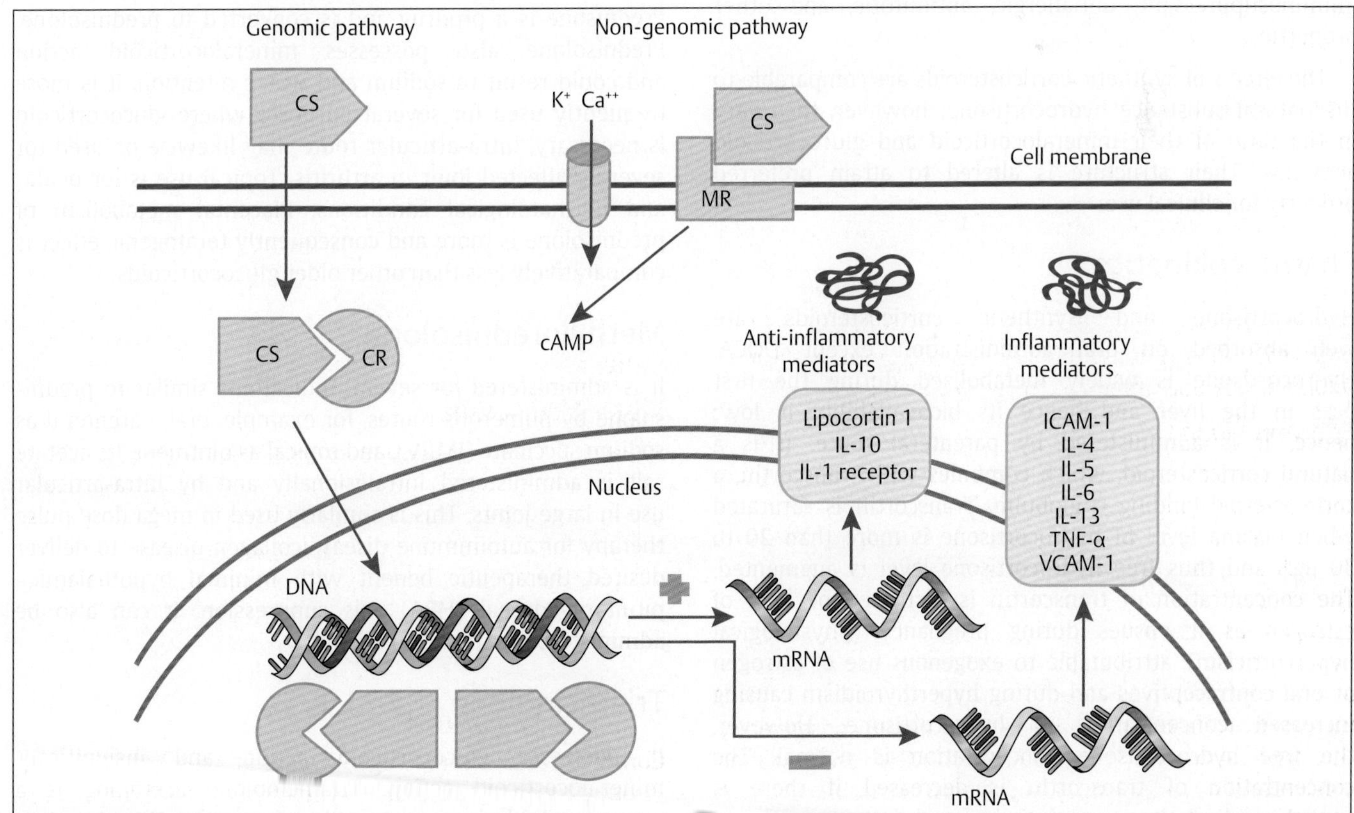

Fig. 78.2 Intracellular mechanism of corticosteroids. cAMP, cyclic adenosine monophosphate; CS, corticosteroid; CR, corticoid receptor; IL, interleukin; MR, mineralocorticoid receptor; VCAM, vascular cell adhesion molecule.

(nongenomic effect) and is a prompt effect. The stimulation of phospholipase A2 is gradual and leads to an inflammatory effect and hence the onset of anti-inflammatory action of corticosteroids is slow and deferred for few hours. Nevertheless, the effect continues even when plasma concentration of steroids decreases.

Suppression

Numerous transcription factors such as activator protein 1 and nuclear factor κB assist transcription and stimulate genes, for example, genes for COX-2, cytokines, and NO synthase (inducible). SR dimer + GRE complex suppresses these proteins and such effect furthers the anti-inflammatory and immunosuppressant action.

Mineralocorticoid Receptor

The MR is not consistently distributed unlike the GR but is limited to tissues. It is chiefly present or expressed in the kidneys. Moreover, it is also existent in the salivary gland, sweat glands, and colon and in the hippocampus in the central nervous system. The mechanism of the MR is comparable to that of the GR. Steroids combine with the MR and, after translocation to nucleus, combine with a DNA sequence, mineralocorticoid-responsive element (MRE), similar to GRE.

Synthetic Corticosteroids

Corticosteroids possessing noticeable glucocorticoid action have been manufactured to be used for an extensive range of conditions exploiting their anti-inflammatory, immunosuppressant, antiallergic, antimitotic, and other properties.

The effects of synthetic corticosteroids are comparable to the natural substance hydrocortisone; however, they vary in the ratio of their mineralocorticoid and glucocorticoid activities. Their structure is altered to attain preferred property for clinical use.

Pharmacokinetics

Hydrocortisone and synthetic corticosteroids are well absorbed on oral administration except DOCA. Hydrocortisone is widely metabolized during the first pass in the liver and hence its bioavailability is low; hence, it is administered by parenteral route. It is a natural corticosteroid, which combines with transcortin, a corticosteroid-binding α-globulin. Transcortin is saturated when plasma level of hydrocortisone is more than 20 to 30 µg% and thus free hydrocortisone level is augmented. The concentration of transcortin is increased because of estrogen as it ensues during pregnancy (physiological hypercorticism), attributable to exogenous use of estrogen or oral contraceptives and during hyperthyroidism causing increased concentration of hydrocortisone. However, the free hydrocortisone concentration is normal. The concentration of transcortin is decreased if there is hypothyroidism, hypoproteinemia, or defect in synthesis. Transcortin possesses a high affinity for hydrocortisone but low affinity for aldosterone and conjugated metabolites of glucocorticoids. Protein binding of hydrocortisone is around 90%. All the synthetic corticosteroids bind with albumin. Cortisone and prednisone are prodrugs and are converted to active drugs hydrocortisone and prednisolone, respectively. They are metabolized primarily in the liver by microsomal enzymes. The metabolites produced are conjugated with sulfate or glucuronide conjugation and eliminated in the urine.

Individual Agents

The relative potencies, anti-inflammatory dose, and duration are given in **Table 78.1**. Other clinically pertinent characteristics of individual agents are briefly stated in the following.

Cortisone and Hydrocortisone (Cortisol)

Cortisone is a prodrug and is converted to hydrocortisone. Hydrocortisone hemisuccinate is a water-soluble ester and can be administered by IV route, whereas hydrocortisone acetate is an insoluble ester (suspension) and is administered by intramuscular (IM) or intra-articular route. Hydrocortisone is rapidly acting and hence is appropriate for emergency situations such as status asthmaticus and to overcome acute adrenal insufficiency; however, the duration of action is short. Hydrocortisone hemisuccinate is given at a dose of 100 mg four times a day. It also has noticeable mineralocorticoid action.

Prednisone and Prednisolone

Prednisone is a prodrug and is converted to prednisolone. Prednisolone also possesses mineralocorticoid action and could result in sodium and water retention. It is more frequently used for several purposes where glucocorticoid is necessary. Intra-articular route may likewise be used for severely affected joint in arthritis. Topical use is for ocular and dermatological conditions. Placental metabolism of prednisolone is more and consequently teratogenic effect is comparatively less than other older glucocorticoids.

Methylprednisolone

It is administered for several indications similar to prednisolone by numerous routes, for example, oral, parenteral as sodium succinate (IM/IV), and topical as ointment. Its acetate salt is administered intralesionally and by intra-articular use in large joints. This is similarly used in mega dose pulse therapy for autoimmune disease/collagen disease to deliver desired therapeutic benefit with minimal hypothalamic–pituitary–adrenal (HPA) axis suppression. It can also be administered as retention enema.

Triamcinolone

It possesses glucocorticoid action and insignificant mineralocorticoid action. Triamcinolone acetonide is a water-insoluble ester and is administered by IM route. It is also administered intra-articularly and topically.

Table 78.1 Relative potencies, anti-inflammatory dose, and duration of corticosteroids

Base	Anti-inflammatory potency relative to cortisol	Mineralocorticoid[a] potency relative to cortisol	Duration of action (h)	Equivalent dose (mg)
Cortisol	1	1	8–12	20
Short-acting				
Hydrocortisone	1	1	12	20
Cortisone	0.8	1	12	25
Intermediate-acting				
Prednisone	3.5	0.8	12–36	6
Prednisolone	4	0.8	12–36	5
Methylprednisolone	5	0–0.5	12–36	4
Triamcinolone[b]	5	0	12–36	4
Fludrocortisone	10–15	125–150	24–48	–
Long-acting				
Betamethasone	25	0	36–72	0.75
Dexamethasone	30	0	36–72	0.75

[a]Mineralocorticoid activity is defined as Na^+/H_2O retention.
[b]Triamcinolone acetonide: $C_{24}H_{31}FO_6$.

Betamethasone and Dexamethasone

Both are comparable and possess glucocorticoid action. They are most potent and longest-acting agents. They lead to a significant inhibition of the HPA axis. They are utilized for various purposes where glucocorticoids are indicated. Sodium and water retention do not occur as they lack mineralocorticoid action. They are administered orally, parenterally, and topically. Dexamethasone sodium phosphate is a water-soluble ester and is administered by IM/IV route. Betamethasone and dexamethasone are less protein bound and undergo a lesser amount of placental metabolism and maternal protein binding as compared to hydrocortisone.

Fludrocortisone

It is an orally effective mineralocorticoid and possesses some glucocorticoid activity. It is utilized for replacement therapy in Addison's disease and in patients with congenital adrenal hyperplasia with salt wasting. Moreover, it is also indicated for idiopathic postural hypotension. In patients with hypotension due to autonomic neuropathy, it is difficult to maintain vasomotor tone (vasoconstriction) and in such cases circulatory volume can be increased by using fludrocortisone.

Deoxycorticosterone Acetate

It has mineralocorticoid action but no glucocorticoid action. It can be administered sublingually for Addison's disease. It is also indicated for inducing hypertension in animals for research purposes.

Aldosterone

It is an endogenous mineralocorticoid with short action. It is promptly inactivated on oral administration because of extensive and rapid first-pass metabolism. Hence, it was earlier administered for acute adrenal insufficiency by IM route but is not currently used. Instead, orally effective fludrocortisone is used.

Deflazacort

It is a newer orally effective agent, similarly efficacious as prednisolone and with comparable uses. Its use has been associated with a lower risk of osteoporosis, has less effect on growth in children, less chances of Cushing's syndrome, and lower hyperglycemic activity, thus proving to be advantageous.

Clinical Uses of Corticosteroids

Corticosteroids could be used for therapeutic or diagnostic purposes. Therapeutic uses might be either to overcome the deficiency states or to treat conditions not related to the deficiency of hormones (**Fig. 78.3** and **Table 78.2**).

Endocrine Uses (due to Deficiency of Corticosteroids)

For this purpose, corticosteroids are given exogenously, and the ideal agent is one that retains both glucocorticoid and mineralocorticoid action, for example, hydrocortisone. The doses necessary are lesser than those essential for the nonendocrine uses.

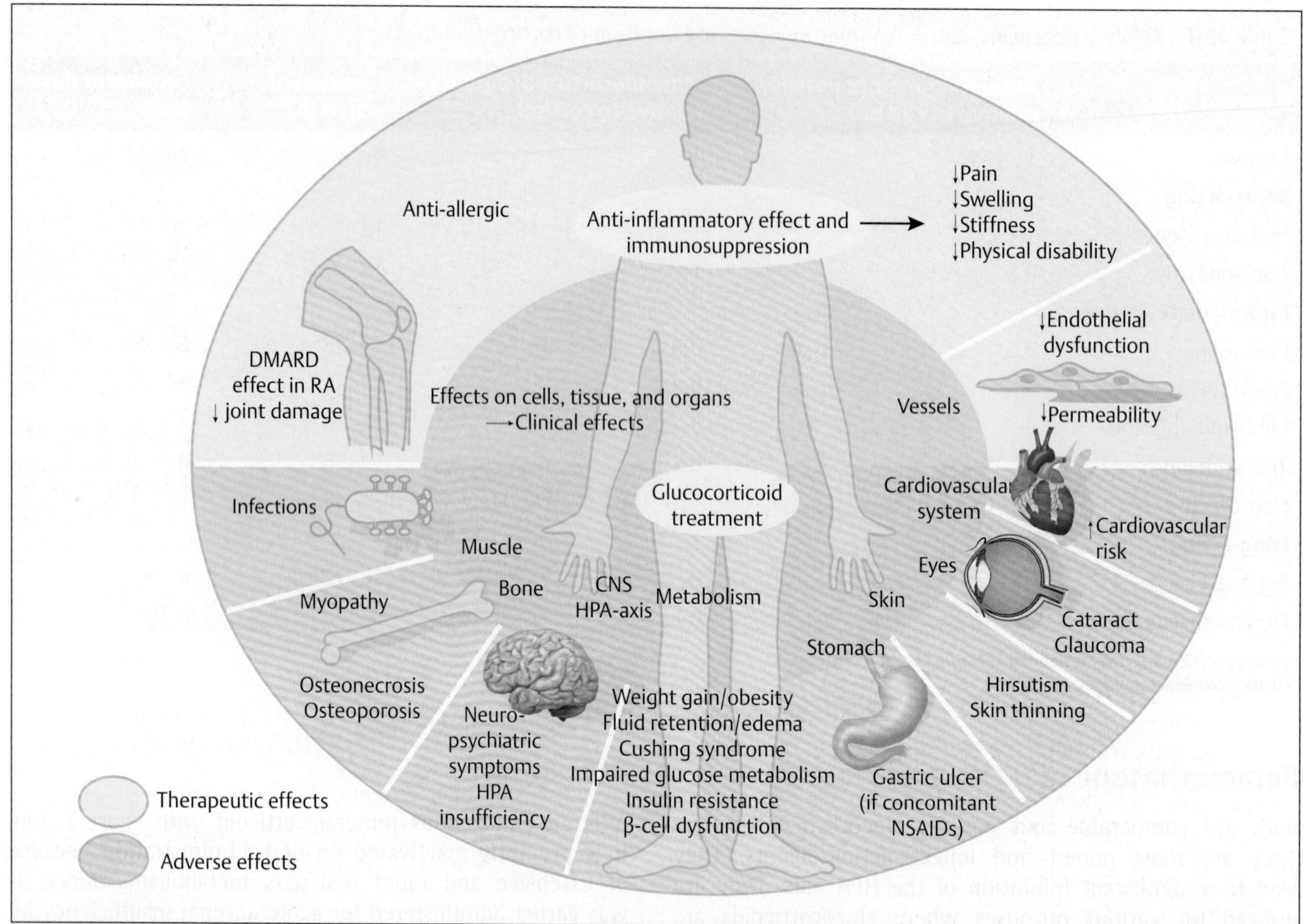

Fig. 78.3 Clinical uses of corticosteroids.

Table 78.2 Uses of individual corticosteroids

Corticosteroid drugs	Treatment for
Betamethasone	Dermatitis
Budesonide	Asthma, noninfectious rhinitis, nasal polyposis
Cortisone	IgE-mediated allergies
Dexamethasone	Inflammation, rheumatoid arthritis
Hydrocortisone	Dermatitis
Methylprednisolone	Arthritis, bronchial inflammation
Prednisolone	Asthma, rheumatoid arthritis, ulcerative colitis, Crohn's disease
Prednisone	Systemic lupus erythematosus, Bell's palsy, asthma, dermatitis
Triamcinolone	Eczema, diabetic retinopathy

Adrenal Insufficiency

Acute

Acute adrenal insufficiency is an emergency condition, and in this, drugs have to be given via IV route. For this situation, hydrocortisone sodium succinate 100 mg must be administered by IV route instantly after the diagnosis, followed by the IV infusion. Once the condition of the patient is restored to normal, oral hydrocortisone could be administered. The dose is progressively decreased and when the daily dose of hydrocortisone is decreased to 50 mg or less, then mineralocorticoids may be supplemented. This is because even when adequate doses of hydrocortisone are administered, hyperkalemia continues. For this reason, fludrocortisone 0.1 to 0.2 mg per day is sufficient. Precaution must be taken to govern the quantity of IV fluid to reestablish the water and electrolyte balance, as these patients could have increased water load. The reason of crisis should be treated. In several circumstances it is due to infection, which can be taken care of by the administration of suitable antibiotics. Also, dexamethasone with supplementation of mineralocorticoid such as fludrocortisone could be used.

The salt-retaining activity of fludrocortisone is 20 times more than its anti-inflammatory activity.

Chronic

Chronic Primary Insufficiency

This is also termed Addison's disease and the treatment is oral administration of hydrocortisone. The dose is generally 20 to 40 mg per day, of which two-thirds could be administered in the morning to mimic the normal secretion and the remaining dose in the evening. Proper salt and water intake ought to be confirmed.

Chronic Secondary Insufficiency

It is because of hypopituitarism, and the best treatment would be supplementation of ACTH; however, it has to be administered frequently by injection and hence it is inconvenient. Instead, hydrocortisone can be used effectively similar to the case of primary deficiency, but the dose necessary is less. Mineralocorticoids are not typically necessary since the pituitary has little control over the secretion of aldosterone and thus an optimum level of aldosterone is secreted.

Congenital Adrenal Hyperplasia (Adrenogenital Syndrome)

It is a disorder of genetic basis due to lack of enzyme(s) responsible for adrenal steroidogenesis. A lack of primarily 21β-hydroxylase is stated. Because of deficit of corticosteroids, ACTH secretion is increased, which may result in hypertrophy of adrenal glands to overcome the insufficiency. Generally, the deficiency is overcome and normal quantity of glucocorticoid and mineralocorticoid might be produced if deficiency is partial (most cases), that is, hormone production may be near-normal. However, there is excess secretion of androgens, which may lead to precocious puberty in children and masculinization (virilization) in young females. Complete deficiency of enzyme results in salt wasting. Hydrocortisone is favored because of both its glucocorticoid and mineralocorticoid action. It is administered in the dose of 10 to 20 mg per day (0.6 mg/kg per day) and can be given in divided doses. Two-thirds of the dose can be administered in the morning. Fludrocortisone must be supplemented orally at a dose of 0.1 to 0.2 mg per day in cases of salt wasting due to total absence of enzyme 21β-hydroxylase. Additional salt could be supplemented to avoid salt wasting and preserve the electrolyte balance, BP, and plasma renin activity.

Deficiency in Fetus (Immature Fetal Lungs)

The maturation of lungs in the fetus is controlled by the secretion of sufficient quantity of hydrocortisone (cortisol) in the fetus. In the premature infant, that is, delivered prematurely (before 34 weeks) because of any reason, there is respiratory distress in the newborn. This can be avoided and/or diminished by the administration of glucocorticoid to mother.

Nonendocrine Uses (Treatment of Other Diseases)

Principles of Uses

The use of corticosteroids in the nonendocrine diseases is largely empirical. Corticosteroids are administered based on wide clinical experience and the principles with respect to use are stated in the following:

1. A single dose, even if higher, is not generally harmful and a short course of up to 1 week is less likely to be harmful, except if there is some contraindication for the use of corticosteroids.
2. Abrupt withdrawal might result in acute adrenal insufficiency and hence gradual tapering of the dose is essential.
3. Short course of corticosteroids must be used, and corticosteroids must be slowly tapered and discontinued: for example, prednisolone 40 mg for days 1 and 2, then 30 mg for days 3 and 4, 20 mg for days 5 and 6, and then 5 mg for two days and then stopped. Likewise, if the treatment is for protracted period, try gradual withdrawal.
4. The choice to administer corticosteroid is of extreme significance and founded on the possibility for the serious side effects. All cases must be deliberated individually with respect to relative risk and benefits.
5. They are beneficial in nonendocrine conditions primarily because of their anti-inflammatory and immunosuppressive property.
6. The correct dose for a specific therapeutic effect is customarily governed by trial and error and this must be assessed from time to time as complications could ensue on persistent use and the underlying disease development may vary as the time progresses.
7. The minimum possible dose ought to be administered for the desired effect (relief of pain) if long-term use is essential. Administration of anti-inflammatory agents such as aspirin is useful in tapering the dose without deterioration of the symptoms. Nonetheless, in life-threatening diseases such as pemphigus, large doses must be administered for quick control of the condition. This dose could be doubled or tripled if the required benefit does not occur and subsequently this dose must be decreased under close scrutiny. It is very critical to evaluate the relative danger of therapy and the disease.
8. When administered for nonendocrine disorders, that is, other than replacement therapy, corticosteroids do not cure the disorder and additionally their effect is nonspecific.

Therapeutic Uses

The nonendocrine conditions where glucocorticoids are more commonly used are stated in the following and the dose of corticosteroid is influenced by the nature and the severity of the disease.

Rheumatic Disorders

Corticosteroids are the mainstay for the treatment of serious inflammatory rheumatic fever with carditis and arthritis, systemic lupus erythematosus, polyarteritis nodosa (vasculitis), and giant cell arteritis. The purpose of treatment is to promptly control the disease and curtail the damage; accordingly, sufficient doses must be administered even if the doses are higher for this purpose.

Arthritis

Rheumatoid Arthritis

Corticosteroids must be administered in advanced disease if the first-line treatment (nonsteroidal anti-inflammatory drugs [NSAIDs] and physiotherapy) fails to achieve the anticipated response. It would be better if corticosteroids are administered along with the disease-modifying agents (e.g., methotrexate, gold salts) till the effect of these agents is obtained. Subsequently, corticosteroids can be gradually tapered and discontinued. For this reason, minimal possible dose must be administered during the acute exacerbation of the disease.

Osteoarthritis, Bursitis, and Tendonitis

Local administration of corticosteroids is highly effective in these conditions, where one or more joints are severely affected and there is acute exacerbation. The regularity of the intra-articular injection must be minimal (at least a gap of 3 months). Else, the recurrent administration could result in painless damage of the joint.

Gout

Patients with acute gout not responding to NSAIDs could be treated with a short course of corticosteroid.

Allergic Disorders

Anaphylactic Shock (Acute Hypersensitivity Reaction)

Corticosteroids have adjuvant importance and enhance the sensitivity of adrenaline. Adrenaline is the mainstay of the treatment and is lifesaving if administered promptly at the right time in the appropriate doses.

Other Allergic Reaction

For particular allergic reactions of short duration, for example, hay fever, serum sickness, urticaria, angioneurotic edema, insect bite (bee stings), and drug reaction, corticosteroids are valuable in inhibiting the manifestations along with the main treatment. Antihistaminics are beneficial if the situation is not severe. In severe circumstances, IV administration of corticosteroids might be necessary (methylprednisolone IV four times a day).

Respiratory Diseases

Bronchial Asthma

Corticosteroids are highly valuable in chronic severe asthma. Bronchial asthma is considered as both allergic and inflammatory disorder. In severe asthma, IV administration of corticosteroid is suggested in hospitalized patients, though the response is delayed for few hours (6–12 hours). If IV administration is essential, the patient is later maintained on oral drug, which is gradually withdrawn after tapering the dose. A short course of oral treatment is likewise administered. For better effect and to curtail the systemic adverse effects, it is better to administer it by the inhalational route. The preparations commonly administered by the inhalational route are beclomethasone valerate, beclomethasone dipropionate, budesonide, triamcinolone acetonide, and ciclesonide.

Chronic Obstructive Pulmonary Disease

They are beneficial in reversible chronic obstructive airway disease, and frequently short courses are administered. In severe cases, long course may be administered, but the purpose should be very clear (e.g., improvement of the lung function test). When long-term treatment is necessary, precautions must be taken while withdrawing the drug and minimal possible doses must be administered.

Ocular Diseases

Allergic Conditions

Corticosteroids are beneficial in allergic conjunctivitis. However, they must be avoided in patients with diabetes mellitus.

Inflammatory Conditions

If administered correctly in inflammatory eye disorders, they could inhibit inflammation efficiently and could thwart blindness. For inflammation of the anterior chamber, topical administration is beneficial. However, if the posterior segment of the eye is involved, they should be administered by the systemic route or subconjunctival and retrobulbar route. Topical administration of corticosteroids in the eye increases the intraocular tension in normal persons and worsens the glaucoma. This may or may not be reversible on stopping the drug. Thus, precaution should be taken while using the steroids in patients with glaucoma. It would be better if intraocular tension is checked all through the treatment in patients with glaucoma.

Infective Conditions

Corticosteroids must be avoided in conjunctivitis because of bacterial, viral, or fungal infection since steroids mask the spread of infection. The infection could advance to such a level that there is irreversible loss of vision. In herpes simplex keratitis, steroids are contraindicated since it could result in permanent loss of vision. This occurs because of the progressive clouding of cornea due to continuous administration of corticosteroids.

Skin Diseases

Inflammatory and Allergic Skin Disorders

In cases such as eczema, corticosteroids are highly effective. They are administered topically and occasionally by occlusive dressing to increase efficacy. However, in occlusive dressing, the chances of systemic absorption and toxicity could also increase. For topical application, a wide variety of preparations in different strengths are available. Hydrocortisone 1% ointment is highly effective in eczema, but the effect is lost on stopping the drug treatment.

Systemic use of corticosteroid is lifesaving in cases of pemphigus, exfoliative dermatitis, Stevens–Johnson syndrome, etc., though higher doses are essential.

Gastrointestinal Disease

Glucocorticoids are beneficial in particular circumstances of inflammatory bowel diseases such as ulcerative colitis and Crohn's disease. In patients unresponsive to drugs, dietary changes, and rest, steroids are usually beneficial during acute exacerbation of these diseases.

Renal Diseases

Corticosteroids are valuable in patients with nephrotic syndrome due to minimal change glomerulonephritis and it is the first-line agent for this condition. However, in patients with nephrotic syndrome because of other types of glomerulonephritis, the use of corticosteroid is not very satisfactory.

Infections

Corticosteroids are immunosuppressants and hence must be avoided. However, in some infections they are beneficial. One example is *Pneumocystis jirovecii* pneumonia in AIDS patients as they may have some degree of hypoxia. In such circumstances, administration of steroids is useful by improving the oxygenation, lowering the incidence of respiratory failure, and, thus, decreasing the mortality. Another example is meningitis due to *Haemophilus influenzae* (type B) in children older than 2 years. In these patients, steroids decrease the long-term neurological injury. Evidently suitable antimicrobial agents are used in these infections.

Hepatic Diseases (IM5.16)

Corticosteroids are beneficial in the treatment of auto-immune chronic active hepatitis. In such cases, it results in remission in the majority of the patients, as indicated by the histological changes, and in fall in the serum transaminase level. However, in other types of hepatitis and cirrhosis of the liver (alcoholic hepatic disease), corticosteroids are of not much benefit. In patients with hepatic encephalopathy, prednisolone might be effective to a certain degree and could be tried. Prednisone, which is a prodrug and converted into the active drug prednisolone in the liver, should be avoided in liver diseases.

Malignancies

Corticosteroids are beneficial in patients with acute lymphatic leukemia and lymphoma as one of the agents of the combination therapy due to the antilymphocytic action (lympholytic). In hypercalcemia due to malignancy, corticosteroids were used earlier. However, currently bisphosphonates are used, which are more effective.

Miscellaneous Uses

Organ Transplantation (SU13.2)

Corticosteroids are administered in higher doses in organ transplantation to avert graft rejection. Steroids are combined with other immunosuppressants for this purpose. Subsequently, the dose of corticosteroids is reduced and the patient is put on the maintenance dose of steroids.

Cerebral Edema

Because of parasites or brain tumors, mostly metastatic ones, in patients with cerebral edema, corticosteroids are beneficial in decreasing the edema as well as in preventing the edema. The role of corticosteroids in edema due to cerebrovascular accidents (stroke) or trauma is not clear.

Other Autoimmune Diseases

Corticosteroids demonstrate a partial response to several autoimmune diseases, for example, thrombocytopenia (autoimmune and idiopathic), autoimmune destruction of erythrocytes (hemolytic anemia), and myasthenia gravis, because of their immunosuppressant action.

Sarcoidosis

It is managed with an initial high dose and subsequently on maintenance dose. Patients getting doses higher than the physiological concentration could develop secondary tuberculosis. Therefore, depending on the positive tuberculin reaction or chances of tuberculosis, prophylactic antitubercular treatment can be administered in these patients.

Spinal Cord Injury

Corticosteroids lead to a decrease in neurological deficit in patients with spinal injury if treated within 8 hours of injury with heavy doses of steroids. The benefit could be because of the inhibition of free radical–mediated cell injury as a result of ischemia and reperfusion. Additionally, because of their anti-inflammatory action, decrease in the spasm due to inflammation may also add to valuable effect in the spinal injury.

Shock

The basis of use of corticosteroids in shock is empirical and probably they enhance the receptiveness of the catecholamines. They could be used in septicemic, cardiogenic, and other types of shock.

Vomiting due to Cancer

Glucocorticoid (e.g., dexamethasone) has adjuvant importance in cases of vomiting due to cancer. The possible mechanism is their anti-inflammatory effect reducing inflammation around the tumor (cancer cells).

For Lung Maturation

In patients with premature labor, the lungs of fetus are not matured. Thus, when tocolytic agents are administered to inhibit premature labor, glucocorticoids are also used together with it for lung maturation (to reduce respiratory distress). Betamethasone is favored since it has less binding to maternal proteins and reduced placental metabolism. This results in increased placental transfer as compared to hydrocortisone and prednisolone. Consequently, use of corticosteroids to mother before the expected premature delivery results in fetal maturation of the lungs and, on this basis, corticosteroids are used for this purpose.

Thyroid Storm

It is frequently associated with adrenal insufficiency. Hydrocortisone can be used since it is fast acting; besides, corticosteroids inhibit conversion of T4 to T3.

Diagnostic Uses

To Test Adrenal–Pituitary Axis Functioning

For this reason, dexamethasone is administered in a dose that does not affect the urinary excretion of the corticosteroid metabolites in the urine but suppresses the adrenal–pituitary axis and so reduces ACTH production.

Diagnosis of Cushing's Syndrome (Dexamethasone Suppression Test)

For this condition, dexamethasone 1 mg is administered orally at 11 p.m. and plasma cortisol level is measured in the morning. In normal individuals, the plasma cortisol concentration is generally less than 3 µg/dL, whereas in patients with Cushing's syndrome it is more than 5 µg/dL.

Adverse Effects

The adverse effects or toxic effects of corticosteroids are of two varieties. These are either because of long-term administration in the higher doses as compared to the physiological concentration or due to withdrawal of corticosteroid therapy. Adverse effects ensuing from both the reasons could be life-threatening. The adverse effects on protracted uses are of more significance since they might be serious and could be due to both the mineralocorticoid action and glucocorticoid action (**Fig. 78.3**).

Due to Mineralocorticoid Action

Fluid and water retention results in increased circulatory volume and rise in BP. Hypochloremic alkalosis also follows due to loss of potassium. Muscle weakness can occur due to hypokalemia. However, such side effects are not common with the use of glucocorticoid that lacks or has minimal mineralocorticoid action. Nevertheless, prolonged use of agents with only glucocorticoid action or very high dose can also result in elevation of BP.

Due to Glucocorticoid Action

Cushing's Syndrome/Habitus

It has distinctive characteristics features which are diagnostic such as buffalo hump (supraclavicular), fish mouth, obesity of trunk, and thin limbs in comparison to other body parts.

Hyperglycemia

Persistent use might lead to hyperglycemia and even frank diabetes mellitus with glycosuria.

Infection and Healing of Wound

Predisposition to develop any infection is increased due to immunosuppression. Frequently, opportunistic infections due to *Candida* can occur. Likewise, if the patient previously has some infection, it could spread, for example, pulmonary tuberculosis can be converted to military tuberculosis. Immunosuppression is more possible when it is used for 3 weeks or more, whereas it is less expected if it is administered for 1 week or less. Glucocorticoids may be administered for infections, if warranted, but always with suitable antibiotic cover. Wound healing including those due to surgical incision can be delayed because of inhibition of fibroblasts and effect on other constituents necessary for healing.

Osteoporosis and Osteonecrosis

Osteoporosis is more frequent in the elderly, and the bones affected are mainly the flat bones. This may result in vertebral fracture. Glucocorticoid must be withdrawn if substantial osteoporosis occurs as indicated by radiological changes. Avascular necrosis of femur head might ensue and long bone fracture is also likely.

Peptic Ulceration

Sustained administration or high dose might exacerbate existing ulcer or cause ulcer. This could possibly be due to increased release of gastric acid and pepsin along with decreased local immune response against *H. pylori*. Complications are expected in patients with peptic ulcer, such as bleeding and silent perforation.

Growth Retardation

Even in the comparatively lesser doses, corticosteroids administered to children might lead to growth retardations that can be overcome by administration of growth hormone. Growth hormone causes increased collagen synthesis and linear growth.

Mental Changes

Insomnia, restlessness, and mood alteration might happen on extended use. Although rare, some patients might develop depression and/or psychosis.

Ocular Side Effects

Glaucoma

Increase in intraocular tension and glaucoma can occur on long-term use.

Cataract

After protracted use, glucocorticoids can lead to posterior subcapsular cataract, particularly in children.

Dermal Changes

Persistent administration can lead to fragile skin, telangiectasia, contusion, and bleeding. Topical use is more expected to cause thin skin and atrophy.

Myopathy

Skeletal muscle weakness and fatigue can occur on prolonged treatment because of skeletal muscle wasting (steroid myopathy).

HPA Axis Suppression

Suppression of the HPA axis results in acute adrenal insufficiency on sudden withdrawal or reduction of the dose if the patient is maintained on high doses and/ or for prolonged period. HPA axis suppression could be reduced by administering pulse therapy; for example, methylprednisolone high dose (1 g) every 6 weeks by IV infusion may be used for chronic autoimmune disease such as rheumatoid arthritis and pemphigus. Aldosterone does not inhibit the HPA axis since its production is independent of the ACTH.

Contraindications

Depending on the side effects of corticosteroids as stated earlier, precautions should be taken while using corticosteroids for the conditions mentioned in **Table 78.3**. These are relative contraindications because corticosteroids are frequently lifesaving in serious situations. However, herpes simplex keratitis and pregnancy are absolute contraindications.

Corticosteroids Withdrawal

Withdrawal of steroids has two foremost complications:

1. Exacerbation/relapse of the disease for which it was used: for example, rheumatoid arthritis and eczema.
2. Acute adrenal insufficiency: It occurs because of rapid withdrawal of therapy after prolonged treatment. Individual disparity is there in the amount and duration of adrenal suppression. Recovery from HPA axis suppression is dependent on this and generally recovery ensues in weeks to months and seldom it takes 1 year or more for the complete recovery.

In order to avert the above-mentioned complications, that is, exacerbation of disease and acute adrenal insufficiency, it is recommended to gradually taper the dose and then withdraw the corticosteroids and follow the guidelines as cited earlier for nonendocrine uses. If the patient is on protracted corticosteroid therapy mainly with higher doses, then severe withdrawal syndrome might occur. It is manifested as fever, malaise, arthralgia, and myalgia. If it is used for arthritis, then it is difficult to distinguish it from the exacerbation of disease. Rarely, reducing the dose or withdrawing the steroids could cause increased intracranial tension with papilledema and this is called pseudotumor cerebri.

Topical Steroids

Topical steroids administered for ocular disorders are betamethasone, dexamethasone, clobetasone, fluorometholone, prednisolone, and loteprednol. Several formulations are used for dermatological conditions. Corticosteroids administered by inhalational route (bronchial asthma) include beclomethasone, budesonide, and fluticasone. Glucocorticoids administered by intra-articular route include hydrocortisone acetate, prednisolone acetate, and triamcinolone acetonide.

Corticosteroid Inhibitors

Synthesis Inhibitors

The following agents are inhibitor of synthesis of corticosteroids:

1. Adrenocorticolytic agent, for example, mitotane.
2. Inhibitor of enzyme cytochrome P450, for example, metyrapone, aminoglutethimide, and ketoconazole.
3. Inhibitor of enzyme 11β-hydroxylase, for example, metyrapone.
4. Inhibitor of 3β-hydroxysteroid dehydrogenase, for example, ketoconazole, and trilostane.

Aminoglutethimide

It suppresses all classes of steroids since it inhibits the conversion of cholesterol to pregnenolone, a rate-limiting step. It is beneficial in decreasing corticosteroid secretion in patients with Cushing's syndrome due to adrenocortical carcinoma not responding to mitotane. It is also valuable in patients with carcinoma breast along with hydrocortisone or dexamethasone. However, currently tamoxifen (estrogen antagonist) is favored over aminoglutethimide. Adverse effects such as maculopapular rash and gastrointestinal and neurological side effects might occur, especially at higher doses. Aminoglutethimide can lead to adrenal insufficiency that may necessitate glucocorticoid replacement. For the replacement purpose, dexamethasone should not be administered in patients taking aminoglutethimide, since the metabolism of dexamethasone is hastened by aminoglutethimide. Some other glucocorticoid must be used.

Ketoconazole

It is an antifungal agent; however, at a little higher dose, it is a nonselective inhibitor of adrenal steroid synthesis. The enzymes inhibited are several cytochrome P450 and 3β-hydroxysteroid dehydrogenase. It similarly inhibits the cleavage of cholesterol. Inhibition of adrenal and gonadal steroidogenesis is the side effect when it is used for the antifungal action. However, this is utilized for the treatment of Cushing's syndrome due to any cause.

Table 78.3 Contraindications of corticosteroids

Contraindications	Reason
Hypertension, congestive heart failure, and renal failure	Due to increased circulatory volume
Diabetes mellitus	Due to hyperglycemic action
Majority of infections (fungal, viral, mycobacterial)	Spread of infection may occur
Psychiatric and epileptic diseases	Aggravation of psychiatric diseases
Peptic ulcer	Aggravation of ulcer and silent perforation may occur
Osteoporosis	May cause the pathological fracture

Metyrapone

It suppresses the synthesis of primarily corticosteroids by inhibiting the conversion of deoxycortisol to cortisol by inhibiting the enzyme 11β-hydroxylase. Thus, it is relatively selective for corticosteroids. There is noticeable increase in the level of 11-deoxycortisol (steroid precursor). Dependent on the above-mentioned effect, metyrapone can be used to assess HPA function. For this use, metyrapone is administered at midnight and, the following morning, the concentrations of cortisol and 11-doxycortisol are measured. Metyrapone is also beneficial in distinguishing the causes of Cushing's syndrome. The adverse effects are salt and water retention and hirsutism due to conversion of 11-deoxycortisol to deoxycorticosterone and androgen. All agents that inhibit the action of corticosteroids are capable of causing acute adrenal insufficiency. Hence, extreme precaution is essential while using these agents. It is also imperative to measure the HPA axis status before starting therapy with these agents.

Inhibitors of the Action of Corticosteroids

1. GR antagonist: for example, mifepristone at higher dose (progesterone antagonist at lower dose).
2. Mineralocorticoid receptor antagonist (aldosterone antagonist): for example, spironolactone, eplerenone, and drospirenone.

Glucocorticoid Receptor Antagonist

Mifepristone

It is a progesterone antagonist and indicated primarily for the termination of early pregnancy because of its antiprogestin action. It has been observed that at higher doses it also blocks the GR and feedback regulation of the HPA axis. As a result, it causes increased ACTH and cortisol level. It could be beneficial for the treatment of hypercorticism due to its antiglucocorticoid action.

Mineralocorticoid Receptor Antagonist

Spironolactone and Eplerenone

These are discussed in Chapter 29.

Drospirenone

It also inhibits the MR and antagonizes the effect of aldosterone. It has progestational activity and used in oral contraceptive pills.

Multiple Choice Questions

1. The drug prednisolone is known to be a powerful anti-inflammatory agent. This is true due to the action of the drug on which of the following enzymes?

A. Cyclooxygenase.
B. Lipoxygenase.
C. Phospholipase A.
D. Phosphodiesterase.

Answer: C

Steroids have inhibitory effects on cytokine transcription and synthesis, especially the ones relevant in chronic inflammation. Steroids increase the synthesis of lipocortin (annexin) I, a phospholipase A_2 inhibitor, decreasing the production of inflammatory mediators.

2. Glucocorticoids act in inflammation by:

A. Decreasing lipocortin.
B. Increasing IL-2.
C. Increasing lipocortin.
D. Increasing C-reactive protein.
E. Increasing leukotrienes.

Answer: C

Steroids have inhibitory effects on cytokine transcription and synthesis, especially the ones relevant in chronic inflammation. Steroids increase the synthesis of lipocortin (annexin) I, a phospholipase A_2 inhibitor, decreasing the production of inflammatory mediators.

3. Which of the following disorders is not aggravated by corticosteroid therapy?

A. Congenital adrenal hyperplasia.
B. Diabetes mellitus.
C. Hypertension.
D. Peptic ulcer.

Answer: A

Corticosteroids are used for the management of congenital adrenal hyperplasia.

4. Steroids are contraindicated in all, except:

A. Diabetes mellitus.
B. Hypertension.
C. Eczematous skin disease.
D. Peptic ulcer disease.

Answer: C

Since steroids may have to be used as a life-saving measure, all of these are relative contraindications. Topical corticosteroids are highly effective in eczematous skin diseases.

5. Toxic effects of long-term administration of a glucocorticoid include:

A. Hepatotoxicity.
B. Osteoporosis.
C. Precocious puberty.
D. Lupus-like syndrome.

Answer: B

Glucocorticoids have a lot of adverse effects on long-term use. These can lead to Cushing's syndrome, hyperglycemia, osteoporosis, delayed wound healing, increased susceptibility to infections, cataract, glaucoma, and many other adverse effects.

6. A glucocorticoid with mineralocorticoid activity is seen in:

A. Triamcinolone.
B. Betamethasone.
C. Cortisol.
D. Dexamethasone.

Answer: C

Glucocorticoids are chiefly produced in the zona fasciculata of the adrenal cortex, whereas mineralocorticoids are synthesized in the zona glomerulosa. Cortisol (or hydrocortisone) is the most important human glucocorticoid.

7. Which of the following antifungal drug can be used in the treatment of Cushing's syndrome?

A. Ketoconazole.
B. Fluconazole.
C. Itraconazole.
D. Miconazole.

Answer: A

Ketoconazole is effective for long-term control of hypercortisolism of either pituitary or adrenal origin. Its effect appears to be mediated by inhibition of adrenal 11-β-hydroxylase and 17,20-lyase, and it, in some unknown way, prevents the expected rise in ACTH secretion in patients with Cushing's disease.

8. A 46-year-old male patient has Cushing's syndrome that is due to the presence of an adrenal tumor. Which of the following drugs would be expected to reduce the signs and symptoms of this man's disease?

A. Betamethasone.
B. Cortisol.
C. Fludrocortisone.
D. Ketoconazole.
E. Triamcinolone.

Answer: D

Ketoconazole inhibits many types of cytochrome P450 enzymes. It can be used to reduce the unregulated overproduction of corticosteroids by adrenal tumors.

9. A 56-year-old woman with systemic lupus erythematosus had been maintained on a moderate daily dose of prednisone for 9 months. Her disease has finally gone into remission and she now wishes to gradually taper and then discontinue the prednisone. Which of the following requires a gradual tapering of glucocorticoid for recovery?

A. Depressed release of insulin from pancreatic B cells.
B. Hematopoiesis in the bone marrow.
C. Normal osteoblast function.
D. The control by vasopressin of water excretion.
E. The hypothalamic–pituitary–adrenal system.

Answer: E

Exogenous glucocorticoids act at the hypothalamus and pituitary to suppress the production of corticotropin-releasing factor and ACTH.

10. A 45-year-old woman was suspected of having Cushing's syndrome. To confirm the diagnosis, the patient was given an oral medication late in the evening and had blood drawn the following morning for laboratory testing. which of the following was the oral medication?

A. Dexamethasone.
B. Fludrocortisone.
C. Glucose.
D. Ketoconazole.
E. Propylthiouracil.

Answer: A

Cushing's syndrome is a consequence of too much steroid production and is most commonly due to an ACTH-secreting pituitary adenoma. Dexamethasone will suppress ACTH production and thus can be used diagnostically to separate pituitary Cushing's from those with ectopic ACTH-producing tumors. As a result, adrenal production of endogenous corticosteroids is suppressed. On discontinuance, the recovery of normal hypothalamic–pituitary–adrenal function occurs slowly. Glucocorticoid doses must be tapered slowly, over several months, to prevent adrenal insufficiency.

11. A 34-year-old woman with ulcerative colitis has required long-term treatment with pharmacologic doses of a glucocorticoid agonist. Which of the following is a toxic effect associated with long-term glucocorticoid treatment?

A. A "lupus-like" syndrome.
B. Adrenal gland neoplasm.
C. Hepatotoxicity.
D. Osteoporosis.
E. Precocious puberty in children.

Answer: D

One of the adverse metabolic effects of long-term glucocorticoid therapy is a net loss of bone, which can result in osteoporosis.

12. A 54-year-old man with advanced tuberculosis has developed signs of severe acute adrenal insufficiency. Which of the following signs or symptoms is this patient most likely to exhibit?

A. A moon face.
B. Dehydration.
C. Hyperglycemia.
D. Hypertension.
E. Hyperthermia.

Answer: B

In acute adrenal insufficiency, there is loss of salt and water that is primarily due to reduced production of aldosterone. The loss of salt and water can lead to dehydration.

13. The patient in the previous question should be treated immediately. Which of the following combinations is the most rational?

A. Aldosterone and fludrocortisone.
B. Cortisol and fludrocortisone.
C. Dexamethasone and metyrapone.
D. Fludrocortisone and metyrapone.
E. Triamcinolone and dexamethasone.

Answer: B

A rational combination of drugs should include agents with complementary effects (i.e., a glucocorticoid and a mineralocorticoid). The combination with these characteristics is cortisol and fludrocortisone. (Note that although fludrocortisone may have sufficient glucocorticoid activity for a patient with mild disease, a patient in severe acute adrenal insufficiency needs a full glucocorticoid such as cortisol.)

14. Which of the following is a drug that, in high doses, blocks the glucocorticoid receptor?

A. Aminoglutethimide.

B. Beclomethasone.

C. Ketoconazole.

D. Mifepristone.

E. Spironolactone.

Answer: D

Mifepristone is a competitive antagonist of glucocorticoid and progesterone receptors. Ketoconazole and aminoglutethimide also antagonize corticosteroids; however, they act by inhibiting steroid hormone synthesis.

Chapter 79 Agents Affecting Calcium Balance

Janakidevi C. H.

PH1.36: Describe the mechanism of action, types, doses, side effects, indications, and contraindications of drugs used in endocrine disorders (diabetes mellitus, thyroid disorders, and osteoporosis).

Learning Objectives

- Calcium.
- Parathormone.
- Calcitonin.
- Vitamin D.
- Bisphosphonates.

Introduction

From the past two decades, the importance of bone mineral ion homeostasis has been increasing steadily, as cases of osteoporosis are increasing among the middle aged and elderly persons.

Calcium

Elemental calcium is an essential constituent for many biological functions in the human body. The adult human body contains about 1,300 g (in male) and 1,000 g (in female) of calcium, of which 99% is present in bones and teeth. The normal serum calcium level ranges from 8.5 to 10.4 mg/dL (4.25–5.2 mEq/L, 2.1–2.6 mm) in three different chemical forms: (1) ionized form (50%), which mediates all cellular functions; (2) protein-bound (40%); and (3) complexed form (10%), with phosphate and citrate. Recommended daily allowance is given in **Table 79.1**.

Sources of Calcium

Milk and milk products are the richest sources of calcium, which assimilates in intestine easily. Although green leafy vegetables and cereals are rich in calcium, the presence of phytates and oxalates inhibits the absorption of calcium.

Pharmacokinetics

Calcium enters the body only through the intestine. Most of the calcium is absorbed passively in the small intestine by the jejunum and the ileum whenever there is adequate intake of calcium. However, when there is a reduced intake of calcium, vitamin D helps in the absorption of calcium through the proximal duodenum. Calcium is excreted through the urine, feces, and sweat. As much as 99% of the calcium will be reabsorbed from the proximal convoluted tubule (PCT). It is regulated by parathyroid hormone (PTH). Of the total intake, 60% of calcium is excreted through the feces. Thus, during starvation, there will be inadequate intake of calcium and continuous loss of calcium through the feces, resulting in hypocalcemia. The loss of calcium through the sweat is minimal, but excess loss of calcium through the sweat is seen in tropical countries.

Physiological Functions of Calcium

Calcium is essential for the formation of milk, bones, and teeth. Ionic calcium acts as a cofactor for most of the enzymes in biochemical reactions. It maintains integrity and regulates permeability of the cell membrane. Ionic calcium regulates excitability and contractions of smooth, skeletal, and cardiac muscles. It acts as an intracellular second messenger for release of hormones and neurotransmitters from storage vesicles of the nerve terminal. It is essential for coagulation of blood, mainly in activation of the prothrombin to thrombin. It is also required for automaticity of cardiac pacemakers.

Regulation of Plasma Calcium Levels by Parathormone, Calcitonin, and Calcitriol

Regulation of calcium homeostasis (**Figs. 79.1** and **79.2**) is maintained by three hormones (PTH, vitamin D, and calcitonin) and three organs (intestine, kidney, and bone). Low calcium levels stimulate release of PTH from parathyroid

Table 79.1 Recommended daily allowance of calcium

Life stage group	Dose (mg/d)
Infants, 0–6 mo	200
Infants, 6–12 mo	260
1–3 years old	700
4–8 years old	1,000
9–13 years old	1,300
14–18 years old	1,300
19–30 years old	1,000
31–50 years old	1,000
51–70 years old males	1,000
51–70 years old females	1,300
70 years old	1,200
14–18 years old, pregnant/lactating	1,300
19–50 years old pregnant/lactating	1,000

Source: NIH office of dietary supplements.

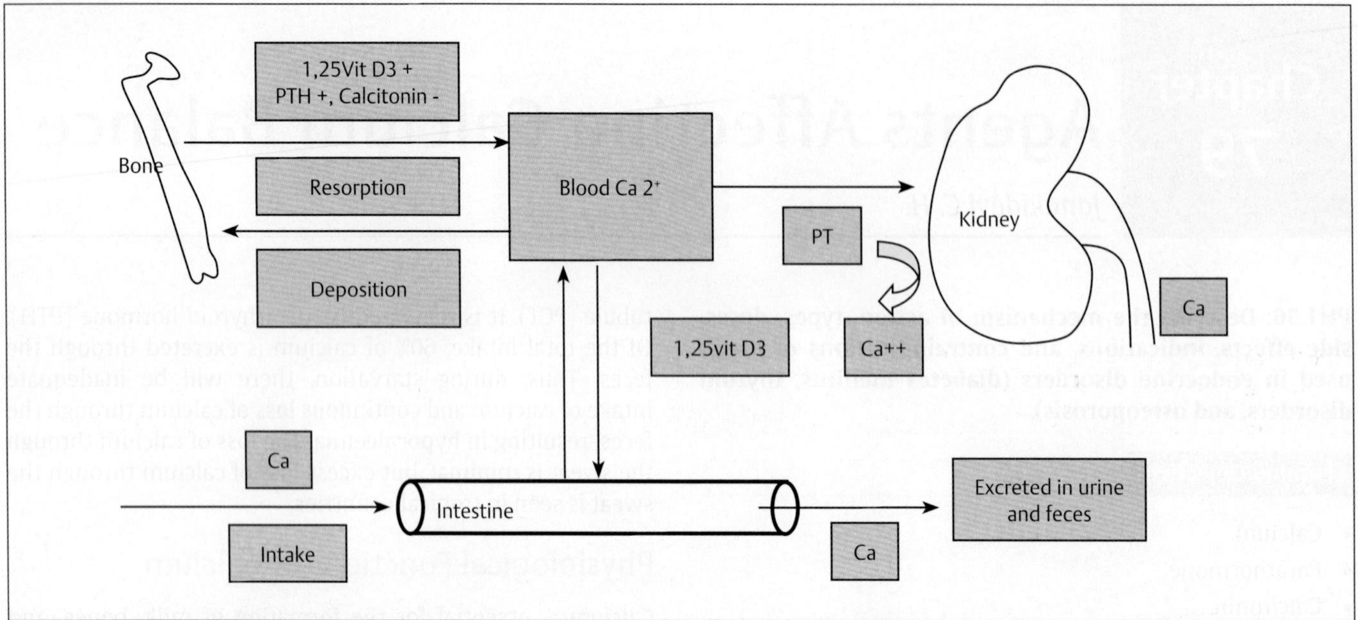

Fig. 79.1 Calcium homeostasis. PTH- Parathormone (+) – Stimulation, (-) – Inhibition, Ca^{++}- Calcium.

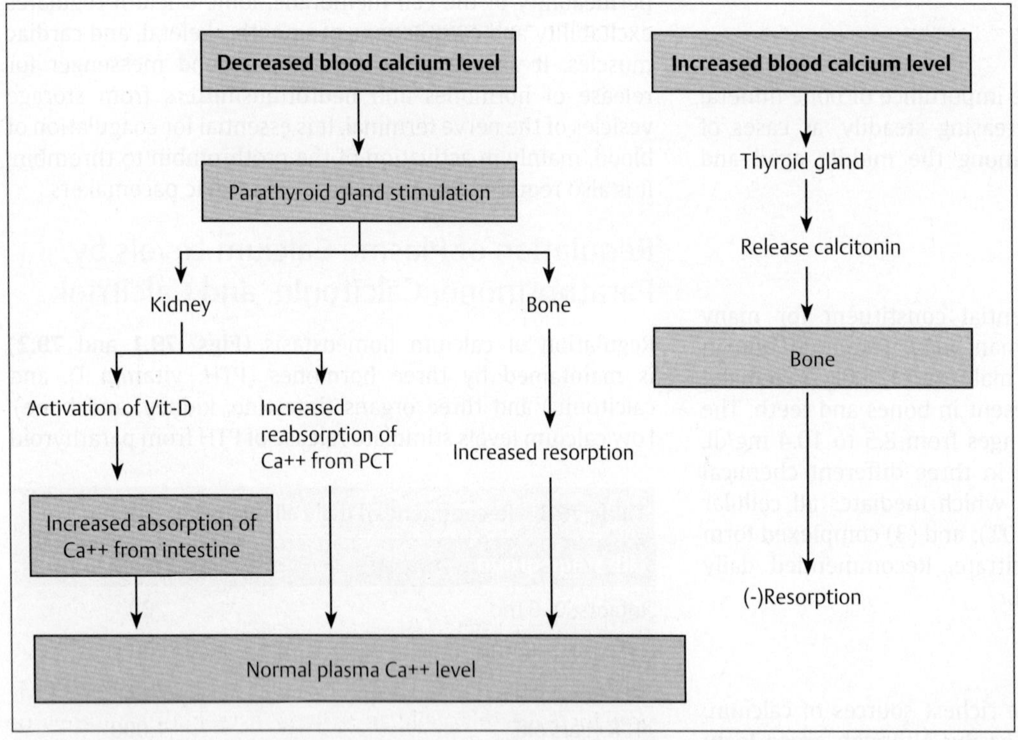

Fig. 79.2 Regulation of plasma calcium levels by parathormone, calcitonin, and calcitriol.

gland. PTH has stimulatory action on the kidney and bone. PTH stimulates the kidney to increase the reabsorption of calcium from PCT and distal convoluted tubule (DCT) of the kidney and increase excretion of phosphate. It also stimulates 25(OH) hydroxylase and activates calcitriol (vitamin D); thus, it enhances the calcium absorption from the intestine. In addition, PTH increases resorption from the bone and mobilizes calcium into the circulation. When the calcium levels are high, calcitonin is released from the thyroid. Calcitonin inhibits resorption and shunts the excess calcium to the bone and aids in bone formation. Thus, it maintains normal plasma calcium levels. The different calcium preparations are mentioned in **Fig. 79.3**.

1. Calcium gluconate (10% Ca): This is the most commonly preferred intravenous (IV) preparation, as it does not cause irritation to the gastrointestinal (GI) mucosa and vascular endothelium. It is administered only through the IV route and not the intramuscular (IM) route, as abscess formation occurs. For oral intake, it is available as 0.5- and 1-g tablets.
2. Calcium carbonate (40% Ca): It is the most commonly used oral preparation. It is well-absorbed in acidic pH and is less expensive.

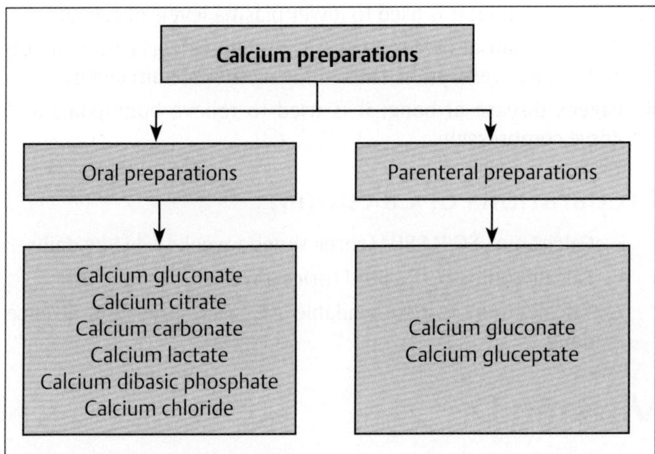

Fig. 79.3 Calcium preparations.

3. Calcium citrate tetrahydrate (21% Ca): It is used in a manner similar to calcium carbonate.
4. Calcium gluceptate (10%): It can be administered via IV and also deep IM routes.
5. Calcium dibasic phosphate (23% Ca): It is used in a manner similar to calcium carbonate.
6. Calcium lactate (13% Ca): It is used orally.
7. Calcium chloride dihydrate (27% Ca): It is no longer used via any route due to its irritant nature.

Uses

1. Tetany: In severe hypocalcemia, calcium gluconate 10% solution is given as infusion.
2. Osteoporosis: Calcium supplement is given in combination with vitamin D in osteoporosis.
3. Antacid: Calcium carbonate is used as antacid.
4. Dietary supplement to prevent hypocalcemia or calcium deficiency in children, pregnant women, and lactating women as well as in hormone replacement therapy.
5. IV calcium is used to treat black widow spider envenomation and also to manage magnesium toxicity.
6. Combination of calcium carbonate and calcium acetate is used in patients with chronic kidney disease (CKD) to avoid absorption of phosphate.
7. Calcium is used in inflammatory bowel disease to inhibit the absorption of oxalates.

Treatment of Hypocalcemia

In severe hypocalcemic tetany, 10% calcium gluconate injected slowly (not more than 1 mL/min) is the treatment of choice: 10 to 15 mg of Ca^{2+} /kg body weight over 4 to 6 hours. Mild hypocalcemia can be treated by oral calcium supplements.

Treatment of Hypercalcemia (IM22.3)

Hypercalcemia is a life-threatening condition. Patients suffering from hypercalcemia are severely dehydrated, and hence immediate fluid resuscitation with large volumes of isotonic saline should be carried out early (6–8 L/d). Loop diuretics are used to increase the Ca^{2+} excretion only after volume repletion. IV bisphosphonates are used for normalizing serum calcium levels, as they inhibit osteoclastic bone resorption. Calcitonin IM acts rapidly by inhibiting osteoclastic resorption and increasing excretion of calcium via urine.

Parathyroid Hormone

PTH is a single polypeptide chain with 84 amino acids, secreted by C cells of parathyroid gland. The primary function of PTH is to maintain constant calcium and phosphate concentration. To maintain calcium levels, the target organs are the bone, kidney, and intestine. PTH is stimulated by low levels of plasma calcium by calcium-sensing membrane receptors in the chief cells of the parathyroid gland.

Physiological Actions

Bone

PTH has both catabolic and anabolic effects on the bone. Prolonged high PTH levels increase the osteoclastic resorption from the bone and mobilize calcium into the extracellular fluid. On the other hand, intermittent exposure of PTH promotes anabolic actions, that is, it helps in bone formation and growth.

Kidney

PTH acts rapidly on the kidney in comparison to the bone. It promotes calcium reabsorption from PCT and DCT and inhibits absorption of phosphate; rather, increased excretion of phosphate, sodium, potassium, and biocarbonate is seen. It also stimulates calcifediol to convert to active form calcitriol by stimulating 1α hydroxylase enzyme.

Intestine

PTH increases the synthesis of 1, 25-$(OH)_2$ vitamin D in the kidneys, which enhances the absorption of calcium from the intestine when Ca^{++} levels are depleted.

Mechanism of Action

PTH acts mainly through PTH receptors, which are G protein–coupled receptors (GPCRs). PTH_1 receptor binds to PTHr protein, while PTH_2 receptors, which are present in the vascular tissues, placental, brain, and pancreas, binds only to PTH. As these are GPCRs, they act by stimulating cAMP and increase intracellular Ca^{2+} on osteoblasts but not on osteoclasts. Once they act on osteoblasts receptors, RANKL are activated, which helps in the formation of bone.

Preparations and Therapeutic Uses

Teriparatide

Teriparatide acts in a manner similar to PTH. Peak concentrations are seen within 30 minutes after the injection, and serum Ca^{2+} peaks at 4 to 6 hours after administration. It is used in the treatment of patients with severe osteoporosis who are at high risk of fractures. In postmenopausal women, it increases the bone mineral density (BMD) and reduces the risk of vertebral and nonvertebral fractures. It is administered once daily (20 μg) via subcutaneous (SC) injection into the thigh or abdomen.

Abaloparatide

Abaloparatide acts in a manner similar to teriparatide. It is available as injector pen with 30 daily doses administered subcutaneously into the periumbilical region of the abdomen, with a starting dose of 80 μg.

Recombinant Human PTH

This agent causes dose proportional increase in serum Ca^{2+} levels, and its peak levels will be attained 10 to 12 hours after injecting subcutaneously. It is approved for the treatment of hypocalcemia in hypoparathyroidism when serum concentration of calcium cannot be controlled by supplementation of calcium and active vitamin D.

Calcimimetic Compounds

Calcimimetics enhance the sensation of parathyroid gland on calcium-sensitizing receptors (CaSR). High levels of calcium will be sensed by CaSR, and this stimulates parathyroid gland to inhibit secretion of PTH. These are of two types: type I and type II.

Type I Calcimimetics

These are agonists and include organic and inorganic compounds along with aminoglycosides and polybasic amino acids.

Type II Calcimimetics

These are allosteric activators that activate the receptor indirectly, for example, cinacalcet.

Uses

Calcimimetics are used in the treatment of secondary hyperparathyroidism in adults with CKD on dialysis, hypercalcemia in adults with parathyroid carcinoma, and hypercalcemia in primary hyperparathyroidism. They should be used with caution when dealing with hypocalcemia.

Calcitonin

Calcitonin is secreted from the parafollicular C cells of thyroid. It is a calcium-lowering hormone. It is synthesized and released when serum Ca^{2+} levels are elevated.

Mechanism of Action

It opposes the action of PTH, that is, it inhibits the osteolysis and osteoclastic bone resorption induced by PTH and helps during periods of calcium stress such as growth, pregnancy, and lactation. Thus, it is useful in the treatment of hypercalcemia, osteoporosis. and Paget's disease.

Uses

1. Diagnosis of medullary carcinoma of thyroid: there will be abnormal increase in calcitonin levels as seen in thyroid C cell hyperplasia and medullary thyroid cancer.
2. Hypercalcemia: it is used to lower plasma levels of calcium.
3. Postmenopausal osteoporosis: it inhibits osteoclastic function and reduces resorption, thus reducing the calcium levels.
4. Paget's disease of bone: it is used to relieve bone pains and nerve compression.

Preparations of Calcitonin

- Calcitonin–SC/IM 80 U three times a week to 4 U/kg daily.
- Salcalcitonin–SC/IM 50 U thrice a week.
- Salcalcitonin is also available as nasal spray 200 U once daily.

Vitamin D

Vitamin D is actually a prohormone rather than a vitamin. Vitamin D is a family of compounds. It gets activated in the body as calcitriol. Important members of this family are vitamin D_2 and vitamin D_3. Vitamin D_2 (ergocalciferol) is obtained from ergosterol (a plant sterol); on exposure to the sunlight, ergosterol becomes ergocalciferol (vitamin D_2). Vitamin D_3 (cholecalciferol) and its precursor, 7-dehydrocholesterol, are present on the human skin; on exposure to the sun, the latter is converted to its active form, vitamin D_3. Both vitamin D_2 and vitamin D_3 are nothing but vitamin D, and these are the medicinal forms of vitamin D. The daily requirement of vitamin D is mentioned in **Table 79.2**.

Physiological Actions

1. Vitamin D facilitates absorption of calcium and phosphate from the intestine through calcium-binding protein or calbindin.
2. It enhances tubular reabsorption of calcium and phosphate from PCT.
3. It facilitates bone mineralization by maintaining adequate plasma concentration of calcium and phosphate.
4. Vitamin D regulates cell division and apoptosis.
5. It inhibits epidermal proliferation and facilitates differentiation; thus, it is useful in psoriasis.
6. It activates stem cells, creates new hair follicles, and allows hair to grow.
7. It allows maturation and differentiation of T-cells and aids in boosting immunity.
8. It improves insulin sensitivity.

Table 79.2 Variations in the daily requirement of vitamin D with exposure to light

Age	RDA/day
Birth: 12 mo	400 IU (10 μg)
Children: 1–13 y	600 IU (15 μg)
Teens: 14–18 y	600 IU (15 μg)
Adults: 19–70 y	600 IU (15 μg)
>71 y	800 IU (20 μg)
Pregnancy and lactation	600 IU (15 μg)

Abbreviation: RDA, recommended daily allowance.
Source: NIH office of dietary supplements.

Metabolic Activation of Vitamin D

On adequate exposure to the sun, vitamin D_3 is monohydroxylated in the liver with 25-hydroxylase enzyme to form monohydroxycholecalciferol or 25-hydroxycholecalciferol. Subsequently, in the kidney, with the help of PTH, 1 OH radical with 1 α hydroxylase enzyme converts to 1, 25, dihydroxycholecalciferol or calcitriol, which is the active form (**Fig. 79.4**).

Mechanism of Action

Calcitriol binds to cytoplasmic vitamin D receptors (VDRs). It is located in various tissues and over 230 VDRs in the nucleus of most tissues. As a nuclear receptor, it regulates gene expression for protein synthesis.

Uses

1. Prophylaxis: It is used in those who are at risk of developing rickets (children who are not properly exposed to the sunshine).
2. Nutritional rickets: The classical rickets of childhood. A combination of vitamin D and calcium is supplemented. The daily dose of 400 IU of vitamin D is given for prophylaxis and a daily dose of 4,000 IU for treatment.
3. Osteomalacia: To remineralize the bone, a combination of vitamin D_3, 50,000 to 100,000 IU/day orally for 1 to 2 weeks, and calcium, 1,000 to 1,500 mg/day, is given and sun exposure is ensured.

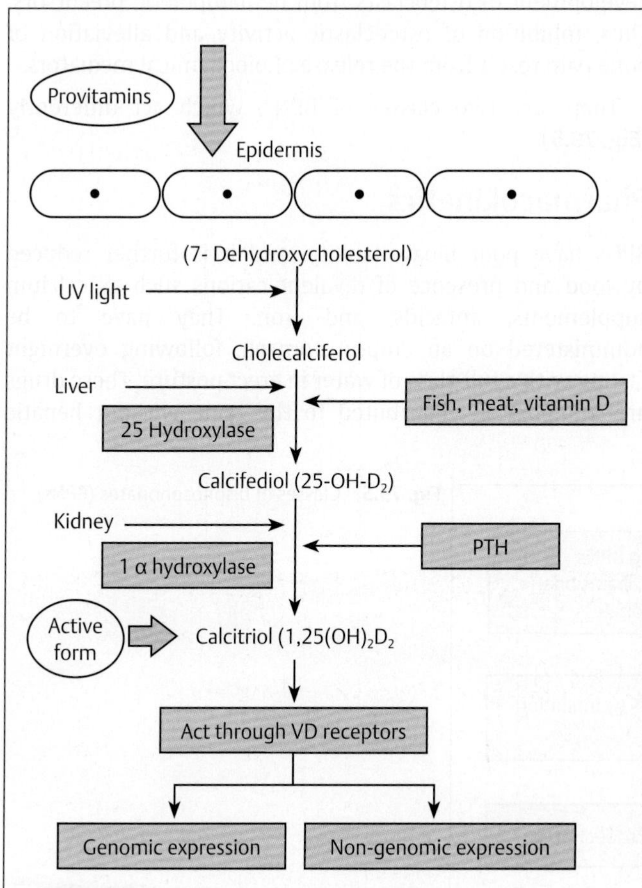

Fig. 79.4 Metabolic activation of vitamin D.

4. Vitamin D–dependent rickets:
   a. Type 1: Autosomal recessive disorder with deficient 25(OH) D_3 and calcitriol in the kidney. Alfacalcidol is provided in required doses.
   b. Type 2: Hereditary resistance to 1,25$(OH)D_3$ and defective calcitriol receptor; hence, it requires huge doses of vitamin D with parenteral calcium administration.
   c. Renal rickets: The conversion of 1,25$(OH)D_3$ to calcitriol is hindered by renal disease; thus, alfacalcidol is administered, as it does not require activation in the kidney.
5. Hypoparathyroidism: Dihydrotachysterol or alfacalcidol are helpful; also, conventional preparations of vitamin D_3 are helpful in high doses.
6. Senile osteoporosis: Small dose of vitamin D is helpful but larger doses may be counterproductive.
7. Psoriasis: Calcipotriol is used as local application.
8. Fanconi's syndrome: Vitamin D is given to increase serum phosphate levels.

Vitamin D Analogs

Cholecalciferol

It is an inactive form, which has to be activated in the liver and kidney.

Dose: granules (60,000 IU in 1 g), IM injection in oily base 5,000 to 50,000 IU daily, or single large dose of 1 to 5 lac IM.

Calcitriol

This is an active form of vitamin D, which does not require activation in the liver or kidney; thus, it is safely utilized in liver and renal disorders. It has a rapid onset of action with shorter half-life of 6 hours. It is an expensive preparation, available as 1 µg in 1 mL aqueous solution given intravenously on alternate days. The recommended dose is 0.25 to 1 µg orally/day/alternate day. It produces hypercalcemia.

Alfacalcidol

It is a synthetic derivative of vitamin D_3. It is a prodrug and has rapid onset of action and a half-life of 2 to 3 weeks. It does not require hydroxylation in the kidney but requires hydroxylation in the liver only; thus, it can be prescribed safely in patients with renal diseases and also in those with renal rickets, hypoparathyroidism, or osteoporosis.

Dose: 1 to 2 µg orally/day. Hypercalcemia may be seen in some cases.

Dihydrotachysterol

It is a synthetic analog of vitamin D_2 with rapid action and shorter duration of action. It directly mobilizes calcium from the bone. It is preferred in patients with renal diseases and hypoparathyroidism, as it does not require PTH-dependent activation of the kidney with 1α hydroxylase.

Dose: 0.25 to 0.5 mg/day.

Paricalcitol

It is an analog of vitamin D_2. It is used in secondary hyperparathyroidism associated with CKD.

Calcipotriol

It is an analog of calcitriol; however, it does not produce hypercalcemia and is effective in psoriasis. It is also used in alopecia areata.

Dose: 0.005% ointment for local application.

22-Oxa-calcitriol

It is an analog of calcitriol. It has lower affinity for vitamin D–binding protein. It has a shorter half-life with potent suppressive action on PTH genes.

Hypervitaminosis D

Excess (> 150 ng/mL) intake of vitamin D results in hypervitaminosis D. Patients with hypervitaminosis D present with hypercalcemic features such as hypercalcemia, overcalcification of bones, soft-tissue, heart, and kidney, hypertension, dehydration, and muscle weakness. Treatment involves withdrawing the vitamin, low calcium diet, administration of glucocorticoids, and fluid support.

Bisphosphonates

Bisphosphonates (BPNs) are also called diphosphonates. They mainly prevent loss of bone mass and regulate bone resorption.

Classification

BPNs are classified into three generations:

- **First generation**
  - Etidronate
  - Clodronate
  - Tiludronate
- **Second generation**
  - Alendronate
  - Ibandronate
- **Third generation**
  - Risedronate
  - Zolendronate
  - Pamidronate

First-Generation Bisphosphonates

First-generation BPNs have simple side chains with chlorophenyl group, which are metabolized into a nonhydrolyzable adenosine triphosphate (ATP) analog. It accumulates within osteoclast and induces apoptosis. These are least potent.

Second-Generation Bisphosphonates

These drugs contain nitrogen group in the side chain and these primarily inhibit resorption of bone. They act by inhibiting mevalonate pathway of cholesterol synthesis and isoprenoid lipids. They are 10 to 100 times more potent than the first-generation BPNs.

Third-Generation Bisphosphonates

Third-generation BPNs contain a nitrogen atom within a heterocyclic ring, and they are 10,000 times more potent than the first-generation BPNs.

Mechanism of Action

BPNs have high affinity toward sites of active remodeling, remain in hydroxyapatite crystals (matrix) until the bone is remodeled and released in acidic environment along with osteoclast, and induce apoptosis. They inhibit the development of osteoclasts, induce osteoblastic activity, and reduce osteoclastic activity. They also prevent the development of osteoclasts from hematopoietic precursors. Thus, inhibition of osteoclastic activity and alleviation of bone pain result from the release of biochemical mediators.

There are two classes of BPNs, which act differently (**Fig. 79.5**).

Pharmacokinetics

BPNs have poor bioavailability, and it is further reduced by food and presence of divalent cations such as calcium supplements, antacids, and iron. They have to be administered on an empty stomach, following overnight fasting with a full glass of water in erect posture. These drugs are immediately distributed to the bone without hepatic

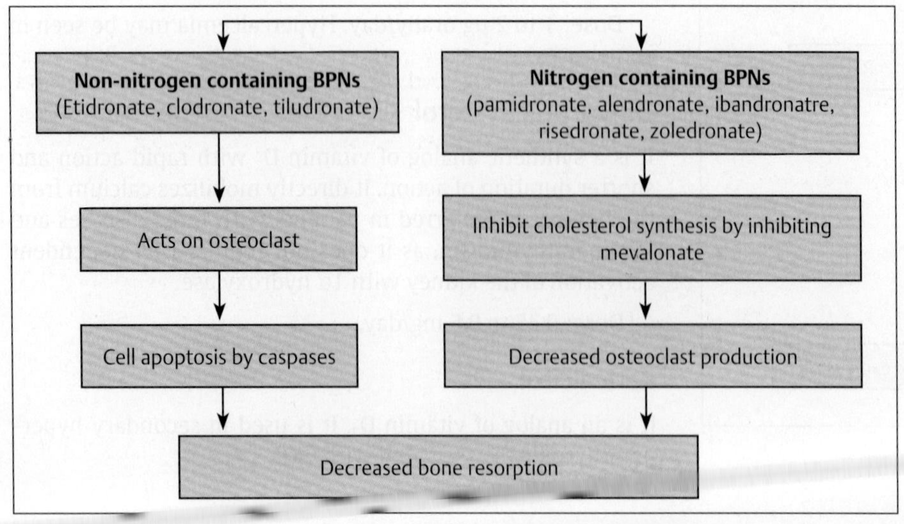

Fig. 79.5 Classes of bisphosphonates (BPNs).

clearance and are excreted unchanged through the kidney. Thus, BPNs are not recommended in patients with renal diseases unless serum creatinine clearance levels are above 30 mL/min.

Adverse Effects

Oral BPNs cause heart burn, esophagitis, or irritation of the esophagus. Other GI side effects include abdomen pain and diarrhea, which are more severe with pamidronate. These side effects can be abated to some extent by taking the drug after overnight fasting with filtered water (not mineral water) and remaining in upright posture for at least 30 minutes before breakfast. These symptoms of side effects can be overcome by IV infusion of pamidronate, but flulike syndrome may be seen, that is, skin flushing, muscle ache, bone aches, and GI disturbances. Zoledronate causes severe hypocalcemia, renal toxicity, and deterioration of kidney function. Before and during the therapy, periodic assessment of kidney function will reduce the risk.

Therapeutic Indications

Osteoporosis

BPNs are prescribed primarily in fracture in high-risk cases, in established cases of osteoporosis, and also in chronic glucocorticoid therapy. Alendronate is the drug of choice, given orally once in a week or daily in addition to calcium supplements and vitamin D_3. Risedronate or etidronate is also given. Zoledronate is given annually as infusion but is an expensive treatment.

Paget's Disease

In focal osteolytic lesion, initially the patient will be asymptomatic and will only present with bone pain, deformities, or fractures. Etidronate and pamidronate are given intermittently, and serum phosphate, alkaline phosphatase and urinary hydroxyproline, which are markers for collagen turnover, should be monitored.

Hypercalcemia of Malignancy

BPNs are given to minimize the bone damage, bone pain, and hypercalcemia.

Contraindications

Absolute: achalasia cardia, esophageal strictures, hypocalcemia, and hypersensitivity.

Relative: gastroesophageal reflux disease, peptic ulcer, GI disorders.

Caution: in renal insufficiency (in cases of renal clearance < 30 mL/min)

Other Drugs Used in the Treatment of Osteoporosis (PH1.36)

Raloxifene

This is a selective estrogen receptor modulator used in postmenopausal osteoporosis, as there is a decline in estrogen levels. Raloxifene acts on bone, stimulates osteoblast, helps in bone formation, and also has inhibitory actions on osteoclast, thus reducing vertebral and nonvertebral fractures. It has agonistic action on the cardiovascular system and antiestrogenic action on the mammary gland and uterus; thus, there are rare chances of breast and uterine cancers and a beneficial action on the heart.

Strontium Ranelate

It inhibits bone resorption, stimulates bone formation, and prevents the vertebral and nonvertebral fractures. It is an alternative to BNPS in postmenopausal osteoporosis.

Denosumab

It is a human monoclonal antibody, which binds to the RANK ligand with high affinity. It blocks osteoclast formation and activation, increases BMD, and decreases bone turnover markers when given subcutaneously, 60 mg once every 6 months.

Multiple Choice Questions

1. A 75-year-old woman with femoral neck fracture presents with a 2-day history of altered sensorium and decreased urinary output. Serum calcium level is 15.5 mg/dL, urea level is 140 mg/dL, and creatinine level is 2 mg/dL. How will you manage the case?

A. Normal saline, furosemide, dialysis.

B. Bisphosphonates, cinacalcet.

C. Calcitonin.

D. Calcium gluconate.

Answer: A

This is a case of hypercalcemia (15.5 mg/dL), and it has to be treated with plenty of fluids to reduce calcium levels.

2. A 34-year-old male patient came to the skin OPD with chief complaints of itchy plaques over trunk, elbows, and knees for the last 5 years. These lesions exacerbate in winter and decrease in summer. On examination, white plaques ++ < 10% body surface area (BSA) and Auspitz's sign positive were found. Which of the following is the underlying treatment?

A. Moisturizers.

B. Clobetasol propionate ointment + salicylic acid.

C. Vitamin D analogs.
D. All the above.

Answer: D

This is a case of skin psoriasis. Vitamin D is necessary in addition to moisturizers and steroids.

3. A 20-year-old woman presented with concerns about intermittent numbness and tingling of the perioral area and her extremities. She reported having had one episode where she lost control of her right leg and fell. On investigation, serum calcium level and serum phosphate level were found to be 6.5 and 6 mg/dL, respectively. What is the correct treatment option?

A. Calcium gluconate IV.
B. Oral calcium supplements.
C. Vitamin D analog.
D. Calcitonin.

Answer: A

The patient has severe hypocalcemia (< 6.5 mg/dL), which has to be corrected immediately.

4. The parents of a 5-year-old boy complain that their boy shows signs of weakness and inability to concentrate and lack of interest in playing. Investigations show normal calcium levels and reduced vitamin D, phosphorus, and hemoglobin levels, with normal total leukocyte count (TLC). X-ray of the wrist and knee shows epiphyseal spraying, metaphyseal cupping, and wide epiphysis. Choose the treatment line for this patient.

A. Vitamin D_3
B. Calcium supplements
C. Phosphorus
D. All of the above

Answer: A

Here the is child presenting with rickets i.e epiphyseal spraying, cupping of metaphyses and wide epiphysis thus the child should be given with vitamin D3 supplements.

5. A 70-year-old man, who had a trivial fall, complains of back pain. X-ray shows wedge fracture of T11 and T12. What will you prescribe?

A. Calcium only.
B. Vitamin D + calcitonin.
C. Teriparatide.
D. Teriparatide + calcitonin+ bisphosphonates.

Answer: D

Here, the patient is suffering from osteoporosis, and with the trivial fall, he has suffered a fracture. He needs bisphosphonates to increase the activity of osteoclasts, and teriparatide and calcitonin to reduce serum calcium levels, inhibit osteoclastic activity, and increase bone mineral density.

6. A 45-year-old diabetic man has a habit of smoking and alcohol consumption for the past 10 years. Also, he is on regular dialysis. He complains of general weakness, and examination shows pallor. Investigation shows reduce hemoglobin (Hb) and vitamin D levels. How will you manage the case?

A. α-calcidol
B. Vitamin D + Hb.
C. α-calcidol + Hb.
D. Vitamin D

Answer: A

Vitamin D has to be prescribed, but as the patient is already on dialysis, vitamin D cannot be converted to vitamin D_3 in the kidney. Therefore, α-calcidol, which does not require conversion in the kidney, is prescribed.

Chapter 80 Drugs Acting on the Uterus: Oxytocics and Tocolytics

Vaishali Undale

PH1.41: Describe the mechanisms of action, types, doses, side effects, indications, and contraindications of uterine relaxants and stimulants.

Learning Objectives

- Oxytocin.
- Ergometrine/methylergometrine.
- Prostaglandins.
- Ritodrine.
- Calcium channel blockers.

Drugs Acting on the Uterus

Drugs acting on the uterus mainly affect the myometrium and/or endometrium.

The uterine wall is composed of three layers of tissues:

1. Outermost serous layer (the perimetrium).
2. Middle muscular layer (the myometrium).
3. Innermost glandular epithelial layer (the endometrium).

The myometrium is innervated by the autonomic, sympathetic, and parasympathetic nerves. Therefore, drugs acting directly or indirectly on the autonomic nervous system can affect myometrial motility.

Estrogens, progestins, and their antagonists are the drugs affecting endometrium.

Drugs acting on the uterus are classified as follows:

1. Uterine stimulants: They are also used as oxytocics/abortifacients.
2. Uterine relaxants/tocolytics.

Oxytocics/Uterine Stimulants/Abortifacients

Oxytocics are defined as drugs that increase uterine motility, especially at the term, that is, at the end period of pregnancy. These drugs are also used to induce abortion to terminate the pregnancy when needed; hence, they are also known as abortifacients.

Classification

There are four classes of oxytocics:

1. *Posterior pituitary hormones*: oxytocin, desamino-oxytocin.
2. *Ergot alkaloids*: ergometrine, methylergometrine.
3. *Prostaglandins*: PGE2, PGF2, 15-methyl PGF2 α, misoprostol.
4. *Miscellaneous*: ethacridine, quinine.

Oxytocin

Oxytocin, a peptide comprising nine amino acids and having a molecular mass of 1,007 Da, is secreted by the posterior pituitary gland. The sequence of amino acids in the oxytocin molecule involves cysteine, tyrosine, isoleucine, glutamine, asparagine, cysteine, proline, leucine, and glycine. Cysteine residue is involved in the formation of the sulfur bridge.

In 1953, du Vigneaud separated oxytocin and antidiuretic hormone (ADH) from pituitary extract and determined their chemical structures and synthesized them (**Fig. 80.1**).

Oxytocin is synthesized in hypothalamic nerve cell bodies and then carried down the axon and stored in the nerve endings in the posterior pituitary, that is, neurohypophysis. It is released by appropriate stimuli such as coitus, parturition, and suckling.

Mechanism of Action

The oxytocin receptors are G protein–coupled receptors. Oxytocin binds to oxytocin receptors and activates an enzyme phospholipase C. The activated phospholipase C converts phosphatidylinositol 4,5-bisphosphate (PIP_2) to inositol triphosphate (IP_3) and diacylglycerol (DAG). IP_3 increases intracellular calcium by opening calcium channels, following which there is an influx of calcium and release from sarcoplasmic reticulum. The calcium binds to protein calmodulin. This complex activates myosin light chain (MLC) kinase activation, inducing contraction in the muscle. DAG formed also activates protein kinase C, which further activates myosin-activated protein kinase (MAPK). MAPK

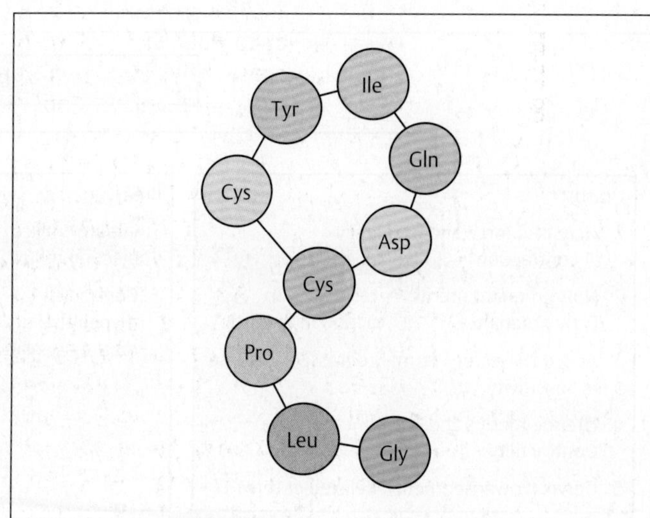

Fig. 80.1 Structure of oxytocin.

activates phospholipase A2 and MLC, contracting the muscle (**Fig. 80.2**).

Pharmacological Actions

The pharmacological actions of oxytocin are described in **Fig. 80.3**.

Pharmacokinetic

It is inactive orally (being a peptide hormone, it is degraded in the gastrointestinal (GI) tract). Thus, it is administered by intramuscular (IM) or intravenous (IV) routes.

Metabolism takes place rapidly in the liver and kidney. Plasma $t_{1/2}$ is approximately 6 minutes, which further decreases at term.

Adverse Effects

Inappropriate use of oxytocin may produce maternal as well as fetal soft-tissue injury, breakdown of the uterus, fetal asphyxia, and death.

Water Intoxication

Oxytocin in high dose with IV fluids produces water intoxication due to ADH like action (antidiuretic hormone) of oxytocin. It is serious and may be fatal.

Indications

Induction of Labor

In cases of postmature or premature toxemia of pregnancies in diabetic mother, erythroblastosis, punctured membrane,

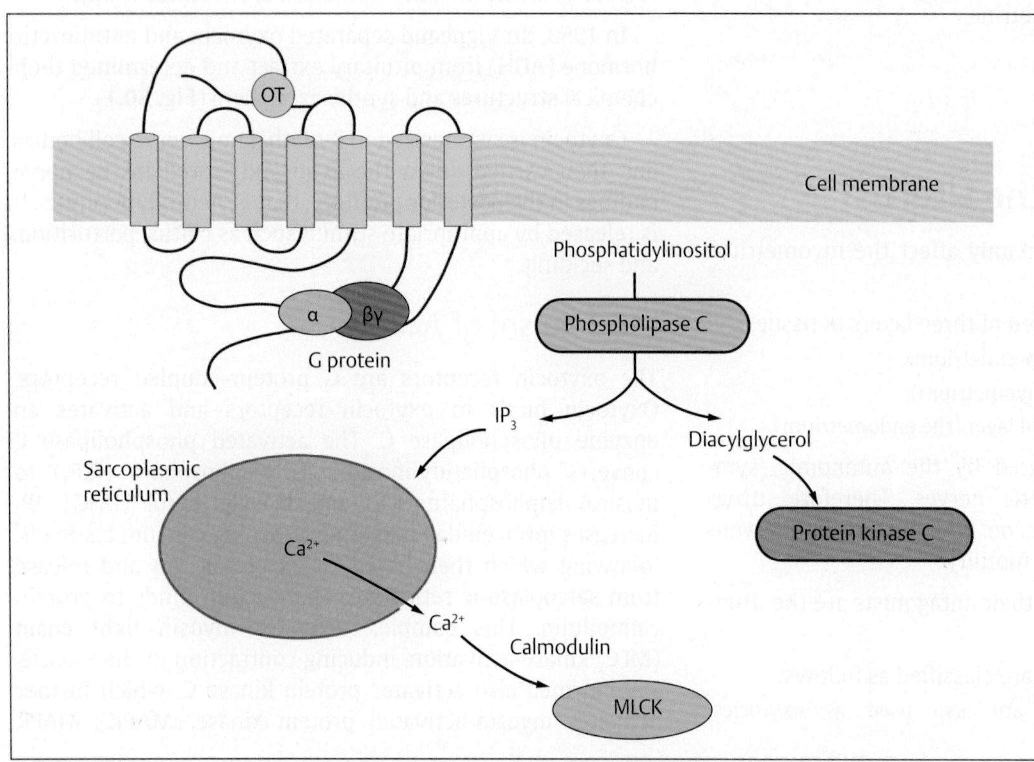

Fig. 80.2 Mechanism of action of oxytocin.

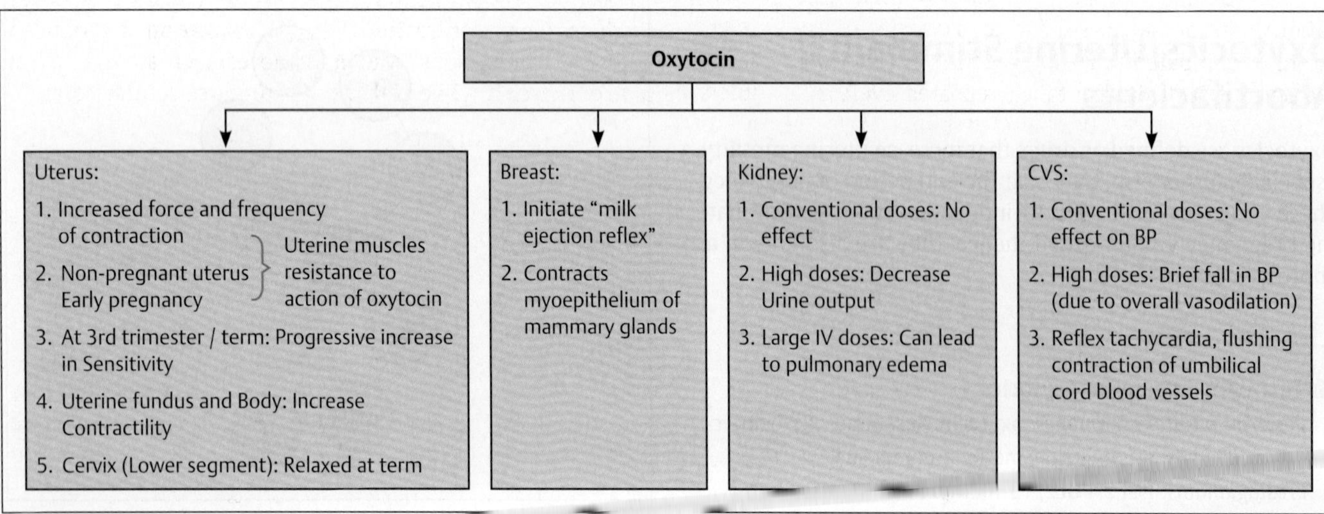

Fig. 80.3 Pharmacological actions of oxytocin.

or placental inadequacy, labor needs to be induced. Oxytocin is given as IV infusion for induction of labor. An infusion of 5 IU of oxytocin mixed with 500-mL glucose or saline solution is started at slow rate and progressively increased. Contractions produced in the uterus are monitored, and the infusion is stopped when sufficiently powerful contractions are induced.

Uterine Inertia

When uterine contractions are feeble and labor is not developing reasonably, it may be used to increase contractions. It should be used only in selected cases and by an experienced person.

Postpartum Hemorrhage

Oxytocin forcefully contracts uterine muscles, constricting uterine blood vessels and thus decreasing hemorrhage during placental separation. Immediately after birth of infant, 5 IU of oxytocin may be injected by IM or IV infusion to decrease hemorrhage. It is a suitable alternative in hypertensive pregnancy cases with ergometrine contraindication.

Breast Engorgement

When milk ejection reflex is inefficient, oxytocin is administered as an intranasal spray.

Oxytocin Challenge Test

This test is risky and rarely done in high-risk pregnancy to diagnose uterine-placental adequacy. Profound increase in fetal heart rate suggests uteroplacental inadequacy. Very low concentration of oxytocin is intravenously infused till uterine contractions are seen every 3 to 4 minutes. Unit/µg: 1 IU = 2 µg of pure hormone

Marketed preparation

Oxytocin, Syntocinon, Pitocin.

Other oxytocin derivatives are discussed as follows.

Desamino-oxytocin

This formulation has been developed in a buccal form. Although its action is similar to oxytocin, it is less consistent as compared to it. It is used in the induction of labor in a dose of 50 IU buccal tablet repeated every 30 minutes, with a maximum of 10 tablets. It is also indicated in the management of uterine inertia in a dose of 25 IU every 30 minutes. This formulation is also beneficial in the promotion of uterine involution and breast engorgement (25–50 IU just before breast-feeding).

Carbetocin

This is a recently introduced formulation, which is a long-acting analog of oxytocin. It is used in the prevention of uterine atony after cesarean section and to control postpartum hemorrhage (PPH).

Contraindications

1. High blood pressure (BP).
2. Placenta previa.
3. A pregnancy with more than one fetus.
4. Previous C-section.
5. Grand multiparity.
6. Malposition or malpresentation of fetus.
7. Fetal distress.

Ergometrine/Methylergometrine

Ergometrine and its derivative methylergometrine are alkaloids obtained from a fungus *Claviceps purpurea.* This fungus cultivates on rye, millet, and some grains.

Ergot had been used since the Middle Ages by midwives to quicken labor. In the 19th century, the use of ergot was sanctioned medically, but due to its advantages identified in the 20th century, its use was suggested after the childbirth. In 1906, Dale and Barger isolated ergot alkaloid and studied pharmacological actions of these derivatives.

Ergometrine, which is also known as ergonovine, was discovered in 1932, while methylergometrine is a synthetic derivative of ergometrine.

Ergometrine and methylergometrine are used in obstetrics.

Mechanism of Action

Ergometrine and methylergometrine are partial agonist/antagonist of serotonergic (5-HT_2) receptors. The stimulation of 5-HT receptors stimulates IP_3–DAG pathway (same as described earlier for oxytocin) and increases intracellular calcium, thereby inducing contraction in the uterine smooth muscles.

Pharmacological Actions

Uterus

The force and frequency of uterine contraction are increased by ergot derivatives.

Dose-dependent action is seen on the uterus. Low doses produce phasic contractions, that is, relaxation is produced between contractions. Moderate doses increase the basal tone of muscles, while higher doses produce contractions.

Cardiovascular System

Weak vasoconstrictions can be produced by ergometrine and methylergometrine, and chances of endothelial damage due to vasoconstriction are less. They can also increase BP at higher dose, but it is nonsignificant at the dose used in obstetrics.

Central Nervous System

At usual doses, no significant effects are seen, but at high doses, complex effects can be seen due to agonistic and antagonistic action on adrenergic, serotonergic, and dopaminergic receptors.

Gastrointestinal Tract

Peristalsis is induced by high doses of ergometrine/methylergometrine.

Pharmacokinetics

Ergometrine and methylergometrine are entirely and quickly absorbed through the oral route. Action is seen quickly. Oral action is seen in about 15 minutes; action is produced in about 5 minutes if given intramuscularly and immediately if given intravenously.

Partial metabolism takes place in the liver and metabolites are excreted in the urine. Plasma $t_{1/2}$ is approximately between 1 and 2 hours. The duration of action is between 3 and 4 hours.

Adverse Effects

The correct use of ergot derivatives does not produce any complication in obstetrics. However, occasionally, nausea, vomiting, and rise in BP can occur. If used in high doses after postpartum for many days, it leads to decrease in milk secretion due to inhibition of prolactin release (action on dopaminergic receptor).

Indications and Doses

1. To control and prevent PPH in doses of 0.2 to 0.3 mg IM.
2. To prevent uterine atony after cesarean section or instrumental delivery.
3. To ensure normal involution.
4. Diagnosis of variant angina.

Marketed preparations

Ergometrine, Methergine, Metherone, Ergomet.

Drug Interactions

With General Anesthetics

Especially with halothane, peripheral vasoconstriction may be enhanced by simultaneous administration with ergometrine/methylergometrine. Halothane concentration of more than 1% interferes with oxytocic action of ergonovine production, causing severe uterine hemorrhage.

With Bromocriptine

Occasionally, hypertension, stroke, seizures, and myocardial infarction may be produced in certain conditions due to combined use with ergot alkaloid.

With Nicotine (Smoking, Tobacco)

Increased nicotine absorption due to profound smoking may increase vasoconstriction.

With Nitroglycerin/Antianginal Drugs

Ergot alkaloids might produce coronary vasospasm, decreasing the effectiveness of nitroglycerin or other antianginal agents.

With Vasopressin/Adrenaline

The vasopressor effect might be enhanced, leading to severe hypertension, headache, and disruption of cerebral blood vessels.

With Dopamine

Simultaneous infusion of dopamine and ergonovine may lead to the formation of gangrene.

Contraindication

Contraindications for ergometrine include patients with vascular diseases, hypertension, toxemia, sepsis, and liver and kidney diseases. It should not be used during gestation period and before the third phase of labor.

Prostaglandins (PGE2, PGF2, 15-Methyl PGF2)

Prostaglandin (PG) derivatives PGE2, PGF2α, and 15-methyl PGF2α are effective as uterine stimulants, particularly in the last phase of gestation, and produce ripening of the cervix. Misoprostol, a PG analog, is also used in obstetrics.

PG misoprostol binds to PG E1 receptor, which is a G protein–coupled receptor. This stimulates adenylyl cyclase enzyme to convert adenosine triphosphate (ATP) to cyclic adenosine monophosphate (cAMP). cAMP increases intracellular calcium by increasing influx of calcium and release from sarcoplasmic reticulum, thus inducing contraction in the myometrial muscles.

Pharmacological Actions

PGE2 and PGF2α uniformly contract both pregnant and nonpregnant uterus. The responsiveness to contractions increases with progression of pregnancy. Both the basal tone and amplitude of contractions are increased by PGs. They cause softening of cervix at low doses and make it compliant when administered intravaginally. In cases of unfavorable uterus, it has achieved good results.

Pharmacokinetic Features

After vaginal insertion, the drug disperses gradually into maternal circulation. Small portion of dose is also absorbed locally in lymphatic and circulatory vessels. Contractions are observed within 10 minutes after dosing, with maximal activity in 17 hours; however, activity is not related with plasma concentrations. The PG derivatives are distributed extensively in maternal blood circulation. They are metabolized in the lungs, liver, kidneys, spleen, and maternal tissues, and metabolites as well as unmetabolized fraction are excreted mainly in the urine, with small amounts in the feces.

Adverse Effects

In mother, diverse adverse effects are seen, for example, central nervous system effects such as headache, dizziness, anxiety, hot flashes, paresthesia, weakness, syncope, and fever, cardiovascular effects such as chest pain, arrhythmias, blurred vision, and eye pain, and GI adverse effects such as nausea, vomiting, diarrhea, vaginal pain, vaginitis, and endometritis in women. Musculoskeletal adverse effects such as nocturnal leg cramps, backache, and muscle cramps may also be produced. Respiratory adverse effects, such cough and dyspnea, and dermatological effects, such as diaphoresis and rashes, are also seen. Shivering, chills, and breast tenderness are some other adverse effects produced by PGs.

In fetus, PGs produce neurological adverse effects such as fetal depression and hyperstimulation with or without fetal distress. Bradycardia, fetal acidosis, and other adverse effects such as amnionitis and intrauterine fetal sepsis are also seen with PGs.

Indications and Doses

Abortion or Termination of Pregnancy

Although the transcervical suction is the procedure of choice for termination of pregnancy in the first trimester, intravaginal administration of PGE2 pessary 3 hours before the procedure can reduce trauma to the cervix. Mifepristone administration in dose of 600 mg orally 2 days before a single oral dose of 400 µg of misoprostol has been found to be effective in aborting pregnancy of up to 7 weeks. It is now a valuable substitute for suction evacuation procedure. Intravaginal administration of misoprostol produces less side effects and is the preferred route of administration. Before administration, the location of conceptus should be confirmed to rule out ectopic pregnancy, and even absolute removal of conceptus should be checked after procedure.

For Midterm Abortion, Missed Abortion, and Molar Gestation

PGs are used as they convert the midterm uterus nonresponsive to oxytocin to responsive. An extra-amniotic injection of PGE2 followed by IV infusion of oxytocin or intra-amniotic (PGF2α) with hypertonic solution produces second trimester abortion without side effects.

Induction/Augmentation of Labor

As compared to oxytocin, PGs are not advantageous for induction of labor at term. However, in rare cases of toxemia and patients with renal failure, they may be used as they do not cause fluid retention.

Cervical Priming (Ripening)

PGE2 in low doses is applied intravaginally or in the cervical canal to induce softening in cervical tissue, thereby increasing compliance with abortion procedure.

Postpartum Hemorrhage

In patients with insensitivity to ergometrine and oxytocin, especially due to uterine atony, carboprost (15-methyl PGF2α) by IM route of administration is an optional drug for controlling PPH.

Dosage of PGE2 (Dinoprostone) Prostin-E2 9

For initiation/augmentation of labor and midterm abortion:

1. Vaginal gel (1 or 2 mg in 2.5 mL) inserted into the posterior fornix, and repeated administration of 1 to 2 mg after 6 hours, if needed.
2. Vaginal tab (3 mg) placed into the posterior fornix, and readministration of 3 mg if labor is not induced within 6 hours.

Interaction of Prostaglandins

Oxytocin

Oxytocin augments efficacy of PGs. The simultaneous use of PG gel for cervical softening and oxytocin infusion is not recommended due to risk of cervical ulceration and trauma. Treatment with oxytocin should be initiated after a time interval of 6 to 12 hours of gel application or 30 minutes after removal of PG insert.

Contraindication

Gel formulation is not recommended in patients with hypersensitivity to PGs or excipients of gel. Likewise, even vaginal bleeding during pregnancy or vaginal pregnancy is a contraindication. Other contraindications include vasa previa or active herpes genitalia.

Suppository form should not be used in patients with hypersensitivity, acute pelvic inflammatory disease, or active cardiac, pulmonary, renal, or hepatic disease.

Vaginal inserts should not be used in patients with hypersensitivity, those with vaginal bleeding due to unknown cause during pregnancy, women with a history of six or more previous term pregnancies, or when oxytocics are not recommended or the patient is administered an IV oxytocic drug.

A comparison of ergometrine and oxytocin is given in **Table 80.1**.

Uterine Relaxants (Tocolytics)

Drugs that decrease uterine motility are called tocolytics or uterine relaxants.

Table 80.1 Comparison between oxytocin and ergometrine

Properties	Oxytocin	Ergometrine
Nature of contractions	Contractions resemble normal physiological contractions	Contractions are tetanic, do not resemble physiological contractions
Onset of action	2–3 min	6–7 min
Duration of action	Shorter (10–20 min)	Longer (3–4 h)
Adverse effects	Minimal	More (from nausea and vomiting to rise in BP)
Contraindications	Hypersensitivity to oxytocin	Hypertension
Efficacy	Highly effective	Moderately effective
Frequency of administration	Continuous	Every 2–4 h, up to five doses in 24 h
Choice	Drug of choice	Use is discouraged now
Uses	To induce and augment labor Postpartum hemorrhage	Only in postpartum hemorrhage

Abbreviation: BP, blood pressure.

Classification

The following categories of drugs are used as uterine relaxants:

1. Adrenergic agonist: ritodrine.
2. Calcium channel blockers (CCBs): nifedipine.
3. Magnesium sulfate.
4. Miscellaneous: ethyl alcohol, nitrates, progesterone, general anesthetics.

Ritodrine

Ritodrine is a β_2-selective agonist.

Mechanism of Action

A β receptor is a G protein–coupled receptor. Its binding stimulates membrane-bound enzyme adenylyl cyclase. This induces conversion of ATP to cAMP at the inner face. The cAMP phosphorylates cAMP-dependent protein kinases, thereby inducing a series of reactions in the cell. Depending on the tissue, variable responses are produced. In uterine smooth muscles, it causes relaxation of smooth muscles, accompanied by hyperpolarization produced in them.

Pharmacological Actions

Uterus

Ritodrine produces prominent uterine relaxation. It is the drug of choice to repress premature labor and postpone delivery when required. It is not recommended in diabetic mothers and in women with heart ailment or on β blockers or steroid therapy.

Pharmacokinetic Features

It is quickly absorbed from the GI tract (oral). Its oral bioavailability is about 30%. It crosses the placental barrier About 5% is metabolized in the liver by conjugation with glucuronic acid or sulfate, while about 70 to 90% of a dose is excreted in the urine within 10 to 12 hours.

Adverse Effects

The adverse effects produced by ritodrine are cardiovascular effects such as hypotension, tachycardia, arrhythmia, and pulmonary edema. Metabolic complications such as hyperglycemia, hypokalemia, and hyperinsulinemia are also seen. Anxiety, restlessness, and headache can occur frequently. It is found to increase maternal morbidity if used to arrest labor. Fetal pulmonary edema can develop. Neonates may develop hypoglycemia and ileus.

Indications and Doses

To Delay or Postpone Labor

Labor needs to be suppressed to allow fetus to mature or to shift the mother in labor to proper facilities. However, a suitable drug does not exist. The labor should not be adjourned if membranes have disrupted, in severe antepartum hemorrhage, toxemia of pregnancy, intrauterine infections, or fetal death. It is also used to arrest threatened abortion. It is also used in the treatment of dysmenorrhea

Dosage

The therapy is initiated with a dose of 50 μg/min IV as infusion; every 10 minutes, the rate of administration is augmented till uterine contractions terminate or the heart rate of mother increases to 120/min. Continuous IV infusion or 10 mg by IM every 4 to 6 hours, followed by 10 mg oral every 4 to 6 hours, is administered to maintain repressed contractions. Administration after 48 hours is not recommended as it might endanger the mother's life.

Calcium Channel Blockers

Calcium plays an important role in contractions of myometrium.

Table 80.2 Contraindications and side effects of uterine relaxants

Class/drug Uterine relaxants	Side effects		Contraindications
	Maternal	Neonatal	
β agonists: ritodrine, terbutaline	Cardiac arrhythmias, pulmonary edema, myocardial ischemia, hypotension, hyperglycemia, hypokalemia, tremors, etc.	Tachycardia, fetal, neonatal hyperglycemia, hypocalcemia, hypotension, myocardial ischemia	Cardiac arrhythmia, diabetes mellitus, poorly controlled hypothyroid disorders
CCBs: nifedipine	Headache, flushing, nausea, transient hypotension, tachycardia	Sudden fetal death and distress	Cardiac disease, caution in renal impairment, maternal hypotension, and with use of $MgSO_4$
Prostaglandin inhibitors: indomethacin, ketorolac, sulindac	Heartburn, nausea, gastritis, renal dysfunction, increased PPH, and dizziness	Narrowing of ductus arteriosus, pulmonary hypertension, intraventricular hemorrhage, necrotizing enterocolitis	Renal and hepatic impairment, active peptic ulcer disease, coagulation disorder
NO donors	Headache, hypertension	Neonatal hypotension	Headache

Abbreviations: CCB, calcium channel blocker; PPH, postpartum hemorrhage; NO, nitric oxide.

Mechanism of Action

CCBs reduce the calcium influx in muscle by blocking the calcium channels and thus reduce tone of myometrium as well as contractions. Nifedipine prominently relaxes smooth muscles and can delay labor if used in the early phase of contractions. Nifedipine 10 mg every 20 to 30 minutes is used till uterine contractions subside.

Adverse Effects

The adverse effects of CCBs are tachycardia, hypotension, and fetal hypoxia.

Miscellaneous

Magnesium sulfate and other miscellaneous drugs, ethyl alcohol, nitrates, and PG inhibitors such as indomethacin, ketorolac, and sulindac progesterone also suppress uterine contractions. But their use is restricted due to safety issues.

Limitations of Tocolytics Therapy

The limitations of tocolytic therapy are as follows:

1. Shorter or moderate duration of action is a limitation of use of tocolytics. Labors or uterine contractions cannot be controlled for longer duration.
2. Long-term use is not advocated.
3. The tocolytics available are associated with certain contraindications and maternal and fetal adverse effects, limiting their use.

Table 80.2 describes the contraindications and side effects.

Multiple Choice Questions

1. A 30-year-old woman in her 41st week of pregnancy had been in labor for 12 hours. Although her uterine contractions had been strong and regular initially, they had diminished in force during the past 1 hour. Which of the following agents would be used to facilitate this woman's labor and delivery?

A. Dopamine.
B. Leuprolide.
C. Oxytocin.
D. Prolactin.
E. Vasopressin.

Answer: C

In this case, initially for 12 hours of labor, the uterine contractions were normal and strong, but later they became weak in the past 1 hour. Oxytocin is routinely utilized to enhance labor. When uterine contractions are weak and labor is not progressing satisfactorily, oxytocin can be used to increase contractions.

2. A 23-year-old woman, primigravida, comes in labor room for induction of labor. The cervix is closed and 3 cm long. Which of the following medicine will be given to her for cervical ripening?

A. Methergine.
B. Salbutamol.
C. Prostaglandin E2.
D. Paracetamol.
E. Methyldopa.

Answer: C

A "primigravida" is a person who is pregnant for the first time or has been pregnant one time. The case here is primigravida, and the cervix is closed. Therefore, before induction of labor, it is necessary to soften the cervix, so as to make expulsion of fetus easy after induction of contractions of uterine muscles. Prostaglandin derivatives cause softening of the cervix at low doses and make it compliant when administered intravaginally. Here, prostaglandin E2 is an appropriate option.

3. A 25-year-old woman P2 comes to emergency after home delivery with heavy bleeding per vaginum. After evaluation and emergency resuscitation, she is diagnosed with uterine

atony. What is the appropriate medicine in the management in this case?

A. Oxytocin.
B. Salbutamol.
C. β blockers.
D. Magnesium sulfate.
E. Hydralazine.

Answer: A

In this case, oxytocin is the most appropriate medicine to treat the woman. Oxytocin forcefully contracts uterine muscles and constricting the blood vessels passing through it, thus decreasing hemorrhage during placental separation.

4. Oxytocin produces following actions except:

A. Vasoconstriction.
B. Increased water reabsorption in renal collecting ducts.
C. Contraction of mammary myoepithelium.
D. Release of prostaglandins from endometrium.

Answer: A

Oxytocin causes overall vasodilation; only uterine blood vessels are constricted. All other actions are produced by oxytocin.

5. Oxytocin is necessary for:

A. Initiation of labor.
B. Formation of milk.
C. Milk ejection reflex.
D. Both "A" and "C" are correct.

Answer: C

Oxytocin facilitates milk ejection from the mammary gland during lactation. The release of oxytocin from the posterior pituitary is stimulated by tactile sensory inputs from the nipple.

6. Oxytocin is chosen over ergometrine for augmenting labor as:

A. It has brief and titratable action.
B. It is less likely to cause fetal anoxia.
C. It is less likely to impede fetal descent.
D. All of the above.

Answer: D

Oxytocin is relatively safer as compared to ergometrine as it does not produce adverse effects on fetus such as fetal anoxia.

7. Which of the following drugs is preferred for controlling postpartum hemorrhage (PPH)?

A. Oxytocin.
B. Methylergometrine.
C. Dihydroergotamine.
D. Prostaglandin E2.

Answer: B

Methylergometrine is a weak vasoconstrictor and produces less damage to endothelial tissue. It is the drug of choice of PPH.

8. Ergometrine is used in the following conditions except:

A. Postpartum hemorrhage (PPH).
B. Insufficient uterine involution.
C. Uterine inertia during labor.
D. Uterine atony after cesarean section.

Answer: C

Oxytocin is preferred for uterine inertia rather than ergometrine.

9. .... is the drug that has been used to suppress labor:

A. Atropine.
B. Ritodrine.
C. Prostaglandin E2.
D. Progesterone Aa.

Answer: B

Ritodrine is a β_2 agonist that causes relaxation of uterine muscles and is used to suppress labor.

10. A young woman begins to bleed extensively after delivering a healthy infant due to failure of uterine contraction. Which of the following drugs should be administered to this woman?

A. Prednisone.
B. Desmopressin.
C. Leuprolide.
D. Oxytocin
E. Prolactin.

Answer: D

Oxytocin contracts uterine smooth muscle. It is used to enhance labor and, here in this situation, it is used to treat postpartum uterine atony.

Part XII

Miscellaneous

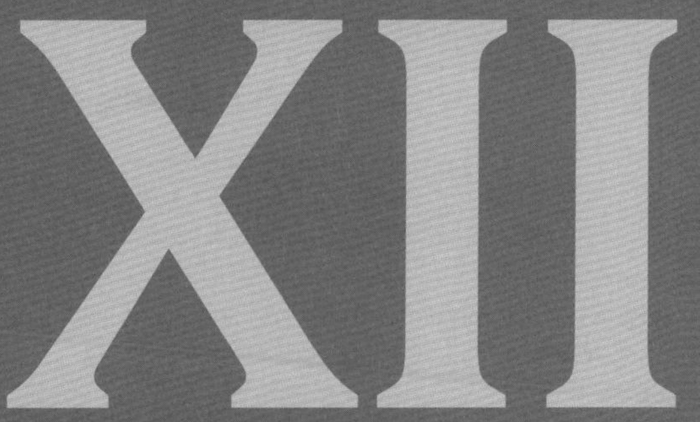

Chelating Agents and Heavy Metal Poisoning

Rupali A. Patil, Shubhangi H. Pawar, Sunil V. Amrutkar, and Rajendra S. Bhambar

PH1.53: Describe heavy metal poisoning and chelating agents.

Learning Objectives

- Heavy metals commonly associated with poisoning.
- Chelating agents.

Heavy Metals Commonly Associated with Poisoning (FM9.3)

Lead (PE14.1)

Circumstances

Although lead is known for occupational and environmental hazards, it is widely used in many commercial products, including storage batteries, metal alloys, shells, fuse, glass, plastics, etc.

Increase in lead concentration of tap water may be due to corrosion of plumbing in old buildings.

Exclusion of lead as an additive in gasoline in the last three decades has decreased environmental lead exposure in air, water, and food. In humans, lead has no useful purpose. Lead is a highly poisonous metal. It affects almost every organ in the body. Even low blood lead concentrations may adversely affect blood pressure and neurocognitive function. Hence, low-level lead exposure also has substantial concern.

This effect of low lead concentration on blood pressure and neurocognitive functions formerly was not recognized as harmful. The toxicity in children is of greater concern as their tissues are softer than in adults. Low levels of lead may be responsible for behavioral problems, learning deficits, and lowered IQ.

Along with these health issues and decreased incidences of serious lead poisoning, low levels of lead exposure are a major concern.

The reason for the collapse of the Roman empire was considered to be lead poisoning, as lead acetate was used as a sweetener of wine, causing dementia to many Roman emperors. Prolonged exposure of lead inhibits porphobilinogen synthesis and incorporation of iron into protoporphyrin IX, preventing heme synthesis or causing ineffective heme synthesis and subsequently microcytic anemia (**Fig. 81.1**).

Mode of Action

Lead is a metal existing as divalent or tetravalent cation. Divalent lead exists as primary environmental form. Tetravalent lead compounds do not exist naturally. Organolead complexes include the gasoline additive tetraethyl lead. Divalent metals are also responsible for lead toxicity. Lead is responsible for alteration of protein structure and inappropriate activation or inhibition of protein function due to size and electron affinity.

Inorganic Lead Oxide and Salts

1. Major route of absorption: gastrointestinal tract (GIT) and respiratory tract.

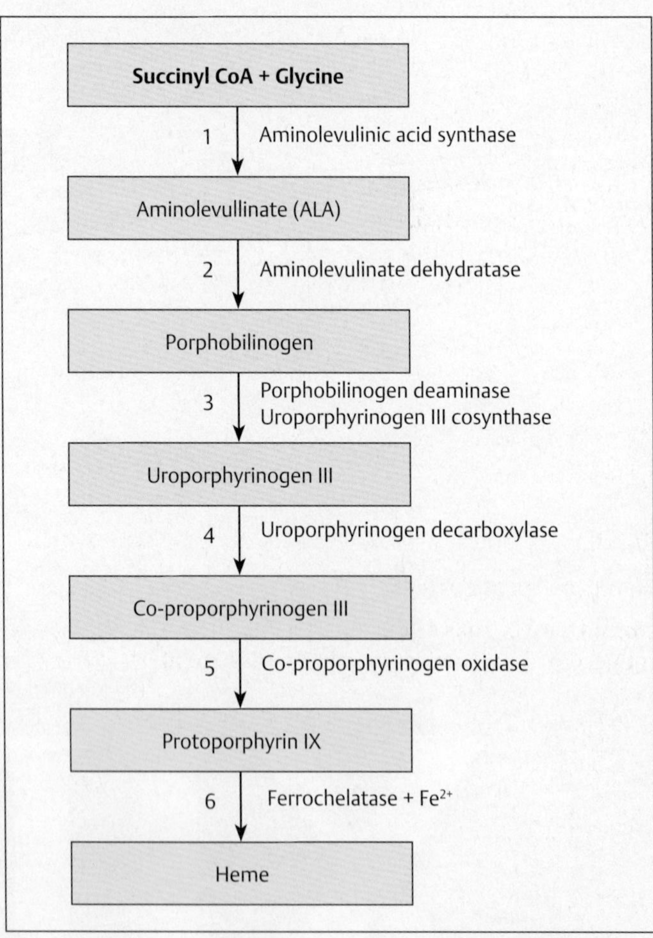

Fig. 81.1 Heme biosynthesis and actions of lead. Lead inhibits steps 1, 2, 5, and 6.

2. Distribution: soft tissues; redistributed to skeleton (> 90% of adult body burden).
3. Major effects: anemia, hypertension, nephropathy, reproductive toxicity, neuropathy.
4. Mechanism: alters structure of membrane and also works through enzyme inhibition.

Organic (Tetraethyl Lead)

1. Major route of absorption: GIT, respiratory tract, skin.
2. Distribution: soft tissues, especially the liver and the central nervous system (CNS).
3. Major effects: encephalopathy.
4. Mechanism: fast dealkylation in the liver to form trialkyl metabolites and then its dissociation to lead.

Major Systems of the Body Affected

Nervous System

Toxic effects of lead are predominantly observed in children as they have developing nervous system. Lead interferes with thinning of synapses, neuronal migration, and the interactions between neurons and glial cells, altogether resulting in decreased IQ, poor performance, and behavioral problems such as distractibility, impulsivity, short attention span, and inability to follow simple sequences of instructions. Low-level lead exposure even below the CDC (Centers for Disease Control and Prevention) action level of 10 mg/dL may result in cognitive delays and behavior changes in children.

Cardiovascular and Renal System

Lead may generate reactive oxygen species (ROS), which further interact with nitric oxide (NO), resulting in elevated blood pressure, by reducing NO-induced vasodilation, and causing cardiovascular toxicity through formation of peroxynitrite. Lead is also involved in the formation of inclusion bodies in the kidney with various proteins such as metallothionein, increasing lead concentration in the kidney. Lead reduces glomerular filtration rate, although it is involved in targeting kidney mitochondria and interfering with the electron transport chain. Lead exposure also increases risk of death due to cerebrovascular and cardiovascular disease.

"Saturnine gout" (recurrent bouts of gouty arthritis) may occur due to alteration in uric acid excretion by the kidney.

Hematological System

Normocytic or microcytic and hypochromic anemia may be induced by low-level lead exposure due to interference with heme synthesis. Lead inhibits enzyme ferrochelatase and thus blocks iron incorporation into protoporphyrin IX; zinc gets incorporated in place of iron, forming highly fluorescent zinc protoporphyrin. Lead also increases membrane fragility of red blood cells (RBCs) and decreases its survival span.

Lead imparts changes in helper T-cell and macrophages, causing inflammation and immunosuppression.

Gastrointestinal System

A persistent metallic taste, malaise, headache, muscle discomfort, loss of appetite constipation, and, sometimes, diarrhea are observed after moderate lead poisoning. At high doses, severe colic pain ("lead colic") occurs, which may be due to spasmodic contraction of intestinal smooth muscles.

Reproductive Organs

Low-level lead exposure in prenatal stage decreases physical and cognitive development in neonates and children. High-dose lead exposure is responsible for stillbirth or spontaneous abortion. High-lead levels (> 40 μg/dL) in males are associated with diminished or abnormal sperm production.

Major Forms of Lead Intoxication

Inorganic Lead Poisoning

Acute

Very uncommon forms of lead poisoning include, largely, inhalation of industrial lead oxide fumes, large ingestion of paint chips (which are lead-based) in small children, lead-contaminated food or drink, or chewing toys fabricated from or coated in lead.

The diagnosis of acute inorganic lead poisoning depends on the presenting symptoms. Subacute symptoms include fatigue, headache, abdominal cramps, arthralgias, and myalgias associated with recent ingestion of lead-containing paint chips, glazes, or weights as per radiographical examination of abdomen.

Chronic

Symptoms of chronic lead poisoning include anorexia, fatigue, malaise, weakness, arthralgias, myalgias, GI symptoms, and neurologic complaints such as headache, concentrating inability, behavioral irritation, and depressed mood. Children show neurocognitive deficits, growth retardation, or developmental delay.

Level of lead in whole blood is the confirmatory test for lead poisoning, but it is not a reliable marker for cumulative lead exposure. Noninvasive K X-ray fluorescence measurement may be correlated with long-term cumulative lead exposure. Concentration of lead in blood at level 30 μg/dL or more, with no simultaneous elevation in zinc protoporphyrin, suggests that there is lag time period after lead exposure and lead-induced elevations in circulating heme precursors.

Organolead Poisoning

Replacement of tetramethyl and tetraethyl lead as antiknock additives in gasoline minimizes the occurrence of organolead poisoning. Some commercial processes still use organolead compounds such as lead naphthenate or lead stearate. These compounds easily get absorbed through the respiratory tract or the skin due to volatility or lipid solubility. They act dose dependently mainly on the CNS to produce neurocognitive deficits, hallucinations, delirium, insomnia, tremors, convulsions, and death.

Mercury

Circumstances

Metallic mercury is also known as "quicksilver." It is the only metal that exists in liquid form under normal conditions.

According to the World Health Organization (WHO), exposure to mercury occurs from dental amalgam, ingestion of contaminated fish, or occupational exposure in humans.

Outgassing from rock or volcanic activity results in atmospheric exposure. Human activities such as coal burning and mining (specifically mercury and gold) are major sources of atmospheric mercury contamination. Elemental mercury in atmosphere settles in water, and microorganisms convert it into organic (methyl or ethyl) mercury. This organic mercury is consumed by smaller creatures, which are eventually consumed by larger fish. Larger fish (e.g., swordfish, shark, or tuna) on the top of the food chain may have considerable concentration of mercury in their tissues.

According to WHO and Berglund et al, mercury exposure in humans due to outgassing from amalgam fillings is at a rate of 2 to 28 µg per facet surface per day, of which about 80% gets absorbed. Spilled mercury is a less common source of mercury vapor. It may cause idiopathic thrombocytopenic purpura (thereby producing a major acute exposure to mercury vapor).

Mercury shows known toxicities and has induced public health disasters in Minamata Bay, Japan, and in Iraq. In the early 1950s, in a Japanese fishing village, Minamata, curious and widespread birth defects and neurological defects occurred due to ingestion of seafood, contaminated with methylmercury. This was discharged into sea by nearby industries.

Mercury is used in many electrical equipment, thermometers, fluorescent lamps, and dental amalgam. It is also used in electrolytic production of chlorine and caustic soda. Artisanal gold with mercury is receiving increasing attention in many developing countries. Recently, mercury is being used in pharmaceuticals and biocides but rarely used in antiseptics and folk medicines. Removal of thiomersal (an organomercurial preservative), which is metabolized into ethylmercury, from vaccines is a major development.

Mode of Action

Toxic effects produced by mercury ions are due to protein precipitation, enzyme inhibition, and generalized corrosive action. Mercury binds with sulfhydryl, phosphoryl, carboxyl, and amide and amine groups. Mercury inhibits enzymes and changes cell membranes after binding with sulfhydryl groups in vivo. Proteins (including enzymes) containing these groups are susceptible to reaction with mercury. After binding with mercury, many proteins become inactive. Toxicity by mercury is associated with the oxidative state and chemical form (organic vs. inorganic).

In organic form, GI absorption is 90%, while in inorganic form absorption is only 10%. High lipid solubility makes it easier for elemental mercury to cross across cell membrane. Elemental mercury gets oxidized to the mercuric state. Mercuric salts form more soluble divalent compounds with more toxicity than mercurous salts forming monovalent mercury compounds. After ingestion, they get rapidly absorbed to produce more toxicity. Short-chained alkyl compounds such as methylmercury are most completely absorbed from the GI, showing greater hazard than long-chained aryl compounds. Methylmercury-like compounds are distributed to the brain, kidney, and liver. They get excreted in the feces. Excretion of aryl mercury compounds is in the form of mercuric ions.

Major Systems of Body Affected by Mercury

Mercury is toxic to fetus in all forms. Methylmercury easily passes through the placenta. Spontaneous abortion or retardation is possible after exposure of pregnant women.

Major Forms of Mercury Intoxication

The chemical form of the metal and the severity of exposure largely determine the pattern of clinical intoxication from mercury. The oxidative states of mercury are elemental mercury (HgO), mercurous (Hg^{1+}), or mercuric (Hg^{2+}). Inhalation of vapor, injection, ingestion, and absorption through the skin are different routes for mercury poisoning.

Acute

Inhalation of elemental mercury vapors:

1. Initial signs and symptoms are chills, shortness of breath, fever, metallic taste, and pleuritic chest pain.
2. Stomatitis.
3. Lethargy.
4. Confusion.
5. Vomiting.
6. Pneumonitis.
7. Pulmonary edema (noncardiogenic).
8. Acute gingivostomatitis.
9. Neurologic sequelae.

Ingestion of inorganic mercury salts (mercuric chloride), which occurs mostly through oral route:

1. Corrosive, potentially life-threatening hemorrhagic gastroenteritis, followed within hours to days by acute tubular necrosis and oliguric renal failure.
2. Ashen-gray mucous membranes secondary to precipitation of mercuric salts.
3. Hematochezia (bloody stool).
4. Vomiting, severe abdominal pain, and hypovolemic shock.
5. Systemic effects: gingival irritation, foul breath, loosening of teeth, mucosal inflammation, metallic taste.

Chronic

Chronic inhalation of elemental mercury vapors causes:

1. Tremor: begins as a fine intention tremor of hand and face.
2. Tremors progress to choreiform movements of the limbs.
3. Neuropsychiatric disturbances: memory loss, fatigue, anorexia, insomnia.

Change in mood to shyness, withdrawal, and depression, as well as explosive anger or blushing (erethism).

1. Gingivostomatitis: may be with loosening of teeth after high-dose exposure.
2. Also includes: peripheral nerve damage, headache, salivation, ataxia, visual disturbances (tunnel vision), and acrodynia (pink disease) in children. Symptoms of pink disease include the following: painful erythema of the extremities and, rarely, hypertension, diaphoresis, anorexia, insomnia, irritability or apathy, and military rash.

Chronic ingestion of inorganic mercury salts, sometimes through topical application in cosmetic creams, diuretics, or cathartics containing mercury:

1. Neurological symptoms.
2. Renal toxicity.

Methylmercury Intoxication

After exposure, it may take several weeks or months to show signs and symptoms.

1. CNS effects: paresthesia, hearing impairment, ataxia, dysarthria, progressive constriction of visual fields.
2. Reproductive system:
   a. High dose: mental retardation and a cerebral palsy–like syndrome in the offspring.
   b. Low dose: subclinical neurodevelopmental deficits.

Arsenic

Circumstances

Arsenic is one of the most toxic metals derived from the natural environment. Human arsenic toxicity is mostly due to contamination of drinking water from natural geological sources rather than from smelting, mining, or agricultural sources (pesticides or fertilizers). Arsenic is naturally present in the earth's crust and has been used since a long time in cosmetics, pharmaceuticals (as a deliberate poison), and agricultural products. Lewisite, dichloro(2-chlorovinyl)arsine, was used as a chemical warfare agent. It was used as a popular murder weapon. In industry, it is used in manufacturing fungicides, pesticides, insecticides, herbicides, paints, wood preservatives, and cotton desiccants. Semiconductors, light-emitting diodes, transistors, and lasers contain gallium arsenide or crystals of aluminum gallium arsenide. Arsenic is an essential trace element for animals and thus is present as an additive in some animal feed.

"Paris green," a pigment in paints, contains arsenic as copper acetoarsenite.

Before the use of electricity for illumination, hydrogen liberated from coal fires and from gas for lighting combined with Paris green used in wallpaper to form a toxic gas, arsine. Conversion of arsenic in Paris green to arsine occurs due to a fungus, *Scopulariopsis brevicaulis*, present in damp wallpaper.

An arsenious hydride gas, arsine (AsH_3), has potent hemolytic effects. It is used in the semiconductor industry. It gets generated accidentally after arsenic-containing ores come in contact with acidic solutions. In the 20th century, organoarsenicals were extensively utilized as an antimicrobial; later, it was replaced by sulfonamides and other more efficacious and less toxic drugs. As per United States Pharmacopoeia, arsenic trioxide is used as an orphan drug for the treatment of relapsed acute promyelocytic leukemia.

Mode of Action

Arsenic exists in two oxidation states: arsenite (As III), a trivalent form (As_2O_3), is 60 times more toxic than arsenate (As V), a pentavalent form (As_2O_5). Inorganic arsenic is toxic and organic arsenic is nontoxic. Arsenic compounds show their toxic effects by several mechanisms. Arsenic toxicity inactivates around 200 enzymes involved in cellular energy pathways and DNA replication and repair.

Trivalent arsenic interferes with enzyme function by binding with sulfhydryl group or by substitution for phosphate. It gets substituted for phosphate in high-energy compounds such as adenosine triphosphate (ATP). Toxicity by unbound arsenic is due to generation of reactive oxygen intermediates during their redox cycling and metabolic activation processes, causing lipid peroxidation and DNA damage. Arsenite, especially, binds thiol or sulfhydryl groups in tissue proteins of the liver, lungs, kidney, spleen, GI mucosa, and keratin-rich tissues (skin, hair, and nails). Arsine, after oxidation in body, causes changes in ionic permeability across the RBC membrane and gives hemolytic effect.

Arsenite inhibits formation of acetyl-CoA and enzyme succinic dehydrogenase, while arsenate forms glucose 6-arsenate in vitro, which may be associated with muscle weakness in chronic arsenic poisoning. Submitochondrial particles synthesize adenosine-5′-diphosphate-arsenate from adenosine diphosphate (ADP) and arsenate in the presence of succinate.

Major Forms of Arsenic Intoxication

Acute Inorganic Arsenic Poisoning

High-dose exposure for minutes to hours:

1. **GIT**: nausea, vomiting, diarrhea, abdominal pain.
2. **Cardiovascular system**: hypotension, shock, death, pancytopenia, cardiogenic or noncardiogenic pulmonary edema, congestive cardiomyopathy, ventricular arrhythmias.
3. **CNS**: delirium, encephalopathy, coma, an ascending sensory-motor peripheral neuropathy after 2 to 6 weeks with proximal musculature and neuromuscular respiratory failure. Transverse white striae in nails after acute exposure for months.

Chronic Inorganic Arsenic Poisoning

1. Noncarcinogenic effects after chronic absorption of arsenic (> 0.01 mg/kg/g): symptoms are dose- and person-dependent—fatigue, weight loss, weakness in association with anemia, other GIT complaints, sensorimotor peripheral neuropathy.
2. After years of exposure, patients show skin changes—hyperpigmentation in "raindrop" pattern and hyperkeratosis of hands and feet.
3. Other symptoms included are peripheral vascular disease and noncirrhotic portal hypertension; long exposure to even low dose shows lung cancer, skin cancer, bladder cancer, and cancer at other sites.
4. It may also be associated with hypertension, diabetes, chronic nonmalignant respiratory disease, and adverse reproductive outcomes.
5. When arsenic is used in cancer chemotherapy at low dose, it has shown ECG changes in the form of prolongation of QT interval, which may lead to malignant ventricular arrhythmias.

Arsine Gas Poisoning

After 2 hours to 24 hours postinhalation, arsine shows massive intravascular hemolysis.

Other symptoms include fatigue, dyspnea, headache, malaise, nausea, emesis, abdominal cramps, jaundice, and hemoglobinuria. Deposition of hemoglobin in renal tubules results in oliguria and further renal failure. Heavy exposure shows lethal effects on cellular respiration before renal failure

Cadmium

Cadmium is present in food and also found in tobacco. Cadmium is resistant to corrosion. It shows useful electrochemical properties and is used in electroplating, galvanization, paint pigments, and nickel–cadmium batteries. Workers in ore mines and metal-processing industries may get exposed to high levels of cadmium due to inhalation. Cadmium is available as a divalent cation. It does not undergo oxidation–reduction reactions.

Mode of Action

The exact mode of action is not well understood. However, it may replace zinc in zinc-finger domain of proteins and disrupt them. It is responsible for lipid peroxidation and glutathione depletion through formation of ROS. It also disrupts beneficial effects of nitric oxide by upregulation of inflammatory cytokines.

Major Forms of Cadmium Toxicity

Acute

After Inhalation

Respiratory tract irritation with severe, early pneumonitis, along with chest pain, dizziness, nausea, and diarrhea progressing to fatal pulmonary edema.

After Ingestion

Salivation, abdominal cramps, nausea, vomiting, and diarrhea (mostly bloody).

Chronic

Symptoms depend on the route of exposure.

Inhalation

1. Lung: long-term exposure due to inhibition of synthesis of antitrypsin: decreased lung function, bronchitis, fibrosis leading to emphysema, increased mortality due to chronic obstructive pulmonary disease (COPD).

It also increases risk of lung cancer.

Inhalation and Ingestion

1. Kidney: increased excretion of small-molecular-weight protein: macroglobulin and retinol-binding protein, decrease in filtration due to glomerular injury.
2. Renal failure and death after chronic occupational exposure.
3. Bones: increased risk of fractures and osteoporosis as a result of vitamin D deficiency.

Cadmium increases mutations and impairs DNA repair in human cells.

There is substitution of zinc in DNA repair proteins and polymerases. It also inhibits nucleotide excision repair, base excision repair, and DNA polymerase required for repairing of single-stranded breaks. Cadmium also alters cell signalling pathways, disrupts cellular controls of proliferation, and acts as a nongenotoxic carcinogen.

Copper

Copper is a transition metal and is essential for various physiological processes. Copper in healthy humans is mainly associated with enzyme prosthetic groups or is bound to proteins. Copper is found in different cells and tissues, majorly in the liver and brain. In biological systems, copper exists as cupric form (Cu^{2+}).

Copper is available as elemental form in nature and in a wide range of compounds. It exists in both oxidized, cupric (Cu^{2+}), and reduced, cuprous (Cu^{+}), forms. In aqueous environment, the cuprous ion can rapidly disproportionate to form Cu (II) and Cu (0). Generally, cupric, the oxidized state of copper, is encountered in water and is coordinated with six water molecules in solution.

Circumstances

Copper is extensively utilized in many machineries, constructions, transportation, and military weapons, because it is less corrosive and more flexible. It also possesses high electrical and thermal conductivity and alloying ability. It is important in imitation jewelry, as it is a component of white gold and other alloys used for this purpose. It is also used in dental products and various cosmetic products. Copper is small sized with high nuclear charge and high ionization potential; therefore, it has low reactivity.

Natural sources of copper are environmental dust, forest fires, and volcanoes. Manmade resources are copper smelters, iron and steel production plants, and municipal incinerators.

Environmental sources are copper pipes, drinking water, copper cookware, birth control devices, intrauterine devices, vitamin and mineral supplements, fungicides, and copper in swimming pools and foods.

Most of the copper remains in bound form with organic matter. Plumbers, welders, and machinists have risk of copper toxicity due to their occupational exposure. Other sources include exposure to metals such as iron, arsenic, or mercury and use of chemicals such as ethanol and polychlorinated biphenyls. Also, use of pesticides can give copper exposure.

It becomes difficult to determine the upper intake level of Cu due to health consequences from both Cu deficiency and Cu excess.

Copper status can be influenced by dietary intake, environmental exposure, vitamins and mineral supplements, and adrenal activity. Hormones of adrenal gland stimulate production of copper-binding protein, ceruloplasmin, in the liver.

Copper accumulates in the tissues due to malfunction of the liver and adrenal gland insufficiency.

In the absence of ceruloplasmin, copper becomes bio unavailable. Dietary zinc is an antagonist of copper, and zinc deficiency leads to accumulation of copper in various organs.

Major Forms of Copper Toxicity

Deficiency of or excessive exposure to copper is not easily recognized due to lack of sensitive and specific indicators. Ceruloplasmin is a biomarker of copper status, as in the liver its synthesis is regulated by the availability of copper. Chaperone of Cu, Zn-SOD may also be used as potential markers of copper status. Copper deficiency impairs catalytic functioning of Cu, Zn-SOD in tissues.

Effects of mild copper deficiency or excess copper are not well explained. Some effects include decreased activities of several cuproenzymes. Certain clinical diseases such as liver cirrhosis can lead to excess copper effects.

High-dose effects include increase in alanine aminotransferase (ALT), aspartate aminotransferase (AST), triglyceride, total bilirubin, total bile acid levels, and scattered, dotted hepatocytic necrosis in male Wistar rats.

Copper is an essential component for the formation and maintenance of myelin. It is also required for the formation of melanin pigment in skin, hair, and eyes. It is also a component of cytochrome-c oxidase involved in the catalysis of reduction of oxygen to water. It is also a part of Cu, Zi-SOD which scavenges superoxide free radicals. Cytochrome P450 monooxygenase enzyme activity is modified by nonspecific catalytic binding of Cu^{2+} to thiol. Dopamine β-hydroxylase, an essential enzyme for the synthesis of catecholamines, also contains copper.

Thus, alterations in copper may play an important role in the development of disorders of the liver and nervous system. Copper homeostasis is maintained by metal regulation at transcriptional, translational, and enzymatic levels; thus, it prevents cellular damage. Disruptions of copper homeostasis results in tissue damage and, further, a number of diseases.

Properties of Ideal Chelating Agent

Although the concept of chelation is based on simple coordination chemistry and the choice of the ideal chelator is crucial to specific and complete removal of toxic metal from the tissue without any adverse effects. This is a process that is considered as base for drug design process.

Following are the properties of ideal chelator:

1. Water-soluble.
2. Capability to form nontoxic complexes with a variety of heavy metals, which are easily excreted from the body.
3. Ability to cross cell membrane (physiological barrier) to reach site of toxic metal deposition.
4. Easy to formulate it in the oral, intravenous (IV), or intramuscular (IM) formulations to be used, as per the type of metal intoxication.
5. Show more affinity toward toxic metal than the essential metals of the host.
6. Have appropriate pharmacokinetics.
7. Ability to form a stable complex with the metal.

As a medicament, chelating agent (CA) should have limited adverse effects and avoid disturbances in metal homeostasis.

Mechanism of Action of Chelating Agent

Chemistry

CAs (endogenous enzymes) generally contain two or more reactive groups (ligands), having capacity to hold the metal from at least two sides, so that a ring is formed, preferably 5 to 7 membered, having maximum stability. Ligand, a functional group, has a capacity to form coordinate bond and/or a covalent bond. Both the shared electrons are donated by the ligand itself. Ligands generally contain oxygen, nitrogen, or sulfur atoms in –SH, –S–S, –NH2, =NH, –OH or >C=O groups. Toxic effects of heavy metals occur after combining with and inactivating ligands of enzymes or other critical biomolecules. CAs show difference in their affinity for different metals. They compete with body ligands for the heavy metal.

The concept of chelation involves coordination chemistry. An ideal chelator and chelation therapy are both parts of an integrated drug design approach. CAs may be inorganic or organic in nature, and they bind with metal ions to form chelate, that is, a complex ringlike structure. If a metal ion and the two-ligand atoms are attached to the metal to form a ringlike structure, it is known as a bidentate or multidentate ligand (**Fig. 81.2**).

In the physiological environment, such complexes are formed by metal cations, namely, Na^+, Mg^+, Cu^+, Cu^{2+}, and Zn^{2+}. Stability of these complexes depends on the characteristics of both the metal and the CA.

CAs bind with ligands through metal covalent or coordinate covalent bonds, to decide CA as mono, bi-, tri-, or polydentate.

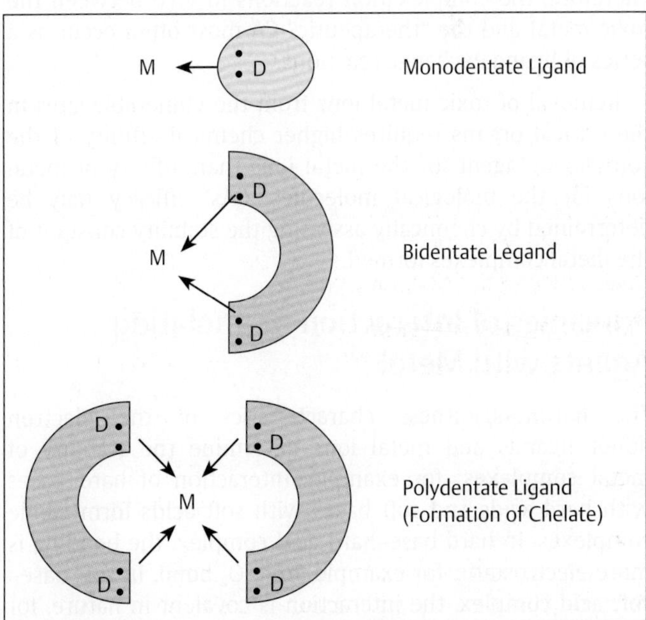

Fig. 81.2 Metal ligand complexes (monodentate, bidentate, and polydentate ligands).

Principles of Use of Chelating Agents

Heavy metals are considered as the oldest form of toxin in humans. But many heavy metals are active centers of various enzymes and thus are essential for all organisms. In body, when their level exceeds optimal level, they are toxic.

Recently, several developments have occurred in the clinical treatment of acute and chronic metal poisoning, and chelation therapy is one of them. Chelation therapy, medically, is used to reduce the toxic effects of metal ions, from acute metal poisoning to genetic metal intoxication.

Chelation therapy is a method of changing the concentration of metals in the body. Chelation (Greek: *chele*, meaning crab claws), the term first used by Sir Gilbert T. Morgan and H. D. K. Drew in 1920, characterizes a way of bonding by firm grasping. They proposed this term for groups that act as a means of linking and are linked to the central atom to avail the formation of a heterocycle. CAs may be inorganic or organic compounds and possess the capability to bind with a metal ion in the complex ring structures known as chelates.

Principle

Toxicity of heavy metals results from combining metal ions with one or more ligands which are required for normal physiological functions. CAs compete with these groups for metals, prevent or reverse toxic effects of metals, and promote their excretion. Heavy metals in the transition series may react with ligands in the body containing oxygen, sulfur, (¾SH, ¾S¾S¾), and nitrogen.

In the biological system, biological ligands are abundant; thus, often, free concentration of toxic metal is very low. Therefore, the complexation reactions in vivo between the toxic metal and the "therapeutic" CA most often occur as a series of ligand exchange reactions.

Removal of toxic metal ions from the vulnerable sites in the critical organs requires higher chemical affinity of the complexing agent for the metal ions than affinity of metal ions for the biological molecules. CAs' efficacy may be determined by chemically assessing the stability constant of the metal complexes formed.

Principles of Interaction of Chelating Agents with Metal

The hardness/softness characteristics of the electron donor ligands and metal ions determine the stability of metal complexes; for example, interaction of hard bases with hard acids and soft bases with soft acids form stable complexes. In hard base–hard acid complex, the bonding is more electrostatic, for example, iron–O_2 bond. In soft base–soft acid complex, the interaction is covalent in nature, for example, Hg–SH bond.

Effective chelation can be optimized by combination of the basic properties of the metals, CAs, and formed complexes. Stability of a formed complex depends on coordination positions of a metal ion occupied by CA. It means when more positions of metal are occupied by CA, a more stable complex is formed. However, the net ionic charge of the chelator governs its absorption, distribution, and binding capabilities. Similarly, the ionic charge of the complex governs its elimination from the specific site and excretion from the body.

Metal excretion from endogenously formed multidentate chelate occurs through many steps; hence, therapeutic chelation of toxic metal in body is a slow process. The efficacy of a chelator depends on its ability to penetrate the site of metal deposition; for example, as the penetration of chelators or chelates across blood–brain barrier (BBB) is restricted, the removal of iron, copper, or lead deposits proceeds slowly from the brain.

Chelation therapy is used for the removal of heavy elements from the body by the formation of a chelate complex with suitable chelating ligands in such a way that the complex must be water-soluble and stable, have less affinity to essential metal and less side effect, and is easily removed from the body system. CAs can decrease metal intoxication by renal excretion of toxic metal. Chelating ligands play an important role in the removal of heavy metal ions such as cadmium, copper, cobalt, zinc, nickel, and lead through the formation of the stable complex.

Advantages of Chelation Therapy

Chelation therapy is a very simple process; however, it can make you feel physically tired and mentally foggy. In this process, the patient is free from risk of heart attack, stroke, pain, swelling, and any other syndromes. The toxic contributor responsible for constant illness can be recognized. Conducting a study to assess chelation strategies and protocols in toxic metal bioaccumulation is possibly low-cost. These are secure therapies focusing on the main originating causes of today's most costly, prevalent persistent diseases.

Pharmacology of Different Chelating Agents

Types of Metal Poisoning

1. **Acute**: It develops rapidly, is easily identifiable, and may be recovered with immediate medical attention.
2. **Subacute:** It may be converted to chronic poisoning. It may be less defined and not identifiable.
3. **Chronic**: It develops slowly and may be reversible or irreversible. Later, it may lead to development of cancer or teratogenic malformations.

Basic Principles of Metal Toxicity Management

Steps involved are as follows:

1. Prevention of further metal absorption into the system, applicable in acute metal poisoning.

2. Elimination of metal from the circulation, applicable in acute metal poisoning.
3. Inactivation of metal bioavailable in the system → sub-chronic–chronic metal toxicity.

Characteristics of toxicity for a number of metals are presented earlier in this text. While the exact tissue and molecular site of the toxic action of each metal is different, CAs are always preferred for the medical treatment of acute metal poisonings. The basis for the use of chelation therapy is the scavenging of toxic metal ions from the organism, or attenuation of their toxicity by converting them into less toxic compounds. Following are the most advanced and clinically important CAs.

British Anti-Lewisite

British anti-Lewisite (BAL), chemically 2,3-dimercaprol, is an older CA. It was first made during World War II. It was developed by British biochemists at Oxford University. Chemically, it is described as having a 3-carbon backbone with two –SH (sulfhydryl) groups and a –OH (hydroxyl) group. Since 1949, BAL has been used clinically in mercury, arsenic, and cadmium toxicity.

In preclinical and clinical experiments, it is shown that when BAL is administered immediately after metal ingestion, its antidote efficacy is more effective. Although it causes rapid excretion of arsenic and mercury from the body, it leads to significant deposition of arsenic and mercury compounds in the brain.

Pharmacological Profile

BAL is not orally absorbed because of its oily nature. Its administration requires deep IM injection, which is very painful and allergenic. It was found to deposit lead into the brain, causing neurotoxicity. During treatment of cadmium toxicity, it increases renal cadmium concentration along with cadmium excretion; thus, BAL is avoided in the treatment of cadmium toxicity.

Disadvantages

1. Narrow therapeutic index (hence, it has small margin of safety).
2. Redistribution of arsenic to the testes and brain.
3. Painful IM injection.
4. Unpleasant odor (like rotten eggs).

Side Effects

Side effects include fever, conjunctivitis, lacrimation, headache, paresthesias, tremor, nausea, and constricted feeling in the chest, limbs, jaw, and abdomen.

More serious complications include abscess at the site of injection, hepatotoxicity, hypertension, tachycardia, and hemolysis in patients with glucose 6-phosphate deficiency.

Calcium Disodium Ethylenediamine Tetra-Acetic Acid

Calcium disodium ethylenediamine tetra-acetic acid ($CaNa_2EDTA$) is the most commonly used CA. Chemically, it is synthetic polyamino-polycarboxylic acid EDTA.

EDTA chelates calcium from plaque deposited in blood vessels and also releases some hormones, causing calcium and cholesterol removal; thus, it is useful in vascular diseases. It is also suggested that EDTA therapy may decrease the oxidative stress and associated injury and inflammation.

$CaNa_2EDTA$ is significant in the treatment of heavy metal poisoning, because it has higher affinity for CA than Ca^{2+}. In lead poisoning, it is significantly used because of its capacity to displace calcium by lead from the chelate. Its initial derivative, sodium EDTA, resulted in hypocalcemia due to excessive calcium excretion through kidney; thus, it was associated with the risk of tetany. To avoid this adverse effect, $CaNa_2EDTA$ is used in the treatment of lead poisoning. The lead–EDTA complex has high stability, and it is easily excretable, leaving calcium in blood.

Pharmacological Profile

Due to poor absorption through GIT, $CaNa_2EDTA$ should be administered by parenteral route only. IV administration gives good bioavailability, but it is very painful; therefore, it is given as IV infusion after dilution in 5% dextrose or saline. $CaNa_2EDTA$ is distributed mainly in the extracellular fluids. It redistributes lead from other tissues to the brain.

$CaNa_2EDTA$ is less metabolized and is excreted unchanged in urine. The elimination $t_{1/2}$ is 1.4 to 3 hours in adults, and its complete excretion occurs within 24 hours.

Adverse Effects

Headache, weakness, fever, nasocongestion, arrhythmias, hypotension, renal failures, bone marrow depression, increased bleeding time, convulsions, respiratory arrest, lacrimation, glycosuria, myalgia, hepatotoxicity, increased urinary frequency, and alterations in ECG. It is contraindicated in pregnancy, active renal diseases or anuria, hepatitis, and hypersensitivity.

D-Penicillamine

Chemically, D-penicillamine (DPA) is β-β-dimethyl-cysteine or 3-mercapto-D-valine, a degradation product of penicillin. Only D-isomer is clinically used, as L-isomer causes optic neuritis. It is used in the treatment of heavy metal toxicity, namely, lead, mercury, and copper poisoning (Wilson's disease).

Pharmacological Profile

DPA is administered orally or IV. Its oral absorption is about 50%. It is extracellularly distributed. After oral administration, the highest plasma concentration (C_{max}) is achieved in between 1 and 4 hours. A part of the dose undergoes hepatic metabolism to form disulfide metabolites. It is majorly excreted unchanged in urine. Elimination half-life is more than 7 hours.

Severe Adverse Effects

Leukocytopenia and thrombocytopenia are adverse effects of DPA. In rare cases, aplastic anemia may also occur. Long-term treatment with DPA can result in anorexia, nausea, and vomiting. In rats, it is reported to cause ulcers through the release of histamine.

Other side effects are GI disturbances, loss of taste, alopecia, and proteinuria. It may stimulate autoimmune phenomenon, resulting in lupus erythematosus, glomerulopathy, and hypersensitivity pneumonitis. DPA is teratogenic in nature. It is contraindicated in cases of penicillin allergy and renal impairment.

Deferoxamine/Desferrioxamine

Chemically, deferoxamine/desferrioxamine (DFO) is trihydroxamic acid, which is a siderophore secreted by a bacteria named *Streptomyces pilosus*. It has strong binding affinity for trivalent iron and less affinity for other metals, so that it is specific for treating iron-related diseases such as thalassemia and also in aluminum poisoning occurring after chronic renal dialysis.

Pharmacological Profile

Orally, DFO is poorly absorbed, so it is administered as IV injection or as an infusion. It shows good extracellular distribution, but less plasma protein binding. It forms ferrioxamine complex with iron and shows rapid renal excretion. Minor routes of its excretion are the bile and feces. It is well tolerated and thus has fewer side effects, for example, ototoxicity, opthalmotoxicity, allergic reactions, and superinfections. The total IV dose should not exceed 80 mg/kg/24 hours.

Deferiprone (L1)

Chemically, deferiprone (L1) is 1,2-dimethyl-3-hydroxypyrid-4-one. It is used as an alternative to deferoxamine in iron toxication, being an iron chelator. Compared to DFO, it is less expensive. Clinical studies have shown that the combination of DFO and L1 is very effective to decrease iron toxicity, with improved cardiac function in thalassemic patients. L1 is very well known for reversal of cardiac dysfunction and is also cardioprotective in nature, which may be because of its capacity to decrease iron overload. Exact mechanism for this is not known. However, treatment with L1 should be carefully monitored, as it leads to higher incidences of agranulocytosis.

Pharmacological Profile

It has rapid absorption through GIT, so it is majorly administered orally. It forms glucuronide conjugates after metabolism and is mainly excreted through the kidney. L1 has a half-life of 47 to 134 minutes. Its reported adverse effects are arthropathy, GI disturbances, headache, and moderate zinc deficiency, which are diminished by discontinuation of the drug. Rarely, most severe complications such as agranulocytosis or neutropenia can occur.

TETA (Trientine)

Tetraethylenetetraamine (TETA) or trientine is specifically used in acute copper intoxication. Nowadays, due to less use of copper utensils, exposure to copper is minimized as compared to ancient times. Administration of TETA leads to increase renal excretion of copper.

Pharmacological Profile

In spite of absorption of TETA being less, it is administered by oral route. The 5 to 18% of absorbed fraction of TETA is significantly metabolized and excreted through the kidney. Now, TETA is preferably used to treat Wilson's disease, as TETA is better chelator with lesser side effects than others. Wilson's disease is a genetic disorder due to altered copper homeostasis, and this dyshomeostasis results in progressive accumulation of copper, which may be fatal also.

Meso-2,3-Dimercaptosuccinic Acid/ Succimer

Meso-2,3-dimercaptosuccinic acid (DMSA) is a derivative of dimercaprol (BAL); chemically, it is dithiol compound with two –SH (sulfhydryl) groups. Its effective use as an antidote in heavy metal poisoning started 40 years ago.

Pharmacological Profile

DMSA is hydrophilic in nature, so it is well absorbed through GIT and therefore administered orally. This is its advantage over BAL. Ninety-five percent of DMSA is bound to plasma protein. One –SH group specifically binds to albumin and the other –SH group binds to metal, in order to form chelate. DMSA is a broad therapeutic window drug, so it is less toxic. It does not lead to loss of any essential metals from the body; however, it alters metabolism of copper. Adverse effects of DMSA includes GI disturbances, increased liver enzymes, skin reactions, and mild neutropenia.

Limitations of Current Chelation Therapy

Possible major and minor adverse effects and contraindications of available CAs are highlighted in earlier in this chapter. Here, we focus on the mechanisms of their limitations. $CaNa_2EDTA$ is commonly used and is considered a general CA, as it can form complex with many metal ions and can also be used with less risks. However, after chelate formation, removal of chelate in the extracellular fluid is restricted due to its impermeability through cell membrane. Similarly, DMSA, which is another commonly used succimer, is safer to use but has limitations of extracellular distribution. Hence, in case of metal reaching organs behind physiological barriers such as the BBB, these cannot be used. DPA, being derivative of penicillin, causes anaphylactic reaction in patients allergic to penicillin, so its use is quite risky here.

The success of any treatment depends on the properties of the CAs used. CAs with the following characteristics are preferred: (1) fast-acting, (2) long half- and shelf lives, (3) minimal side effects, and (4) ease of application.

The need to discover new antidotes is due to the following: (1) nonavailability of preventive, effective and safer pretreatment to avoid and treat metal exposure, (2) the available and suggested treatments have many major side effects or few are contraindicated in various heavy metal toxication, (3) available CAs are extensively administered by IV route, so self-medication is not possible by patients, and (4) fast-acting antidote for immediate removal of toxic metal from blood and soft tissues is unavailable. Thus, conventionally available CAs have many drawbacks; currently, there is no safe and effective treatment available for heavy metal poisoning.

Newer Strategies: Combination Therapy

Combined use of structurally different CAs is a novel approach in chelation therapy. The principle behind this is two different CAs acting through different mechanisms produce addition effect. They support the action of each other through synergism. Different CAs tend to mobilize toxic metals from different tissue compartments; thus, when they are combined, mobilization of toxic metal from the body could be enhanced. This may reduce required dose of chelators and reduce incidences of adverse reactions.

The combination of DMSA and MiADMSA (monoisoamyl DMSA) has shown to protect hepatic DNA damage in chronic arsenic poisoning. This greatly supported the assumption that combined administration of two different CAs could be more efficacious in arsenic-induced oxidative stress and also help in dose reduction of toxic chelator to minimize adverse effects.

Chapter 82 Immunosuppressants and Stimulants

Prince Allawadhi, Sachin Karkale, Amit Khurana, and Kala Kumar Bharani

PH1.50: Describe mechanisms of action, types, doses, side effects, indications, and contraindications of immunomodulators and management of organ transplant rejection.

Learning Objectives

- Immune system.
- Immunosuppressants.
- Immunostimulants.

Immune System

The immune system is a natural host defense system in the body that discriminates self from nonself and protects the body against harmful foreign substances (microorganisms, growth of tumor cells, and a transplanted organ). The immune responses are of two types: innate (or natural or nonspecific or rapid) and acquired (or adaptive or specific or delayed). Innate immunity is present since birth, and major components include barriers (mucous membrane, skin, saliva, tears, stomach acid, normal flora, and digestive enzymes) and mediators (macrophages, neutrophils, monocytes, complement, natural killer cells, dendritic cells, eosinophils and basophils, etc.). In innate immunity, there is no involvement of memory cells. Acquired immunity depends upon specific foreign substances known as antigens, and in response to antigens, body develops specific antibodies that boost the immune system. They are classified into two categories: one is humoral and another is cellular, both of which involve the role of memory cells.

B and T lymphocytes play a central role in acquired immunity. B lymphocytes are involved in humoral immunity; when they get exposed to specific antigens, they produce plasma cells in the bone marrow (pluripotent stem cells), leading to differentiation of antibodies. Moreover, these differentiated antibodies finally inactivate the antigens. The pluripotent stem cells travel into thymus and develop into mature T cells, which are involved in cell-mediated immunity. T lymphocytes recognize antigens on the surface of antigen-presenting cells (APCs) such as macrophages, dendritic cells, and other cell types expressing major histocompatibility complex (MHC) antigens and get differentiated to helper T-cells ($CD4^+$ cells) and cytotoxic T-cells ($CD8^+$ cells). All these cells are important in organ transplantation, immunological diseases, and autoimmunity (**Fig. 82.1**).

Immune system is broadly affected by two distinct categories of drugs: the first one consists of immunostimulant drugs that act by stimulating the immune system by promoting antigenic properties, and the second one comprises immunosuppressants that slow down the

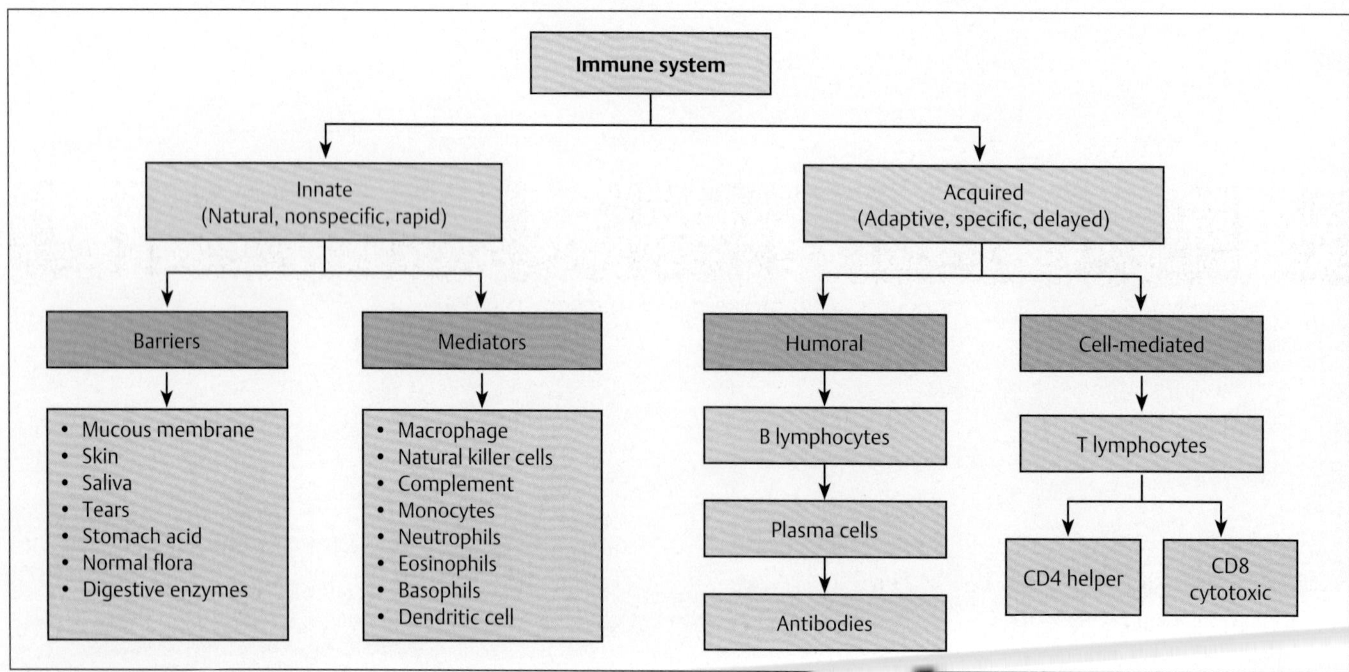

Fig. 82.1 The classification of immune system and the various cellular components.

hyperactive immune system by suppressing the immune signaling pathways, specifically or nonspecifically (**Fig. 82.2**).

Immunosuppressants

Immunosuppressants are drugs that control the pathological immune response and suppress the hyperintense immune responses. Immunosuppressants are commonly used in the treatment of autoimmune diseases, cancer, allergy and lupus, and also to prevent and/or treat transplant rejection. Classification of immunosuppressants is given in **Table 82.1**.

Calcineurin Inhibitors

Calcineurin inhibitors block the activity of calcineurin, an enzyme involved in T-cell activation, and thus suppress cell-mediated immunity. Calcineurin inhibitors are the first-line treatment during organ transplantation surgeries. Some of the important calcineurin inhibitors are cyclosporine and tacrolimus.

Cyclosporine

Cyclosporine (ciclosporin) is a cyclic polypeptide consisting of 11 amino acids. It is naturally occurring and is obtained from the fungus *Beauveria nivea*. Cyclosporine is a highly lipophilic compound with potent immunosuppressive activity.

Mechanism of Action

Cyclosporine selectively suppresses T-cell-dependent immune (cell-mediated) mechanisms. The main action involves inhibition of interleukin (IL)-2 gene transcription and T lymphocyte proliferation. Normally, antigens interact with T-cell receptor (T-helper cell), which leads to activation of T-cell receptor and phosphorylation of the phospholipase (PLc) in the presence of protein kinase, resulting in the release of Ca^{2+}. Moreover, the released Ca^{2+} activates a phosphatase (calcineurin), and activated calcineurin is responsible for dephosphorylation of "nuclear factor of activated T-cell" (NFAT). Dephosphorylated NFAT translocates into the

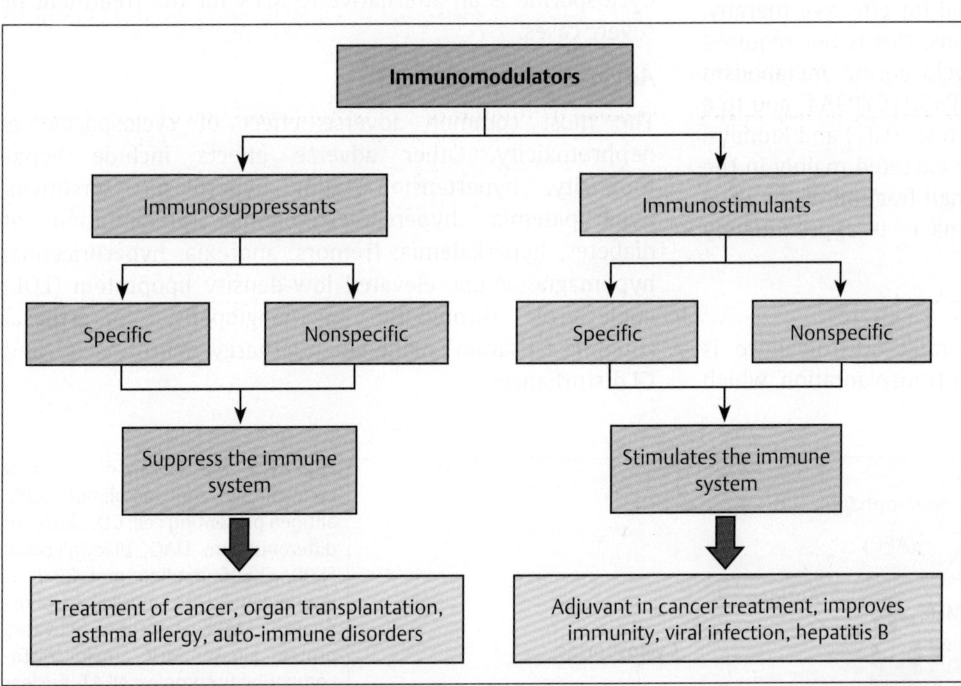

Fig. 82.2 Broad overview of immunomodulators, which encompass the immunosuppressants and immunostimulants.

Table 82.1 Classification of immunosuppressants

Mechanism of action	Examples
Calcineurin inhibitors	Cyclosporine (ciclosporin), tacrolimus (FK506)
mTOR inhibitors	Sirolimus, everolimus
Cytotoxic immunosuppressants	Azathioprine, methotrexate, MMF, cyclophosphamide, chlorambucil
Drugs inhibit cytokine gene expression	Glucocorticoids
TNF-α inhibitors	Etanercept, adalimumab, infliximab
IL-1 receptor antagonist	Anakinra
Monoclonal antibodies	Muromonab (OKT-3), daclizumab, basiliximab, alemtuzumab (Campath-1H), efalizumab
Polyclonal antibodies	ATG
Small molecule agent	Fingolimod (FTY720)
Miscellaneous	Rho (D) immune globulin

Abbreviations: ATG, antithymocyte globulin; IL, interleukin; MMF, mycophenolate mofetil; mTOR, mammalian target of rapamycin; TNF-α, tumor necrosis factor α.

nucleus and triggers the transcription of cytokine, complete T-cell activation, which initiates production of IL-2 and other cytokines. Cyclosporine enters into target cells and forms a complex with cyclophilin (immunophilin cytoplasmic receptor protein). This complex binds to and inhibits calcineurin, which leads to inactivation of dephosphorylated NFAT, decreases T-cell activation, and subsequently inhibits IL-2 or other cytokine production (**Fig. 82.3**). Cyclosporine also increases expression of transforming growth factor beta (TGF-β).

Pharmacokinetics

Cyclosporine can be given orally or as an intravenous (IV) infusion. Oral absorption of cyclosporine is variable because it has low oral bioavailability of about 20 to 50%. After oral administration of cyclosporine, peak plasma concentrations are achieved at approximately 3 to 4 hours. The microemulsion formulation of cyclosporine has more bioavailability as compared to other traditional preparations. Its administration with food decreases absorption. Monitoring of serum concentration of the drug is essential for effective therapy, but in case of autoimmune conditions, this is not required because lower doses are used. Cyclosporine metabolism occurs in the liver by a cytochrome P450 (CYP3A4) and to a lesser extent in the gastrointestinal tract (GIT) and kidneys. Cyclosporine and its metabolites are excreted mainly in the bile and then in feces but only a small fraction of the drug is excreted in the urine. The plasma $t_{½}$ is approximately 24 hours.

Dose

Orally, 10 to 15 mg/kg/day with milk or fruit juice is recommended, till 1 to 2 weeks after transplantation, which is gradually reduced to a maintenance dose of 2 to 6 mg/kg/day, and for IV infusion, it is 3 to 5 mg/kg.

Therapeutic Uses

Cyclosporine is usually used to prevent rejection of heart, kidney, hepatic, bone marrow, and other transplantations. It is effective in autoimmune diseases (rheumatoid arthritis, atopic dermatitis, endogenous uveitis, psoriasis, etc.), inflammatory bowel disease, graft-versus-host disease, and Behçet's acute ocular syndrome. It is also used for xerophthalmia and other skin diseases as well. Cyclosporine is given 4 to 12 hours before transplantation and then continued for as long as needed, and during organ rejection, it can be given IV. The dose varies usually, depending on the organ being transplanted. It is also used in combination with other agents such as glucocorticoids or methotrexate (MTX) and azathioprine or mycophenolate mofetil (MMF). In some cases, if a drug shows adverse effect in that condition, treatment starts with low dose to reduce adverse effects. Cyclosporine is an alternative to MTX for the treatment of severe cases.

Adverse Effect

The most common adverse effect of cyclosporine is nephrotoxicity. Other adverse effects include hepatotoxicity, hypertension, gum hyperplasia, hirsutism, hyperlipidemia, hypercholesterolemia, precipitation of diabetes, hyperkalemia, tremors, anorexia, hyperuricemia, hypomagnesaemia, elevated low-density lipoprotein (LDL) cholesterol, thrombotic microangiopathy, paresthesia (tingling sensation), malignancy, lethargy, neurotoxicity, and GI disturbances.

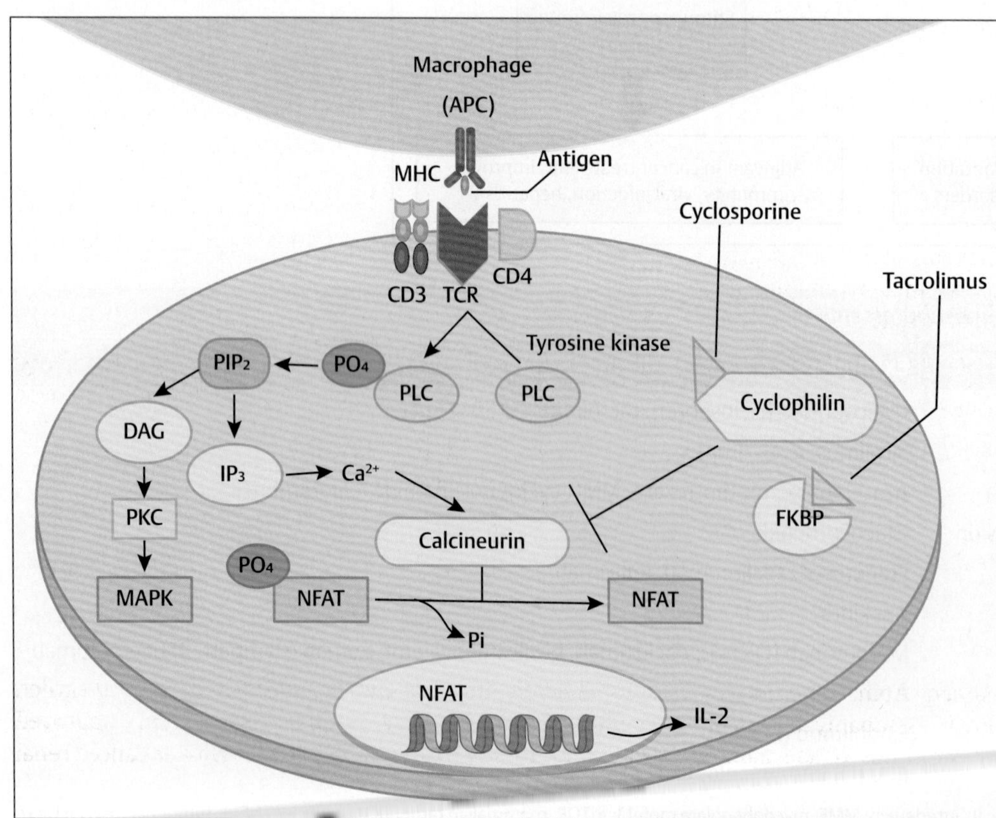

Fig. 82.3 Mechanism of action of cyclosporine and tacrolimus. APC, antigen presenting cell; CD, cluster of differentiation; DAG, diacylglycerol; FKBP, FK506 binding protein; IL-2, interleukin 2; IP3, inositol trisphosphate; MAPK, mitogen-activated protein kinase; MHC, major histocompatibility complex; NFAT, nuclear factor of activated T-cell; PIP2, phosphatidylinositol 4,5-bisphosphate; PKC, protein kinase C; PLC, phospholipase C; PO4, phosphate; TCR, T-cell receptor.

Drug Interactions

Cyclosporine interacts with different types of drugs such as rifampin, nafcillin, carbamazepine phenobarbital, phenytoin, ticlopidine, octreotide, and other enzyme (CYP3A4) inducers as well, which increase cyclosporine metabolism and decrease blood concentrations. In contrast, enzyme (CYP3A4) inhibitors such as ketoconazole, fluconazole, erythromycin, methylprednisolone, allopurinol, cimetidine, verapamil, nicardipine, diltiazem, norethisterone, grapefruit, indinavir, and related drugs reduce cyclosporine metabolism and increase blood concentrations, thus leading to toxicity. Coadministration with drugs such as nonsteroidal anti-inflammatory drugs (NSAIDs), aminoglycoside antibiotics, vancomycin, and amphotericin B can enhance its nephrotoxicity. Angiotensin-converting enzyme (ACE) inhibitors, potassium supplements, and K^+-sparing diuretics increase the risk of hyperkalemia.

Tacrolimus (FK506)

Tacrolimus (FK506) is a macrolide antibiotic from the fungus *Streptomyces tsukubaensis*. Tacrolimus is chemically different from cyclosporine but has a similar mechanism of action. Tacrolimus is 10 to 100 times more potent than cyclosporine. Tacrolimus binds to different intracellular protein labeled FK-binding protein (FKBP), called immunophilin A complex (tacrolimus-FKBP), which inhibits the phosphatase action of calcineurin, thereby suppressing nuclear translocation of NFAT to nucleus, prevents transcription of IL-2, and inhibits T-cell activation. Tacrolimus may be administered orally or as an IV infusion. Tacrolimus is poorly and incompletely absorbed orally. Serum drug concentration monitoring is also required for tacrolimus. Absorption is decreased if the drug is taken with food. It is metabolized in the liver by CYP3A4 prior to elimination. Tacrolimus is eliminated primarily via the liver, with an elimination half-life of approximately 7 to 8 hours, and is excreted in the bile. Therapeutic use, drug interactions, and adverse effects are similar to cyclosporine. Tacrolimus is used for liver and kidney transplantation, prophylaxis of solid-organ allograft rejection, atopic eczema, and fistulating Crohn's disease. Toxicity of tacrolimus includes neurotoxicity, alopecia, and insulin-dependent diabetes mellitus (type 1 diabetes). Nephrotoxicity, hypertension, hyperkalemia, hyperuricemia, hyperlipidemia, and hyperglycemia are less prominent toxicities as compared to cyclosporine (**Fig. 82.1**).

Mammalian Target of Rapamycin Inhibitors

Mammalian target of rapamycin (mTOR) is a serine/threonine-protein kinase enzyme, which belongs to the phosphatidylinositol-3 kinase (PI3K) family of kinases. It plays a crucial role in cellular growth and proliferation. It is the target of immunosuppressant drug rapamycin.

Sirolimus (Rapamycin)

It is a macrolide antibiotic obtained from *Streptomyces hygroscopicus* and was earlier known as rapamycin, but it has now been assigned the name sirolimus (trade name: Rapamune).

Mechanism of Action

Sirolimus is a potent immunosuppressive agent whose mechanism of action is different from calcineurin-inhibiting agents. Sirolimus inhibits T-cell proliferation and differentiation activated by IL-2 and other cytokines. Sirolimus binds to immunophilin (FKBP) and forms a complex. However, formed complex (sirolimus-FKBP) binds to mTOR instead of tacrolimus-binding site (calcineurin) and inhibits the activity of mTOR, like T lymphocyte activation and proliferation activated by IL-2, resulting in arrest of cell-cycle progression at the G1 to S-phase (**Fig. 82.4**).

mTOR signaling pathway is an important signaling cascade, which leads to the activation and proliferation of T-cells activated by IL-2 and other cytokines. Sirolimus (rapamycin) and everolimus work at a later stage in T-cell activation. Sirolimus and everolimus bind to immunophilin (FKBP) and form a complex. However, formed complex (sirolimus or everolimus-FKBP) binds to mTOR instead of tacrolimus-binding site (calcineurin) and inhibits the activity of mTOR, like T lymphocyte activation and proliferation activated by IL-2, resulting in arrest of cell-cycle progression at the G1 to S-phase.

Pharmacokinetics

Sirolimus is given orally and reaches peak blood concentrations in approximately 2 hours after administration in renal transplant recipients. Absorption of sirolimus may be reduced in the presence of high-fat food. The systemic bioavailability of sirolimus is 15 to 20%. Sirolimus is metabolized by CYP3A4 isozyme and is eliminated through biliary/feces route. Elimination half-life ($t_{½}$) of sirolimus is approximately 62 hours. Therapeutic drug monitoring is required for sirolimus.

Therapeutic Uses

Sirolimus is approved for use in renal transplant but can be used with lower dose of cyclosporine and corticosteroids, thereby lowering their toxic potential. It is also used in graft rejection, stem cell transplant, and halting graft vascular disease. Sirolimus-coated stents are used in coronary artery restenosis by preventing proliferation of the endothelial cells.

Adverse Effect

Sirolimus causes hyperlipidemia, myelosuppression (bone marrow suppression), and thrombocytopenia. Other adverse effects are nausea, diarrhea, GI effects, headache, leucopenia, anemia, and pneumonitis.

Everolimus

Everolimus has the same mechanism of action, clinical efficacy, and toxicity as sirolimus but differs in pharmacokinetics. Everolimus is administered orally and rapidly absorbed. The elimination half-life ($t_{½}$) is approximately 40 hours and steady state is achieved earlier. The U.S. Food and Drug Administration (FDA) approved everolimus for the treatment of patients with advanced renal cell carcinoma (RCC) as well (**Fig. 82.4**).

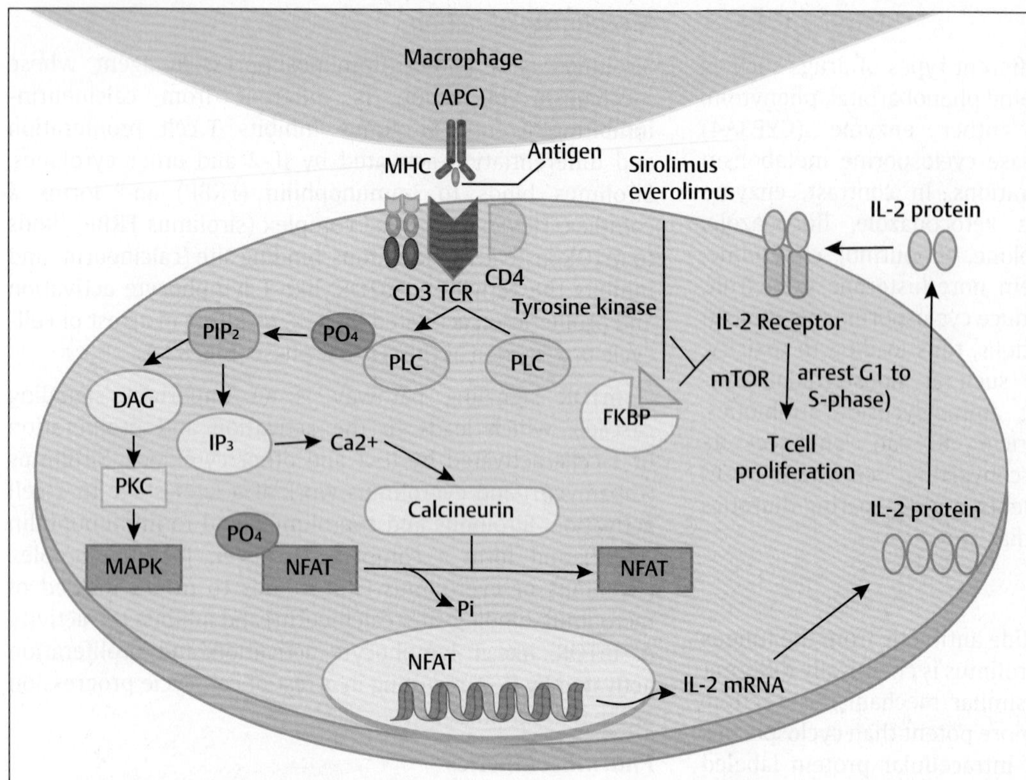

Fig. 82.4 Mechanism of action of sirolimus and everolimus. APC, antigen presenting cell; CD, cluster of differentiation; DAG, diacylglycerol; FKBP, FK506 binding protein; IL-2, interleukin 2; IP3, inositol trisphosphate; MAPK, mitogen-activated protein kinase; mTOR, mammalian target of rapamycin; MHC, major histocompatibility complex; NFAT, nuclear factor of activated T-cell; PIP2, phosphatidylinositol 4,5-bisphosphate; PKC, protein kinase C; PLC, phospholipase C; PO4, phosphate; TCR, T-cell receptor.

Cytotoxic Immunosuppressants

This class of immunosuppressants is primarily cytotoxic and are mainly used for anticancer activity. Due to their strong immune-inhibiting potential, some of the cytotoxic agents are used for the immunosuppressant activity. Some of the major drugs of this class include azathioprine, MTX, cyclophosphamide, and chlorambucil.

Azathioprine

Azathioprine is a purine antimetabolite; chemically, it is an imidazolyl derivative of 6-mercaptopurine (6-MP). Azathioprine is a prodrug and was first synthesized in 1957. It is converted into 6-MP in the presence of glutathione S-transferase, which, in turn, is converted to additional metabolites to inhibit de novo purine synthesis. 6-MP is again converted into 6-thiosine 5′-monophosphate (6-TIMP), and 6-TIMP, a fraudulent nucleotide, is converted into 6-tioguanine metabolites (6-TGM), which are incorporated into DNA, leading to inhibition of cell proliferation and impairment of lymphocytes function.

Azathioprine is given orally and reaches maximum blood levels within 1 to 2 hours after administration. Azathioprine is bound to plasma proteins, metabolized in the liver (oxidation or methylation), and the metabolites are excreted by renal route. The elimination half-life ($t_{½}$) is approximately 10 hours. Azathioprine is oxidized by "xanthine oxidase"; its metabolism is inhibited by allopurinol. Azathioprine was initially used for renal allografts. It is used in autoimmune diseases (rheumatoid arthritis, ulcerative colitis), inflammatory bowel disease, and organ transplant rejection. Adverse effects include depression of the bone marrow, GI toxicity, skin eruptions, alopecia, increased risk of neoplasia, pancreatitis, nausea, vomiting, and mild hepatotoxicity.

Methotrexate

MTX is a folate antagonist. It has immunosuppressant and anti-inflammatory property, which markedly depresses cytokine production and cellular immunity. MTX was originally used for chemotherapy in high doses, but in low doses, it is the first-line therapy for the treatment of rheumatoid arthritis, psoriasis, Crohn's disease, and other autoimmune diseases. Low doses of MTX are generally safe and well tolerated.

Mycophenolate Mofetil

MMF can be derived from fungi, and it is a prodrug of mycophenolic acid (MPA). MMF is rapidly hydrolyzed to active form, MPA, which is a selective, noncompetitive, and reversible inhibitor of inosine monophosphate dehydrogenase enzyme. This enzyme is essential for de novo synthesis of guanosine nucleotides in both T- and B-cells. B and T lymphocytes are dependent on de novo synthesis pathway for cell proliferation, whereas other cells generate purines through another pathway. Therefore, MPA selectively inhibits lymphocyte proliferation, antibody production, DNA replication in T- and B-cells, and cellular adhesion and migration.

MMF is given orally and is completely absorbed and highly bound to plasma albumin. MMF is completely metabolized to MPA, and the latter is slowly inactivated by glucuronidation. The elimination half-life ($t_{½}$) is approximately 16 hours. The glucuronide metabolite is excreted in urine. MMF is used in prophylaxis of transplant rejection. It is used in combination with glucocorticoids and cyclosporine in kidney transplantation but not with azathioprine. MMF is also used in combination with glucocorticoids, and sirolimus is a nonnephrotoxic combination that is utilized in patients developing renal toxicity with cyclosporine/tacrolimus. Diarrhea, leucopenia, nausea, vomiting, anemia, sepsis associated with cytomegalovirus (CMV), predisposition to CMV infection, and GIT disturbance are some of the adverse effects. MMF when administered with antacids containing aluminum or magnesium hydroxide impairs absorption, and in combination with cholestyramine reduces plasma concentration.

Cyclophosphamide and Chlorambucil

Cyclophosphamide and chlorambucil are alkylating agents with cytotoxic effect and are mainly used to treat cancer. Chlorambucil has weak immunosuppressant action. Cyclophosphamide is used in the treatment of severe systemic lupus erythematosus, idiopathic thrombocytopenic purpura, vasculitides such as Wegener's granulomatosis, bone marrow transplantation, and management of rheumatoid disorders.

Drugs Inhibiting Cytokine Gene Expression

This class of immunosuppressants act by inhibition of cytokines. Classical examples include glucocorticoids and antibodies directed against specific cytokines such as tumor necrosis factor-α (TNF-α) and IL-1β inhibitors.

Glucocorticoids

Glucocorticoids have immunosuppressant and anti-inflammatory activity. It rapidly reduces lymphocyte populations and inhibits several components of the immune response. Glucocorticoids suppress cell-mediated immunity and to a lesser extent show effect on humoral immunity as well. They inhibit proliferation of T lymphocytes by reducing transcription of cytokine genes IL-2 and many other interleukins. Glucocorticoids are commonly used in combination with other immunosuppressants in organ transplantation.

It is used in various autoimmune disorders (refractory rheumatoid arthritis, systemic lupus erythematosus, and temporal arthritis) and asthma. High doses of IV corticosteroids are used in graft rejection and in autoimmune diseases during exacerbation. In addition, glucocorticoids are also efficacious for treatment of chronic graft-versus-host disease.

Tumor Necrosis Factor-α Inhibitors

TNF-α receptors are generally transmembrane proteins (TNFR1, TNFR2), but many of them can also be secreted as soluble form (sTNFR1, sTNFR2). TNF-α is primarily generated by macrophages, monocytes, and other immune cells. TNF-α plays a vital role in the production of immune inflammation by releasing different cytokines and enzymes. TNF-α inhibitors are used in rheumatoid arthritis, polyarticular idiopathic juvenile arthritis, ankylosing spondylitis, plaque psoriasis, Crohn's disease, etc.

Etanercept

Etanercept is a recombinant fusion protein composed of human TNF receptor and Fc portion of human immunoglobulin G1 (IgG1) and binds to TNF-α, thereby preventing its interaction with cell surface TNF receptors. Etanercept is mostly used for treatment of rheumatoid arthritis either alone or in combination with MTX. It is approved for polyarticular idiopathic juvenile arthritis, ankylosing spondylitis, and plaque psoriasis. Etanercept is given by subcutaneous route; some injection-site reactions include swelling, itching, pain, and erythema.

Adalimumab

Adalimumab is a recombinant monoclonal antibody with specificity to TNF-α, which inhibits its interaction with cell surface TNF receptors. It alters biological responses that are regulated by TNF. After treatment with adalimumab, reductions in level of C-reactive protein, serum cytokines (IL-6), and serum levels of matrix metalloproteinases (MMP-1 and MMP-3) in different diseases are observed. Adalimumab is used in rheumatoid arthritis either alone or in combination with MTX or other conventional drugs. It is indicated for Crohn's disease, psoriatic arthritis, and ankylosing spondylitis. Adalimumab is given via subcutaneous route.

Infliximab

Infliximab is a chimeric anti-TNF-α monoclonal antibody composed of human and murine regions. Infliximab neutralizes the biological activity of TNF-α by binding with specificity to TNF-α and inhibits its effective binding of TNF-α with its receptors. Infliximab is approved for use in rheumatoid arthritis either alone or with MTX. It is also used in treatment of plaque psoriasis, ulcerative colitis, Crohn's disease, psoriatic arthritis, and ankylosing spondylitis. Infliximab is infused IV for at least 2 hours.

IL-1 Receptor Antagonist

Macrophages, fibroblasts, monocytes, and other cells produce IL-1, which plays a main role in the regulation of immunological and inflammatory response.

Anakinra

Anakinra is a recombinant IL-1 receptor antagonist. It competitively inhibits IL-1 binding to the IL-1 type I receptor. It is approved for therapy in patients with rheumatoid arthritis. Anakinra can be given along with MTX or TNF-α antagonist.

Monoclonal Antibody

Monoclonal antibodies are one of the most important classes of drugs used against cancer and chronic inflammatory diseases such as rheumatoid arthritis. They specifically target only one antigen to elicit biological response. The classical monoclonal antibodies were derived from mouse hybridomas. However, most of the currently used monoclonal antibodies are either humanized or chimeric with low immunogenicity. Some of the important immunosuppressant monoclonal antibodies include muromonab, daclizumab, basiliximab, and alemtuzumab.

Muromonab (Anti-CD3, OKT-3)

Muromonab-CD3 is a murine monoclonal antibody, often referred to as OKT-3, against the glycoprotein CD3 antigen of human T-cells (T lymphocytes). CD3 is a glycoprotein, trimeric molecule, and T-cell coreceptor found on the surface of human T-cell and involved in antigen recognition and T-cell activation and proliferation. Muromonab-CD3 binds to the CD3, thereby interfering with antigen recognition and inducing rapid internalization of the T-cell receptor. Following antibody binding, it depletes T-cells and decreases the T-cell activity. Muromonab is used in the treatment of acute organ transplant rejection. It is effective in the treatment of rejections resistant to conventional treatment; however, it has shown efficacy in steroid-resistant cases as well. Muromonab is given via IV bolus. Adverse effects include cytokine release syndrome (typically associated with initial dose of muromonab), high fever, chills, tremor, wheezing, nausea/vomiting, malaise, rigor, aseptic meningitis, pulmonary edema, skin reactions, seizures, etc.

Daclizumab and Basiliximab (Anti-CD25, IL-2 Receptor Antagonist)

Daclizumab is a humanized murine monoclonal antibody, which consists of 90% human protein. Basiliximab is a murine–human chimeric monoclonal antibody, which consists of 75% human protein. CD25 molecule is a protein expressed on the surface of IL-2 receptor alpha chain. IL-2 receptor is present on activated T-cells. Daclizumab and basiliximab are anti-CD25 antibodies, which bind to the α-chain of the IL-2 receptor on activated T-cells and act as an IL-2 receptor antagonist. The net effect involves interfering with the proliferation of these cells and reduction of T-cell responses. Both compounds are used for prophylaxis of acute organ rejection. Daclizumab has been used in combination with calcineurin antagonists, corticoids, and/or azathioprine/MMF, and basiliximab has been used in combination with calcineurin antagonists and corticoids. Both antibodies are given via IV route. The half-life of daclizumab plasma is 3 weeks and that of basiliximab plasma is 1 week. Both daclizumab and basiliximab can cause anaphylaxis, lymphoproliferative disorders, and opportunistic infections.

Alemtuzumab (Anti-CD52, Campath-1H)

Alemtuzumab is a humanized monoclonal antibody. CD52 is a cell-surface glycoprotein expressed on lymphocytes, monocytes, macrophages, and natural killer cells. Alemtuzumab binds to the CD52 antigen present on lymphocytes and causes extensive lympholysis of targeted cells and reduction of lymphocyte populations. It is used to treat chronic lymphocytic leukemia and multiple sclerosis (MS), as well as in renal transplantation. It can be given by IV injection.

Efalizumab (Anti-CD11a, LFA-1 Inhibition)

Efalizumab is a humanized monoclonal antibody. CD11a is a subunit of the lymphocyte function–associated antigen 1 (LFA-1), which is present on lymphocytes and causes activation, proliferation, and migration of lymphocytes. Efalizumab binds to CD11a, a subunit of LFA-1, and inhibits the binding of LFA-1 to the intercellular adhesion molecule-1 (ICAM-1), thereby preventing lymphocyte activation and cell migration. Efalizumab is approved for treatment of severe plaque psoriasis. It is given as weekly subcutaneous injections. Adverse effects include fever, headache, muscle hypersensitivity reactions, nausea, and fatigue.

Polyclonal Antibody

Polyclonal antibodies cause modulation of all types of lymphocytes, thus causing generalized immunosuppression. They not only affect the T-cells but also may modulate other cell types such as B-cells, natural killer cells, and monocytes. Antithymocyte globulin is an important polyclonal immunosuppressant antibody.

Antithymocyte Globulin

Antithymocyte globulin is a polyclonal antibody preparation derived from rabbits or horses immunized with human thymocytes or T-cells. Antithymocyte globulin binds to multiple T-cell markers, CD2, CD3, CD4, CD8, CD11a, CD18, CD25, CD44, and CD45, as well as human leukocyte antigens (HLA) markers and other tissue antigens on the surface of human T lymphocytes and depletes them. It depletes circulating lymphocytes by cytotoxicity (complement-mediated destruction, cell-mediated apoptosis, and opsonization) and prevents lymphocyte function. Antithymocyte globulin is used in the treatment of acute allograft rejection episodes or corticosteroid-resistant acute rejections in combination with other immunosuppressive agents. It is given by slow IV injection. Adverse effects include fever and chills, anaphylaxis, serum sickness, thrombocytopenia, glomerulonephritis, leukopenia, and risk of infection.

Small Molecule Agents

Small molecule–based immunosuppressants are small-sized synthetic chemicals which exhibit their pharmacological effects mainly by inhibition of T lymphocytes. Fingolimod is an important representative of this class and helps in reducing the use of calcineurin inhibitors and steroids.

Fingolimod (FTY720)

Fingolimod is a structural analog of sphingosine produced from myriocin (ISP-1), a metabolite of the fungus *Isaria sinclairii*. Fingolimod is a prodrug and sphingosine 1-phosphate (S1P) receptor modulator. Fingolimod is phosphorylated by sphingosine kinases in the cell. Phosphorylated fingolimod causes the internalization of S1P receptors, which reduces recirculation of lymphocytes from lymphoid tissues (lymphatic nodes), thus preventing them from taking part in an autoimmune response. Fingolimod is mostly used for treating MS by reducing the rate of relapses.

Miscellaneous

The miscellaneous class agents act by a variety of mechanisms and include the Rho immune globulin, described in the following.

Rho (D) Immune Globulin

It is human IgG containing a higher titer of antibodies against the Rho (D) antigen. Rh factor is a part of the red blood cell. A person has either Rh-positive or Rh-negative blood. If a person receives the opposite type of blood, the person's body will create antibodies that can destroy the red blood cells. Rho immune globulin binds to Rho antigens and predominantly prevents the antibody formation in Rh-negative individuals. Rho (D) immune globulin is also used to prevent antibodies from forming if a person with Rh-negative blood receives a transfusion with Rh-positive blood or during pregnancy when a mother has Rh-negative blood and the baby is Rh-positive. Rho (D) immune globulin is used to treat immune thrombocytopenic purpura in patients with Rh-positive blood. It can be given by intramuscular or IV injection.

Role of Immunosuppressants in Prevention and Treatment of Organ Transplantation Rejection (SU13.2)

The body, due to its highly sophisticated immune system, has the ability to sense the foreign substance (allograft) after transplantation, which leads to the development of antigenic antibody reaction followed by organ rejection, thus resulting in failure of organ transplantation. Human body rejects the allografts by two distinct mechanisms (**Fig. 82.5**), namely, direct and indirect, both of which focus on the source of the APCs (recipient vs. donor). Direct pathway works by migration of dendritic cells from the graft to secondary lymphoid tissues to activate T-cells that distinguish intact nonself MHC molecules present on the surface of donor cells. The indirect pathway of allograft recognition describes the ability of T-cells to recognize donor MHC molecules that are processed and presented as peptides by self-MHC molecules.

The identification of intact donor MHC molecules provokes a highly intense antigraft immune reaction, whereas processed MHC peptides and minor histocompatibility antigens generate a reduced amount of intense immune response. Herein, the role of immunosuppressant comes into picture by suppressing the antigen–antibody reaction by downregulating the host immunogenic defense system, which reduces the immune system's capability to recognize the allograft-mediated antigenic property, making the transplantation successful. Therefore, the use of immunosuppressants plays a critical role in successful organ transplantation, and depending upon the stage of transplantation, generally three types of drug regimens are employed in clinical practice:

1. Induction regimen.
2. Maintenance regimen.
3. Antirejection regimen.

Induction Regimen

This type of regimen is given just prior to organ transplantation and lasts about 2 to 12 weeks after transplantation. Organ rejection develops generally in two ways, accelerated and acute. Accelerated rejection develops in the first week of transplant, whereas acute rejection develops within 2 to 12 weeks. The most common drugs

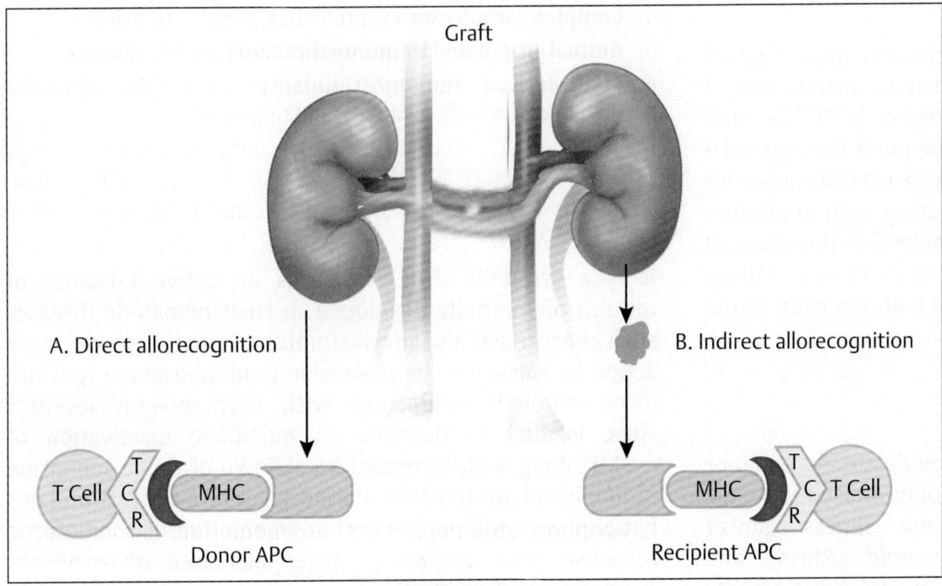

Fig. 82.5 Two different pathways of allorecognition. A. Direct pathway of allorecognition: DCs migrate from the graft to secondary lymphoid tissues to activate T cells. B. Indirect pathway of allorecognition: graft proteins are processed by recipient DCs and then presented to T-cells. APC, antigen-presenting cells; MHC, major histocompatibility complex.

given in this regimen include triple therapy, covering prednisolone + MMF/azathioprine + tacrolimus/sirolimus/ cyclosporine. To avoid renal toxicity in patients with compromised renal function, the combination of MMF/ sirolimus + prednisolone is used in clinical application. As many of the immunosuppressant drugs produce severe adverse effects during treatment phase, this limits their use and time course of duration as well. Cyclosporine produces nephrotoxicity, especially in renal transplantation cases, so, in such cases, cyclosporine is not given until and unless it is highly required. The dose regimen is reduced in a gradual manner after 2 weeks if rejection does not develop in due time, and this induction phase indiscernibly joins with maintenance phase of regimen.

Maintenance Regimen

This is prescribed for a prolonged duration, which could even last for a lifetime as well. In this regimen, the chances of drug-induced toxicities are less as the drugs given in these phases are of low dose just for maintenance purpose. Triple-drug regimen most commonly includes the choices of any three drugs from cyclosporine/tacrolimus, prednisolone, sirolimus, MMF, and azathioprine. There is no doubt that lifelong treatment with these drugs causes adverse effects on host body; out of many adverse effects, cyclosporine/ tacrolimus-induced nephrotoxicity is a common adverse event, which is a limiting factor so also prolonged steroid use. Drugs that produce more adverse effects are dropped off from the treatment regimen, and two-and one-drug regimen are implicated in treatment course but doing so may result in increased incidence of acute rejection. Normally, after 1 year, cyclosporine is discontinued, as its continuous use can be related to fewer acute rejections. In case of intolerance to the first line of drugs (tacrolimus, sirolimus, cyclosporine, MMF, prednisolone, and azathioprine), second line of drugs such as chlorambucil, cyclophosphamide, daclizumab, or MTX could be taken into consideration as a treatment option.

Antirejection Regimen

To curb the episodes of acute organ rejection, drug regimen of this category is prescribed, which includes mainly steroid pulse therapy (methylprednisolone 0.5–1 g IV for 3–5 days). In case no response is seen to the pulse therapy, then antithymocyte globulin and muromonab CD3 are given as rescue therapy or steroids in combination with antibodies can be used. Cyclosporine can be employed in this phase if it is not prescribed earlier, but by doing so, there are likely chances of developing renal toxicity of high intensity to the transplanted kidney.

Immunostimulants

These are the class of drugs that modulate or enhance the immune response of immunocompromised patients to help them fight against chronic illness, cancer malignancies, AIDS, COVID-19, rheumatoid arthritis, and lepra reaction by inducing activation or increasing activity of any of its components. This is yet an emerging field of immunopharmacological research, which is growing vigorously, especially in the wake of the coronavirus crisis. In healthy persons, they serve as prophylactic or immune-promoting agents as immune potentiators by enhancing the basal level of immune response and in immunocompromised patients it acts as immunotherapeutic agent. Mechanistically, they act by increasing humoral antibody response, by enhancing phagocytic action of macrophages or by modulating cell-mediated immune response. Immunostimulants are classified under two major categories as follows:

1. **Specific immunostimulants**: These act by stimulating the body immune function specifically toward antigen injected to patients, such as vaccines or antigens.
2. **Nonspecific immunostimulants**: These augment the immune response nonspecifically without antigenic specificity, for example, adjuvants and immunostimulators. Many endogenous cell metabolites are nonspecific immunostimulators, for example, female sex hormones are known to stimulate both adaptive and innate immune responses. Some autoimmune diseases such as lupus erythematosus strike women preferentially, and their onset often coincides with puberty. Other hormones appear to regulate the immune system as well, most notably vitamin D, prolactin, and growth hormone.

On the basis of their source of origin and mechanism of action, they are classified as immunoenhancing drugs, bacterial products, complex carbohydrates, vaccines (adjuvants and antigens), recombinant cytokines, colony-stimulating factors, nutritional factors, animal extracts, and plant extracts (**Fig. 82.6**).

Classification of Immunostimulants Based on Their Origin

1. **Immunostimulatory drugs**: levamisole, thalidomide, lenalidomide, immunocyanin, bestatin, isoprinosine.
2. **Bacterial products**: bacillus Calmette–Guérin (BCG) vaccine.
3. **Recombinant cytokines**: interferon α-2b (IFN α-2b), IFN-b1, IFN-γ, IL-2.
4. **Complex carbohydrates**: prebiotics, glucans, trehalose.
5. **Animal-originated immunostimulants**: chitin, chitosan.
6. **Plant-derived immunostimulants**: flavonoids, pigments, phenolics, steroids, alkaloids, and terpenoids.

Immunostimulant Drugs

Levamisole

It is a synthetic drug, which is an active L-isomer of tetramisole, initially developed to treat nematode diseases such as ascariasis and ancylostomiasis. It mainly produces its action by raising cyclic guanosine monophosphate (c-GMP) levels through interaction with thymopoietin receptor sites, leading to decrease in metabolic inactivation of c-GMP along with increased breakdown of cyclic adenosine monophosphate (c-AMP). Raised level of c-GMP stimulates lymphocyte proliferation and augmentation of chemotactic response. This altogether causes increased phagocytosis, antibody, and lymphokine production that ultimately enhances the host immunity.

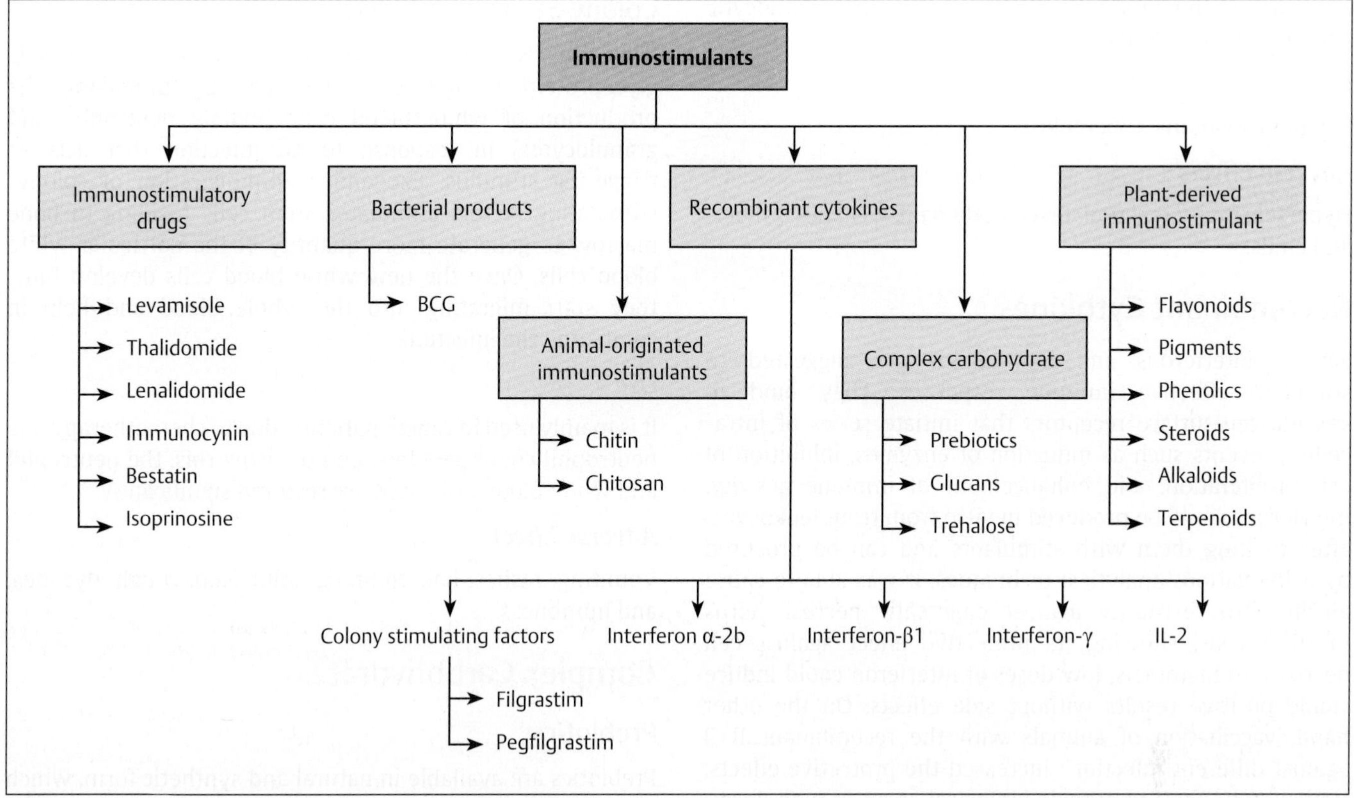

Fig. 82.6 Schematic classification of immunostimulant drugs.

Use

It is used as an adjuvant with 5-fluorouracil for the treatment of colon cancer, malignant tumors, ulcers, dermatological disorders, recurrent herpes, and rheumatoid arthritis.

Adverse Effects

Nausea, muscle pain, abdominal pain, allergy, fatigue, lightheadedness, and agranulocytosis.

Thalidomide

Thalidomide, which is chemically related to barbiturates, was introduced in 1958 for morning sickness and banned in 1960 due to its highly teratogenic property that caused phocomelia in newborn babies. However, it made a comeback into the market with new applications, of which immunomodulatory potential is a major claim. It sensitizes immune system by decreasing TNF-α level, reducing phagocytosis by neutrophils and IL-2 modulation, and enhancing cell-mediated immunity through T-cells. These cumulatively result in its anti-inflammatory effect as well. It also blocks the synthesis of prostaglandins via inhibition of COX-2 that inhibits angiogenesis, which retards tumor growth. It is also prescribed as adjuvant for tumor malignancies. Lenalidomide, which is a derivative of thalidomide, is used for multiple myeloma and myelodysplastic syndrome. It also has teratogenic property.

Use

It is the drug of choice in symptomatic treatment of moderate-to-severe erythema nodosum leprosum, refractory cutaneous lupus lesions, Crohn's disease, treatment of cachexia, and weight loss in HIV.

Adverse Effect

It causes nausea, vomiting and anorexia, hypothyroidism, peripheral neuropathy, teratogenic potential, mood changes, and tremors.

Isoprinosine

It stimulates the production of cytokines such as IL-1, IL-2, and IFN-γ by increasing the proliferation of lymphocytes. It has been also reported that it increases the numbers of IgM/IgG spleen antibody-forming cells in response to mitogenic or antigenic stimuli that collaborate to its immune-strengthening property.

Bacterial Products

Bacillus Calmette–Guérin

It is sourced from bacillus of Calmette and Guérin strain of *Mycobacterium bovis* and was discovered by Robert Koch in 1882 for the treatment of tuberculosis. It is available as live unlyophilized or killed lyophilized form. It is a nonspecific immunoenhancer, which is used to stimulate intact immune system of the body. BCG and its methanolic extract filtrate have muramyl dipeptide as an active immunostimulant. T and B lymphocytes are principal target cells for the action of BCG vaccine. It stimulates macrophage function, improves phagocytic activity, lysosomal enzyme activity, and chemotaxis mechanisms, which induce the production of lymphocyte activity factor, resulting in induction of a granulomatous reaction at the site of administration. It is active against tumor antigen and is found beneficial in the treatment of lung and breast cancer and acute lymphocytic and myelogenous leukemia.

Use

Bladder carcinoma, tuberculosis.

Adverse Effects

Hypersensitivity reaction, fever, body pain, weakness, shock, and chills.

Recombinant Cytokines

Several interferons and interleukins are suggested to stimulate effective immune responses. They bind to specific cell-surface receptors that initiate series of intra-cellular events such as induction of enzymes, inhibition of cell proliferation, and enhancement of immune activity. Interferons could be produced in vitro from trout leukocytes after treating them with stimulants and can be procured by using various analytical techniques. It was able to cause an in vitro resistance against pancreatic necrosis virus in trout cells, showing its protective effect against cell necrosis. In mammals, low doses of interferon could induce stable positive results without side effects. On the other hand, vaccination of animals with the recombinant IL-2 against different infections increased the protective effects. However, IL-2 is a very toxic biological agent in high doses, causing side effects such as fever and diarrhea.

Interferon α-2b

This is a low-molecular-weight glycoprotein cytokine produced by host cells in response to viral infections. They produce immunomodulatory activity by binding to cell-surface receptors. This in turn triggers intracellular events such as enzyme induction and inhibition of cell proliferation. Additionally, they also affect viral replication, and protect against respiratory syncytial virus, influenza virus, and herpes simplex virus.

Use

Hairy cell leukemia, malignant melanoma, hepatitis B, and viral infection.

Adverse Effect

Hypotension, arrhythmia, flulike symptoms (fever, chills, headache), depression, confusion, and dizziness.

Interleukin

It is a protein that regulates the activities of white blood cells, which play a critical role in immune system. IL-2 is a part of the body's natural response to microbial infection and in discriminating between foreign and self.

Use

Metastatic RCC, melanoma, toxicity, hypotension.

Adverse Effects

The interleukin-2 infusion (the high dose regimen) can cause a reaction that may include low blood pressure, increased heart rate or arrhythmias, shortness of breath, rash, nausea, diarrhea, and joint and muscle stiffness.

Colony-Stimulating Factors

Filgrastim is a classic example of this subclass that is glycoprotein in nature, which acts by provoking the production of white blood cells (mainly neutrophil and granulocytes) in response to an infection that acts as triggering stimulus. Exogenous administration of colony-stimulating factors stimulates stem cells residing in bone marrow to generate more quantity of the particular white blood cells. Once the new white blood cells develop fully, they start migrating into the whole blood and help in combating the infection.

Use

It is mainly used in cancer patients; due to chemotherapy, the neutrophil count gets low, and by using this, the neutrophil and white blood cell count are restored significantly.

Adverse Effect

Vomiting, rashes, hair thinning, joint pain, cough, dyspnea, and numbness.

Complex Carbohydrates

Prebiotics

Prebiotics are available in natural and synthetic form, which are marketed as food products with indigestible fibers that boost beneficial gut commensal bacteria, resulting in improvement of the host's overall health. Prebiotics, such as mannan-oligosaccharide, insulin, fructo-oligosaccharide, and β-glucan, are called immunosaccharides. They produce their action by inducing phagocytic mechanism and neutrophil activation, activating the alternative complement system, and augmenting the lysozyme activity. Immunosaccharides directly activate the innate immunity by interaction with pattern recognition receptors, which are expressed on innate immune cells. They may also react with microbe-associated molecular patterns to stimulate innate immune cells.

Animal-Origin Immunostimulants

Animal-based immunostimulants have potent antigenic potential that stimulates the host immune system, which results in the release of defensive biochemical messengers inside the body. Based on this property, they are interestingly used in immunopharmacology. The typical examples of this class are chitin and chitosan, which are obtained from exoskeleton of arthropods and the cell walls of fungi. Chitosan, the deacetylated derivative of chitin, has shown strong antimicrobial activity, depending on its degree of deacetylation and molecular weight. Both oligomers of chitin and chitosan were effective in enhancing the migratory activity of macrophages. Furthermore, chitosan could activate the production of cytokines, and now chitosan is being employed in nanoparticle-based formulation due to its different therapeutic properties.

Plant-derived Immunostimulants

Plant and plant-based products are vital source for many phytoconstituents such as alkaloids, flavonoids, pigments, phenolics, terpenoids, steroids, and essential oils, which have proven pharmacological action in different diseases such as cardiac complications, cancer, diabetes, inflammation, epilepsy, and many more. Besides their application in the treatment of different diseases, they are also used to boost the immune power of the body. Medicinal plants have been known to be immunostimulant and growth promoters, where they act as antibacterial and antiviral agents to the host immune system, but the mechanism behind their immunostimulant action is unexplored. Leaves and seeds of *Ocimum sanctum* (*tulsi*) contains water-soluble phenolic compounds and various other constituents that may act as an immunostimulant by specific and nonspecific mode of action. Leaves extract of *O. sanctum* affects both specific and nonspecific immune responses. It stimulates both antibody response and neutrophil activity. It has been also observed that the immunostimulant action might act directly on the immunopoietic cells to enhance immunity. *Phyllanthus emblica* (*amla*) has rich antioxidant, antiemetic, antifungal, antiseptic, antimicrobial, and anti-inflammatory activities. *Amla* fruit pulp contains a large amount of vitamin C, which works as potent antioxidant that scavenges the reactive oxygen species and acts as an immunostimulant. Likewise, there are many plant-based products such as *ashwagandha, shilajeet, sarpagandha,* black pepper, cardamom, ginger, and turmeric that have been reported to be used as immunostimulants, but due to lack of toxicity profile and bioavailability data, their use in clinical application is challenging.

Multiple Choice Questions

1. A 45-year-old female patient was presented with rheumatoid arthritis. Suggest a drug that is both immunosuppressive and anti-inflammatory:

A. Cyclosporine.
B. Azathioprine.
C. Methotrexate.
D. Sirolimus.

Answer: C

Methotrexate has both immunosuppressive and anti-inflammatory action by increasing adenosine, an endogenous anti-inflammatory mediator.

2. A 58-year-old executive suffering from inflammatory bowel disease (IBD) was presented for treatment. The most likely candidate drug with immunosuppressant activity will be:

A. Azathioprine.
B. Leflunomide.
C. Methotrexate.
D. Anakinra.

Answer: A

Azathioprine is used in IBD.

3. A drug with hitherto teratogenic properties and now repurposed in the treatment of systemic lupus erythematosus is:

A. Cyclosporine.
B. Thalidomide.
C. Leflunomide.
D. Mycophenolate.

Answer: B

Thalidomide is a derivative of glutamic acid, with sedative and antiemetic activity, introduced in the 1950s as a sedative for its rapid action and apparent safety. However, teratogenicity of the drug was described, estimating that 5,000 to 6,000 children suffered phocomelia secondary to its use during pregnancy. It was demonstrated in 1965 to possess beneficial effects on erythema nodosum leprosum. Since then, there have been progressively more studies demonstrating the immunomodulatory and anti-inflammatory effect of thalidomide and its possible application in immune-mediated inflammatory diseases and skin disorders such as chronic refractory prurigo nodularis, *erythema multiforme*, Behçet's syndrome, and cutaneous lupus erythematosus (CLE).

4. A 54-year-old woman diagnosed with carcinoma of the mammary gland. Which of the following colony-stimulating factors is/are likely to be prescribed?

A. OKT-3.
B. Filgrastim.
C. Thalidomide.
D. Fingolimod.

Answer. B

The cytotoxicity of chemotherapeutic drugs results in neutropenia. Filgrastim restores white blood cell count and improves neutrophil count.

5. Which of the following drugs should be prescribed as an adjuvant along with 5-FU for a patient with colon cancer?

A. Methotrexate.
B. Levamisole.
C. Leflunomide.
D. Cyclosporine.

Answer: B

Levamisole is an anthelminthic and immunostimulant prescribed along with 5-FU.

Chapter 83 Vaccines and Sera

Arshiya Sehgal and Vijay Kumar Sehgal

PH1.54: Describe vaccine and their uses.

Learning Objectives

- Vaccines.
- Antisera.
- Immunoglobulins.

Common Terms

- Vaccine—It is a biological product that acts as an antigen and is used to stimulate the production of antibodies without induction of disease. They impart active immunity.
- Serum—The clear liquid that can be separated from clotted blood.
- Antiserum—A blood serum containing antibodies against specific antigens, which is injected to treat or protect against specific diseases. It imparts passive immunity.
- Toxin—A poison of plant or animal origin, especially one produced by or derived from microorganisms and acting as an antigen in the body.
- Antitoxin—An antibody that counteracts toxin.
- Herd immunity—Herd immunity is the indirect protection from a contagious infectious disease that occurs when a population is immune either through vaccination or through immunity developed through previous infection. Once herd immunity has been established for a while, and the ability of the disease to spread is hindered as buffer is created between infected and normal individual, the disease can eventually be eliminated, for example, smallpox.

Role of Immune System

Vaccines and sera act by modulating the immune mechanism of the body. Immunology is the study of how normal body defenses resist and overcome invasion from infectious agents and foreign substances. Vaccination has made an enormous contribution to global health. Two major infections, smallpox and rinderpest, have been eradicated. Global coverage of vaccination against many important infectious diseases of childhood has been enhanced dramatically since the creation of the World Health Organization's (WHO's) Expanded Programme on Immunization in 1974 and the Global Alliance for Vaccines and Immunization in 2000. Polio has almost been eradicated, and success in controlling measles makes this infection another potential target for eradication. The WHO suggests that vaccination prevents 2 to 3 million deaths each year. For many essential vaccines, coverage is now much higher than 80%. However, the rates of vaccination are still not sufficient. The coverage of the first dose of diphtheria–pertussis–tetanus (DPT) vaccine was 90%, indicating that 13.5 million children were not vaccinated in 2018. When foreign substances invade the human body and breach the host's natural barriers such as skin, then the innate immunity plays its role. If still the pathogen is not controlled, then the specific defense system plays its role.

Specific defenses can be divided into:

1. Active immunity:
   a. Humoral immunity.
   b. Cellular immunity.
   c. Combination.
2. Passive immunity:
   a. Normal human immunoglobulins.
   b. Animal antitoxins or antisera.

Active Immunity

Active immunity is developed due to infection or by specific immunization. It is specific for a particular disease. It depends on humoral and cellular responses of host. It can be acquired in three ways:

1. By clinical infection; for example, chickenpox, rubella, and measles.
2. By subclinical or inapparent infection; for example, polio and diphtheria.
3. By immunization with antigen.

Humoral Immunity

It is mediated by B-cells (bone marrow-derived lymphocytes). After antigen presentation by macrophages, B-cells proliferate and produce specific antibodies. These antibodies are immunoglobulins—IgG, IgM, IgA, IgD, and IgE—which act directly by neutralizing the microbe and making it susceptible to polymorphonuclear leucocyte and monocyte. IgM is initially secreted, and after some days, IgG, which has enhanced neutralizing capacity, is secreted. IgA is concentrated in mucous secretions, breast milk, and tears. IgE is important in the elimination of parasitic infections. IgG antibodies are the targets of vaccine design, as they undergo rigorous selection process. Once the pathogen is eliminated during primary response, pathogen-specific B- and T-cells survive long term—sometimes, for the entire life of the host as memory B- and T-cells. When reinfection occurs, memory cells use their specific antigen receptors to recognize the pathogen. This results in their activation, and they directly kill infected cells or generate antibodies that will neutralize the pathogen. Vaccine works on this principle, so uninfected individuals are given controlled infection and memory B- and T-cells neutralize the microbe.

Cellular Immunity

When infection is not controlled by humoral response or pathogen (e.g., *Mycobacterium leprae, Mycobacterium tuberculosis, Candida albicans*), cellular immunity plays a role. When an antigen comes in contact with body, a chain of responses is initiated by T-cells; for example, macrophage's activation and release, then release of cytotoxic factors, mononuclear inflammatory reaction and delayed hypersensitivity reactions. $CD4^+$ T-cells stimulate B-cells to produce antibodies. $CD8^+$ T-cells kill infected cells.

Combination

B- and T-cells work together with macrophages and human T-cells. They together constitute complex events of immunity. Antibody-dependent cell-mediated cytotoxic cells recognize membrane viral antigens through specific antibody. Natural killer (NK) cells destroy nonspecific virus-infected target cells.

Disorders of Immunological Function

It includes hypersensitivity reaction, autoimmunity, and transplant rejection.

Hypersensitivity Reaction

Hypersensitivity is an immunological state in which the immune system "overreacts" to foreign antigen such that the immune response itself is more harmful than the antigen. All types of hypersensitivity involve the adaptive immune response, that is, highly specific reactions via T- or B-cells and prior exposure to the antigen.

Types of Hypersensitivity Reaction

Type 1 (Allergic Reactions)

It involves the activation of mast cells or basophils through the binding of antigen to IgE on the cell surface, which triggers the release of histamine, prostaglandins, and leukotrienes. The release of these mediators causes redness, swelling, itching, mucus, etc., which characterize allergic reactions. It includes hives in the skin, mucus, sneezing, and anaphylactic shock by animal venoms or certain foods.

Type 2 (Cytotoxic Reaction)

It involves destruction of cells bound by IgG or IgM antibodies via the activation of complement, and destroys the target cell. It takes 5 to 12 hours to develop this reaction, for example, blood transfusion (ABO blood group incompatibility) and Rh incompatibility.

Type 3 (Immune Complex)

This is caused by high levels of antigen–antibody complexes (due to foreign or self-antigen) that are not cleared efficiently by phagocytes and tend to deposit in certain tissues and blood vessel endothelium in kidneys, lungs, and joints. This can result in local cell damage via complement activation, attraction of phagocytes, and other cells involved in inflammation (e.g., neutrophils), for example, Arthus reaction and serum sickness.

Type 4 (Delayed Hypersensitivity)

In this, antigens activate T_C cells that kill target cells, for example, reaction of transplanted tissue, poison ivy, and tuberculosis.

Autoimmunity

Autoimmunity refers to the generation of an immune response to self-antigens. Normally, T-cells with receptors that bind self-antigens are eliminated in the thymus, and B-cells with antibodies that bind self-antigens are eliminated or rendered anergic in the bone marrow or even in the periphery. However, in rare cases, T- and/or B-cells that recognize self-antigens survive and are activated; for example, type 1 diabetes mellitus, lupus, rheumatoid arthritis, and multiple sclerosis.

Transplant Rejection

Transplanted organs and tissues are rejected as foreign by the immune system due to the presence of nonself major histocompatibility complex (MHC) class I molecules. The recipient has no tolerance to donor MHC: recipient T-cells that bind strongly to donor MHC molecules and recognize their target antigen that is presented by MHC class II molecules. This leads to major cytotoxic T-lymphocytes (CTLs) attacking and killing donor cells, activating B-cells and producing donor MHC-specific antibodies.

Passive Immunity

It involves transfer of preformed antibodies from immune individual to nonimmune individual to confer temporary immunity. For example:

1. Maternal antibodies are transferred across the placenta. Human milk contains IgA, which is protective in nature.
2. Infection of antivenom antibodies in neutralization of venom toxin.

Passive immunity is beneficial if after active immunization, the host cannot form antibodies or who takes time to form antibodies.

Table 83.1 highlights the differences between active and passive immunity.

Vaccines

A vaccine is an immunobiological substance that stimulates a person's immune system to produce immunity to a specific disease, protecting the person from that disease. Effective vaccines activate both innate and adaptive immune system. There are three types of vaccines:

1. Live attenuated.
2. Killed or inactivated.
3. Subunit vaccines:
   a. Polysaccharide.
   b. Surface protein.
   c. Toxoids.

Live Attenuated

It uses a weakened virus that contains antigens that stimulate immune response. These organisms retain their immunogenicity, but they do not cause disease. Memory cells are developed after repeated doses.

Table 83.1 Differentiation between active and passive immunity

Active immunity	Passive immunity
It is acquired because of infection or by specific immunization. It is specific for a particular disease	It involves transfer of preformed antibodies from immune individual to nonimmune individual to confer temporary immunity
It takes time to develop	It takes less time to develop
It is long-lasting	It is short-living
Efficacy is more	Efficacy is less
Severe reactions are rare	Severe reactions are more
It is less expensive	It is more expensive
Examples include vaccine	Examples include antisera and immunoglobulins

For example, bacillus Calmette–Guérin (BCG), measles, oral polio, mumps, cholera, varicella, rubella, yellow fever, and rotavirus.

The advantage of live vaccines is that they are more efficient as they provide lifelong immunity. Disadvantages of live vaccines include: (1) they must be refrigerated to retain their activity; (2) they cannot be utilized in immunocompromised individuals (cancer, HIV, corticosteroids); and (3) pregnancy is another contraindication.

Inactivated/Killed Vaccines

Pathogens are killed by heat, chemicals, or radiations, but they retain their immunogenicity. They usually require two or three doses to produce adequate antibodies and "booster" injections are required.

For example, typhoid, cholera, plague, pertussis, influenza, inactivated poliomyelitis vaccine, rabies, and Japanese encephalitis.

Advantages of these vaccines are that: (1) they can be freeze-dried and transported without refrigeration; (2) they are killed vaccines and hence can be given in immunodeficient individuals; and (3) they are highly stable. Disadvantages of these vaccines include: (1) multiple doses are required and (2) they are less efficacious.

Subunit Vaccines

In this, component of a microorganism is used as vaccine antigen to mimic exposure to the organism. The advantage is that they are relatively safe. The disadvantage is that they are less efficacious, as immunity is not guaranteed.

Polysaccharide Vaccine

This vaccine utilizes polysaccharide antigen to induce an immune response. Bacterial cell wall contains a polysaccharide, which acts as a target of host immune response. Antibodies to polysaccharide clear the bacteria by complement-mediated killing and opsonophagocytosis, for example, pneumococcus, meningococcus, *Haemophilus influenzae* B (HiB), and typhoid.

The advantage of this vaccine is that it provides more long-term protection in young children and adults. The disadvantage is that immune response is serotype specific.

Conjugate vaccines are vaccines such as polysaccharide vaccines, but antigens are recognized by T-cells—chemically linked to protein. They are serotype-specific, for example, streptococcal, pneumococcal, and meningococcal.

Toxoids

Some organisms such as *Clostridium tetani* and *Corynebacterium diphtheriae* produce exotoxins. Therefore, vaccines against toxins are called toxoid vaccines. Antibodies are produced that neutralize toxic moiety produced during infection, for example, diphtheria, tetanus, acellular pertussis, anthrax, and influenza subunit. The advantage is that it is safe, since inactivated toxin is used as immunogen.

Surface Protein Subunit Vaccine

In this, immune response is produced by purified proteins from the pathogen. Since these proteins may not be presented in natural form, antibodies may not bind efficiently to live pathogen, for example, acellular pertussis and hepatitis B.

Recombinant Protein Vaccine

In this type of vaccine, with the help of recombinant deoxyribonucleic acid, protective protein antigens in heterologous expression system such as mammalian cells and yeast are expressed—for example, hepatitis B virus (HBV), Lyme disease, cholera toxin B, and human papilloma virus (HPV). The advantage is that it is safe. The disadvantage is that there is reduced immunogenicity, which may require addition of adjuvant.

Combined Vaccine

Combined vaccine is a vaccine which has more than one kind of immunizing agent—for example, DPT, diphtheria–tetanus (DT), measles–mumps–rubella (MMR).

Immunization Schedule of Children, Adults, and Pregnant Women

Vaccines that can be given after discussion with parents (**Table 83.2**):

1. Varicella—15 months (or after 1 year).

Table 83.2 National immunization schedule

Vaccine	Due age	Maximum age	Dose	Route	Site
For pregnant women					
TT-1	Early in pregnancy		0.5 mL	Intramuscular	Upper arm
TT-2	4 wk after TT-1		0.5 mL	Intramuscular	Upper arm
TT booster	If TT doses in a pregnancy within the last 3 y received		0.5 mL	Intramuscular	Upper arm
For infants					
BCG	At birth	Till 1 y	0.05 mL until 1 mo 0.1 mL beyond age 1 mo	Intradermal	Upper arm—left
Hepatitis B	At birth	Within 24 h	0.5 mL	Intramuscular	Anterolateral side of midthigh—left
OPV 0	At birth	Within 15 d	Two drops	Oral	Oral
OPV 1, 2, 3	At 6, 10, 14 wk	Till 5 y	Two drops	Oral	Oral
Pentavalent 1, 2, and 3 (diphtheria + pertussis + tetanus + hepatitis B + HiB)	At 6, 10, 14 wk	1 y of age	0.5 mL	Intramuscular	Anterolateral Side of midthigh—left
Fractional IPV	At 6 and 14 wk	1 y of age	0.1 mL	Intradermal	Upper arm—right
Rotavirus (where applicable)	At 6, 10, and 14 wk	1 y of age	Five drops	Oral	Oral
PCV	At 6 and 14 wk At 9 completed months—booster	1 y of age	0.5 mL	Intramuscular	Anterolateral side of thigh—right
Measles/rubella (first dose)	At 9 completed months to 12 mo	5 y of age	0.5 mL	Subcutaneous	Upper arm—right
Japanese encephalitis 1	9–12 mo	15 y of age	0.5 mL	Subcutaneous	Upper arm—left
Vitamin A (first dose)	At 9 mo	5 y of age	1 mL	Oral	Oral
For children					
DPT booster 1	16–24 mo	7 y of age	0.5 mL	Intramuscular	Anterolateral side of midthigh—left
Measles/rubella (second dose)	16–24 mo	5 y of age	0.5mL	Subcutaneous	Upper arm—right
OPV booster	16–24 mo	5 y of age	2 drops	Oral	Oral
Japanese encephalitis 2 (where applicable)	16–24 mo	Till 15 y of age	0.5 mL	Subcutaneous	Upper arm—left
Vitamin A (second–ninth dose)	At 16 mo, then 1 dose every 6 mo	Up to 5 y of age	2 mL	Oral	Oral
DPT booster 2	5–6 y	7 y of age	0.5 mL	Intramuscular	Upper arm
TT	10 and 16 y	16 y	0.5 mL	Intramuscular	Upper arm

Abbreviations: BCG, bacillus Calmette–Guérin; DPT, diphtheria, pertussis, tetanus; HiB, *Haemophilus influenzae* B; IPV, inactivated polio vaccine; OPV, oral polio vaccine; PCV, pneumococcal conjugate vaccine; TT, tetanus toxoid.

2. Hepatitis A—high-risk infants, 18 months and 6 months later.
3. Pneumococcal conjugate vaccine—6 weeks.
4. Influenza vaccine—6 months to high-risk infants annually.

Vaccines for Bacteria

BCG Vaccine

1. It is live attenuated vaccine.
2. It is used to prevent disease due to *M. tuberculosis*.
3. Given by intradermal route to infants at the time of birth.
4. Dose—0.05 mL for neonate and 0.1 mL for older individual.
5. Site—left deltoid region.

Before immunization, tuberculin testing is done in children and adults, and it is given to negative responders. In 7 to 10 days, papule of 8 mm appears; in 5 weeks, swelling of axillary lymph node occurs; thereafter, it may ulcerate, but it later scales and dries in 3 months, and is restored in 6 months.

Precaution: Tuberculin sensitivity test is a must to prevent hypersensitivity reaction.

Typhoid Vaccine (MI3.3)

Typhoid is an acute illness caused by *Salmonella typhi*. Three types of vaccines are as follows:

Typhoid–Paratyphoid A, B (TAB Vaccine)

TAB vaccine is a suspension containing *S. typhi* and *Salmonella paratyphi*. The recommended dose is 0.5 mL subcutaneously, two to three injections at an interval of 2 to 4 weeks. Adverse effects include local tenderness, fever, and malaise. It protects from enteric fever for up to 1 year.

V Typhoid Polysaccharide Vaccine

It contains purified Vi capsular antigen of *S. typhi*. However, it offers no protection against *S. paratyphi*. It is given at a dose of 0.5 mL subcutaneously or intramuscularly. Adverse effects are less than TAB vaccine. It is contraindicated in children younger than 2 years and also in pregnant women.

Typhoid-Typ21a Oral Vaccine

It is a live vaccine prepared from Vi polysaccharide lacking Typ21 strain of *S. typhi*, which is nonpathogenic. Three doses are given on alternate days in the form of capsules. Side effects include diarrhea, abdominal pain, and rashes. The advantage is that it is convenient, safer, and long-acting.

Whooping Cough (Pertussis) Vaccine

It is a killed/inactivated vaccine containing *Bordetella pertussis* organism. The recommended dose is 0.25 to 0.5 mL subcutaneously or intramuscularly three times at a 4-week interval in infants and children younger than 5 years. Side effects include local pain, induration, high fever, and hypotonic-hyporesponsive child.

Toxoid Vaccines

Tetanus Toxoid Vaccine

Tetanus is caused by *C. tetani*, which enters host through wounds. Tetanus toxin inhibits the inhibitory neurotransmitter from the nerve cells and results in uninhibited skeletal muscle contraction. There are two types of preparation–fluid toxoid and adsorbed toxoid. The recommended dose is 0.5 mL intramuscularly or subcutaneously. For primary immunization, two doses 4 to 6 weeks apart are to be given. Booster is given after 1 year and then at every 10 years. In nonimmunized, it is to be given after every injury. Side effects include local erythema, pain, fever, chills, malaise, and pain.

Diphtheria Toxoid Vaccine

Diphtheria is caused by *C. diphtheriae* toxin, which damages the myelin sheath in the nervous system, leading to loss of sensation or motor control. The throat becomes swollen. The vaccine is indicated in infants and children younger than 6 years. For primary immunization, the recommended dose is 0.5 mL, via intramuscular injection two to three times 4 to 6 weeks apart. Booster dose to be given after 1 year and then at school entry.

Mixed Antigens

Double Antigen (DT-DA)

A 0.5-mL ampule consists of toxoids of tetanus and diphtheria. It is given at a dose of 0.5 mL intramuscularly and is indicated in children older than 5 years.

Triple Antigen (DPT)

It is a mixture comprising toxoids of tetanus and diphtheria along with pertussis vaccine. It is given at a dose of 0.5 mL intramuscularly on the anterolateral aspect of midthigh or right deltoid. It is indicated at 3 to 9 months and at 18 months.

Pentavalent Vaccine

It contains toxoids of tetanus and diphtheria along with pertussis vaccine, HBV, and HiB vaccine. The recommended dose is 0.5 mL intramuscularly. It is indicated at 6, 10, and 14 weeks. It reduces the total number of infections.

Other vaccines are meningococcal vaccine, antiplaque vaccine, and *H. influenzae* vaccine.

Vaccines for Viruses

Poliovirus Vaccine

Polio is characterized by acute flaccid paralysis. There are two types of vaccine.

Oral Poliovirus Vaccine (Sabin Vaccine)

It is a live attenuated vaccine produced in monkey kidney cell culture. It provides active immunity in the intestine. The recommended dose is two drops directly in the mouth. It is indicated at birth and at 6, 10, and 14 weeks. Booster is given between 15 and 18 months and at school entry. It is contraindicated in vomiting and diarrhea.

Inactivated Poliomyelitis Vaccine (Salk Vaccine)

It induces humoral immunity. Three doses of 1 mL are given subcutaneously in the deltoid region at 4- to 6-week interval. The fourth dose is given 6 to 12 months later. Booster is given every 5 years. It is indicated in adults. Adverse effects include fever and local pain.

Rabies Vaccine

Lyssavirus transmits rabies from bite of infected mammals. Three types of vaccines are used: purified chick embryo vaccine, human diploid vaccine, and purified new cell rabies vaccine.

Use as Preexposure Prophylaxis

Rabies vaccine is used among veterinary doctors, animal handlers, spelunkers or laboratory workers involved in production of rabies biological. It is given at a dose of 0.1 mL intradermally. It is indicated at 0, 7, and 28 days. Booster can be given to those who are repeatedly exposed to rabies.

Postexposure Prophylaxis in Nonimmunized

It is used in emergency situations following a bite or close exposure to animal, for example, rats. According to the WHO regimen, wound washing, and post-exposure prophylaxis should be instituted immediately. For postexposure prophylaxis, human rabies immunoglobulin and cell culture– or embryonated egg–based rabies vaccines should always be used. Intramuscular or intradermal is the route of administration.

Intramuscular Regimens

For postexposure vaccination, a five-dose and a four-dose intramuscular regimens are recommended, but the five-dose regimen is more commonly used:

1. The five-dose regimen: It is administered on days 0, 3, 7, 14, and 28 into the deltoid muscle.
2. The four-dose regimen: It is administered as two doses on day 0 on the right and left deltoid, and then one dose each on days 7 and 21 into the deltoid muscle.

For people who are previously exposed, previously immunized, healthy, and who were able to get wound care immediately. rabies immunoglobulin and WHO-prequalified rabies vaccines are administered intramuscularly on days 0, 3, 7, and 14.

Intradermal Regimens

In developing countries unable to afford five- or four-dose intramuscular schedules, intradermal administration of cell culture– and embryonated egg–based rabies vaccines has been used. One intradermal injection of 0.5 mL is administered at two sites on days 0, 3, 7, and 28.

Hepatitis A Vaccine

Hepatitis A is caused by fecal–oral route. It causes acute liver disease. The vaccine is an inactivated/killed one. The dose is 0.5 mL and is administered intramuscularly. It is indicated for children at 1 year of age; booster is given at 6 months. It is contraindicated if there is allergic reaction to any vaccine component.

Hepatitis B Vaccine

HBV causes hepatitis B, cirrhosis, and hepatocellular cancer. Contact with body fluids and sexual contact are modes of transmission. The vaccine is prepared by recombinant DNA technique in yeast cells. The recommended dose is 1 mL, given intramuscularly in the deltoid. It is indicated at 0,1, and 6 months. Adverse effects include fever, malaise, and induration. A neonate whose mother has active infection is treated with the vaccine and hepatitis B immunoglobulin.

Measles–Mumps–Rubella (MMR) Vaccine

It is a live attenuated vaccine. It is given as a single dose over the right deltoid subcutaneously. It is indicated in children older than 12 months. Adverse effects include fever, rash, and swelling of lymph nodes and parotid glands. It is contraindicated in pregnancy.

Measles Vaccine

It is a live attenuated vaccine containing 1000 $TCID_{50}$ of Edmonston–Schwartz strain or Edmonston–Zagreb strain. It is administered as a single subcutaneous dose over the right deltoid. No booster is required, as immunity lasts for 8 years. It is indicated in children older than 9 months. It is contraindicated in children who have a history of febrile convulsions or whose parents have a history of epilepsy. Adverse effects include fever, rash, and coryza.

Mumps Vaccine

Mumps is a disease of the parotid glands. The vaccine is a live attenuated one. A single dose is given. Measles, mumps, and rubella vaccines are administered together. Mild febrile reaction is an adverse effect.

Rubella Vaccine

Rubella is transmitted through respiratory droplets. It is harmful only to fetuses. During pregnancy, it causes miscarriage, preterm, stillbirth, or various birth defects. A dose of 0.5 mL of the vaccine is administered subcutaneously or intramuscularly. It is indicated from 1 year to puberty. It is contraindicated in pregnancy and febrile illness. Adverse drug reactions include fever, malaise, throat and joint pain, and enlargement of lymph nodes.

Human Papilloma Virus Vaccine

HPVs cause cervical and anal cancer. The vaccine protects against vaginal and vulvar cancer in women, and against genital warts and anal cancer in both men and women. It is indicated in those who are older than 11 and 12 years, women between 13 and 26 years, and men who are 13 to 21 years. It is given through a three-dose regimen at 0, 1, 2, and 6 months.

Influenza Virus Vaccine

It is available in two forms: injection and nasal form. Injection contains inactivated influenza virus A and B. It is given by intramuscular route. The recommended dose is 0.5 to 1 mL via two injections 1 to 2 months apart. It is indicated in all persons older than 6 months, infants, young children, pregnant women, and immunodeficient persons. Nasal spray contains trivalent or quadrivalent live attenuated virus vaccine. It is indicated in persons 2 to 49 years old. It is contraindicated in patients with life-threatening allergic reaction.

New Vaccines

Dengue Virus Vaccine

Dengue is a mosquito-borne flavivirus disease. It is characterized by mild systemic illness and can cause death. There is currently no dengue vaccine approved but CYD-TDV developed by Sanofi Pasteur is a recombinant live vaccine used in individuals of 9 to 45 years of age. It is given in three doses at 0, 6, and 12 months.

Malaria Vaccine

It is a recombinant protein-based vaccine with AS01 (comprised of liposomes,3-o-desacycl-4'mono phosphoryl lipid A(MPL) and QS-21 (Quilleja saponaria extract) adjuvant against *Plasmodium falciparum*. It is under trials and has completed efficacy trial testing.

Coronavirus Vaccine

Due to the pandemic, many vaccines have been given emergency approval. In India, AstraZeneca, Oxford's Covishield (recombinant viral vector vaccine), Bharat Biotech's Covaxin (inactivated virus vaccine), Gamaleya Institute Moscow's Sputnik-V (recombinant viral vector vaccine), Moderna by USA (m-RNA vaccine) and Johnson &Johnson single-dose vaccine. Expected vaccines to be given approval in near future are Biological -E `S Corbevax and Serum Institute of India's Covovax.

Vaccine Adjuvants

Adjuvants are substances that are added to vaccine to elevate the immune response. Live attenuated vaccines usually do not contain adjuvants. Commonly used examples are aluminum salts. Approved adjuvants are as follows.

Antibiotics

They are used to prevent bacterial contamination of tissue culture, for example, neomycin in MMR vaccine.

Preservatives

These are added in a vial to prevent contamination from bacteria and fungi, for example, 2-phenoxyethanol, benzethonium chloride, phenol, and thimerosal.

Stabilizers

For confirming quality, a variety of compounds are added to control acidity, and stabilize antigens for preventing loss of immunogenicity, for example, potassium or sodium salts, lactose, human serum albumin, gelatin, and bovine serum albumin.

Vaccine Myths

There are several myths about the use of vaccines such as the following.

Vaccine Causes Autism

Some studies claimed that vaccination causes autism. Many studies in different parts of world with large cohorts and rigor found no evidence that vaccine causes autism.

Vaccines Causes Diseases

Common adverse effects include minor local reactions, such as pain, swelling, and redness, and systemic reactions, such as fever, rash, irritability, and drowsiness. Other adverse events are as follows.

Allergic Reaction

Allergy to component of vaccine formulation can cause itching, angioedema, breathlessness, and redness. It can cause anaphylactic shock. For example, patients allergic to eggs should not be given influenza vaccine.

Fainting

It is common after HPV and Tdap vaccination. It is triggered by pain or anxiety rather than the contents of vaccines. Head injury is a serious concern with regard to fainting.

Febrile Seizure

It can occur after MMR vaccine. It is characterized by fever of 102°F and body spasm and jerky movements. Viral infections such as roseola and ear infections can also cause febrile seizures.

Guillain–Barré Syndrome

Studies have shown that swine flu vaccine is associated with Guillain–Barré syndrome, which is characterized by muscle weakness and paralysis when one's own immune system injures the neurons.

Vaccine Causes Sudden Infant Death Syndrome

It peaks when babies are between 2 and 4 months. Although there was a temporal overlap of peak sudden infant death syndrome (SIDS) incidence and vaccination, numerous studies failed to detect any association of vaccines and SIDS.

Future of Vaccine Technology

There is dire need to improve vaccine technology, as the WHO reports that over 40% of deaths are caused by infectious diseases, highlighting the need to improve existing vaccines, develop new vaccines, and enhance delivery methods to increase efficacy. Viruses, bacteria, parasites, and antigens on cancerous cells are future vaccine targets. Pregnant and elderly people will have better access to vaccines. Investigations are under clinical trials for new edible vaccines using microneedles or dermal patches. Vaccines targeting both antibodies and T-cell responses are in the pipeline against chronic viral infections when the host is immunocompromised. In autoimmunity, the goal of vaccine is to dampen immune function to prevent self-destruction of tissue.

The Adverse Events Following Immunization (AEFI) Surveillance program is an integral immunization program in India to monitor vaccine safety in the postmarketing phase. The Indian AEFI program depends on passive surveillance and reporting by practitioners. In the last decade, there had been strengthening of AEFI surveillance, which resulted in escalation of AEFI reports in the country. Distinctive features of this program are the establishment of National AEFI Secretariat, National Technical Collaborating Centre, and development of risk communication strategy as well as quality management certification. Causality assessment of all serious AEFI reports is done by trained committees, according to WHO algorithm. The Vaccine Adverse Event Reporting System (VAERS) is cosponsored by Food and Drug Administration (FDA) and Centers for Disease Control and Prevention (CDC). Also, their official website is present, where physicians, nurses, and other health workers can report their adverse drug reports. Reporting of serious AEFIs is much less than expected, so it is the biggest challenging part of this program.

Antisera and Immunoglobulins

Antisera

These are readymade antibodies produced by nonhuman sources such as horses that have been immunized and transferred to recipient. They provide passive immunity. They are discussed in the following.

Tetanus Antitoxin

After injury, prophylactic dose of 1,500 units of horse antitetanus immunoglobulin or tetanus antitoxin (ATS) can be administered subcutaneously or intramuscularly.

Gas Gangrene Antitoxin

It is a polyvalent antitoxin, and it is used in wounds against *Clostridium perfringens* and *Clostridium septicum*. It is given as 30,000 to 750,000 IU subcutaneously, intravenously, and intramuscularly at a therapeutic dose.

Diphtheria Antitoxin

It is given in patients with diphtheria where it counteracts the exotoxin, which is discharged at the site of infection. It is given at a dose of 20,000 to 40,000 IU intramuscularly or intravenously for pharyngeal disease.

Antirabies Serum

It is a refined and concentrated serum that is given after suspected exposure. It is given intramuscularly at a dose of 40 IU/kg within 72 hours; it is best when given within 24 hours of exposure.

Antisnake Venom Polyvalent

It is given to patients after cobra bite or Russell's viper bite to neutralize the venom. It is given at a dose of 1 mL/min repeated at 1- to 6-hour intervals till symptoms disappear.

Adverse Effects

Immediate Anaphylactic Shock

It is characterized by urticaria, angioedema, breathlessness, increase in heart rate, and decrease in blood pressure. Treatment involves adrenaline (1:1,000 amp intramuscularly).

Serum Sickness

Serum sickness occurs 7 to 12 days later and is characterized by fever, rash, joint pain, and lymphadenopathy.

Immunoglobulins

To counter the adverse effects, human immunoglobulins are used. They have longer half-life and less adverse effects. Immunoglobulins are derived from humans who carry antibodies. They may be specific or nonspecific. Immunoglobulins can be prepared in the following ways.

Normal Human Gamma Globulin

It is a nonspecific, antibody-rich fraction obtained from a pool of 1,000 donors. It is used to prevent measles, hepatitis A, hepatitis B, poliomyelitis, and chickenpox. It can be given via the intravenous route. Live vaccine is not to be given for 12 weeks after normal human gamma globulin.

Anti-D Immune Globulin

It is an IgG antibody against Rh (d) antigen. It prevents antibody formation in Rh-negative individual. Indication is in avoidance of Rh hemolytic disease in future offspring by giving within 72 hours, and prevention of neonatal hemolytic jaundice at 28 weeks of pregnancy.

Tetanus Immune Globulin

It is given to nonimmunized individuals who get contaminated wound and can develop tetanus. It is efficacious and longer-acting. The recommended dose is 250 to 500 IU as prophylaxis and 3,000 to 6,000 IU intramuscularly as a therapeutic dose.

Rabies Immunoglobulin Human

It is used in individuals suspected to be infected with rabies. It is given at a dose of 20 IU/kg on day 0, infiltrated around the bite. It is superior to antirabies serum, as it has longer half-life.

Hepatitis B Immunoglobulin

It is a human immunoglobulin containing titer of antibody to hepatitis B surface antigen. Target population includes those who have had percutaneous or mucosal exposure, neonates of mothers with hepatitis B surface antigen (HBsAg), and sexual contacts of acute hepatitis B patients. It is given at a dose of 0.05 to 0.07 mL/kg body weight, repeated in 1 month.

Multiple Choice Questions

1. A vaccine can be:

A. An antigenic protein.
B. Weakened pathogen.
C. Live attenuated pathogen.
D. All of these.

Answer: D

Vaccine can be live attenuated, killed, or protein.

2. Passive immunization includes:

A. Introduction of antibodies directly.
B. Transfer of maternal antibodies across placenta.
C. Transfer of lymphocyte directly.
D. All of these.

Answer: D

Passive immunization is directly giving preformed antibodies and cells to body.

3. Which of the following statements is true regarding vaccination?

A. Vaccination is a method of active immunization.
B. Vaccination is a method of passive immunization.
C. Vaccination is a method of artificial passive immunization.
D. Vaccine is a method of natural passive immunization.

Answer: A

Vaccine involves stimulating immune response by giving weakened antigen.

4. Vaccines against viruses are usually:

A. Given at birth.
B. Expensive.
C. Either live attenuated or killed.
D. Mainly polysaccharide.

Answer: C

They are live attenuated or killed vaccines.

5. Immunoglobulins are prepared:

A. From viruses and bacteria which are not active or killed.
B. In the acute phase of infection from plasma.
C. From the pooled plasma of blood donors.
D. In a laboratory artificially from proteins.

Answer: C

They are obtained from human blood donors.

6. Live vaccine should be delayed in:

A. Breastfeeding patients.
B. Patients on systemic high-dose steroids.
C. Premature infant.
D. History of epileptic patients.

Answer: B

Prolonged intake of steroids makes person immunocompromised.

7. Patients with no spleen or dysfunctional spleen should not have:

A. Meningitis B vaccine.
B. *Haemophilus influenzae* B (HiB)/meningitis C vaccine.
C. Varicella vaccine.
D. Pneumococcal vaccine.

Answer: C

The spleen is responsible for phagocytosis of bacteria such as *H. influenzae*, pneumococcus, and meningococcus; therefore, when the spleen is removed, immunization against these pathogens is must.

8. Which of the following is contraindication to give repeated dose or further dose of vaccine?

A. Pain, swelling, or redness of site.
B. Irritability.
C. Headache.
D. Cardiovascular collapse or anaphylactic reaction.

Answer: D

These are life-threatening conditions and thus vaccine dose should not to be given in these cases, whereas others are mild reactions.

9. By which route of administration, adrenaline (epinephrine) 1:1,000 should be given in suspected patient of anaphylactic reaction?

A. Intradermally.
B. Subcutaneously.
C. Intramuscularly
D. Intravenously.

Answer: C

It is a life-threatening condition, and therefore adrenaline (epinephrine) should be administered intramuscularly.

10. Which of following infection with oral poliovirus vaccine is false?

A. Is killed/inactivated vaccine.
B. Promotes antibody formation in gut.
C. Vaccine-associated paralytic polio may occur.
D. Is being used in the national immunization schedule.

Answer: A

It is a live vaccine.

11. An immunocompetent, previously unimmunized individual at high risk of rabies who sustained an exposure yesterday will require:

A. Two doses on days 0 and 3
B. Four doses on days 0, 3, 7, and 14.

C. Two doses of rabies vaccine on days 0 and 3 plus hyperimmune rabies immunoglobulin on day 2.

D. Four doses of rabies vaccine on days 0, 3, 7, and 14 with hyperimmune rabies immunoglobulin on day 0.

Answer: D

In nonimmunized patient, four doses with hyperimmune globulin are to be given.

12. A 10-year-old child who sustained a high-risk tetanus wound got vaccinated with a total of three doses will further require:

A. Two doses of vaccine.

B. One dose of vaccines and one dose of human tetanus immunoglobulin.

C. Only one dose of human tetanus immunoglobulin.

D. One reinforcing dose of vaccine.

Answer: B

In contaminated wound, both vaccine and immunoglobulin are to be given.

13. Which of the following is true about bacillus Calmette–Guérin (BCG) immunization?

A. Tuberculin skin test is mandatory for those who had prior contact with a person with TB.

B. It is a killed vaccine.

C. It is given subcutaneously.

D. It is given normally to the lateral aspect of arm at the origin of deltoid muscle.

Answer: A

Tuberculin sensitivity is must to prevent allergic reaction.

14. Which of following vaccine is presently not in the national immunization schedule?

A. Human papilloma virus (HPV).

B. Japanese encephalitis vaccine.

C. Vitamin A.

D. Pneumococcal conjugate vaccine (PCV).

Answer: A

HPV is not present in the national immunization schedule.

15. A contraindication to influenza vaccine is:

A. Established anaphylactic reaction to egg allergy.

B. A rash after previous immunization.

C. Pregnancy.

D. Age less than 2 years.

Answer: A

Anaphylactic reaction to egg allergy is fatal.

Chapter 84 Antioxidants

Tuhin Kanti Biswas, Mayank Kulshreshtha, and Shivam Yadav

Learning Objectives

- Free radicals and reactive oxygen species.
- Fundamentals of antioxidants.

History

The concept of antioxidants and their application in different fields of medical science is very recent. The idea of antioxidants was first introduced by the great American chemist Linus Pauling (1901–1994), who won the Nobel Prize twice and is considered one of the distinguished scientists of the twentieth century. In 1970, Pauling published a book titled *Vitamin C and the Common Cold*, where he wrote that regular daily dosage of vitamin C would produce an increased feeling of well-being as well as strikingly decrease the numbers of cold caught and their severity. Pauling explained one of the causes of common cold is oxidative reaction, and vitamin C plays an important role as a strong antioxidant agent. This evidence was later on well documented after an extensive research on vitamin C at the Linus Pauling Institute of Oregon State University, USA.

Apart from vitamin C as source of antioxidant, vitamins A and E are also considered as potent antioxidants. In due course, elaborate research works were also conducted with other synthetic natural agents such as glutathione, carotenoids, and various cofactors, for example, zinc, copper, thiamine, etc., for their antioxidant activities in different diseases.

Although the modern concept of antioxidant was first introduced by Linus Pauling by establishing the effect of vitamin C in combating common cold, the hint of antioxidative activities is found long back in the Indian system of medicine, the *Ayurveda*, about 5,000 years back describing the therapeutic module in the name of *Rasayana*. Strong documentation on the potent natural source of vitamin C in *amla* (*Phyllanthus emblica*) and its various uses are described in *Charaka Samhita* (ca. 3000 BC), including antiaging property, thereby corroborating its antioxidant activity.

Free Radicals and Reactive Oxygen Species

Free radicals are reactive chemical substances that have unstable single unpaired electron in their outer orbit. This unstable configuration creates energy, which reacts with molecules such as proteins, lipids, carbohydrates, and nucleic acids. Most of the free radicals that cause harm to living organism are reactive nitrogen species (RNS) and oxygen free radicals. The oxygen free radical is more common than RNS, and it is known as reactive oxygen species (ROS) or superoxide. There are many chemical and biological ways for generating ROS from both exogenous and endogenous sources. Exogenous sources such as exposure to UV light irradiation, exposures to X-rays, gamma rays, metal catalyzed reaction, and exposure to atmosphere pollutants are considered as important factors (**Box 84.1**). Endogenous sources of generation of ROS include mitochondrial damage, metabolism of cytochrome P450, peroxisomes, and inflammatory cell activation (**Box 84.2**). Besides, there are a number of metabolic reactions that may accelerate the generation of ROS.

Cellular sources of superoxide such as xanthine oxidase catalyze the reaction of hypoxanthine to xanthine and xanthine to uric acid, respectively. Production of ROS is also common in several other diseases such as diabetes mellitus, respiratory disorders like chronic obstructive pulmonary disorder (COPD), cancer, and neuromuscular disorders (**Box 84.3**). The pathological condition like hyperuricemia and/or gout directly acts against ROS production in biological system. The amount of ROS generation varies, depending upon the influence of specific factors.

Box 84.1 Exogenous source of ROS

- X-ray exposure
- Gamma irradiation
- Xenobiotics (toxins, pesticides, herbicides)
- Drugs (bleomycin, adriamycin)
- Foods containing peroxides and aldehydes
- Air pollutants (cigarette, car exhaust, industrial contaminants)

Box 84.2 Endogenous source of ROS

- Mitochondria
- Endoplasmic reticulum
- Peroxisomes

Box 84.3 Oxidative stress–induced diseases

- Diabetes mellitus
- Chronic obstructive pulmonary disorder and relevant respiratory disease
- Cardiovascular diseases
- Neurodegenerative disorders
- Chronic kidney diseases
- Cancer
- Ageing

Physiological Effect of ROS

Regulation of Vascular Diameter

Mitochondrial ROS, particularly superoxide anion and hydrogen peroxide, play an important role in coronary resistance from arterial damage due to shearing of external stress, influenced by risk factors such as hyperlipidemia and smoking.

Oxygen-Sensing Activities of ROS

Oxygen-sensing is a vital process for healthy cells, as it allows cells to start an adaptive response that increases survival in anticipation of limited oxygen availability.

Regulation of Immune System

ROS regulates both the innate and acquired immune response by activating phagocytes under inflammatory situations. Stimulation of phagocytic activity in acquired immunity by ROS is mediated by T-lymphocytes, while the role of ROS in innate immunity is partial, depending upon the nature of host pathogens.

Maintenance of Skeletal Muscle Physiology

Skeletal muscle requires continuous energy for proficient contraction and therefore needs a large supply of oxygen; thus, it becomes most vulnerable to oxidative stress, resulting in excess mitochondrial ROS.

Role of ROS in Wound Healing

Healing of wound involves several factors, out of which collagen synthesis is one of the most important. Collagen is a triple-helix structure formed with three major proteins: as proline, hydroxyproline, and glycine. Conversion of proline into hydroxyproline needs hydroxylation, which can be regulated by ROS.

Role of ROS in Genomic Stability, Regulation of Transcription, and Signal Transduction

Cellular redox condition is considered to be an emerging regulatory factor for genomic stability and transcription. Several physiological processes, namely, cell cycle regulation, response to DNA damage, controlling intermediary metabolism, and apoptosis are identified to be regulated at transcription level of related genes. In oxidative stress, ROS plays a primary role in transcription regulation and thereby might affect essential processes such as glucose homeostasis, inflammation, cellular lifespan, and multiple geriatric diseases including cancer.

ROS-Induced Cellular Damage

ROS and other oxidative radicals are being continuously formed in the body for maintaining different cellular functions in small concentration, but this may damage the cellular integrity due to their higher concentration and higher activities. Due to the presence of unpaired electron, the ROS has a tendency to attract electron of other biological materials and may directly react with protein, lipid, and DNA. ROS may directly harm mitochondria and influence living cells via mitochondria-dependent or mitochondria-independent pathways by targeting these biomolecules. Multiple diseases and/or pathological conditions may develop due to ROS-induced mitochondrial damage, some of which are describing in the following.

ROS-induced Aging

The physiological process of aging may accelerate due to mitochondrial DNA (mtDNA) damage by ROS in mitochondria. ROS may participate in manifestation of cardiovascular diseases, malignancy, and autoimmune diseases, due to rapid mutation of mtDNA and lipid peroxidation.

Neurodegenerative Diseases

Increased level of ROS in neurodegenerative processes may influence normal mitochondrial reactions such as adenosine triphosphate (ATP) production, membrane potential, mitochondrial permeability transition pore (mPTP) activation, and calcium uptake. Functional or sensory loss of neuron occurs due to ROS activation in older age, and as a result, there is manifestation of neurodegenerative diseases such as Parkinson's disease, Alzheimer's disease, amyotrophic lateral sclerosis, or Huntington's disease.

Diabetes Mellitus

In type 2 diabetes mellitus (T2DM), there is an increased production of ROS, leading to progression of insulin resistance, β-cell dysfunction, and impaired glucose tolerance. These types of pathological changes help in acceleration of the disease process, especially with advancement of age, due to overproduction of advanced glycation end-products. Diabetic complications, particularly diabetic retinopathies and glaucoma, develop in T2DM, with the involvement of ROS.

Acceleration of Cancer

ROS increases the process of transformation of healthy cell into abnormal cells during the pathogenic pathway of carcinogenesis. Initiation, promotion, and progression of cancer by overexpression of genetic mutation are mediated through the ROS.

Cardiovascular Diseases

It has been observed that balance between proinflammatory and anti-inflammatory defense mechanisms plays a critical role in the development of atherosclerosis. Free radicals, particularly ROS, play an important role in vascular proliferation and inflammation in vascular occlusive disease. ROS oxidizes low-density lipoprotein (oxLDL), which accumulates within plaques and contributes to atherosclerosis and vasoconstriction. Cardiovascular diseases such as coronary artery disease, cardiovascular accident, myocardial infarction, and hypertension may be developed in this pathogenic way.

Urolithiasis

Lipid peroxidation mediated by oxalate anions under oxidative stress might produce urolithiasis, which causes membrane disruption due to decreased activity of superoxide dismutase (SOD).

Respiratory Diseases

Bronchial asthma, COPD, and asthma–COPD overlapping syndrome (ACOS) are characterized by common features such as inflammation of airway, hyperresponsiveness, airway obstruction, and bronchospasm. There is evidence that oxidative stress plays a crucial role in the development of airway inflammation, induction of mucin secretion, and increased airway hyperresponsiveness. ROS act as a messenger, inducing NF-κB activator which, in turn, induces proinflammatory cytokine IL-4 in certain respiratory diseases like asthma, COPD, and ACOS.

Oxidative Stress in Rheumatoid Arthritis

In rheumatoid arthritis, oxidative stress prompted by NAD(P)H oxidase and uncoupled endothelial nitric oxide synthase (eNOS) results in production of nitrotyrosine, lipid peroxidation, and 4-hydroxy-2-nonenal (HNE). Nitrotyrosine, lipid peroxidation, and HNE are factors associated with collagen damage in rheumatoid arthritis.

Cataract

There is a close interrelationship between ROS and development of cataract. The pathophysiology of cataract is attributed to oxidative stress playing a central role in both onset and progression of cataract. In the cataractogenous process, proteins in the lens cross-links with disulfide bonds, forming insoluble aggregates, which affect lens transparency. Increased levels of serum malondialdehyde and decreased levels of SOD and glutathione peroxidase are found in patients with cataract as marker of ROS.

Immune Deficiency

It is reported that the ROS has an indirect role in the development of immune deficiency. Increased level of oxidative stress leads to deficiency of the immune system, followed by flaring up of diseases such as COPD, pulmonary tuberculosis, and diabetes mellitus.

Fundamentals of Antioxidants

Antioxidant can be described as, "any substance that, when present in low concentrations compared to that of an oxidisable substrate, significantly delays or inhibits the oxidation of that substrate." Physiologically, an antioxidant prevents cellular damage by reacting with ROS to convert it into partial or completely inactive substance. Free radicals such as ROS are barely attracted to a magnetic field and are supposed to be paramagnetic. Mostly, radicals are highly reactive and can either donate an electron to or extract an electron from other molecules, thus behaving as oxidants or reductants. As a result of this high reactivity, most radicals have a very short half-life (10^{-6} seconds or less) in biological systems. Antioxidants can block the unpaired electron of the ROS, so that it can become inactive sharply. Antioxidants readily absorb and quench free radicals by chelating redox metals at physiologically applicable levels. They work in both aqueous and/or membrane domains and affect gene expression in an affirmative way. Different types of antioxidants work in different ways for specific biological purposes.

Types of Antioxidants

Antioxidants can be broadly classified on the basis of nature and the mode of action into four classes as: (1) antioxidant enzymes, (2) chain-breaking antioxidants, (3) transition metal–binding proteins, and (4) antioxidant minerals (**Fig. 84.1**). Catalase, glutathione peroxidases, and SOD are characterized under antioxidant enzymes. The chain-breaking antioxidant is again subdivided into two categories, according to their mode of action: (1) lipid phase chain–breaking antioxidants such as vitamin E or α-tocopherol, carotenoids, flavonoids, and ubiquinol-10 (a reductase form of co-enzyme Q10) and (2) aqueous phase chain-breaking antioxidants such as vitamin C (ascorbic acid), uric acid, and plasma protein (albumin) bound thiol groups. The third category of antioxidants (transition metal–binding proteins) are those that have the capability of binding mainly iron and copper, such as ferritin, transferrin, lactoferrin (iron-binding antioxidants), and caeruloplasmin (copper-binding antioxidant). The fourth group is composed of minerals such as copper, zinc, magnesium, and selenium, which act as antioxidants (**Box 84.4**).

Antioxidant enzymes

Catalase

Catalase has four protein units, each containing a heme group and a molecule of NADPH. It is largely located within the cell in the peroxisomes, particularly in the liver and erythrocytes. Peroxisome contains major enzymes that generate hydrogen peroxide (H_2O_2). Catalase degrades H_2O_2 into water and oxygen.

Glutathione Peroxidases

There are two forms of glutathione peroxidases: selenium-dependent and selenium-independent or glutathione *S*-transferase (GST). Selenium-dependent glutathione peroxidase acts in association with tripeptide glutathione (GSH), which is present in high concentrations in cells and catalyzes the conversion of hydrogen peroxide or organic peroxide to water or alcohol while simultaneously oxidizing GSH. The role of GST as antioxidant is doubtful.

Superoxide Dismutase

This type of intracellular antioxidant has enzymatic action in the conversion of superoxide anions into dioxygen and hydrogen peroxide. SOD exists in several isoforms, linking with specific metals such as Zn, Mn, and Cu. SOD neutralizes superoxide ions by going through successive oxidative and reductive cycles of transition metal ions at its active site. Cu- and Zn-linked SODs specifically catalyze the dismutation of the superoxide anions to oxygen and water, while Mn-linked SOD mainly exists in mitochondria and works in a similar way. Besides intracellular SODs, there is a certain extracellular SOD which has mild activity on ROS for its dismutation.

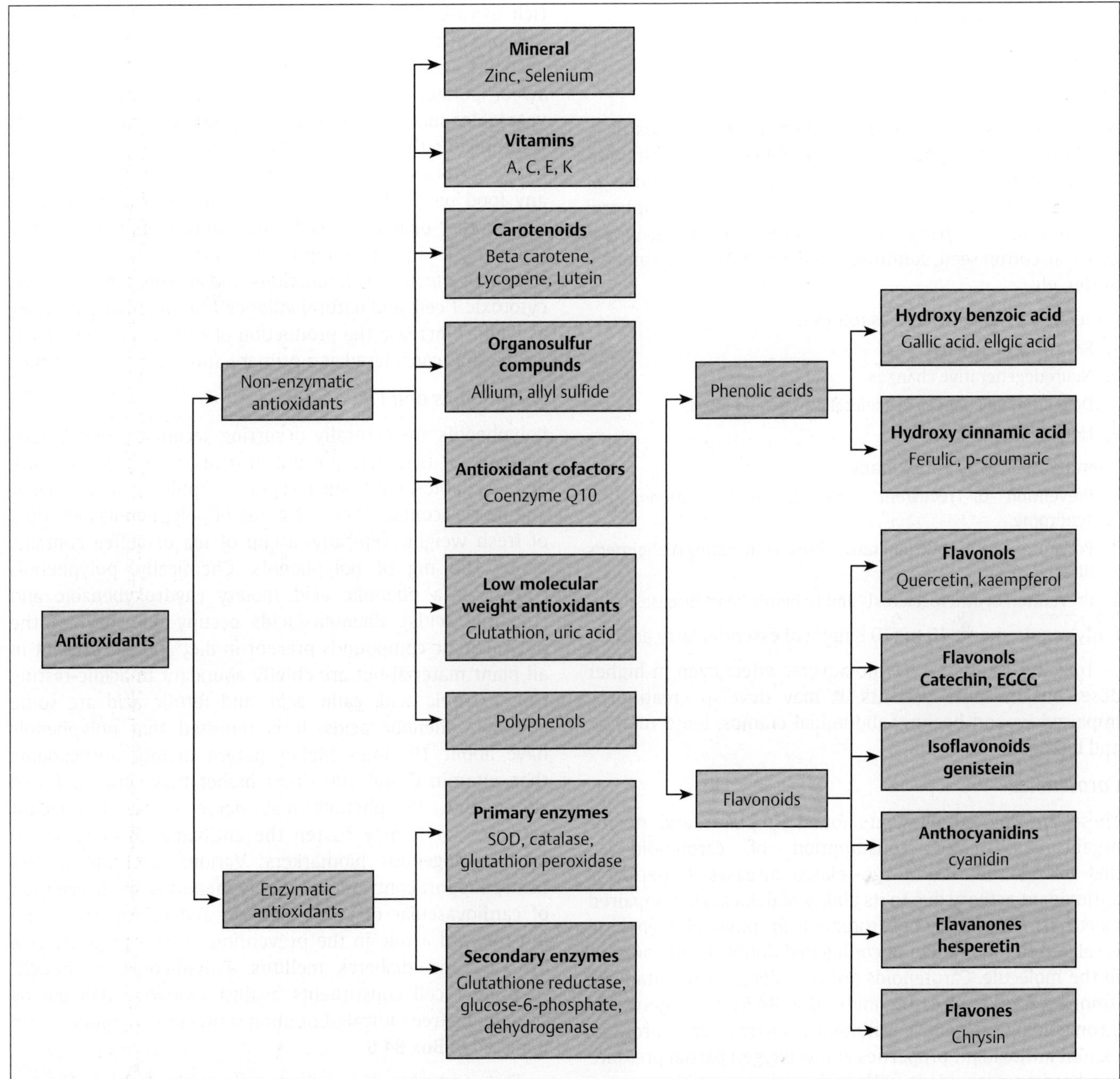

Fig. 84.1 Classification of antioxidants.

Box 84.4 Classification of antioxidants

Class I: Antioxidant enzymes: catalase, glutathione peroxidases, superoxide dismutase

Class II: Chain-breaking antioxidants:

- Lipid phase chain-breaking antioxidants: vitamin E (α-tocopherol), carotenoids, polyphenols and flavonoids, ubiquinol-10
- Aqueous phase chain-breaking antioxidant: ascorbic acid (vitamin C), uric acid, protein-bound thiol

Class III: Transition metal-binding protein

- Fe-binding antioxidant: ferritin, transferrin, lactoferrin
- Cu-binding antioxidant: ceruloplasmin

Class IV: Mineral antioxidant: Cu, Mg, Zn, Se

Chain-Breaking Antioxidant

Lipid Chain–Breaking Antioxidant

Vitamin E

Among the many tocopherols, vitamin E exists mostly in the form of α-tocopherol, which is found to be abundant in mammalian tissues and is potent. The D isomer of α-tocopherol is more potent than the L isomer. α-tocopherol is a naturally occurring vitamin E, found in cereals, wheat germ oil, cotton seed, sunflower seed, egg yolk, nuts, spinach, butter, etc.

Deficiency syndromes are as follows:

1. Recurrent abortion.
2. Neurodegenerative changes.
3. Degenerative changes of skeletal muscle and heart.
4. Hemolytic anemia.

Therapeutic use as antioxidant

1. Prevention of recurrent abortion, sterility, menopausal syndrome.
2. Prevention of neurodegenerative diseases including Alzheimer's disease.
3. Prevention of atherosclerosis and ischemic heart disease.

Daily requirement: 10 mg (0.8 mg/g of essential fatty acid).

Toxicity: Vitamin E has no adverse effect even in higher dose, but in some patients, it may develop creatinuria, impaired wound healing, abdominal cramps, loose motion, and lethargy.

Carotenoids

These are colored pigments found in plants and micro-organisms. Greater consumption of carotenoid-rich diet lowers the risk of age-related diseases. It performs antioxidant activity due to its ability of delocalizing unpaired electrons. The efficacy of carotenoids for physical quenching is related to the number of conjugated double bonds present in the molecule. Carotenoids are considered as provitamins. Among varieties of carotenoids (**Box 84.5**), β-carotene has strong biological value. Carotenoids, in particular β-carotene, exhibit antioxidant properties at low oxygen partial pressure but become prooxidant with high oxygen partial pressure, causing an increased lipid peroxidation, and are converted into vitamin A. They can also scavenge peroxy radicals, thus preventing damage in lipophilic compartments. Some foods rich in carotenoids are pumpkins, carrots, corn, tomatoes, salmon, lobster, shrimp, etc. β-carotene is specifically available in orange-yellow vegetables such as pumpkins, sweet potato, carrots, and winter squash, and in green vegetables such as spinach, collard green, and turnip green. It is interesting that the diet of flamingos is rich in carotenoids. Dried carrots contain the highest amount of carotene of any food per 100 g. It has been reported that β-carotene can protect phagocytic cells from auto-oxidative damage, improve T and B lymphocyte proliferative responses, stimulate effector T cell functions, and augment macrophage, cytotoxic T cell, and natural killer cell tumoricidal capacities, as well as increase the production of certain interleukins. It can be thus considered as a primary anticancer supplement.

Polyphenols and Flavonoids

Polyphenols are naturally occurring secondary metabolites of plants. It is largely present in fruits, vegetables, cereals, and vegetables. Fruits such as grapes, apples, pears, cherries, and berries contain 200 to 300 mg of polyphenols per 100 g of fresh weight. Typically, a cup of tea or coffee contains about 100 mg of polyphenols. Chemically, polyphenols consist of a phenolic acid moiety (hydroxybenzoic and cinnamic acids). Phenolic acids occupy one-third of the polyphenolic compounds present in diet and are present in all plant material but are chiefly abundant in acidic-tasting fruits. Caffeic acid, gallic acid, and ferulic acid are some common phenolic acids. It is reported that polyphenols have about 10 times higher potent dietary antioxidants than vitamin C and 100 times higher than vitamin E and carotenoids. Polyphenols may serve direct antioxidant activities, or it may hasten the antioxidative activities of other endogenous biomarkers. Various scientific studies firmly support contribution of polyphenols to the prevention of cardiovascular diseases, cancers, and osteoporosis, and put forward a role in the prevention of neurodegenerative diseases and diabetes mellitus. Polyphenols is thought to protect cell constituents against oxidative damage by scavenging free radicals. Common sources of polyphenols are depicted in **Box 84.6**.

The most abundant polyphenols in the human diet are flavonoids, having a common basic structure consisting of two aromatic rings bound together by three carbon atoms that form an oxygenated heterocycle.

Box 84.5 Carotenoids family members and their sources

- **Antheraxanthin**: e.g., maize
- **Astaxanthin**: e.g., salmon, shrimp, lobster, flamingo
- **α-carotene**: e.g., carrots, most green plants
- **β-carotene**: e.g., carrots, beetroot, cantaloupe, pumpkin, sweet potato, tomato, watermelon, mango, papaya, peaches, orange, broccoli, cabbage, kale, lettuce, spinach, capsicum, peas
- **Capsanthin**: e.g., peppers, paprika
- **Diatoxanthin**: e.g., algae, corals
- **Lycopene**: e.g., tomato
- **Neoxanthin**: e.g., chloroplast of many plants
- **Zeaxanthin**: e.g., many plants, particularly maize

Box 84.6 Polyphenols and their sources

- **Flavonoids**: These accounts for 60% of all polyphenols. Common flavonoids are quercetin, kaempferol, catechins, and anthocyanins. Common sources are apples, onions, and red cabbage.
- **Phenolic acids**: This group occupies about 30% of all polyphenols and common examples are stilbenes and lignans present in fruits, vegetables, whole grains, and seeds.
- **Polyphenolic amides**: This category includes capsaicinoids in chili peppers and avenanthramides in oats.
- **Other polyphenols**: This group includes resveratrol in red wine, ellagic acid in berries, curcumin in turmeric, lignans in sesame seeds, etc.

N.B.: Concentration of polyphenols in food depends on its source, ripeness, storing, and preparation process.

Flavonoids are the most abundant compounds of polyphenols, which exist in nature through foods, vegetables, and medicinal plants. There are about 6,000 flavonoids that contribute to colorful pigments of herbs, fruits, vegetables, and medicinal plants. The antioxidant activities of flavonoids include: (1) superoxide radical scavenging, (2) suppressing generation of ROS by inhibition of enzymes and chelating trace elements, and (3) upregulating antioxidant defense mechanisms.

Flavonoids have been proven to be effective against several oxidative stress-induced diseases in the elderly such as cancer, diabetes, cardiovascular diseases, Alzheimer's disease, and other dementia-oriented diseases. Some of the common foods are highly enriched with different types of flavonoid compounds and are beneficial for preventing some specific diseases, as described in the following.

1. Apple: Apples are one of the main sources of flavonoids in the Western diet, along with onion, red wine, tea, and chocolate. Procyanidins, a heterogeneous group of polymeric catechin, is present in apples, which has strong antioxidant properties. Evidentially, it is reported that the antioxidant property of apple is responsible for prevention of lung cancer, myocardial infarction, bronchial asthma, obesity, and hyperlipidemia.
2. Tea: Tea is a common drink across the world. Black and green tea is specifically proven as a potent antioxidative agent. Fresh tea leaves are rich in flavanol monomers known as catechin. Tea is, therefore, recommended to prevent diseases such as atherosclerosis and tumors of lung, digestive tract, prostate, bladder, mammary glands, and skin. In many countries, tea is commonly consumed by adding milk to it, but it is reported that tea along with milk diminishes antioxidant activity in vitro. However, in human clinical trials, it was observed that adding milk to black tea does not diminish its antioxidant activity.
3. Alcoholic beverages: Red wine is a complex mixture of flavonoids such as anthocyanins and flavonols, which have potent antioxidant activity, as they reduce LDL cholesterol oxidation, modulate cell signaling pathway, and reduce platelet aggregation. Therefore, red wine has significant cardioprotective activity. Beer is another alcoholic beverage that is enriched with many nutrients such as carbohydrates, amino acids, minerals, vitamins, and several polyphenols. Major raw materials of beer are hop (*Humulus lupulus* L.) and dried hop cones, which contain about 14.4% polyphenols, mainly phenolic acids prenylated chalcones, flavonoids, catechins and proanthocyanidins. The compounds found in beer have diverse biological effects demonstrated in vitro as antioxidant, anticarcinogenic, anti-inflammatory, estrogenic, and antiviral. Both red wine and beer have cardiovascular disease–protective activities, owing to potent antioxidant property. Although red wine and beer have cardioprotective properties, general recommendations are one drink (150 mL of wine or 10 g of alcohol) per day for women and two drinks (300 mL of wine or 20 g of alcohol) daily for men; individual precision may vary based on age, gender, genetics, body type, and drug/supplement use.

Ubiquinol-10

It is a derivative and oxidative form of ubiquinone (UQ) or coenzyme Q10 (CoQ10) and is abundantly found in animal protein, particularly fish and meat. It is a potent antioxidant, which neutralizes the ROS and protects the inner lining of the lymph, blood vessels, and endothelium, thereby preventing cardiovascular diseases particularly congestive heart disease. Besides dietary sources, a synthetic form of the drug is also available.

Aqueous Phase Chain-Breaking Antioxidant

Ascorbic Acid

Ascorbic acid, also known as vitamin C, is one of the most ubiquitous hydrosoluble antioxidants. Ascorbic acid acts as a cofactor for many enzyme-catalyzed reactions, for example, preserving connective and vascular tissue integrity, enhancing collagen biosynthesis followed by stepping up of wound healing and iron absorption, modulating leukocyte and hematopoiesis functioning, neuroprotection, and hydroxylation of lysine and proline. Ascorbic acid has strong antiaging property by providing ascorbate in different tissues, which increase cellular uptake, turnover, and also increase absorption of essential micronutrients.

Source

They are present in almost all citrus fruits and vegetables such as lemons and oranges, tomatoes, green chilies, cabbage, and potato. Human milk is richer in vitamin C (25–50 mg/L) than cow's milk. *Amla* fruit (*Phyllanthus emblica* L.) is the richest natural source of ascorbic acid (5.38 mg/g) along with other polyphenolic compounds such as ellagic acid and gallic acid. Ascorbic acid contents of other dietary sources are shown in **Box 84.7**.

Adverse Effect

Mega dose (2–6 g/day) may have risk of urinary oxalate stone formation.

Uric Acid

The end-product of purine nucleotide metabolism in humans is uric acid. After undergoing kidney filtration, 90% of the uric acid is reabsorbed by the body, proving that it has

Box 84.7 Dietary sources of vitamin C and concentration

Source group	Dietary items	Concentration (mg/100g)
Fruits	Amla	600
	Guava	212
	Lime	63
	Orange	30
	Tomato	27
Germinated pulse	Bengal gram	16
Vegetables	Cabbage	124
	Amaranth	99
	Cauliflower	56
	Spinach	28
	Brinjal	12
	Potatoes	17
	Radish	15

important functions within the body. Uric acid prevents lysis of erythrocytes by peroxidation and is a potent scavenger of singlet oxygen and hydroxyl radicals. It is also known to prevent the overproduction of oxo-heme oxidants that result from the reaction of hemoglobin with peroxides.

Transition Metal-Binding Protein

Fe-Binding Antioxidant

There are a number of Fe-binding biological agents such as lactoferrin, ferritin, and transferrin, which may act as natural antioxidants. Lactoferrin belongs to the iron transporter or transferrin family of glycoproteins. It is mainly found in whey and exocrine secretions of mammals and is released from neutrophil granules during inflammation. Human breast milk may contain as much as 15% lactoferrin, while cow's milk may have only 0.5 to 1.0%. It has two important roles: (1) it shows antibacterial, antiviral, antifungal, anti-inflammatory, antioxidant, and immunomodulatory activities and (2) it plays an important role in the uptake and absorption of iron through the intestinal mucosa. Its ability to bind iron probably contributes to both its antioxidant properties and its antibacterial action. Ferritin is an intracellular protein that serves as storage for iron and regulates its release. Ferritin is synthesized by almost all living organisms, including algae, bacteria, higher plants, and animals. Ferritin converts ferrous (Fe^{2+}) to ferric (Fe^{3+}) by ferroxidase activity, thereby reducing the chance of deleterious reaction that occurs between ferrous iron and hydrogen peroxide, better known as the Fenton reaction, producing highly damaging hydroxyl radical. Transferrin (iron-binding blood plasma glycoprotein) binds iron very tightly but reversibly and hence controls the level of free iron in biological fluids. Transferrin acts as an antioxidant by virtue of its reducing properties. It reduces the concentration of free ferrous ions, which is responsible for conversion of hydrogen peroxide into lethally toxic hydroxyl radical via the Fenton reaction. Transferrin is a universal iron carrier and is able to deliver iron to cells without formation of free radicals.

Cu-Binding Antioxidant: Ceruloplasmin

Ceruloplasmin, an α-2-glycoprotein, is a naturally occurring antioxidant present in serum that contains six atoms of copper within it and plays an important role in the mobilization and oxidation of iron into transferrin. Ceruloplasmin mobilizes iron into plasma from iron storage cells in the liver. Ceruloplasmin has antioxidant properties that prevent production of harmful ROS via the Fenton reaction. Ceruloplasmin is a ferroxidase that also plays a role in iron efflux from cells. It can thus help to regulate cellular iron homeostasis. It plays a specific neuroprotective role in cerebral ischemia manifested after cerebral stroke and Wilson's disease.

Mineral Antioxidant

Selenium

Selenium is an essential element for antioxidative reactions, which is needed in small amounts in humans and animals. Selenoproteins (proteins containing selenium) are significant antioxidant enzymes. The antioxidant properties of selenoproteins aid in controlling thyroid function, play a key role in the immune system, and prevent cellular injury from free radicals. Low level of selenium may cause a form of heart disease, hypothyroidism, and a weakened immune system. Deficiency of selenium, along with vitamin E deficiency, may lead to reduction of antibody production.

Zinc

As antioxidant, zinc takes part in regulation of glutathione metabolism, inhibition of nicotinamide adenine dinucleotide phosphate-oxidase (NADPH-oxidase) enzyme, and modulation of metallothionein, and acts as a cofactor for SOD enzyme. Zinc is required for the synthesis of insulin by the pancreas and for immunity. The average adult body contains about 1.4 to 2.3 g of zinc. Adequate zinc supplementation is necessary for the maintenance of the immune system.

Copper

Deficiency of copper enhances cytochrome P450 activity in microsomes of the liver and lungs, and thus amplifies generation of ROS and iNOS expression. The amount of copper in an adult is 100 to 150 mg. On the one hand, deficiency may cause neutropenia; on the other hand, hypercupremia is common in patients with nephrosis and those who eat food prepared in copper vessels. Estimated copper requirement for adults is about 2.0 mg per day. Natural sources of copper are seafood, mushroom, sesame seeds, cashews, chickpeas, oysters, coconut milk, etc.

Magnesium

Magnesium serves as a cofactor for SOD enzymes. Mg is one of the important constituents of bones and is present in all the body cells. Human adult contains about 25 g of magnesium of which about half the amount is found in skeletal system. Mg deficiency may occur in chronic alcoholism, cirrhosis of liver, protein-energy malnutrition, and pregnancy, and may lead to manifest mental irritability, tetany, hyperreflexia, etc. Daily requirement of Mg in adult is about 340 mg. Mg is available naturally in many foods such as green leafy vegetables (spinach), fruits (figs, banana, raspberry), nuts and seeds, legumes (black beans, kidney beans), vegetables (peas, cabbage, brussels sprouts), and seafood (salmon, tuna).

Multiple Choice Questions

1. Which of the following can reduce the effect of "bad" cholesterol and lessen its harmful effect on our arteries?

A. Papaya.
B. Sweet potato.
C. Nuts.
D. All the above.

Answer: D

Each of these fruits contains a high amount of antioxidants. A current health study conducted on diets of more than 73,000 nurses revealed that vitamin E–rich diet (found in nuts) lowered the risk of heart attack by 52%, followed by diet laden with vitamin C (abundant in papaya), which reduced the chance by 43%, and a diet loaded with β-carotene (plentiful in sweet potatoes), which diminished the risk by 38%. Nurses who habitually taken this trio-nutrients were found to be 63% less vulnerable to heart attacks than those who did not.

2. As a precautionary measure, professionals suggest to get antioxidants from food as well as to rely on supplements because:

A. Supplements generally have therapeutic levels of antioxidants, whereas foods have maintenance quantity.
B. Supplements lack range of naturally occurring phytochemicals that fruits and vegetables have.
C. Quite often, people do not remember to take medication.
D. Supplements have to be taken in extra-large doses to show their effect.

Answer: B.

One bite of a carrot, for example, can get you β-carotene along with uncountable other carotenoids, present in orange and yellow fruits and veggies. This myriad of phytochemicals cannot be found in supplements.

3. Which of the following drinks bestows the most heart-healthy antioxidant power?

A. Red wine.
B. Green tea.
C. Pomegranate juice.
D. Cranberry juice.

Answer: C

When it comes to antioxidant squall, pomegranate juice is the best choice. Studies reveal that a glass of this fruit juice is packed with a huge amount of polyphenols, which no other juice has.

4. A free radical is:

A. A cell that helps in maintaining the well-being of the body.
B. A naturally occurring or synthetic molecule that causes disease if not checked.
C. A vitamin that is available without any charge at health food outlets and natural medicine clinics.
D. A nutrient that acts to correct any imbalance in the human body.

Answer: B.

Free radicals lose an electron and become unstable. Antioxidant compounds lend electrons to these free radicals, thus neutralizing their harmful effects to guard against circumstances such as heart disease, premature aging, and cancer.

5. Which of the following actions will cause free radicals to generate, potentially putting you at greater risk of heart disease?

A. Eating Pie à la Mode.
B. Breathing.
C. Taking high amounts of a single antioxidant.
D. All of the above.

Answer: D

Unbelievably, all of these actions can act towards producing free radicals. Not to worry: generation of free radicals in the body is a natural phenomenon, through metabolic processes; if we could follow a proper diet regime with antioxidants and regular habit of certain level of physical exercise, those free radicals cannot do any harm and their detrimental effects can easily be overpowered.

6. Which of the following is true relating to genes and free radical activity in your body?

A. Your DNA is unaffected by free radicals.
B. Free radicals can cause genetic mutations.
C. Free radicals cause cancer.
D. Both B and C.

Answer: D

Free radicals can cause base pairs, causing building blocks of DNA to switch and mutate, which in turn ignite early phases of carcinoma.

7. Which statement is false?

A. More colored fruits and vegetables indicate greater antioxidant activity.
B. Consuming different colored fruits and vegetables in a meal generally ensures a broad variety of nutrients.
C. One should go for three servings of fruits and vegetables a day.
D. Eating lots of antioxidant-rich fruits and vegetables will also fill you up, preventing you from overeating.

Answer: C

Actually speaking, three servings are also not enough, but of course it is better than nothing. Ideally, five to nine servings of fruits and veggies daily are required, for optimum protection. According to the Dietary Guidelines for Americans, released

jointly by the U.S. Department of Agriculture and the U.S. Department of Health and Human Services, children between 2 and 6 years ought to eat five servings of fruits and vegetables a day; children older than 6 years, active women, and teens should eat seven servings; and active teen boys and men require nine servings. Our heart can be protected well if we go for a rainbow eating habit with lots of colorful fruits and veggies.

8. Which is not an antioxidant enzyme?

A. Superoxide dismutase.

B. Glutathione peroxidase.

C. Catalase.

D. Renin.

Answer: D

Renin is a hormone that deals with blood pressure through rennin angiotensinogen system.

9. Function of catalase enzyme:

A. Protecting the cell.

B. Deal with digestion.

C. Both of them.

D. None of the above.

Answer: A

Catalase is a common enzyme found in nearly all living organisms exposed to oxygen (such as bacteria, plants, and animals). It catalyzes the breakdown of hydrogen peroxide to water and oxygen. It is a very important enzyme that guards cells from oxidative damage by reactive oxygen species (ROS).

Chapter 85 Physiological Functions of Essential Bioelements in Humans

Srinivasa Reddy Yathapu, Narendrababu Kondapalli, and B. Dinesh Kumar

Learning Objectives

- Principal anions.
- Microelements.

Introduction

The chemical elements that make up the matter of living organisms are known as "bioelements" or "biogenic elements." The bioelements contribute to biologically active complexes in which they exist, as nanoparticles, ions, and atoms with organic compounds.

Living matter is composed of four major organic macromolecules (biomolecules), that is, proteins, carbohydrates, lipids, and nucleic acids. The organic matter is composed of C, H, O, N, P, and S, which are known as "organogens." Other than the organogens, more than 20 essential elements were classified into either macro- or microminerals (**Fig. 85.1**). Each of these elements is required in certain quantities for normal physiological functions, which take place at different life stages of human beings. Dietary intake either lower or higher than the required level of a particular element may result in deficiency or toxicity, respectively, which alters the physiological functions. In view of this, the recommended dietary allowances (RDAs) are defined as "the average daily dietary nutrient intake level that is sufficient to meet the nutrient requirements of nearly all (97–98%) healthy individuals in a particular life stage and gender group." Wherever the data are insufficient to derive the RDAs, the adequate intake is used, which is defined as "the recommended average daily intake level based on observed or experimentally determined approximations or estimates of nutrient intake by a group (or groups) of apparently healthy people that are assumed to be adequate."

The daily requirement of macroelements of an adult human being is generally above 100 mg/day. Microelements are required less than 100 mg/day. There are certain elements (e.g., silicon, nickel) whose function is not established, but their presence was noted in various tissues. Another group of elements does not have any proven essential role in human body; instead, they cause toxicity upon exposure. Examples of such elements are arsenic (As), lead (Pb), mercury (Hg), cadmium (Cd), etc.

For details on macroelements, please refer to Chapter 86, "Minerals."

Principal Anions

Phosphorus

Phosphorus exists as anionic phosphate (PO_4^-) in the biological system. Phosphate is an essential component of bone mineral hydroxyapatite, $Ca_{10}(PO_4)_6(OH)_2$, where the ratio of calcium to phosphorus is about 1:2. In adults, major percentage (85%; equivalent to ~700 g) of total phosphorus is distributed in the bones, whereas the remaining is

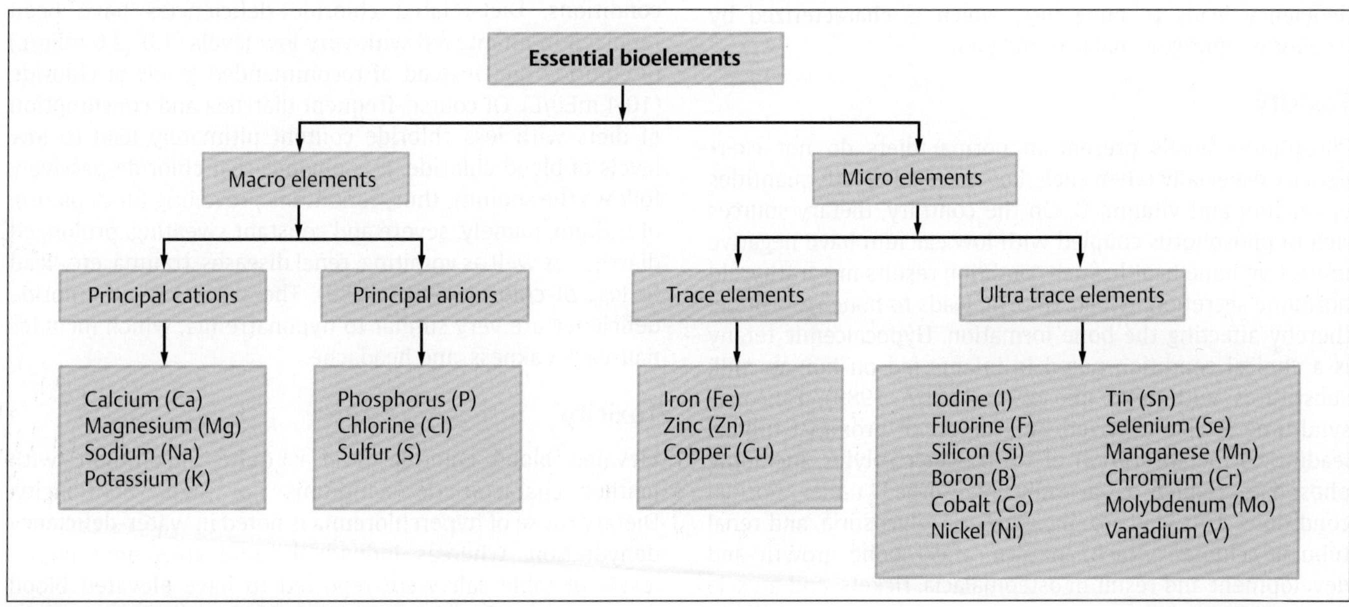

Fig. 85.1 Schematic categorization of essential bioelements: macro- and microelements.

distributed in soft tissues (~15%) and extracellular fluid (ECF) (~1%). The phosphate groups are chemically attached to a variety of macromolecules, which perform key physiological functions.

The free phosphate form of phosphorus is efficiently absorbed by the small intestine. Further, its absorption is either dependent on or independent of calcium and vitamin D. A higher percentage of phosphorus absorption was noted in infants fed with human milk (85–90%) compared with those fed with cow's milk (65–70%). Children and adults absorb 50 to 70% of the phosphorus in normal diets and as much as 90% when the intake is low.

RDA

Twice the RDA of phosphorus is essential for pregnant and lactating women in comparison to nonpregnant/nonlactating women.

Dietary Sources

Cereal grains and protein-rich foods are the major dietary sources of phosphorus. Cereal products contribute about 12%, whereas convenience foods prepared with food additives possess 20 to 30 % phosphorus. A 15- to 20-fold higher phosphorus than calcium is present in fish, poultry, and meats, especially bone. Similarly, the level of phosphorus is twice the level of calcium in eggs, nuts, grains, peas, lentils, and dry beans. On the contrary, higher calcium than phosphorus is noted in green leafy vegetables, natural cheese, and milk.

Deficiency

Hypophosphatemia, a condition of low levels of serum phosphate, does not usually occur, as almost all foods contain phosphorus. In the case of small premature infants, human milk's phosphorus content is insufficient for normal bone mineralization. Failure of additional phosphorus supply results in hypophosphatemic rickets. In adults, hypophosphatemia leads to rhabdomyolysis, respiratory failure, hemolysis, and cardiac failure. Further, phosphorus deficiency leads to bone loss, which is characterized by weakness, anorexia, malaise, and pain.

Toxicity

Phosphorus levels present in normal diets do not exert toxicity especially when such diets have adequate quantities of calcium and vitamin D. On the contrary, dietary sources rich in phosphorus coupled with low calcium have negative impact on bone health. Such condition results in parathyroid hormone secretion, which, in turn, leads to bone resorption, thereby affecting the bone formation. Hypocalcemic tetany is a clinical condition noted in infants fed on human milk substitutes with high phosphorus (RDA 1989). Fanconi's syndrome is characterized by a defect of proximal tubule, leading to malabsorption of various electrolytes, including phosphate, which is actually reabsorbed under normal conditions. This leads to phosphaturia, glycosuria, and renal tubular acidosis, which, in turn, affect bone growth and development and result in osteomalacia, rickets, and muscle weakness.

Chlorine

Chlorine exists in an anionic form called chloride, which is the primary anion of ECF. Chloride plays a critical role in maintaining various activities such as acid–base balance, electroneutrality in serum, osmotic pressure, fluid homeostasis, renal function, and production of hydrochloric acid (HCl) in gastrointestinal (GI) tract. In addition, chloride ions are essential for "general electrical activity" involved in muscular action. The chloride ions move across the cell membrane through protein channels, that is, chloride channel encoded by *CFTR* (cystic fibrosis transmembrane conductance regulator) gene. The synthesis, structure, and/or stability of the chloride channel are affected by the mutations in the *CFTR* gene; as a result, the transport of chloride ions as well as water movement into the tissues is prevented from cells. Consequently, the epithelial cell lining of airway passages, GI tract (the pancreas and biliary system), and other organs produce thickened and sticky mucus; such a condition is known as cystic fibrosis.

RDA

The RDAs of chloride for different age groups of population vary from 1,500 to 2,300 mg/day.

Dietary Sources

The majority of chloride in the diet comes from sodium chloride (NaCl—table salt). A teaspoon (5,600 mg) of table salt has about 60% chloride, which is equivalent to 3,400 mg of chloride and 2,200 mg of sodium. Similarly, the contribution of chloride from human milk is higher than sodium level, as human milk contains 11 mEq of chloride per liter. An alternate form of table salt chloride is KCl. All foods possessing NaCl serve as good sources of dietary chloride. In addition, wholegrain, tomatoes, celery, lettuce, rye, olives, and seafoods possess chloride.

Deficiency

Dietary chloride deficiency is uncommon under normal conditions. Diet-related chloride deficiencies have been reported in infants fed with very low levels (1.0–2.0 mEq/L) of chloride diet instead of recommended levels of chloride (10.4 mEq/L). Of course, frequent diarrhea and consumption of diets with less chloride content ultimately lead to low levels of blood chloride. It is obvious that chloride passively follows the sodium; thus, conditions prevailing for depletion of sodium, namely, severe and constant sweating, prolonged diarrhea as well as vomiting, renal diseases, trauma, etc., lead to loss of chloride (RDA 1989). The symptoms of chloride deficiency are very similar to hyponatremia, which includes nausea, weakness, and headache.

Toxicity

Elevated blood chloride level is quite uncommon, with neither characteristic symptoms nor signs of toxicity. Dietary cause of hyperchloremia is noted in water-deficiency dehydration, whereas individuals who consumed higher levels of table salt were reported to have elevated blood pressure.

Sulfur

Sulfur is one of the essential elements for both humans and animals; it is another important principal anion. The sulfur-containing amino acids (SAAs), including methionine and cysteine, are the main sulfur sources for human beings. These amino acids are exclusively obtained through plant-based foods. Plants and bacteria convert sulfate (SO_4^{2-}) to organic sulfur compounds. Organosulfur compounds such as alliin, isothiocyanates, and diallyl sulfides present in garlic, onions, and other vegetables are well known for their beneficial actions. Of the SAAs, methionine is essential, which acts as parent compound for synthesis of a variety of necessary sulfur-containing compounds except the two "S-containing" vitamins: thiamin (vitamin B_1) and biotin (vitamin H or coenzyme R). Cysteine can be synthesized by the human body by utilizing the methionine through transsulfuration pathway, but the reverse is not possible. Glutathione and other thiol compounds present in the plasma are known to have antioxidant functions.

RDA

There are no RDAs for sulfur, as the required "S" is met through various dietary sources. Further, the severe form of sulfur deficiency is impractical, unless there is extreme protein deprivation.

Dietary Sources

The sulfur requirement of the human body is met through the organic sulfur-containing complexes, especially the SAAs—cysteine and methionine. The legume proteins are comparatively less in SAAs than the cereal and animal proteins. Further, the ratio of methionine to cysteine is higher among animal proteins compared with plant sources. Dairy products, eggs, fish, meats, legumes, cabbage, garlic, nuts, raspberries, onions, soft water, and wheat germ are the sources of sulfur compounds.

Deficiency

As mentioned, the severe form of "sulfur deficiency" is a very uncommon condition, since protein from plant and animal origin possesses adequate quantities of SAAs.

Toxicity

Excessive intake of SAAs is known to cause depressed growth. Nonetheless, an elevated level of sulfur-rich substances in the domestic ruminants causes the polioencephalomalacia along with secondary metabolic disorders.

Microelements

These included trace elements and ultratrace elements. The trace elements include iron, zinc, and copper.

Iron

(Refer to Chapter 86.)

Zinc

About 2.6 g of zinc is present in the human body, of which 80 to 120 µg/dL exists in the plasma. Zinc proteins play a role in a majority of molecular and cell biology functions, through maintenance of protein structure and enzyme catalysis. Zinc ions (Zn^{2+}) are part of the active sites of all the six major classes of metalloenzymes, namely, oxidoreductases, isomerases, hydrolases, transferases, lyases, and ligases. Zinc is essential for sperm production, development, and maturation, along with genomic integrity of sperm. It is responsible for organogenesis, neurotransmission, normal development of thymus, healing process of wound, sense of taste, and secretion processes of pancreatic juices as well as gastric enzymes.

Dietary Sources

Except in individuals with acrodermatitis enteropathica, an autosomal recessive genetic disorder (caused by a defect in the absorption of Zn), Zn get absorbed very well across the GI tract. Animal-based dietary products such as meat, liver, eggs, and seafoods (especially oysters) are good sources of available Zn, whereas wholegrain products contain the element in a less available form. Phytates and dietary fibers of plant-based products affect the bioavailability of zinc. The simultaneous supplementation of ferrous sulfate and zinc to humans has shown less absorption of the latter.

Deficiency

Zinc deficiency primarily affects many enzymes involved in gene expression, thus influencing cell growth and repair. The deficiency symptoms include acidosis, intoxication of alcohol, blockage of protein biosynthesis, and transmutation. The vulnerable groups include pregnant and lactating women; adolescents, children, and infants are at higher risk of Zn depletion in comparison to adults.

Toxicity

Ingestion of ≥ 2 g of zinc sulfate results in acute toxicity with characteristic features of GI irritation and vomiting. Zinc intakes of 18.5 to 25 mg/day are known to influence the copper status. Zinc supplementation to patients at a dose of 10- to 30-fold higher than RDA for several months resulted in hypocupremia, microcytosis, and neutropenia. In addition, such higher doses of zinc supplementation for weeks together are known to result in diminishing spectrum of immune responses along with lowering of high-density lipoproteins. Thus, any dose more than 15 mg/day of zinc supplements is recommended under the medical supervision only.

Copper

The average adult (70 kg) human being may contain approximately 100 mg of copper. Of the entire blood copper content, 60% exist in erythrocytes as Cu–Zn metalloenzyme superoxide dismutase (SOD), and the rest in loosely bound form to various amino acids and proteins. Over 90% of the plasma Cu is in ceruloplasmin-bound form—a major Cu-carrying protein of blood. The role of ceruloplasmin in iron metabolism is also well established through animal models, suggesting that it is involved in transportation of iron between the plasma and cells. Cu is an important constituent of several metalloenzymes, namely, lactase, tyrosinase, catalase, and SOD, and a variety of oxidases such as cytochrome oxidase, ferroxidase, monoamine oxidase, peroxidase, and ascorbic acid oxidase.

Dietary Sources

The major sources of copper are animal-based diets, such as liver, shellfish, milk, and milk products, and plant-based compounds, such as dried fruit, tahini, sunflower seeds, sun-dried tomatoes, and sesame seeds. Human milk contains higher quantity (~0.3 mg/L) of copper than cow's milk (~0.09 mg/L). Healthy individuals require 2 to 5 mg of copper per day, of which 50% gets absorbed from the GI tract and the rest is excreted through bile and kidney.

Deficiency

In the case of adult human beings, the severe form of Cu deficiency is very rare, whereas in children a prolonged dietary Cu deficiency during active growth phase results in growth retardation, anemia, defective keratinization, and skeletal defects. In addition, it also leads to defects in pigmentation and structure of hair, hypothermia, mental retardation, reproductive failure, myocardial degeneration, and decreased arterial elasticity. Hypocupremia is probably unrelated to dietary copper intake alone; various other conditions such as protein-calorie malnutrition, sprue, and nephrotic syndrome are also considered as the potential contributors. In certain malignancies, reduced copper levels are noted.

Toxicity

Excessive Cu intake through either dietary or other sources leads to increased Cu levels in serum and tissue, which, in turn, causes nausea, vomiting, diarrhea, profuse sweating, oxidative stress, and renal dysfunction and affects several immune functions.

Iodine

Iodine, which predominantly exists as iodide, is an essential micronutrient for human beings and all other animal species. It is an important component of thyroid hormones, that is, thyroxine (T4) and triiodothyronine (T3). These hormones regulate several biochemical reactions such as protein synthesis, an enzymatic activity. Thyroid gland attains 20 to 50 times higher iodide concentration than plasma iodide levels through its sodium/iodide transporter.

Dietary Sources

Iodine is high in seafood in comparison to other food sources. Most foods provide 3 to 75 mg of iodine per serving. Processed foods may also contain higher levels, as they were either added to or fortified with iodine, for example, iodized salt. Iodate, a form of iodine, is used in fortification processes, which upon ingestion rapidly reduced to iodide form and get absorbed completely.

Deficiency

Iodine deficiency causes a range of manifestations such as mental retardation and enlargement of the thyroid, that is, goiter. Endemic goiter and the more severe forms of iodine deficiency disorders continue to be a worldwide problem. The thyroid gland is able to concentrate the iodine from the plasma during iodine deficiency; further lower levels of dietary iodine lead to manifestations. In addition, iodine deficiency leads to impaired reproductive outcome, increased childhood mortality, decreased learning ability, and economic stagnation.

Toxicity

The acute toxic studies in animals with iodide and iodate in a range of 200 to 500 mg/kg per day resulted in the death of laboratory animals. No adverse physiological reactions were noted in healthy adults and children who consumed as high as 2 and 1 mg/day iodine, respectively.

Fluorine

Vast controversial reports have been debated over essentiality of fluorine in human physiology. However, fluoride is vital for certain calcified tissues such as teeth and bones. Fluoride has higher affinity with calcium, thus approximately 99% of fluoride is associated with calcified tissues, which is known to prevent dental caries and stimulate new bone formation. Endemic fluoride toxicity is prevalent in some of the geographical regions of India, wherein the drinking water, agricultural products raised with such water, and livestock are the contributory factors.

Dietary Sources

Fluoridated water, beverages, especially tea, and marine fish such as sardines (when consumed with bones) are the primary sources of dietary fluoride. Tea leaves have the tendency to accumulate fluoride (as high as 10 mg/100 g of dry weight); thus, brewed tea may possess 1 to 6 mg/L fluoride, depending on the quantity of dried tea leaves. In regions where the fluoride content of water is very low, children are advised to use fluorinated dental products such as toothpaste and mouthwashes.

Deficiency

An association has been reported between inadequate fluoride intake and risk of dental caries. No exact mechanisms were reported, whereas it was proposed that fluoride replaces hydroxyl ions in developing enamel prior to tooth eruption, thereby forming an apatite crystal that is less susceptible to solubilization by acid and, hence, more resistant to caries formation.

Toxicity

If growing children prior to eruption of teeth take excess of fluoride, it leads to discolored/pitted teeth and skeletal fluorosis, a very rare effect characterized by elevated bone-ash fluoride concentrations. Chronic toxic effects of fluorosis are altered bone health, kidney, muscle, and nerve functions.

Selenium

The human body contains approximately 13 to 20 mg of selenium. Selenium exists in the selenocysteine form at active sites of selenoproteins and plays a vital function in human health. Antioxidant enzymes such as glutathione peroxidase and thioredoxin reductase possess selenium. Selenoproteins regulate thyroid hormone actions and the redox status of vitamin C and other molecules. The role of selenium in the immune system has been well established, especially through T-lymphocyte response. An association has been shown between low levels of selenium in blood and mortality related to cardiovascular disease.

Dietary Sources

Seafood, kidney, liver, other meats, some vegetables, and wholegrain are some of the good dietary sources of selenium. Selenium content in cooked and processed foods is lesser than in raw foods.

Manganese

Manganese, another essential element, involved in formation of bone and in certain reactions related to amino acid, cholesterol, and carbohydrate metabolism. Metalloenzymes of Mn are arginase, phosphoenolpyruvate decarboxylase, glutamine synthetase, and manganese superoxide dismutase.

Dietary Sources

In comparison to fruits and vegetables, wholegrain and cereal products are good sources of manganese. Further, lower levels of Mn were noted in dairy products, meat, fish, and poultry. Tea is a rich source of manganese, but typical drinking water consumed at the rate of 2 L daily contributes only about 40 to 64 µg, or about 2 to 3% of the amount furnished by diet.

Deficiency

In general, dietary-associated Mn deficiency is not reported in healthy individuals. However, experimentally induced Mn depletion in humans has shown scaly dermatitis and hypocholesterolemia.

Toxicity

Excess intake of Mn through diet/food is not reported, whereas the toxicity of Mn reported in occupationally exposed individuals has shown similar effects of Parkinson's disease. Manganese toxicity exerts its effects on the central nervous system. An association was established between higher blood Mn levels and neurotoxicity in both humans and animals.

Chapter 86 Minerals

Arpita Shrivastav and Neeraj Shrivastav

Learning Objectives

- Major minerals.
- Microminerals.

Introduction

Minerals are elements/inanimate substances, extant in all body tissues, fluids, and drinking water. They originate in the soil and are required for all normal life processes. Minerals found in the diet are unswervingly obtained from plants, fruits, and vegetables, or circuitously from animal sources and cannot be created by living things. Minerals are required in relatively huge amounts, and trace minerals are required in very small quantities.

Classification

As per the requirement of the body, minerals/essential minerals are grouped as follows:

1. Macrominerals/major minerals: These are minerals that are needed in larger amounts: more than 100 mg/dL or more than 50 mg/day. Amounts needed in the body are not an indication of their importance. Some of the important major minerals are sodium, potassium, calcium, phosphorus, and magnesium.
2. Microminerals/trace minerals: They are required in smaller amounts than major minerals: less than 100 mg/dL or less than 50 mg/day. Some examples are iron, copper, cobalt, iodine, zinc, manganese, molybdenum, fluorine, chromium, selenium, and sulfur.

Major Minerals

Sodium

Source and Chemistry

Sodium has a bright silver color and is an extremely reactive, basic, metallic element. Normal salt comprises 40% sodium, and 5 g of it (one teaspoonful) holds 2 g of sodium. Sodium is found in rock and sea salt, baking soda, soy sauce, some preservatives, monosodium glutamate, vegetables including dry lotus stems, leafy vegetables, pulses, legumes, fruits, fish, milk, breads, unprocessed meats, and processed food.

Requirement

An adult's average requirement is 2 g/day (equal to 3.3–4.0 g/day NaCl).

Physiological Role/Functions

It maintains fluid balance along with muscle and nerve activity control. As a constituent of extracellular fluid, it regulates the osmotic pressure of the extracellular fluid. It also stimulates amylase enzyme.

Pharmacokinetics

Absorption of sodium starts 3 to 6 minutes after intake and is completed within 3 hours.

Mechanism of Action

Sodium is mainly present in body fluids. It plays a vital role in regulating blood volume and blood pressure by attracting and holding water. Sodium is also vital in regulating osmotic pressure and in conducting nerve impulses through cells. It is an electrolyte that is essential in regulating adenosine triphosphate (ATP) and potassium.

Deficiency

Hyponatremia involves reduction in serum sodium concentration less than 136 mEq/L due to excess of water in comparison to solute. Common causes of deficiency are use of diuretics, diarrhea, heart failure, liver and renal ailment, and abnormal ADH secretion (i.e., syndrome of inappropriate antidiuretic hormone secretion [SIADH]). Sodium deficiency does not occur normally. During long and heavy exercises, sweating may lead to loss of sodium or its deficiency. Cramps, weakness, fatigue, nausea, and thirst are common signs of sodium deficiency.

Therapeutic Uses

Sodium is a crucial element, and a certain quantity of it is desirable for regular body function. The recommended daily intake of sodium is 0.9 to 2.3 g, and in distinct situations like profuse sweating and diarrhea, more sodium may be desirable.

Calcium

Refer to Chapter 79 Agents Affecting Calcium Balance.

Magnesium

Source and Chemistry

Magnesium is found in plant chlorophyll as well as in tissues and bones. It is present in various enzymes, including thymine pyrophosphate. Green vegetables, legumes and seeds, peas, beans, nuts, shellfish, spices, and soya flour are rich in magnesium. Unrefined cereal grains are rational sources. Many highly refined flours, tubers, fruits, fungi, and most oils and fats contribute little dietary magnesium (< 100 mg/kg fresh weight). Corn flour, cassava and sago flour, and polished rice flour have an extremely low magnesium content. Alfalfa, bladderwrack, catnip, cayenne, chamomile, chickweed, dandelion, eyebright, fennel seed, fenugreek, hops, horsetail, lemongrass, licorice, mullein, nettle, oat straw, paprika, parsley, peppermint, raspberry leaf, red, clover, sage, shepherd's purse, yarrow, and yellow dock are good sources of magnesium.

Requirement

As per the National Research Council's recommendation, the minimum daily consumption of magnesium should be 250 mg for children younger than 10 years, 300 to 400 mg for adults, and 450 mg for pregnant and lactating women.

Physiological Role/Functions

Magnesium is a constituent of bones, teeth, and enzyme cofactor. It activates phosphate-transferring enzymes, pyruvic acid carboxylase, pyruvic acid oxidase, and other enzymes used in the citric acid cycle. Magnesium is required for enzymes involved in energy metabolism, protein synthesis, RNA and DNA synthesis, and maintenance of the electrical potential of nervous tissues and cell membranes.

Most of the body magnesium is located in the bone (50% and 60%) of body where it is thought to form a surface constituent of the hydroxyapatite (calcium phosphate) mineral component, this magnesium is readily exchangeable with serum and therefore represents a moderately accessible magnesium store used in times of deficiency.

Deficiency

Primary magnesium deficiency results in intestinal hypoabsorption, urinary leakage, reduced magnesium bone uptake and mobilization, hyperglucocorticism, insulin resistance, and adrenergic hyporeceptivity.

Secondary magnesium deficiency occurs in various pathological conditions such as noninsulin-dependent diabetes, high intake of alcohol, ingestion of hypermagnesuric diuretics, etc.

In chronic magnesium deficiency, hyperexcitability related to central and peripheral nerves and muscles is seen, as in latent tetany, chronic fatigue, asthenia, idiopathic Barlow's disease, and preeclampsia convulsions. Eclampsia decreases activity of taurine and glutaurine. There is increased susceptibility to peroxidation, with increased activity of the excitatory neuromediators acetylcholine and catecholamines.

Effects on the cardiovascular system result in change in electromyography (EMG), irregular heartbeat, and increased sensitivity to cardiac glycoside. It impairs the release of nitric oxide, a potent nitrovasodilator and inhibitor of platelet aggregation, from the coronary endothelium.

Magnesium deficit can influence fiber and collagen structures, lipid content, and hormones. Acidosis and muscle contraction result in decrease in plasma volume and the shift of cellular magnesium into the extracellular fluids. Its deficit in elderly people is also seen to be affecting magnesium metabolism.

Therapeutic Uses

Magnesium is used in eclampsia and preeclampsia, arrhythmia, severe asthma, and migraine. It helps in relieving the symptoms of dysmenorrhea. It is also useful in stroke, where depressed extracellular magnesium results in vasoconstriction and infusion of magnesium sulfate results in dilatation of cerebral arterioles and venules.

Association between hypomagnesemia and chronic obstructive lung disease, as well as improvement in the respiratory parameters after magnesium therapy, is observed. Parenteral magnesium therapy has traditionally been used in the treatment of toxemias of pregnancy. Magnesium improves leg cramps in pregnant women and ischemic heart disease.

Hypomagnesemia is associated with diabetes mellitus. Magnesium lowers the risk of metabolic syndrome and improves glucose and insulin metabolism; therefore, magnesium supplementation proves to be very useful.

Chronic alcoholics become magnesium deficient as a result of increased renal excretion, poor intake, and secondary aldosteronism due to cirrhosis. Correction of magnesium deficiency is effective in correcting the neuromuscular and cardiac disorders associated with chronic alcoholism.

Potassium

Source and Chemistry

Potassium is present mainly as blood mineral and is required for both cellular and electrical function. Spinach, parsley, lettuce, broccoli, peas, lima beans, tomatoes, potatoes, and herbs such as red clover, sage, catnip, hops, horsetail, nettle, plantain, and skullcap are all good sources of potassium. Oranges, bananas, apples, avocados, raisins, and apricots, especially dried, also contain potassium. Whole grains, wheat germ seeds, nuts, flounder, salmon, sardines, cod, and meat foods are rich in potassium.

Around 4 to 5 mg of the total potassium is present per 100 mL of blood serum; the red blood cells contain 420 mg.

Requirement

Adults should take 4,700 mg of potassium per day. There is no specific recommendation for potassium; 2 to 2.5 g per day is the minimum amount needed.

Physiological Role/Functions

Potassium and sodium control water and acid–base balance in the blood and tissues. It activates the sodium–potassium exchange across the cell membranes. This sodium–potassium flux generates the electrical potential and helps in the conduction of nerve impulses, which help in muscle contractions, regulate heartbeat, and prevent the swelling of cells.

Potassium participates actively in the metabolism of glycogen and glucose by changing glucose to glycogen, which is stored in the liver, thus affecting carbohydrate metabolism. It is significant for normal growth and for structuring muscle. It is also required for the heart, nervous system, and electrolyte balance.

Deficiency

Potassium level in the blood and cells is very important for normal body functions. Reduction in the potassium level leads to hypertension, congestive heart failure, cardiac arrhythmia, depression, and mood swings.

In chronic deficiency, fatigue is most commonly observed. Initially, lower potassium causes muscle weakness, slow reflexes, and dryness of skin or acne, which may further progress to nervous disorders, insomnia, slow or irregular heartbeat, and loss of gastrointestinal tone. Cardiac arrhythmia is seen with sudden decrease in potassium level, and glucose metabolism is affected by increased blood sugar.

Therapeutic Uses

Potassium supplements can be used for the treatment of high blood pressure, fatigue, and weakness in elderly people. Colic in newborns and cases of allergies and headache can be cured by the use of potassium chloride. Loss of potassium during diarrhea needs replacement therapy. Potassium is useful during weight-loss programs and is also used to prevent hangover symptoms after alcohol drinking. It helps in rehydration of body after fluid losses.

Microminerals

Iron

(Refer to Chapter 48 Hematinics and Treatment of Anemia.)

Molybdenum

Source and Chemistry

Molybdenum is classified as a trace metal among human nutrients. It is essential for good health, but there is no evidence that molybdenum deficiency is responsible for any human disease. It is present in meat and beef liver (1.5 ppm), green beans, eggs, sunflower seeds, wheat flour, lentils, cucumbers, and cereal grain.

Requirement

Normally, 0.07 mg/kg of molybdenum is found in the human body. Daily amount of molybdenum taken is 0.12 and 0.24 mg.

Physiology/Functions

Molybdenum is a chief constituent of the iron-containing enzyme xanthine oxidase, which breaks down purines to uric acid and is also involved in the mobilization of ferritin, storage iron, from reserves in the liver. It is essential for xanthine oxidase activity and also for the actions of the enzymes sulfite oxidase and aldehyde oxidase. Excretion takes place in the bile and urine.

Molybdenum is secreted in the bile and then recirculated into the liver by an enterohepatic circulation, with the excess appearing in the feces. About half of the total intake may be excreted in the urine. Urinary levels vary with environmental exposure to the metal and do not regulate tissue levels.

Deficiency

Molybdenum is a copper antagonist. Like zinc, excess molybdenum interferes with copper absorption. In livestock, copper and molybdenum prevent the uptake of excessive amounts of each other, but only in the presence of inorganic sulfate. Molybdate absorption is inhibited by sulfate. It is suspected that the relatively high copper intake in humans also inhibits both molybdenum and iron absorption. There is no spontaneous molybdenum deficiency syndrome in humans. In various experimental situations, the following signs and symptoms have been reported: tachycardia, night blindness, irritability, headaches, nausea, lassitude and lethargy, coma, decreased xanthine oxidase activity in the intestine and liver, and impaired purine metabolism.

A molybdenum deficiency syndrome in a young man shows severe headache, nyctalopia, tachycardia, tachypnea, nausea, vomiting, central scotoma, lethargy, disorientation, and coma. Hypouricemia is accompanied by raised plasma methionine levels.

Therapeutic Uses

Molybdenum is a crucial trace element plentiful in food, and a balanced diet will provide all the molybdenum needed for normal function at all levels of activity. Multivitamin supplements commonly contain the metal, typically 15 μg, in the form of yeast, per tablet or capsule. This practice is unnecessary. A high normal daily intake of molybdenum (0.54 mg) compromises copper balance and, therefore, molybdenum supplementation may be harmful.

Chromium

Source and Chemistry

Chromium holds importance among overweight people. Grains, broccoli, mushrooms, liver, processed meats, egg yolks, beef, molasses, cheese, grape juice, bread, honey, potatoes, chicken, spinach, bananas, carrots, and blueberries are common sources of chromium.

Requirement

In young males, more than 35 g/day of chromium is required, and in young females, more than 25 g/day of chromium is required.

Physiology/Functions

Chromium controls blood sugar and fat levels of the body. It is required for glucose tolerance factor, helping to reduce blood glucose through insulin assistance and uptake of glucose by the muscle and other tissues. Insulin resistance leads to diabetes.

Deficiency

Chromium deficiency results in mood changes due to hypoglycemia, particularly after rich carbohydrate meals. In chronic cases, it leads to diabetes, high blood pressure, heart disease, stroke, and obesity. Increased intake of white flour, white pasta, white rice, potatoes, and processed foods may use up chromium, resulting in its deficiency.

Therapeutic Uses

No specific therapeutic use.

Multiple Choice Questions

1. A 50-year-old woman comes to you complaining about the pains in the legs, weakness, and difficulty in lifting heavy objects and fast movement. What would you suggest?

A. Calcium.
B. Multivitamins.
C. Iron.
D. Both A and C are correct.

Answer: D

Women older than 50 years are more likely to suffer from calcium and iron deficiency. This mainly occurs due to menopause and imbalance between the hormone estrogen and progesterone, which play a major role in calcium metabolism.

2. A young lady showing symptoms of early tiredness, lack of concentration, puffing in the body, poor physical strength, and pale mucous membrane should increase the intake of:

A. Pulses and legumes.
B. Ascorbic acid.
C. Polyphenols and calcium.
D. Both A and B are correct.

Answer: D

Such symptoms appear in case of low hemoglobin and iron deficiency. Pulses and legumes are very good sources of iron and folates. Ascorbic acid promotes iron assimilation.

3. In Congo, Africa, as a result of cassava diet, there is an overload of thiocyanate. The cause of deficiency of minerals can be overcome by:

A. Increase iodine intake.
B. Increase copper intake.
C. Increase calcium intake.
D. All of the above.

Answer: A

Cassava, being a staple diet in Africa, is consumed in high amount. This acts as goitrogens and affects the proper utilization of iodine by the thyroid gland. Iodine intake in increased amount in the form of iodized salt can overcome this problem.

4. Newborn and infants with less or deficient iron intake are more likely to suffer from the toxicity of:

A. Sulfur.
B. Manganese.
C. Zinc.
D. Fluoride.

Answer: B

Individuals with increased iron absorption have increased manganese absorption as well. Normal adult population appears to be protected by the intestinal and blood–brain barriers, which is not the case in Fe-deficient patients and most likely in newborns and infants. This may lead to its toxicity.

5. If a growing child shows delayed development, protruding abdomen (tummy), scoliosis, floppy limbs and body because of muscle weakness, teeth taking longer than usual to come through, weak tooth enamel, and painful bones, he is likely to be suffering from:

A. Goiter.
B. Rickets.
C. Osteomalacia.
D. Anemia.

Answer: B

Rickets is a softening of bones in growing children due to deficiency or impaired metabolism of vitamin D, phosphorus, or calcium, potentially leading to fractures and deformity. The predominant cause is vitamin D deficiency, but lack of adequate calcium in the diet may also lead to rickets.

6. Which mineral is the second most abundant cation, acts as a calcium antagonist and vasodilator, and plays a role in metabolism and cellular function?

A. Phosphorus.
B. Iodine.
C. Manganese.
D. Magnesium.

Answer: D

Calcium metabolism is correlated with the metabolism of both magnesium and phosphorus, and any change in the level of these two minerals will indirectly affect the level of calcium.

7. Copper deficiency is more frequent in preterm infants, especially those with very low birth weights, because of the following reason(s):

A. Reduced copper stores at birth.
B. The smaller relative size of the liver.
C. Higher requirements determined by their high growth rate.
D. All of the above.

Answer: D

In neonates, specifically premature infants, less is known about required copper intakes to accumulate copper stores and meet increased demands during rapid growth. During fetal development, copper accretion is approximately 50 µg/kg/d, an amount believed to provide the appropriate copper reserve to term infants in the first stages of postnatal life. Babies who are born prematurely will begin life with incomplete copper stores as the majority of copper is accumulated during the third trimester of pregnancy.

Chapter 87 Dermatopharmacology

Rahul Kumar and Vinita Awasthi

PH1.57: Describe drugs used in skin disorders.

Learning Objectives

- Topical antibacterial, antiviral, and antifungal agents.
- Acne vulgaris.
- Psoriasis.
- Alopecia.
- Pigment disorders.
- Sunscreens.

Introduction

Skin is the largest organ of the body, with a surface area of 1.6 to 1.8 m^2, and acts as a barrier to the external environment. It permits and limits inward and outward movement of water and electrolytes across it. It provides protection against various microorganisms, toxic substances, and ultraviolet (UV) radiation, and also acts as a source of vitamin D. The various layers of skin play the role of barriers for drugs diffusion.

The stratum corneum is the outermost lipophilic keratinous layer, which consists of dead cells that shed every 4 weeks. It is considered to be a part of the epidermis and the main barrier for absorption of drugs.

Other layers of the epidermis such as the stratum lucidum, stratum granulosum, stratum spinosum, and stratum basale consist of viable cells intercalated with neutrophils, lymphocyte, Langerhans cells, melanocytes, drug-metabolizing enzymes, and transporter proteins (OATP, MDR, P-glycoprotein).

The dermis is located between the epidermis and the subcutaneous tissue and consists of collagen, elastin, sweat glands, sebaceous glands, hair follicles, and blood vessels. It is the main site of absorption of drugs into the systemic circulation through the capillary plexus.

The hypodermis or subcutaneous tissue is well vascularized and consists of loose connective tissue and adipose tissue.

Factors Affecting Cutaneous Drug Absorption (PH1.3, PH1.11)

Topical agents are available in the form of sprays, powders, lotions, creams, ointments, pastes, and aerated foams. Their absorption across the skin depends on various factors.

1. Molecular mass of drug–Smaller molecules can cross the skin barrier easily, and topical drugs with molecular weight above 500 Da are usually not absorbed.
2. Region of skin the drug is applied–Thickness of the stratum corneum varies in different regions of the body, as it is easily permeable in face, axilla, scrotum, and scalp.
3. Drug concentration–Drug penetration increases with the rise in drug concentration gradient.
4. Dosing schedule or duration of contact–It affects the amount of available drugs to be absorbed.
5. Condition of skin (normal or with disease)–Burns, abrasions, wounds, and skin diseases increase the absorption of drugs.
6. Type of vehicle (water- or oil-based, newer liposomes, and microgel)–Vehicles may vary in terms of drug release rate and moistening/drying effect on the stratum corneum. Lipophilic agents are readily absorbed than hydrophilic ones.

Principles of Selection of a Topical Formulation (PH1.3, PH1.11)

Topical dermatologic formulations are classified as creams, lotions, ointments, gels, tinctures, pastes, aerosols, powders, wet dressings, and foams. Their selection depends upon various factors such as the type of disease and the main aim of drug application.

1. Acute inflammation–Drying preparations such as lotions and tinctures are preferred.
2. Chronic inflammation–Diseases with xerosis and scaling are best treated with lubricating preparations such as ointments and creams.
3. Retard evaporation–Ointments are the best option to prevent evaporation from skin.
4. Skin with hairs–Gels, lotions, tinctures, foams, and aerosols are preferred, as they are convenient.
5. Intertriginous areas (in axilla, anogenital region, skin folds of the breasts, and digits)–Vanishing cream ("oil in water"-type emulsion) is preferred, as it does not cause maceration and disappears quickly.

Topical Antibacterial Agents (DR15.3)

Antimicrobial agents are used topically for several common skin infections such as folliculitis, cellulitis, fasciitis, abscesses, and impetigo (**Table 87.1**). Bacitracin and mupirocin are used for gram-positive infections (e.g., *Staphylococcus aureus* and *Streptococcus pyogenes*). Polymyxin B and neomycin are effective against gram-negative infections, while silver sulfadiazine, gentamycin, and mafenide acetate are used in mixed infections.

Impetigo

This is a common and highly contagious skin infection that affects children on face, arms, and legs. Initially, it appears

Table 87.1 Antimicrobial agents used topically

Topical antibacterial agents	Spectrum
Bacitracin	Gram-positive infections (such as *Staphylococcus aureus* and *Streptococcus pyogenes*)
Mupirocin	Gram-positive infections
Retapamulin	Gram-positive infections
Polymyxin B	Gram-negative bacteria such as *Pseudomonas aeruginosa*
Neomycin	Staphylococci and most gram-negative bacilli
Colistin	Gram-negative bacteria such as *P. aeruginosa*
Silver sulfadiazine	Gram-positive bacteria such as MRSA, and gram-negative bacteria such as *P. aeruginosa*
Gentamycin	*S. aureus* and gram-negative bacteria such as *P. aeruginosa*
Mafenide acetate	Broad-spectrum bacteriostatic action against some anaerobes, many gram-positive and gram-negative organisms

Abbreviation: MRSA, methicillin-resistant Staphylococcus aureus.

as red sores, which burst and develop into honey-colored crusts. Gram-positive bacteria such as *S. aureus* or *S. pyogenes* infect the superficial layers of the epidermis.

This is treated with mupirocin—2% ointment or cream applied topically twice daily for 5 days. Retapamulin is topically applied as 1% ointment twice daily for 5 days in patients 9 months or older.

Furuncle (Boil)

It is a painful infection with pus collection in perifollicular tissues, which mainly affects thighs, armpits, buttocks, face, and neck. It starts as a red tender lump. Topical antibiotics are helpful in treating the condition when the number of lesions is limited. But if systemic symptoms such as fever, lymphadenitis, or cellulitis appear, systemic antibiotics are used for treating folliculitis and boils. Available preparations include:

1. Fusidic acid 2% cream twice daily
2. Clindamycin 2% gel twice daily.
3. Mupirocin 2% ointment applied two to three times daily.
4. Benzoyl peroxide 2 to 10% gel applied twice daily.
5. Dicloxacillin (250 mg four times daily).
6. Cefadroxil 500 mg twice daily.
7. Ciprofloxacin 400 to 500 mg twice daily for gram-negative folliculitis.

Topical Antiviral Agents (DR8.7)

Common viral infections of the skin are caused by human papillomavirus, herpes simplex virus, molluscum contagiosum virus, and varicella zoster virus. Topically active antiviral drugs are acyclovir, valacyclovir, penciclovir, and famciclovir.

Genital Herpes Simplex

This (caused by type-2 virus) can be treated by topical, oral, or parenteral acyclovir, depending on the stage and severity of disease. Topical acyclovir (5% ointment, six times a day for 10 days) is effective in early and mild cases; otherwise, oral therapy is advised. Acyclovir provides symptomatic relief and rapid healing of lesions, but recurrence is not prevented.

Mucocutaneous Herpes Simplex

In this (type-1 virus), usually lips and gums are affected and resolve itself without any treatment but acyclovir skin cream (alone or in combination with hydrocortisone) may be used for some relief. Other topical agents available are docosanol and penciclovir. In immunocompromised patients, oral agents are used.

Herpes Simplex Keratitis (Type-1 Virus)

Acyclovir and idoxuridine (eye ointment applied five times daily till 3 days after healing) are equally effective in superficial corneal ulcer and for deep stromal infections because of good corneal penetration.

Anogenital Warts (by Human Papillomavirus)

Anogenital warts can be treated by applying topical cidofovir (1% gel) once daily for five consecutive days every other week for a maximum of six cycles. Topical use of cryotherapy, podophyllin, and trichloroacetic acid may be considered. Topical immunomodulatory therapies such as imiquimod and sinecatechins are other options.

Topical Antifungal Agents

Dermatophyte Infections

These infections of the skin (tinea corporis, cruris, and pedis) can be treated with topical antifungal agents, for example, clotrimazole, miconazole, econazole, ketoconazole, luliconazole, oxiconazole, sulconazole, sertaconazole, ciclopirox olamine, naftifine, terbinafine, butenafine, and tolnaftate. Topical naftifine, terbinafine, and butenafine provide sustained cure in comparison to azole antifungals, but azoles have some antibacterial effect and can be considered in lesions with bacterial superinfection.

Cutaneous Candidiasis

Localized lesion can be treated with topical applications of clotrimazole, miconazole, econazole, ketoconazole, oxiconazole, ciclopirox olamine, nystatin, or amphotericin B. Severe cases require systemic fluconazole or itraconazole. For oropharyngeal candidiasis, clotrimazole gel is applied in the mouth.

Vaginal Candidiasis

Clotrimazole is preferred due to its long-lasting residual effect after once daily application. Miconazole is also highly efficacious (> 90% cure rate) drug for tinea, cutaneous, and vulvovaginal candidiasis.

Onychomycosis (Fungal Infection of the Nails)

Oral therapy (terbinafine or itraconazole) is preferred in mild cases (when nail matrix is spared); ciclopirox nail lacquer, efinaconazole, and tavaborole may be used as a 48-week treatment course.

Agents for Ectoparasitic Infections (DR5.3)

Pediculus capitis (head louse), pediculosis corporis (body louse; by *Pediculus humanus humanus*), *Pthirus pubis* (pubic or crab louse), and scabies (by *Sarcoptes scabiei*) are infestations that specifically affect humans.

1. Lindane is a cyclohexane derivative and causes paralysis of parasites (pediculicide and scabicide) by neuronal hyperstimulation. It is not a preferred drug due to neurotoxicity as an adverse effect.
2. Permethrin is neurotoxic to lice (1%) and scabies (5%), as it interferes with insect Na^+ transport. However, it should not be used in infants younger than 2 months.
3. Pyrethrins (with piperonyl butoxide, which prevents the lice from metabolizing the pyrethrins) is the drug of choice for pediculosis.
4. Malathion causes paralysis in lice by inhibiting acetylcholinesterase.
5. Benzyl alcohol is available as 5% lotion, which asphyxiates lice.
6. Crotamiton is used in scabicide with antipruritic action (less effective than other topical treatments for scabies and lice).
7. Ivermectin 0.5% lotion is used to treat lice. Oral ivermectin 200 µg/kg is used for both scabies and lice. It causes few local irritant effects after application, but after oral administration it can cause dizziness, somnolence, vertigo, and tremor.

Acne Vulgaris

It is the formation of comedones (clogged hair follicles), which can be opened (blackhead) or closed (whitehead), pustules, nodules, and cysts due to *Propionibacterium acnes* (a gram-positive rod, part of the normal skin flora), which cause obstruction and inflammation of pilosebaceous units (hair follicles and their accompanying sebaceous gland). Commonly used drugs for acne are retinoids, benzoyl peroxide, salicylic acid, azelaic acid, and antibiotics such as erythromycin and clindamycin.

Retinoids

Retinoids are used for moderate-to-severe cystic acne. They are derivatives of vitamin A and all are topical agents (except isotretinoin, which is administered orally and reserved for severe cystic acne) (**Table 87.2**). Retinoids are also used for psoriasis and photoaging.

Retinoids bind to the nucleic retinoic acid receptors and function as transcription factors. They are used in disorders of differentiation and proliferation such as acne, psoriasis, and photoaging. Retinoids have several adverse effects such as irritation, dryness, skin peeling, erythema, and photosensitivity (severe sunburn may occur, so wearing sunscreen for protection is recommended). Oral isotretinoin may result in hair loss, hypothyroidism, and altered mood. It is also teratogenic. All retinoids are contraindicated in pregnancy. Acitretin is esterified with alcohol into etretinate, whose $t_{1/2}$ is about 3 months. Female patients are advised to avoid pregnancy due to the risk of retinoid-induced embryopathy for at least 3 years.

Benzoyl Peroxide

It is a topical agent used as antiseptic (also opening of pores) against mild-to-moderate acne. Concomitant use of benzoyl peroxide with tretinoin is not recommended because it inactivates tretinoin. Common adverse effects are dry skin, peeling, and irritation.

Table 87.2 Uses and routes of administration of retinoids

Retinoid generation	Drugs	Route
First generation (decrease sebum production)	Retinol (vitamin A)	Topical
	Tretinoin (all-*trans*-retinoic acid)	Topical
	Isotretinoin (13-*cis*-retinoic acid)	Oral
	Alitretinoin (9-*cis*-retinoic acid)	Topical
Second generation	Acitretin	Topical
Third generation (comedolytic, anti-inflammatory, less irritating, and more effective than other retinoids)	Adapalene	Topical
	Tazarotene	Topical

Salicylic Acid

It penetrates the pilosebaceous unit and works as an exfoliant to clear comedones by comedolytic and anti-inflammatory activity. It is effective for mild acne and also acts as a keratolytic at higher concentrations. It can cause mild skin peeling, dryness, and local irritation.

Azelaic Acid

It is available as topical preparation for mild-to-moderate acne, with antibacterial activity against *P. acnes*. It also possesses anti-inflammatory and anticomedogenic effects. It may cause mild skin irritation.

Antibiotics

These are effective for moderate-to-severe acne with inflammatory lesions. Topical erythromycin and clindamycin are the preferred drugs. Other drugs such as topical dapsone or oral preparations of minocycline, doxycycline, and erythromycin can be used. Topical preparations of antibiotics are available in combination with benzoyl peroxide or retinoids.

Psoriasis

Psoriasis is an immunological disorder with involvement of T-cell-mediated immune components and genetic factors. Psoriasis is manifested as localized/widespread erythematous scaling lesions/plaques with excessive epidermal proliferation, dermal inflammation, and periodic flare-ups.

Retinoids (Tazarotene, Acitretin)

Tazarotene is a topical acetylenic retinoid prodrug, which converts to active metabolite tazarotenic acid. It is useful in plaque psoriasis due to anti-inflammatory and antiproliferative actions.

Acitretin, used orally in pustular psoriasis, is metabolized to etretinate (with half-life of 120 days) by transesterification. As ethanol ingestion increases transesterification, it is better to avoid drinking while on acitretin. Acitretin is teratogenic, so a 3-year gap is needed between acitretin therapy and pregnancy. Other side effects are pruritis, skin peeling, cheilitis, and hyperlipidemia.

Topical Corticosteroids

Corticosteroids are used topically in the treatment of psoriasis, eczema, and contact dermatitis, as they possess immunosuppressive and anti-inflammatory actions due to the inhibitory effects on the arachidonic acid cascade. They decrease cytokines and inhibit epidermal cell mitosis. Tolerance may occur with continuous use. Possible adverse effects are skin atrophy, dermatitis, local infections, striae, purpura, acneiform eruptions, and hypopigmentation. Systemic toxicity occurs if applied on large surface area, which can cause hypothalamic-pituitary-adrenal (HPA) axis depression.

Keratolytic Agents (Coal Tar and Salicylic Acid)

They have anti-inflammatory effects, inhibit excessive skin cell proliferation, and thus also improve corticosteroid penetration. Coal tar is cosmetically unappealing.

Calcipotriene and Calcitriol

Calcipotriene is available as 0.005% cream and scalp lotion alone or in combination with betamethasone dipropionate. It is a synthetic vitamin D_3 derivative and is used in the treatment of plaque-type psoriasis vulgaris by suppressing proliferation and enhancing differentiation. Improvement starts after regular 2 weeks of therapy. Its combination with betamethasone dipropionate is more effective. Common adverse drug reactions include burning, itching, erythema, irritation, and dryness.

Calcitriol contains 1,25-dihydroxycholecalciferol and is available as 3 µg/g ointment. It is effective topically in plaque-type psoriasis and is better tolerated in intertriginous and sensitive areas of the skin.

Keratolytic Agents

Salicylic acid, propylene glycol, urea, sinecatechins, podophyllum resin, and podofilox are used to treat hyperkeratosis conditions such as calluses, verrucae, and xerosis.

Salicylic Acid

It solubilizes cell surface proteins and intercellular proteins, resulting in desquamation of keratotic debris. Elimination of the stratum corneum starts from the outermost level. Salicylic acid is keratolytic in concentrations of 3 to 6%. In concentrations greater than 6%, it can be destructive to tissues. Topical use may be associated with local irritation, acute inflammation, and ulceration. Urticaria, anaphylactic, and erythema multiforme reactions may occur in allergic patients.

Propylene Glycol

It acts as keratolytic agent in 40 to 70% concentrations and is a commonly used vehicle for various topical preparations. It is also an effective humectant and increases the water content of the stratum corneum. Propylene glycol alone or with 6% salicylic acid is used for the treatment of ichthyosis, palmar and plantar keratodermas, psoriasis, pityriasis rubra pilaris, keratosis pilaris, and hypertrophic lichen planus. It may cause allergic contact dermatitis, so patients having eczematous dermatitis are recommended a patch test with 4% aqueous propylene glycol solution.

Urea

Topical application of urea has many effects on the stratum corneum such as softening, moisturizing, proteolytic, keratolytic, epidermis-thinning, and antipruritic action. Urea reduces epidermal hyperproliferation and induces cell differentiation. It is used to treat dry/rough skin conditions (e.g., eczema, psoriasis, corns, callus). Urea has hygroscopic characteristics and increases the water content of the stratum corneum (humectant as 2–20% creams and lotions). Keratolytic effect (as 20% creams or lotions) of urea may be due to interfering with the quaternary structure of keratin and breaking of hydrogen bonds. Thus, by denaturizing, keratin urea is used in ichthyosis vulgaris, hyperkeratosis of palms and soles, and xerosis.

Sinecatechins

It is a water extract of green tea leaves from *Camellia sinensis*. It is indicated for the topical (15% ointment) treatment of external warts around the genital and rectal areas in immunocompetent patients. Sinecatechins ointment should be applied three times daily to warts until complete clearance, but the therapy should not exceed 16 weeks. It may sensitize the skin to sunlight, so sinecatechins-treated area should not be exposed to sunlight.

Podophyllotoxin (Podofilox)

This is purer and more stable form of podophyllin and is approved for use as 0.5% solution or gel for the treatment of genital warts. It acts as antineoplastic, keratolytic, microtubule destabilizing agent and prevents cell division. Only 70 µL per application of podofilox is sufficient to treat penile warts. Treatment cycles consist of twice-daily application for three consecutive days, which is followed by a four-day drug-free period. Local adverse effects are inflammation, erosions, burning pain, and itching. Podofilox used in low concentration reduces the potential for systemic toxicity, as seen with podophyllum resin, which is a crude form.

Alopecia

Minoxidil

This is available as topical foam and solution and used for the treatment of androgenic alopecia. It stops hair loss in both men and women and can also induce hair growth, but at least 6-month treatment is required, and medication needs to be continued to retain benefits. Minoxidil works by shortening the rest phase of hair cycle.

Finasteride

It is a 5α-reductase inhibitor and is administered orally as 1 mg once daily for androgenic alopecia. It blocks conversion of testosterone to the potent androgen 5α-dihydrotestosterone, which is responsible for atrophy of hair follicle. Among sexual side effects, erectile dysfunction is the most common, followed by ejaculatory dysfunction and loss of libido. If used during pregnancy, it can cause hypospadias in male children.

Bimatoprost

Bimatoprost is a prostaglandin analog used to treat eyelashes hypotrichosis and is available as 0.03% ophthalmic solution. Eyelashes hypotrichosis occurs as a part of alopecia areata totalis. Bimatoprost is applied to upper eyelid margins at the base of the eyelashes, using a separate disposable applicator for each eyelid. It increases eyelash length, thickness, and darkness. Side effects include pruritus, conjunctival hyperemia, skin pigmentation, and erythema of the eyelids. Bimatoprost ophthalmic solution when instilled in the eyes may result in increased brown iris pigmentation.

Pigmentation Disorders

Hyperpigmentation Conditions Such as Melasma and Photoaging

Hydroquinone (Whitening Agent)

It reduces hyperpigmentation associated with freckles and melasma. It is also used for treating photoaging. Melanin synthesis is decreased by inhibition of the tyrosinase enzyme. Irritation is the most common complication. Other adverse effects are erythema, contact dermatitis, transient hypochromia, and paradoxical postinflammatory hypermelanosis.

Monobenzone

It is benzyl ether of hydroquinone. It makes vitiligo discoloration even, but can cause permanent discoloration.

Azelaic Acid

It is used in acne treatment and is found to be effective in hyperpigmentary disorders, as it inhibits tyrosinase enzyme. Azelaic acid also acts by reducing free-radical production. It specifically affects abnormal melanocytes, and normally pigmented skin remains unaffected.

Kojic Acid

It is hydrophilic fungal product with potent antioxidant and tyrosinase-inhibiting action. It is equally effective as hydroquinone but can cause irritation, erythema, and contact dermatitis.

Hypopigmentation Condition Such as Vitiligo

Methoxsalen

It is a repigmentation agent, which stimulates melanocytes. It is photoactivated by UV radiation and inhibits cell proliferation and promotes cell differentiation of epithelial cells. It takes months for repigmentation of the affected skin. Adverse effects are skin aging and carcinogenicity.

Sunscreens

UV light is associated with certain skin disorders, as mentioned in **Table 87.3**. To protect the skin, sunscreens are applied topically to give temporary protection against sunlight and absorb UV light. Most of the sunscreens absorb the UVB wavelength in the range of 280 to 320 nm. *p*-Aminobenzoic acid (PABA) is the most effective against

Table 87.3 Skin disorders associated with UV rays

Ultraviolet light	Wavelength	Skin problem
UVA	320–400 nm	Skin aging, drug-induced photosensitivity, cutaneous lupus erythematosus, skin cancer
UVB	280–320 nm	Erythema, sunburn, skin aging, skin cancer

Abbreviation: UV, ultraviolet.

Table 87.4 Ingredients effective against UV rays

Sunscreen ingredients	Effective against
Zinc oxide and titanium dioxide	UVA and UVB
Dibenzoylmethane (avobenzone)	UVA
PABA	UVB
Benzophenones (oxybenzone, dioxybenzone, and sulisobenzone)	UVB
Cinnamates (cinoxate, octinoxate)	UVB
Salicylates (trolamine salicylate, homosalate, octisalate)	UVB
Octocrylene and ensulizole	UVB

Abbreviations: PABA, p-aminobenzoic acid; UV, ultraviolet.

UVB exposure. In 2019, FDA designated over the counter sunscreen products as generally recognized as safe and effective (GRASE). Major active ingredients of sunscreens are organic agents that absorb UV rays in the range of UVB or UVA and convert them to heat energy (**Table 87.4**). Others are inorganic agents/physical blockers (known as sunshades), which contain particulate materials that scatter visible, UV, and infrared radiation to reduce its transmission to the skin. Sunshades are opaque materials reflecting sunlight, for example, titanium dioxide.

Sun Protection Factor

Sun protection factor (SPF) is defined as the ratio of the minimal erythema dose of incident sunlight on the sunscreen-protected skin to the minimal erythema dose on the sunscreen unprotected skin. It is the measure of sunscreen effectiveness in absorbing UV light.

It primarily measures UVB protection.

New guidelines for labeling and effectiveness testing of sunscreens were published by Food and Drug Administration (FDA) in 2011. Continuous wave (CW) method is used to assess UVA protection. Products with a CW of 370 nm or greater may be labelled as "broad spectrum," referring to UVA radiation protection in relation to the amount of UVB protection.

In 2019, FDA proposed to increase the claimed maximum SPF value from 50+ (of 2011) to 60+ on the basis of benefits from clinical evidence. Moreover, the marketing of Sunscreens with SPF upto 80+ is being proposed. Sunscreens with SPF 2 to 14 prevent only sunburn. Sunscreens with SPF 15 or higher give a wide coverage of protection against sunburn, skin cancer, and early skin aging. Sunscreens should be applied 15 to 30 minutes before exposure to sun and needs to be applied again every 2 hours. If doing activities like swimming or sweating, water-resistant sunscreens should be used and reapplied every 40 or 80 minutes.

Deodorants and Anhidrotics

Deodorants

They are topically applied products with body odor-masking fragrance. The underarms are the most common site of application. Deodorants minimize the odor caused by the bacterial breakdown of perspiration. Deodorants are classified under cosmetics and available as solid, aerosol, or liquid base.

Anhidrotics or Antiperspirants

The primary function of anhidrotics or antiperspirants is to inhibit perspiration, which is an essential component for the growth of malodor-causing bacteria. They are classified as over-the-counter drugs. Their main active ingredients are aluminum-based compounds that form a temporary plug within the sweat duct, which stops the sweat flow to the skin's surface. Commonly used antiperspirant active ingredients are aluminum chloride, aluminum chlorohydrate complexes, and aluminum zirconium complexes. They have no impact on the body's natural ability to control its temperature by sweating.

Topical Corticosteroids

They have anti-inflammatory, immunosuppressant, and antimitotic actions and are locally administered as topical and intralesional preparations. They are classified on the basis of potency (**Table 87.5**), which is measured by vasoconstrictor assay (assessment of an area of skin blanching after the application of topical agent on skin under

Table 87.5 Potency of topical corticosteroids

Potency	Corticosteroids
Mild potent	Hydrocortisone
Moderate potent	Clobetasone butyrate, alclometasone dipropionate
Potent	Beclomethasone dipropionate, fluticasone propionate, mometasone furoate, triamcinolone
Very potent	Betamethasone dipropionate, clobetasol propionate

Table 87.6 Absorption of hydrocortisone solution through normal skin of different regions

Area	Extent of absorption (%)
Ventral forearm	1
Plantar foot arch	0.15
Palm	0.80
Scalp	3.5
Forehead	6
Vulvar skin	9
Scrotal skin	42

Table 87.7 Ranking of dermatologic disorders responsiveness to topical corticosteroids

Very responsive	Less responsive	Least/no response topically responsive: intralesional injection required
Atopic dermatitis	Discoid lupus erythematoses	Keloids
Psoriasis	Pemphigus	Hypertrophic scars
Seborrheic dermatitis	Necrobiosis lipoidica diabeticorum	Alopecia areata
Pruritus ani	Sarcoidosis	Acne cysts

occlusion), psoriasis bioassay (to assess the effect of the agent on psoriatic lesions), and other assays (inflammation is induced experimentally and then suppression of erythema and edema by the topical agent is assessed).

Absorption of topically applied corticosteroids varies to a great extent across skin of different body parts (**Table 87.6**). Absorption increases several folds in inflammatory conditions. A ranking of dermatologic disorders, responsiveness to topical corticosteroids is provided in **Table 87.7**.

Topical corticosteroids possess the potential to cause several adverse effects. Generalized flare occurs in sensitive individuals; hence, hypersensitive individuals should avoid corticosteroids. Short-term use of low-potency members of the class is safe. Applying potent corticosteroids to extensive areas of the body for prolonged period may cause growth retardation in children. Long-term use can lead to skin atrophy (cigarette paper appearance), telangiectasia, striae, purpura, and acneiform eruptions. This is partially reversible when the treatment is discontinued. Application of fluorinated compounds on face leads to perioral dermatitis and rosacea (steroid rosacea), with erythema, telangiectatic vessels, pustules, and papules; hence, these compounds should not be used here. There is an increased risk of HPA axis suppression on occlusion. Other adverse effects are hypopigmentation, hypertrichosis, increased intraocular pressure, allergic contact dermatitis, and alteration of cutaneous infection, with possible reactivation of a coexisting infection.

Multiple Choice Questions

1. A 25-year-old woman presents with complaint of acne. She is already using erythromycin 3% cream for the last 3 months, but there is no visible improvement. Now, her prescription changed to capsule isotretinoin. What may be the reason for no improvement in this case of acne?

A. Concentration of erythromycin is less.
B. Topical erythromycin is not effective enough in acne.
C. She should wait for 1 more month.
D. Clindamycin may be the better option instead of erythromycin.

Answer: B

Topical antibiotics such as erythromycin and clindamycin are not effective enough to treat acne. They are more suitable for inflamed papules. Erythromycin is available as 2 to 4% cream, lotion, ointment, and gel. Within 3 months of regular use of topical erythromycin, some effects are usually visible. Retinoids are added to topical antibiotic preparations for treating acne effectively.

2. In the above-mentioned case, even if no improvement is visible, it is not rational to shift her on oral isotretinoin from erythromycin cream because:

A. Isotretinoin is less effective in women.
B. Isotretinoin is less effective than erythromycin.
C. Isotretinoin should be the first drug to start in acne.
D. Isotretinoin is avoided in women of childbearing age.

Answer: D

Isotretinoin is very teratogenic (can cause craniofacial, heart, and central nervous system abnormalities) and is avoided in women of childbearing age. Isotretinoin is very effective, but due to its adverse effects, it should be reserved for unresponsive severe acne cases.

3. A 4-year-child attended the OPD for scabies. What would be the most appropriate treatment for him?

A. Permethrin.
B. Lindane.
C. Crotamiton.
D. Mupirocin.

Answer: A

Permethrin and lindane are more effective scabicidal than crotamiton. Concerning neurotoxicity, permethrin is safer than lindane. Mupirocin is used in scabies for secondary bacterial infections.

4. A couple is planning for Goa tour. What would you like to suggest them about sunscreen?

A. SPF of sunscreen should be in the range of 2 to 14.
B. SPF of sunscreen should be in the range of 15 to 50.
C. SPF of sunscreen should be in the range of 50 to 80.
D. Sunscreen should be applied once in the morning for full-day protection.

Answer: C

In 2019 FDA proposed to increase the claimed maximum SPF value from 50+ to 60+ on the basis of benefits from clinical evidence and the marketing of Sunscreens with SPF upto 80+ is being proposed.

5. A 30-year-old engineering student attended the OPD for the problem of alopecia areata. What would be the most appropriate treatment for him?

A. Minoxidil lotion.
B. Dutasteride.
C. Finasteride.
D. Triamcinolone intralesional injection.

Answer: D

Intralesional corticosteroids are preferred for adults with isolated patches of hair loss. Triamcinolone treatment results in hair regrowth in more than 50% patients.

Chapter 88 Gene Therapy

Nilofer Sayed, Prince Allawadhi, Amit Khurana, and Kala Kumar Bharani

Learning Objectives

- Gene therapy.
- Gene transfer techniques.
- Applications and future perspectives of gene therapy.

Introduction

As the field of medicine has advanced, pharmacological treatment strategies have progressed tremendously. However, the small molecules, biologics, and peptide-based drugs cannot be applied to all disease settings due to specific limitations such as uncertain effect on genetic level to cure or repair the disease related to gene alteration. Treatment options now aim to curb the underlying factors than ameliorate the symptoms of a disease by employing different biomedical approaches, out of which gene therapy is a promising tool for disease treatment in the modern era. Gene therapy involves introduction or entry of genes in the cells of humans. It not only consists of treatment strategies in single gene disorders where an alteration in gene occurs, but also aids in diseases where more than one gene is involved and environment interacts, as in coronary artery disease and diabetes, and diseases having an alteration in acquired genes such as cancer and AIDS. In the last few years, along with gene therapy strategies, clinical trials have also been accepted for offering promising results. Genetic disorders in metabolism, cell cycle regulation, ligand/receptor function, cytoskeleton, and extracellular proteins cause serious diseases, wherein gene therapy can offer a solution.

Gene therapy can be defined as the strategy to insert, remove, or correct the altered (mutated) genes that target therapeutic treatment. Gene therapy has shown exciting results in laboratory settings in the form of preclinical in vivo experiments. However, its successful application in clinical settings is under trials. Most of these trials are being conducted in the United States, EU, China, Japan, and Australia. Gene therapy is attempted in recessive gene disorders such as cystic fibrosis, hemophilia, muscular dystrophy, and sickle cell anemia. Among the acquired genetic diseases, cancer is remarkably targeted through gene therapy. Certain viral infections and AIDS are also being investigated for treatment through gene manipulation. Gene therapy is also applied in plant biotechnology by using *Agrobacterium tumefaciens*, a pathogen of dicotyledonous (broad-leafed) plants, which is used as a vector that transfers target gene into the plant genome. Although, conceptually, gene therapy opens up new avenues in the field of medicine and biomedical engineering, large-scale formulation, production, and successful clinical translation are still in their nascent stage.

Gene Therapy

As defined earlier, gene therapy involves suppression of gene expression, overexpression, or gene modification. RNA interference (RNAi) technology can suppress the gene expression at the mRNA level (posttranscriptional gene silencing). The antisense oligonucleotides (ASOs), microribonucleic acid (miRNA), small interfering ribonucleic acid (siRNA), and short hairpin ribonucleic acid (shRNA) can be delivered within the cell to bring about the reduction in the protein turnover by silencing the mRNA in the cytosol, resulting in reduced or no effect by the targeted gene. Overexpression of gene can be achieved by direct delivery of the gene (in the form of plasmid DNA) to the cell (gene replacement therapy). This facilitates a transient or persistent production of the abnormal or deficient protein within the diseased body, which tends to restore the altered function of body.

Corrective gene therapy involves the use of engineered or bacterial nucleases to bring about targeted modification of genomic sequences in all eukaryotes. The programmable nucleases are zinc finger nucleases (ZFNs), transcription activator–like effector nucleases (TALENs), and clustered regularly interspaced short palindromic repeat (CRISPR)-Cas-associated nucleases. **Fig. 88.1** shows the two major methods by which gene therapy is carried out clinically.

Gene Transfer

For the success of gene therapy, it becomes imperative to select a safe and efficient method to transfer the manipulated DNA/gene into the targeted cells or tissues. Gene transfer thus can be defined as a process where gene copies are inserted into the living cells to induce synthesis of the gene's product. The desired gene can be transferred into the cells either directly or through vectors. A delivery system is required to transfer the desired gene to the target cell, since the hydrophilic nature of the naked DNA molecules and the large size and anionic charge due to the phosphate groups hamper the entry into the cell. Additionally, these DNA molecules are easily destroyed by nuclease enzymes.

The ideal characteristics of successful gene delivery system comprise certain assets such as: (1) it should shield the transgene from intracellular nucleases; (2) it should carry the transgene from cell membrane to the target nucleus; and (3) it should be capable of overcoming the barriers involved at each phase of the gene delivery process. It should not cause any toxic effect and should exhibit minimal inflammatory response.

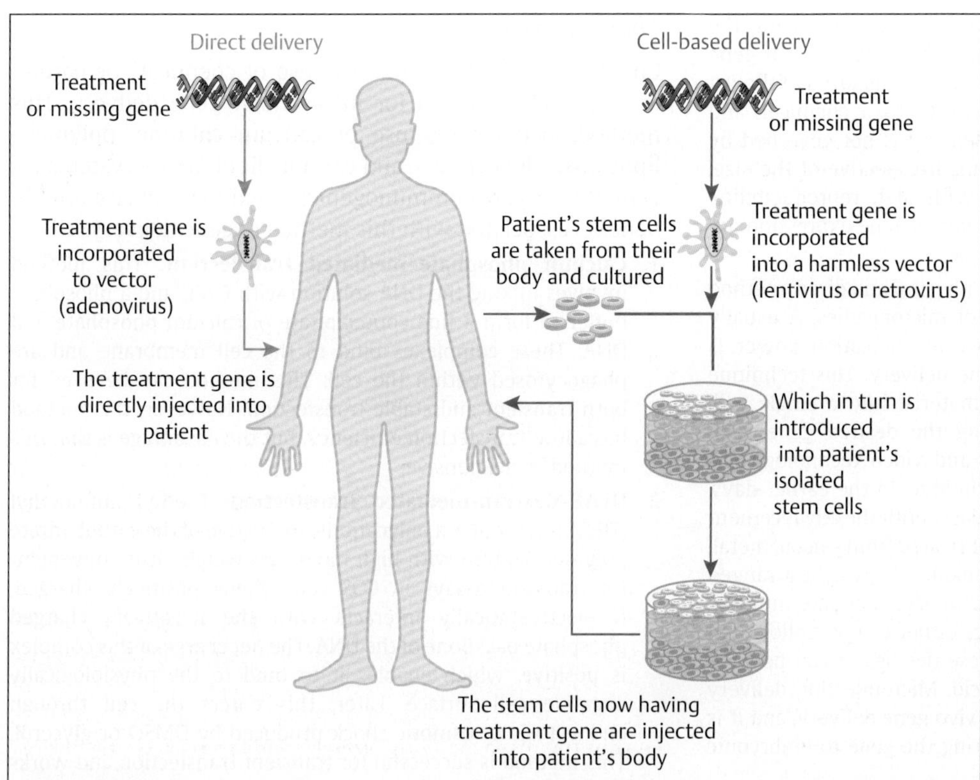

Fig. 88.1 Two distinct methods of incorporating the treatment gene into the patient's body.

Methods of Gene Transfer

Several techniques can be used for intracellular DNA transfer. However, no single method can be universally adopted. The chances of success of a gene therapy vary depending on the gene targeted for therapy, the organ site of delivery, surrounding environment of the organ, and many more. Factors that determine the choice of method include efficiency, affordability, reproducibility, safety, gene delivery technique, and ease of use.

Physical Methods

Physical methods are associated with employing physical force to enhance the permeability of the cell membrane and deliver the desired gene. The advantage of physical methods is convenience and reliability. However, the major disadvantage is the injury to cells during the process. This reduces the cell count of viable transfected cells drastically. Physical methods are electroporation, biolistic, microinjection, laser, elevated temperature, ultrasound, and hydrodynamic applications.

1. **Electroporation**: DNA can be transfected into any cell by subjecting it to controlled short electric impulses of high voltage to carry DNA across the cell membrane. Electric field transiently alters the structure and physiology of the cell membrane, thereby enabling exogenous nucleic acids to enter inside the cell. Factors affecting the efficiency of transfection and cell viability are strength of the applied electric field, exposure time of the host cell to the electric impulse, temperature, DNA conformation, DNA concentration, and ionic composition of the transfection medium. This method can be used for both in vivo and in vitro gene delivery. It is a cost-effective and quick method. It is highly reliable and can be as effective as viral transfection. However, considerable optimization of conditions is needed, as the death rate of cells subjected to this method is high. There are certain drawbacks of using this method, such as: limited effective range of working is approximately 1 cm between the electrodes; surgical procedure is needed to place the electrodes deep inside the internal organs where target genes have to be delivered; and as the high voltage is applied to target location, it causes thermal heating that results in irreversible tissue damage.
2. **Thermal-assisted gene transfer**: This method is based on the hypothesis that cell membrane permeability responds to changes in temperature. Change in the surrounding temperature of cell causes increase in the permeability under external force, and during this phase, the desired gene with suitable vector gets inside the host cell and produces the desired effects. This method is usually used in combination with other methods such as electroporation. High voltages applied during electrotransfer of gene may cause tissue damage. To deal with this, heat can be supplied exogenously, so that the same effect is obtained in lower voltages. Targeted application of heat could also help in plasmid localization.
3. **Biolistic**: The gene gun evolved from a modified Crosman air pistol that was invented at Cornell University by John C. Sanford, Ed Wolf, and Nelson Allen. Delivery with gene gun method is also termed ballistic DNA delivery or DNA-coated particle bombardment. A gene construct comprises a DNA cassette carrying all required regulatory elements for a proper expression within the target organ. Depending on the target and on the desired outcome of the transformation process, a gene construct may be altered in its design. Typically, all constructs consist of a promoter sequence, a terminator sequence, gene of interest, and the reporter gene. In this method, DNA or RNA adheres to the biological inert particles such as gold or tungsten. Using this transfer method, the DNA–particle complex is placed on the surface of the target tissue and is accelerated

by a powerful shot into the tissue, thereby introducing the DNA effectively into the target cells. The advantages of gene gun over other in vivo gene delivery systems are as follows: being a physical method of gene delivery, toxic chemicals and biological systems are not used; delivery is not governed by receptor interaction; DNA fragments, irrespective of the size, are transported within the cells with high reproducibility. However, short-term and low amounts of gene expression are the major drawbacks of this technique

4. **Microinjection**: Microinjection is a physical and direct method of gene delivery through the use of microneedles. A usually inverted microscope with a proper magnification power is used to attain a precise desire gene delivery. This technique is mainly used to insert genetic material into a single cell. Handling the pipette and injecting the desired gene with the help of computerized control and video technology has increased the efficiency of this technique. In the earlier days, these microneedles were made of glass. With the advancement of technology, now microneedles fabricated from silicon, metal, and biodegradable polymers are available. They can be arranged in arrays and can be manufactured to accommodate multiple delivery applications. These needles either can be hollow and contain the nucleic acid within these needles or can be solid needles coated with the nucleic acid. Microinjection delivery can be used in both in vitro and in vivo gene delivery, and it is an important technique for delivering the gene to embryonic cells.
5. **Laser-assisted transfection**: Light amplification by stimulated emission of radiation (LASER)-assisted transfection is also known as phototransfection, laserfection, or optoporation. The underlying principle of this method is that transient modulation of the cell membrane permeability is possible through a laser pulse. The subsequent pore formation leads to a difference in the osmotic pressure between the medium and the cytosol, thereby facilitating the entry of genetic materials and macromolecules into the desired cell.
6. **Ultrasound-assisted gene transfer**: This method is known as sonoporation. The ultrasound waves lead to the formation of cavitation bubbles in the cell membrane. These microbubbles expand and contract under the influence of ultrasound radiation. Collapsing of the bubble ruptures the cell membrane, generating a pore that facilitates the entry of DNA/RNA into the cell. The cell membrane permeability has direct correlation with the formation of pores. Ideally, this method is used for delivering the plasmid and/or fragments and can be used in both in vitro and in vivo gene transfer. Compared to retroviral and adenoviral vectors, sonoporation is associated with lower incidence of carcinogenesis. It is potentially a suitable method of gene delivery, as it supports real-time tracking of irradiated fields. However, this procedure has low-transfection efficiency and could lead to cell injury.
7. **Hydrodynamic gene transfer**: This system is based on the hydrodynamic principles of blood flow within the capillaries and is known as hydroporation. Injecting large volumes of DNA solution creates a hydrodynamic pressure, eventually increasing the capillary wall permeability, forming pores in the plasma membrane, and encircling the parenchyma cells. Membrane pores are eventually closed, and the molecules are retained within the cell. Success of the hydrodynamic procedure depends on the structure of the capillary, the cells encircling the capillaries, and the hydrodynamic force applied. This method is superior to other gene delivery systems due to its simplicity, versatility, and efficiency.

Chemical Methods

Chemical methods include the use of chemicals or natural and synthetic carriers for intracellular gene delivery. This method includes the use of calcium chloride, polymers, liposomes, dendrimers, and cationic lipid–based systems for gene delivery. Nonimmunogenicity and low toxicity are the benefits associated with this method of gene delivery.

1. **Calcium phosphate–mediated transfection**: This method involves mixing the DNA solution with $CaCl_2$ and a phosphate buffer to form a fine coprecipitate of calcium phosphate and DNA. These complexes bind to the cell membrane and are phagocytosed within the cell. This method can be used for both transient and stable transfection. However, this method has a low-transfection efficiency, but the advantage is that this method is inexpensive.
2. **DEAE–dextran-mediated transfection**: Diethyl aminoethyl (DEAE)-dextran is a polycationic derivative of the carbohydrate polymer dextran with high molecular weight. It is convenient for transient assays in COS cells. Being positively charged, it electrostatically interacts with the negatively charged phosphate backbone of the DNA. The net charge of this complex is positive, which enables it to bind to the physiologically negative cell surface. Later, this enters the cell through endocytosis or osmotic shock produced by DMSO or glycerol. This method is successful for transient transfection and works best with BSC-1, CV-1, and COS cell lines. This method is simple, cheap, and can be employed in transient cells that cannot survive even a short exposure to calcium phosphate. However, this polymer is very toxic, cannot be used to transfect cells that are sensitive to serum-free media, and is inefficient for the production of stable transfectants.
3. **Cationic lipid–mediated transfection**: These lipids comprise a hydrophilic cationic head group (these are most commonly primary, secondary, tertiary amine, or quaternary amine salts). The hydrophobic tail consists of aliphatic chain, cholesterol, or steroid rings. Ether, ester, carbamate, and amide are the linker groups that connect the hydrophilic and hydrophobic sections of the lipid. The nature of these groups determines the biodegradability. These are usually unilamellar structures and the positively charged head group strongly associates with the negatively charged phosphate backbone. The overall positive charge of the transfection complex aids in the interaction with the cell membrane. This complex then fuses with the cell membrane and is internalized through endocytosis. Intracellularly, this complex should escape the endosomal pathway, diffuse through the cytoplasm, and reach the nucleus to complete the process and initiate gene expression. Cationic lipid–based transfection systems are easy to synthesize and reproduce, irrespective of the size of DNA to be transported; they also have low immunogenicity, and are efficiently taken up by cells through endocytosis. However, their structural instability and heterogeneity, toxicity, inactivation due to enzymes in the circulation, and lack of targeted delivery are some of the disadvantages when compared to other systems.
4. **Polymers**: Cationic polymers lack a hydrophobic moiety; hence, they are easily miscible in water.
   a. These are long-chained structures made up of small units called monomers. Cationic polymers form stable complexes with the DNA material and have higher transfection efficiency when compared to DEAE–dextran complex. However, they are cytotoxic. Higher molecular-weight

polymers are nonbiodegradable and hence are toxic compared to low-molecular-weight polymers, but these also show higher transfection efficiency due to their increased polymer-to-nucleic acid charge ratio. This method limits the exposure of DNA to heavy encapsulation conditions and also enhances its rapid release. This method is nonimmunogenic, simple, and cheap. However, low-transfection efficiency, cytotoxicity, and instability of the complex limit its use in gene therapy.

b. Dendritic polymers: Dendrimers are repeating, branched, large spherical molecules with nanocavities within. They possess a large number of terminal functional groups on their surface. These functional groups determine the variability of dendrimers, whereas branching facilitates growth of the structure. Their size, degree of branching, and functionality can be controlled and adjusted by the synthetic approaches. These structures possess a high ratio of multivalent surface moieties to molecular volume, making them good candidates for transporters of gene to the cell of interest. Just as other delivery systems, these are also based on the electrostatic interaction between the DNA molecule and dendritic polymers. Dendrimers are highly efficient in targeted delivery of the genetic material. However, the size of the dendrimers (generations), the nature, and density of the charged groups determine the toxicity of the delivery system.

Biological Methods

Transduction using viral vectors: The very infective nature of viruses can be exploited for the delivery of transgenes to the cell of interest. The other genes must then be deleted from the viral genome to reduce its pathogenicity and immunogenicity and, finally, the transgene can be inserted into the viral construct and the vector is ready for use. Recombinant-deficient viral vectors (viruses that are replication deficient or lack any harmful effect) are used to transduce the dividing and postmitotic cells, and then they have been developed to facilitate powerful, regulatable, long-term, and cell-specific expression. Viral vectors can be used to bring about both the types of transfection, namely, transient and stable transfection. For example, viruses such as adenoviruses do not integrate within the host cell genome and have an episomal expression. Hence, these viruses bring about a transient gene expression. However, lentiviruses integrate within the host genome and bring about a stable and permanent expression of gene and its products. Viral systems have advantages of high-transfection efficiency and constant expression of therapeutic genes. However, there are limitations in large-scale virus production, immunogenicity, toxicity, and insertional mutagenesis.

Other biological methods used are bactofection, bacteriophages, viruslike particles, erythrocytes, and exosomes.

Types of Cells Suitable for Gene Transfer

Every cell contains genes; thus, theoretically, all cells can be treated through gene therapy. These cells can be divided into two major types: somatic cells and germline cells (eggs or sperm).

Germ Line Cells

Gene therapy using germ line cells results in permanent changes that are transferred to the subsequent generations. Gene manipulations can be done in gametes during in vitro fertilization and also during early embryologic development. It is also termed as embryo manipulation. Germline gene therapy is done in order to circumvent a genetic disease or to introduce an "enhancing" genetic variation. The beauty of germ line gene therapy lies in its potential to offer a permanent therapeutic effect. However, there is a possibility that genetic change propagated by germ line gene therapy can also turn deleterious and harmful, and may also have unforeseen negative effects on future generations. Recently, some new genes also have been successfully introduced into the germ cells of other mammals, but with very less efficiency. Moreover, manipulating the genes in the germ line cells has a great potential to be misused, as we see the idea of designer babies, where genes are engineered to get desired traits in the child. Hence, a lot of ethical issues are involved when it comes to editing genes in the germ line cells.

Somatic Cells

Somatic cells are nonreproductive, such as hepatocytes, neurons, and blood cells. Somatic cell therapy is safer as the genetic alteration is limited to the targeted cells in the patient and is not transferred to future generations. However, this type of therapy also has some limitations, one being the short-term effect of the therapy, since cells of most tissues ultimately die and are replaced by new cells; therefore, multiple treatments are required to maintain the therapeutic effect. Gene delivery to the target cells or tissue is also problematic due to the many physiological barriers such as inadequate cellular and tissue targeting and unprecise control over processing and trafficking. Despite these challenges, gene therapy has been a ray of hope in cystic fibrosis, muscular dystrophy, cancer, and certain infectious diseases.

Ex Vivo and In Vivo Gene Transfer

Somatic gene therapy can be categorized into ex vivo and in vivo.

Ex Vivo

When gene manipulation is done on cells outside the body, in external environment, and then transplanted back into the patient, such a strategy is called ex vivo gene therapy or gene transfer. While treating hematological diseases, peripheral blood mononuclear cells or bone marrow is harvested from the patient and the cells are cultured in the laboratory. These cells are then exposed to the virus carrying the desired gene. The gene is delivered to the cells through the viral vector; upon entry into the cell, the virus integrates its nucleic acid with the host genome. The transfected cells are grown in the laboratory and are then returned to the patient through intravenous (IV) route. This is called ex vivo gene therapy.

In Vivo

When genes are modified within the patient body itself, it is called in vivo gene transfer. The liver is the most preferred organ for in vivo gene therapy, as it consists of highly metabolic active and long-living hepatocytes, which can receive and release the substance to bloodstream. The methods usually employed for in vivo gene transfer are electroporation, gene gun, microinjection, laser-assisted transfection, and sonoporation for the direct transfer of DNA to target cell. However, sometimes these are used in combination with other viral or nonviral vectors to increase the transfection efficiency in vivo.

Applications and Future Perspectives of Gene Therapy

Nucleic acid therapeutics have attracted scientists worldwide due to their potential in mitigating dreaded inherited and acquired genetic diseases. Gene therapy–related clinical trials in different cardiovascular and neurodegenerative diseases and also in a variety of cancers are conducted by a number of research organization and companies. Gene therapy is less likely to face the problem of being resistant, as we see in the case of chemotherapeutics. Moreover, this technique could be a permanent alternative for a patient born with a genetic disease to live a healthy life. However, formulation of the gene therapy in conventional dosage form is a major challenge.

Severe Combined Immunodeficiency (SCID)

Gene therapy was first approved for this disease. The first trial was done on a 4-year-old girl in the United States on September 14, 1990. Severe combined immunodeficiency is caused due to a defective adenosine deaminase (ADA) gene. In the therapy, the patient's T-lymphocytes were isolated through aphaeresis and then these cells were subjected ex vivo to a genetically engineered live nonvirulent retrovirus carrying the normal ADA gene. These genetically modified T-cells were then transfused back into the patient's blood circulation. This initial trial had a remarkable success, which opened up bright avenues for further research in this area of therapeutics.

Leber's Congenital Amaurosis or Retinitis Pigmentosa

This disease is due to mutations in gene RPE65 that lead to blindness. Luxturna is an adeno-associated virus (AAV)–mediated gene therapy used to cure this disease where the mode of gene transfer is in vivo. It was developed by Spark Therapeutics and first approved in 2017.

Hemophilia A

This is a bleeding disorder due to a defect in the gene of human coagulation factor VIII. An AAV-mediated gene therapy called Valrox (Valoctocogene Roxaparvovec), also known as BMN 270, developed by BioMarin Pharmaceuticals, has been approved for treatment in patients in 2020. It is a single-dose IV administration therapy.

Spinal Muscular Atrophy (SMA)

In 2019, Novartis received a historic U.S. Food and Drug Administration (FDA) approval for gene therapy Zolgensma in spinal muscular atrophy. This therapy uses an AAV9 viral vector to deliver a copy of SMN1 gene into the motor neurons of afflicted patients, thereby curing them of this debilitating disease.

Heart Failure

Various targets have been identified and employed in clinical trials of gene transfer. The transgenes include sarcoplasmic/endoplasmic reticulum calcium ATPase 2a (SERCA2a), adenylyl cyclase 6 (AC6), and stromal cell–derived factor-1 (SDF-1)

Similarly, clinical trials are ongoing for a number of cardiovascular and neurodegenerative diseases as well as cancer. Both ex vivo and in vivo gene therapy products are termed *human gene therapy products* in the United States and *advanced therapy medicinal products* (ATMPs) in the EU. **Fig. 88.2** shows the major applications of gene therapy.

Summary

Gene therapy proves to be a promising therapeutic strategy that circumvents the limitations of pharmacological treatments such as chemoresistance and inability to rectify the genetic defects. However, the challenge lies in the delivery of plasmid gene or modified gene to the cell of interest. Discovery of safe gene delivery system that is scalable and also possess high-transfection efficiency with low toxicity is the rate-limiting step in the clinical translation of this therapeutic strategy.

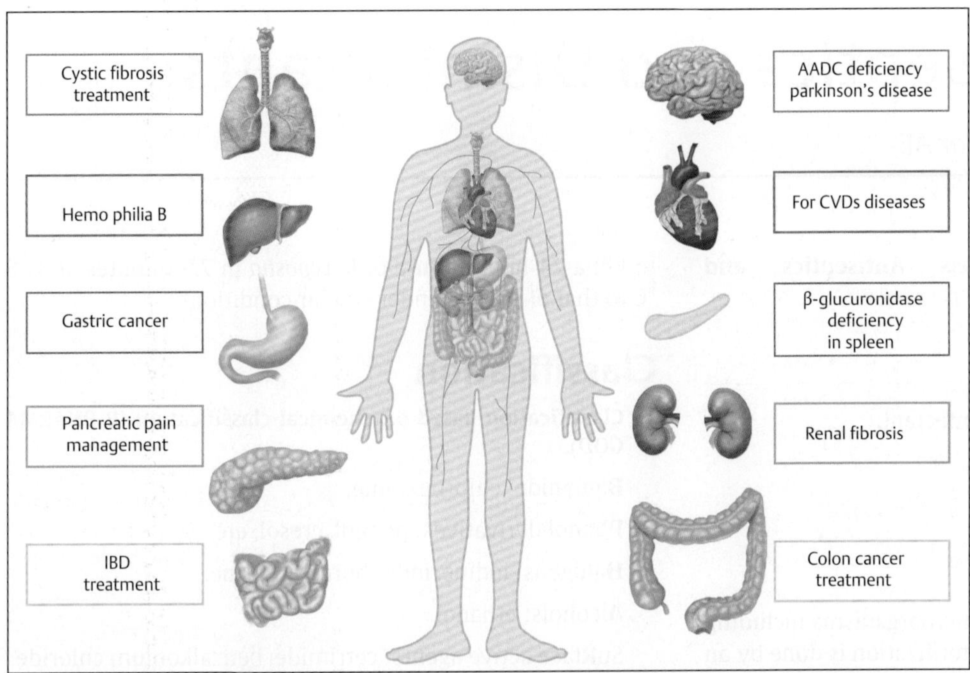

Fig. 88.2 Therapeutic applications of gene therapy. AADC, aromatic l-amino acid decarboxylase; CVD, cardiovascular disease; IBD, inflammatory bowel disease.

Multiple Choice Questions

1. A 34-year-old male patient was diagnosed with type II diabetes mellitus 10 years ago and has been on oral hypoglycemic drugs since then. The patient has now turned resistant to all the pharmacological interventions and refuses to take insulin injections and wishes to try gene therapy. What type of gene therapy will you advise him?

A. Delivery of plasmid DNA having the transgene that encodes for human insulin.
B. Isolate the β-cells that are responsible for insulin secretion. Edit the genes and transplant them back into the patient.
C. Advise not to go for gene therapy.
D. None of the above.

Answer: A

Although the majority of gene therapy studies have been performed with viral vectors, they have serious limitations in terms of immunogenicity and pathogenicity. Non-viral (primarily plasmid-based) gene therapy raises fewer safety concerns and is not hampered by immunogenicity to vector-specific sequences or products, permitting readministration. Overexpression of gene can be achieved by direct delivery of the gene (in the form of plasmid DNA) to the cell (gene replacement therapy). This facilitates a transient or persistent production of the abnormal or deficient protein within the diseased body, which tends to restore the altered function of body.

2. Which of the following statements, if any, is false?

A. Gene therapy is defined as replacement or modification of a defective gene for therapeutic benefit.
B. Current gene therapy is targeted only for somatic cells.
C. Only ex vivo gene therapy has been successful.
D. Gene therapy is meant only for recessively inherited disorders.

Answer: C

3. Which of the viral vectors will be best suited for gene delivery in hematopoietic stem cells?

A. Adenovirus.
B. Lentiviruses.
C. Adeno-associated viruses.
D. None of the above.

Answer: B

Since it is an integrating vector, the modified gene gets incorporated into the hematopoietic stem cells and persistent therapeutic effect is achieved.

4. What is the best disease among the options to be treated with nonintegrating viruses or nonviral vectors?

A. Cancers.
B. Parkinson's disease.
C. Hemophilia A.
D. None of the above.

Answer: B

As neurons do not divide in Parkinson's disease, episomal expression will also last for a prolonged period of time.

Chapter 89 Antiseptics and Disinfectants

Vijayakumar AE

PH1.62: Describe and Discuss Antiseptics and Disinfectants.

Leaning Objectives

- Ideal properties of antiseptic/disinfectant.
- Classification.
- Individual antiseptic uses.

Introduction

Sterilization is a process that kills microorganisms including spores, viruses, and fungi. Usually, sterilization is done by an autoclave. Other methods used are infrared, ultraviolet, and gamma radiations.

Germicides kill microorganisms, except bacterial spores, by using chemical methods. Germicides are further classified into disinfectants and antiseptics.

Disinfectants are the chemical substances that eliminate microorganisms from inanimate objects like instruments and scopes.

Antiseptics are the chemical substances that eliminate microorganisms from living tissues like skin and mucous membrane.

In 1847, Ignaz Semeelweis proposed hand washing techniques and fingernail scrubbing. In 1862, Louis Pasteur proposed the germ theory of disease transmission. In 1867, Joseph Lister did antiseptic surgery using phenol.

Ideal Properties of Antiseptic/ Disinfectant

- Chemically stable.
- Cheap.
- Cidal and not merely static.
- Ability to kill the vegetative form of pathogenic organisms.
- It should be effective even on short exposure.
- Active in room temperature.
- Active in presence of blood, pus, etc.
- Disinfectants should not corrode/rust instruments.
- Nonirritating to tissues.
- Should not interfere with healing.

Phenol Coefficient or Rideal–Walker Coefficient

It measures the potency of germicide. It is defined as the ratio of the minimum concentration of the test drug required to kill a 24-hour culture of *B. typosha* in 7.5 minutes at 37.5 °C to that of phenol under similar conditions.

Classification

1. **Classification based on chemical classification (B PHARMA GOD).**

   Biguanide: chlorhexidine.

   Phenol derivatives: phenol, cresol, etc.

   Halogens: iodine, iodophores, chlorine.

   Alcohols: ethanol.

   Su**R**face active agents: cetrimide, benzalkonium chloride.

   Metallic salts: zinc sulfate, calamine, zinc oxide.

   Aldehydes: formaldehyde; glutaraldehyde **a**cids, boric acid, acetic acid.

   Gases: ethylene oxide.

   Oxidizing agents: $KMnO_4$, H_2O_2, benzyl peroxide.

   Dyes: gentian violet, acriflavine.

2. **Classification based on mechanism of action.**

   Denaturing bacterial proteins:

   Phenol: phenol, cresol, etc.

   Alcohol: ethanol.

   Aldehydes: formaldehyde, glutaraldehyde.

   Oxidizing the sulfhydryl (SH) groups of bacterial enzymes:

   Halogens: iodine, iodophores, chlorine.

   Oxidizing agents: KMnO4, H202, benzyl peroxide.

   Alters the properties of the bacterial membrane:

   Su**R**face active agents: cetrimide, benzalkonium chloride.

   Miscellaneous agents:

   Dyes: gentian violet, acriflavine.

A summary of the mechanism of action of antiseptics and disinfectants is provided in **Fig. 89.1.**

Individual Agents

Phenols

The chemical name of phenol is carbolic acid. It is the oldest surgical antiseptic but is seldom used as a disinfectant due to its corrosive action, toxicity, and carcinogenicity. It was discovered by Lister. The most commonly used phenolic agents are p-phenylphenol, o-benzyl p chlorophenol, and p tertiary amylphenol. They are weak antiseptic and poor

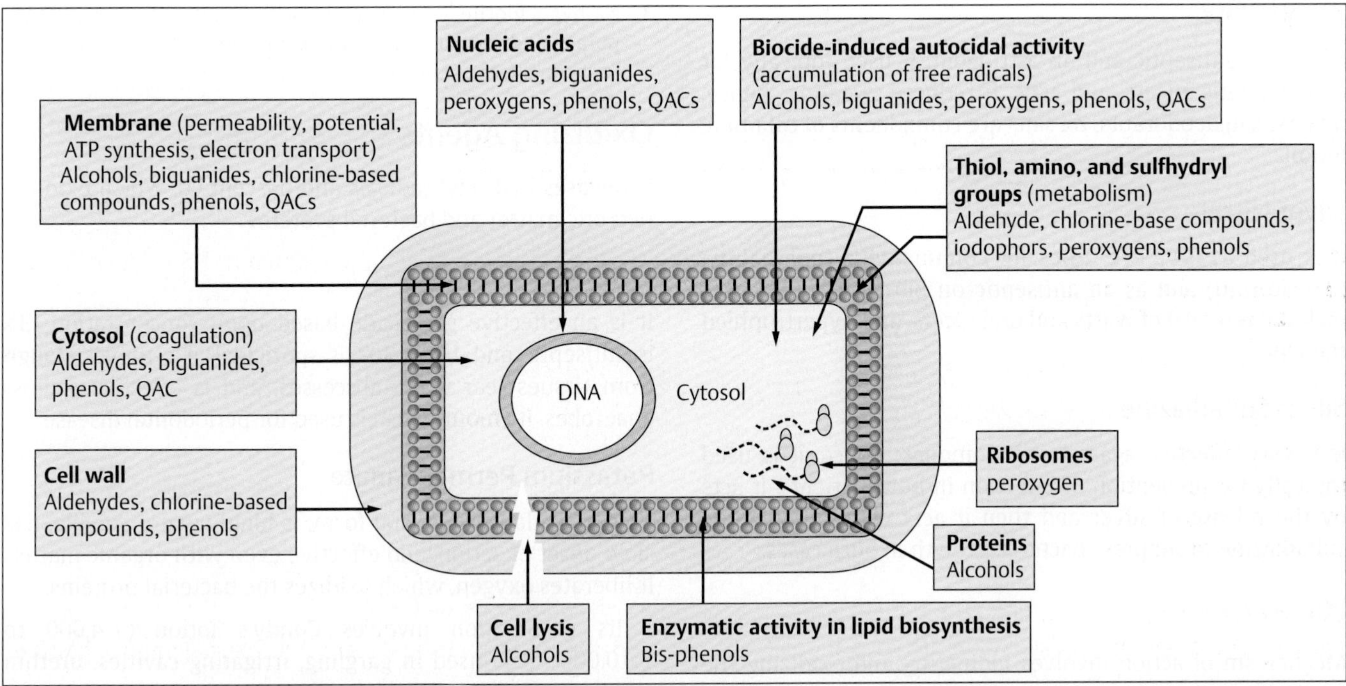

Fig. 89.1 Summary of the mechanism of action of antiseptics and disinfectants.

sporicidal agents. In high concentration, it causes skin burns and is caustic. It has mild local anesthetic action. It is used to disinfect urine, feces, pus, and sputum.

Cresols and Xylenols

They are derived from cold tar distillates and are more active and have less toxicity than phenol. It is used as a surface disinfectant.

Lysol is a 50% soapy emulsion of cresol. It is one of the most commonly used disinfectant in hospitals.

Chloroxylenol

It has equal efficacy as phenol but does not have corrosive, irritant properties of phenol. Dettol is made of 4.8% chloroxylenol and is used as a surgical disinfectant. It precipitates (denaturation) bacterial proteins by disrupting walls and membrane. It is a broad-spectrum germicide with bactericidal activity including mycobacterium, it is fungicidal, and it inactivates lipophilic viruses. It has no action on bacterial spores.

Triclosan is nonirritating, nonstaining, and has low sensitization. Listerine mouthwash is used for halitosis and gingivitis.

Aldehydes

Their mechanism of action involves denaturing bacterial proteins. It is a broad-spectrum germicidal agent which is active against Gram-positive bacteria, Gram-negative bacteria, bacterial spores, tubercle bacilli, viruses, and fungi.

Formaldehyde

This is a pungent gas used for fumigation. 37% aqueous solution of formalin diluted into 4% is used for preserving dead tissues. It is volatile, irritating, and causes sensitization. It is also occasionally used to disinfect instruments, excreta, and glassware.

Its disadvantages are its pungent odor and skin reaction (eczematoid reaction).

2% Glutaraldehyde

This is less volatile, less pungent, and less irritating. It is used to disinfect surgical instruments, glassware, endoscopes, etc. It used in dentistry as an immersion agent for instruments that cannot be autoclaved. The disadvantages are that it should not be used to disinfect working surfaces, as repeated inhalation can cause asthma. Alkalization activates glutaraldehyde activity.

Alcohols

These are commonly used for antiseptic purposes. They denature and precipitate bacterial proteins. The commonly used alcohols for germicide purpose are ethanol and isopropyl alcohol. In ethanol, the concentration used is 70 to 90%, and in isopropyl alcohol, the concentration used is 90%. It is a poor disinfectant and poor sporicidal agent. It is an irritant (hence not applied on mucous membrane, ulcers, open wounds, scrotum), and it is used as an antiseptic before intramuscular (IM) or intravenous (IV) injections (cotton swab soaked in 70% alcohol). It is used to sanitize working surfaces in dentistry. Isopropanol is the most potent agent which is used to disinfect thermometers.

Heavy Metal Salts

Mercury metal salts are obsolete as disinfectants. Only thiomersal (0.001–0.001%) is used as a preservative.

Zinc Sulfate

It is mild antiseptic and an astringent. It used topically for conjunctivitis, ulcers, and acne. It reduces sweating; hence, it is used in deodorants. Zn salts are components of calamine lotion.

Silver Nitrate

It is used as 0.1% eye drops for conjunctivitis (ophthalmia neonatorum) and as an antiseptic on burns. Its other uses include: removal of warts and oral ulcers, and hypertrophied tonsillitis.

Silver Sulfadiazine

It is very effective against pseudomonas; hence, it is used topically for prevention of infection in burn patients. It acts by the release of silver and then it acts with sulfonamide sulfadiazine to suppress bacterial growth in burn cases.

Halogens

Mechanism of action involves iodinating and oxidizing the protoplasm.

Iodine

Its advantages are that it acts rapidly and belongs to a broad spectrum (bacteria, viruses, and fungi). It has few disadvantages such as coloring of skin and materials, odor, and painful on open wounds. Its organic matter retards germicidal action.

Iodophores

They are soluble complexes of iodine or tri-iodide complexed with polymers (polyvinyl pyrrolidone) which release iodine slowly. The advantages are little or no odor and no discoloration of the surfaces. The most commonly used iodophore is povidone iodine. Other preparations include tincture iodine, Mandl's paint, iodex, betadine, etc.

1. 1% povidone iodine oral rinse for gingivitis.
2. 5% povidone iodine used on boils, burns, and bacterial infections.
3. 10% solution can be used endoscopes and surgical instruments.

Chlorine

At the concentration of 0.25 ppm, it kills most pathogens except M. tuberculosis and is mostly effective in acidic medium. It is most commonly used to disinfect water. Hypochlorous acid (HOCL) is responsible for its disinfectant action.

Chlorophores

These are salts of hypochlorite in the form of chloride lime. They slowly release HOCI.

1. Chlorinated lime–It contains 30 to 35% w/w available chlorine. It exposes chlorine on moisture. It is short-acting. It is used as a disinfectant in swimming pools and water tanks.
2. "EUSOL"–chlorinated lime (1.25%) + boric acid (1.25%) to clean infected wounds.
3. Na hypochlorite solution 2% loosens and dissolves dead tooth pulp in addition to exerting rapid antisepsis; hence, it is used in root canal treatment.

Oxidizing Agents

It releases hydroxyl radicals and nascent O_2, which oxidizes necrotic matter and bacterial proteins.

Hydrogen Peroxide

It is an effective germicide based upon concentration; 3% is antiseptic and 10 to 30% is sporicidal. It removes slough from tissues (ear wax), abscesses, and is effective against anaerobes. Its mouthwash is used for periodontal disease.

Potassium Permanganate

This is available in crystal form, is highly water soluble, has slow onset of action, and effective even with organic matter. It liberates oxygen, which oxidizes the bacterial proteins.

Its preparation involves Condy's lotion (1:4,000 to 1:10,000). It is used in gargling, irrigating cavities, urethra and wounds, disinfecting water (wells and ponds), and stomach wash in alkaloidal poisoning. The disadvantages of $KMnO_4$ are it is irritating, causes blisters, promotes rusting of surgical equipment, and stains tissues.

Biguanides

They alter the properties of bacterial cell wall.

Chlorhexidine

It is highly effective against Gram-positive bacteria (bactericidal), Gram-negative bacteria, Mycobacterium tuberculosis (MTB), fungi, and spores which are resistant. The common preparations are "Savlon" (chlorhexidine gluconate 1.5% + cetrimide 3%). It is widely used as sanitizers, antiseptic, and disinfectant for surgical instruments, surgical scrubs, neonatal baths, mouthwashes, obstetrics, and general skin antiseptics. This is most widely used as an antiseptic in dentistry in the form of oral rinses and toothpastes. It is also effective as antiplaque and antigingivitic agent (ANUG) for prevention and treatment. The major disadvantages are brownish discoloration of teeth and tongue, unpleasant aftertaste, alteration of taste perception, and, rarely, oral ulcers.

Cationic Surface-Active Agents: (Alters the Properties of Bacterial Cell Membrane)

This group contains quaternary ammonium or pyridinium or piperidinium group. Its mechanism involves detergent action (cationic surface-active agents), which lowers the surface tension and damages the bacterial cell membrane. It is bacteriostatic in nature. These agents are highly effective against Gram-positive bacteria. They have moderate effect on Gram-negative, MTB, and fungi. Spores, MTB, and viruses are resistant to this.

Benzalkonium Chloride

It is a good cleansing agent and is often combined with other agents to serve as a broad-spectrum disinfectant. The disadvantage is that their activity is greatly reduced in the presence of organic materials. It is used as sanitizer and disinfectant for surgical instruments and gloves.

1. 1:1,000 solution of benzalkonium chloride is used for preoperative disinfection of skin.
2. 1:2,000 solution is used for wound cleaning.
3. 1:10,000 solution is used for irrigation of the bladder.

Cetrimide

1 to 3% solution is used for roadside wound cleaning. Savlon (cetrimide with chlorhexidine) is one of the most commonly used antiseptics for surgical instruments.

Acids

They have antibacterial activity. They are fungistatic and bacteriostatic. The common ones are boric acid and sodium borate (borax).

Boric Acid

They are used as eye and ear drops, 2 to 4% solution as mouthwash, and 10% ointment for cuts and abrasions. It is also a component of prickly heat powder. Boroglycerine paint is used for stomatitis and glossitis, irrigating the bladder, cleaning wounds, and for burn dressings. The disadvantage is systemic absorption, which causes diarrhea, vomiting, and renal toxicity.

Benzoic Acid

It is antibacterial and antifungal. Whitfield's ointment–6% benzoic acid + 3% salicylic acid–is used for ringworm infections.

Dyes

Acriflavine

It is an orange-yellow acridine dye. It is active against Gram-positive bacteria and gonococci. Its effect is enhanced in alkaline medium. It is used in chronic ulcers, wounds, and simple burn dressings. It is available in 0.1 to 0.5% cream. It causes staining.

Aminacrine has the advantage of being nonirritating and nonstaining; its other properties are similar to acriflavine.

Gentian Violet

This is rosaniline dye. It is active against Gram-positive bacteria and fungi. Its 0.5 to 1% alcoholic solution is used in gingivitis, oral thrush, bed sores, chronic ulcers, and burns, but it causes staining of the skin.

Furan Derivatives

Nitrofurazone

This is bactericidal to Gram-positive bacteria, Gram-negative bacteria, and aerobic and anaerobic bacteria. It works by inhibiting the enzymes involved in carbohydrate mechanism, involved in bacteria, and it is used as 0.2% cream for burn dressing and skin grafting. The disadvantage is sensitization of the skin.

Methylene Blue

It is used in cyanide poisoning.

Table 89.1 depicts the actions and uses of common antiseptics and disinfectants.

Table 89.1 Summary of actions and uses of common antiseptics and disinfectants

Common antiseptics and disinfectants		
Chemical	**Action**	**Uses**
Ethanol (50–70%)	Denatures proteins and solubilizes lipids	Antiseptic used on skin
Isopropanol (50–70%)	Denatures proteins and solubilizes lipids	Antiseptic used on skin
Formaldehyde (8%)	Reacts with NH_2, SH, and COOH groups	Disinfectant, kills endospores
Tincture of Iodine (2% in 70% alcohol)	Inactivates proteins	Antiseptic used on skin
Chlorine (Cl_2) gas	Forms HClO, a strong oxidizing agent	Disinfect drinking water; general disinfectant
Silver nitrate ($AgNO_3$)	Precipitates proteins	Antiseptic and used in the eyes of newborns
Mercuric chloride	Inactivates proteins by reacting with SH groups	Disinfectant, occasionally used as an antiseptic on skin
Detergents (e.g., quaternary ammonium compounds)	Disrupts cell membranes	Skin antiseptics and disinfectants
Phenolic compounds (e.g., lysol, hexylresorcinol, hexachlorophene)	Denature proteins and disrupt cell membranes	Antiseptics at low concentrations; disinfectants at high concentrations
Ethylene oxide gas	Alkylating agent	Disinfectant used to sterilize heat-sensitive objects (plastics)

Multiple Choice Questions

1. A 30-year-old man with alleged history of road traffic accident had abrasion in the arm and ankle. Duty medical officer advised tetanus toxoid (TT) injection. Nursing staff used alcohol disinfectant before giving TT injection. Maximum antiseptic potential of alcohol is observed at .... concentration?

A. 100%.
B. 90–100%.
C. 70–90%.
D. 40–60%.

Answer: C

Major alcohols used as antiseptics are ethyl alcohol and isopropyl alcohol. It acts by mainly precipitating bacterial proteins. Antiseptic action rapidly increases at 70 to 90%; below 70% and above 90%, its action decreases. Disadvantage of alcohol antiseptics: does not kill spores and promotes rusting.

2. Formalin is one of the most commonly used disinfectants for preservation of the body. Composition of formalin is?

A. 27% w/v aqueous solution of formaldehyde diluted to 6%.
B. 37% w/v aqueous solution of formaldehyde diluted to 4%.
C. 20% w/v aqueous solution of formaldehyde diluted to 10%.
D. 70% aqueous solution of formaldehyde diluted to 2%.

Answer: B

Formalin is used for hardening and preserving dead tissues. It is a 37% aqueous solution of formaldehyde diluted to 4%.

3. Ideal agent of choice for noncorrosive metallic surgical instruments sterilization?

A. Formaldehyde 10%.
B. Glutaraldehyde 4%.
C. Formaldehyde 4%.
D. Glutaraldehyde 2%.

Answer: D

Formaldehyde is a pungent gas, which is irritant in nature and can cause eczematous reaction; hence, it is not used. Glutaraldehyde is the most commonly used to disinfect noncorrosive metallic surgical instruments. The concentration used is 2%.

4. A 45-year-old woman having dental caries. Dental surgeon wants to do root canal treatment. What is the antiseptic mainly used in root canal treatment in dentistry?

A. Gentian violet.
B. Povidone iodine.
C. Sodium hypochlorite solution.
D. Silver sulfadiazine.

Answer: C

4 to 6% sodium hypochlorite is a powerful disinfectant used in root canal treatment.

5. Chlorine is one of the most commonly used disinfectants. It acts by oxidizing protoplasm. Antiseptic action of chlorine is due to?

A. HCl.
B. Chloride ions.
C. Hypochlorous acid.
D. Hypochlorite ions.

Answer: C

Chlorine is used to disinfect urban water supplies. Its disinfectant action is due to hypochlorous acid (HOCl).

6. A 30-year-old man with abrasions in the arm and leg uses Savlon antiseptic liquid. Savlon antiseptic liquid contains?

A. Chlorhexidine plus chloroxylenol.
B. Cetrimide with cresol.
C. Chlorhexidine with cetrimide.
D. Lysol with benzalkonium chloride.

Answer: C

"Savlon" (chlorhexidine gluconate 1.5% + cetrimide 3%). It is widely used as sanitizers, antiseptics, and disinfectants for surgical instruments, surgical scrubs, neonatal baths, mouthwashes, obstetrics, and general skin antiseptics. This is most widely used as an antiseptic in dentistry in the form of oral rinses and toothpastes.

Chapter 90

Drug Therapy of Medical Emergencies

Sachin Parab, Snehal Lonare and Prasan R. Bhandari

Learning Objectives

- Shock.
- Status epilepticus.
- Status asthmaticus.
- Tetany.
- Acute addisonian crisis.
- Diabetic ketoacidosis.

Introduction

Medical emergencies generally include, but are not limited, to the following:

1. Shock: anaphylactic, cardiogenic, septic, hypovolemic.
2. Status epilepticus.
3. Status asthmaticus.
4. Tetany.
5. Acute addisonian crisis.
6. Diabetic ketoacidosis (DKA).

Shock

It is a state of acute circulatory collapse, leading to inadequate tissue perfusion and hypoxia. The different types of shock with their general causes include the following:

1. Anaphylactic shock: severe allergic reaction.
2. Cardiogenic: myocardial infarction.
3. Septic: bacteremia.
4. Hypovolemic: hemorrhage, burns, dehydration, severe vomiting, diarrhea.

Anaphylactic Shock

The drug of choice is adrenaline, 0.3 to 0.5 mL of 1:1,000 solution, injected subcutaneously, which is to be repeated after 20 minutes if necessary. For persistent anaphylaxis, add 1-mg adrenaline to 500 mL of 5% dextrose, and administer with an infusion rate of 1 mL/min. This is to be supplemented by ECG, blood pressure (BP) monitoring, and airway management. Other treatment modalities include antihistaminic agent pheniramine maleate 22.75 mg/mL and hydrocortisone 500 mg intravenously (IV) stat and 100 mg IV hourly. Bronchodilators could be administered if there is persistent bronchoconstriction.

Cardiogenic Shock

Inotropes such as dopamine are administered at a dose of 2 to 20 μg/min by IV route with 5% dextrose. Dobutamine 1 to 20 μg/kg/min can be added to improve the cardiac contractility. The end point is improved perfusion, BP, and urine output. Diuretics such as furosemide can also be administered. Other measures include taking care of airway, breathing, and circulation (ABC).

Septic Shock

This could be due to multiorgan system failure, leading to coma, acute respiratory distress syndrome (ARDS), congestive heart failure (CHF), renal failure, ileus or gastrointestinal (GI) hemorrhage, and disseminated intravascular coagulation (DIC). The more organ systems involved, the worse is the prognosis. Therapy includes taking care of ABC, fluid administration, inotropes, and vasoconstrictors. Appropriate antibiotics should be administered and treatment of underlying cause should be carried out.

Hypovolemic/Hemorrhagic Shock

Always begin with ABC. Replace circulating blood volume rapidly and blood products as soon as available for hemorrhagic shock. Replace ongoing fluid/blood losses and treat the underlying cause. Vasopressors may be considered for persistent hypotension after restoring blood volume.

Status Epilepticus

Administer IV diazepam 10 to 20 mg over 2 to 4 minutes and repeat after 30 minutes *or* clonazepam 1 mg over 30 seconds and repeat if necessary. Administer lorazepam 4 mg IV stat and repeat after 10 minutes. Phenytoin 20 mg/kg up to 25 to 50 mg/min can be administered or fosphenytoin 15 to 20 mg phenytoin equivalents (PE)per kg can be infused at a rate as high as 150 mg PE/min. Because 1.5 mg of fosphenytoin is equivalent to 1 mg of phenytoin, the dosage, concentration, and infusion rate of intravenous fosphenytoin are expressed as PE. Phenobarbital typically is used after a benzodiazepine or phenytoin has failed to control status epilepticus. The normal loading dose is 15 to 20 mg/kg. Because high-dose phenobarbital is sedating, airway protection is an important consideration, and aspiration is a major concern. Parenteral valproate is used primarily for rapid loading and when oral therapy is impossible. It has a broad spectrum of efficacy and may be useful in patients with absence or myoclonic status epilepticus. Adverse effects include local irritation, gastrointestinal distress, and lethargy. This drug is not FDA-approved for the treatment of status epilepticus. General anesthetic agents and skeletal muscle relaxants with positive pressure ventilation should be administered.

Status Asthmaticus

Intermittent humidified oxygen is administered to the patient along with salbutamol 2.5 to 5 mg by nebulizer or terbutaline 5 to 10 mg. If there is no improvement, then give 250 μg of salbutamol by IV route. In addition, give hydrocortisone 200 mg IV every 4 hours for 24 hours and prednisolone 60 mg orally daily. Ipratropium 0.5 mg can be added to α-agonist by nebulizer. Alternatively, aminophylline 5 mg/kg diluted in 20 to 50 mL of 5% glucose by IV infusion could be used. Antibiotics can be added, depending on the presence of infection, if at all. Simultaneously, correct the dehydration and acidosis.

Tetany

It is managed by injecting calcium gluconate10 to 20 mL (elemental calcium 90–180 mg) by IV route over 10 minutes, followed by slow infusion (total 0.45–0.9 g calcium over 6 hours is needed); this is along with the supportive measures.

Acute Addisonian Crisis

It is treated by injecting hydrocortisone 100 mg by IV route three times daily along with IV infusion of normal saline until the patient is stable. Additionally, correct fluid and electrolyte balance. Subsequently, the dose of cortisol is gradually tapered to a maintenance dose of 50 mg/day. Fludrocortisone tablet can be added at a dose of 0.1 to 0.2 mg/day.

Diabetic Ketoacidosis

This emergency is managed by giving regular insulin with a bolus dose of 0.1 to 0.2 U/kg IV, followed by 0.1 U/kg/hour infusion, till glucose level falls to 300 mg/dL. Fluid loss averages approximately 6 to 9 L in DKA. The goal is to replace the total volume loss within 24 to 36 hours, with 50% of resuscitation fluid being administered during the first 8 to 12 hours. A crystalloid fluid is the initial fluid of choice. Current recommendations are to initiate restoration of volume loss with boluses of isotonic saline (0.9% NaCl) IV based on the patient's hemodynamic status. Thereafter, IV infusion of 0.45% NaCl solution, based on corrected serum sodium concentration, will provide further reduction in plasma osmolality and help water to move into the intracellular compartment. Hyperosmolar hyponatremia due to hyperglycemia is a frequent laboratory finding in DKA and is usually associated with dehydration and elevated corrected sodium concentrations.

KCL is administered at a dose of 0 to 20 mEq/hour to the IV fluid. Sodium bicarbonate and phosphate are not routinely needed. Antibiotics should be administered if needed. For the management of hyperosmolar nonketotic syndrome, the general principles of treatment are identical to DKA, except that fluid replacement should be faster and prophylactic heparin therapy is recommended.

Chapter 91 Drugs Used in Ocular Disorders

Shrikant V. Joshi and Sapna D. Desai

PH1.58: Describe drugs used in ocular disorders.

Learning Objectives

- Autonomic drugs on pupil.
- Topical antimicrobial agents used for treatment of ophthalmic infections.
- Glucocorticoids.
- Antihistamines and mast-cell stabilizers.
- Glaucoma.

Ocular Disorders

The diseases or disorders of the human eye vary considerably in their etiology. Refractive errors, which are age-related, are the most common and include myopia (nearsightedness), hyperopia (farsightedness), astigmatism (distorted vision at all distances), and presbyopia (gradual loss of ability of eyes to focus on near objects). Glaucoma is a group of heterogeneous diseases developed due to elevated intraocular pressure (IOP) and characterized by optic neuropathy and visual disturbances. A cataract is a clouding of the lens of the eye, leading to decreased vision. Age-related macular degeneration is blurring of sharp and central vision due to degeneration of macula in older people. Uveitis, blepharitis, dacryocystitis, conjunctivitis, keratitis, endophthalmitis, and corneal ulcers are the inflammatory conditions, which may be due to noninfectious or infectious causes. Diabetic retinopathy is a complication associated with uncontrolled diabetes, characterized by damage to blood vessels supplying blood to retina, leading to problems ranging from mild visual disturbances to permanent blindness. Amblyopia is a partial or complete loss of vision in one eye due to loss of coordination between the eye and brain. Strabismus is an abnormal alignment of the eyes or imbalance in the positioning of the eyes. It is of two types: (1) esotropia, where one or both eyes are crossed in or turned inward and (2) exotropia, where one or both eyes are turned outward. Besides this, strabismus also leads to diplopia (double vision) or amblyopia (reduced vision).

Autonomic Drugs on Pupil

Autonomic drugs are used extensively for various purposes in ophthalmology, namely, to produce or reverse mydriasis, as topical anesthetic, cycloplegic retinoscopy, and funduscopic examination, and for the treatment of glaucoma, uveitis, and strabismus.

Mydriasis can be reversed by muscarinic cholinergic agonists, anticholinesterases, and α_2-adrenergic agonists, while muscarinic antagonists are used to induce cycloplegia for retinoscopy or fundoscopy.

Glaucoma is a chronic and progressive condition with prominent features such as optic nerve fiber degeneration, optic disk cupping, and notching of neuroretinal rims, which leads to irreversible blindness. Increased IOP is the chief cause for glaucoma and hence the therapies are targeted to decrease the production of aqueous humor at the ciliary body and to increase outflow through the trabecular meshwork and uveoscleral pathways. Nonselective β-adrenergic receptor antagonists and α_2-adrenergic agonists are used for the treatment. (Glaucoma, types of glaucoma, and treatment are explained in subsequent portions of this chapter.)

Uveitis is an inflammation of the uvea due to infectious and noninfectious causes. Antimuscarinic agents are frequently used to prevent posterior synechia formation (adhesion between iris and lens) and to relieve ciliary muscle spasm and associated pain. In the case of already formed synechiae, α-adrenergic agonist may break it by enhancing pupillary dilation.

Strabismus, or ocular misalignment, has numerous causes. Whenever amblyopia is developed (mostly in one eye), atropine is used to produce cycloplegia in the other eye (i.e., in eye without amblyopia) to induce cycloplegia, which forces the patient to use the eye with amblyopia.

The autonomic agents used in ophthalmology mainly affect the pupil diameter, ciliary muscles, and outflow of aqueous humor through trabecular meshwork and uveoscleral pathways. The drugs preferred are summarized in **Table 91.1**.

Topical Antimicrobial Agents Used for Treatment of Ophthalmic Infections

Ocular infections, both superficial and deep, such as conjunctivitis, corneal ulcers, and endophthalmitis, are caused by a diverse group of bacterial, viral, and fungal pathogens. Accordingly, the armamentarium of available antimicrobials used in the prevention and treatment of these infections includes antivirals, antifungals, and antibacterials.

Table 91.1 Autonomic drugs used for ophthalmic conditions

Generic name	Strength and formulation	Mechanism of action	Indications	Side effects
Cholinergic agonists				
ACh	10 mg/mL (after reconstitution) intraocular solution	Circular muscles of iris and ciliary muscles possess muscarinic M_3 receptor, while radial muscles of iris do not have parasympathetic supply. Muscarinic M_3 receptor is a G-protein-coupled receptor, which is stimulatory in action and acts by increasing the production of IP_3 and DAG from PIP_2. Cholinergic agonists cause constriction in circular muscles of iris, leading to constriction of pupil (miosis). Stimulation of M_3 receptors on ciliary muscles leads to loosening of suspensory ligaments of the lens, which brings about bulging of the lens or the lens becomes more convex (focal length reduced). This leads to accommodation of eye's focus for near vision. Ciliary muscle contraction along with stretching of pupil due to miosis, facilitates drainage of aqueous humor by opening the pores of the canal of Schlemm, causing reduction in intraocular pressure (especially in glaucoma patients). Carbachol is a carbamic acid ester of choline, which is resistant to hydrolysis by AChE as well as pseudocholinesterases. Therefore, it has longer duration of action as compared to acetylcholine. Pilocarpine is an alkaloid obtained from *Pilocarpus jaborandi*, having dominant muscarinic M_3 receptor agonistic action.	Intraocular injection for rapid and complete miosis during and after cataract surgery, penetrating keratoplasty, iridectomy, and other anterior segment surgery	Corneal edema
Carbachol	0.01–3% w/v intraocular injection			Corneal edema, miosis, induced myopia, decreased vision, brow ache, retinal detachment
Pilocarpine	0.25–10% w/v eye drops		• Initial treatment of open-angle glaucoma. Reduces intraocular pressure within short span of time and effect lasts for 4–8 h. • To counteract mydriasis produced by atropine • In iridocyclitis to separate adhesion between iris and the lens (instilled alternatively with homatropine)	
Anticholinesterase agents				
Physostigmine (available in combination with pilocarpine)	2% w/v eye drops	Anticholinesterases act by inhibiting AChE in synaptic cleft. At higher concentrations, these drugs can also inhibit pseudocholinesterases. These enzymes bring about rapid hydrolysis of ACh in synaptic cleft and responsible for inhibition of actions of ACh. AChE such as physostigmine and echothiophate inhibit the hydrolysis of ACh and increases availability as well as prolongs the actions of ACh on target organs.	• After refraction testing to counteract mydriasis • In cases of iritis, iridocyclitis and corneal ulcers to prevent adhesion of iris with lens (along with homatropine) • Treatment of OAG and closed-angle glaucoma	Retinal detachment, miosis, cataract, pupillary block glaucoma, iris cysts, brow ache, punctal stenosis of the nasolacrimal system

(Continued)

Table 91.1 (*Continued*) Autonomic drugs used for ophthalmic conditions

Generic name	Strength and formulation	Mechanism of action	Indications	Side effects
Echothiophate		Physostigmine is a reversible and competitive inhibitor of AChE, which increases availability of ACh at site of action, i.e., circular muscles of iris and ciliary muscles, leading to miosis and bulging of lens. Also, it decreases IOP and is used to prevent adhesion of iris with lens. Echothiophate is a quaternary ammonium compound having low local irritancy. It is an irreversibly acting AChE inhibitor, which is potent and longer acting (keep intraocular pressure decreased for 1–2 wk).	Used as miotic and in treatment of glaucoma	
Muscarinic antagonists				
Atropine	0.01–1% w/v eye drops, eye ointment	Muscarinic antagonists compete with ACh and other muscarinic agonists for M_3 receptors present in papillary constrictor muscles in the eye. This inhibition of M_3 receptors leads to unopposed sympathetic dilator activity on radial muscles of iris through a_1 adrenoceptors, eventually leading to mydriasis. Hence, mydriasis caused by these drugs is called passive or indirect mydriasis. As responses to cholinergic stimulation are blocked, eyes become unresponsive to light (loss of light reflex). Muscarinic antagonists also block M_3 receptors present on ciliary muscles, leading to tightening of suspensory ligaments, flattening of lens (i.e., lens becomes convex), thereby setting the eyes for distant vision. As responses to cholinergic stimulation are blocked, the eyes cannot respond to the attempt of accommodation for near vision, termed as paralysis of accommodation or cycloplegia.	▪ As mydriatic for ophthalmoscopic examinations (cycloplegic retinoscopy, dilated fundoscopy) ▪ To prevent adhesion of iris to lens in iridocyclitis, iritis, or uveitis ▪ Atropine and homatropine used as supportive therapy, to prevent spasm of ciliary muscle in corneal ulcer	Photophobia, Photosensitivity, blurred vision
Scopolamine	0.5% w/v eye drops			
Homatropine	1–2% w/v eye drops			
Cyclopentolate	0.5–1% w/v eye drops			
Tropicamide	0.5–1% w/v eye drops			
Sympathomimetic agents				
Dipivefrin	0.1% w/v eye drops	Sympathomimetics produce mydriasis by stimulating a_1 receptors present on radial pupillary dilator muscle of iris. a_1 receptors, when stimulated, contract the radial muscle, leading to dilatation of pupil. This is active mydriasis.	Dipivefrin, epinephrine, apraclonidine, and brimonidine are used for the treatment of glaucoma. Phenylephrine is used to produce mydriasis.	Photosensitivity, conjunctival hyperemia, hypersensitivity
Epinephrine	0.1, 0.5, 1, and 2% w/v eye drops	Ciliary muscles exhibit presence of β_2 receptors, which are also blocked but effect on accommodation of eye	Cocaine is used as topical anesthetic.	

(Continued)

Table 91.1 (*Continued*) Autonomic drugs used for ophthalmic conditions

Generic name	Strength and formulation	Mechanism of action	Indications	Side effects
Phenylephrine	0.12, 2.5, 5, and 10% w/v eye drops	is insignificant. This is because ciliary muscles show predominance of parasympathetic system. As cholinergic responses are unaffected, there will be no cycloplegia and blurring of vision. Light reflex also remained unaffected. α_1 agonists decrease the IOP by increasing the outflow of aqueous humor. Hence, they are used for treatment of glaucoma. Dipivefrine is a prodrug of epinephrine, having enhanced corneal permeability. Epinephrine stimulates both α- and β-adrenergic receptors, decreases IOP through β_2 receptors, and increases uveoscleral outflow (perhaps via prostaglandin production). Phenylephrine and naphazoline are α_1 selective agonists. Apraclonidine and brimonidine are selective α_2 agonists, which reduce aqueous humor production and enhance uveoscleral outflow, thereby lowering IOP.	Hydroxyamphetamine and cocaine are used to evaluate anisocoria.	
Apraclonidine	0.5 and 1% w/v eye drops			
Brimonidine	0.1, 0.15, 0.2% eye drops			
Cocaine	1–4% solution			
Hydroxyamphetamine	1% w/v eye drops			
Naphazoline	0.012–0.1% w/v eye drops			
Tetrahydrozoline	0.05% eye drops			
α- and β-adrenergic antagonists				
Dapiprazole	0.5% w/v eye drops	Selective α_1 adrenergic antagonist responsible for reversal of mydriasis by blocking α_1 adrenergic receptors present on radial muscles of iris	Reverse the mydriasis	Conjunctival hyperemia
Betaxolol	0.25 and 0.5% w/v, eye drops	Selective β_1 adrenergic receptor blocker	Glaucoma	Blurred vision, temporary stinging, or burning sensation in eyes
Carteolol	1% w/v eye drops	Nonselective β-blocker; decreases production of aqueous humor. Timolol is the most frequently used drug from this category.	Glaucoma	Blurred vision, photosensitivity
Levobunolol	0.25 and 0.5% w/v eye drops		Glaucoma	Blurred vision, temporary stinging or burning sensation in eyes
Metipranolol	0.3% w/v eye drops		Glaucoma	Blurred vision, photosensitivity
Timolol	0.25 and 0.5% w/v eye drops		Glaucoma	Blurred vision, bradycardia, orthostatic hypotension, syncope

Abbreviations: ACh, acetylcholine; AChE, acetylcholinesterase; IOP, intraocular pressure; OAG, open-angle glaucoma.

Host Defense

The eye's natural defense against foreign invasion is multilevel. The first level is physical barriers, which include orbital rim, eyebrows, eyelids, and eyelashes. The blinking of the eye prevents entry of smaller particles. The tear film along with various antimicrobial components forms the second barrier against microorganisms. Goblet cell mucus traps the bacteria. The tear film washes off the invasion along with chemical degradation by lysozyme, beta-lysin, lactoferrin, immunoglobulins (primarily IgA), complement, and cathelicidin. Adaptive immune responses regulated by conjunctiva-associated lymphoid tissue and low temperature of ocular surface lead to inhibition of the growth of microorganisms.

Antibacterial Agents

Ocular infections or orbital infections account for a large number of impaired vision or blindness cases worldwide. These are preventable and treatable. The bacteria accountable for a range of ocular infections can be classified as gram-positive or gram-negative (depending on staining with Gram stain), cocci or bacilli (depending on shape), and aerobic or anaerobic (depending on the need for oxygen) (**Fig. 91.1**).

Bacteria may infect periorbital or orbital structures such as periorbital skin (includes preseptal and postseptal), eyelids, conjunctivae, and lacrimal apparatus. Dacryoadenitis is an inflammatory response of lacrimal glands toward bacterial infection. It is secondary to the obstruction of the nasolacrimal duct and common in children and adolescents. Hordeolum and blepharitis are the infectious processes of the eyelids. A hordeolum is an infection of the glands in the eyelid margin such as meibomian, Zeis, or Moll glands, while inflammatory responses such as irritation and burning sensation in the eyelids are known as blepharitis. Conjunctivitis is an irritation or inflammation of the conjunctiva due to bacterial or other infections. The severity varies from mild hyperemia to severe purulent discharge. Keratitis is a corneal inflammation which may involve epithelium, subepithelium, stroma, and endothelium and may be due to noninfectious or infectious causes. Endophthalmitis is an infection to intraocular tissues, leading to severe inflammation. Panophthalmitis is the inflammation of all coats of the eye including intraocular structures. The pathological conditions and bacteria responsible for it are listed in **Table 91.2**.

Common topical antibacterials used in the treatment of ocular infectious diseases include sulfonamides, aminoglycosides, polymyxin-based combinations, and fluoroquinolones (**Table 91.3**). The selection of drug and the route of administration depend on symptoms of patients, clinical examination, and culture/sensitivity results. The local side effects of topical preparations are milder and include eye irritation, redness, itching, burning sensation, etc. Systemic side effects are rare.

Antifungal Agents

Fungi are ubiquitous organisms found in soil and decaying organic matters. Generally, they are saprophytes but become pathogens to cause opportunistic infection when the person is immunocompromised. Various fungi causing infections are shown in **Fig. 91.2**. Filamentous infection is treated with natamycin. Other alternatives are amphotericin B, miconazole, and voriconazole. There are various ophthalmic antifungal preparations available in the market along with the oral and intravenous preparations. Systemic antifungal agents can be administered in severe cases. Various topical preparations are listed in **Table 91.4**.

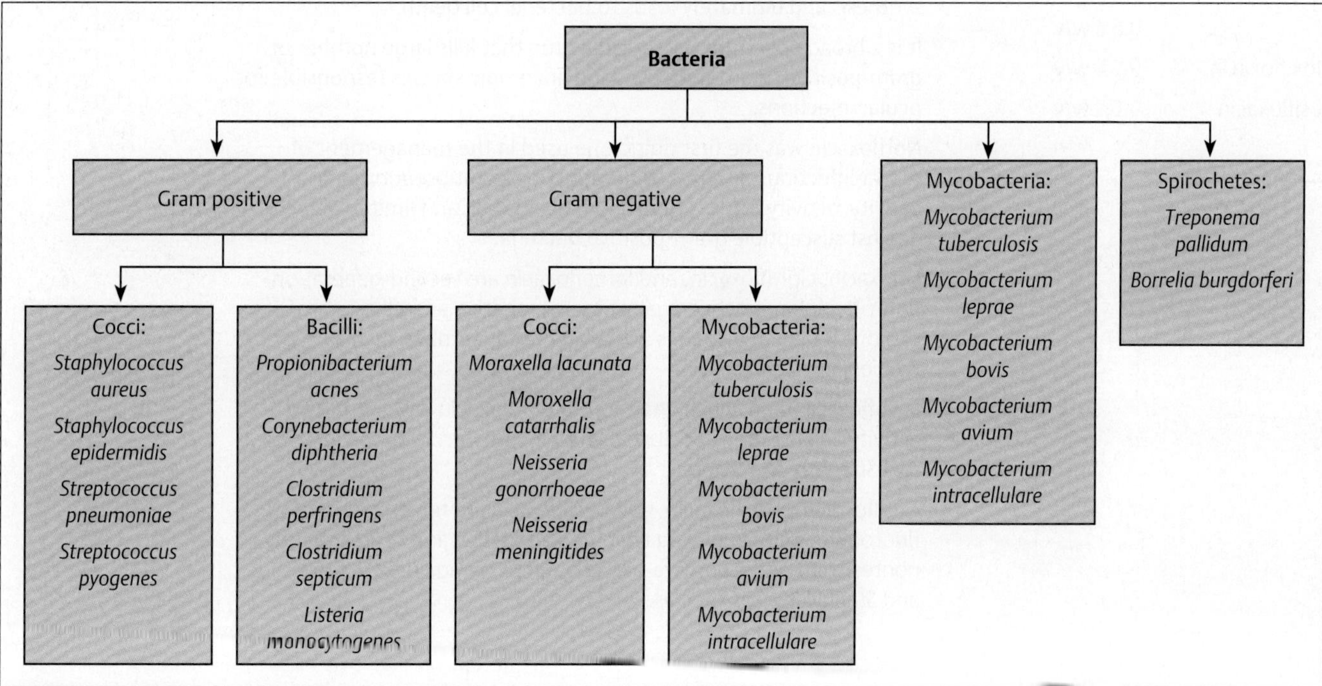

Fig. 91.1 Classification of bacteria leading to ocular infections.

Table 91.2 Pathological condition and causative bacteria

Pathological condition	Causative bacteria
Blepharitis	*Staphylococcus aureus, Staphylococcus epidermidis, Streptococcus pyogenes, Pseudomonas aeruginosa, Moraxella lacunata*
Dacryocystitis	*S. aureus, Staphylococci, P. aeruginosa, Escherichia coli*
Conjunctivitis	*S. aureus, S. epidermidis, Streptococcus pneumoniae, P. aeruginosa, Klebsiella pneumonia, E. coli, M. lacunata, Moraxella catarrhalis, Neisseria gonorrhoeae, Neisseria meningitides, Chlamydia trachomatis*
Keratitis	*P. aeruginosa, S. aureus, Corynebacterium diphtheria, M. catarrhalis*
Endophthalmitis	*S. aureus, S. epidermidis, Streptococcus viridians, Streptococcus pneumonia, K. pneumonia, Propionibacterium acnes, C. diphtheria, Clostridium perfringens, Clostridium septicum, Listeria monocytogenes*
Corneal ulcers	*S. epidermidis*

Table 91.3 Antibacterial drugs used for ophthalmic infections

Generic name	Strength	Mechanism of action	Uses
Bacitracin (available in combination with neomycin and polymyxin B)	500 IU (400 IU in combination with other drugs)	Bacitracin is a polypeptide synthesized by *Bacillus subtilis*. It is a bactericidal drug that interferes cell wall synthesis by inhibiting peptidoglycan production. Active against gram-positive organisms (both cocci and bacilli), *Neisseria*, and *Haemophilus influenzae*. Poorly absorbed orally and hence preferred topically. Used along with neomycin and polymyxin B to cover broad range of gram-positive and gram-negative bacterial eye infections.	Infectious conjunctivitis, anterior blepharitis
Norfloxacin Ofloxacin Ciprofloxacin Lomefloxacin Levofloxacin Gatifloxacin Moxifloxacin Besifloxacin	0.3% 0.3% w/v 0.3% w/v 0.3% w/v 0.5% w/v 0.3% w/v 0.5% w/v 0.5% w/v 0.6% w/v	These are fluoroquinolone derivatives that inhibit bacterial DNA gyrase and topoisomerase IV. DNA gyrase helps in separation of daughter DNA by introducing de-coiling in bacterial DNA double helix at the time of replication, while topoisomerase IV is responsible for decatenation, i.e., removing the interlinking of daughter chromosomes. Inhibition of these enzymes results in inhibition of bacterial DNA replication/ synthesis and ultimately leads to bacterial cell death. It is a broad-spectrum bactericidal drug that kills large number of gram-positive, gram-negative, and anaerobic species responsible for ocular infections. Norfloxacin was the first quinolone used in the management of ocular infectious diseases. It demonstrated antipseudomonal activity, activity against gram-negative bacilli, and limited activity against susceptible gram-positive bacteria. Ofloxacin, ciprofloxacin, and lomefloxacin are second-generation fluoroquinolones active against gram-negative as well as gram-positive bacteria. Also, it is active against anaerobes such as *Propionibacterium acnes*. Levofloxacin is an active enantiomer of ofloxacin with improved activity against gram-positive including *Streptococcus pneumoniae* and *Streptococcus viridans*. Gatifloxacin, moxifloxacin, and besifloxacin are fourth-generation fluoroquinolones active against gram-negative and resistant and nonresistant gram-positive bacteria. Effective against *Streptococcus* and *Staphylococcus* species.	Infectious conjunctivitis, bacterial keratitis, endophthalmitis

(Continued)

Table 91.3 (*Continued*) Antibacterial drugs used for ophthalmic infections

Generic name	Strength	Mechanism of action	Uses
Chloramphenicol	1% w/w ointment	It is a broad-spectrum antibiotic that inhibits bacterial protein synthesis by binding to 50S ribosomal subunit (bacterial ribosome has 30S and 50S subunits). It prevents binding of aminoacyl-tRNA to 50S ribosomal subunit, thereby acting as bacteriostatic. Less used as many organisms are resistant to it. Useful for treating infection of *Haemophilus* species resistant to other antibiotics.	Ocular surface infections, anterior blepharitis
Gentamicin sulfate	0.3% w/v	These are broad-spectrum bactericidal aminoglycosides, which prevent protein synthesis. As they act on protein-synthesizing assembly, they have to cross bacterial cell wall and cytoplasmic membrane. They diffuse through porin channels present in cell wall of gram-negative bacteria. Transportation across cytoplasmic membrane needs carrier proteins linked to electron transport chain and oxygen-dependent active process. Hence, they are ineffective against anaerobes as they are unable to cross cytoplasmic membrane. Once they enter cytoplasm, they bind with 30S subunits of bacterial ribosomes and 30S-50S interface, thereby preventing protein synthesis. Gentamicin is preferred as a first-line treatment for gram-negative organisms, including *Pseudomonas aeruginosa*.	Infectious conjunctivitis, anterior blepharitis, bacterial keratitis
Tobramycin	0.3% w/v		
Sulfacetamide	10% w/v 20% w/v 30% w/v	It inhibits folic acid synthesis and acts as bacteriostatic drug. It is a sulfa drug which inhibits bacterial enzyme and dihydropteroate synthetase, thereby preventing the conversion of *p*-aminobenzoic acid to folic acid. Unavailability of folic acid in bacteria leads to inhibition of synthesis of nucleic acids (DNA and RNA).	Infectious conjunctivitis, bacterial keratitis

Table 91.4 Antifungal agents for ophthalmic infections

Drug class/agent	Strength	MOA	Indications	Side effects
Polyenes				
Amphotericin B	0.15% (w/v) eye drops 5–10 mg/0.1 mL injection	Polyene antibiotics bind to ergosterol (a fungal cell membrane sterol) and poke holes in the fungal cell membrane, thereby altering the membrane permeability. Through these pores, Na^+, K^+, Mg^{2+}, H^+, and other macromolecules are leaked out, leading to death of fungi.	Yeast and fungal keratitis, fungal postoperative endophthalmitis, cutaneous, and mucocutaneous mycotic infections caused by candida species	Skin irritation, dryness, redness, itching, severe blistering, peeling
Natamycin	5% w/v eye drop	Amphotericin B can be injected intravitreally to treat chronic fungal infection.	Fungal infection of eye	Eye irritation
Imidazole				
Fluconazole	0.3% w/v eye drops	This class of drugs acts by inhibiting cytochrome P450-dependent 14-α-demethylase enzyme, thus preventing conversion of lanosterol to ergosterol and thereby inhibiting the synthesis of ergosterol which leads to damaged leaky fungal cell membrane. It is also proposed to inhibit respiratory electron transport chain, which is considered to be more plausible alternative mechanism for antifungal effects.	Fungal corneal, ulcers, or keratitis only	Eye irritation, stinging in the eyes
Voriconazole	1% w/v eye drop		Severe fungal infections	Headache, nausea, rash, vomiting, altered vision, slow heart rate, hallucination, abnormal liver function tests
Itraconazole	1% w/v eye drop		Fungal infection of eye	Eye irritation, Burning sensation
Ketoconazole	2% eye drop		Fungal infection of eye	Loss of appetite, headache, paresthesia, rashes, and hair loss. It also causes hormonal effects

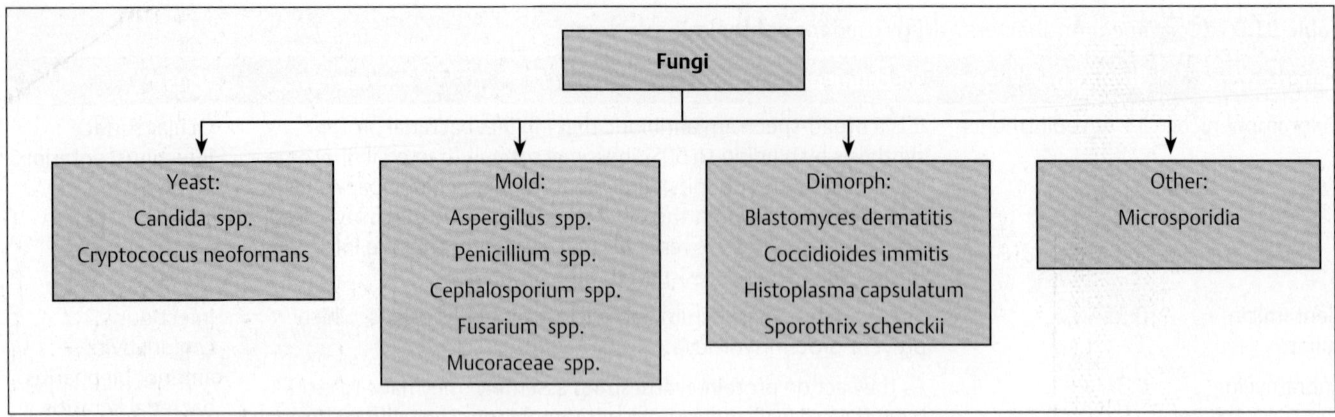

Fig. 91.2 Classification of fungi leading to ocular infections.

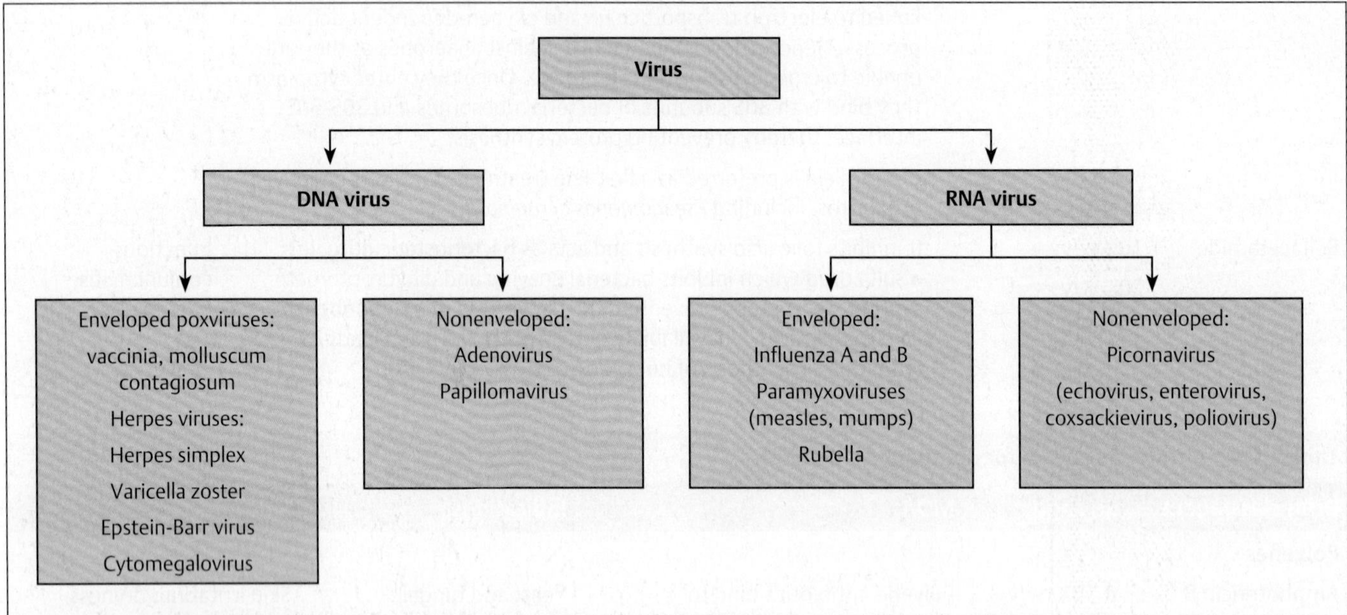

Fig. 91.3 Classification of viruses leading to ocular infections.

Antiviral Agents

Viruses are capable of causing ocular infections, attacking the surface or interior of the eye (**Fig. 91.3**). Adenovirus causes the viral conjunctivitis commonly associated with cold. These are probably the most common causes of acute viral infections of the eye. It manifests as one of the three classic forms: pharyngoconjunctival fever, epidemic keratoconjunctivitis, and nonspecific follicular conjunctivitis. Antibiotic treatment is ineffective in viral conjunctivitis. Herpes infection caused by herpes simplex virus 1 (HSV-1) can sometimes affect the eye and cause keratoconjunctivitis. This condition is generally referred to as herpes keratitis. The various other viral infections affecting the eye are herpes zoster ophthalmicus (it is reactivation of varicella zoster virus infection, i.e., shingles residing within the first division of the trigeminal nerve) and uveitis (a well-known complication of varicella infection); less common infections are HSV-2, Epstein–Barr virus, and cytomegalovirus (CMV) retinitis (DNA virus of herpes virus group; the primary ocular manifestation is chorioretinitis). Molluscum contagiosum is a mild viral disease caused by DNA virus of poxvirus group. The other virus-associated disease of eye, especially affecting the lid margin, is verruca. It is also caused by DNA virus of papovavirus group. The lesions produced are asymptomatic or associated with a chronic conjunctivitis, usually resistant to treatment. There are various antiviral agents used to treat these ocular viral infections. General treatment measures include discontinuation of topical steroids and topical application of antiviral agents.

Patients infected with viral keratitis who are treated with topical antivirals must be followed very closely, as antiviral agents have narrow therapeutic index and have toxic effect on the cornea. In disciform keratitis, epithelial and endothelial surfaces can be involved concurrently, with the latter being associated with marked central thickening. The use of topical glucocorticoids accelerates the recovery in disciform keratitis. Weak topical steroids along with antiviral therapy can be used for the treatment of stromal keratitis, which protect it against secondary dendritic ulcers. Topical steroids should be used judiciously, as they can enhance herpetic keratitis, but they might not lead to reactivation of latent virus. Highly active antiretroviral therapy (HAART) can be used for the treatment of viral retinitis if the specific anti-CMV therapy is not continued but CMV retinitis does not appear to progress even then; uveitis is observed in some patients who show immune recovery. Long-term antiviral therapy via various routes is usually followed for treatment. Oral steroids should be considered in case of optic nerve involvement. Various drugs along with their mechanism of action, dosage forms, side effects, and indications are listed in **Table 91.5**.

Table 91.5 Antiviral agents for ophthalmic use

Generic name	Strength	Mechanism of action	Indications	Side effects
Trifluridine	1% topical solution	It is a trifluoromethyl derivative of idoxuridine, which gets incorporated into viral DNA and inhibits viral DNA polymerase. It is comparatively more potent than idoxuridine. It inhibits HSV-1, HSV-2 and CMV infection.	Herpes simplex keratitis and conjunctivitis.	Blurred vision, dryness of eye, irritation of eye, itching, redness, swelling, lid edema
Vidarabine	3% ophthalmic ointment	Vidarabine acts by inhibiting DNA polymerase by formation of vidarabine triphosphate. It is formed in the presence of viral thymidine kinase and host enzymes. It then inhibits DNA polymerase and terminates the chain in DNA replication.	Herpes simplex keratitis and conjunctivitis	Lacrimation, pain, Eye irritation, superficial keratitis, photophobia, punctal occlusion, and sensitivity
Acyclovir	3% w/w eye drops, eye ointment	Acyclovir is as a DNA polymerase inhibitor. It penetrates cornea well.	H. simplex (type 1) keratitis, H. simplex encephalitis, Herpes zoster, Genital herpes simplex	Irritation, mild stinging in eye, conjunctivitis, swollen eyelids.
Idoxuridine	0.1% eye drops, eye ointment	It is 5-IUDR, which acts as a thymidine analog. It gets incorporated in DNA, competes with thymidine, and forms faulty DNA which breaks down easily. It shows its activity only against DNA viruses. Idoxuridine eye drops are more potent than acyclovir eye ointment.	Herpes simplex keratitis	Ocular irritation
Valacyclovir	500 mg tab, 1000 mg tab	Valacyclovir is an ester prodrug of acyclovir. Famciclovir is an ester prodrug of a guanine nucleoside analog penciclovir.	Herpes simplex keratitis, Herpes zoster ophthalmicus	Headache, nausea, abdominal pain
Famciclovir	250 mg tab 500 mg tab	Both drugs are DNA polymerase inhibitor and nucleoside analog. They show their antiviral activity against HSV-1 and HSV-2 and VZV. Famciclovir also have activity against HBV.	Herpes zoster ophthalmicus, Herpes simplex keratitis	Rashes, redness, peeling of skin, tightness in chest or throat, difficulty in breathing, swallowing, swelling in mouth, face, lips, tongue or throat.
Foscarnet	24 mg /mL IV solution	It is inorganic pyrophosphate derivative which does not require phosphorylation for its action. It blocks pyrophosphate-binding site and inhibits DNA polymerase activity. It also suppresses reverse transcriptase. It selectively inhibits herpetic DNA polymerase.	CMV retinitis, HSV	Anemia, phlebitis, tremor, convulsions and toxic doses can lead to Kidney damage.
Ganciclovir	0.15% w/w, ophthalmic gel	It is an acyclovir analog that is active against herpes simplex, herpes zoster, EBV and CMV. Ganciclovir inhibits viral DNA polymerase by formation of triphosphate nucleotide in presence of virus-specific thymidine kinase. This leads to inhibition of DNA replication. IV infusion prevents blindness in AIDS patients with CMV retinitis.	CMV retinitis	Pain in eye, redness, swelling, itching of eyes change in vision, white patches on eye, cloudiness in pupil or iris, crusting of eyes, sudden vision loss.

(Continued)

Table 91.5 (*Continued*) Antiviral agents for ophthalmic use

Generic name	Strength	Mechanism of action	Indications	Side effects
Cidofovir	75 mg/mL Cidofovir injection	Cidofovir is a monophosphate nucleotide analog of cytidine. It inhibits most DNA viruses including HSV, CMV, pox and adenoviruses. It selectively inhibits viral DNA polymerase.	CMV retinitis	Common side effects are decreased urination, increased thirst, and urination. Rare side effects are decreased vision or any change in vision.
Valganciclovir	450 mg tablet	Valganciclovir, is a valine ester prodrug of ganciclovir. Valganciclovir is hydrolyzed to valine and ganciclovir during corneal absorption and ganciclovir, after phosphorylation, inhibits replication of DNA.	Treatment of inflammatory disease due to herpes viruses (HSV, varicella zoster, etc.), adenoviruses and HBV, hypertensive anterior uveitis associated with CMV iritis	Ocular side effects are retinal detachment, blurred vision, macular edema, vitreous floaters and eye pain.

Abbreviations: 5-IUDR, 5-iodo-2-deoxyuridine; CMV, cytomegalovirus; DNA, deoxyribonucleic acid; EBV, Epstein–Barr virus; HBV, hepatitis B virus; HSV, Herpes simplex virus; IV, intravenous; VZV, varicella zoster virus.

Antiprotozoal Agents

Parasitic eye infections do not always cause symptoms, which can make them hard to recognize. When symptoms do occur, they can include various severe forms of eye-related problems that can range from pain in eye to loss of vision and blindness.

Acanthamoebiasis is caused by a protozoan parasite. *Acanthamoeba* is a very common organism within freshwater and marine environments worldwide. *Acanthamoeba* keratitis occurs mainly in 80% of contact lens users because of poor hygiene, wearing lenses in pool, and ocular trauma. Severe pain due to neuritis is its characteristic. It can progress to severe scleritis. Various drugs are given in combination for the treatment of infection. Some of the examples include topical antibiotics (polymyxin B sulfate, bacitracin zinc, and neomycin sulfate) and in certain cases imidazole (clotrimazole, miconazole, or ketoconazole) are used. Aromatic diamidines (0.08% polyhexamethylene biguanide [PHMB] ophthalmic solution) and 0.1% propamidine isethionate along with 0.02% PHMB are evaluated for efficacy, safety, and tolerability among patients affected by *Acanthamoeba* keratitis in the UK. Propamidine isethionate, Brolene 0.1% w/v eye drop, hexamidine diisethionate (Desomedine 0.1% eye drops), and dibromopropamidine (GoldenEye ointment) are used in 0.1% concentration for treating keratitis, a relatively resistant infection. An alternative to PHMB is topical 0.02% chlorhexidine. In addition to topical medications, oral itraconazole or ketoconazole is often used. Oral and topical voriconazole also have been used for patients who were not responsive to PHMB, chlorhexidine, and hexamidine. *Acanthamoeba* keratitis needs a long time of treatment. If toxoplasmosis is not treated at initial stage, it can lead to blindness. Drugs are prescribed in different regimens with concomitant use of systemic steroids: (1) pyrimethamine, sulfadiazine, and folinic acid; (2) pyrimethamine, sulfadiazine, clindamycin, and folinic acid; (3) sulfadiazine and clindamycin; (4) clindamycin; and (5) trimethoprim-sulfamethoxazole with or without clindamycin.

Glucocorticoids

Glucocorticoids play an important role in managing ocular inflammatory diseases. These are given via three routes: topical application, periocular injection, and systemic administration. Topical application is used for anterior inflammatory diseases such as conjunctivitis, keratitis, or anterior uveitis. Currently, the glucocorticoids formulated for topical administration are listed in **Table 91.6**.

Antihistamines and Mast-Cell Stabilizers

In inflammation and allergic reactions, mast cells play a pivotal role. Mast-cell mediators, specifically histamine, are targeted successfully by antiallergic therapies. Histamine receptors are present on many cells, and antihistaminic agents interact with these receptors, whereas mast-cell stabilizers such as disodium cromoglycate act by inhibiting degranulation of mast cells. Certain most successful compounds developed recently show both antihistaminic and mast cell-stabilizing activities. Allergic conjunctivitis is the most common ocular event of allergy. It occurs because of hypersensitivity response caused after exposure of ocular surface to airborne antigens. Various antihistaminics and mast-cell stabilizers used for treating ocular allergy are listed in **Table 91.7**.

Table 91.6 Glucocorticoids for ophthalmic use

Generic name	Strength	Mechanism of action	Uses	Side effects
Dexamethasone	0.1% eye drops	It acts as an anti-inflammatory agent by suppressing neutrophil migration, decreases production of inflammatory mediators, reverses the increased capillary permeability, and suppresses immune response. It has minimal sodium-retaining properties.	Eye inflammation caused by allergies, shingles (herpes zoster), severe acne, iritis, uveitis, eye injury, radiation, chemical burns, or certain other conditions and to prevent rejection of grafts in the eye.	Blurred vision, do not drive or operate machinery until drug has worn off, dry or watery eyes, irritation, itching, or redness of the eyes, sensitivity to bright light, crusting on the eyelids, unusual taste
Prednisolone	0.125 and 1% w/v ophthalmic suspension, eye drops	Blocks the production of inflammatory chemical messengers that make the eye red, swollen, and itchy.	It relieves redness and swelling by infection or allergy. It provides relief from redness, itchiness, and soreness. Used for severe anterior uveitis.	Burning sensation, eye irritation, watery eyes
Fluorometholone	0.1% w/v ophthalmic suspension, eye drop	It acts by the induction of phospholipase A2 inhibitory proteins, collectively called lipocortins. It controls the biosynthesis of prostaglandin and leukotrienes, the potent mediators of inflammation by inhibiting the release of their common precursor, arachidonic acid. Their primary target is the cytosolic glucocorticoid receptor. After binding the receptor, the newly formed receptor-ligand complex translocates itself into the cell nucleus, where it binds to many GRE in the promoter region of the target genes. The DNA bound receptor then interacts with basic transcription factors, causing the increase in expression of specific target genes.	Used to treat redness and swelling in the eyes that may be due to infection or allergy. It reduces swelling, itching, and soreness after any eye injuries or eye surgery	Eye irritation, burning sensation, watery eyes
Loteprednol etabonate	0.5% w/v eye drop, ophthalmic suspension	It is a steroid that blocks the production of certain chemical messengers (prostaglandins) that make the eye red, swollen, and itchy.	Redness and swelling in the eye	Eye irritation, watery eyes, burning sensation
Medrysone	1% ophthalmic solution/drops	It inhibits the edema, fibrin deposition, capillary dilation, and phagocytic migration of the acute inflammatory response as well as capillary proliferation, deposition of collagen, and scar formation.	Allergic conjunctivitis, vernal conjunctivitis, episcleritis, and epinephrine sensitivity	Common side effects include burning, stinging, irritation, itching, redness, blurred vision, or sensitivity to light. Rare side effects are an increase in the pressure inside of the eye, formation of cataracts, or perforation of the cornea

(Continued)

Table 91.6 (*Continued*) Glucocorticoids for ophthalmic use

Generic name	Strength	Mechanism of action	Uses	Side effects
Rimexolone	1% ophthalmic suspensions	Rimexolone is a glucocorticoid receptor agonist. The anti-inflammatory actions of corticosteroids are thought to involve lipocortins and phospholipase A2 inhibitory proteins which, through inhibition of arachidonic acid, control the biosynthesis of prostaglandins and leukotrienes. By binding to the glucocorticoid receptor, this drug ultimately leads to changes in genetic transcription involving the lipocortins and prostaglandins.	Postoperative inflammation following ocular surgery and in the treatment of anterior uveitis	Change in eyesight, eye pain, or very bad eye irritation, eye discharge
Betamethasone	0.10% w/v eye drops	It inhibits neutrophil apoptosis and demargination and also inhibits NF-kappa B and other inflammatory transcription factors. They also inhibit phospholipase A2, leading to decreased formation of arachidonic acid derivatives.	Used to reduce redness and swelling caused by infections, allergies, and injuries. It is sometimes used after eye surgery and in mild anterior uveitis	Eye irritation, watery eyes, bitter taste

Abbreviation: GRE, glucocorticoid response elements.

Table 91.7 Antihistaminics for ophthalmic use

Generic name	Strength	Mechanism of action	Uses	Side effects
Pheniramine and naphazoline	Naphazoline (0.05% w/v) + phenylephrine (0.12% w/v) eye drops	Naphazoline is a vasoconstrictor. It acts by narrowing swollen blood vessels in the eyes to reduce eye redness. Pheniramine is an antihistamine that reduces the effects of natural chemical histamine in the body. Histamine can produce symptoms of itchy or watery eyes.	Allergic diseases of the eye. Relieves redness and swelling of the eye	Stinging in the eyes, eye pain, blurred vision, photophobia
Antazoline and naphazoline	Antazoline phosphate (0.5%) and naphazoline hydrochloride (0.05%)	The combination of naphazoline and antazoline produces significant whitening and inhibition of itching in all eyes challenged by histamine. The combination of the two drugs was more effective than either component alone in preventing redness. Antazoline, an antihistaminic agent, and naphazoline, a sympathomimetic agent (α-receptor agonist), work in the eye to decrease congestion. Both are equally effective in arresting itching.	Relives itching and redness caused by pollen and animal hair	Change in eyesight, eye pain, eye irritation
Antazoline and xylometazoline	Xylometazoline 0.05% w/v and antazoline 0.5% w/v	Antazoline is an ethylenediamine derivative with histamine H_1 antagonistic and sedative properties. Antazoline antagonizes histamine H_1 receptor and prevents the typical allergic symptoms caused by histamine activities on capillaries, skin, mucous membranes, and gastrointestinal and bronchial smooth muscles. Antazoline is used to provide symptomatic relieve of allergic symptoms.	Redness and itching of the eyes due to seasonal and perennial allergies such as hay fever or house dust allergy	Slight transient local stinging on instillation, occasionally reported side effects are blurred vision, mydriasis, headache, drowsiness, and reactive hyperemia. Local allergic reactions (e.g., rash, edema, pruritus) and eye irritation

(Continued)

Table 91.7 (*Continued*) Antihistaminics for ophthalmic use

Generic name	Strength	Mechanism of action	Uses	Side effects
Emedastine difumarate	0.05% ophthalmic solution	It is the difumarate salt form of emedastine, a second-generation, selective histamine H_1 receptor antagonist with antiallergic activity. It reversibly and competitively blocks histamine by binding to H_1 receptors. As a result, this agent interferes with mediator release from mast cells either by inhibiting calcium ion influx across mast cell/basophil plasma membrane or by inhibiting intracellular calcium ion release within the cells. It may also inhibit the late-phase allergic reaction mediated through leukotrienes or prostaglandins, or by producing an antiplatelet-activating factor effect. Ocular administration of drug causes a dose-dependent inhibition of histamine-stimulated vascular permeability in the conjunctiva.	It is used to relieve redness, itching, and swelling of the eyes from allergic conjunctivitis	Blurred vision, headache, dry eyes, eye discomfort, staining of the eyes, a bad taste of mouth, weakness, and unusual dreams may occur
Levocabastine hydrochloride	0.05% ophthalmic suspension	It is a synthetic piperidine derivative with antihistamine properties. Second-generation histamine-1 receptor antagonist. It inhibits the release of chemical mediators from mast cells and on the chemotaxis of polymorphonuclear leukocytes and eosinophils. Both histamine- and antigen-induced conjunctivitis can be inhibited by drug.	Allergic conjunctivitis	Visual disturbances, dry mouth, fatigue, pharyngitis, eye pain, dryness, somnolence, red eyes, lacrimation, cough, nausea, erythema, eyelid edema, and dyspnea
Cromolyn sodium	4% ophthalmic solution	Cromolyn sodium is a mast-cell stabilizer with anti-inflammatory activity. It probably interferes with the antigen-stimulated calcium transport across the mast cell membrane, thereby inhibiting mast cell release of histamine, leukotrienes, and other substances that cause hypersensitivity reactions. It also inhibits eosinophil chemotaxis.	For treatment of certain allergic eye conditions, e.g., vernal keratoconjunctivitis, vernal conjunctivitis, vernal keratitis	More common side effects are burning or stinging of the eye. Less common or rare effects are dryness or puffiness around the eye, watering, or itching of eye
Lodoxamide tromethamine	0.1% ophthalmic solution	Lodoxamide is a synthetic mast-cell stabilizing compound with anti-inflammatory activity. Lodoxamide appears to inhibit the antigen-stimulated calcium transport across the mast cell membrane, thereby inhibiting mast cell degranulation and the release of histamine, leukotrienes, and other substances that cause hypersensitivity reactions. Lodoxamide also inhibits eosinophil chemotaxis	Vernal keratoconjunctivitis, vernal conjunctivitis, and vernal keratitis	Transient burning, stinging, or discomfort upon instillation
Pemirolast	0.1% ophthalmic solution	Pemirolast binds to the histamine H_1 receptor. This blocks the action of endogenous histamine, which subsequently leads to temporary relief of the negative symptoms brought on by histamine. Pemirolast has also been observed to inhibit antigen-stimulated calcium ion influx into mast cells through the blockage of calcium channels. Pemirolast inhibits the chemotaxis of eosinophils into ocular tissue and prevents inflammatory mediator release from human eosinophils.	For the prevention of itching of the eyes caused by allergies, such as hay fever, and allergic conjunctivitis	Headache, rhinitis and cold or flu. Less common side effects: burning, dry eye, foreign body sensation, and ocular discomfort

(*Continued*)

Table 91.7 (*Continued*) Antihistaminics for ophthalmic use

Generic name	Strength	Mechanism of action	Uses	Side effects
Nedocromil	2% eye drops	Nedocromil has been shown to inhibit the in vitro activation of, and mediator release from, a variety of inflammatory cell types associated with asthma, including eosinophils, neutrophils, macrophages, mast cells, monocytes, and platelets. Nedocromil inhibits activation and release of inflammatory mediators such as histamine, prostaglandin D_2 and leukotrienes C_4 from different types of cells in the lumen and mucosa of the bronchial tree. These mediators are derived from arachidonic acid metabolism through the lipoxygenase and cyclo-oxygenase pathways. The mechanism of action of nedocromil may be due partly to inhibition of axon reflexes and release of sensory neuropeptides, such as substance P, neurokinin A, and calcitonin-generated peptides. The result is inhibition of bradykinin-induced bronchoconstriction. Nedocromil does not possess any bronchodilator, antihistamine, or corticosteroid activity.	Itchy eyes due to allergies	Headache, burning, stinging, eye irritation, stuffy nose, and bad taste in your mouth. Bright lights can make you feel uncomfortable
Olopatadine hydrochloride	0.2% w/v ophthalmic eye solution, eye drop	Olopatadine is a dual-action selective histamine H_1 receptor antagonist and mast-cell stabilizer with antiallergic activity. Olopatadine stabilizes mast cells and prevents histamine release from mast cells. In addition, this agent also blocks histamine H_1 receptors, thereby preventing histamine from binding to these receptors.	Ocular itching associated with allergic conjunctivitis	Blurred vision, eye irritation or pain, swelling of the eyelids
Ketotifen fumarate	0.025% ophthalmic solution	It is a cycloheptathiophene derivative with antiallergic activity. Selective histamine receptors blocker. It interferes with the release of inflammatory mediators from mast cells involved in hypersensitivity reactions, thereby decreasing chemotaxis and activation of eosinophils.	Itching of the eye due to allergic conjunctivitis	Allergic reactions, burning or stinging, conjunctivitis, discharge, dry eyes, eye pain, itching, keratitis, lacrimation disorder, mydriasis, photophobia, and rash
Azelastine	0.05% ophthalmic solution	Acts as H_1-receptor antagonist, acts by inhibiting the release of histamine and other mediators involved in the allergic response.	Itching of the eye associated with allergic conjunctivitis	Causes temporarily sting or burning sensation in eyes for a minute or two after use. Temporary blurred vision, headache, or a bitter taste in your mouth may also occur
Epinastine	0.05% ophthalmic solution	It inhibits the allergic response in three ways: (1) it stabilizes mast cells by preventing mast-cell degranulation to control the allergic response, (2) it prevents histamine binding to both the H_1- and H_2-receptors to stop itching and provide lasting protection, and (3) it prevents the release of proinflammatory chemical mediators from the blood vessel to stop progression of the allergic response	Prevents itching associated with allergic conjunctivitis	Causes burning sensation in the eye, folliculosis, hyperemia, and pruritus

Glaucoma

Glaucoma is a group of heterogeneous diseases that differ in etiology, pathogenesis, risk factors, duration, symptoms, and treatments. It is a chronic and progressive condition characterized by optic neuropathy and visual disturbances. Optic nerve fiber degeneration, optic disk cupping, and notching of neuroretinal rims are the prominent features of glaucoma, which lead to irreversible blindness. Despite various etiological factors (**Table 91.8**), increased IOP remained the predominant cause for glaucoma. The increased pressure in the eyeball can cause blindness within days or even in hours by compressing the axons of the optic nerve in the region of optic disk.

Eye pressure less than 21 mm Hg is considered normal. In glaucoma, IOP increases to more than 21 mm Hg. Retina and optic nerve damage starts when IOP crosses 40 mm Hg. If the rise persists and crosses 60 mm Hg, permanent damage may be seen in the optic nerve or retina.

Intraocular Pressure

The intraocular fluid, present in the eyeball, maintains sufficient pressure to keep the eyeball distended. Unlike vitreous body, aqueous humor is synthesized and released, flows freely through various chambers, and is removed out of the eye. Production of aqueous humor mostly remains constant.

The prominent mechanisms responsible for removal of aqueous humor from the anterior chamber are resorption through the trabecular network and removal through the canal of Schlemm. The trabecular meshwork is a spongy tissue area located near the base of the cornea, which drains the aqueous humor from the anterior chamber. The canal of Schlemm is the cylindrical vessel, which drains the aqueous humor to the episcleral veins. The flow of aqueous humor from the canal of Schlemm to episcleral veins is governed by the gradient of IOP to episcleral venous pressure. These two pathways clear almost 80% of the aqueous humor, while 20% of resorption is achieved by the uveoscleral route. This route consists of two segments, that is, the uveal portion and the scleral portion. Aqueous humor passes through the uveal portion (comprising longitudinal muscle bundles) and reaches the suprachoroidal space. Further, it flows through the scleral portion, that is, from suprachoroidal space to the lymphatics in the orbit outside the eye.

Resistance to aqueous humor outflow is the major cause of increased IOP. Almost 75% of resistance is localized in trabecular meshwork region, while 25% of resistance occurs in the Schlemm's canal. The extracellular matrix of the trabecular meshwork is made up of glycosaminoglycans. Osmotic pressure exerted by these glucosaminoglycans leads to edema in the trabecular meshwork which obstructs the flow of humor. Increased thickness of extracellular matrix in the inner walls of the canal of Schlemm and juxtacanalicular meshwork also obstruct the drainage. Deposition of debris and proteins such as cochlin along with mucopolysaccharides are found extensively in glaucomatous eye, obstructing the trabecular meshwork. Resistance by iris and ciliary muscles to aqueous outflow has also been contemplated. Contractions in anterior tendons lead to inward movement of ciliary muscle. It spreads the trabecular meshwork and dilates the canal of Schlemm, thus increasing drainage. During relaxation, trabecular meshwork shows contraction and the diameter of Schlemm's canal decreases, which leads to outflow resistance.

Besides IOP, other factors such as blood supply to the eyeball, foreign materials, intraorbital or extraorbital bleeding, local anesthetics, and extraocular muscle tone may also lead to increase in IOP.

Epidemiology

Glaucoma is one of the leading causes of blindness worldwide. Approximately, 80 million people of the globe will suffer from glaucoma in 2020. Among these, 56 million will develop open-angle glaucoma (OAG) and 24 million will develop angle-closure glaucoma. In 2010, bilateral blindness from glaucoma was found in 8.4 million individuals worldwide, and it will further increase to 11 million by 2020. India alone will have 20% of the global burden of glaucoma with 12 million cases. Two-thirds of the cases are of OAG among the Caucasian population, while equal proportion of OAG and closed-angle glaucoma cases are seen in the Indian population. As compared to Caucasians, African-Americans are 15 times more likely to be visually impeded from glaucoma.

Table 91.8 Etiological factors for glaucoma

Increased IOP	Vitreoretinal disorders
Congenital anomalies	Ocular surgery
Raised episcleral venous pressure	Ocular trauma
Corneal endothelial disorders	Ocular neovascularization
Inflammatory ocular conditions	Drugs
Pigment dispersion syndrome	Systemic diseases
Lens abnormalities	Intraocular tumors

Abbreviation: IOP, intraocular pressure.

Types of Glaucoma

Glaucoma can be categorized using two schemes: (1) anatomic or mechanistic (**Table 91.9**) and (2) based on etiology of the disease. The former classifies the glaucoma depending on whether the angle formed between the iris and cornea is open or closed **(Fig. 91.4)**, while the latter classifies it depending on the underlying ocular or systemic disorder.

Open-Angle Glaucoma

OAG is a multifactorial and progressive optic neuropathy that leads to loss of vision. It exhibits optic nerve cupping, damage to retinal nerve fibers, and progressive visual field loss. It occurs predominantly in adults and is usually bilateral and not necessarily symmetrical. Elevated IOP is seen in majority of the OAG patients (i.e., > 21 mm Hg).

Those who never exhibit such rise (IOP below 21 mm Hg), but shows other symptoms of glaucoma, are categorized as the cases of normotensive or low-tension glaucoma. Patients whose IOP levels are above 21 mm Hg, but exhibit no damage optic nerve, are considered to be the cases of ocular hypertension.

OAG can be categorized as primary open-angle glaucoma (POAG) and secondary open-angle glaucoma (SOAG). POAG occurs independently without other ocular diseases, while SOAG is caused by eye injury, inflammation, drugs (e.g., steroids), cataract, diabetes, etc.

POAG accounts for 90% of overall disease burden. The angle formed between the iris and cornea remains wide open in patients with POAG. Slow and progressive clogging of drainage canals leads to rise in IOP. It is a chronic condition devoid of easily identifiable symptoms and usually remained unnoticed.

The etiology of POAG can be explained by two theories: mechanical and vascular theory. Mechanical theory suggests involvement of damage to the optic nerve axons by compression due to elevated IOP. Vascular theory states that the damage produced is due to decreased blood flow to optic nerve head. It is still uncertain whether mechanical or vascular or both processes lead to apoptosis of ganglion cell axons in lamina cribrosa.

SOAG includes pigmentary glaucoma and pseudo-exfoliation glaucoma. Pigmentary glaucoma is due to pigmentary dispersion syndrome in which pigments released from iris get deposited in anterior and posterior chambers of the eye. Trabecular endothelium phagocytosed this pigment, leading to damage and drop-off of the trabecular lamellae. The denuded trabeculae functions improperly and collapses, causing obstruction to aqueous outflow and increased IOP.

Various basement membranes of the eye releases amyloidlike grayish-white exfoliative material in the anterior and posterior chambers of the eye, conjunctiva, and orbit, leading to pseudoexfoliative syndrome and pseudoexfoliation glaucoma. This pseudoexfoliative material probably gets deposited and obstructs the aqueous outflow from the anterior chamber, leading to increased IOP.

Table 91.9 Mechanistic and clinical classification of glaucoma

Anatomic (mechanistic) classification	Clinical (etiology-based) classification
Open-angle glaucoma Closed-angle glaucoma	**Primary glaucomas** ▪ Primary open-angle glaucoma ▪ Primary angle-closure glaucoma ▪ Childhood glaucoma **Secondary glaucomas** ▪ Elevated episcleral venous pressure ▪ Disorders of corneal endothelium ▪ Steroid-induced glaucoma ▪ Pigmentary glaucoma ▪ Traumatic glaucoma ▪ Neovascular glaucoma ▪ Lens-induced glaucoma ▪ Glaucoma from vitreoretinal disorders ▪ Glaucoma from ocular surgery ▪ Glaucoma from intraocular tumors ▪ Glaucoma from ocular inflammation ▪ Glaucoma associated with systemic diseases

Angle-Closure Glaucoma

Angle-closure glaucoma is a less common form of glaucoma caused by adhesion of the iris to the cornea, thereby blocking the flow of aqueous humor. It is of two types: primary (independent of other ocular abnormalities) and secondary (associated with various diseases such as diabetes, retinal vein occlusion, uveitis, phacomorphic glaucoma, aphakic and pseudophakic pupillary block, or iridocorneal endothelial syndrome).

Relative papillary block and plateau iris syndrome are the two mechanisms for primary angle-closure glaucoma. Relative pupillary block is a resistance produced by critical pupillary diameter (4–6 mm) and tight iridolenticular contact (junction of pupillary margin of iris and anterior surface of lens) to aqueous drainage from posterior chamber. The pressure thus generated pushes peripheral iris toward trabecular meshwork, causing appositional angle closure, which may progress to permanent synechial angle closure.

In plateau iris syndrome, the iris remains in flat position instead of convex (**Fig. 91.5**) and also remains apposed to the trabecular meshwork. When the pupil dilates, the iris tissue is pushed toward the trabecular meshwork and closes the angle. Iridectomy resolves relative papillary block but is unable to resolve block due to plateau iris syndrome.

Childhood Glaucoma

It is a group of disorders mostly seen in children and characterized by developmental abnormalities in the

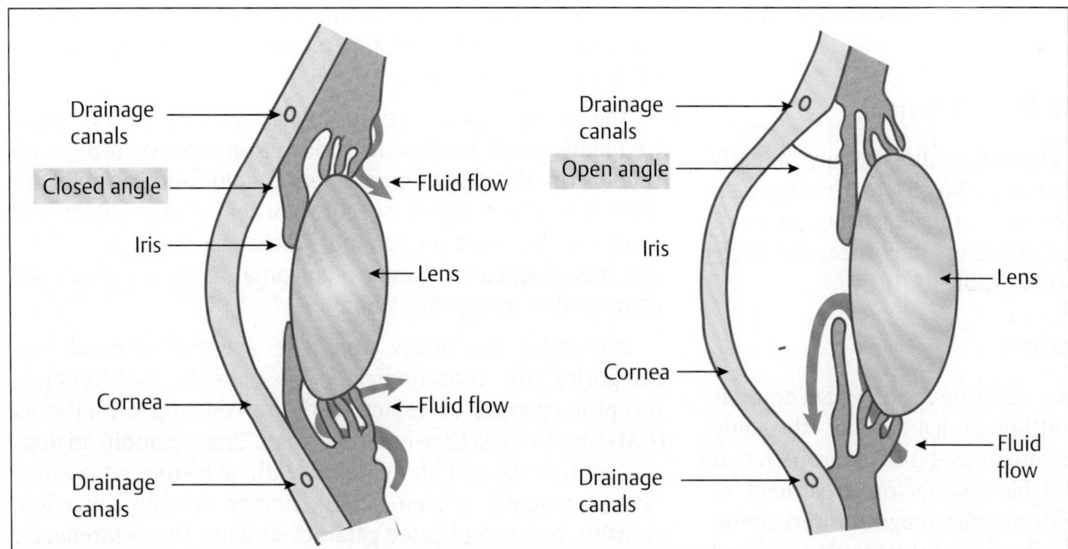

Fig. 91.4 Open-angle and angle-closure in eye.

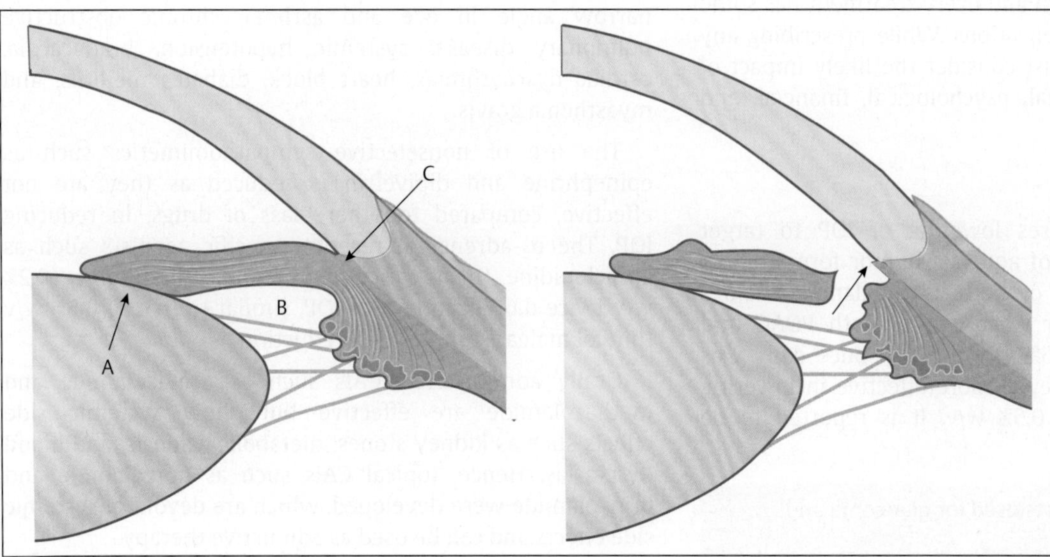

Fig. 91.5 Plateau iris syndrome.

aqueous outflow system of the eye. It is classified on the basis of associated anatomic defects.

1. Primary congenital glaucoma, characterized by developmental anomalies in trabecular meshwork.
2. Secondary congenital glaucoma, caused due to acquired ocular diseases.
3. Glaucoma caused by other ocular or systemic congenital anomalies.

Increased IOP is due to obstruction to aqueous flow through trabecular sheets. No blockade was seen in Schlemm's canal.

Secondary Glaucoma

Glaucomas precipitated due to other ocular or systemic diseases/disorders are classified as secondary glaucomas. The "red eye" glaucoma or the glaucoma due to raised episcleral venous pressure is a secondary glaucoma precipitated by obstruction to venous drainage, arteriovenous fistula, or ocular episcleral venous anomalies. Episcleral vein serves as prominent drainage pathway for aqueous humor. Increased episcleral pressure will elevate IOP, leading to glaucoma and damage.

Disorders of corneal endothelium such as iridocorneal endothelial syndrome and posterior polymorphous dystrophy cause glaucoma. Conditions such as keratitis, scleritis, uveitis, and episcleritis compromise outflow and elevate IOP.

Pigment deposition on cornea, dense pigmentation on trabecular meshwork, and defects in radial midperipheral iris transillumination lead to pigmentary glaucoma. The IOP remains normal but extensive optic nerve damage is seen in such patients.

Ocular trauma may increase IOP and precipitate glaucoma, which is known as traumatic glaucoma. However, posttraumatic elevation of IOP is not always necessary. Formation of newer blood vessels in the angle also leads to glaucoma, which is termed neovascular glaucoma. This neovascularization is due to hypoxia, which is a common end-stage feature of ophthalmic disorders.

Lens disorders such as ectopia lentis, cataract, exfoliation syndrome, and aphakia and pseudophakia also lead to glaucoma. Moreover, ocular surgery, intraocular tumors, vitreoretinal disorders, and various systemic diseases are also found to elevate IOP and cause damage to optic nerve, leading to glaucoma.

Glaucoma Detection Techniques

Successful management of glaucoma relies heavily on early and accurate detection of glaucoma (**Box 91.1**). The diagnosis is based on identification of change in IOP, shape and color of optic nerve, field of vision, thickness of cornea, and angle formed between iris and cornea (**Table 91.10**).

Treatment of Glaucoma

The rationale behind the treatment of glaucoma is controlling/reducing IOP. Although IOP is not the only factor contributing to glaucomatous optic neuropathy, it is the only clinically modifiable risk factor. Treatment of glaucoma usually begins with pharmacological intervention (**Table 91.11** and **Fig. 91.6**), followed by laser therapy and surgery when required. Each and every treatment has some sort of side effects or complications. While prescribing any treatment, the clinician must consider the likely impact of the treatment from a social, psychological, financial, and convenience point of view.

Open-Angle Glaucoma

The treatment strategy uses lowering of IOP to target range either by reduction of aqueous humor formation or by enhancing its outflow, or both. Prostaglandin analogs are the preferred drug for treatment of both POAG and SOAG. Latanoprost in 0.005% w/v instilled once daily was found to be equivalent or even more effective in lowering IOP than timolol maleate 0.5% w/v. It is reported to be more efficacious if given in the evening. Bimatoprost, travoprost, and unoprostone are newer analogs with similar pharmacological profile.

The β-adrenergic receptor blockers are the next most frequently used treatment option. Nonselective β-blockers such as timolol, levobunolol, metipranolol, and carteolol are more efficacious than β_1-specific blocker betaxolol. Betaxolol is devoid of pulmonary and cardiovascular side effects but less efficacious against glaucoma, as β_2 receptors are expressed more on ciliary body.

Whenever the drugs from the above-mentioned two categories are contraindicated in patients, a_2-adrenergic receptor agonists or topical carbonic anhydrase inhibitors (CAIs) are used as first-line treatment. Prostaglandin analogs are contraindicated in patients with a history of uveitis, cystoid macular edema (CME), herpes simplex infection, keratitis, and complicated cataract surgery. The β-adrenergic receptor blockers are contraindicated in patients with narrow angle in eye and asthma, chronic obstructive pulmonary disease, systemic hypotension, bradycardia, cardiac dysrhythmias, heart block, diabetes mellitus, and myasthenia gravis.

The use of nonselective sympathomimetics such as epinephrine and dipivefrin is reduced as they are not effective, compared to other class of drugs, in reducing IOP. The α_2-adrenergic receptor-specific agonists such as apraclonidine (0.5% thrice daily) and brimonidine (0.2% w/v twice daily) can reduce IOP, similar to that of 0.5% w/v timolol maleate (almost 22% reduction).

Orally administered CAIs such as acetazolamide and methazolamide are effective but show systemic side effects such as kidney stones, metabolic acidosis, and blood dyscrasias. Hence, topical CAIs such as dorzolamide and brinzolamide were developed, which are devoid of systemic side effects and can be used as adjunctive therapy.

Topical mitotic agents are less commonly used due to their numerous side effects and inconvenient dosing.

Drugs are also preferred in combination, for example, 2% dorzolamide and 0.5% timolol maleate. This combination was found to be more efficacious than monotherapy. It lowers IOP by almost 33% against monotherapy with dorzolamide, that is, 15 to 20% and timolol maleate 22%. Another combination used is 0.2% brimonidine tartrate and 0.5% timolol maleate.

Table 91.10 Diagnostic tests used for glaucoma and parameters assessed

Diagnostic test	Parameter assessed
Tonometry	Intraocular pressure
Ophthalmoscopy	Shape and color of optic nerve
Perimetry	Field of vision
Gonioscopy	Angle between iris and cornea
Pachymetry	Thickness of cornea

Box 91.1 Suggestions for medical management of glaucoma

- Appropriately diagnose the glaucoma.
- Determine the appropriate target IOP to be achieved and readjust the target as and when required.
- Try to use fewest medication in lowest concentration to achieve desired target IOP.
- Substitute rather than adding medication, if the treatment is ineffective.
- Check and regularly insist the patient for treatment compliance.
- Make the convenient treatment regimen, according to the need of patients.
- Counsel the patient about medicine, dosage regimen, clinical outcomes, time required to obtain desired outcomes, correct method of instilling eye drops, expected side effects, and adverse effects.

Abbreviation: IOP, intraocular pressure.

Table 91.11 Medication used for management of glaucoma

Generic name	Strength and formulation	Mechanism of action	Indications	Side effects
Sympathomimetics	Refer to **Table 91.1**			
Dipivefrin				
Epinephrine				
Apraclonidine				
Brimonidine				
β-adrenergic blockers				
Betaxolol				
Carteolol				
Levobunolol				
Metipranolol				
Timolol				
Cholinergic agonists				
Pilocarpine				
Carbachol				
Prostaglandin analogs				
Bimatoprost	0.01 and 0.03% w/v eye drops	Prostaglandin analogs act by stimulating various prostanoid receptors. Latanoprost, bimatoprost, travoprost, and unoprostone are PGF2α derivatives and acts by stimulating FP receptors. The FP receptors are G-protein-coupled receptors which act via Gq protein, i.e., stimulating production of IP3 and DAG as a secondary messenger system. These agents appear to lower IOP by facilitating aqueous outflow through the accessory uveoscleral outflow pathway. Due to potent IOP-lowering effects, less systemic side effects, and once daily dosing, these agents are used as first-line treatment against glaucoma. Latanoprost is the first drug of this class that is stable and has long-acting derivative; it has shown efficacy similar to timolol in reducing IOP. 0.005% w/v given once a day lowers IOP by 27–35%. It is more effective when administered in the evening. Bimatoprost, travoprost, and unoprostone are newer analogs with similar pharmacological profile as latanoprost. Both bimatoprost 0.03% and travoprost 0.004% can lower IOP up to 33%. Unoprostone isopropyl 0.12% used twice daily lowers IOP by 11–23%.	Glaucoma, first-line treatment of OAG	Blurred vision, stinging, burning, hyperemia, foreign body sensation, itching, increased iris pigmentation, eyelash changes, punctate epithelial keratitis, cystoid macular edema, iritis, herpes simplex keratitis
Latanoprost	0.005% w/v eye drops			
Travoprost	0.004% w/v eye drops			
Unoprostone	0.15% w/v eye drops			

(Continued)

Table 91.11 (*Continued*) Medication used for management of glaucoma

Generic name	Strength and formulation	Mechanism of action	Indications	Side effects
Carbonic anhydrase inhibitors				
Acetazolamide	Oral—200 and 500 mg capsule, tablet, or sustained release formulation Systemic —500 mg/5 mL reconstituted solution	Ciliary body of eye possesses carbonic anhydrase (isoenzyme II), which secretes sodium bicarbonate into aqueous humor. Inhibition of carbonic anhydrase decreases the formation of humor and thereby decreases IOP. These agents when administered orally can lower IOP by about 20–40%. Topical CAIs such as dorzolamide (2% w/v used three times daily) and brinzolamide (1% w/v two or three times daily) lowers IOP by 3–5 mm Hg for 1 year.	Glaucoma	Malaise, depression, confusion, metallic taste, anorexia, diarrhea, paresthesias, kidney stones, metabolic acidosis, leading to tachypnea, blood dyscrasia
Dichlorphenamide	50 mg tablet			
Methazolamide	25 mg and 50 mg tablet			
Dorzolamide	2% w/v eye drops			Stinging, burning sensation, allergic sensitivity, blurred vision, superficial punctate keratitis, corneal edema
Brinzolamide	1% w/v eye drops			
Hyperosmotic agents				
Glycerol	50% glycerol administered orally, 1–1.5 g/kg	These agents create osmotic gradient between blood and the ocular fluids, leading to water loss from eye to hyperosmotic plasma, thereby decreasing IOP. The blood osmolality increased by 20 to 30 mOsm/L after the use of these agents. Glycerol is contraindicated while isosorbide is preferred in diabetic patients. Mannitol is more effective than glycerol in lowering the intraocular pressure. Mannitol should be warmed to room temperature before intravenous administration to avoid formation of crystals.	As hyperosmotic agent for treatment of acute angle-closure glaucoma To lower IOP prior to surgery in secondary and OAG	Nausea, vomiting
Mannitol	20% mannitol administered intravenously, 1–2 g/kg			Cellular dehydration, diuresis
Isosorbide	Orally, 1.5–2.0 g/kg			Cellular dehydration, dieresis, nausea, and vomiting

Abbreviations: IOP, intraocular pressure; OAG, open-angle glaucoma; CAI, carbonic anhydrase inhibitors.

Angle-Closure Glaucoma

Patients diagnosed with acute primary angle closure should be treated immediately with (if not contraindicated):

1. Oral 500 mg acetazolamide.
2. One drop of 0.5% timolol.
3. One drop of 2% pilocarpine.
4. One drop of 1% apraclonidine.

Check IOP at interval of 15 to 30 minutes. If the attack is not resolved (i.e., IOP not decreased to normal, pupil not miotic, and angle closed) within 1 hour of treatment, oral hyperosmotics (50% glycerin in a dose of 1.5 mL/kg body weight) should be added to the treatment. If the patient is diabetic, glycerin can be replaced with 45% isosorbide. If the attack is still not resolved after 2 hours, the patient should undergo argon laser gonioplasty. If the patient remains in angle closure for up to 4 to 6 hours after initiation of treatment, laser peripheral iridotomy (LPI) or surgical iridectomy should be performed. Perform gonioscopy to confirm angle opening if IOP falls to 20 mm Hg. The angle should be opened, as decreased IOP may not be the confirmation that attack is resolved. The patient should be maintained on 2% pilocarpine four times a day bilaterally, 1% prednisolone acetate four times daily, and timolol 0.5% two times a day in the affected eye until an LPI is performed. Atropine and cyclopentolate should not be administered

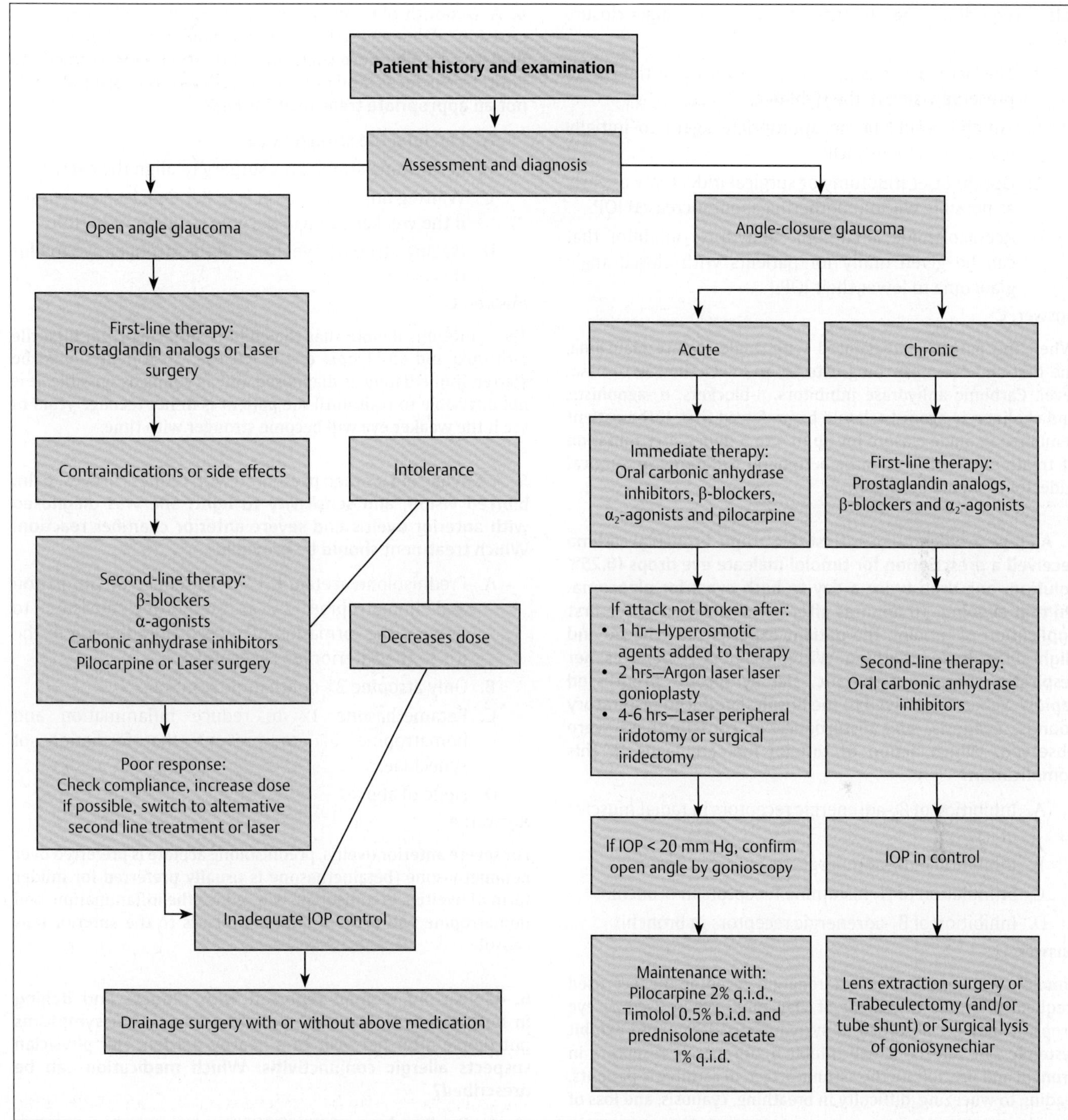

Fig. 91.6 Treatment algorithm for glaucoma

for ciliary muscle relaxation and pupil dilatation (for ocular fundus examination) in patients with primary angle-closure glaucoma, as it precipitates angle closure.

Pharmacological intervention of chronic angle-closure glaucoma includes prostaglandin analogs, β-blockers, and a_2-agonists, keeping the target of reduction of IOP to its basal value. CAIs can replace these agents if contraindicated in patients. Once IOP is reduced less than 20 mm Hg, lens extraction surgery, trabeculectomy (and/or tube shunt), or surgical lysis of goniosynechiae can be opted

Multiple Choice Questions

1. A 75-year-old man presented in emergency department with blurred vision and pain in the right eye. He reported to have feeling of nausea. Upon examination, the right eye was found to have cloudy cornea and conjunctival hyperemia. The right pupil was semidilated and fixed to light. Gonioscopy revealed closed anterior angle of the right eye. Intraocular pressure (IOP) of the right eye was 60 mm Hg. The patient was diagnosed with closed-angle glaucoma. Which of the following statements is

false regarding the treatment of acute angle-closure crisis?

A. The patient needs immediate lowering of the IOP to preserve vision in the right eye.
B. Timolol would be an appropriate agent to initially lower the patient's IOP.
C. Opt for laser iridotomy or surgical iridectomy as early as possible without bothering about increased IOP.
D. Acetazolamide is carbonic anhydrase inhibitor that can be given orally for patients with closed-angle glaucoma to lower their IOP.

Answer: C

When the patient is diagnosed with angle-closure glaucoma, the first and foremost thing is to try to lower the IOP to basal level. Carbonic anhydrase inhibitors, β-blockers, α_2-agonists, and cholinergic agonists should be preferred first. If the patient remained in angle closure for up to 4 to 6 hours after initiation of treatment, then only laser peripheral iridotomy or surgical iridectomy should be opted.

2. A 60-year-old woman with stable atopic bronchial asthma received a prescription for timolol maleate eye drops (0.25% solution, one drop twice a day to both eyes) for glaucoma. On that evening, 10 minutes after administration of the first application of timolol, the patient experienced wheeze and slight difficulty in breathing. Within the next 10 minutes, her respiration became asthmatic. Her symptoms progressed rapidly. When she arrived to the hospital, reduced respiratory sounds, cyanosis, and disturbance of consciousness were observed. Which action of timolol maleate leads to this complication?

A. Inhibition of β_2-adrenergic receptors in radial muscles of iris.
B. Inhibition of β_1-adrenergic receptors in heart.
C. Stimulation of H_1 histamine receptors in bronchi.
D. Inhibition of β_2-adrenergic receptors in bronchi.

Answer: D

Timolol is a nonselective β-adrenergic receptor blocker used frequently for the treatment of glaucoma. When used as eye drops, it may get absorbed in systemic circulation and exhibit systemic side effects. It will inhibit b_2-adrenergic receptors in bronchi and precipitate the asthma attack in asthmatic patients, leading to wheezing, difficulty in breathing, cyanosis, and loss of consciousness.

3. Brinzolamide decreases intraocular pressure (IOP) by:

A. Increasing aqueous humor outflow through the trabecular meshwork.
B. Decreasing uveoscleral outflow.
C. Increasing aqueous humor production.
D. Decreasing aqueous humor production.

Answer: D

Brinzolamide is a carbonic anhydrase inhibitor, which acts by inhibiting carbonic anhydrase enzyme in ciliary body, thereby decreasing aqueous humor formation and lowering IOP.

4. A 6-month-old female infant presents with occasional crossing of her eyes. Her parents believe that her left eye deviates nasally more than the right. The infant responds to light, tracks faces, and plays with toys without issue. What is not an appropriate treatment for her?

A. Patching the stronger eye.
B. Performing strabismus surgery to align the eyes.
C. Waiting until the patient is in her teenage years to see if the weaker eye will become stronger with time.
D. Placing atropine eye drops in the stronger eye to blur this eye.

Answer: C

The symptoms denote that the child is suffering from infantile esotropia and amblyopia of the left eye. Treatment should be started immediately as diagnosed and as young as possible. It is not advisable to wait until the patient is in her teenage years to see if the weaker eye will become stronger with time.

5. A 23-year-old woman presented with redness in eyes, pain, blurred vision, and sensitivity to light. She was diagnosed with anterior uveitis and severe anterior chamber reaction. Which treatment should be provided?

A. Prednisolone acetate 0.125% to reduce inflammation and homatropine 2% as supportive measure to prevent the formation of synechiae (adhesion of the iris to the anterior lens capsule).
B. Only atropine 2% ophthalmic solution.
C. Betamethasone 1% to reduce inflammation and homatropine 2% to prevent the formation of synechiae.
D. None of above.

Answer: A

For severe anterior uveitis, prednisolone acetate is preferred over betamethasone (betamethasone is usually preferred for milder form of uveitis). Prednisolone will reduce the inflammation, and homatropine will prevent adhesion of iris to the anterior lens capsule.

6. 48-year-old woman reported with redness and itching in both the eyes. Over the past few weeks, her symptoms got worse after her visit to a nearby garden. Her physician suspects allergic conjunctivitis. Which medication can be prescribed?

A. Prednisolone acetate 0.125%.
B. Antazoline phosphate (0.5%) and naphazoline hydrochloride (0.05%).
C. Gatifloxacin 0.3%.
D. Atropine 2%.

Answer: B

The case may be of allergic conjunctivitis due to allergy of pollen grains as the symptoms got worse after her visit to a nearby garden. Prescribing antihistaminics will be more relevant than glucocorticoid, antibacterial agent, or atropine. Antazoline, an antihistaminic agent, and naphazoline, a sympathomimetic agent (α-receptor agonist), relieve itching and redness caused by pollen and decrease congestion in eyes.

7. Following are the etiological factors for glaucoma except:

A. Increased intraocular pressure (IOP).

B. Ocular trauma.

C. Bacterial infection.

D. Systemic diseases.

Answer: C

Direct involvement of bacterial infection is not there in the etiology of glaucoma.

8. A 65-year-old man reported with blurred vision, eye pain, and decreased visual acuity. He had successful cataract surgery a few weeks before. Culture test confirms Candida infection. Which antifungal should be preferred for the treatment?

A. Amphotericin B 10 mg/0.1 mL intravitreal injection.

B. Fluconazole 0.3% w/v eye drops.

C. Itraconazole 1%w/v eye drops.

D. Ketoconazole 2% eye drops.

Answer: A

The patient showed symptoms such as blurred vision, eye pain, and decreased visual acuity after a few weeks of cataract surgery. It directs toward possible postoperative endophthalmitis. The culture test confirms *Candida* infection. For the treatment of fungal postoperative endophthalmitis, the preferred antifungal drug is amphotericin B administered by intravitreal injection.

9. A 45-year-old woman presents with itchy, irritable eyes. She finds it is generally worse in the morning. Although there is no obvious discharge, she occasionally finds herself cleaning dandruff-like particles from her lashes. The swab test from eye confirmed staphylococcal infection. Lid hygiene is maintained by warm compresses and lid scrubs. The topical antibacterial chloramphenicol in the form of ointment can be applied to lid margins. What is the mechanism of action of chloramphenicol?

A. Bactericidal that binds with 30S subunit of ribosomal subunit.

B. Bacteriostatic that inhibits bacterial protein synthesis by binding to 50S ribosomal subunit.

C. Inhibits folic acid synthesis and acts as bacteriostatic drug.

D. Inhibits bacterial DNA gyrase and topoisomerase IV.

Answer: B

Chloramphenicol is a broad-spectrum antibacterial agent, which is a bacteriostatic and acts by binding to 50S ribosomal subunit, thereby inhibiting bacterial protein synthesis.

10. The treatment strategy that uses lowering of IOP to target range in open-angle glaucoma (OAG) involves:

A. Reduction of aqueous humor formation.

B. Enhancing aqueous humor outflow.

C. Induction of miosis.

D. Both A and B.

Answer: D

The treatment strategy that uses lowering of IOP in OAG includes reduction of aqueous humor formation or enhancement of aqueous humor outflow or both.

11. Topical atropine is contraindicated in:

A. Retinoscopy in children.

B. Iridocyclitis.

C. Corneal ulcer.

D. Primary angle-closure glaucoma.

Answer: D

Atropine should not be administered for ciliary muscle relaxation and pupil dilatation (for ocular fundus examination) in patients with primary angle-closure glaucoma, as it precipitates angle closure.

12. An appropriate counseling statement for timolol is:

A. This medication has no significant systemic effects.

B. This medication may cause mydriasis.

C. Do not use this medication if you are allergic to sulfonamides.

D. This medication may cause bradycardia.

Answer: D

Timolol is a nonselective β-blocker, which decreases production of aqueous humor and is most frequently used for the treatment of glaucoma. Although administered topically, it may show systemic side effects by blocking β_1-adrenergic receptors. The side effects include bradycardia, orthostatic hypotension, and syncope. Hence, patients should be warned about side effects such as bradycardia while counseling.

13. Which of the following statements is/are true about systemic drugs used in the treatment of glaucoma?

A. Acetazolamide causes tachypnea.

B. Acetazolamide should be avoided in patients with hepatic failure.

C. Mannitol should be warmed to room temperature before intravenous administration to avoid formation of crystals.

D. All of the above.

Answer: D

Acetazolamide and mannitol are administered systemically for the treatment of acute angle-closure glaucoma. The carbonic anhydrase inhibitor acetazolamide produces metabolic acidosis, which leads to tachypnea, and it should be avoided in patients with renal or hepatic failure, as it can cause fatal acid–base imbalance. Mannitol can form crystals in blood and hence should be warmed to room temperature before intravenous administration.

14. In the treatment of open-angle glaucoma (OAG), bimatoprost is a first-line drug used for the treatment, which acts by of the following mechanisms:

A. Inhibition of carbonic anhydrase decreases the formation of humor and thereby decreases intraocular pressure (IOP).

B. It is a PGF2α derivative and acts by stimulating FP receptors and facilitates aqueous outflow through the accessory uveoscleral outflow pathway.

C. It creates osmotic gradient between blood and the ocular fluids, leading to water loss from eye to hyperosmotic plasma and thereby decreasing IOP.

D. It stimulates muscarinic M3 receptor, causing miosis.

Answer: B

Bimatoprost is a prostaglandin analog ($PGF_{2\alpha}$ derivative) and it acts by stimulating FP receptors and facilitates aqueous outflow through the accessory uveoscleral outflow pathway.

15. The care that should be taken while managing glaucoma includes:

A. Try to use least medication in lowest concentration to achieve desired target intraocular pressure (IOP).

B. Substitute rather than adding medication if the treatment is ineffective.

C. Monitor and try to increase patient compliance.

D. All of the above.

Answer: D

Drugs are a double-edged sword which have the potential to produce undesired effects. Hence, the use of multiple medication (polypharmacy) or higher doses should be avoided as much as possible. If the patient is not responding to the treatment provided, substitute the medication rather than adding a newer one. It will prevent unnecessary exposure of the patient to drugs. Patient compliance is of utmost importance in any therapy. Effectiveness or potency of drug does not matter unless patients instill/swallow it. While managing glaucoma, all of these points should be addressed or taken care of.

Chapter 92 Essential Medicines, Fixed-Dose Combinations, Over-the-Counter Drugs, and Herbal Medicine

R. S. Ray and R. Srinivasa Rao

PH1.59: Describe and discuss the following: essential medicines, fixed-dose combinations, over-the-counter drugs, herbal medicines.

Learning Objectives

- Essential medicines.
- Fixed-dose combinations.
- Over-the-counter drugs.
- Herbal medicine.

Essential Medicines (CM19.1)

Medicines are one of the most significant discoveries used by modern society for basic health care and therapeutic resource. Access to safe, affordable, and appropriately prescribed medicines by all is an important goal of national health care systems. Essential medicines play an indispensable role in health care systems, which satisfy the health care needs of the majority of population. Essential medicines are intended to be available at all times in sufficient quantities, in the required dosage forms, with assured consistency and adequate details, and at a price that can be afforded by the person and the community. Essential medicines lists (EMLs) are necessary to promote cost-effective therapy, rational use of medications, and evidence-based learning in health care systems to help attain universal health coverage. They serve as a model for selecting cost-effective and high-quality medicines considering public health relevance and proven efficacy and safety. Therefore, these drugs should always be available in reasonable quantities in the appropriate dosage forms at all times. Essential medicines are those drugs that fulfill the population's primary health care needs, according to the World Health Organization (WHO). Essential medicines treat most chronic and acute diseases with due regard to disease prevalence, efficacy, protection, and comparative cost-effectiveness.

History of Essential Medicines

The first country in the world to devise its EML was Tanzania in 1970. The idea of defining essential medicines was taken up during the 1975 World Health Assembly to expand the scope and availability of medicines for populations with limited access. The WHO Expert Committee on the Use of Essential Medicines was set up to assist member states in the selection and procurement of essential medicines. Back in 1977, the first WHO list of critical drugs was published, with 205 items based on people's health needs, which was reviewed every 2 years by experts in the chosen field after duly ascertaining that they have no conflict of interest. A model list of essential medicines is maintained by the WHO and serves as a reference to help countries choose drugs and medical devices that best meet their population's public health needs. This EML definition has been practically implemented at state, regional, district, and hospital levels in more than 150 countries. This idea of essential drugs helps countries rationalize the procurement and distribution of medicines, and by allowing one to get the best medicines at low cost, it proves useful particularly in poor-resource environments.

The WHO Expert Committee on the Selection and Use of Essential Medicines meets every 2 years to review and update the model list, and the most recent biennial meeting happened in April 2019 at the WHO headquarter, Geneva, Switzerland. In June 2019, the WHO released the most recent 21st WHO Model List of Essential Medicines and the 7th Model List of Essential Medicines for Children, which includes 433 medications. The recent list contains 28 new medicinal products for adults and 23 new medicinal products for children, and 9 previously listed products for use for a new condition have also been specified. The 21st list also included new formulations of 16 medicines already listed and introduced a range of essential and appropriate measures in response to the additional indications for medicines already listed and the removal of 9 medicines. The concept of EML serves as an excellent public health tool, which has been adopted in principle by some 156 countries today. In February 2020, the WHO also released the first-ever digital edition of its model EML.

National List of Essential Medicines

At present, the EML is adopted by over 150 countries, including India. Every person in India has an equal right to have access to public health care facilities. Health services operate at multiple levels in India, such as subcenters, primary health centers, community health centers, and district-level hospitals, superspecialty hospitals, or medical institutes, to meet the need of its large populations. For a specific indication, the list is deemed to contain the most cost-effective drugs. It is established according to the standard guidelines for care, taking into account the health needs of the majority of the population.

The national list of essential medicines plays an important role in providing an efficient health care system by ensuring that all primary, secondary, and tertiary levels of health care are safe, effective, and accessible in terms of quality medicine. The Ministry of Health and Family Welfare (MoHFW), Government of India, is committed to providing quality health care system for all its population. The first national list of essential medicines (NLEM) of India was prepared and released in 1996 and subsequently revised in 2003, 2011, and 2015. The drugs listed in the NLEM include drugs used in different national health systems as well as in the treatment of new and reemerging diseases.

Primary Objectives of NLEM

1. To promote rational use of medicines, taking into account the three important aspects, that is, cost, safety, and efficacy.
2. To serve as a guidance manual for safe and effective treatment of priority disease conditions of a population.
3. To promote prescription by generic names.
4. To help monitor the price of drugs.
5. To serve as a reference guide for proper dosage form and strength for prescribing.
6. To help optimize the available health resources of a country.
7. To act as a public education and training tool for health care providers.

The Ministry of Health and Family Welfare, Government of India, updates and reviews the NLEM from time to time in order to address the issues of changing disease incidence, treatment modalities, the implementation of new drugs, and the recognition of an inappropriate risk–benefit profile as well as the therapeutic profile of certain medicines. The NLEM revision was also based on two essential national reference documents, that is, Indian Pharmacopeia and National Formulary of India; the former deals with medicinal standards of identity, purity, and power, while the latter provides information on the rational use of medicines, particularly for health care professionals.

The NLEM has been prepared carefully after several rounds of consultation with experts from various fields across the country and belonging to different organizations. Careful NLEM-based selection of drugs has contributed to a significant reduction in the number of important medicinal products, not only improving the rational use of medicines but also reducing the overall expenditure on medicinal products. The NLEM is a dynamic document and receives feedback from all stakeholders to assist in its revision on a regular basis. In addition, several states in India have their own EMLs, including Karnataka, Tamil Nadu, Rajasthan, and Kerala. The most recent edition of NLEM is the one revised in 2015.

The criteria for inclusion of a medicine in NLEM are as follows:

1. The medicine should be approved/licensed in India.
2. The medicine should be useful in a disease that is a public health problem in India.
3. The drug should have a proven profile of effectiveness and protection, based on credible clinical evidence.
4. The drug should be cost-effective.
5. The medicine should be aligned with the current treatment guidelines for the disease.
6. The medicine should be stable under normal storage conditions in India.
7. If more than one medicine is available from the same therapeutic class, after due deliberation and careful consideration of their relative protection, efficacy, and cost-effectiveness, preferably one prototype/medically best suited medicine of that class should be included.
8. The cost of overall treatment should be taken into account and not the unit price of a drug.
9. Fixed-dose combinations (FDCs) are usually not used unless the mixture has an undeniably proven benefit in terms of increasing effectiveness, reducing adverse effects, and/or enhancing compliance over individual ingredients administered separately.
10. In NLEM, the listing of medication is based on the standard of health care, that is, primary (P), secondary (S), and tertiary (T), since treatment facilities, training, expertise, and availability of health care personal vary at these levels.

The criteria for deletion of a medicine from NLEM are as follows:

1. Medicine banned in India.
2. Available concerns on the safety profile of a medicine.
3. A medicine with improved efficacy or favorable safety profiles and better cost-effectiveness than currently available products.
4. The burden of illness for which a medication is indicated is no longer a national health issue in India.
5. In case of antimicrobials, if drug resistance rendered a medicine ineffective in the Indian population.

Salient Features of NLEM 2015

In NLEM 2015, a total of 376 essential medicines are listed with regard to the different levels of health care, namely, primary (P), secondary (S), and tertiary (T). There are 209 formulations of medicines listed for all levels of health care (P, S, T), 115 formulations of medicines for secondary and tertiary levels (S, T), and 79 formulations of medicine for tertiary levels (T). NLEM 2015 was prepared to adhere to the basic principles of efficacy, protection, and cost-effectiveness, considering diseases in India as problems of public health.

Despite the fact that NLEM is designed to ensure safe and effective medicines for all, there are many obstacles that affect NLEM's efficient implementation, including

1. Nonavailability of standard treatment guidelines.
2. Nonavailability of trained staff in procurement.
3. Lack of market data.
4. Insufficient fund allocation.
5. Lack of confidence in the quality of the drugs supplied by the framework of public health care.
6. Medicine shortages in Indian public health centers push patients to buy higher-cost goods from the open market.

Fixed-Dose Combinations

FDCs are a combination of two or more active pharmaceutical ingredients in a single dosage form in fixed ratio of doses, typically for the same indication. FDCs are aimed to increase the therapeutic effectiveness of each component of the medication while reducing the adverse drug reactions. FDCs play an important role in the public health perspective and are commonly used in the treatment of various conditions, including pain, inflammation, hypertension, diabetes, malaria, tuberculosis, HIV/AIDs, etc.

Criteria for FDCs

An FDC should fulfill the following characteristics:

1. The drugs must act through different mechanisms of action.
2. It is important to have a similar pharmacokinetic profile of the drugs.
3. The drugs should not cause additive toxicity.
4. Superiority of using FDCs over individual drugs should be present.

Advantages of FDCs

1. Reduce the pill burden by reducing the number of pills to be taken by patients, especially in the treatment of infectious diseases such as HIV, influenza, and tuberculosis.
2. Reduce the risk of adverse reaction compared to higher dose of monotherapy.
3. Safe and efficacious.
4. Lower the cost of medication compared to individual drugs.
5. Simple dosing schedule.
6. Ease of administration.
7. Improve patient compliance and treatment outcomes.
8. Improved therapeutic efficacy compared to higher dose of monotherapy.
9. More economical than monotherapy.
10. Ease in transport and reduction in packing cost.
11. Reduce risk of medication errors.
12. Reduce treatment cost.
13. Simplified drug supply management, shipping, and distribution.
14. Help upscale national health programs such as National Tuberculosis Elimination Program (NTEP) (earlier known as Revised National Tuberculosis Control Program) and National AIDS Control Programme (NACP).

Disadvantages of FDCs

1. Pharmacodynamic incompatibility between the two components with additive/antagonistic effect of one drug, leading to decreased efficacy or increased toxicity.
2. Incompatible pharmacokinetics of constituent drugs having peak efficacy at different times likely to pose problem in frequency of administration of formulation.
3. Chemical incompatibility of ingredients leading to decreased shelf-life of FDC.
4. Dosage alteration of one drug is not possible and cannot be regulated based on patient needs, especially as in the case of age, weight, and comorbidity, which may alter the metabolism and effect.
5. Increased chance of adverse drug reactions and drug interactions.
6. Contraindication of one component will restrict the utility of the FDC.
7. FDCs make it difficult to identify the causal relationship of adverse effect of any one component, which limits their use.
8. If used irrationally, it can lead to antimicrobial resistance, especially in case of anti-TB and antiretroviral medications.

The therapeutic categories with high number of FDCs are analgesics, antipyretics, muscle relaxants, antimicrobials, antihypertensive drugs, vitamins and minerals, drugs used in the management of cough and cold, antidiabetic drugs, and psychotropic medications. The FDC formulation contains up to five or even more ingredients, with or without rationality. Although FDCs are available in almost all therapeutic categories, many of them are bizarre combinations.

Examples of rational FDCs

1. Sulfamethoxazole + trimethoprim (cotrimoxazole).
2. Amoxicillin + clavulanic acid.
3. Levodopa + carbidopa.

Examples of some irrational FDCs banned in Indian market

1. Aceclofenac SR + paracetamol.
2. Azithromycin + cefixime.
3. Ciprofloxacin + fluticasone + clotrimazole + neomycin.
4. Metformin + pioglitazone + glimepiride.

Regulation of FDC Products in India

The criteria for the production/import approval and marketing of different types of FDCs are specified in Appendix VI of Schedule Y to the Drugs and Cosmetics Rules 1945. In India, FDC is classified as a new drug, according to the Drugs and Cosmetics Rules of Rule 122 E. This is due to the fact that the safety, effectiveness, and bioavailability of the individual active pharmaceutical ingredient can be changed by combining two or more drugs. As notified under Section 21 (b) of the Drugs and Cosmetics Act, the national regulatory body, the Central Drugs Standard Control Organization (CDSCO), issues necessary approval after due consideration of data on rationality, protection, and efficacy. On the basis of this, the State Licensing Authority gives the manufacturing and marketing permission.

In India, 24 of the 376 drugs included in the 2015 NLEM are FDC drugs. Majority of FDCs belong to antimalarial, antitubercular, and antiretroviral drugs, which stress the importance of the use of FDC in the adherence to care and prevention of drug resistance. The Indian medicine market has been the world leader in FDCs, with India's estimated number of FDCs being over 6,000. On March 10, 2016, the CDSCO banned 344 FDCs under Section 26A of the Drugs and Cosmetics Act, 1940, in order to curb irrational FDCs, based on the findings of the expert panel.

Over-the-Counter Medications

Medications taken without a doctor's prescription by patients for the treatment of common illnesses are known as over-the-counter (OTC) or nonprescription medications. The easy availability of these OTC medications enables the consumers to treat numerous ailments without the supervision of a health care professional. The use of OTC medicines has grown steadily in the recent past few years and the easy availability, affordability, and increased awareness among patients are responsible for this trend. It is commonly believed that OTC preparations are safe and suitable for use without health care practitioners' supervision. OTC medications are used to treat wide range of conditions such as musculoskeletal pain, fever, cough, common cold, heartburn, diarrhea, and allergies. The formulations widely used as OTC preparations are analgesics, laxatives, antacids, cough and cold preparations, antihistamines, dermatologicals, throat preparations, nasal preparations, and antidiarrheals. OTC medicines are effective when used as directed, and the label information instructs consumers on how to properly choose and use them.

Common Concerns about OTC Medications

OTC medications can act as a double-edged sword, and inappropriate use of OTC drugs can lead to serious health implications, especially in pediatric and geriatric population, pregnant and lactating mothers, and patients with comorbidities. The most common risks associated with the use of OTC medications are misuse, adverse effects including dependence (especially to sedatives, analgesics, antacids, laxatives), drug resistance, improper self-diagnosis, inappropriate dosage, delayed diagnosis of underlying conditions owing to the use of OTC medicines, adverse drug reactions, and drug interactions. Inappropriate self-medication of OTC products often results in overuse or misuse, which is often seen as a growing public health concern. Owing to insufficient awareness, lack of accessibility to medical information, inadequate facilities, and poor laws and regulations, improper use of OTC drugs is also often seen as a public health concern. Despite the fact that OTC medications are used inappropriately, leading to adverse effects, their number in the market and incidence of their usage are increasing. Furthermore, the overwhelmed OTC use is attributed to the direct-to-patient advertising by pharmaceutical industries, and easy availability at pharmacies increases the exposure of medications to patients. Many countries recognize OTC medicines as a separate category of drugs and have established regulations for their use. However, in India, there are no specific unifying regulations related to use and sale of OTC products in India.

Herbal Medicine

Herbal medicine is used by mankind since ages. Throughout ancient civilization, mankind depended on nearby plants and herbs for food and relief from ailments. These ancient practices assimilated into codified indigenous medicinal systems on a regional basis (e.g., traditional Indian medicine—*ayurveda*, traditional Chinese medicine [TCM], etc.). Asia is at the forefront of codified herbal medicine systems (India, China, Korea, Japan, etc.).

WHO reports 70% of population in developing countries depend on herbal medicine for their primary health care needs. In the recent COVID-19 pandemic, China could successfully integrate TCM and conventional medicine and claimed superior control of the pandemic. This strategy shows importance of herbal medicine even in today's contemporary world, wherein advanced drugs such as biotechnology-derived products, gene therapeutics, and large protein are critically acclaimed for their role in public health. In few parts of the globe, these codified herbal medicinal systems are grouped under complementary and alternative medicine.

Often, communities use multiple products (e.g., prescription drugs, herbal medicinal products, dietary supplements, functional foods, products from *ayurveda*, *unani*, and *siddha*, homeopathy, TCM, etc.) to cure/mitigate their health problems. Universally, people are living longer, due to improving health care infrastructure. As people become old and live longer, many of them suffer from multiple ailments and thus they use combination therapies. In the current age of polypharmacy, herb–drug interactions are bound to increase exponentially. In few, herbs may interfere with absorption of conventional drugs, leading to variability in bioavailability. This variability in absorption may result in unpredictable efficacy or increased side effects. Patients, while visiting their health care professionals, may not reveal about other products they are using, unless asked for. This is the context that makes it imperative for every healthcare professional to be aware of other therapies including herbal medicine.

It is estimated that about 25% of all modern medicines are directly or indirectly derived from plants sources. Few leads from herbal medicine that gave birth to conventional drugs include metformin (diabetes), paclitaxel (anticancer), aspirin (heart attack, stroke prevention), digoxin (heart failure), quinine (malaria), and artemisinin (malaria). For the discovery of artemisinin, Chinese scientists were awarded the Nobel Prize for physiology/medicine in 2015. Few plant actives from TCM are in advanced clinical use in China after extensive clinical trials—huperzine A (treats memory dysfunction) and paeoniflorin (treats cardiovascular disease). Notably, these compounds are developed as single-moiety drugs instead of complex herbal mixtures.

In India, similar R&Ds resulted in phytopharmaceuticals such as guggulipid (*guggulu*, cholesterol lowering), *arteether* from the plant *Artemisia annua* (severe *Plasmodium falciparum* malaria), *brahmi* (*Bacopa monnieri*, age-associated memory impairment in adults, and children with attention-deficit hyperactive disorder), *vijayasar* (heart wood of *Pterocarpus marsupium* Roxb.) for diabetes mellitus, *shakotak* (stem bark of *Streblus asper* Lour. antifilariasis), and *Picrorhiza kurroa* Royle ex Benth. (designated as Picroliv) for viral hepatitis. An AYUSH (*ayurveda*, yoga and naturopathy, *unani*, *siddha*, and homoeopathy) formulation for dengue is under clinical evaluation. Several other drug candidates (phytopharmaceutical/AYUSH) are under evaluation by the Central Drug Research Institute (CDRI), CSIR, Lucknow, India.

Herbal medicine products consist of herbs, herbal materials, herbal preparations, and finished herbal products, which include parts of plants, other plant materials, or mixtures thereof as active ingredients. Herbs comprise crude plant material, for instance, leaves, flowers, fruit, seed, root, and stems. Herbal materials , in addition, comprise herbs, fresh juices, gums, fixed oils, essential oils, resins, and dry powders of herbs. Herbal preparations are the source for complete herbal products, which could incorporate either comminuted or powdered herbal materials or extracts, tinctures, and fatty oils of herbal materials. Finished herbal products contain herbal preparations prepared with one or more herbs.

Generally, herbal medicines are consumed by mouth only, an exception being China, wherein few injectables are in use. The common belief is conventional medicine works well for acute illness, whereas herbal medicine acts slowly, thus, works well against chronic ailments such as joint pains and skin problems, which may not be completely true.

Conventional medicine works through a single, highly potent active ingredient, whereas herbal medicine acts through multiple active moieties due to synergy. To cite an example, many of the herbal formulae do have certain ingredients (e.g., piperine, pepper in *ayurveda*), which increase availability of other plant actives when taken by mouth.

Selected medicinal plants and dietary constituents possessing functional characteristics are spices such as onion, garlic, mustard, red chili, turmeric, clove, cinnamon, saffron, curry leaf, fenugreek, and ginger. Several fruits and vegetables such as *amla*, wheat grass, soybean, and *Garcinia cambogia* have antitumor effects. Other medicinal plants with such functional properties comprise *Aegle marmelos*, *Allium cepa*, *Aloe vera*, *Andrographis paniculata*, and *Azadirachta indica*.

Herbal medicine is used in other forms such as dietary supplements, food supplements, nutraceuticals, functional foods, and natural health products. All these terms represent similar products that are used for either prevention of ailments or mitigating mild symptoms associated with them. In the United States, dietary supplements and functional foods are preferred terms, whereas in Europe terms such as nutraceuticals and food supplements are in use. Canada labels these products as natural health products. Japan regulates these products under FOSHU (food for specified health uses). A noteworthy point is every country has its own rules and regulations (definition, scope, control, need of prior approval before sale, etc.). Hence, there is *no* harmonization in terms of regulating these products across the globe. Lack of harmonization, adds another layer of complexity into herbal medicine, which already have several intrinsic variabilities. All these products, in general, are composed of herbs, vitamins, minerals, etc. For these products, no cure claims are allowed. These products may be prescribed by herbal medicine physicians sometimes, where in other places, patients buy and use these products on their own, over the trade (OTC).

In India, these products are categorized and regulated under three categories: (1) food products, regulated by Food Safety and Standards Authority of India (FSSAI); (2) *ayurveda/unani/homeopathy* drug, regulated by department of AYUSH; and (3) phytopharmaceuticals drug, regulated by CDSCO. Point to note is these three regulating agencies are independent from each other, have their own perceptions of rules, regulations, leading to flooding of products into market place. Each product will fall into one of the three categories, depending on source, composition, and associated claims. If the product claims cure of any ailment, it is considered a drug product and has to comply with all relevant rules and regulations prescribed for drugs.

Intrinsic Problems Associated with Herbal Medicine

As herbs are soil-dependent, there could be soil contamination with pesticides and other pollutants, which are accumulated in herbs and then transferred to herbal formulations, too. For instance, some Indian regions are polluted with arsenic in the soil (e.g. east India), and plants/herbs grown in such soil are bound to have higher arsenic content, sometimes beyond permissible limits by WHO.

As herbs depend on soil fertility of those areas, same plant grown in varied climates and environments, can have variable plant actives. Collection timing and other practices may add to this variability. Furthermore, there could be seasonal variability. Hence, the herbal medicinal products have variable phytoactive content, based on season. Considering this intrinsic variability associated with herbal medicine, it is important and crucial to follow the quality control standards. In a nutshell, all these factors contribute to variability in terms of product standardization. This variability may sometimes lead to variability in efficacy and safety.

Herbal medicine depends on natural sources such as forests, and these primary sources are continuously exploited for herbs, because of which sustainability of these resources is critical and challenging now, for example, Himalayan and Western Ghats plant resources are depleting fast.

Conducting Clinical Trials in Herbal Medicine

Conducting clinical trials in herbal medicine is challenging, due to intrinsic variabilities, as described. Furthermore, it is very difficult, impracticable, or sometimes impossible to have active and control groups with identical color, smell, and taste. Also, the use of placebo involves similar difficulties as the herbal study drug may exhibit its strong aroma and a specific distinguished taste; hence, these cannot be exactly imitated while manufacturing a placebo. Quite often, the problems are multiplied when working with formulations containing more than one plant extracts. Special attention must also be paid on standardization of the compounds using bioactive markers. There are difficulties in estimation of "active" molecules in body fluids in the pharmacokinetic studies in early phytopharmaceutical development (phase I), especially in multiactive herbal formulation.

India is very rich in natural resources and the knowledge of traditional medicine and the use of plants as a source of medicine is an innate and very important component of the health care system. The Indian system of medicine has identified 1,500 medicinal plants, of which 500 are commonly used.

Ayurveda

Ayurveda (the science of life) is one of the branches of *vedas*. It is considered as *upaveda* of *rigveda* or *atharvaveda*. It is a stream of the knowledge passed down from generation to generation since eternity, parallel to the *vedic* literature.

Hence, its emergence has been said to be from the creator (*Brahma*) himself, prior to the creation. It is termed eternal, since nobody knows when it was not there. All this demonstrates its long tradition and deep attachment to the Indian culture.

As per *ayurveda*, every human being is a unique phenomenon of cosmic consciousness, manifested through the five basic elements—ether, air, fire, water, and earth. *Vata* (a combination of ether and air), *pitta* (a combination of fire and water), and *kapha* (a combination of water and earth) are called the *tridosha*. These are the three humors or the three organizations of the body, which are also derived from consciousness. Each individual constitution or psychosomatic temperament is determined by the relative proportions of these three *doshas* at the time of fertilization. When the embryo is formed, the constitution is determined. There are seven basic constitutions with one or more *doshas* predominant, according to *ayurveda*. They are: *vata*, *pitta*, or *kapha* predominant, *vata-pitta*, *pitta–kapha*, or *kapha–vata* predominant, and *vata-pitta-kapha* in equal balance, a rare occurrence.

Pharmacological Basis of Ayurveda

Ayurveda herbal medicine has certain principles to which pharmacological actions of individual herbs are attributed to. They are five in number and are as follows:

1. *Rasa* (taste, six in number, each *rasa* is said to aggravate/pacify relevant humors).
2. *Guna* (physiological properties, 20 in number, each *guna* is said to aggravate/pacify relevant humors).
3. *Veerya* (potency, two in number, each is said to aggravate/pacify relevant humors).
4. *Vipaka* (postdigestive effects, two in number, each is said to aggravate/pacify the relevant humors).
5. *Prabhava* (idiosyncrasy, due to which a herb may behave extraordinarily, other factors being equal).

Herbal formulations are prescribed depending on humors and bodily tissues. *Ayurveda* believes cosmos is composed of five basic elements—air, space, water, fire, and earth. It states the same elements constitute human body also. In diseases, correction of these five elements in unison with humors and bodily tissues is the core concept of *ayurveda*. Herbs are the primary modality through which this balance is acquired. Ancient classical *ayurveda* treatises such as *Charaka Samhita*, *Susruta Samhita*, and *Astanga Hridayam* describe thousands of herbal formulations that are suggested for many diseases/ailments.

Homeopathy

This medicine originated in Germany by Samuel Hahnemann (1755–1843). Homeopathy believes in 'like cures like', which is often called the 'principle of similars.' (drugs that cause disease symptoms cure similar diseases, when given in ultrasmall dosing). In this medicine, herbs are used in small dilutions and prescribed in the forms of pills and tinctures.

TCM

Originated in China over two thousand years ago and developed in the following centuries. The Five elements theory in TCM, named as wood, fire, earth, metal, and water, divides human body into five systems. Each system has its own specific features that can be inferred by analyzing those natural materials. The movement and interchange among the five elements are used to explain human body's physiology. During the formation and development of TCM, there are two ideological ideas that fully penetrate into the whole process. The first is the homeostasis idea that focuses on the integrity of human body and emphasizes the close relationship between human body and its social and natural environment (integrity between human and cosmos). The second is the dynamic balance idea that takes emphasis on the movement in the integrity.

Unani

This medical system is believed to have originated from the Middle East. However, some others believe *ayurveda* traveled to the Middle East and was renamed *unani*. It practices principles similar to *ayurveda*. *Unani* uses a lot of herbal formulations, which are prescribed for various ailments.

Siddha

Siddha medicine is one of the most ancient medical systems of India, originated from ancient Tamils/Dravidians of peninsular South India. The ancient scholars, named Siddhars, recorded their mystic findings in medicine, yoga, and astrology in Tamil. Fundamental principles of Siddha include theories of five elements (Aimpootham), and three forces/faults (Mukkuttram). The eight methods of examination (Envakai Thervukal) is used to determine diagnosis, etiology, treatment, and prognosis. Siddha has safe herbal and herbomineral treatment for skin ailments, hairfall, diabetic ulcer, warts, leprosy, and many more very common and rare diseases. Lifestyle modifications including diet are important.

Herbs as Food/Dietary Use

Herbs used in food, for example, Indian spices, turmeric, ginger, garlic, cinnamon, cardamom, pepper have digestive, assimilative properties and thus aid proper functioning of digestive system. Ayurveda believes digestive fire is critical for human well-being and thus stresses importance of foods both in preventive and curative aspects. Recently Department of AYUSH has released food preparations, based on Indian traditional medicine. This is a right step towards preventing various ailments, through our dietary interventions/modification.

Traditional Knowledge Digital Library

With growing demand for traditional medicine, bioresources all over the world are under the threat of biopiracy and many cases of misappropriation of traditional knowledge regularly make headlines in the media. *Ayurvedic* medicines, herbs, and formulations which find an incognito description in *classical ayurveda* texts are nonetheless in common use in India. This situation has often led to wrong patents being granted by authorities becuase they are aware that the claims and compositions fall under traditional medicines, under use since many years. The case in point is that of a patent granted by United States Patent and Trademark Office (USPTO) on turmeric, which is used in India as an essential ingredient in Indian meals as well as for a variety of *ayurvedic* treatments including simple cuts, wounds, minor burns etc. Encouraged by the success of getting this patent revoked as a result of public outrage, India launched the project on the Traditional Knowledge Digital Library (TKDL).

TKDL is a pioneering joint initiative of India's Council of Scientific and Industrial Research and Department of AYUSH to prevent misappropriation of country's traditional medicinal knowledge at international patent offices. Its software translates the information contained in ancient Sanskrit classical texts of *ayurveda* as well as that of other non-English Indian systems of medicine to half a dozen international languages comprehensible and accessible to patent examiners in Europe and the United States. It also has its own elaborate classification system, which is compatible with International Patent Classification (IPC).

On herb–drug interactions, data available refer to plants used in TCM, and phytomedicine of Europe and the United States. Data on Indian traditional medicine is minuscule. Most of the herbs are tested using in vitro CYP interference on metabolism of conventional drugs, but clinical evidence is minimal. Few of the important clinical interactions are mentioned in **Table 92.1**.

Gums, mucilages, pectins, or fibers contained in several medicinal plants have the ability to bind, trap, and form viscous matrices with concurrently administered drugs. Hence, they may reduce their absorption.

Characteristics of the patient, such as age, frailty, infrequent genotypes, ethnicity, gender, and comorbidity, should be taken into account when considering herb-to-drug interactions.

System-wise Herbal Drugs with Evidence

1. Cardiovascular system: *arjuna, forskolin.*
2. Pulmonary bronchodilator: *vasa, kantakari, yastimadhu.*
3. Metabolism: *guggulu*–guggulipid (cholesterol lowering).
4. Immune boosters/immunomodulator: ginger, *ashwagandha, guduchi.*
5. Gynecological: *shatavari, asoka.*
6. Brain boosters: *brahmi, saraswati.*
7. Bone and joints: *shallaki, asthisamhara, nirgundi, haridra* (curcumin).
8. Diabetes: *vijayasara, karela, gymnema, stevia.*
9. Dermatological: *neem.*
10. Eye disorders: Berberine from daruharidra.
11. Gastrointestinal system: *dadima*–diarrhea, *kutaja*–dysentery.
12. Liver ailments: Picroliv, *katukarohini, bhuyamlaki, sarapunkha, kalmegha.*
13. Renal system: *punarnava, pashanbhed.*

Table 92.1 Important clinical herb–drug interactions

Herb name	Latin name	Use	Remarks
St. John's-wort	*Hypericum perforatum*	Alternative to conventional antidepressant drugs for mild to moderate forms of depressive disorders	Well-documented and clinically relevant interactions include: (1) reduced blood cyclosporine concentration associated in some cases with rejection episodes; (2) reduced efficacy of the oral contraceptive pill, resulting in unwanted pregnancy; (3) reduced plasma concentration of antiretroviral (e.g., indinavir, nevirapine) and anticancer drugs (e.g., imatinib, irinotecan)
Danshen	*Salvia miltiorrhiza*	Prevent and treat cardiovascular conditions, such as acute ischemic stroke and myocardial infarction, TCM	Case reports have highlighted the possibility of interactions between warfarin and danshen, resulting in an increased anticoagulant effect
Dong quai	*Angelica sinensis*	Preparations from its roots are used mainly for dysmenorrhea, amenorrhea, or excessive menstrual flow. TCM	Two well-documented case reports suggest excessive anticoagulation following coadministration of warfarin and dong quai
Licorice	*Glycyrrhiza glabra*	Treatment of peptic ulcer and catarrhs of the upper respiratory tract	Glycyrrhizin is known to increase the plasma prednisolone concentration in humans
Peppermint	*Mentha piperita*	Peppermint oil may be effective in relieving some of the symptoms of irritable bowel syndrome	Some clinical data suggest that peppermint might increase the levels of drugs metabolized by CYP3A4 such as felodipine

Abbreviation: TCM, traditional Chinese medicine.

Multiple Choice Questions

1. Essential drugs are:

A. Life-saving drugs.
B. Drugs that meet the priority health care needs of the population.
C. Drugs that must be present in the emergency bag of a doctor.
D. Drugs that are listed in the pharmacopoeias of a country.

Answer: B

2. The organization that fixes ceiling price of essential medicines in India is:

A. CDSCO.
B. Drug Pricing Control Organization.
C. Indian Pharmacopeia Commission.
D. National Pharmaceutical Pricing Authority.

Answer: D

3. National Pharmaceutical Pricing Authority was established in the year:

A. 1990.
B. 1985.
C. 1962.
D. 1997.

Answer: D

4. How are prescription medicines different from over-the-counter (OTC) ones?

A. They contain much smaller amounts of active ingredients.
B. They do not contain dyes or preservatives.
C. They are unsafe for use without medical supervision.
D. They can be toxic.

Answer: C

5. .... is known as the pharmacy of the world:

A. Japan.
B. United States of America.
C. India.
D. China.

Answer: C

6. Adverse drug reactions should be reported to:

A. Central Drugs Standards Control Organisation.
B. State Licensing Authority.
C. Indian Pharmacopoeia Commission.
D. Food and Drug Administration.

Answer: A

7. National list of essential medicines (NLEM) is prepared by:

A. MoHFW.
B. CDSCO.
C. FSSAI.
D. FDA.

Answer: A

8. A herb shown to have beneficial effects in treating depression is:

A. St. John's wort.
B. Danshen.
C. Dong quai.
D. Licorice.

Answer: A

9. This medicine originated in Germany:

A. *Ayurveda*.
B. Unani.
C. Homeopathy.
D. Siddha.

Answer: C

10. This medical system is believed to have originated in the Middle East:

A. *Ayurveda*.
B. Unani.
C. Homeopathy.
D. Siddha.

Answer: B

Index